Handbuch der experimentellen Pharmakologie

Handbook of Experimental Pharmacology

Heffter-Heubner New Series

Volume XXV

Bradykinin, Kallidin and Kallikrein

Contributors

D. Armstrong · K. F. Austen · G. A. Brecher · G. F. Brobmann · H. O. J. Collier
R. M. Daugherty · C. R. Diniz · V. Eisen · D. F. Elliott · T. E. Emerson · E. G.
Erdös · E. Habermann · F. J. Haddy · S. M. Hilton · S. Iwanaga · E. D. Jacobson
J. Lecomte · G. P. Lewis · M. Mares-Guia · H. Moriya · J. V. Pierce · J. J. Pisano
J. L. Prado · M. Schachter · E. Schröder · J. B. Scott · F. Sicuteri · J. Spragg
J. M. Stewart · T. Suzuki · R. C. Talamo · I. Trautschold · V. Trčka · R. Vogel
W. Vogt · E. J. Walaszek · M. E. Webster · E. Werle · H. Y. T. Yang
G. Zickgraf-Rüdel

Editor

Ervin G. Erdös

Technical Editor

Anne F. Wilde

With 117 Figures

Springer-Verlag Berlin · Heidelberg · New York 1970

ISBN-13: 978-3-642-46224-5 e-ISBN-13: 978-3-642-46222-1
DOI: 10.1007/978-3-642-46222-1

Softcover reprint of the hardcover 1st edition 1970

Title No. 3863

Preface

Bradykinin is frequently referred to as an elusive substance; the editor of a comprehensive volume dealing with kinins thus has a difficult task. The complexity of the issues calls for a large number of contributors who approach the topics from the various angles that are dictated by the sometimes divergent views of the individuals. The editor saw no reason to prescribe the mode of presentation, which was left to the authors and accounts for the variety of approaches.

Contributors from nine countries were asked to participate in the volume. The chapters were organized to present, first, the history of the discoveries and methods of approach to kinin research. Then follows a discussion of the enzymes that release kinins, their substrates, and other enzymes that inactivate the peptides. If the release of kinin is important, then the inhibition of the releasing enzymes is of obvious interest and is described. Since the measurement of kininogen levels in blood has been frequently used as an indicator of kinin liberation, in addition to a separate chapter, kininogens are also mentioned where the functions of kinins are discussed. The conclusions drawn from establishing structure-action relationships for many analogs and the actions of kinins are indicated and summarized.

The role of kinins in functional vasodilatation in the salivary gland has been debated for decades; the two opposing views on this subject are summarized in separate articles. The available information on the importance of kinins in pathological processes was presented in detail in different articles. The discussion of the mechanism of pain production is followed by a description of the effects of kinins on the intracranial circulation and by the clinical pharmacology of the peptides. The participation of kinins in inflammation, anaphylactic phenomena and several other pathological conditions are separately surveyed. Sources of kinins other than plasma are dealt with subsequently.

Although most articles on kinins have been published in English or German, the literature from other languages is quite considerable, and papers published in Czech, French, Italian, Japanese, Polish, Portugese, Russian, Slovak, and Spanish journals are summarized. These reviews indicate the extent of kinin research in other countries and summarize articles, abstracts, and theses in English. This chapter should help settle priorities in discoveries, even though the findings were not first published in international journals of wide circulation. The nomenclatures compiled in the Appendix should provide further guidelines for authors and may help to establish standard values.

The original discovery of the hypotensive action of urine clearly goes back to the nineteenth century (C. BOUCHARD: *Traité de Pathologie Générale*, vol. 3, Paris, 1900). Although its effects were described in the middle 1920s, kallikrein still continues its career by being rediscovered over and over again. Synthetic kinins and highly purified kallikreins have become available only during the 1960s, and the progress made during that decade is remarkable. Although the pioneering observations of WERLE and ROCHA E SILVA were made with very crude extracts, they are still valid today.

Bradykinin, kallidin, and kallikrein are among the most potent endogenous substances, but no single well defined mechanism offers a generally accepted explanation for their presence in the body. To complicate matters, kinins occur in man in potentially large quantities in the protein precursor, kininogen; they are rapidly inactivated after their release and the breakdown products are indistinguishable from other body constituents. Kinins in plasma are part of a very complex system that regulates their release and inactivation. When this homeostatic balance is disturbed, kinins may contribute to some pathological syndromes. In research, as elsewhere, it is risky to argue for future developments from past experiences, but study of several decades of investigation seems to indicate that the presence of plasma kinins in mammals is primarily related to their roles in pathological processes.

January 1970, Oklahoma City, Oklahoma E. G. Erdös

Table of Contents

Chapter 1: Introduction

Chapter 2: Methods Used in Kinin Research

Chapter 3: Kininogenases

Chapter 4: Kininogens

Chapter 5: Kininases

Chapter 6: Kinins

Section A: Physiological and Pharmacological Actions

Chapter 7: Urinary Kinins

Chapter 8: Non-Mammalian Kinins

Chapter 9: Summary of Literature Published in Various Languages

Appendix

Glossary of Frequently Used Abbreviations and Terms

ATEe	= acetyl-L-tyrosine ethyl ester
ATP	= adenosine triphosphate
BAA	= benzoyl-L-argininamide
BAEe	= benzoyl-L-arginine ethyl ester
BAL	= 2,3-dimercaptopropanol
BAMe	= benzoyl-L-arginine methyl ester
BANA	= benzoyl arginine-*p*-nitroanilide
Bk	= bradykinin
Bzd	= benzamidine
C-terminal	= carboxyl-terminal
CM	= carboxymethyl
CNS	= central nervous system
CSF	= cerebrospinal fluid
DEAE	= diethylaminoethyl
DFP	= diisopropylfluorophosphate
EACA	= ε-amino-n-caproic acid
EDTA	= ethylenediaminetetraacetate
EU	= esterase unit
FU	= Frey Unit for kallikrein
HF	= Hageman factor
HLA	= hippuryl-L-arginine
HLAa	= hippuryl-L-argininic acid
HLL	= hippuryl-L-lysine
HMW	= high molecular weight
5-HT	= 5-hydroxytryptamine
I_{50}	= concentration of inhibitor that inhibits 50% of enzyme activity
K_9, K_{10}, K_{11} enzymes	= enzymes that liberate bradykinin, kallidin or Met-Lys-bradykinin resp.
Kd	= kallidin
Kk	= kallikrein
Kininase	= See appendix
Kininogenase	= See appendix
KIU	= kallikrein inhibitor unit
LBTI	= Lima bean trypsin inhibitor
LMW	= low molecular weight
LSD	= lysergic acid diethylamide
MLBr	= methionyllysylbradykinin
N-terminal	= amino terminal
OMTI	= ovomucoid trypsin inhibitor
PF/dil	= permeability factor
PKFL	= Met-Lys-bradykinyl-Ser-Val-Gln
PKFS	= Met-Lys-bradykinyl-Ser-Val-Gln-Val-Met
PTI	= pancreatic trypsin inhibitor
SBTI	= soybean trypsin inhibitor
SRS-A	= slow reacting substance of anaphylaxis
TAMe	= p-toluenesulfonyl-L-arginine methyl ester
TCA	= trichloroacetic acid
TLCK	= 1-chloro-3-tosylamido-7-amino-2-heptanone
Tris	= tris (hydroxymethyl) aminomethane
TPCK	= α-L-(1-tosylamido-2-phenyl)ethylchloromethyl ketone

List of Contributors

Armstrong, Désirée A. J., 6020 Cannon Hill Road, Fort Washington, Pennsylvania, U.S.A.

Austen, K. Frank, Harvard Medical School, Robert B. Brigham Hospital, Boston, Massachusetts, U.S.A.

Brecher, Gerhard A., Department of Physiology and Biophysics, University of Oklahoma Medical Center, Oklahoma City, Oklahoma, U.S.A.

Brobmann, Günther F., Department of Physiology and Biophysics, University of Oklahoma Medical Center, Oklahoma City, Oklahoma, U.S.A.

Collier, H. O. J., Miles Laboratories, Ltd., Stoke Court Research Department, Stoke Court, Stoke Poges, Slough, Buckinghamshire, England.

Daugherty, Robert M., Jr., Department of Physiology, Michigan State University, East Lansing, Michigan, U.S.A.

Diniz, Carlos R., Departamento de Bioquimica, Faculdade de Medicina, Uni versidade Federal de Minas Gerais, Belo Horizonte, Brasil.

Eisen, V., Rheumatology Research Department, The Middlesex Hospital Medical School, London, England.

Elliott, D. F., CIBA Laboratories, Ltd., Horsham, Sussex, London, England.

Emerson, Thomas E., Department of Physiology, Michigan State University, East Lansing, Michigan, U.S.A.

Erdös, E. G., Department of Pharmacology, University of Oklahoma Medical Center, Oklahoma City, Oklahoma, U.S.A.

Habermann, E., Pharmakologisches Institut der Justus Liebig-Universität, Giessen, Germany.

Haddy, Francis J., Department of Physiology, Michigan State University, East Lansing, Michigan, U.S.A.

Hilton, Sidney M., Department of Physiology, The Medical School, University of Birmingham, Birmingham, England.

Iwanaga, Sadaaki, Division of Plasma Proteins, Institute for Protein Research, Osaka University, Osaka, Japan.

Jacobson, Eugene D., Department of Physiology and Biophysics, University of Oklahoma Medical Center, Oklahoma City, Oklahoma, U.S.A.

Lecomte, Jean, Physiologie, Institut Leon Fredericq, Université de Liege, Liege, Belgium.

Lewis, G. P., Research Division, CIBA Laboratories, Ltd., Horsham, Sussex, England.

Mares-Guia, Marcos, Departamento de Bioquimica, Faculdade de Medicina, Universidade Federal de Minas Gerais, Belo Horizonte, Brasil.

Moriya, Hiroshi, Laboratory of Physiological Chemistry, Science University of Tokyo, Tokyo, Japan.

Pierce, Jack V., Experimental Therapeutics Branch, National Heart and Lung Institute, N.I.H., Bethesda, Maryland, U.S.A.

PISANO, JOHN J., Experimental Therapeutics Branch, National Heart and Lung Institute, N.I.H., Bethesda, Maryland, U.S.A.

PRADO, JOSE LEAL, Department of Biochemistry and Pharmacology, Escola Paulista de Medicina, Sao Paulo, Brazil.

SCHACHTER, M., Department of Physiology, University of Alberta, Edmonton, Alberta, Canada.

SCHRÖDER, EBERHARD, Abteilung für Arzneimittelchemie, Schering AG, Berlin, Germany.

SCOTT, JERRY B., Department of Physiology, Michigan State University, East Lansing, Michigan, U.S.A.

SICUTERI, F., Clinica Medica Dell'Università, Firenze, Italy.

SPRAGG, JOCELYN, Harvard Medical School, Robert B. Brigham Hospital, Boston, Massachusetts, U.S.A.

STEWART, JOHN M., University of Colorado School of Medicine, Denver, Colorado, U.S.A.

SUZUKI, TOMOJI, Division of Plasma Proteins, Institute for Protein Research, Osaka University, Osaka, Japan.

TALAMO, RICHARD C., Harvard Medical School, The Massachusetts General Hospital, Boston, Massachusetts, U.S.A.

TRAUTSCHOLD, I., Institut für Klinische Biochemie und Physiologische Chemie, Medizinische Hochschule, Hannover, Germany.

TRČKA, VÁCLAV, Research Institute for Pharmacy and Biochemistry, Prague, Czechoslovakia.

VOGEL, ROSMARIE, Institut für klinische Chemie und klinische Biochemie der Universität, München, Germany.

VOGT, W., Max-Planck-Institut für experimentelle Medizin, Göttingen, Germany.

WALASZEK, EDWARD J., Department of Pharmacology, University of Kansas Medical Center, Kansas City, Kansas, U.S.A.

WEBSTER, MARION E., Experimental Therapeutics Branch, National Heart and Lung Institute, N.I.H., Bethesda, Maryland, U.S.A.

WERLE, EUGEN, Institut für klinische Chemie und klinische Biochemie der Universität, München, Germany.

YANG, H. Y. T., Department of Pharmacology, University of Oklahoma Medical Center, Oklahoma City, Oklahoma, U.S.A.

ZICKGRAF-RÜDEL, GERTRUD, Institut für klinische Chemie und klinische Biochemie der Universität, München, Germany.

Chapter 1: Introduction

Discovery of the Most Important Kallikreins and Kallikrein Inhibitors

EUGEN WERLE

A. Discovery of Kallikrein from Urine

In the course of research on the connection between heart action and function of the kidneys in 1925 E. K. FREY (1926) found that intravenous injection of dog urine to another dog decreased the blood pressure, which could be registered by measuring the pressure in the carotid artery with a Ludwig mercury manometer. Using the Frank-Petter spring manometer, FREY saw an initial decrease of the pulse amplitude, which was followed by an increase. Thus there was a difference in pressure during systole and diastole and an increase of heart rate, which were dependent on the dose given. Also human urine caused the same reactions. Yet there were quantitative differences, as a greater volume of human urine than dog urine had to be used to cause the same effects. FREY was convinced that he had discovered a hitherto unknown substance, which had a physiological function on heart action. As a surgeon he was not trained in this field; he therefore asked a well-known physiological chemist to isolate and chemically characterize this substance. But the chemist, who was pharmacologically well informed, declined, since he thought the action of urine on blood pressure would be the sum of the actions of substances normally contained in the urine, which were known to be more or less toxic. He assumed that it was histamine—known to be formed in the intestine as a product of decomposition and excreted with urine.

If the active substance were really histamine, it would be lost during dialysis and preserved during boiling, for it was generally known that histamine has a low molecular weight and is heat stable. Examination by FREY showed that the active substance was destroyed by boiling and was not lost during dialysis. When rabbit instead of dog was used as the experimental subject, the difference between the effect of boiled and not boiled urine was small. This way it became more obvious that the material was a hitherto unknown substance.

At this point FREY asked RICHARD WILLSTÄTTER, the professor of chemistry at the University of Munich, a Nobel Laureate, for help. After considering the arguments WILLSTÄTTER became convinced that these substances were worth further examination. He could not do it himself, but he promised to ask the cooperation of a skilled co-worker, the university lecturer in chemistry, HEINRICH KRAUT, who from this time worked with FREY on this new substance. KRAUT had worked in WILLSTÄTTER's research group on isolation of enzymes and had already had experience in the purification of thermolabile, high molecular weight substances. He had also contributed to the development of adsorbents for enzyme isolation, especially of different aluminum hydroxides, of which aluminum hydroxide Cγ proved to be very selective. KRAUT's primary aim was to prepare a stable preparation. This substance—first called "F-Stoff" (F-substance, for

Frey) could then be used as standard for measuring the effectiveness of further isolation. A biological unit of the F-substance was fixed as the amount in a 5-ml sample taken from 50 liters of pooled human urine after dialysis through parchment membranes for 48 hours. A dried powder was prepared from human urine by means of benzoic acid adsorption, which stabilized the F-substance. Enriched preparations of the F-substance, which were kept in aqueous solution under toluol in a closed bottle in a refrigerator, were also stable without time limit. The F-substance was thought to be a circulation hormone. Because during isolation of the effective substance there were no indications of separation into several active components, and because the mode of action on blood pressure remained unchanged, the uniformity of the F-substance was assumed (Frey and Kraut, 1928; Kraut et al., 1928).

B. Discovery of the Kallikrein Inhibitor of Blood Serum

A very high concentration of F-substance in urine was thought to occur after a so-called postoperative reflex anuria. When Frey injected such urine into a dog, it was completely inactive. The urine, however, was much contaminated with blood, which led Frey and Kraut (1928) to the assumption that the blood could have made the substance ineffective. Examining this, they found that the F-substance was indeed inactivated by blood plasma or serum. Sera of other mammals were also able to inactivate the substance. This principle was then called "serum inactivator" (Kraut et al., 1928).

C. Discovery of F-Substance in Pancreas

In 1930 my part of the work was the search for the origin of F-substance in organs of mammalian body. During this work Frey, Kraut, and Schultz (1930) found that the content of a surgically removed human pancreatic cyst caused a marked decrease of blood pressure on injection to dog. This observation drew our attention to the pancreas. We prepared pancreas of men and various animals (Kraut et al., 1930a) and found such great amounts of F-substance that the pancreas could be taken for its site of origin. The substance was therefore named kallikrein. It is formed from the word *καλλικρεας* from the Greek, term for pancreas.

According to experiments of Frey et al. (1930), which demonstrated that extirpation of the pancreas caused the excretion of kallikrein in the urine to be markedly decreased, it seemed to be logical to call kallikrein a hormone of the pancreas. Pursuing these experiments, I found that after extirpation of the pancreas in dogs the excretion of kallikrein in urine was not diminished—contrary to expectation—as long as the dogs were in sufficiently good condition. First it was deduced from this observation that kallikrein was produced by other organs besides the pancreas. During these experiments it was found that the external secretion of the pancreas of dog, and also of man, contains kallikrein (Frey and Werle, 1933; Werle, 1934). This finding should have refuted the theory that F-substance is a hormone.

D. Discovery of Kallikrein in Salivary Glands and Saliva

In the search for other organs which produce kallikrein, the salivary glands had to be considered. It was known that intravenous injection of saliva and extracts of salivary glands of cats and dogs causes a marked decrease of blood pressure; acetylcholine was thought to be the active substance. Yet there were hints that the hypotension could not or could only partly be caused by acetylcholine. We therefore examined saliva and salivary glands for kallikrein. We found in all species examined and also in humans a principle of high molecular weight, with the capacity to lower blood pressure, which possessed all the qualities of kallikrein (WERLE and VON RODEN, 1936, 1939).

E. Discovery of Kallikreinogen in Pancreas and Pancreas Secretion and in Other Organs

In experiments done to improve methods of extracting kallikrein from pancreas, it was striking that extracts which were prepared under conditions that prevented autolysis contained especially little kallikrein (WERLE, 1937). First it was assumed that kallikrein occurred in the gland in a lyo- and in a desmo-form. The real facts emerged later: according to MIGAY and PETROFF (1936) the effect of pure pancreatic secretion in lowering blood pressure is markedly increased on mixing it with intestinal fluid. This we could confirm. Because we had proved that the spontaneous action of pancreatic juice on blood pressure was caused by kallikrein, we wanted to know whether the increase in activity that occurred after mixing pancreas secretion with intestinal fluid could be caused by newly formed kallikrein. This proved to be true (WERLE, 1937). Further, I succeeded by mild extraction of pancreas of dog, pig, and cattle, in obtaining a solution of inactive kallikrein. This we could activate by adding an extract from small intestine. Later we achieved this also by adding crystallized trypsin to the kallikrein solution (WERLE and URHAHN, 1940).

We named the inactive precursor of kallikrein, kallikreinogen. According to the suggestions of the commission on nomenclature the substance is now called prekallikrein. Pancreas contains two different prekallikreins (FIEDLER and WERLE, 1967).

F. Discovery of Plasma Kallikrein

On the assumption that inactivation of urinary kallikrein consists of a reversible binding of serum inactivator to kallikrein, we tried to disrupt this by mild acidification. Indeed, a small amount of the primary added kallikrein could be shown to be reactivated.

When serum was treated the same way, it had the effect of lowering blood pressure, especially if papain was added. The active principle could be identified as kallikrein by its behavior during dialysis, boiling, or at addition of fresh plasma (KRAUT et al., 1928).

For the purification of plasma kallikrein a stable source of starting material was necessary. This was obtained by drying human serum with acetone and ether. The solution obtained by dissolving the dried preparation in water or phosphate buffer (pH 7.5) or in 0.02 M sodium bicarbonate showed a marked activity on blood pressure. The activity per milliliter of human plasma corresponded to 6 KU. It was later established that 7 ml plasma mixed with 2 ml acetone produced the same activity on blood pressure within hours (KRAUT et al., 1933; WERLE, 1936). As the active principle was a thermolabile, high molecular weight substance which could be inactivated by fresh serum, it was called serum or plasma kallikrein.

After it had been proved that the kallikreinogen of pancreas could be transformed by trypsin into active kallikrein, we found that trypsin also liberates active kallikrein from the kallikreinogen of blood plasma (WERLE et al., 1953).

According to Rocha e Silva et al. (1949) trypsin liberates from the kininogen of blood plasma bradykinin, which contracts the intestine and lowers the blood pressure. When we incubate such a mixture containing human plasma for 20 minutes, contraction of guinea pig ileum is no longer demonstrable, because bradykinin has meanwhile been degraded by the kininase of plasma. Yet if this mixture is injected intravenously into an anaesthetized dog, a marked lowering of blood pressure can be shown in spite of the fact that such an amount of trypsin or plasma, if injected separately, would be without effect. Further examination proved the active substance to be plasma kallikrein (Werle et al., 1955). Therefore trypsin transforms kallikreinogen from pancreas and plasma in the active form.

Plasma kallikreinogen and pancreas kallikreinogen are not identical, because the kallikreins which are liberated from them by trypsin are different. The kallikreinogen of plasma is *not* an inactivated pancreas kallikrein bound to the serum inhibitor, because from this complex neither trypsin nor addition of acetone sets free active kallikrein. We do not know yet to what extent this inactivation is achieved by enzymatic degradation (Werle and Schmal, 1968).

G. Discovery of the Kallikrein Inhibitor of Bovine Organs (Trasylol)

This was done in connection with the discovery of kallikrein in the pancreas. The research group of Frey, Kraut, and Werle had developed a hypothesis according to which active kallikrein was transferred from pancreas to the blood stream where it became bound to the inactivator and was liberated in other parts of the body, for example, by lowering the pH. That kallikrein occurs in the gland in the form of kallikreinogen was not known then. Working with bovine pancreas from a slaughterhouse, I found attached to one pancreas a small gland which differed from the yellow-brown pancreas in consistency and color. I surmised that if kallikrein were transferred in active form to the blood stream, it would impair the circulation. It might be that kallikrein passes through this gland in order to become inactivated there; and only then is it transferred to the blood stream. I argued that inactivator might originate in this gland. I therefore examined extracts of such glands and found a very large amount of inactivator (Kraut et al., 1930b). The reversibility of kallikrein inactivation by means of *this* inactivator could be well demonstrated. Later I found that this inhibitor occurs only in organs of cattle and some other ruminants and that it is not identical with the inhibitor of blood plasma.

H. Discovery of Kallidin and the Enzymatic Nature of Kallikrein

During our research work on kallikrein I was soon impressed by the similarities of kallikrein and enzymes. It occurred to me that I was dealing with an enzyme, but this really was no progress since it was impossible to predict what specific function the enzyme kallikrein could exert. In any case, a dilatation of blood vessels should be achieved by means of an event catalyzed by kallikrein. This dilatation was not caused by nervous impulses but by a direct action on vessels. Today one would argue that the substrate of the enzyme could occur in the wall of blood vessels or in blood. But at that time such considerations were unknown and therefore I had to look for this enzymatic process by analyzing the pharmacological actions of kallikrein.

In 1936 I found that kallikrein preparations from human urine contracted the isolated dog intestine (WERLE, 1936a). If kallikrein was the active substance here and not a contamination, the action on intestine should be abolished by incubation of the kallikrein with suitable amounts of blood serum. This proved to be true. Yet the identity of the substances that lower blood pressure and contract the intestine could be shown only when the velocity of inactivation was be the same for both substances. I therefore registered the time course of both activities, starting with the moment of mixing kallikrein with blood serum and ending with total inactivation. I found that the activity on intestine was not diminished at first but increased markedly. Because these solutions stimulated the isolated guinea pig ileum, which kallikrein alone did not do, formation of a new substance had to be considered. This substance could be concentrated. Its pharmacological actions were the same as those of kallikrein, but it was of low molecular weight and thermostable. It was not a split product of kallikrein but a split product of a serum protein. The substance, which we thought to be a polypeptide, we called DK at first (WERLE et al., 1937) and kallidin later. The inactive form was named kallidinogen (WERLE, 1948). Kallikrein therefore should be a proteolytic enzyme. Our idea of the enzymatic process turned out to be the right one and formed the basis for future findings. From the fact that substance DK migrates in a broad pH range toward the cathode we concluded that basic amino acids would share in its composition (WERLE and DÄUMER, 1940).

J. Detection of Kallidin-Inactivating Enzymes

Formation of substance DK was easy to demonstrate by means of submandibular kallikrein, but not with pancreas kallikrein. Even highly purified pancreas kallikrein is contaminated with an enzyme (a peptidase) that inactivates DK even faster than chymotrypsin. We found that cysteine inactivates this enzyme and we could produce kallidin also with pancreas kallikrein. Such kininases were also found in plasma in pancreas and in extracts of many organs (WERLE et al., 1937).

References

FIEDLER, F., WERLE, E.: Vorkommen zweier Kallikreinogene im Schweinepankreas und Automation der Kallikrein- und Kallikreinogenbestimmung. Hoppe-Seylers Z. physiol. Chem. **348**, 1087 (1967).

FREY, E. K.: Zusammenhänge zwischen Herzarbeit und Nierentätigkeit. Langenbecks Arch. klin. Chir. **142**, 663 (1926).

— KRAUT, H.: Ein neues Kreislaufhormon und seine Wirkung. Naunyn-Schmiedebergs Arch. exp. Path. Pharmak. **133**, 1 (1928).

— — SCHULTZ, F.: Über eine neue innersekretorische Funktion des Pankreas. Naunyn-Schmiedebergs Arch. exp. Path. Pharmak. **158**, 334 (1930).

— WERLE, E.: Kallikrein im inneren und äußeren Pankreassekret. Klin. Wschr. **12**, 600 (1933).

KRAUT, H., FREY, E. K., BAUER, E.: Über ein neues Kreislaufhormon. II. Mitt. Hoppe-Seylers Z. physiol. Chem. **175**, 97 (1928).

— — WERLE, E.: Der Nachweis eines Kreislaufhormons in der Pankreasdrüse. Hoppe-Seylers Z. physiol. Chem. **189**, 97 (1930a).

— — — Über die Inaktivierung des Kallikreins. Hoppe-Seylers Z. physiol. Chem. **192**, 1 (1930b).

— — — Über den Nachweis und das Vorkommen des Kallikreins im Blut. VIII. Mitt. Hoppe-Seylers Z. physiol. Chem. **222**, 73 (1933).

MIGAY, TH. J., PETROFF, J. R.: Untersuchungen über die Wirkung des Pankreassaftes auf den Organismus bei parenteraler Einführung. Z. ges. exp. Med. **36**, 457 (1936).

ROCHA E SILVA, M., BERALDO, W. T., ROSENFELD, G.: Bradykinin, a hypotensive and smooth muscle stimulating factor released from plasma globulin by snake venom and by trypsin. J. Physiol. (Lond.) **109**, 488 (1949).

WERLE, E.: Zur Kenntnis des Haushaltes des Kallikreins. Biochem. Z. **269**, 415 (1934).
— Über Kallikrein aus Blut. Biochem. Z. **287**, 235 (1936).
— Die Wirkung des Kallikreins auf den isolierten Darm. Klin. Wschr. **1936** a, 848.
— Über den Aktivitätszustand des Kallikreins der Bauchspeicheldrüse und ihres äußeren Sekretes beim Hund. Biochem. Z. **290**, 129 (1937).
— Zur Kenntnis des Kallikreins. Angew. Chem. **60**, 53 (1948).
— DÄUMER, J.: Über das Verhalten des Kallikreins, des Inaktivators aus Lymphdrüsen, der Substanz DK, sowie der Histidindecarboxylase bei der Kataphorese. Biochem. Z. **304**, 377 (1940).
— FORELL, M., MAIER, L.: Zum Mechanismus der Blutdruckwirkung des Trypsins. Naturwissenschaften **40**, 627 (1953).
— — — Zur Kenntnis der blutdrucksenkenden Wirkung des Trypsins. Naunyn-Schmiedebergs Arch. exp. Path. Pharmak. **225**, 369 (1955).
— GÖTZE, W., KEPPLER, A.: Über die Wirkung des Kallikreins auf den isolierten Darm und über eine neue darmkontrahierende Substanz. Biochem. Z. **289**, 217 (1937).
— RODEN, P. VON: Über das Vorkommen des Kallikreins in den Speicheldrüsen und im Mundspeichel. Biochem. Z. **286**, 213 (1936).
— — Über das Vorkommen von Kallikrein in den Speicheldrüsen und im Mundspeichel und über eine blutdrucksteigernde Substanz in der Submaxillardrüse des Hundes. Biochem. Z. **301**, 328 (1939).
— SCHMAL, A.: Über ein Kallikrein-abbauendes Enzym im Blutplasma der Ratte. Hoppe-Seylers Z. physiol. Chem. **349**, 521 (1968).
— URHAHN, K.: Über den Aktivitätszustand des Kallikreins in der Bauchspeicheldrüse. Biochem. Z. **304**, 387 (1940).

The Discovery and Characterization of Bradykinin

D. F. Elliott

With 1 Figure

"We came into the world like brother and brother,
And now let's go hand in hand, not one before another."
The Comedy of Errors

To pharmacology goes the credit for the discovery of bradykinin this active principle which, for a time, remained a monopoly interest and challenge to pharmacological investigators. In the early 1950s chemical methodology had not advanced to the point where the isolation and characterization of the pure substance would have been possible, and later progress in this respect could be seen to be made almost in step with advances in the techniques of polypeptide chemistry.

The pharmacological effects of the venom of *Bothrops jararaca* and of trypsin had been under investigation in Brazil by Rocha e Silva and his co-workers and led to the finding that incubation of the venom or trypsin with the pseudoglobulin fraction of plasma resulted in the formation of a potent vasodilator and smooth-muscle-stimulating substance (Rocha e Silva et al., 1949) (see also p. 634). Their experiments indicated that these pharmacological actions were due to a substance whose destruction by enzymes in the plasma or by chemical means was consistent with the hypothesis that it was a polypeptide. The guinea pig ileum responded slowly to the substance compared to histamine or acetylcholine, hence the name bradykinin was derived to describe this slow action. The action of bradykinin was not antagonized by atropine or antihistamines and both hypotensive and smooth-muscle-stimulating actions progressed in parallel when the substance was passed through a number of purification procedures (Rocha e Silva, 1960). These observations, among others, led to the belief that the new principle was a single substance. Bradykinin became known as the slow-acting principle, not antagonized by atropine or antihistamines, formed by the action of trypsin or snake venom on plasma or a globulin fraction therefrom. In the early 1950 period it was not possible to decide whether or not it was chemically identical with certain substances formed from plasma by other means which eventually became known under the generic name of plasma kinins (Lewis, 1960a).

The first significant advance toward the isolation of a pure substance was the work of Andrade and Rocha e Silva (1956). These workers used as a substrate the protein precipitate formed from ox plasma at an ammonium sulfate concentration of 25%. The enzyme source was whole snake venom. Preliminary purification was on columns of paper pulp and aluminium oxide. The final step was ion-exchange chromatography on Amberlite IRC-50. An overall increase in biological activity of about 1,000-fold was achieved, and the authors produced evidence indicating that the substance might have been pure. Conclusive proof by the recognized techniques of peptide chemistry was, however, not possible because the substance could not be separated from the involatile buffers used in the ion-exchange column procedures. The very high biological potency of bradykinin was revealed by these experiments, and the amounts of material isolated were only fractions of a milligram, most of which were consumed in the analytical determinations.

Elliott et al. (1959b) used as a substrate the protein precipitate formed from ox serum between 33% and 45% of saturation with ammonium sulfate. It was heated in solution at pH 1, 37°, for 30 minutes in order to destroy kininase and was then digested with trypsin at pH 7.5 for 6 hours. Purification of the peptide mixture which resulted from alcoholic precipitation of the digest was carried out first by countercurrent distribution in a butanol:water:TCA system, and this was followed by gradient elution ion-exchange chromatography on CM-cellulose with volatile ammonium acetate buffers. The technique of ion-exchange chromatography and the use of appropriately substituted cellulose powders was, at the time, a new technique developed by Peterson and Sober (1956). The availability of a simple and reliable biological assay method using guinea pig ileum greatly facilitated the chemical isolation work. Nevertheless the work was not without its difficulties; on the one hand on account of substances used in the chromatographic procedures that interfered with the bioassay; on the other hand on account of chelation of the peptide with metal ions, particularly magnesium ions. Bioassay was available with a minimum of delay at every stage of the investigation, and the importance of close collaboration between chemist and pharmacologist, preferably in the same laboratory, should be emphasized.

In the early phase of this investigation, CM-cellulose chromatography did not give a completely pure product, but purity was finally achieved by paper chromatography. The first sample of completely pure bradykinin was obtained in this way and weighed about 50 μg. During the course of the purification it was observed that the steady rise in biological potency was accompanied by a fall in the number of different amino acids produced on acid hydrolysis. The number eventually fell to five (arginine, glycine, serine, proline, and phenylalanine), and then appeared to be at a minimum; this encouraged us to believe that the substance was pure. By this time it had become generally known that our experiments at Mill Hill had almost reached fruition, and we were asked to speak about this work at a symposium in London in 1959. In view of the short time available before the symposium was held, and the minute amount of pure material obtained, it was decided to use it all in a quantitative amino acid analysis in the belief that if molar ratios close to whole numbers were obtained for the constituent amino acids, this would provide good, but of course not conclusive, evidence that the preparation was pure. The analysis was carried out by a paper chromatographic technique (Mandelstam and Rogers, 1959) which was the most sensitive method available at the time. The result announced at the symposium (Elliott, 1960) was that the five constituent amino acids—arginine, phenylalanine, proline, glycine, and serine—were present in the molar proportions 2:2:2:1:1. Unfortunately, an error had been made in the molar proportion of proline, which was actually 3 and not 2 as found. This led to further errors in what should have been a simple structural problem but developed into a situation as complicated as a Shakespearean plot.

During the few months following the symposium, supplies of the pure peptide were at all times critical as we had to satisfy the demands of the structural investigations and the pharmacological evaluation of the pure material, as well as trying to meet requests from outside investigators for the pure substance for comparison studies. It was fortunate that improvements in our isolation techniques had enabled us to prepare pure bradykinin by means of CM-cellulose chromatography at the final stage, thus eliminating preparative paper chromatography (ELLIOTT et al., 1961; ELLIOTT, 1963). Nevertheless it was never possible to standardize the isolation procedure, probably on account of the very large scale of the initial steps which made accurate control impossible. As a result, the yield of pure material sometimes fell far below expectations, the yield of 3.5 mg from 90 liters of ox blood being about the maximum ever obtained, and this was only 25% of the amount originally present in the tryptic digest.

The structural work was pressed forward with all possible speed and would have been a simple problem, consideration of shortage of pure material apart,

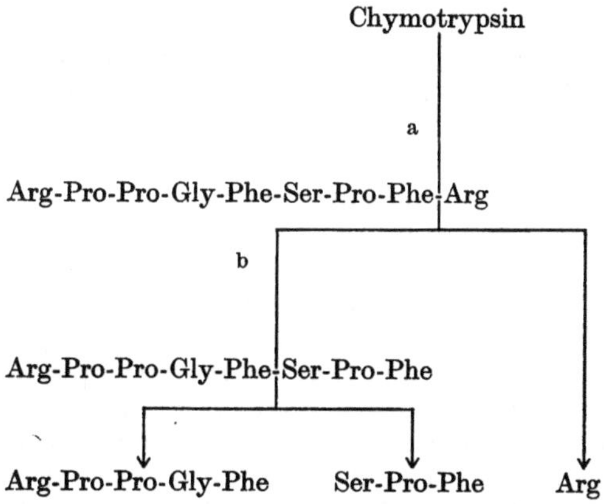

Fig. 1. Chymotryptic scission of bradykinin

were it not for the error made in the amino acid analysis, as already mentioned. The well-known and widely used technique of EDMAN for stepwise degradation yielded the sequence of the first five residues in bradykinin, the structure of which is given in Fig. 1, and required only 0.5 mg of material. SANGERS' fluorodinitrobenzene end-group technique, when used in conjunction with chymotrypsin, gave all the necessary information for the determination of the complete sequence of bradykinin, and these experiments were possible with amounts of peptide varying between 0.2 and 1 mg according to the particular type of experiment. The dinitrophenyl derivative of bradykinin, prepared by SANGERS' method, yielded DNP-arginine on acid hydrolysis, whereas when it was digested with chymotrypsin a second residue of arginine was released as the free amino acid. This was demonstrated by application of SANGERS' technique to the digest itself. Thus the molecule of bradykinin was shown to contain a residue of arginine at each end. Prolonged chymotryptic digestion of bradykinin itself yielded three substances which were separable by paper electrophoresis. The fastest moving component was arginine from the C-terminal end; this was followed by a peptide, which, on acid hydrolysis, yielded the amino acids arginine, proline, phenylalanine, and glycine in the proportions 1:2:1:1. Clearly this pentapeptide had come from the N-terminal portion and there remained only the peptide from the center portion of the molecule as the third component. This peptide, after conversion to the dinitrophenyl derivative, gave DNP-serine on acid hydrolysis. The only free amino acid found in the acid hydrolysate by paper chromatography was phenylalanine; thus the peptide appeared to be Ser-Phe and this fitted with all other data obtained.

Unlike pharmacologists, who are forced by the very nature of their work to clear away experimental material and tidy the laboratory each day, chemists are afforded a much greater latitude and frequently hoard the remains of past experiments under the guise that further reference may be necessary when the fact may often be that it is just a case of sentimental attachment to a satisfactory experiment. Every peptide laboratory where the occupants are not imbued with excessive zeal for tidiness will have a pile of paper chromatograms in some odd corner away from the light, slowly bleaching, nevertheless, and exuding that rich mixture of odors which is strangely attractive to those who work within. It so happened that the paper chromatogram showing the single spot of phenylalanine from the supposedly Ser-Phe peptide remained in the writer's laboratory for several days during which time a small yellow spot appeared in the position expected of proline. This seemed an impossible result, as the two residues of proline had already been accounted for by independent experiments, and it provoked lengthy discussions as to whether it was due to proline, and, if so, how it could be present in that particular peptide. Unfortunately it was not possible to repeat the experiment, for by that time all available pure material had been consumed, and the state of our isolation experiments was such that fresh material would not be available for at least one month.

Eventually it was decided that the yellow spot was an artefact and a communication to the Biochemical Society was accordingly given (ELLIOTT et al., 1960a). The structure proposed was that in which the proline residue number 7 in Fig. 1 was missing. Contributory factors in our undue haste were the many requests received from other research groups, including pharmaceutical companies, to impart the structure as soon as it was known. Several of these groups were informed simultaneously shortly before publication of the preliminary communication. Fortunately the missing proline residue did not long remain uncovered. The group of Dr. BOISSONNAS at Sandoz had, within ten days, synthesized the octapeptide sequence and had shown that it was biologically inactive. This information was communicated privately to us on April 14, 1960, by Dr. BOISSONNAS. It soon became obvious that the mysterious yellow spot on the paper chromatogram was, in fact, due to proline, particularly in view of the finding of the Sandoz group that the octapeptide, Arg-Pro-Gly-Phe-Ser-Pro-Phe-Arg had weak biological activity, whereas two other analogs composed of the same numbers of amino acid residues but with serine joined directly to phenylalanine were inactive. The Sandoz group were following certain ideas of their own which were based on the observation that the synthetic octapeptide Arg-Pro-Pro-Gly-Phe-Ser-Phe-Arg was split by chymotrypsin more rapidly in the middle than at the end of the molecule (BOISSONNAS et al., 1960a), whereas in natural bradykinin exactly the opposite was true (bond a in Fig. 1 was split faster than bond b). This was taken as an indication that the sequences in natural bradykinin and the octapeptide differed in some way in those parts away from the extremities. It was logical, therefore, to prepare some of the analogs in which the four central residues were rearranged.

We were informed of these results on May 21, 1960, and in our reply of May 26 the possibility of the nonapeptide structure was again mentioned. It had previously been raised in a letter of ours dated May 11 but discounted because the sequence did not fit the experimental data, particularly the amino acid analyses on bradykinin itself and on the pentapeptide formed on chymotryptic digestion (scission of bond b in Fig. 1), which showed two residues of proline in both cases. One June 7, Dr. BOISSONNAS informed us that he had synthesized the nonapeptide and had obtained biological data suggesting that it was probably identical with bradykinin (BOISSONNAS et al., 1960b, 1960c, 1963). Owing to a shortage of pure material, much of which had been used in studies in man, confirmation of the nonapeptide sequence in the natural material was not possible until a few weeks later when it was shown conclusively that a proline residue must be present between serine and phenylalanine (ELLIOTT et al., 1960b).

Almost at the same time as the activities just referred to, workers from CIBA reported the isolation of bradykinin from bovine plasma after its treatment with venom from *B. jararaca* (ZUBER and JAQUES, 1960). The amino acid analysis was the same that as reported by us at the symposium; in particular, two residues of proline were also found by these workers. Preliminary degradative evidence also indicated the probable identity of the bradykinin formed in this way with the bradykinin formed by trypsin. Unfortunately, Dr. SCHWYZER's group from the same laboratories (SCHWYZER et al., 1960) were also misled into synthesizing the inactive octapeptide and at about the same time also, a group from Parke, Davis laboratories (NICOLAIDES et al., 1960) reported the synthesis of the same inactive octapeptide. The reason why two independent groups should obtain low values for proline in bradykinin prepared in different ways has never been explained convincingly, but it could be simply a case of pushing the existing methodology to the limits of sensitivity on account of the very small amounts of material available. This is a common enough experience to those who work with the polypeptide hormones. In the intervening years, however, the limits of sensitivity of chemical methods have been lowered still further, probably by the order of ten times or more, and a similar mistake would not be likely today. It should also be mentioned that another group (HAMBERG et al., 1961), while confirming that bradykinin from ox blood was the same whether liberated by trypsin or snake venom, found no loss of proline on acid hydrolysis of their preparations.

The full characterization of bradykinin required the careful comparison of natural and synthetic material in a number of biological preparations, and it was also necessary to answer the question whether the pure substance showed all the biological actions of the crude material. The latter was answered in the affirmitive by the finding that pure natural bradykinin did possess all these actions, that is, smooth muscle stimulation, vasodilation, increased capillary permeability, and pain production (ELLIOTT et al., 1959a, 1960c). Comparison of the actions of pure natural bradykinin with those of synthetic bradykinin on eleven different biological preparations was made by LEWIS (1960b). The natural bradykinin was that isolated at Mill Hill, and the synthetic material came from the Sandoz laboratories or from the laboratories of Parke, Davis (NICOLAIDES and DE WALD, 1961).

All these preparations of the active substance were found to be identical within the limits of experimental error. Similar comparisons of Mill Hill material with synthetic material were carried out in the Sandoz laboratories (KONZETT and STÜRMER, 1960) and in the Parke, Davis laboratories (SHORLEY and COLLIER, 1960). Bradykinin was an extremely potent vasodilator in man; close intra-arterial injection of as little as 0.1 μg sometimes produced an increase of blood flow in the hand or forearm (FOX et al., 1960). Comparison of natural bradykinin, prepared at Mill Hill with synthetic bradykinin from the Sandoz laboratories demonstrated their identity also in these studies in the human (FOX et al., 1961). Human bradykinin is almost certainly identical with ox bradykinin, although complete structural proof is still lacking (PIERCE and WEBSTER, 1961; HAMBERG, 1961, 1962). Apart from the release by trypsin or snake venom, bradykinin can be formed by the action of the enzyme kallikrein from the human (PIERCE and

WEBSTER, 1961) or the ox (WERLE et al., 1961) on the homologous plasma fraction, or by "spontaneous" generation from human plasma (HAMBERG, 1961) and ox plasma (HABERMANN and OKON, 1961; ELLIOTT et al., 1963; ELLIOTT and LEWIS, 1965).

It is not intended in this chapter to provide a general review of later work; by the end of 1961 the characterization was complete in every respect. Bradykinin was discovered through the brilliant observations of a pharmacologist, but its characterization took more than ten years and required the concerted efforts of chemists, biochemists, and pharmacologists. Methodology has now improved so much that had it been discovered in 1967, the synthetic material would have been available less than twelve months later. One has to admit that this would have been very dull, for the bradykinin problem provided diversion and interest for a large number of people and, as in classical comedy, the story had a happy ending and honor was satisfied all round in spite of a near-tragedy in the middle.

References

ANDRADE, S. O., ROCHA E SILVA, M.: Purification of bradykinin by ion-exchange chromatography. Biochem. J. **64**, 701 (1956).

BOISSONNAS, R. A., GUTTMANN, S., JAQUENOUD, P.-A.: Synthèse de la L-arginyl-L-prolyl-L-prolyl-glycyl-L-phénylalanyl-L-seryl-L-phénylalanyl-L-arginine. Distinction entre cet octapeptide et la bradykinine. Helv. chim. Acta **43**, 1481 (1960a).

— — — Synthèse de la L-arginyl-L-prolyl-L-prolyl-glycyl-L-phénylalanyl-L-seryl-L-prolyl-L-phénylalanyl-L-arginine, un nonapeptide présentant les propriétés de la bradykinine. Helv. chim. Acta **43**, 1349 (1960b).

— — — KONZETT, H., STÜRMER, E.: Synthesis and biological activity of peptides related to bradykinin. Experientia (Basel) **16**, 326 (1960c).

— — — PLESS, J., SANDRIN, E.: The synthesis of bradykinin and of related peptides. Ann. N. Y. Acad. Sci. **104**, 5 (1963).

ELLIOTT, D. F.: Discussion, in: Polypeptides which affect smooth muscles and blood vessels, p. 266, ed. by M. SCHACHTER. Oxford-London-New York-Paris: Pergamon Press 1960.

— Bradykinin and its mode of release. Ann. N. Y. Acad. Sci. **104**, 35 (1963).

— HORTON, E. W., LEWIS, G. P.: Biological activity of pure bradykinin—a plasma kinin from ox blood. J. Physiol. (Lond.) **150**, 6P (1959a).

— — — Actions of pure bradykinin. J. Physiol. (Lond.) **153**, 473 (1960c).

— — — The isolation of bradykinin, a plasma kinin from ox blood. Biochem. J. **78**, 60 (1961).

— LEWIS, G. P.: Methionyl-lysyl-bradykinin, a new kinin from ox blood. Biochem. J. **95**, 437 (1965).

— — HORTON, E. W.: The isolation of bradykinin: A plasma kinin from ox blood. Biochem. J. **74**, 15P (1959b).

— — — The structure of bradykinin. Biochem. J. **76**, 16P (1960a).

— — — The structure of bradykinin—a plasma kinin from ox blood. Biochem. biophys. Res. Commun. **3**, 87 (1960b).

— — SMYTH, D. G.: A new kinin from ox blood. Biochem. J. **87**, 21P (1963).

FOX, R. H., GOLDSMITH, R., KIDD, D. J., LEWIS, G. P.: Bradykinin as a vasodilator in man. J. Physiol. (Lond.) **154**, 16P (1960).

— — — — Bradykinin as a vasodilator in man. J. Physiol. (Lond.) **157**, 589 (1961).

HABERMANN, E., OKON, M. E.: Identifizierung eines „spontan“ aus Serumglobulin entstehenden Peptids mit Bradykinin. Hoppe-Seylers Z. physiol. Chem. **326**, 171 (1961).

HAMBERG, U.: Isolation and amino acid composition of human bradykinin. Suom. Kemist. **34**, 168 (1961).

— Isolation and molar activity of human bradykinin. Biochem. biophys. Res. Commun. **7**, 95 (1962).

— BUMPUS, F. M., PAGE, I. H.: Isolation and amino acid composition of bradykinin released by venom of *Bothrops jararaca* from bovine plasma. Biochim. biophys. Acta (Amst.) **52**, 533 (1961).

KONZETT, H., STÜRMER, E.: Synthetic bradykinin: Its biological identity with natural pure trypsin bradykinin. Nature (Lond.) **188**, 998 (1960).

LEWIS, G. P.: Active polypeptides derived from plasma proteins. Physiol. Rev. **40**, 647 (1960a).

— Natural and synthetic bradykinin. Nature (Lond.) **188**, 999 (1960b).

MANDELSTAM, J., ROGERS, H. J.: The incorporation of amino acids into the cell-wall mucopeptide of staphylococci and the effect of antibiotics on the process. Biochem. J. **72**, 654 (1959).

NICOLAIDES, E. D., DEWALD, H. A.: Studies on the synthesis of polypeptides. Bradykinin. J. org. Chem. **26**, 3872 (1961).

— — SHORLEY, P. G., COLLIER, H. O. J.: Synthesis and biological properties of L-arginyl-L-prolyl-L-prolyl-glycyl-L-phenylalanyl-L-seryl-L-phenylalanyl-L-arginine, an octapeptide related to bradykinin. Nature (Lond.) **187**, 773 (1960).

PETERSON, E. A., SOBER, H. A.: Chromatography of proteins. I. Cellulose ion-exchange adsorbents. J. Amer. chem. Soc. **78**, 751 (1956).

PIERCE, J. V., WEBSTER, M. E.: Human plasma kallidins: Isolation and chemical studies. Biochem. biophys. Res. Commun. **5**, 353 (1961).

ROCHA E SILVA, M.: Biochemistry and pharmacology of bradykinin. In: Polypeptides which affect smooth muscles and blood vessels, p. 210, ed. by M. SCHACHTER. Oxford-London-New York-Paris: Pergamon Press 1960.

— BERALDO, W. T., ROSENFELD, G.: Bradykinin, a hypotensive and smooth muscle stimulating factor released from plasma globulin by snake venoms and by trypsin. Amer. J. Physiol. **156**, 261 (1949).

SCHWYZER, R., RITTEL, W., SIEBER, P., KAPPELER, H., ZUBER, H.: Synthese von L-Arginyl-L-prolyl-L-prolyl-glycyl-L-phenylalanyl-L-seryl-L-phenylalanyl-L-arginin (Bradykinin ?). Helv. chim. Acta **43**, 1130 (1960).

SHORLEY, P. G., COLLIER, H. O. J.: Direct comparisons of the synthetic nonapeptide with trypsin bradykinin. Nature (Lond.) **188**, 999 (1960).

WERLE, E., TRAUTSCHOLD, I., LEYSATH, G.: Isolierung und Struktur des Kallidins. Hoppe-Seylers Z. physiol. Chem. **326**, 174 (1961).

ZUBER, H., JAQUES, R.: Isolierung von Bradykinin aus Rinderplasma nach Einwirkung von Schlangengift (*Bothrops jararaca*). Helv. chim. Acta **43**, 1128 (1960).

The Kinins: Methods of Chemical Synthesis

J. M. Stewart

With 4 Figures

The chemical synthesis of bradykinin has a remarkable history, for this peptide hormone was successfully synthesized before the completed structure of the natural material had been determined, and the molecule has been synthesized since by many different methods. Indeed it has more than once served as a model for the demonstration of new methods of peptide synthesis. The other mammalian kinins, kallidin and methionyl-lysyl-bradykinin, have been synthesized several times. *Polistes* kinin and phyllokinin, two kinins of nonmammalian origin, have also been synthesized. The structures of these peptides are given in Fig. 1.

Arg-Pro-Pro-Gly-Phe-Ser-Pro-Phe-Arg
bradykinin

Lys-Arg-Pro-Pro-Gly-Phe-Ser-Pro-Phe-Arg
kallidin

Met-Lys-Arg-Pro-Pro-Gly-Phe-Ser-Pro-Phe-Arg
methionyl-lysyl-bradykinin

$$\begin{array}{r}OSO_3H\\ |\\ \text{Arg-Pro-Pro-Gly-Phe-Ser-Pro-Phe-Arg-Ile-Tyr}\end{array}$$
phyllokinin

Pyroglu-Thr-Asn-Lys-Lys-Lys-Leu-Arg-Gly-Arg-Pro-Pro-Gly-Phe-Ser-Pro-Phe-Arg
polistes kinin

Fig. 1. Structures of kinins

In this review of the chemical synthesis of these peptides, we shall consider first some of the techniques and problems of peptide synthesis, and then see how these apply to the individual kinins.

A. Methods of Peptide Synthesis

Since every amino acid has both an amino and a carboxyl group, the primary requirement for successful synthesis of peptides of defined sequence is that one of these functional groups be covered with a protecting group while the other is brought into reaction. The protecting group used must be such that it can be subsequently removed selectively without any damage to the amide, or peptide, bonds which have been formed. Since the carboxyl group of one amino acid must be made to react with the amino group of another for the formation of a peptide bond, it follows that selectively removable protecting groups must be available for both amino and carboxyl groups. The development of a variety of protecting groups removable under a wide range of conditions has been one of the major accomplishments of peptide chemists.

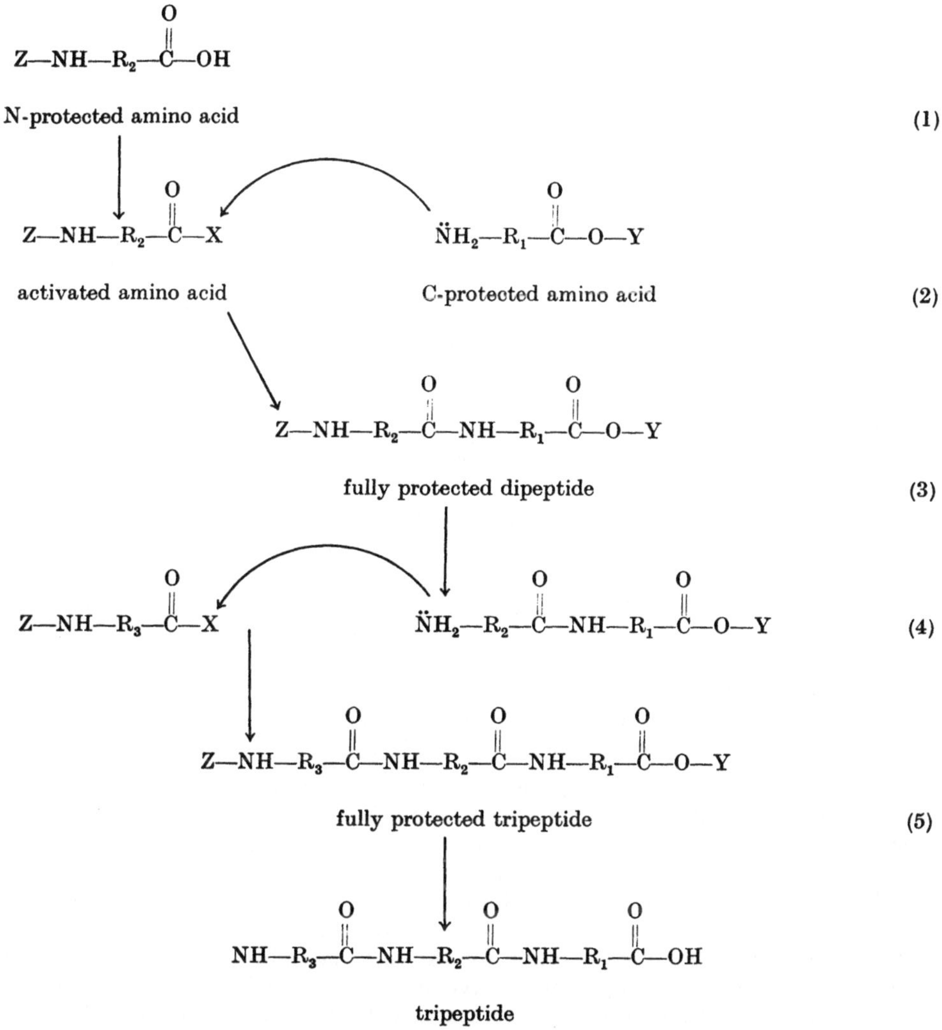

Fig. 2. Peptide synthesis

Another major development in peptide chemistry has been the discovery of a number of good methods to activate amino acids to cause them to couple together to form peptides. This is most generally done by conversion of the carboxyl group to some energy-rich derivative that can then be attacked by the amino group of another amino acid. These points are illustrated in Fig. 2. An amine-protected amino acid is first converted (reaction 1) to an activated derivative, which is then brought into reaction with a carboxyl-protected amino acid (reaction 2) to yield the protected dipeptide. The activating group X is one that withdraws electrons from the carboxyl carbon of amino acid R_2 and makes that carbon subject to facile attack by the free electron pair of the amine group of amino acid R_1 (nucleophilic attack). This is the most commonly used scheme of peptide synthesis.

Before the peptide chain can be elongated, one of the protecting groups (Z or Y) must be removed selectively (reaction 3) to expose one functional group for further reaction. In order to minimize racemization, as discussed below, peptides are generally lengthened at the amine end, as shown in reaction 4. Such a sequence of reactions can be repeated at will, adding each time N-protected amino acids or peptides, until the desired peptide sequence is assembled. Then in a final deprotection, or deblocking, step or steps (reaction 5) all protecting groups are removed to yield the desired peptide. At the present time, the most commonly used amine-protecting groups are the carbobenzoxy (Z) and *t*-butyloxycarbonyl (Boc) groups, and carboxyl groups are usually protected as methyl (Me), benzyl (Bzl) or *t*-butyl (Bu) esters. For the synthesis of peptides containing trifunctional amino acids, another category of blocking groups must generally be used to prevent the involvement of these side-chain functional groups in peptide-forming reactions. In the kinins, the trifunctional amino acids encountered are arginine, lysine, and serine. The guanidine group of arginine is usually protected as the nitro (NO_2) or toluenesulfonyl (Tos) derivative. The ε-amino group of lysine is protected as the carbobenzoxy, *t*-butyloxycarbonyl, or toluenesulfonyl derivative, and the hydroxyl group of serine has been protected as the benzyl or *t*-butyl ether.

One great concern of peptide chemists is that of avoiding racemization during synthesis. All amino acids but glycine are optically active and occur in the kinins in their L forms. There is risk of destruction of this optical activity of these amino acids when they are activated for coupling reactions. Generally, Z- or Boc-amino acids can be activated in a variety of ways without risk of racemization, but when peptide carboxyl groups are activated, only the azide (N_3) coupling reaction is universally racemization-free. For the coupling of Z- or Boc-amino acids, *p*-nitrophenyl esters (ONP), dicyclohexyl-carbodiimide (DCC), and mixed anhydrides are most widely used.

Two general methods of peptide synthesis are available: (1) the fragment condensation method, and (2) the stepwise method. In the first, small peptides representing fragments of the desired sequence are made, and then these fragments are coupled together to give the final product. With this method the synthetic attack can be carried out on several fronts at once, and the risk of total loss from a single bad reaction is not so great. However, the chemist is generally limited to the azide-coupling reaction for the final assembly unless the assembly points involve the carboxyl groups of glycine or proline, which do not racemize. In the stepwise method, the chemist starts with the carboxyl-terminal amino acids and adds N-protected amino acids, one at a time, until the desired sequence is assembled. In this method, all the effort is concentrated in a single channel, and a single bad reaction near the end of the sequence can destroy the entire effort. However, a much wider variety of coupling reactions can be used.

A dramatic new approach to the stepwise method is that of "solid-phase peptide synthesis," developed principally by R. B. Merrifield (1968). In this method, the C-terminal amino acid is esterified to an insoluble support (a synthetic resin bead), and the peptide chain is then assembled, in the stepwise manner, while still attached to the support. Finally a reagent is used which will cleave the finished peptide from the support and liberate it into solution. The solid-phase method is outstanding because of its great speed, which has been further increased by the construction of an automatic instrument (MERRIFIELD et al., 1966). A recent book (STEWART and YOUNG, 1969) describes this method in detail.

The considerations outlined above will determine the strategy used to assemble peptides such as the kinins. There are excellent treatises on peptide synthesis (GREENSTEIN and WINITZ, 1961; SCHRÖDER and LÜBKE, 1965) for the reader who wishes to study more deeply this general subject.

B. Syntheses of Bradykinin

The first synthesis of bradykinin was accomplished by the fragment condensation method (BOISSONNAS et al., 1960), and is outlined in Fig. 3. This synthesis

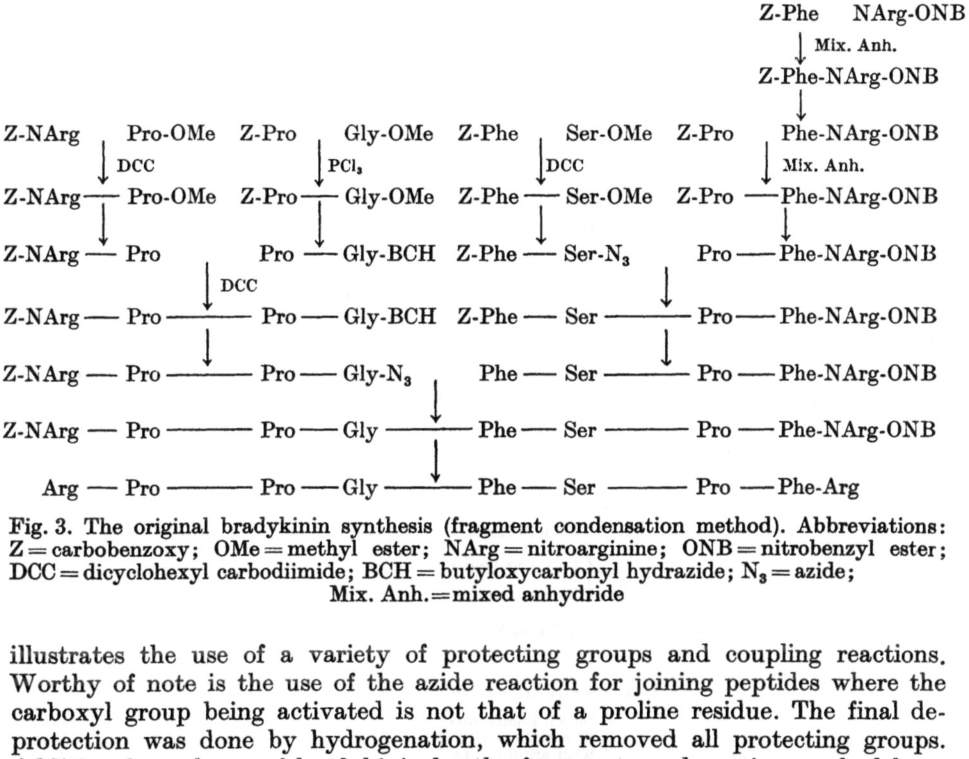

Fig. 3. The original bradykinin synthesis (fragment condensation method). Abbreviations: Z = carbobenzoxy; OMe = methyl ester; NArg = nitroarginine; ONB = nitrobenzyl ester; DCC = dicyclohexyl carbodiimide; BCH = butyloxycarbonyl hydrazide; N_3 = azide; Mix. Anh. = mixed anhydride

illustrates the use of a variety of protecting groups and coupling reactions. Worthy of note is the use of the azide reaction for joining peptides where the carboxyl group being activated is not that of a proline residue. The final deprotection was done by hydrogenation, which removed all protecting groups. Additional syntheses of bradykinin by the fragment condensation method have been reported by GUTTMANN et al. (1962), SIEMION (1964), SHCHUKINA et al. (1965, 1966), and SAKAKIBARA and INUKAI (1966).

Very shortly after the original synthesis of bradykinin, NICOLAIDES and DEWALD (1961) showed that the stepwise method is applicable to the synthesis of bradykinin. Beginning with nitroarginine methyl ester, the chain was lengthened by coupling each new amino acid as its carbobenzoxy derivative. For introduction of the final arginine residue, tricarbobenzoxy arginine was used. The nitrophenyl estercoupling method was used for all the amino acids except serine, which was coupled by the azide method. Deprotection of the finished peptide was by saponification and hydrogenation. SUZUKI et al. (1966) reported a stepwise synthesis which differed from that of NICOLAIDES and DEWALD chiefly in that the final two amino acids were incorporated as a dipeptide.

A radically different approach was reported by MERRIFIELD (1964a, b), who used the synthesis of bradykinin to demonstrate the feasibility of his new solid-phase method of peptide synthesis. The solid-phase method is a stepwise synthesis, but the novel feature is that the first (carboxyl-terminal) amino acid is esterified to an insoluble support. The peptide is then assembled on this solid support, one amino acid at a time, until the desired sequence is completed. All the chemical reactions are thus carried out in the solid phase, rather than in solution in the usual manner. At the end of the synthesis a reagent is applied to the insoluble product, which will cleave the bond linking the peptide to the support and liberate the peptide into solution. The great advantage of this method is that it eliminates all the laborious purification of intermediates, which is the most time-consuming part of classical peptide synthesis. Once conditions have been found which will assure that all reactions go fully to completion, the only purification needed during the synthesis is washing of the support with the attached peptide. A consequence of this simplification is that it is very rapid: MERRIFIELD's synthesis of bradykinin by this method required only 8 days, including purification. In addition, the synthesis of peptides by the solid-phase method can be automated, and an instrument has been constructed (MERRIFIELD and STEWART, 1965) which carries out all the coupling reactions in the synthesis of bradykinin in 32 hours. Additional time is required for the attachment of the first amino acid to the support and for cleavage and purification of the product. The bradykinin thus synthesized was indistinguishable from a standard sample. This method has also been used for the synthesis of all-D-bradykinin (STEWART and WOOLLEY, 1965) as well as many bradykinin analogs and a wide range of other peptides.

The solid-phase synthesis of bradykinin is outlined in Fig. 4. The support used for the synthesis is a synthetic resin, consisting of minute beads of a copolymer

Boc-NArg + Cl—CH_2-resin
↓
Boc-NArg-resin
↓ HCl-Dioxane (1)
HCl·NArg-resin
↓ Triethyl amine (2)
Boc-Phe NArg-resin
↓ DCC (3)
Boc-Phe-NArg-resin
↓ Seven repetitions of reactions 1, 2, 3 with appropriate amino acids
Boc-NArg-Pro-Pro-Gly-Phe-BzlSer-Pro-Phe-NArg-resin
↓ HF
Arg-Pro-Pro-Gly-Phe-Ser-Pro-Phe-Arg

Fig. 4. Solid-phase synthesis of bradykinin. Abbreviations as in text

of styrene and divinylbenzene, which is made reactive by chloromethylation. Butyloxycarbonyl nitroarginine is then esterified to this chloromethyl resin. The ester bond thus formed is a substituted benzyl ester and can be cleaved by reagents which normally cleave benzyl esters. The butyloxycarbonyl (Boc)-protecting group is removed from the Boc-nitroarginyl resin by treatment with anhydrous hydrogen chloride in an organic solvent (acetic acid or dioxane), and, after washing, the hydrochloride of the arginine is neutralized with triethylamine.

Boc-Phenylalanine is then coupled to the nitroarginine resin by means of dicyclohexyl carbodiimide (DCC). This sequence of deprotection, neutralization, and coupling is repeated with the appropriate amino acids until the protected bradykinin is assembled on the resin. The peptide resin is then treated with anhydrous hydrogen bromide in trifluoroacetic acid to cleave the peptide from the resin. LENARD and ROBINSON (1967) have applied anhydrous hydrogen fluoride for this purpose and reported a satisfactory synthesis of bradykinin by this modification of the solid-phase method. After hydrogen bromide cleavage, a hydrogenation step is needed to remove the nitro-protecting group from the arginine residues, but if hydrogen fluoride is used for cleavage this is not necessary, since HF also removes nitro groups. A simple purification procedure then yields pure bradykinin in high yield.

The most recent bradykinin synthesis (FRIDKIN et al., 1968) uses insoluble active esters of all the necessary amino acids in a stepwise synthesis starting with nitroarginine nitrobenzyl ester. While this approach offers some advantages over classical solution methods for the synthesis of bradykinin, it does not afford the speed, simplicity, and high yields of the solid-phase method.

C. Syntheses of Kallidin

Since the structure of kallidin is that of bradykinin with an additional lysine residue attached to the amino end, it follows that kallidin can be synthesized by coupling a suitable lysine derivative to a suitable derivative of bradykinin. The first syntheses were accomplished in just this way (PLESS et al., 1962). In one synthesis these authors used dicarbobenzoxy lysine nitrophenyl ester for coupling with a dinitrobradykinin ester, and in another synthesis toluenesulfonyl-protecting groups were used. In two additional syntheses by classical methods (NICOLAIDES et al., 1961; SCHRÖDER and GIBIAN, 1964), a derivative of the dipeptide lysyl-arginine was coupled to a derivative of the carboxyl-terminal octapeptide of bradykinin. Kallidin has also been synthesized by the solid-phase method (STEWART, unpublished); in this case the bradykinin resin was merely carried through an additional coupling step with a lysine derivative and diimide. After cleavage of the peptide from the resin and purification, kallidin was obtained in good yield.

D. Syntheses of Methionyl-Lysyl-Bradykinin

This undecapeptide kinin has been synthesized by both classical and solid-phase methods. SCHRÖDER (1964) coupled the butyloxycarbonyl derivative of methionyl-lysine with free bradykinin by the azide method. MERRIFIELD (1964) extended his solid-phase synthesis of bradykinin by two additional coupling steps with suitable derivatives of lysine and methionine. Satisfactory yields of the desired peptide were obtained in each case.

E. Syntheses of Nonmammalian Kinins

Phyllokinin A (Fig. 1), obtained from the skin of *Phyllomedusa rohdei* and characterized by ANASTASI et al. (1966), was synthesized by BERNARDI et al. (1966) by a fragment condensation method. The sulfate residue was attached to the tyrosine by reaction of the final protected peptide with a pyridine-sulfur trioxide complex. During this reaction the hydroxyl group of serine was protected as the acetyl derivative. Removal of protecting groups and purification yielded the desired undecapeptide sulfate.

Polistes kinin (Fig. 1), the kinin obtained from the venom of the paper wasp *Polistes* (Pisano, 1968), has been synthesized by the solid-phase method (Stewart, 1968). Bradykinin resin was carried through nine additional coupling steps with the appropriate amino acid derivatives. Dicyclohexyl carbodiimide was used for all coupling reactions except that of asparagine; it was introduced by the nitrophenyl ester method. Pyroglutamic acid was used without any protecting group. Treatment of the octadecapeptide resin with anhydrous hydrogen fluoride removed the peptide, and preparative electrophoresis yielded a pure product.

These results show that many different methods can be successfully applied to the synthesis of kinins. These syntheses have made these peptides available for a wide variety of biological studies.

References

Anastasi, A., Bertaccini, G., Erspamer, V.: Pharmacological data on phyllokinin (bradykininyl-isoleucyl-tyrosine O-sulphate) and bradykininyl-isoleucyl-tyrosine. Brit. J. Pharmacol. **27**, 479 (1966).

Bernardi, L., Bosisio, G., De Castiglione, R., Goffredi, O.: Synthesis of phyllokinin, a natural bradykinin analog. Experientia (Basel) **22**, 425 (1966).

Boissonnas, R. A., Guttmann, S., Jacquenoud, P. A.: Synthèse de la L-arginyl-L-prolyl-L-prolyl-glycyl-phénylalanyl-L-seryl-L-prolyl-L-phénylalanyl-L-arginine, un nonapeptide présentant les propriétés de la bradykinine. Helv. chim. Acta **43**, 1349 (1960).

Fridkin, M., Patchornik, A., Katchalski, E.: Use of polymers as chemical reagents. II. Synthesis of bradykinin. J. Amer. chem. Soc. **90**, 2953 (1968).

Greenstein, J. P., Winitz, M.: Chemistry of the amino acids. New York: Wiley 1961.

Guttmann, S., Pless, J., Boissonnas, R. A.: Nouvelle synthèse de la bradykinine. Helv. chim. Acta **45**, 170 (1962).

Lenard, J., Robinson, A. B.: Use of hydrogen fluoride in Merrifield solid phase peptide synthesis. J. Amer. chem. Soc. **89**, 181 (1967).

Merrifield, R. B.: Solid-phase peptide synthesis. III. An improved synthesis of bradykinin. Biochemistry (ACS) **3**, 1385 (1964a).

— Solid-phase peptide synthesis. IV. The synthesis of methionyl-lysyl-bradykinin. J. org. Chem. **29**, 3100 (1964b).

— Automatic synthesis of proteins. Sci. Amer., March 1968, p. 56.

— Stewart, J. M.: Automated peptide synthesis. Nature (Lond.) **207**, 522 (1965).

— — Jernberg, N.: An instrument for automatic synthesis of peptides. Anal. Chem. **38**, 1905 (1966).

Nicolaides, E. D., DeWald, H. A.: Synthesis of polypeptides. Bradykinin. J. org. Chem. **26**, 3872 (1961).

— — McCarthy, D. A.: The synthesis of a biologically active decapeptide having the structure proposed for kallidin. II. Biochem. biophys. Res. Commun. **6**, 210 (1961).

Pisano, J.: Vasoactive peptides in venoms. Fed. Proc. **27**, 58 (1968).

Pless, J., Stürmer, E., Guttmann, S., Boissonnas, R. A.: Kallidin, Synthese und Eigenschaften. Helv. chim. Acta **45**, 394 (1962).

Sakakibara, S., Inukai, N.: The trifluoroacetate method of peptide synthesis. II. An improved synthesis of bradykinin. Bull. chem. Soc. Japan **39**, 1567 (1966).

Schröder, E.: Über Peptidsynthesen. Synthese von Methionyl-Lysyl-Bradykinin, einem Kinin aus Rinderblut. Experientia (Basel) **20**, 39 (1964).

— Gibian, H.: Synthese von Orn[1]-Kallidin und Kallidin. Ann. Chem. **673**, 176 (1964).

— Lübke, K.: The peptides. New York: Academic Press 1965.

Shchukina, L. A., Ravdel, G. A., Filatova, M. P., Semkin, E. P., Krasnova, S. N.: Synthesis of bradykinin. Khim. Prirodn. Soedin. Akad. Nauk Uz. S.S.R. **2**, 124 (1966).

— — — Zhuze, A. L.: Depsipeptide analogs of biologically active peptides. II. Synthesis of bradykinin and its depsipeptide analogs. Acta chim. Acad. Sci. hung. **44**, 205 (1965).

Siemion, I. Z.: New synthesis of bradykinin. Rocz. Chem. **38**, 133 (1964).

Stewart, J. M.: Synthesis and pharmacology of polistes kinin, a bradykinin homolog. Fed. Proc. **27**, 534 (1968),

— Woolley, D. W.: All-D-bradykinin and the problem of peptide antimetabolites. Nature (Lond.) **206**, 619 (1965).

— Young, J. D.: Solid phase peptide synthesis. San Francisco: Freeman 1969.

Suzuki, K., Abiko, T., Asaka, M.: Synthesis of 4-L-leucine-6-O-acetyl-L-serine, 4-L-leucine, 6-O-acetyl-L-serine bradykinin, and bradykinin. Chem. pharm. Bull. **14**, 217 (1966).

Purification of Mammalian Kallikreins, Kininogens, and Kinins

Jack V. Pierce

With 1 Figure

A. Introduction

Many reports describing procedures for purifying the components of the kallikrein–kininogen–kinin system have appeared since Frey and co-workers (Frey, 1926; Frey and Kraut, 1926) initiated the work on urinary kallikrein which led to the discovery of this system. However, not until the advent of high-resolution separation methods in the last twelve years has much progress been made toward the isolation of these proteins in pure and biologically active form. The older methods, such as the Cohn alcohol fractional precipitation of plasma proteins (Cohn et al., 1946), tend to be nonspecific by present-day standards and thus inefficient, and to cause denaturation and hence loss of activity. The newer methods usually employ mild conditions of pH, temperature, and solvent, and so favor the retention of biological activity. Such methods also embody a continuous countercurrent principle which magnifies small differences between closely similar compounds, thus making possible high resolution and, as a corollary, high recovery. Outstanding examples are ordinary and recycling gel filtration; gradient elution chromatography on columns of ion exchangers and hydroxyapatite; preparative polyacrylamide gel electrophoresis and isoelectric focusing; and ultracentrifugation in density gradients. Reviews of the theory and applications of these techniques appear in alternate years in *Analytical Chemistry* [see Anal. Chem. **40**, no. 5, IR-620R (1968)]. The reader is referred also to the useful book on chromatography edited by Heftmann (1967). Future progress in the purification of proteins and other macromolecules will probably lie chiefly in the further development of affinity adsorption methods (Cuatrecasas et al., 1968). Examples are the use of immunoadsorbents for the purification of antigens and antibodies and the use of inhibitor and enzyme columns for the purification of enzymes and inhibitors respectively (Fritz et al., 1967b, c, 1968, 1969a, b).

I. Methodological Considerations

The *first fractionation step* is often necessarily a concentration step. An extreme example is furnished by the purification of kallikrein from human urine, estimated to contain between 0.02 and 0.1 microgram of enzyme per milliliter. It is obvious that several hundred liters of this urine must be processed to provide even a few milligrams of pure enzyme.

The *number of steps* should be kept to a minimum, since losses of activity due to handling, denaturation, and the discarding of impure side fractions attend every step.

The *nature of the steps* chosen should be such as to give both high resolution and high recovery of activity, although this may not be feasible at the first step if its main purpose is concentration. For this reason, salt and solvent fractionation steps should generally be avoided. Countercurrent methods are nearly always better than single-stage ones. For example, gradient elution hydroxyapatite chromatography will give, in most cases, far superior results to those obtainable by batch treatment with calcium phosphate gel.

The *order of the steps* is important with regard to economy of material and effort. The early steps should be capable of handling relatively large amounts of material in a minimal space, while the high-resolution, low-capacity techniques should be reserved for the final stages of purification. For example, it is frequently preferable to use the high-capacity cellulose ion exchangers in the early part of the scheme, and to use such methods as hydroxyapatite chromatography, gel filtration, isoelectric focusing, and preparative gel electrophoresis in the later part. Often these latter methods can also be used to assess the degree of homogeneity, as well as to provide estimates of molecular weight (gel filtration, density gradient ultracentrifugation) and of isoelectric point (isoelectric focusing).

In chromatography and gel filtration, *packing of columns* should be done in such a way as to minimize inhomogeneities, which would cause uneven bands with consequent loss of resolution. The column during packing and chromatography should be perfectly vertical, and the top surface of the packed column should be perfectly flat and perpendicular to the vertical axis of the column. *Resolution* is increased by decreased *particle size* and narrowed *range of particle sizes*. However, we are often restricted in practice to the use of larger than ideal particle size, since flow rates decrease with decrease in particle size and since usually only moderate pressures can be used.

The *height:diameter* ratio of the chromatographic column will often have a large effect on the degree of resolution. Generally, a ratio of at least 20:1 and sometimes 40:1 or more (especially in the case of gel filtration) should be used.

The *equilibration* of all columns with starting buffer before adding the sample is essential to successful and reproducible separations in chromatography and gel filtration. Columns should be packed in the presence of starting, or equilibration, buffer, then washed with the same until the properties of the influent and effluent solutions are the same (e.g. the pH). It is advisable to cycle ion exchangers and certain other adsorbents before use and to select a narrow range of particle size by removal of fine and coarse particles by decantation, flotation, or other means. The adsorbent is then suspended in equilibration buffer and the pH of the stirred suspension is adjusted to the desired value with strong acid or alkali. The sample is dissolved in, or equilibrated against, the starting buffer by dialysis or gel filtration on a Sephadex G-25 column, and added to the equilibrated column. The sample solution should always be followed by at least one column volume of starting buffer before developing the column with stronger buffers. It is important to clarify, by filtration or centrifugation, all solutions before applying them to the column, since insoluble particles will clog the top surface of the column and so tend to diminish the flow rate.

Different *flow rates* must be used with columns packed with different materials. For example, recommended flow rates for columns of hydroxyapatite, Sephadex G-200, and cellulose (or Sephadex) ion exchangers are about 5, 2, and 8 ml/cm^2/hour respectively. The use of a too high flow rate for a given adsorbent or gel material will prevent equilibration of the solute between the mobile and stationary phases, thus diminishing the resolution. Columns packed with small particles often force us to use low flow rates, which further increase the efficiency of the column (i.e. the number of theoretical plates) by allowing a closer approach to equilibrium.

In *gradient elution chromatography*, the slope and even the shape of the gradient will frequently have a decisive effect on the degree of resolution. Very often, too steep a gradient is used. In most cases the gradient should be so formed that the material of interest is eluted near the middle of the gradient. A *linear gradient*, being the easiest of all to produce and to interpret, is generally to be recommended.

The *fraction volume* should be small enough in countercurrent methods that the resolution achieved by them is not destroyed. In general, an activity peak should be spread over at least ten fractions, although more may be desirable where two overlapping peaks are present in the region of interest, or fewer in some cases (e.g. isoelectric focusing).

The optimum *sample weight* to be applied to an adsorption column will depend on such factors as the properties of the adsorbent, the compound sought, and the impurities; the composition of the starting buffer; the pH; and the temperature. The amount of starting sample will usually lie between 0.5 and 10% of the adsorbent dry weight. Using the maximum amount of sample consonant with high resolution will increase yields by minimizing losses due to irreversible adsorption and to the tendency of sensitive proteins to denature at low protein concentrations.

Maximum purification of a compound in *gel filtration* is usually achieved by choosing a column material which gives a K_d[1] of about 0.5—i.e. the compound appears halfway through the internal (pore) volume of the column effluent. There are many examples in the literature of the use of Sephadex G-75 or -100 with proteins, including those of the kallikrein system, where the use of G-200 (or Bio-Gel P-200) would have been more appropriate. As a general rule, the use of a neutral salt or *buffer* solution is recommended for gel filtration experiments, in view of the known aberrant behavior of certain proteins, particularly glycoproteins, to which class both hog pancreatic kallikrein and mammalian low molecular weight (LMW) kininogens are known to belong. For example, human LMW kininogens are adsorbed to Sephadex G-200 in the presence of distilled water, but behave normally in a salt or buffer solution above 0.02 M (PIERCE, unpublished data). In many cases, ammonium acetate buffers can be used, both in gel filtration and ion exchange chromatography, so that the fractions need only be lyophilized to obtain the salt-free protein.

The *sample volume* in gel filtration will depend entirely on the size of the column, the nature and solids content of the sample, and the degree of resolution desired. For optimum results, the sample volume should be no more than 1–2% of the column volume. At the same time, the viscosity of the sample should be less than 5 centipoise. The protein concentration corresponding to this value decreases with increasing molecular weight of the dominant species in the sample. In adsorption chromatography, the volume of sample is not very critical, although too concentrated or too viscous starting samples should be avoided. One of the chief advantages of adsorption chromatography is that large volumes of starting material can be applied to the column with the same result as adding the same amount of sample in a much smaller volume. This means that frequently the

1. $K_d = \frac{V_e - V_0}{V_i}$, where V_e = effluent volume to the peak of activity, V_0 = void volume of the column, and V_i = pore volume of the column.

product of the previous step need not be concentrated and desalted, but perhaps only diluted with water.

Relative to other chromatographic techniques, ***hydroxyapatite chromatography*** has been little used, despite a number of reports of high purification factors

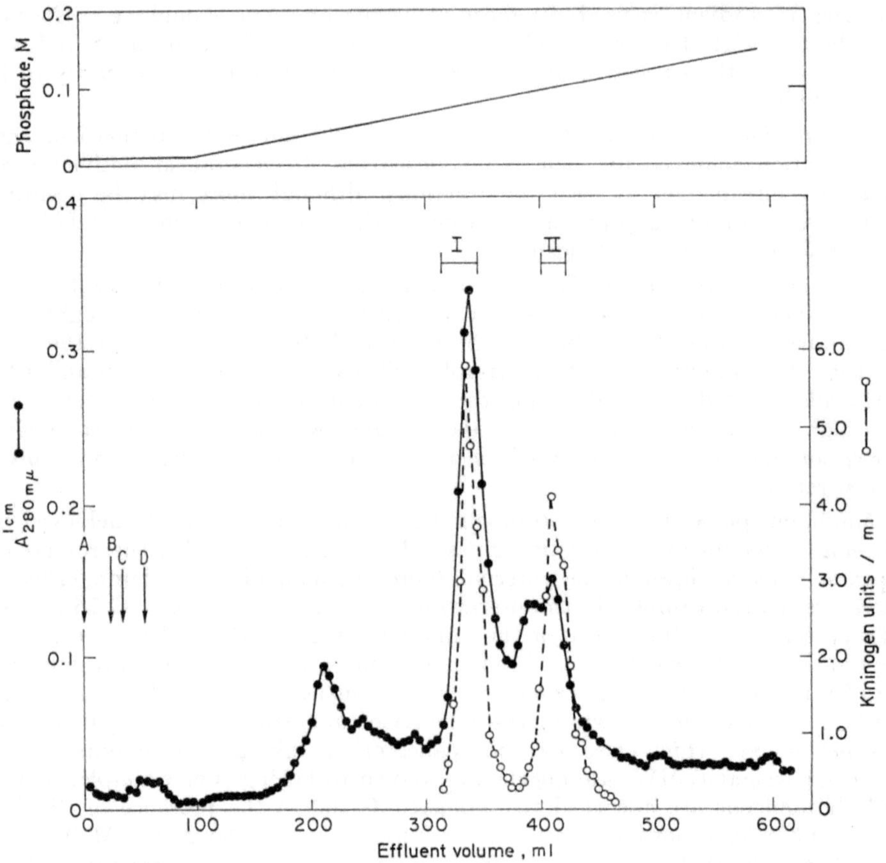

Fig. 1. Hydroxyapatite chromatography of human LMW kininogens (step 5). ***Column:*** **1.25×40 cm (V_t=50 ml).** ***Starting sample*** **(A): Fraction 4b (31.4 mg) in 20 ml of 0.01 M sodium phosphate–0.001 M EDTA, pH 6.15.** ***Eluents:*** **(B) 10 ml of 0.01 M sodium phosphate–0.001 M EDTA, pH 6.0; (C) 20 ml of 1.0 M sodium chloride–0.01 M sodium phosphate–0.1 mM EDTA, pH 6.0; and (D) 550-ml linear gradient of eluent C to 1.0 M sodium chloride–0.12 M sodium-phosphate–0.1 mM EDTA, pH 6.1. Fraction volume: 5 ml. Flow rate: 7 ml/hour. Temperature: 2–4°**

and high yields obtainable with it. When it has been used, often it was not properly exploited—e.g. by employing columns with a too small height:diameter ratio, stepwise rather than gradient elution, a too high flow rate, etc. By means of a linear phosphate gradient in the presence of 1.0 and 3.0 M sodium or potassium chloride, respectively, we have been able to resolve and further purify human LMW kininogens I and II (PIERCE and WEBSTER, 1966) as shown in Fig. 1 and human urinary kallikreins A-1 and A-2 (PIERCE and NUSTAD, in preparation). This modification of hydroxyapatite chromatography may be generally applicable to glycoproteins, as well as to nucleoproteins (FAULHABER and BERNARDI, 1967).

II. Reporting Purification Results

The manner in which a worker reports his purification procedures and results is of great importance both to himself and to his colleagues, who may wish to repeat his methods. Values for the volume, material content (dry weight, A_{280}, ninhydrin color, etc.), specific activity (units of activity should be unequivocally defined and related to those in general use), pH, and other relevant properties should be noted for each major fraction. The material content is preferably given in terms of dry weight; when this is inconvenient or impossible, attempts should be made to relate the measuring unit used to the dry weight, at least for certain key fractions. A summary of the fractionation scheme, based on a definite and constant amount of starting material, in table form is highly desirable. The table should include the following column headings: (1) treatment, (2) total material content, (3) specific activity, (4) purification factor, and (5) percent yield. This pattern is followed below in the tabular summaries for each specific purification procedure. In column chromatography, the following should be reported: source, treatment, and capacity (e.g. of ion exchangers) of column material; the dimensions of the packed column (diameter times height in centimeters); the volume of the starting sample, the fractions collected, and the developing buffer(s); a precise description of the buffers, indicating their points of application; the flow rate; and the operating temperature. Descriptions of gel filtration experiments should also include values for the void and pore volumes (V_0 and V_i) and calculated K_d values.

It has become customary to include many of the above descriptions on the *elution diagram* or in the accompanying legend. The elution diagram should minimally show plots of fraction number or effluent volume against both material concentration and activity concentration. Where applicable (e.g. in gradient elution chromatography), it is helpful also to plot measured values of pH, conductivity, or concentration of important ions of at least some of the fractions, especially in the region of the activity peak(s).

III. Possibility of a Unified Approach to the Purification of Kallikrein and Kininogen Homologs and Kinins

The homologous proteins of the mammalian kallikrein system generally do not exhibit immunological cross-reactivity and hence must differ significantly in structure. Nevertheless, they are sufficiently alike to allow the use of at least some of the same methods in their purification. For example, the LMW kininogens from human, bovine, and rabbit blood behave similarly on ion exchange columns and in disk gel electrophoresis. Also, human and hog pancreatic kallikreins exhibit remarkably similar fractionation behavior and physicochemical properties. Thus, although no two homologous proteins of this system have yet been isolated by exactly the same methods, it seems highly probable that a single purification scheme, with perhaps minor modifications, can be successfully applied to all such homologs.

Since none of the methods used so far for any one homologous class of these proteins of the kallikrein system is flawless, I shall describe usually at least two schemes for each class (e.g. horse and human urinary kallikreins) and indicate those steps which I consider to be the best in each scheme in terms of the general principles given above and which may conceivably be combined into a single scheme applicable to all members of the same class.

In outlining methods for purifying the mammalian kinins (bradykinin-containing peptides), I have assumed that they can be isolated by the same scheme from whatever the source.

B. Plasma Kallikreins

The kallikreins are enzymes found in mammalian plasma and certain glandular tissues which act extremely rapidly on native kininogens to produce bradykinin or kallidin (lysyl-bradykinin) and which resemble trypsin in their ability to hydrolyze N-α-acyl-L-arginine esters and to be inhibited by DFP and certain other trypsin inhibitors (see pp. 156 and 213). So far as is known, plasma kallikrein hydrolyzes only the Lys-Arg and Arg-Ser bonds at either end of the bradykinin sequence in native kininogens. A comparable specificity is shown only by snake venom kinin-releasing enzymes (see SUZUKI, Chapter 3), which may ultimately be classified as salivary kallikreins.[2] Wherever critically tested, glandular kallikreins break only the Met-Lys and Arg-Ser bonds at either end of the kallidin sequence in native kininogens, and thus resemble trypsin even less than the plasma kallikreins. These considerations suggest that the kallikreins and kininogens have an extremely high degree of specificity toward each other. With this possibility in mind, reports that horse urinary kallikrein can hydrolyze Arg-X bonds in salmine (BRANDI et al., 1965, 1967) and Arg-Arg bonds in tetra- and poly-L-arginine (PRADO et al., 1967) and that human kallikrein can convert human plasminogen to plasmin and chymotrypsinogen to chymotrypsin (COLMAN, 1969) should be viewed with some skepticism.

The kallikreins of all mammalian plasmas tested occur in the form of an inactive precursor, prekallikrein. The prekallikreins can be activated by treatment with acetone (KRAUT et al., 1933; WEBSTER and PIERCE, 1963); casein (WERLE, 1936; FREY et al., 1950, 1968; HABERMANN and KLETT, 1966); ammonium sulfate (KRAUT et al., 1933); acid (KRAUT et al., 1933); trypsin (WERLE et al., 1955); papain (KRAUT et al., 1928); and negatively charged surfaces such as glass, kaolin, fused alumina, and Celite (MARGOLIS, 1963). They are activated also by dilution (SCHACHTER, 1960); by brief heating in dilute acid (ROCHA E SILVA and HOLZHACKER, 1959); and by alcohol fractionation (COLMAN et al., 1969a).

Plasma kallikreins have been purified from human (WEBSTER and PIERCE, 1963; COLMAN et al., 1969a; LAUFER et al., 1969); hog (HABERMANN and KLETT, 1966); bovine (NAGASAWA et al., 1967); rabbit (ZYKOVA and PASKHINA, 1965); and horse (HENRIQUES et al., 1966) serum or plasma. Table 1 shows a comparison of some of these kallikreins.

Human. Three human plasma kallikreins were isolated by Cohn fractionation of fresh ACD human plasma, alcohol precipitation of Cohn fraction IV-1 at pH 4.8 in the presence of saline, followed by chromatography on CM-Sephadex C-50 and DEAE-cellulose columns (COLMAN et al., 1969a). Three active peaks were obtained and called kallikreins I, II, and III in the order of their emergence from the DEAE-cellulose column. Further purification of these peaks led to the preparations described in Table 1. Kallikreins I and II were immunologically identical and probably interconvertible. Kallikrein III showed only partial immunological identity with I and II and is the most unstable of the three. Kallikrein I contained two components, as shown by disk gel electrophoresis and ultracentrifugation: the 5.7 S component comprised 87% of the total protein and was identified as kallikrein I; the 8.3 S component (13% of the total protein) was presumably inactive. Consistent with their low specific activities, kallikreins II and III were shown to be much more impure than I by disk gel electrophoresis and by starch block electrophoresis of II, which gave enzyme activity in the fast γ-globulin region with a specific activity of 4.95. Although not stated, one

2. WEBSTER and PIERCE (1963) have reported evidence for the presence in *Agkistrodon contortrix* venom of two kinin-releasing enzymes, one of which forms bradykinin and the other of which forms kallidin from purified human kininogen. The venom did not convert added kallidin to bradykinin. Similar experiments with purified snake venom kinin-releasing enzymes should now be performed.

Table 1. *Comparison of some purified mammalian plasma kallikreins*

Fraction	Source	$s_{20,w}$	Molecular weight	Electrophoretic type	Inhibitors			Specific activity			Yield (%)	Reference
					DFP	SBTI	PTI	(EU[a]/mg)	(pH)	(°C)		
3-3	Human Acetone-activated Cohn fractionation, chromatography				+	+	+	0.25	8.5	37	30	PIERCE and WEBSTER (1963)
	I		99,800[b]	slow γ	+	+	+	9.3	7.6	37	0.08	COLMAN et al. (1969a)
	II		163,000[b]	fast γ	+	+	+	1.53	7.6	37	0.10	COLMAN et al. (1969a)
	III		124,000[b]	α	+	+	+	1.10	7.6	37	0.03	COLMAN et al. (1969a)
2-7	Hog	5.19 S	97,000[c]	fast γ	+	+	+	22	7.8		13	HABERMANN and KLETT (1966)
	Bovine		130,000[d]		+	+	+	4				NAGASAWA et al. (1967)
	Rabbit	6.0–6.5 S		γ		+	+	0.8	8.5	37		ZYKOVA and PASKHINA (1965)

[a] µmoles TAMe hydrolyzed/minute.
[b] Sedimentation equilibrium.
[c] Sephadex G-100 gel filtration.
[d] Sephadex G-150 gel filtration.

can calculate that at least 3.7, 0.27, and 11 liters of plasma were required to provide 11, 6.3, and 102 mg of kallikreins I, II, and III, respectively. The recoveries of these kallikreins by the Colman procedure are extremely low, especially in view of the recent report (Colman, 1969) that maximal kaolin activation (no details given) of human plasma developed 3.48 μmoles TAMe/ml of plasma/min The yields shown in Table 1 were based on this value.

Starting with kaolin-activated plasma, one should be able to recover plasma kallikrein(s) in more nearly native form and in much higher yields than by the Colman procedure. If the specific activity of pure plasma kallikrein is assumed to be about 20 μmoles TAMe/min/mg, as found by Habermann and Klett (1966) for homogeneous hog serum kallikrein, 1 liter of maximally activated human plasma will contain 174 mg of kallikrein. The conversions of plasminogen and chymotrypsinogen to active enzymes mentioned earlier were accomplished with a human plasma kallikrein I preparation with a specific activity of 5.25—i.e. one that may be no more than 25% pure. It will be very important, therefore, to repeat these experiments with more nearly pure human plasma kallikrein, preferably with one isolated by milder methods than used by Colman and coworkers.

Human plasma kallikrein has also been obtained by acetone activation of plasma and subsequent batch adsorption and elution steps, as described in detail below. The stable product had the properties shown in Table 1 (Webster and Pierce, 1963). According to Seidel and Vogt (1969), such a product contains only kininogenase I; they found further that acetone precipitation of human plasma activates both kininogenases I and II, but that II is lost on further treatment.

Hog. Habermann and Klett (1966) have isolated from casein-activated defibrinated hog serum a highly purified kallikrein with a specific activity of 60 FU/mg (Table 2, fraction 7). It was found to be stable and homogeneous in the ultracentrifuge; other properties are shown in Table 1.

Werle and Trautschold (1963) (see Frey et al., 1968, p. 39) have also isolated a highly purified hog serum kallikrein from casein-activated serum. They reported occasionally obtaining a preparation with a purity of 100 FU/mg which was highly unstable, whereas preparations of less than 60 FU/mg were quite stable. Complete experimental details of the purification procedures used have not yet been published.

Bovine. Nagasawa et al. (1967) have partially purified bovine plasma kallikrein by adsorption and activation of a dialyzed pseudoglobulin solution on a glass powder column, elution of the adsorbed activity with 1 M sodium chloride, and gradient elution chromatography on a DEAE-cellulose column.

Two peaks of activity were obtained, the first containing about 80% of the biological activity and 10–20% of the TAMe esterase activity, and the second, about 20% of the biological activity and 80–90% of the esterase activity. The first peak hydrolyzed 4 μmoles of TAMe/min/mg.

Prekallikrein. Only the prekallikrein from bovine plasma has been isolated in highly purified form (Nagasawa et al., 1968). It was nearly homogeneous by disk gel electrophoresis and immunoelectrophoresis. It could be converted to active kallikrein by treatment with trypsin or with bovine Hageman factor (HF, factor XII), purified by the method of Schoenmakers et al. (1965). The prekallikrein content was determined by treating aliquots of fractions with purified bovine HF and measuring the developed TAMe esterase and kinin-releasing activities. A purified bovine high molecular weight (HMW) kininogen, obtained as described later (YANO et al., 1967b), was used in the latter assay. Whereas HF is inhibited by LBTI but not by SBTI (SCHOENMAKERS et al., 1965), plasma kallikrein is inhibited by SBTI but not by LBTI.

I. Hog Serum Kallikrein (Habermann and Klett, 1966)

In the procedure summarized in Table 2, the biological activity is determined by injecting kallikrein samples into the femoral vein of an anesthetized dog, measuring the blood pressure drop in the carotid artery, and comparing this to the effect observed with a standard preparation (fraction 3 S below) defined as having a specific activity of 1.0 unit/mg. Esterolytic (TAMe) activity is determined at pH 7.8 and 25° by measuring the change in $A_{248m\mu}$ for several minutes and calculating the μmoles of TAMe hydrolyzed per minute from the middle, linear part of the curve of $A_{248m\mu}$ versus time.

Table 2. *Purification of kallikrein from 3.0 liters of hog serum* (HABERMANN and KLETT, 1969)

Fraction	Treatment	Protein (mg)	TAMe (μmoles/min/mg)	Biological activity[a] (U/mg)	purification factor	yield (%)
1	Casein precipitate	75,500	0.25	0.4	(1.0)	(100)
2	$(NH_4)_2SO_4$ fraction, 30–60% saturated	32,500	0.325	0.75	1.9	81
3	Supernatant, pH 4.6	20,500	0.63	0.94	2.4	64
4	DEAE-Sephadex A-50 chromatography of fraction 3 (15,150 mg)	1,990		13.7	34	47
5	Sephadex G-200 gel filtration of fraction 4 (1,990 mg)	332		51	128	29
6	P-Cellulose chromatography of fraction 5 (280 mg)	63		120	300	25
7	Sephadex G-100 gel filtration of fraction 6 (19 mg: best fractions)	7.0	22.2	206	515	4.7

[a] Depressor activity in the dog as compared with the standard preparation, fraction 3 S, defined to contain 1.0 unit/mg and later found to have a specific activity of 0.3 FU/mg. Thus the specific activity of fraction 7 would be about 60 FU/mg.

Comments

1. The method of HABERMANN and KLETT is an excellent one and can probably be applied to the purification of human plasma kallikrein. Their experiments are described in gratifyingly complete detail, so that one need not make involved and time-consuming calculations to discover important facts—as is the case with a surprisingly high proportion of the reports dealing with the purification of components of the kallikrein–kinin system. Their yields and purification factors are high at each step; a reasonable number and sequence of steps are used; and the final product, fraction 7, appears to be homogeneous by several criteria.

2. Were I to use this procedure, I would use the P-cellulose chromatography as step 5 and the Sephadex G-200 gel filtration as step 6, replacing the 4×76 cm by a 2×150 cm column. It might thus be possible to eliminate step 7. I would be inclined also to try hydroxyapatite chromatography of the Sephadex G-200 activity peak, despite disappointing results obtained by HABERMANN and KLETT when they failed to adsorb the activity from fraction 5 to a column of hydroxyapatite.

II. Human Plasma Kallikrein (Webster and Pierce, 1963)

The steps are summarized in Table 3.

Table 3. *Purification of acetone-activated plasma kallikrein from 1.0 liter of human plasma* (WEBSTER and PIERCE, 1963)

Fraction	Treatment	Protein (mg)	Esterase activity[a]			Biological activity[b]		
			(U/mg)	Purification	yield (%)	(FU/mg)	purification factor	yield (%)
1	Acetone-activated and dialyzed plasma	67,500	0.0090	(1.0)	(100)	0.074	(1.0)	(100)
2	DEAE-cellulose filtrate	14,700	0.036	4.1	53			
3	IRC-50 eluate, pH 8.4[c]	753	0.25	28	33	2.0	27	30

[a] One unit of esterase activity is defined as 1.0 μmole of TAMe hydrolyzed per minute at pH 8.5 and 37°.

[b] Measured by increased blood flow of dog femoral artery (SARNOFF et al., 1958), with a hog pancreatic kallikrein standard (Padutin).

[c] Dissolve the dry solid with about 20 ml of 0.02 M ammonium acetate, pH 7.5, unstead of with water as in the original report.

Comments

1. In step 3, ammonium acetate can probably be substituted for ammonium formate to advantage: very concentrated solutions of the former will remain frozen during lyophilization, whereas solutions of the latter at concentrations above 0.15 M tend to melt; also, the pH of aqueous solutions of proteins after lyophilization from ammonium formate solutions of pH 7.5–8.0 is generally around 4–5, while the pH of aqueous solutions after lyophilization from comparable ammonium acetate solutions is usually around 6.

2. If I were now to attempt the isolation of human plasma kallikrein, I should be inclined to start with kaolin-activated plasma. COLMAN (1969; COLMAN et al., 1969b) has realized by this means very high levels of TAMe esterase activity, almost all of which appears to be due to liberated plasma kallikrein.

III. Bovine Plasma Prekallikrein (Nagasawa et al., 1968)

The purification steps are summarized in Table 4.

Table 4. *Purification of bovine plasma prekallikrein from 1.0 liter of plasma* (NAGASAWA et al., 1968)

Fraction	Treatment	Protein, (A_{280})	Specific activity (U^a/A_{280})	Purification factor	Yield (%)
1	Pseudoglobulin	19,700			
2	First DEAE-Sephadex A-50 chromatography	674	0.09	(1.0)	(100)
3	Second DEAE-Sephadex A-50 chromatography	11.6	1.31	15	24
4	CM-Sephadex C-50 chromatography of 9.75 mg of fraction 2	1.44	7.92	88	18

[a] 1.0 unit = 1.0 μmole TAMe/min at pH 8.5 and 37° (ROBERTS, 1958).

At step 4 the volume of NaCl was not given; the elution diagram shows activity between 100 and 250 ml of effluent, but the text states that activity is eluted between 0.18 and 0.20 M NaCl; perhaps this is the concentration of salt at the peak.

Comment

1. The authors fail to indicate how they avoided activation of kallikrein by ammonium sulfate fractionation. It would seem that some, and perhaps a large fraction, of the total prekallikrein originally present in the plasma *was* activated, but that enough prekallikrein remained for purification purposes. To avoid or minimize kallikrein activation, it may be desirable to perform the fractionation steps in the presence of hexadimethrine bromide (Polybrene), a known inhibitor of HF (EISEN, 1964); and/or of LBTI, which also inhibits HF (SCHOENMAKERS et al., 1965).

C. Pancreatic Kallikreins

Hog pancreatic kallikrein has been highly purified by HABERMANN (1962), FRITZ et al. (1967a), and MORIYA et al. (1965b, 1969); and human pancreatic kallikrein by MORIYA et al. (1963). Table 5 compares some of the properties of these authors' best preparations. MORIYA found only one hog pancreatic kallikrein, which was homogeneous by several criteria (including disk gel electrophoresis). HABERMANN found two kallikreins by starch column and membrane electrophoresis. FRITZ and co-workers found from one to five variants by membrane electrophoresis, depending on the conditions used (see Table 5). These variants were estimated to contain between 0 and 3 sialic acid residues per molecule: removal of the residues by means of neuraminidase gave two biologically active electrophoretic bands with mobilities corresponding to the two slowest-moving kallikreins before neuraminidase treatment. Evidence for the presence of two prekallikreins in hog pancreas has been provided by FIEDLER and WERLE (1967), who found two prekallikrein peaks by gradient elution DEAE-cellulose chromatography of a fresh extract of pancreas made in the presence of SBTI and without autolysis. However, the two peaks were not separately rechromatographed or otherwise critically compared, so that the question of the natural occurrence of more than one prekallikrein in hog pancreas has yet to be conclusively settled. Thus far, evidence for the existence of only one human pancreatic kallikrein has been obtained (MORIYA et al., 1963).

Table 5. *Comparison of highly purified hog and human pancreatic kallikreins*

Source of enzymes	Activation method	Number of variants	Molecular weight	Specific activity (FU/mg)	Reference
Hog	Autolysis 3 days at 37°	2[a]	24,000[b]	800	HABERMANN (1962)
Hog	Autolysis 3 days at 37°	1[c], 2[d], 5[e]	33,600[f] 29,000[g]	1,400	FRITZ et al. (1967a)
Hog	Autolysis 10–24 hr at 20°	1[h]	25,000[g]	2,400	MORIYA et al. (1969)
Human	pH 4.5 for 16 hr at 12°	1[i]	31,200[g]	550	MORIYA et al. (1963)

[a] Starch column electrophoresis (0.03 M veronal–acetate–HCl, pH 8.7; 10 V/cm).
[b] Calculated from sedimentation and diffusion constants, assuming $\bar{v} = 0.734$.
[c] Electrophoresis in 0.01 M buffer, pH 7–8, 200 V.
[d] Cellulose acetate electrophoresis (0.01 M borate, pH 7.0, 400 V).
[e] Cellulose acetate electrophoresis (0.01 M acetate, pH 4.6, 400 V).
[f] Calculated from amino acid and carbohydrate composition.
[g] Calculated from sedimentation constant ($s_{20,w} = 2.56$ S), assuming $\bar{v} = 0.749$.
[h] Disk gel electrophoresis at pH 9.5 (Tris–glycine).
[i] Gel electrophoresis at pH 8.6–8.8 (Tris–EDTA–borate).

I. Hog Pancreatic Kallikrein (Method 1, Moriya et al., 1965b, 1969)

The steps are summarized in Table 6.

Table 6. *Purification of kallikrein from 1.0 kilogram of hog pancreas* (Moriya, 1965b, 1969)

Fraction	Treatment	Protein (A_{280})	Specific activity (FU/A_{280})	Purification factor	Yield (%)
1	Acetone filtrate, 30%	364,000	0.55	(1.0)	(100)
2	DEAE-cellulose eluate	25,000	4.1	7.4	52
3	Acetone precipitate, 75%	3,300	14	25	23
4	Supernatant, pH 4.2	815	31	56	12.2
5	Acetone precipitate, 67%	170	140	254	11.9
6	Hydroxyapatite chromatography	17	960	1,740	8.2
7	Sephadex G-100 gel filtration	11.5	1,240	2,280	7.1

Since fraction 7 was found to contain 0.5 mg of protein/A_{280}, the specific activity on a weight basis can be calculated to be 2,400 FU/mg. It should be noted that Fritz et al. (1967a) report a molar extinction of 51,000 for their preparation (1,400 FU/mg); assuming a molecular weight of 33,600 one can calculate a value of 0.66 mg/A_{282}. If this factor is used with Moriya's value of 1,200 FU/A_{280}, a weight basis specific activity of 1,820 FU/mg can be calculated. Fraction 7 was homogeneous by ultracentrifugation, disk gel electrophoresis, and immunoelectrophoresis. However, isoelectric focusing indicated the presence of at least four kallikrein isoenzymes (Moriya, personal communication).

Comments

1. Autolysis may be omitted from step 1, in view of the possible presence of neuraminidase in the pancreas. Further, Schultz (1957) has found that heating alone (pH 4.6, 55°) gave a maximum yield of kallikrein, 35 FU/g of pancreas. In agreement with this result, Habermann (1962) obtained yields of between 17 and 34 FU/g by autolysis and methanol precipitation. Thus, the value of 200 FU/g reported by Moriya (1969) seems too high; this point should be carefully checked.

2. Steps 3 and 4 can be omitted, since the purification is only 3.6- and 2.2-fold with recoveries of 45% and 53%, respectively, or 7.6-fold and 24% overall. It is likely that gradient elution DEAE-Sephadex A-50 (or DEAE-cellulose) chromatography[3] would give a better purification, as well as a higher recovery, than these two steps combined.

3. Step 6 might be improved by using a 1.25×40 cm (same volume as 1.6×25 cm) column of hydroxyapatite and a 500-ml linear gradient of 0.01 to 0.12 M potassium phosphate, pH 6–7, in the presence of 1–3 M potassium chloride[3].

4. The use of a longer column—e.g. 1.0×100 cm, a sample volume of less than 0.5 ml, and Sephadex G-200 instead of G-100 should improve the results obtained at step 7, and also provide an independent estimate of the molecular weight. A neutral salt or buffer solution should be substituted for distilled water as developer, e.g. 0.5 M ammonium acetate.

5. Since human pancreatic kallikrein has been partially purified by means of essentially the same procedure originally applied to the purification of hog pancreatic kallikrein (Moriya et al., 1963), it is probable that the scheme ultimately adopted for the latter can be applied with little or no change to the purification of other mammalian pancreatic kallikreins.

3. Either or both of these procedures should reveal the presence of hog pancreatic kallikrein isoenzymes.

II. Hog Pancreatic Kallikrein (Method 2, Habermann, 1962)

The steps are summarized in Table 7.

Table 7. *Purification of kallikrein from 1.0 kilogram of hog pancreas* (HABERMANN, 1962)

Fraction	Treatment	Protein (mg)	Specific activity, (FU/mg)	Purification factor	Yield (%)
0	Pancreas (23,600 FU)	10,000[a]	2.4	(1.0)	(100)
1	Methanol fraction, 33–73%	848	25	10.6	94
2	Starch column electrophoresis	55	300	127	70
3	DEAE-cellulose chromatography	11	800	338	40

[a] Based on the observation that an aqueous extract of thermolyzed pancreas contained about 10 mg of nondialyzable solids per g of wet tissue (PIERCE, unpublished).

Comments

1. Probably autolysis should be replaced by thermolysis for the reasons given in comment 1 above on MORIYA's procedure.

2. Since FIEDLER and WERLE (1967) obtained two biologically active peaks from a crude hog pancreatic kallikrein (Padutin, Bayer) by applying gradient elution (0.1 to 0.8 M ammonium acetate, pH 6.7 at 5°) to a 1×51 cm column of DEAE-cellulose, this procedure is recommended as a replacement for step 3.

3. Both MORIYA (1969) and FRITZ et al. (1967) have achieved dramatic purification of hog pancreatic kallikrein by means of hydroxyapatite chromatography. (See my recommendation in comment 3 on MORIYA's procedure above.)

D. Urinary Kallikreins

Highly purified urinary kallikreins have been isolated from the human (MORIYA et al., 1963), the horse (PRADO et al., 1962, 1963) and the hog (WERLE and TRAUTSCHOLD, 1963). These enzymes, as well as rat urinary kallikrein, will hydrolyze such N-α-acyl-L-arginine esters as TAMe, BAMe, and BAEe. MARES-GUIA and DINIZ (1967a, b) have reported that rat urinary kallikrein[4] will also hydrolyze BAPA. The horse and rat enzymes can be distinguished from trypsin by the use of the trypsin inhibitors benzamidine and TLCK: the kinin-releasing and esterase activities of these kallikreins are inhibited by the former but not by the latter (DINIZ et al., 1965, 1966). They also reported the inexplicable observation that the biological activities of crude human urinary kallikrein preparations, which were found to have little or no BAEe esterase activity, were not inhibited by benzamidine (or by TLCK). In our work with human urinary kallikrein, we have always found a nearly constant ratio of kinin-releasing activity to TAMe esterase activity over a wide range of purification (WEBSTER and PIERCE, 1961, 1963; MORIYA et al., 1963). To verify this point, we determined the esterase and kinin-releasing activities of newly obtained crude and highly purified human urinary kallikrein preparations, as well as a crude preparation of rat urinary

4. The rat urinary kallikrein used by DINIZ and co-workers in these studies was purified 30-fold from dialyzed rat urine by fractionation between 50 and 75% acetone, followed by Sephadex G-100 gel filtration in 0.05 M ammonium acetate, pH 6.7 (MARES-GUIA and DINIZ, 1967a).

kallikrein (PIERCE and NUSTAD, unpublished data). The results are summarized in Table 8, which also includes data reported by PRADO et al. (1962) for purified horse urinary kallikrein (see also Table 9). It is clear that the relationships between the biological activity and the two esterase activities are remarkably similar for the crude and the highly purified human urinary kallikrein preparations. It is interesting that each kind of enzyme differs from the others in the proportions of the different specific activities.

Table 8. *Comparison of the esterase and biological activities of horse, human and rat urinary kallikreins, and trypsin*

Enzyme	Specific activities			Ratios of specific activities		
	Esterase[a]		Biological (U/mg)	TAMe / BAEe	Biological / TAMe	Biological / BAEe
	TAMe	BAEe				
Trypsin, twice crystallized	190	36		5.3		
Urinary kallikreins						
Horse (fraction 4, Table 2)	22	31	330[b]	0.71	15.0	10.6
Horse (fraction 5, Table 2)	(54)[c]	(77)[c]	817[b]			
Human, crude[d]	0.22	0.16	5.1[e]	1.33	23.2	30.9
Human, purified[f]	27	20	ca. 540[e]	1.35	20.0	27.0
Rat, crude[d]	1.1	3.5	7.8[e]	0.31	7.1	2.2

[a] μMoles/min/mg by titration at pH 8.0 and 25° (trypsin, horse urinary kallikrein) or 30° (human and rat urinary kallikreins).

[b] Kinin release measured directly by adding horse urinary kallikrein and heat-treated horse plasma to an isolated guinea pig ileum suspended in Tyrode's solution. The values are given in terms of the unit defined in footnote a, Table 9.

[c] Calculated by means of the factor, 817/330.

[d] Prepared by pressure dialysis of fresh urine as described in Table 10.

[e] Kinin release measured directly by adding kallikreins and a human LMW kininogen fraction to an isolated estric rat uterus suspended in de Jalon's solution. The values are given in Frey units, determined by comparison with a human urinary kallikrein standard (5.0 FU/mg).

[f] Prepared by PIERCE and NUSTAD (unpublished work).

BRANDI et al. (1965, 1967) have reported the hydrolysis of salmine by 500-fold purified horse urinary kallikrein, but WERLE and FIEDLER (see FREY et al., 1968, p. 45) were unable to confirm this. The same enzyme (purified 160-fold), like trypsin, completely hydrolyzes bradykinyl-serine to bradykinin and serine; this reaction is inhibited by benzamidine (BABEL et al., 1968). These workers also found some bradykinin by CM-cellulose gradient elution chromatography when they reacted the 160-fold purified enzyme with methionyl-lysyl-bradykinin and lysyl-lysyl-bradykinin. However, one must be cautious in interpreting the results obtained from the use of impure preparations. Evidence for the presence of an aminopeptidase converting kallidin to bradykinin both in crude human urinary kallikrein and in human plasma was clearly indicated by experiments of WEBSTER and PIERCE (1963): when crude enzyme or substrate was used, often more bradykinin than kallidin was found; but when highly purified enzyme and partially purified human kininogen were reacted, only kallidin was found. These cautionary remarks apply equally to the results of CARVALHO and DINIZ

(1966), who detected only bradykinin in an incubation mixture of a rat kidney extract and dog pseudoglobulin.

Horse urinary kallikrein (250-fold purified; fraction 4, Table 9), like the human enzyme, was inhibited by DFP and PTI but not by SBTI or ovomucoid (PRADO et al., 1963).

PRADO et al. (1965) have reported that 200- to 600-fold purified horse urinary kallikrein requires the presence of Na^+, K^+, Rb^+, or Cs^+ ions at a concentration of about 0.04 M for kinin-releasing but not for BAEe esterase activity.

Since detailed procedures only for the purification of human and horse urinary kallikreins have been published, I shall confine myself to summarizing the steps used to obtain highly purified preparations of these enzymes. WERLE and co-workers (see FREY et al., 1968, p. 37) have prepared hog urinary kallikrein with a specific activity of 670 FU/mg in 4% yield, but have not so far published their results in detail (see RODER, 1967 for experimental details).

I. Horse Urinary Kallikrein (Prado et al., 1962, 1963)

The steps are summarized in Table 9.

Table 9. *Purification of horse urinary kallikrein from 110 liters of urine* (PRADO et al., 1962, 1963)

Fraction	Treatment	Protein (mg)	Specific activity (U/mg)	Purification factor	Yield (%)
0	Horse urine (61,500 units[a])				(100)
1	Ammonium sulfate fractionation, 40–60% saturated	28,400	1.3	1.0	60
2	Acetone fractionation, 60–75% (V/V)	1,025	27	20.8	45
3	DEAE-cellulose chromatography	54.5	260	200	23
4	Acetone fractionation, 60–75%	32.5	330	254	16
5	Sephadex G-75 gel filtration		817	628	

[a] A horse urinary kallikrein standard (UKS) was prepared by twice fractionating horse urine between 40 and 70% saturated ammonium sulfate, dialyzing extensively against distilled water at 4°, and lyophilizing the salt-free protein solution. The ability of 1.0 mg of UKS to form kinin from heat-treated horse plasma was defined as 1.0 unit. The kinin was released directly in the isolated guinea pig ileum bath.

Comments

1. In step 3, a DEAE-cellulose column with a larger height:diameter ratio could probably be used to advantage, as well as gradient rather than stepwise elution. Also, DEAE-Sephadex A-50 might give better results than DEAE-cellulose.

2. Step 4 could be eliminated, since little purification is effected and 30% of the activity is lost. A promising procedure with which to replace this step is hydroxyapatite chromatography, with phosphate gradient elution in the presence of 3.0 M potassium or sodium chloride.

3. Step 5 might be improved by using Sephadex G-100, -150, or -200, depending on which one will give a K_d of 0.5 with horse urinary kallikrein. If it has a molecular weight the same or greater than that of human urinary kallikrein, G-200 should be chosen.

II. Human Urinary Kallikrein (Moriya et al., 1963)

The steps are summarized in Table 10.

Table 10. *Purification of human urinary kallikrein from 200 liters of urine* (Moriya et al., 1963)

Fraction	Treatment	Protein (A_{280} units)	Specific activity (EU^{a}/A_{280})	Purification factor	Yield (%)
0	Human urine[b]	600,000	0.04	(1.0)	(100)
1	IRC-50 eluate	200,000	0.10	2.5	83
2	DEAE-cellulose eluate	6,800	2.2	55	62
3	Acetone fraction, 50–60% (V/V)	750	15	375	47
4	$(NH_4)_2SO_4$ fraction, 69–83% saturated	145	29	725	18
5	Sephadex G-75 gel filtration	53	60	1,500	13
6	DEAE-Sephadex A-50 chromatography	6.3	230	5,700	6

[a] EU = esterase units. Esterase activity was determined by the TAMe colorimetric method of Roberts (1958) (pH 8.5/37°/1.0 hour). One EU was defined as equivalent to one FU for a standard preparation of human urinary kallikrein (6.0 FU/mg), the biological activity of which had been determined by comparison with a standard hog pancreatic kallikrein preparation (Padutin) in the dog assay described by Sarnoff et al. (1958). In the presence of excess TAMe at pH 8.5 and 37°, one human urinary kallikrein EU will hydrolyze about 0.08 μmole of TAMe/min. The titration assay at pH 8.0 and 30° gives 0.05 μmole TAMe/min/EU.

[b] To determine the esterase activity of the starting urine, a 100-ml sample was dialyzed exhaustively against distilled water at 4°, lyophilized, and dissolved in 2.5 ml of 0.01 M potassium phosphate, pH 7.5.

Comments

1. The ammonium sulfate fractionation (step 4) should be eliminated, since only a 2-fold purification in 38% yield was obtained, and replaced by DEAE-Sephadex A-50 chromatography. I suggest using a 1.5 × 60 cm column packed in the presence of and equilibrated with 0.2 M KCl–0.01 M potassium phosphate, pH 7.0; applying the sample (fraction 3) dissolved in about 20 ml of equilibration buffer; washing the column with 200 ml of the same buffer; and developing with a 1-liter linear gradient of 0.20 to 0.60 M KCl in the presence of 0.01 M potassium phosphate, pH 7.0, at a flow rate of 15 ml/hour. Collect 10-ml fractions (see comment 3 below).

2. Sephadex G-200 or Bio-Gel P-200[5] can be advantageously substituted for the Sephadex G-75 of step 5. However, I recommend the use of a longer column—e.g. 1.0 × 100 cm—and a dilute salt or buffer developing solution (e.g. 0.5–1.0 M ammonium acetate, pH 6.0–7.0, which can be removed by lyophilization).

3. Recently we have concentrated urine at 25° in the presence of toluene or, preferably[6a], 0.025% sodium azide by pressure dialysis to about 0.1–0.2% of the original volume, equilibrating against several changes of distilled water during the final stages. The concentrate was removed from the dialysis sacs[6a] with distilled water to give about 1% of the original urine volume, the somewhat viscous aqueous suspension was made with vigorous stirring to 0.15 M ammonium acetate and pH 7.0 with 5 M ammonium acetate, pH 7.2 and ammonia, and stored at 2–4° for 24–48 hours. The inactive, gelatinous precipitate, accounting for about 50% of the nondialyzable solids in urine, was removed by centrifugation at 2° and washed twice with 0.15 M ammonium acetate, pH 7.0. The combined supernatants were concentrated

5. The bead form of Bio-Gel P-200 gives higher flow rates than the bead form of Sephadex G-200 when salt solutions above 1.0 M are used.

6. Visking dialysis tubing (80–100 cm lengths of 1.0 cm flat width) previously expanded (to ca. 1.5 cm flat width) with water at 18 psi nitrogen pressure: one 80-cm length will pass about 1 liter of urine in 24 hours at 25° and 15 psi nitrogen pressure.

6.a Inasmuch as we have recently found that sodium azide slowly destroys kallikrein in human urine, we now avoid its use. We now recommend storing urine at –20° or under toluene at 2–4°.

to about 0.1% of the original urine volume by pressure dialysis and lyophilized. As far as has been ascertained, recovery of kallikrein activity is 100%. The specific activity lies between 3 and 12 EU/mg (2 and 8 EU/A_{280}). Application of 440 mg (from 10 liters of urine) of such material (3.0 EU/mg; 2.3 EU/A_{280}) dissolved in 10 ml of equilibration buffer, to a 1.3×35 cm column of DEAE-Sephadex A-50 (0.20 M potassium chloride–0.01 M potassium phosphate, pH 7.0), washing the column with 70 ml of equilibration buffer, and developing with a 425-ml linear gradient of equilibration buffer to 0.60 M potassium chloride–0.01 M potassium phosphate, pH 7.0, at a flow rate of 15 ml/hr and at 25°, gave a product with a specific activity of 34 EU/mg (31 EU/A_{280}) in 76% yield[7]. In a comparable experiment, the specific activity was increased from 12 EU/mg (8.7 EU/A_{280}) to 55 EU/mg (28 EU/A_{280}) in 80% yield. This degree of purification is reached only after four steps of the procedure described above, but with a loss of 80% of the starting activity—i.e. with the 83% saturated ammonium sulfate precipitate (fraction 4, Table 10).

4. The IRC-50 batch adsorption step is a rather tricky one, however useful it is for concentrating the kallikrein contained in large volumes of urine. The pH must be 4.0 ± 0.05. Below pH 3.9 the activity is destroyed, whereas above pH 4.1 kallikrein is less strongly adsorbed. Furthermore, the resin strongly adsorbs the polyphenolic acids of urine and perhaps modifies them in such a way as to add to the later difficulties encountered in purifying the enzyme. A much smaller fraction of these polymeric contaminants is found in the product obtained by pressure dialysis. Perhaps industrial dialyzers now used for the purification or concentration of pharmaceuticals can be applied to the concentration of large volumes (≥1,000 liters) of human and other mammalian urines.

E. Salivary Kallikreins

The kallikreins present in saliva or submaxillary glands have been relatively little studied. A highly purified hog submaxillary kallikrein (molecular weight, 32,000) has been prepared by Trautschold (1965) and Roder (1967). Their methods are briefly summarized in Frey et al. (1968, p. 34), to which source I was limited in describing the purification scheme below. No criteria of homogeneity were reported. Moriya et al. (1965a, 1966) have obtained a highly purified human salivary kallikrein; although no estimate of the molecular weight is made, a value of 30,000 is consistent with some of the reported gel filtration data. The so-called kinin-releasing enzymes of certain snake venoms are now thought to be salivary kallikreins (Suzuki, Chapter 3).

I. Hog Submaxillary Kallikrein (Trautschold, 1965; Roder, 1967)

The steps are summarized in Table 11.

Table 11. *Purification of hog submaxillary kallikrein from 1.0 kilogram of glands* (Trautschold, 1965; Roder, 1967)

Fraction	Treatment	Protein (mg)	Specific activity (FU/mg)	Purification factor	Yield (%)
1	Dilute acetic acid extract	50,000	0.75	(1.0)	(100)
2	Acetone fraction, 40–60% (V/V)	4,200	8.0	11	90
3	DEAE-cellulose batch adsorption	380	70	93	71
4	DEAE-cellulose chromatography	83	300	400	58
5	Protamine sulfate precipitation				
6	Sephadex G-75 gel filtration	51	330	440	45
7	Column electrophoresis	38	330	440	33
8	Sephadex G-75 gel filtration	15	670	890	27
9	Column electrophoresis	5	1,250	1,160	17

7. Similar results can be obtained with a linear gradient of 0.20 to 0.60 M ammonium acetate, pH 7.0.

No details are given for steps 5 through 9 by FREY et al. (1968). To obtain information, the original work of TRAUTSCHOLD (1965) and RODER (1967) should be consulted.

Comments

1. The first four steps seem to be very good ones in having high purification factors and high yields. However, apparently the best conditions were not used in steps 5, 6, and 7, since almost no purification was realized and significant amounts of activity were lost, and since both steps 8 and 9 (repeats of steps 6 and 7 respectively) gave good purification in reasonable yields.

2. Although no K_d was given for the Sephadex G-75 steps, one would expect it to be about 0.3 for a protein with a molecular weight of 32,000. For such a protein, Sephadex G-150 should give a K_d of about 0.5 and therefore should replace G-75.

II. Human Salivary Kallikrein (Moriya et al., 1965a, 1966)

The steps are summarized in Table 12.

Table 12. *Purification of human salivary kallikrein from 2.0 liters of saliva* (MORIYA et al., 1965a, 1966)

Fraction	Treatment	Protein (mg or A_{280})	Specific activity (FU/mg or A_{280})	Purification factor	Yield (%)
0	Human saliva	21,800	0.156	(1.0)	(100)
1	Acetone precipitate, 75% (V/V)	2,430	1.4	9.0	100
2	DEAE-cellulose batch adsorption	1,530	1.7	10.9	77
3	Acetone fraction, 55–60% (V/V)	50	24	154	35
4	Sephadex G-75 gel filtration	19	41	263	23
5	Sephadex G-100 gel filtration	11	365	2,340	12

Comments

1. These workers gave no clear hint of the volume of starting saliva. A reasonable value of 2.0 liters was arrived at by determining the total A_{280} units recovered in the G-100 gel filtration by measuring the area under the A_{280} curve of the elution diagram (MORIYA et al., 1966) and using this value, 19, as the amount of protein in fraction 4. From the values given for the specific activity and percent yield of this fraction and from the value of 1.7 FU/ml for the starting saliva, one can calculate that the starting volume of saliva must have been about 2 liters.

2. Since the DEAE-cellulose batch method gave very little purification and a 23% loss of activity, step 2 should be replaced by DEAE-cellulose (or DEAE-Sephadex A-50) chromatography, with gradient elution, e.g. 0.2 to 0.8 M ammonium acetate, pH 6.0.

3. I should be inclined to replace step 1 by step 3, thus eliminating step 3.

4. Step 4 should be eliminated, since Sephadex G-75 obviously has a too small pore size for a protein with a presumed molecular weight of about 30,000. A K_d of about 0.5 should be obtained with Sephadex G-150. The Sephadex G-100 column in step 5 is far too short: the length should be at least 100 cm. Also, the flow rate of 11 ml/cm²/hour should be reduced to at least 3 ml/cm²/hour.

These comments and the general principles dealt with in the Introduction suggest the following tentative scheme for purifying salivary kallikreins:

(1) 55–60% acetone fractionation of clarified saliva.

(2) DEAE-cellulose or DEAE-Sephadex A-50 gradient elution chromatography.

(3) Hydroxyapatite chromatography, with a linear phosphate gradient in the presence of 1 or 3 M potassium chloride.

(4) Sephadex G-150 gel filtration in a 100- or 150-cm long column, with 0.5 M ammonium acetate, pH 6.0, as eluent.

(5) Preparative gel electrophoresis or isoelectric focusing.

F. Low Molecular Weight Kininogens

Mammalian kininogens are acidic glycoproteins which, in their native state, are highly specific substrates for the kallikreins and snake venom kinin-releasing enzymes (now considered to be salivary kallikreins). They serve, particularly when denatured, as nonspecific substrates for trypsin. The preponderance of evidence favors the generalization that plasma kallikreins release bradykinin from kininogens and that glandular kallikreins, such as those found in the urine, pancreas, and saliva or submaxillary gland, form kallidin from the same substrates (Webster and Pierce, 1963; Pierce, 1968). The subject is discussed in detail in this volume by Habermann.

Two main classes of kininogens have been found in human, dog, guinea pig, rabbit, and rat plasmas by Jacobsen (1966a, b); in bovine plasma by Yano et al. (1967b); and in horse plasma by Henriques et al. (1967). These classes were first detected by Jacobsen (1966a) by Sephadex G-200 gel filtration. He found the first peak, which he named substrate 1, to be an equally good substrate for plasma kallikrein and salivary kallikrein; but the second peak (substrate 2) to be a poor substrate for plasma kallikrein and a good substrate for salivary kallikrein. I shall refer to substrate 1 as HMW (high molecular weight) kininogens and to substrate 2 as LMW (low molecular weight) kininogens.

Bovine LMW kininogen has been isolated in homogeneous form by Habermann and co-workers (Habermann et al., 1963; Habermann, 1963) and by Suzuki and co-workers (Suzuki et al., 1965; Nagasawa et al., 1966; Yano et al., 1967a). Habermann named his preparation kininogen I, whereas Suzuki called his kininogen II.

Egorova and Paskhina (1967) and Egorova et al. (1969) isolated a highly purified *rabbit LMW kininogen* which shared many of its properties with the bovine LMW kininogen.

Two *human LMW kininogens* have been isolated by Pierce and Webster (1966). Originally they were named kininogens I and II; now they should be called human LMW kininogens I and II. The kinin moiety appears to lie at the carboxyl terminus of I and inside the polypeptide chain of II. The human LMW kininogens I and II are immunologically identical. For additional information about I and II, see Pierce and Webster (1966), Pierce (1968), and Habermann (p. 254).

HMW kininogens have not yet been isolated in pure form. Owing to their high susceptibility to destruction by plasma kallikrein (which is readily activated by various means, such as contact with glass or other negatively charged surfaces), they were not detected until precautions were taken against activation. Using siliconized equipment and working at room temperature rather than in the cold, JACOBSEN and KRIZ (1967) succeeded in isolating a quite highly purified human HMW kininogen with a molecular weight of 197,000 and the electrophoretic mobility of a β-globulin. HMW kininogens from bovine (YANO et al., 1967b) and horse (HENRIQUES et al., 1967) plasmas have been rather less highly purified than human HMW kininogen.

If both HMW and LMW kininogens are desired from the same starting plasma, blood should be collected in polyethylene containers or in siliconized glassware and treated immediately with hexadimethrine bromide, a known inhibitor of Hageman factor (factor XII) (EISEN, 1964) and SBTI, an inhibitor of plasma kallikrein, besides a complexing agent for calcium ion (citrate, oxalate, or EDTA). PASKHINA and EGOROVA (1966) have observed that the addition of SBTI (0.6 mg/ml) to rabbit serum prevents destruction of kininogen.

I. Bovine LMW Kininogen (Suzuki and co-workers)

The steps are summarized in Table 13.

Table 13. *Purification of bovine LMW kininogen from 5.25 liters of plasma* (SUZUKI and co-workers)

Fraction	Treatment	Total protein (mg)	Total protein (A_{280})	Specific activity[a]	Purification factor	Yield (%)
0	Bovine plasma (citrated)		300,000			
1	Ammonium sulfate fraction, 30–50% saturated		66,350	0.246	(1.0)	(100)
2	Zinc filtrate		11,900	0.77	3.1	56.4
3	CM-cellulose chromatography		935	4.3	17.4	24.5
4	DEAE-cellulose chromatography		425	8.2	33.5	21.5
5	DEAE-Sephadex A-50 chromatography		280	10.7	43.5	18.4
6	Sephadex G-100 gel filtration	200	116	20.7	84	14.7

[a] Bradykinin (μg) released per A_{280} of protein by heat-treated *Agkistrodon halys blomhoffii* venom (SUZUKI et al., 1965).

Comments

1. As can be seen in Table 13, the first two steps accounted for the major losses of kininogen activity encountered in this scheme. It seems likely that they can be ascribed to the action of plasma kallikrein activated by the ammonium sulfate fractionation in step 1 and carried over in the 50% saturated ammonium sulfate precipitate to step 2. However, beginning with the CM-cellulose chromatographic step—in which the kininogen activity is recovered in the unadsorbed fraction—the losses are greatly reduced; this can be attributed to adsorption of the basic plasma kallikrein to the ion exchanger. The use of hexadimethrine bromide is suggested to prevent activation of prekallikrein and of SBTI, to inhibit any plasma kallikrein formed.

2. The K_d value calculated for step 6 is too low to give optimum purification. It is therefore advisable to replace Sephadex G-100 by G-200, in about a 2.5–3.0 × 100–150 cm column, to give a K_d closer to 0.5.

3. I would substitute DEAE-Sephadex A-50 for DEAE-cellulose in step 4 and use hydroxyapatite chromatography (linear phosphate gradient in the presence of 1 M potassium chloride) as step 5 or as the step following the Sephadex G-200 gel filtration.

II. Rabbit LMW Kininogen (Egorova and Paskhina, 1967, Egorova et al., 1969)

All chromatographic steps are conducted at 10–12° and are summarized in Table 14.

Table 14. *Purification of rabbit LMW kininogen from one liter of plasma* (Egorova and Paskhina, 1967; Egorova et al., 1969)

Fraction	Treatment	Protein (mg)	Specific activity[a]	Purification factor	Yield (%)
0	Rabbit plasma (citrated)	57,000	0.036	(1.0)	(100)
1	Cohn fraction IV-1	5,300	0.29	8	
2	DEAE-Sephadex A-50 chromatography, pH 6.9	330	4.5	130	72
3	DEAE-Sephadex A-50 chromatography pH 4.0	90	12.6	366	57
4	Sephadex G-200 gel filtration	40	22.0	625	43

[a] Bradykinin (μg) released by means of trypsin per mg of denatured kininogen fraction (Diniz and Carvalho, 1963; Paskhina and Egorova, 1966).

Polyacrylamide disk gel electrophoresis of fraction 4 showed three kininogen bands having nearly thc same specific activity as the starting material, and an albumin band. Ultracentrifugation indicated a purity of about 90% (Egorova et al., 1969).

Comments

1. So far as it goes, the above scheme eminently satisfies all of the criteria being used in this chapter except for the Cohn fractionation in step 1, for which the substitution of a milder method may be desirable.

2. It should be possible to resolve and further to purify the active components found in fraction 4 by phosphate gradient elution in the presence of salt on hydroxyapatite columns or by preparative gel electrophoresis.

III. Human LMW Kininogens I and II (Pierce and Webster, 1966)

The following scheme for purifying LMW kininogens I and II from 1 liter of outdated plasma was derived from the original work in which 5.8 liters were used. The steps are summarized in Table 15. Step 5 is shown in Fig. 1.

Fractions were assayed for kininogen by a direct method (Webster and Gilmore, 1965) by means of an isolated estric rat uterus suspended in a 10-ml bath of de Jalon's solution (Jalon et al., 1945) at 29°. To the bath add the kininogen sample containing about 1 μg of pure kininogen (the amount present in about 0.005 ml of human plasma or serum) in less than 0.2 ml. Wait one minute to test for the presence of free kinin in the sample. Add 0.10 ml of a 5 FU/ml saline solution of a partially purified human urinary kallikrein (3–10 FU/mg) and compare the contraction with that obtained with a kininogen standard or with synthetic bradykinin.

The presence of impurities in both I and II was shown by disk gel electrophoresis and by immunological tests with sheep antiserum to I or II.

Table 15. *Purification of human LMW kininogens I and II from one liter of plasma* PIERCE and WEBSTER, 1966)

Fraction	Treatment	Protein (mg)	Protein (A_{280})	Specific activity[a]	Purification factor	Yield (%)
0	Human plasma (ACD)		56,800	0.056	(1.0)	(100)
1	First DEAE-cellulose chromatography		3,540	0.51	9.2	56
2	Second DEAE-cellulose chromatography	2,270	1,800	0.61	13.5	34
3	Hydroxyapatite chromatography					
	a) First activity peak	168	106	2.1	47	7
	b) Second activity peak	105	76	8.3	138	20
4a	Sephadex G-200 gel filtration of 3a					
	1. Main activity peak (K_d 0.45)		21	4.8	80	3.2
	2. Minor activity peak ($K_d = 0.22$)		31	1.4	24	1.3
4b	Sephadex G-200 gel filtration of 3b	31.4	22.9	14.8	265	11
5	Hydroxyapatite chromatography of 4b					
	a) LMW kininogen I	8.2	5.9	13.2	220	2.4
	b) LMW kininogen II	4.2	3.1	20.7	345	2.0

[a] Kininogen units/A_{280}; 1 kininogen unit is approximately equal to 1 μg of bradykinin.

Comments

1. In step 2, the first and second peaks should be worked up separately, since it is quite likely they correspond to LMW and HMW kininogens respectively.

2. The HMW component of fraction 2 was probably present only in fraction 3a (peak 1 of step 3), since lyophilization of the concentrate of this peak gave a 50% activity loss and since Sephadex G-200 gel filtration of the lyophilized material showed, besides a large peak of LMW kininogens ($K_d = 0.45$) (fraction 4a) a small peak ($K_d = 0.22$) which was probably HMW kininogen. Therefore, lyophilization of fractions suspected of containing HMW kininogens should be avoided—a recommendation made also by JACOBSEN and KRIZ (1967).

Since hydroxyapatite chromatography of either fraction 4a or 4b in the absence of salt gave very broad activity peaks with no purification, and since these fractions gave similar disk gel patterns, it seemed likely that a complex of kininogens with other proteins gave the false peak 1 in step 3. Following a lead provided by ADA (1963), I thought it possible that hydroxyapatite chromatography in the presence of salt would dissociate the complex. Such an experiment not only confirmed this hypothesis but also resolved LMW kininogens I and II.

3. I would no longer use this scheme as it now stands to isolate human plasma kininogens. In the summary at the end of the section on kininogens I have proposed a new scheme incorporating the results from the several methods described in this section.

G. High Molecular Weight Kininogens

I. Human HMW Kininogen (Jacobsen and Kriz, 1967)

JACOBSEN (1966a) found that fresh human plasma lost HMW kininogen activity on storage in untreated glassware or at 4°, whereas the activity was retained on storage at room temperature in siliconed glassware for at least 56 hours.

This confirms the observation of ARMSTRONG et al. (1966) that whole human plasma collected in polyethylene containers rapidly lost kininogen activity at 0° but retained it for long periods, up to several days, at 37°. Therefore the steps (summarized in Table 16) were conducted at 20° rather than in the cold room.

Table 16. *Purification of HMW kininogen from human plasma* (JACOBSEN and KRIZ, 1967)

Fraction	Treatment	Protein (mg/ml)	Bradykinin content[a] (ng/ml)	Specific activity[b]	Purification factor	Yield[c] (%)
0	Human plasma	73.5	500	6.8	(1.0)	
1	DEAE-Sephadex A-50 chromatography	5.2	1,500	288	42	70
2	Sephadex G-200 gel filtration	0.4	300	750	110	80
3	DEAE-Sephadex A-50 concentration	1.2	1,000	870	128	84
4	Preparative gel electrophoresis	0.15	600	4,000	588	66

[a] Bradykinin content is determined by incubating 0.2 ml of HMW kininogen fraction with 0.1 ml of 27 mM disodium EDTA and 0.1 ml of human pseudoglobulin solution at 37° for 1 minute. The amount of kinin released in a suitable aliquot is estimated by comparing the contraction of an estric rat uterus preparation suspended in de Jalon's solution at 29° with that given by a synthetic bradykinin standard. The pseudoglobulin preparation (plasma kallikrein) is made from human plasma by fractionating with ammonium sulfate between 33 and 46% of saturation (LEWIS, 1960), dissolving the 46% precipitate in water, and dialyzing the solution against running tap water for at least 48 hours. The final volume is about one third that of the starting plasma. Aliquots of the pseudoglobulin solution are stored at −20° until used (JACOBSEN, 1966a).

[b] Nanograms bradykinin released/mg protein.

[c] Recovery at each step.

In a parallel series of experiments, JACOBSEN and KRIZ isolated human LMW kininogen with a specific activity of 3.75 μg of bradykinin/mg, a molecular weight of 57,000, and the electrophoretic mobility of an α_1-globulin.

Comments

1. This scheme should be useful for the rapid isolation of small amounts of highly purified human and other mammalian HMW and LMW kininogens.

2. Although the height:diameter ratio of the Sephadex G-200 column in step 2 is too small for best results, JACOBSEN and KRIZ found it adequate to their purposes (JACOBSEN, personal communication). Originally they used columns 150 cm long but obtained impracticably low flow rates with them. We have found that 100- to 150-cm long columns of Bio-Gel P-200 (bead form) give usable flow rates with salt solutions above 1 M. However, to use such conditions would necessitate finding a way to concentrate and desalt the HMW kininogen fractions without losing activity. Perhaps the losses of activity suffered by JACOBSEN and KRIZ during ultrafiltration of such fractions could be mitigated or eliminated in the presence of hexadimethrine and SBTI.

II. Bovine HMW Kininogen (Yano et al., 1967b)

1. *Ammonium Sulfate Fractionation.* Follow the directions given in the first step of the purification of bovine LMW kininogens. The pseudoglobulin fraction (50% saturated ammonium sulfate precipitate) is dissolved in water and heated at 65° for 30 minutes to destroy

plasma kallikrein and other enzymes. From 86 ml of plasma, 10 ml of heated pseudoglobulin fraction (fraction 1) is obtained with 1,300 A_{280} units. Treat this solution with 0.4 mg of SBTI and 10 mg of *o*-phenanthroline to give fraction 1.

2. *DEAE-Sephadex A-50 Chromatography (40)*. Apply fraction 1 to a 2.5×11 cm column of DEAE-Sephadex A-50 equilibrated with 0.02 M phosphate–0.1 M sodium chloride, pH 8.0. Wash the column with about 100 ml of equilibration buffer and start a 750-ml linear gradient of 0.1 to 0.3 M sodium chloride in 0.02 M phosphate, pH 8.0. LMW kininogen is found between 200 and 450 ml of effluent and HMW kininogen between 450 and 600 ml of effluent after starting the gradient. Combine the best HMW kininogen fractions, lyophilize, desalt by Sephadex G-25 gel filtration, and lyophilize the salt-free protein solution (fraction 2). This material released about 1.5 µg of bradykinin per A_{280} of protein, when heat-traeted *Agkistrodon halys blomhoffii* venom, was used and about half of that with bovine plasma kallikrein.

Further steps have not been reported.

Comment

1. The use of hexadimethrine bromide, in being a milder method, would seem preferable to heating the pseudoglobulin fraction. However, the HF inhibitor has not yet been tested for preventing plasma kallikrein activation during fractionation procedures.

Proposed Scheme for the Isolation of Mammalian LMW and HMW Kininogens. Blood should be freshly collected in polyethylene or siliconized containers in the presence of hexadimethrine bromide, SBTI, and a complexing agent, and centrifuged at room temperature. The plasma thus obtained, after being suitably diluted, could be carried through the following steps at room temperature:

(1) DEAE-cellulose or DEAE-Sephadex A-50 gradient elution chromatography to resolve LMW and HMW kininogens.

(2) DEAE-Sephadex A-50 gradient elution chromatography of each peak, with eluents different from those used in the first step.

(3) Sephadex G-200 gel filtration on a long or recycling column.

(4) Hydroxyapatite gradient elution chromatography in the presence of 1 M potassium chloride.

(5) Preparative gel electrophoresis and/or isoelectric focusing.

It may be desirable to use hexadimethrine and SBTI throughout the fractionation or until the last step or two and to add an appropriate bacteriostatic agent to all eluents.

H. Kinins

The kinins are polypeptides containing the bradykinin sequence H-Arg-Pro-Pro-Gly-Phe-Ser-Pro-Phe-Arg-OH and are extremely potent pharmacological agents when the carboxyl-terminal arginine residue has its carboxyl group free.[8] They are typically derived from the kininogens by the action of various kallikreins (Lewis, 1960; Schachter, 1964; Erdös, 1966). The mammalian kinins and kinin-containing fragments so far described are bradykinin (Elliott et al., 1961); kallidin (lysyl-bradykinin) (Pierce and Webster, 1963); methionyl-lysyl-bradykinin (Elliott and Lewis, 1965); Met-Lys-bradykinyl-Ser-Val-Gln (PKFL) and Met-Lys-bradykinyl-Ser-Val-Gln-Val-Met (PKFS) (Habermann, 1966); and Gly (or Ser)-Arg-Met-Lys-bradykinin (Hochstrasser and Werle, 1967). Their structural relationships to one another and to the kininogens have been discussed

8. Phyllokinin (bradykinyl-isoleucyl-tyrosine-*O*-sulfate) is the only known kinin blocked at its carboxyl terminus with pharmacological activity comparable to and occasionally greater than that of bradykinin (Anastasi et al., 1966). Bradykinyl-serine, PKFS, and PKFL have, on a molar basis, a much lower potency than bradykinin; however, treatment with trypsin and certain other enzymes completely releases the inherent kinin activity.

elsewhere (PIERCE, 1968; HABERMANN, p. 250; SCHRÖDER, p. 324). The non-mammalian kinins are dealt with by PISANO in Chapter 8.

It is unfortunate that a systematic attempt to discover a single, economical, and convenient procedure for isolating and resolving kinins from various sources has not been made. The availability of ^{14}C bradykinin, kallidin, and methionyl-lysyl-bradykinin now makes such a study feasible.

Lacking the information this investigation would provide, I shall present a tentative approach to accomplishing this goal by selecting the most promising methods from a number of sources and integrating them into a single, plausible scheme (TRAUTSCHOLD, p. 52). The methods chosen for this purpose have been gleaned from the following observations:

(1) Strong adsorption of bradykinin to IRC-50 below pH 6–7 (ANDRADE and ROCHA E SILVA, 1957).

(2) Elution of bradykinin in high yields from IRC-50 columns with 9 M acetic acid (GUTTMANN et al., 1962) and with a gradient of 1 to 10 M acetic acid (MERRIFIELD, 1964).

(3) Gel filtration of kinins on columns of Sephadex G-25 to give high purification and yield (PIERCE and WEBSTER, 1961; WERLE et al., 1961).

(4) Gradient elution chromatography with volatile buffers on CM-cellulose or CM-Sephadex C-25 columns to purify and/or resolve bradykinin (ELLIOTT et al., 1961); bradykinin and kallidin (PIERCE and WEBSTER, 1961; WERLE et al., 1961); *Polistes* kinin and other kinins (NAKAJIMA et al., in preparation); bradykinin, kallidin, and methionyl-lysyl-bradykinin from human urine (MIWA et al., 1968, 1969); and PKFL and PKFS (HABERMANN, 1966).

(5) Gradient elution chromatography with volatile buffers on P-cellulose columns to purify and resolve PKFL and PKFS (HABERMANN, 1966).

Procedure

I. Preparation of the Extract

Solutions with a relatively low concentration of protein and salt may be suitable for the next step without treatment (e.g. urine). For tissue extracts and plasma it will generally be advisable, sometimes necessary, to dilute with water or to remove the bulk of proteins by precipitating with TCA and removing the TCA from the filtrate by ether extraction. Adjust the pH of the final kinin solution to about 4.

II. IRC-50 Adsorption

a) Batch. It will be advisable to use this method of adsorption for processing large volumes, e.g. urine. First, determine the amount of resin necessary to adsorb all the kinins in the extract by vigorously stirring small aliquots of the step 1 extract with graded levels of IRC-50 at pH 4.0 for several hours at 20–25°. Second, using the minimum level thus determined, stir several aliquots of the extract for different periods of time (e.g. 1, 3, 10 hours) to learn the equilibrium time. The use of a 200–400-mesh resin from which fines have been removed is recommended. Recover the resin by filtering through a coarse fritted-glass funnel. The resin adsorbate, after being thoroughly washed with distilled water, is now ready for elution.

Examples

(1) Human and bovine plasmas, after treatment with human urinary kallikrein (PIERCE and WEBSTER, 1961) and hog submaxillary kallikrein (WERLE et al., 1961), respectively, and dilution with water, were stirred at pH 4.0 and 2 and 15 hours with IRC-50. The former

workers used 2.5 g of resin per liter of plasma; the latter did not specify the amount they used. In both cases, about 10% of the starting biological activity was not adsorbed and therefore was probably not due to unadsorbed kinins.

(2) MIWA et al. (1968, 1969) adsorbed human urinary kinins to IRC-50 (1.0 g/liter of urine) at pH 4–5. The stirring time and temperature were not reported. (Overnight stirring at 20–25° would be advisable in view of the low level of resin being used.)

(3) WEBSTER and GILMORE (1965) adsorbed the kinins present in dog blood to IRC-50. They withdrew 15-ml portions of venous or arterial blood within 20–40 seconds into a syringe containing 2.25 ml of 1 M phosphoric acid and 1.5 mg of SBTI. The expelled mixture (pH 4–5) was transferred with an equal volume of water to a beaker containing 100 mg of IRC-50 (H^+) and stirred at pH 4.0 and 22–26° for one hour.

b) Column. If the volume of the extract is small and protein and salt are present in low concentration, adsorption to an IRC-50 column will be preferable to batch adsorption. Determine the capacity of the resin with respect to the particular extract by percolating it through a small test column at a low flow rate (about 2 ml/cm²/hour) until kinin activity first appears in the effluent. In the main experiment, use less than 80% of the capacity of the column. The choice of sample load will depend on the properties of the sample and on the aims of the experiment.

Examples

(1) GUTTMANN et al. (1962) adsorbed about 1.64 g of crude synthetic bradykinin in 200 ml of 1 M acetic acid to a 300-ml column of IRC-50 previously washed with 1 M acetic acid.

(2) Similarly, MERRIFIELD (1964) adsorbed 70.8 mg of crude synthetic bradykinin in 1 ml of 1 M acetic acid to a 2×98 cm column of IRC-50.

III. IRC-50 Elution

a) With Ammonium Formate or Acetate buffers. PIERCE and WEBSTER (1961), WERLE et al. (1961), WEBSTER and GILMORE (1965), and MIWA et al. (1968, 1969)) eluted adsorbed kinins from IRC-50 with 0.20–0.25 M ammonium formate, pH 8.2–9.0 (presumably, ammonium acetate could be substituted for ammonium formate with similar results). Losses were observed in the first three cases, perhaps caused by kininases which may have been co-adsorbed and co-eluted.

b) With Acetic Acid. Elution with high concentrations of acetic acid appears to be the method of choice: recoveries appear to be very high, large purification can probably be realized in some cases, the acetic acid can be easily removed by lyophilization, and adsorbed kininases can be ignored, as they will certainly be inactive in acetic acid.

Examples

(1) GUTTMANN et al. (1962) eluted synthetic bradykinin from the column described above with 4 liters of 9 M acetic acid after washing the column with 3 liters of 1 M acetic acid. They recovered 1.39 g (85% recovery of solids) of bradykinin which was shown to be pure by several criteria.

(2) MERRIFIELD (1964) (see above) applied 1 to 9 M acetic acid and recovered 57.2 mg (81% of the starting solids) from the main Sakaguchi-positive peak. The presumption is that 100% of the biological activity was recovered in both experiments, the loss of material being attributable to impurities.

(3) To test this point, as well as to see if bradykinin can be separated from kallidin by IRC-50 chromatography, I applied 2 μg of ^{14}C-bradykinin (100,000 cpm) plus 2 μg of ^{12}C-kallidin in 1 ml of 1 M acetic acid to a 0.3×30 cm column of IRC-50 (1 M acetic acid), washed the column with 6 ml of 1 M acetic acid, and started a 40-ml linear gradient of 1 to 10 M acetic acid at a flow rate of 2 ml/hour at 25°. First, the recovery of radioactivity was about 90%, indicating that with 100 times the sample charge—well within the capacity of the column—one could expect a 100% recovery. Second, biological assay of the lyophilized fractions suggested that there was no separation of the two kinins. However, the use of a flatter gradient than used here might resolve them.

IV. Gel Filtration

Although many successful applications of gel filtration to peptide separation and purification have been reported, this technique has yet to be fully exploited with respect to the kinins.

Examples

(1) Gel filtration on a 1.7×72 cm column of Sephadex G-25 (0.002 M hydrochloric acid) gave, in 56% yield, a 10-fold purification of crude kinins (200 mg) isolated from the IRC-50 adsorption and elution steps described above (PIERCE and WEBSTER, 1961). Rechromatography on a 1.25×94 cm column (0.005 M ammonium formate, pH 8.5) gave a further 3-fold purification in 100% yield.

(2) WERLE et al. (1961) also used Sephadex G-25 gel filtration, but the column dimensions and other details are lacking. They performed this step three times to obtain a 25-fold purification in 80% yield.

It may be possible to resolve the several kinins on long or recycling columns of Sephadex G-15, or Bio-Gel P-4 or P-6. Perhaps the use of acetic acid and other solvents as eluents in gel filtration of kinins should be explored.

V. CM-Cellulose and CM-Sephadex C-25 Chromatography

Although there are now a number of reports showing or suggesting that mixtures of kinin homologs can be resolved on columns of CM-cellulose and CM-Sephadex C-25, no systematic study has yet been made—with the sole exception of that reported by HABERMANN and BLENNEMANN (1964; see example 5, below).

Examples

(1) ELLIOTT and co-workers were the first to apply CM-cellulose gradient elution chromatography to the purification of kinins. This method played a very important role in their isolation of bradykinin from trypsin-treated bovine pseudoglobulin (ELLIOTT et al., 1961). They applied 4 g of a crude bradykinin preparation to a 3.2-cm diameter column containing 32 g of CM-cellulose and applied a gradient formed by adding 0.20 M ammonium acetate, pH 6.4, to 250 ml of starting buffer in a constant-volume mixing chamber. The single peak of activity yielded 60–70 mg of product (P 4) purified 40-fold in 60–70% yield. Rechromatography of P 4 (35 mg) gave a further 30-fold purification in 66% yield. In similar fashion, ELLIOTT and LEWIS (1965) were able to effect a high purification of methionyl-lysyl-bradykinin. The first CM-cellulose chromatogram of crude kinin gave three activity peaks. The third yielded methionyl-lysyl-bradykinin. The other two were not identified, although one of them was very likely bradykinin. These workers obtained superior results by performing the CM-cellulose chromatography at 20° rather than at 2°.

(2) PIERCE and WEBSTER (1961) applied 26 mg of the kinin product from the second Sephadex G-25 gel filtration step mentioned above to a 0.67×23 cm column of CM-cellulose. They initiated a gradient by adding 0.50 M ammonium formate, pH 7.5, to 125 ml of 0.01 M ammonium formate, pH 5.0, in a constant-volume mixing chamber. Two peaks of activity were obtained, the first between 50 and 57 ml of the gradient and the second between 75 and 81 ml. Lyophilization of the best fractions from the two peaks gave, respectively, 5.5 and 3.6 mg with purities of 500 and 225 units/mg (starting material was 180 units/mg; one unit is approximately equivalent to 0.8 μg of pure bradykinin). The first peak was identified as bradykinin and the second as kallidin.

(3) In like manner, synthetic kallidin was purified 3.4-fold in 34% yield (total yield 100%) (WEBSTER and PIERCE, 1963) on a column of CM-cellulose. The activity peak appeared between 462 and 502 ml of the gradient and was immediately preceded by a large peak of inactive material. The use of a flatter gradient would undoubtedly give further resolution.

(4) The human urinary kinins eluted from IRC-50 above were adsorbed to a CM-Sephadex C-25 column and eluted with a linear gradient of 0.05 M ammonium formate, pH 5.0, to 0.50 M ammonium formate, pH 7.5 (MIWA et al., 1968, 1969). Three peaks of activity were obtained. The first peak was identified as bradykinin by chromatographing a mixture of peak 1 material and ^{14}C-bradykinin on a CM-Sephadex C-25 column. The second and third peaks were provisionally identified as methionyl-lysyl-bradykinin and kallidin respectively. These workers estimated that 1 liter of fresh, normal urine contains 10–36 μg of bradykinin, 6–7 μg of kallidin, and 13–25 μg of methionyl-lysyl-bradykinin.

(5) Habermann and Blennemann (1964) applied a mixture of bradykinin (10 μg), kallidin (10 μg), and methionyl-lysyl-bradykinin (50 μg) in 0.01 M ammonium formate, pH 4.8, to a 0.7×18 cm column of CM-cellulose and developed the column with a gradient of 0.10 to 0.35 M ammonium formate, pH 4.8. Three peaks of activity were obtained and identified in the order of their emergence from the column as bradykinin, methionyl-lysyl-bradykinin, and kallidin. They were eluted at the following concentrations of buffer respectively: 0.19–0.20, 0.25, and 0.26–0.27 M ammonium formate. This work should now be repeated with radioactive kinins.

VI. P-Cellulose Chromatography

Although P-cellulose chromatography has been widely and successfully used for the resolution of tryptic and chymotryptic peptides, only Habermann (1966) has applied it to the purification of kinin-containing fragments of kininogen.

About 10 mg of PKFL, partially purified by CM-cellulose chromatography and paper chromatography, was adsorbed to a 0.7×10 cm column (pyridine acetate, pH 3.9: 0.05 M acetate), and the column was developed with a gradient obtained by adding a solution composed of glacial acetic acid and pyridine. Two activity peaks resulted; the first and larger was identified with PKFL and the second smaller peak with PKFS.

Since the behavior of both PKFL and PKFS is different on CM-cellulose and P-cellulose columns, a study of the behavior of other kinins on P-cellulose should be rewarding.

References

Ada, G. L.: Purification and properties of avian neuraminidase. Biochim. biophys. Acta (Amst.) **73**, 276 (1963).

Anastasi, A., Bertaccini, G., Erspamer, V.: Pharmacological data on phyllokinin (bradykinyl-isoleucyl-tyrosine-*O*-sulphate) and bradykinyl-isoleucyl-tyrosine. Brit. J. Pharmacol. **27**, 479 (1966).

Andrade, S. O., Rocha e Silva, M.: Purification of bradykinin by ion-exchange chromatography. Biochem. J. **64**, 701 (1957).

Armstrong, D., Mills, G. L., Sicuteri, F.: Physiological influence on the liberation of human plasma kinin at low temperatures. In: Hypotensive peptides, p. 139, ed. by E. G. Erdös, N. Back, and F. Sicuteri. Berlin-Heidelberg-New York: Springer 1966.

Babel, I., Stella, R. C. R., Prado, E. S.: Action of horse urinary kallikrein on synthetic derivatives of bradykinin. Biochem. Pharmacol. **17**, 2232 (1968).

Brandi, C. M. W., Mendes, J., Paiva, A. C. M., Prado, E. S.: Proteolysis of salmine by horse urinary kallikrein. Biochem. Pharmacol. **14**, 1665 (1965).

— Roncada, M. J., Prado, E. S., Prado, J. L.: Observations on the hydrolysis of salmine by kallikreins. In: Vaso-active polypeptides: Bradykinin and related kinins, p. 135, ed. by M. Rocha e Silva and H. A. Rothschild. São Paulo 1967.

Carvalho, I. F., Diniz, C. R.: Kinin-forming enzyme (kininogenin) in homogenates of rat kidney. Biochim. biophys. Acta (Amst.) **128**, 136 (1966).

Cohn, E. J., Strong, L. E., Hughes, W. L., Jr., Mulford, D. J., Ashworth, J. N., Melin, M., Taylor, H. L.: Preparation and properties of serum and plasma proteins. IV. A system for the separation into fractions of the protein and lipoprotein components of biological tissues and fluids. J. Amer. chem. Soc. **68**, 459 (1946).

Colman, R. W.: Activation of plasminogen by human plasma kallikrein. Biochem. biophys. Res. Commun. **35**, 273 (1969).

— Mattler, L., Sherry, S.: Studies on the prekallikrein (kallikreinogen)-kallikrein enzyme system of human plasma. I. Isolation and purification of plasma kallikreins. J. clin. Invest. **48**, 11 (1969a).

— — — Studies on the prekallikrein (kallikreinogen)-kallikrein enzyme system of human plasma. II. Evidence relating the kaolin-activated arginine esterase to plasma kallikrein. J. clin. Invest. **48**, 23 (1969b).

Cuatrecasas, P., Wilchek, M., Anfinsen, C. B.: Selective enzyme purification by affinity chromatography. Proc. nat. Acad. Sci. (Wash.) **61**, 636 (1968).

DINIZ, C. R., CARVALHO, I. F.: A micromethod for determination of bradykininogen under several conditions. Ann. N.Y. Acad. Sci. **104**, 77 (1963).
— PEREIRA, A. A., BARROSO, J., MARES-GUIA, M.: On the specificity of urinary kallikreins. Biochem. biophys. Res. Commun. **5**, 448 (1965).
— — — — Studies of the specificity of kinin-forming enzymes: The inhibition of the kininogenic activity of trypsin and kallikreins by model compounds. In: Hypotensive peptides, p. 175, ed. by E. G. ERDÖS, N. BACK, and F. SICUTERI. Berlin-Heidelberg-New York: Springer 1966.
EGOROVA, T. P., MAKAROVA, O. V., PASKHINA, T. S.: Properties and substrate nature of purified rabbit kininogen. Biokhimiya **34**, 610 (1969).
— PASKHINA, T. S.: Purification of kininogen (bradykininogen) from rabbit's blood plasma and the study of its properties. Biokhimiya **32**, 354 (1967).
EISEN, V.: Effect of hexadimethrine bromide on plasma kinin formation, hydrolysis of *p*-tosyl-L-arginine methyl ester and fibrinolysis. Brit. J. Pharmacol. **22**, 87 (1964).
ELLIOTT, D. F., HORTON, E. W., LEWIS, G. P.: The isolation of bradykinin, a plasma kinin from ox blood. Biochem. J. **78**, 60 (1961).
— LEWIS, G. P.: Methionyl-lysyl-bradykinin, a new kinin from ox blood. Biochem. J. **95**, 437 (1965).
ERDÖS, E. G.: Hypotensive peptides: bradykinin, kallidin, and eledoisin. Advanc. Pharmacol. **4**, 1 (1966).
FAULHABER, I., BERNARDI, G.: Chromatography of calf-thymus nucleoprotein on hydroxyapatite columns. Biochim. biophys. Acta (Amst.) **140**, 561 (1967).
FIEDLER, F., WERLE, E.: Vorkommen zweier Kallikreinogene im Schweinepankreas und Automation der Kallikrein- und Kallikreinogenbestimmung. Hoppe-Seylers Z. physiol. Chem. **348**, 1087 (1967).
FREY, E. K.: Zusammenhänge zwischen Herzarbeit und Nierentätigkeit. Langenbecks Arch. klin. Chir. **142**, 663 (1926).
— KRAUT, H.: Über einen von der Niere ausgeschiedenen, die Herztätigkeit anregenden Stoff. Hoppe-Seylers Z. physiol. Chem. **157**, 32 (1926).
— — WERLE, E.: Kallikrein (Padutin). Stuttgart: F. Enke 1950.
— — — VOGEL, R., ZICKGRAF-RÜDEL, G., TRAUTSCHOLD, I.: Das Kallikrein-Kinin-System und seine Inhibitoren. Stuttgart: F. Enke 1968.
FRITZ, H., BREY, B., SCHMAL, A., WERLE, E.: Verwendung wasserunlöslicher Derivate des Trypsin-Kallikrein-Inhibitors zur Isolierung von Kallikreinen und von Plasmin. Hoppe-Seylers Z. physiol. Chem. **350**, 617 (1969a).
— ECKERT, I., WERLE, E.: Isolierung und Charakterisierung von sialinsäurehaltigem und sialinsäurefreiem Kallikrein aus Schweinepankreas. Hoppe-Seylers Z. physiol. Chem. **348**, 1120 (1967a).
— GEBHARDT, M., FINK, E., SCHRAMM, W., WERLE, E.: Verwendung wasserunlöslicher Enzymharze mit polyanionischer und polyamphoterer Harzmatrix zur Isolierung von Proteaseinhibitoren. Hoppe-Seylers Z. physiol. Chem. **350**, 129 (1969b).
— HOCHSTRASSER, K., WERLE, E.: Nachweis und präparative Trennung von Proteinase-inhibitoren und von Proteinasen mit Hilfe wasserunlöslicher Enzym- bzw. Inhibitorharze. Z. anal. Chem. **243**, 452 (1968).
— HÜLLER, I., WIEDEMANN, M., WERLE, E.: Zur Chemie und Physiologie der spezifischen Trypsininhibitoren aus den Bauchspeicheldrüsen von Rind, Hund, Schwein und Mensch. Hoppe-Seylers Z. physiol. Chem. **348**, 405 (1967b).
— SCHULT, H., HUTZEL, M., WIEDEMANN, M., WERLE, E.: Isolierung von Protease-Inhibitoren mit Hilfe wasserunlöslicher Enzym-Harze. Hoppe-Seylers Z. physiol. Chem. **348**, 308 (1967c).
GUTTMANN, ST., PLESS, J., BOISSONNAS, R. A.: Nouvelle synthèse de la bradykinine. Helv. chim. Acta **45**, 170 (1962).
HABERMANN, E.: Trennung und Reinigung von Pankreaskallikreinen. Hoppe-Seylers Z. physiol. Chem. **328**, 15 (1962).
— Über pH-bedingte Modifikationen des kininliefernden α-Globulins (Kininogen) aus Rinderserum und das Molekulargewicht von Kininogen I. Biochem. Z. **337**, 440 (1963).
— Strukturaufklärung kininliefernder Peptide aus Rinderserum-Kininogen. Naunyn-Schmiedebergs Arch. exp. Path. Pharmak. **253**, 474 (1966).
— BLENNEMANN, G.: Über Substrate und Reaktionsprodukte der kininbildenden Enzyme Trypsin, Serum- und Pankreaskallikrein sowie von Crotalusgift. Naunyn-Schmiedebergs Arch. exp. Path. Pharmak. **249**, 357 (1964).
— KLETT, W.: Reinigung und einige Eigenschaften eines Kallikreins aus Schweineserum. Biochem. Z. **346**, 133 (1966).
— — ROSENBUSCH, G.: Partielle Reinigung und einige Eigenschaften eines Kininogens aus Rinderblut. Hoppe-Seylers Z. physiol. Chem. **332**, 121 (1963).

HEFTMANN, E., Ed.: Chromatography, 2nd ed. New York: Reinhold 1967.
HENRIQUES, O. B., KAURITCHEVA, N., KUZNETSOVA, V., ASTRAKAN, M.: Substrates of kinin-releasing enzymes isolated from horse plasma. Nature (Lond.) **215**, 1200 (1967).
— LAVRAS, A. A. C., FICHMAN, M., PICARELLI, Z. P.: Plasma enzymes that release kinins. Biochem. Pharmacol. **15**, 31 (1966).
HOCHSTRASSER, K., WERLE, E.: Über kininliefernde Peptide aus pepsinverdauten Rinderplasmaproteinen. Hoppe-Seylers Z. physiol. Chem. **348**, 177 (1967).
JACOBSEN, S.: Substrates for plasma kinin-forming enzymes in human, dog, and rabbit plasmas. Brit. J. Pharmacol. **26**, 403 (1966a).
— Substrates for plasma kinin-forming enzymes in rat and guinea-pig plasma. Brit. J. Pharmacol. **28**, 64 (1966b).
— KRIZ, M.: Some data on two purified kininogens from human plasma. Brit. J. Pharmacol. **29**, 25 (1967).
JALON, P. G. DE, BAYO, J. B., JALON, M. G. DE: A sensitive and new method for measuring adrenalin on the isolated rat uterus. Farmacoterap. Actual (Madrid) **2**, 313 (1945).
KRAUT, H., FREY, E. K., BAUER, E.: Über ein neues Kreislaufhormon. II. Mitt. Hoppe-Seylers Z. physiol. Chem. **175**, 97 (1928).
— — WERLE, E.: Über den Nachweis und das Vorkommen des Kallikreins im Blut. VIII. Mitteilung über Kallikrein. Hoppe-Seylers Z. physiol. Chem. **222**, 73 (1933).
LAUFER, A. L., GULIKOVA, O. M., PASKHINA, T. S.: Two kinin-producing enzymes from human plasma. Biokhimiya **34**, 3 (1969).
LEWIS, G. P.: Active polypeptides derived from plasma proteins. Physiol. Rev. **40**, 647 (1960).
MARES-GUIA, M., DINIZ, C. R.: Studies on the mechanism of rat urinary kallikrein catalysis, and its relation to catalysis by trypsin. Arch. Biochem. **121**, 750 (1967a).
— — The specificity of kallikreins, as studied with model compounds. In: Vaso-active polypeptides: Bradykinin and related peptides, p. 149, ed. by M. ROCHA E SILVA and H. A. ROTHSCHILD. São Paulo 1967b.
MARGOLIS, J.: The interrelationship of coagulation of plasma and release of petides. Ann. N.Y. Acad. Sci. **104**, 133 (1963).
MERRIFIELD, R. B.: Solid-phase peptide synthesis. III. An improved synthesis of bradykinin. Biochemistry **3**, 1385 (1964).
MIWA, I., ERDÖS, E. G., SEKI, T.: Presence of three peptides in urinary kinin (Substance Z) preparations. Life Sci. **7**, 1339 (1968).
— — — Separation of peptide components of urinary kinin (substance Z). Proc. Soc. exp. Biol. (N.Y.) **131**, 768 (1969).
MORIYA, H., KATO, A., FUKUSHIMA, H.: Further study on purification of hog pancreatic kallikrein. Biochem. Pharmacol. **18**, 549 (1969).
— MORIWAKI, C., YAMAZAKI, K., AKIMOTO, S., FUKUSHIMA, H.: Human salivary kallikrein and liberation of colostrokinin. In: Hypotensive peptides, p. 161, ed. by E. G. ERDÖS, N. BACK and F. SICUTERI. Berlin-Heidelberg-New York: Springer 1966.
— PIERCE, J. V., WEBSTER, M. E.: Purification and some properties of three kallikreins. Ann. N.Y. Acad. Sci. **104**, 172 (1963).
— YAMAZAKI, K., FUKUSHIMA, H.: Biochemical studies on kallikreins and their related substances. I. Isolation and purification of human saliva kallikrein. J. Biochem. (Tokyo) **58**, 201 (1965a).
— — — MORIWAKI, C.: Biochemical studies on kallikreins and their related substances. II. An improved method of purification of hog pancreatic kallikrein and some of its biological properties. J. Biochem. (Tokyo) **58**, 208 (1965b).
NAGASAWA, S., HORIUCHI, K., YANO, M., SUZUKI, T.: Partial purification of bovine plasma kallikrein activated by contact with glass. J. Biochem. (Tokyo) **62**, 398 (1967).
— MIZUSHIMA, Y., SATO, T., IWANAGA, S., SUZUKI, T.: Studies on the chemical nature of bovine bradykininogen: Determinations of amino acid, carbohydrate, amino and carboxyl terminal residues. J. Biochem. (Tokyo) **60**, 643 (1966).
— TAKAHASHI, H., KOIDA, M., SUZUKI, T.: Partial purification of bovine plasma kallikreinogen, its activation by Hageman factor. Biochem. biophys. Res. Commun. **32**, 644 (1968).
NAKAJIMA, T., TAMURA, Z., PISANO, J. J., UDENFRIEND, S.: *Polistes* kinin, a bradykinin homolog in wasp venom. (In preparation.)
PASKHINA, T. S., EGOROVA, T. P.: Purification and properties of kininogen (bradykininogen) from rabbit blood serum. Biokhimiya **31**, 468 (1966).
PIERCE, J. V.: Structural features of plasma kinins and kininogens. Fed. Proc. **27**, 52 (1968).
— NUSTAD, K.: Resolution of human urinary kallikrein isoenzymes on columns of hydroxyapatite. (In preparation.)
— WEBSTER, M. E.: Human plasma kallidins; isolation and chemical studies. Biochem. biophys. Res. Commun. **5**, 353 (1961).

PIERCE, J. V., WEBSTER, M. E.: The purification and some properties of two different kallidinogens from human plasma. In: Hypotensive peptides, p. 130, ed. by E. G. ERDÖS, N. BACK and F. SICUTERI. Berlin-Heidelberg-New York: Springer 1966.
PRADO, E. S., PRADO, J. L., BRANDI, C. M. W.: Further purification and some properties of horse urinary kallikrein. Arch. int. Pharmacodyn. **137**, 358 (1962).
— STELLA, R. C. R., RONCADA, M. J., PRADO, J. L.: Action of horse urinary kallikrein on arginine and lysine peptides. In: Vaso-active polypeptides: Bradykinin and related kinins, p. 141, ed. by M. ROCHA E SILVA and H. A. ROTHSCHILD. São Paulo 1967.
PRADO, J. L., KATCHBURIAN, A. V., MENDES, J., PRADO, E. S.: Ions and the kininogenic activity of horse urinary kallikrein. Acta physiol. lat.-amer. **15**, 386 (1965).
— PRADO, E. S., BRANDI, C. M. W., KATCHBURIAN, A. V.: Some properties of highly purified horse urinary kallikrein. Ann. N.Y. Acad. Sci. **104**, 186 (1963).
ROBERTS, P. S.: Measurement of the rate of plasmin action on synthetic substrates. J. biol. Chem. **232**, 285 (1958).
ROCHA E SILVA, M., HOLZHACKER, E. L.: Liberation of bradykinin from plasma by treatment with peptone or by boiling with hydrochloric acid. Arch. int. Pharmacodyn. **122**, 168 (1959).
RODER, O.: Diss. Med. Fakultät, Munich, 1967.
SARNOFF, L. C., SUSSMAN, K. E., SARNOFF, S. J.: Observations on the vasodilator properties of urine. II. The problem of reproducibility in blood flow bioassay technics for vasoactive substances. Studies with human urine. Circulat. Res. **4**, 526 (1958).
SCHACHTER, M.: Some properties of kallidin, bradykinin and wasp venom kinin. In: Polypeptides which affect smooth muscles and blood vessels, p. 232, ed. by M. SCHACHTER. London: Pergamon Press 1960.
— Kinins—a group of active peptides. Ann. Rev. Pharmacol. **4**, 281 (1964).
SCHOENMAKERS, J. G. G., MATZE, R., HAANEN, C., ZILLIKEN, F.: Hageman factor, a novel sialoglycoprotein with esterase activity. Biochim. biophys. Acta (Amst.) **101**, 166 (1965).
SCHULTZ, F.: Process for the recovery of callikrein from animal substances. U.S. Patent 2,784,142 (1957).
SEIDEL, G., VOGT, W.: Kininogenspezifität von acetonaktiviertem menschlichem Plasmakallikrein. Naunyn-Schmiedebergs Arch. exp. Path. Pharmak. **262**, 135 (1969).
SUZUKI, T., MIZUSHIMA, Y., SATO, T., IWANAGA, S.: Purification of bovine bradykininogen. J. Biochem. (Tokyo) **57**, 14 (1965).
TRAUTSCHOLD, I.: Habil.-Schr. der Med. Fakultät, Munich, 1965.
WEBSTER, M. E., GILMORE, J. P.: The estimation of the kallidins in blood and urine. Biochem. Pharmacol. **14**, 1161 (1965).
— PIERCE, J. V.: Action of the kallikreins on synthetic ester substrates. Proc. Soc. exp. Biol. (N.Y.) **107**, 186 (1961).
— — The nature of the kallidins released from human plasma by kallikreins and other enzymes. Ann. N.Y. Acad. Sci. **104**, 91 (1963).
WERLE, E.: Über Kallikrein aus Blut. Biochem. Z. **287**, 235 (1936).
— FORELL, M. M., MAIER, L.: Zur Kenntnis der blutdrucksenkenden Wirkung des Trypsins. Naunyn-Schmiedebergs Arch. exp. Path. Pharmak. **225**, 369 (1955).
— TRAUTSCHOLD, I.: Kallikrein, kallidin, kallikrein inhibitors. Ann. N.Y. Acad. Sci. **104**, 117 (1963).
— — LEYSATH, G.: Isolierung und Struktur des Kallidins. Hoppe-Seylers Z. physiol. Chem. **326**, 174 (1961).
YANO, M., KATO, H., NAGASAWA, S., SUZUKI, S.: An improved method for the purification of kininogen-II from bovine plasma. J. Biochem. (Tokyo) **62**, 386 (1967a).
— NAGASAWA, S., HORIUCHI, K., SUZUKI, T.: Separation of a new substrate, kininogen-I, for plasma kallikrein in bovine plasma. J. Biochem. (Tokyo) **62**, 504 (1967b).
ZYKOVA, V. P., PASKHINA, T. S.: Discovery of the kallikrein in the γ-globulin fraction of rabbit serum proteins. Dokl. Acad. Nauk. USSR **165**, 1439 (1965).

Assay Methods in the Kinin System

IVAR TRAUTSCHOLD

With 5 Figures

Introduction

Terms like "tissue hormones" and "local hormones" were created (FELDBERG and SCHILF, 1930; GADDUM, 1936) almost before the class of the pharmacologically polyvalent and potent kinin hormones was discovered. The pioneers in the field of this subdivision of tissue hormones used essentially the same assay methods for the detection of the kinins that we do today. FREY and KRAUT (1928) demonstrated by intravenous injection of urine in the dog the vasodilator activity of kallikrein. The contraction of smooth muscle was used by WERLE et al. (1937) to show for the first time the liberation of a kinin by applying a mixture of human serum and an extract of salivary gland to an isolated segment of guinea pig ileum. The knowledge that the kinins were liberated enzymatically from the serum precursor kininogen was the result of studying the kinetics of the formation of kallidin (WERLE and BEREK, 1948) and of bradykinin (ROCHA E SILVA et al., 1949) by means of isolated smooth muscle preparations.

The kinin system is characterized by various well-known and distinct pharmacological activities, all of which may be used for biological assays. In general the bioassays show a high sensitivity and, owing to different biological receptors, they also have a relatively high specificity. The various receptors which are excitable by the kinins, however, may also show affinity for other biologically active substances. Other tissue hormones share the properties of the kinins; this requires a differentiation of the specific kinin action. Such differentiation is made possible by using different pharmacological parameters to get a ratio of potency which is constant for a given substance, or by using different test objects or species to get the so-called index of discrimination which again characterizes an unknown effector.

In addition, the interfering substances may be eliminated by the use of inhibitors as, for example, antihistamines for the inhibition of histamine, atropine for blocking acetylcholine, or methysergide or other derivatives of lysergic acid to prevent the action of serotonin.

The receptors of the biological system recognize the true biological effector and can not be deceived by artefacts which may originate from chemical isolation methods and differ very little from the original substrate. On the other hand, everyone knows the disadvantages of the biological assay: the poor reproducibility of the results, the great loss of time and money in *in vivo* (whole animal) methods, the varying sensitivity from preparation to preparation, and the change in sensitivity of the same preparation with time. The resulting large standard deviations not infrequently exceed the range of the physiological and even the pathological deviations of the analytical parameters. Since bioassay gives no absolute results, standard and reference preparations must be available. In most cases there are no standardized units and the activity must be compared with that of synthetic preparations. It is not advisable to replace such standard preparations by definitions of biological units, because of the varying responses of tissue.

Another handicap of biological assay methods which is difficult to overcome is the identification of unknown kinins or the differentiation of components of a mixture of several kinins without using chemical methods for separation and structure analysis. The pharmacological and physiological effects of the various kinins are quantitatively nearly identical and show quantitative differences only in some cases. Though the biological assay methods have a high sensitivity they are not efficient enough to detect the very small amounts of kinins *in vivo* which may play a physiological role or to prove the activation of the kinin system in pathological conditions, partly because of the very short half-life of the kinins *in vivo*. Therefore we should try to find more precise and specific analytical methods which are at least as sensitive as the bioassay. Assays using radioimmunological methods show some promise in this direction.

There are better and more practical methods for the identification and quantitative estimation of the enzyme components of the kinin system. For example, with the physiological kininogen substrate method, the specific analytical parameter for kininogenases or kininases is the formation or degradation of certain amounts of kinin per unit of time under fixed conditions. Other analytical techniques use synthetic substrates. These chemical methods are easy to apply but are usually not specific enough. This may be compensated in most cases by the application of specific inhibitors which eliminate other enzyme activities or suppress only the activity of the enzyme to be investigated. We have to synthesize substrates for chemical tests which are similar in structure to the natural substrates and are highly specific for the respective enzymes that participate in the kinin system.

Kinins

A. Isolated Smooth Muscle Preparations Used in the Bioassay of Kinins

I. Guinea Pig Ileum

The name of bradykinin was chosen to indicate the slow effect of this kinin upon the guinea pig ileum, in contrast to the rapid action caused by histamine or acetylcholine. It is about seven times slower than histamine in giving a contraction of the same size (ROCHA E SILVA, 1955). The technique is the same as that used for assaying histamine.

Preparation of the Ileum. Guinea pigs weighing 200–400 g, both sexes, are used. The animals are killed by a blow on the head and bled from the carotid arteries. The lowest piece of the ileum next to the colon is found to be especially sensitive. The gut is freed carefully from the mesenterium and a piece of about 10–15 cm is cut off. The strip is washed with Tyrode's solution through the lumen. Portions of 2–3 cm length are used for the assay. It was sometimes found that the storage of the ileum in Tyrode's solution at 4° for some hours improved its sensitivity to kinins. The ileum strip is suspended in a Tyrode bath of 5–10 ml at 35–37° and the solution is oxygenated by aeration or with 95% O_2, 5% CO_2. The strip is stressed by a counterweight of about 1 g. The contraction of the smooth muscle is generally recorded with about 10-fold magnification in a kymograph with a frontal writing lever or with an electric force transducer.

Irregular spontaneous contractions may be suppressed by addition of 10^{-6}–10^{-7} g atropine sulfate per liter of Tyrode's solution. As potent antihistamines, promethazine hydrochloride (10^{-7}–10^{-9} g/liter) pyrilamine, or diphenhydramine (0.1–1 μg/ml) can be used.

Before starting any assay the muscle is made to contract several times by additions of bradykinin until it gives a fairly steady response to the same submaximal dose of the active material. Histamine may also be used as initial stimulator. When the reaction of the strip reaches constant level to a given dose of standard, the sample is assayed by the four-point method (Rocha e Silva, 1952). There is a linear relationship between intensity of effect (height of contraction in millimeters) and the logarithm of the dose injected into the bath. It is not necessary to measure the slope of the contraction curve since it is correlated with the height. The time between washing the muscle with fresh Tyrode's solution and the addition of the following dose of kinin must be about 3–5 minutes, the contact time about 45–60 seconds (Frey et al., 1950, 1968; Yoshinaga et al., 1963; Habermann et al., 1963; Khairallah and Page, 1963; Miwa, 1965; Abe et al., 1966; Greenbaum and Kim, 1967; Gascon, 1967).

Sensitivity and Specificity. The minimal quantities of bradykinin that were used to obtain standard responses of the ileum ranged from about 1 to 10 ng/ml, but there are preparations which give a response only to more bradykinin (50–100 ng/ml). Dilute solutions of kinins are quite unstable. This is caused in part by the adsorption of the kinin to glass. *p*-Toluene sulfonic acid (0.001 M) was used as additive when samples of the reaction mixture were diluted for assay on the guinea pig ileum. This agent had previously been found to aid against kinin adsorption to glass (Greenbaum et al., 1965; Greenbaum and Kim, 1967). This adsorption is partially avoided by using acid-washed glassware and omitting detergents (Gladner et al., 1963) or by the addition of casein 0,25% as stabilizer (Webster and Gilmore, 1965). Crude kinin preparations used as standard preparations by Werle (Frey et al., 1950; Rocha e Silva, 1955) and others before synthetic material became available are more stable. All the properties of the crude material could be confirmed later with the synthetic substances. Preservatives such as chlorobutanol added to bradykinin solution can interfere with the bioassay (Hamberg, 1964; Collier, 1965; Erdös, 1966). Diluted kinin solution should be kept in polypropylene tubes.

The guinea pig ileum is at least ten times less sensitive than the rat uterus. In addition, the specificity of the response of the ileum is unsatisfactory. It is difficult to find another smooth muscle preparation that is contracted by such a variety of biologically active substances (vasopressin, angiotensin, substance P, eledoisin, physalaemin, histamine, serotonin, prostaglandin, slow-reacting substance, etc.). The influence of hydrogen and calcium ions on the contraction of the guinea pig ileum was studied by Stopp and Jung (1968). Walaszek et al. (1968) discussed the influence of the pH value on the polypeptide receptor mechanism.

The enhancement of the sensitivity by treating the smooth muscle preparation with an application of 0.1–0.5 mg of trypsin was assumed to be caused by digestion of membranes which impede the diffusion (Habermann et al., 1963). Chymotrypsin (100–500 μg) caused after a few seconds a rapid contraction of the ileum, which was prevented by 0.5–1 μg of pyrilamine. After addition of chymotrypsin, the preparation became more sensitive to subsequent applications of kinins. The latent period of the response was shortened and the height of contraction increased. Chymotrypsin not only sensitizes the isolated ileum to the action of synthetic bradykinin but also to kinin liberated by trypsin or kallikrein. After three to five successive applications of 100–300 μg of chymotrypsin most of the preparations responded to as little as 200 pg/ml in the bath. The responses to histamine, acetylcholine, and serotonin were unaffected (EDERY, 1964, 1968). GREENBAUM and KIM (1967) described a two- to fourfold sensitization of the muscle to bradykinin after a 1-minute incubation with 200 μg chymotrypsin. An example of such a magnification is shown in Fig. 1 (EDERY, 1964).

Several substances were found to enhance the response of smooth muscle to bradykinin: dibenamine and phenoxybenzamine (ROCHA E SILVA and LEME, 1963), cysteine (LEWIS, 1960; PICARELLI et al., 1962), BAL or thioglycolic acid

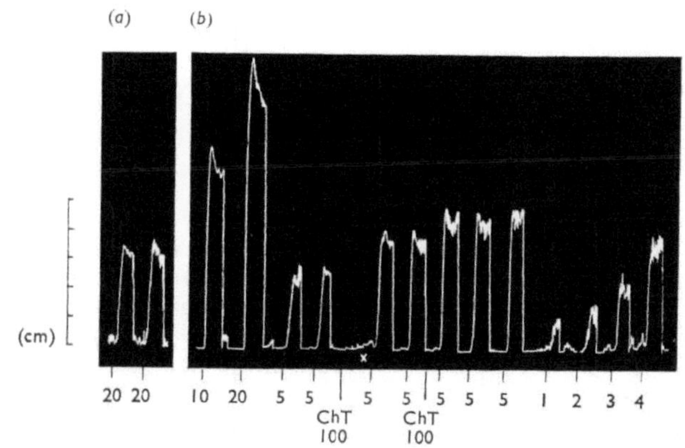

Fig. 1. Guinea pig isolated ileum preparation, suspended in 5 ml of atropinized Tyrode's solution. Time of contact 1 min; time cycle 5 min. Response to synthetic bradykinin (at marks, doses in ng). Between a and b there were three separate doses of 100 μg chymotrypsin (ChT, doses in μg) given in the presence of pyrilamine. At x and after each contraction the organ-bath fluid was changed twice. After chymotrypsin the sensitivity of the preparation increased so much that 1 ng of bradykinin caused a contraction (EDERY, 1964)

(FERREIRA and ROCHA E SILVA, 1962), tetraethylammonium (KHAIRALLAH and PAGE, 1961), fibrinogen split products (GLADNER et al., 1963), a fraction in snake venom (FERREIRA, 1965), trypsin hydrolysates of plasma proteins (AARSEN, 1968). No specific antagonist of bradykinin is at present available. Some analgetic and antipyretic and other drugs inhibit the kinin action partially (ERDÖS, 1966). For the action of kinins on smooth muscle *in vivo* see Table 1, p. 60, ERDÖS (1966) and Chapter 6A, p. 421. The detailed kinetics of the contraction of the ileum revealed that atropine and morphine (WIEGERSHAUSEN et al., 1964) can interfere with the action of bradykinin.

II. Rat Uterus

The Erspamer method (ERSPAMER, 1948; ERSPAMER and ERSPAMER, 1962) is based on the use of young rats (weighing 120–160 g) which are ovariectomized and after a recovery period of one week are treated subcutaneously on two successive days with doses of 100–200 μg of estradiol dipropionate.

The uterus is removed 3–5 days after the first injection and suspended in Tyrode's solution (ERSPAMER, 1966). According to GADDUM (GADDUM and HAMEED, 1954) ovariectomy does not appear to be essential. Stilbestrol (100 μg/kg) is injected subcutaneously 18 hours before use to a virgin rat weighing 160–200 g and the next day the uterus is removed. For the assay the middle 2 cm of one horn is used, or the intact horn is cut off on the proximal side only. The uterus is suspended in a bath (2–10 ml) of oxygenated de Jalon's solution at 29–31°. The uteri can be used on the same day, preferably after a short storage at 4°, or stored at 2° in de Jalon's solution for a day with no deleterious effect. To get a stable preparation atropine (10^{-6} g/liter) is added to the bath and the temperature lowered to 27° or less. The magnification of the lever can be up to 10-fold and the tension should be about 1 g. The time interval between two doses should be at least 5 minutes, the contact with the active material about 1 minute.

The composition of the Tyrode's solution is: sodium chloride 8 g; potassium chloride 0.2 g; calcium chloride 0.2 g; magnesium chloride 0.1 g; sodium bicarbonate 1 g; sodium dihydrogenphosphate 0.05 g/liter. Jalon's solution: sodium chloride 9 g; potassium chloride 0.4 g; calcium chloride 0.06 g; sodium bicarbonate 0.15 g; glucose 1 g/liter.

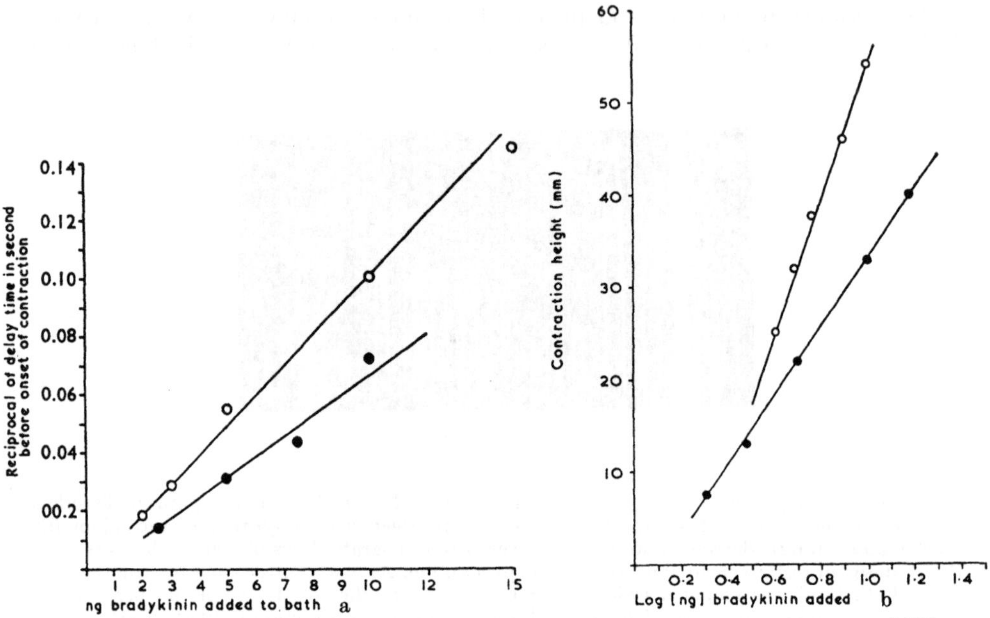

Fig. 2a and b. Dose-response curves obtained for typical rat uterus preparations on addition of standard amounts of synthetic bradykinin (DAVIES et al., 1966). a In terms of concentration. b In terms of reciprocal of contraction time

Response, Sensitivity, and Specificity. After the preparation has been set up the uterus is allowed to obtain an equilibrium for about 1 hour before starting the experiment. The dose-response relationship is determined with a solution of synthetic bradykinin (after an initial stimulation with oxytocin). Generally the active substance is washed out as soon as the first contraction of the uterus has attained its maximum, which is measured in millimeters. The response will be a number of contractions with partial relaxation. The estrous uterus and also the uterus of untreated animals sometimes show no correlation of the maximal height of the first contraction with the amount of kinin added. In these cases the bioassay is based not so much on the amplitude of single contractions as on the maintenance of diastolic tone. Sometimes there is a direct correlation of the amount of kinin added with the height of the minimum after partial relaxation following the first contraction (TRAUTSCHOLD and WERLE, unpublished; ERSPAMER, 1966). A linear dose-response curve is obtained when log weight of kinin added is plotted against height of contraction. A linear relationship is also obtained when the kinin concentration is plotted against the reciprocal of the delay time before contraction (DAVIES et al., 1966) (Fig. 2a, b). The stimulant action of acetylcholine is completely blocked by atropine. The threshold dose of bradykinin is 0.01–0.1 ng/ml. Histamine in higher doses (more than 10 µg) acts as blocking agent as do the catecholamines, tyramine, and dopamine. The response to serotonin is lower than to bradykinin (5 ng/ml); that of angiotensin and oxytocin much higher (0.01 and 0.001 ng/ml). Eledoisin, physalaemin, and substance P are also effectors (GADDUM and LEMBECK, 1949; HORTON, 1959; ERSPAMER and ERSPAMER, 1962; MARGOLIS and BISHOP, 1963; KHAIRALLAH and PAGE, 1963; WEBSTER and GILMORE, 1965; JACOBSEN, 1966b; DAVIES et al., 1966; HABERMANN et al., 1966; ERSPAMER, 1966; BROCKLEHURST and ZEITLIN, 1967; ZACEST and MASHFORD, 1967; BIELTVEDT and BRISEID, 1967; SARDESAI, 1968). To reach a higher sensitivity one can use the superfusion technique of GADDUM (1953). The increase in the response to bradykinin obtained is similar to the enhancement of the guinea pig sensitivity by repeated treatment with 100–250 μg chymotrypsin or 100–500 μg chymotrypsinogen. There is, however, no spontaneous contraction of the uterus by chymotrypsin (EDERY, 1964).

Although the bioassay with isolated smooth muscle preparations is easily performed, it is very susceptible to several biological and physical parameters, including the ionic strength and pH value and nature of the buffer, the calcium concentration, the oxygen saturation, and the time of year. The muscle preparations in springtime, for example, very often show excessive spontaneous contractions. This period is referred to as "spring fever" of the rats and is a frustrating aspect of the bioassay (KELLERMEYER and GRAHAM, 1968). An apparatus for recording isotonic contractions of smooth muscle was described by ERDÖS et al. (1962).

III. Miscellaneous Preparations

Various smooth muscle preparations were reported to be contracted by kinins. Exceptions are the rat duodenum and the hen's rectal caecum which relax after contact with kinins.

Rat Fundus Strip. The pyloric antrum of the stomach is removed and the fundus is cut into strips by opening the fundus along the lesser curvature, preserving the longitudinal musculature. The strip was used by VANE (1957) for the detection of serotonin and later also for bradykinin and eledoisin (VANE, 1964; FERREIRA and VANE, 1967). The strip was suspended in a 10-ml bath containing Tyrode's solution at 37°. A dose cycle of 3–5 minutes with 30–60 second contact was used (ERSPAMER and ERSPAMER, 1962).

Rat Duodenum. The proximal segments of the duodenum (2–3 cm) from rats weighing 150–200 g were first stored at 4° and than suspended in a 5-ml bath with aerated Jalon's solution. Atropine (10^{-6} g/liter) and pyrilamine maleate (10^{-7} g/liter) were added. Test samples were applied every 3 minutes and contact time was 30 seconds (TELLA and MAEGRAITH, 1966; ERSPAMER and ERSPAMER, 1962; JACOBSEN, 1966a; FERREIRA and VANE, 1967). The threshold dose of bradykinin is about 0.1 ng/ml. The response is a relaxation (see Table 1).

Rabbit Large Intestine. A segment of terminal colon 5–6 cm long (the whole narrower smooth portion caudal to the sacculated colon is suitable) is suspended in a 10-ml bath using Tyrode's solution at 37°. The tissue is stored at 4° for 12–48 hours before use. A dose cycle of 5–7 minutes with 2–3 minute contact is used. The gut responds to about 100 ng/ml bradykinin with a contraction (ERSPAMER and ERSPAMER, 1962).

Rabbit Duodenum. This tissue is prepared and handled like the colon. Contraction of the muscle results with about 1 ng bradykinin/ml (STÜRMER and BERDE, 1963a; ERSPAMER et al., 1964; GARBE and VOGT, 1967).

Other Preparations. Different sections of the intestine and the uterus from dog, cat, monkey, rat, and rabbit for the assay of biologically active polypeptides were used by ERSPAMER and ERSPAMER (1962) and by HORTON (1959). Smooth muscle preparations were also taken from the fowl (CLEUGH et al., 1961), frog (ERSPAMER and ERSPAMER, 1962), and spiral strips from isolated sheep and ox carotid artery (KOVALCIK, 1962; KOBOLD and THAL, 1963).

Human Intestine. Longitudinal and circular muscle strips about 20 mm long and 1–2 mm wide were taken from different regions. In gassed Tyrode's at 37° longitudinal strips from the jejunum responded to 0.2–1.0 ng bradykinin/ml with contraction; the circular strips were insensitive. Longitudinal ileum strips contracted with 0.1–0.5 ng/ml whereas the circular relaxed. The taenia coli strips were less sensitive. All preparations were sensitive to acetylcholine (FISHLOCK, 1966).

IV. Superfusion Technique by Vane (1964) and Ferreira and Vane (1967)

According to the superfusion method of Gaddum (1953), Vane assayed circulating substances after their injection or release into the circulation by

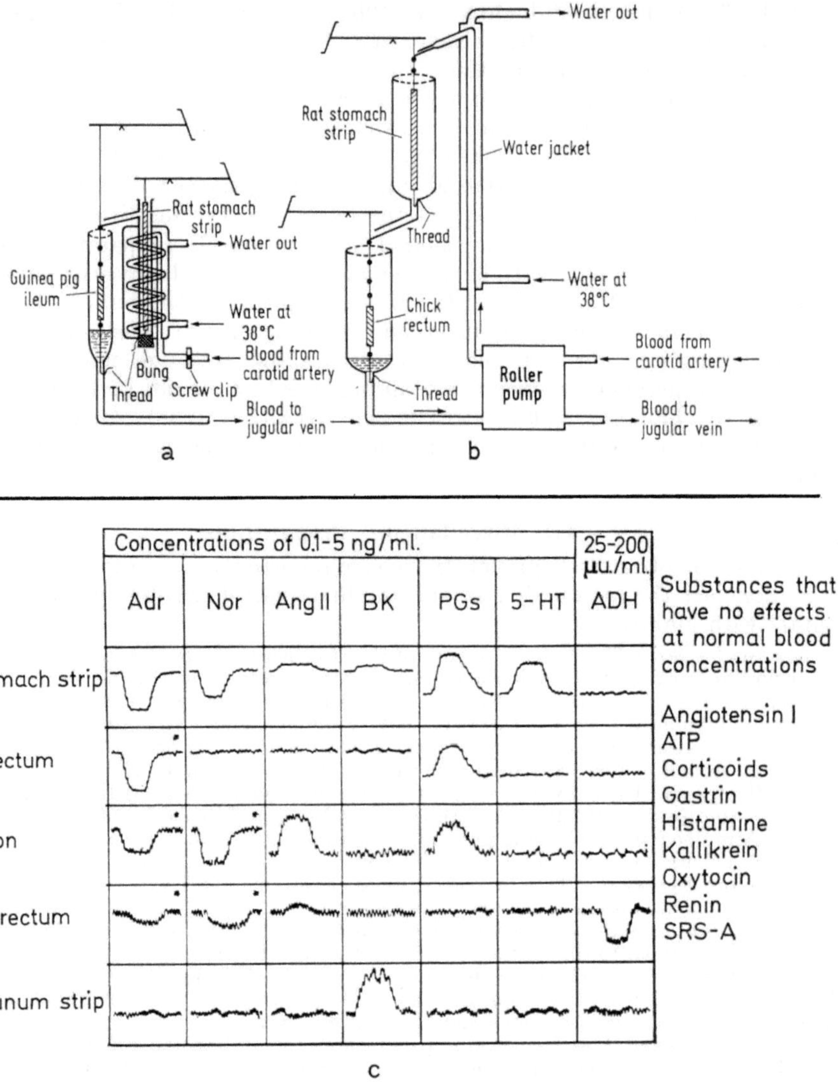

Fig. 3a—c. Diagram of apparatus. a Bathing one tissue in a bath of blood and superfusin another. b Superfusing two tissues with blood (Vane, 1964). c Reaction of some organ preparations to various vasoactive substances (Vane, 1969). Adr = adrenaline; Nor = noradrenaline; Ang II = angiotensin II; BK = bradykinin; PGs prostaglandins; 5-HT = 5-hydroxytryptamine; ADH = vasopressin. Response may be abolished with propranolol or pronethalol

bathing or superfusing isolated smooth muscle preparations in a stream of heparinized arterial blood which passed at 38° the organ bath as extracorporeal circuit (Vane, 1958) (Fig. 3a, b). Calibration of the system is carried out by injection of standards. The differentiation of biologically active material (catecholamines, histamine, 5-hydroxytryptamine, kinin) may be done by using a combination of different smooth muscle preparations. For the identification of bradykinin, which gives a response with a total of 1 μg peptide, e.g., a combination of rat duodenum with rat stomach strip is indicated. Bradykinin coming into the bathing blood relaxes the duodenum and contracts the stomach strip. Catecholamines relax both organs whereas 5-hydroxytryptamine contracts both.

Recently VANE (1969) surveyed the release and fate of vasoactive hormones in the circulation. He suggests the use of the cat jejunum strip for the detection of bradykinin. This organ preparation is not affected by any other hormone. Fig. 3c shows the reactions of various organ preparations to some circulating vasoactive substances.

B. Vascular Effect of the Kinins and Bioassay

Perhaps the most significant action of the kinins is the dilatation of blood vessels. The kallikreins which exert their biological activity by enzymatic release of kinins were first defined in terms of their hypotensive effect. Various vascular beds react differently to the kinin system. Depending on the species and the interaction with other vasoactive substances that may be liberated in pathological conditions or as reactive and physiological action of the body, the systemic blood pressure and the peripheral resistance are lowered by arteriolar dilatation. Kinins are also reported to cause constriction of veins (p. 378).

I. Blood Pressure Recorded from the Carotid Artery

The carotid artery of the anesthetized (pentobarbital) animal (various species) is cannulated with a polyethylene catheter (anticoagulant) which is connected with a mercury manometer. The blood pressure may also be recorded with a Statham transducer. Injections are made into the femoral vein. The samples are washed in with another injection of saline. As in the bioassay with smooth muscle preparations, the response of an unknown kinin sample must be compared with a standard preparation. To assay kallikrein by this method it is necessary to wait for a complete normalization of the blood pressure to the initial steady base line before another injection of kallikrein. Most of the studies of the group of WERLE (FREY et al., 1950, 1968) were carried out on dogs anesthetized with butallylonal (Pernocton). This method is used to study the kinin effect on conscious and on anesthetized dogs (PEARSON and LANG, 1967). The dog responds to about 0.1 μg bradykinin/kg.

The rabbit is most sensitive to intravenous injection of bradykinin; about 0.05 μg/kg is necessary for a good reproducible hypotension (see Table 1). Other animals that react with a transient hypotension to the administration of kinins are the cat and the rat (HORTON, 1959; GREENBAUM and HOSODA, 1963; HABERMANN et al., 1966; TELLA and MAEGRAITH, 1966; GASCON, 1967; LECOMTE and SALMON, 1968).

The kinin system from birds gives no response in the mammalian system. Ornithokinin and ornithokallikrein therefore were tested on the hen blood pressure (WERLE et al., 1966; WERLE and LEYSATH, 1967; FREY et al., 1968).

II. Blood Flow Bioassay Techniques for Vasoactive Substances

SARNOFF et al. (1958) described a simple technique of direct continuous metering of femoral artery flow. This method shows a good reproducibility of response. Dogs were anesthetized with 30 mg pentobarbital per kg and given anticoagulants. A cannula in the left femoral artery conducted blood flow through siliconized Tygon tubing to a Shipley-Wilson rotameter, then through the cuvette of a multiple injection magnetic mixer (into which the samples were injected), and finally back to the distal femoral artery with a bifurcation to record the blood pressure. Flow was recorded on a multichannel writing oscillograph.

Table 1. *Comparison of the relative activities of kinins and eledoisin* (ERDÖS 1966)

Test	Bradykinin[a]	Kallidin	Met-Lys-Bk	Eledoisin	Threshold dose of bradykinin	Reference
In vitro						
Rat uterus	1; contraction	0.6; contraction	0.3; contraction	0.001—0.002; contraction	0.03 ng/ml	1, 2, 3, 5, 9, 13
Guinea pig ileum	1; contraction	0.3; contraction	0.1—0.3; contraction	5; contraction	1 ng/ml	1, 2, 3, 5, 8, 9, 13
Rabbit large intestine	1; contraction			13; contraction	≈100 ng/ml	9
Rabbit duodenum	1; contraction	2; contraction		contraction	1 ng/ml	1, 3, 9
Rabbit uterus	1; contraction			200; contraction	≈0.2 ng/ml	2, 9
Hen rectal caecum	1; relaxation	2; relaxation		contraction		2, 3, 9
Rat duodenum	1; relaxation	0.5; relaxation	0.25; relaxation	contraction	0.1 ng/ml	2, 3, 6, 7, 13
In vivo; in situ						
Guinea pig bronchial muscle	1; contraction	0.3; contraction	0.25; contraction	10; contraction	0.2 μg/kg	1, 2, 4, 6, 13
Cat uterus	1; contraction			15; contraction		2
Rabbit uterus	1; contraction			200; contraction (irregular)		2
Dog blood pressure (iv)	1; decrease	decrease	(decrease)	50—100; decrease	0.2 μg/kg	1, 2, 7, 10
Dog hind leg blood flow (ia)	1; increase	>1; increase	(increase)	5—10; increase	0.01 ng/kg	4, 7, 12
Dog blood pressure (unrestrained; iv)	1; decrease	1; decrease		10—20; decrease		11
Cat blood pressure (iv)	1; decrease	0.6; decrease		8; decrease	0.5 μg/kg	1, 2, 3, 10
Diuresis rat	1; antidiuretic	2.8; antidiuretic				3
Rabbit blood pressure (iv)	1; decrease	1.9; decrease	2—3; decrease	4—50; decrease	0.05 μg/kg	1, 2, 3, 5, 10, 13
Rat blood pressure (iv)	1; decrease	3.3; decrease	1; decrease	10; decrease	0.2—1.0 μg per kg	1, 2, 3, 13
Guinea pig blood pressure (iv)	1; decrease	0.7; decrease		10; decrease	0.2 μg/kg	1, 2, 4, 10
Chicken blood pressure (iv)	1; initial decrease then increase			initial decrease then increase	40/80 μg per kg	1, 2, 10
Guinea pig capillary permeability (id)	1; increase	1; increase	1; increase	1; increase	1 ng	1, 2, 3, 6, 13

[a] Bradykinin = 1.

References: 1. KONZETT and STÜRMER (1960a, b); 2. STÜRMER and BERDE (1963b, c); 3. STÜRMER and BERDE (1963a); 4. NICOLAIDES et al. (1963); 5. SCHRÖDER and HEMPEL (1964); 6. ELLIOTT et al. (1963); 7. BERGAMASCHI and GLÄSSER (1963, 1964); 8. HABERMANN and BLENNEMANN (1964); 9. ERSPAMER and ERSPAMER (1962); 10. ERSPAMER and GLÄSSER (1963); 11. OLMSTED and PAGE (1962); 12. MCCARTHY et al. (1965; 13. ELLIOT and LEWIS (1965).

For long experiments, intravenous infusion and heating are necessary. The semilog plot of amount of vasoactive substance and increase in flow was linear. This method is about ten times more sensitive than the carotid artery method; threshold dose of braykinin is 0.01 μg/kg.

Another modification of the blood flow bioassay was reported by FASCIOLO et al. (1958), who adjusted a fixed blood pressure in the hind limb of a dog by perfusion with a pump. The samples to be tested are injected into the perfusion system near the femoral artery, and the decrease of the perfusion pressure is registered electrically or by means of a mercury manometer. The biological measurement of a sample is performed by finding a dose of the standard that will produce an equivalent depressor effect (FASCIOLO, 1963; BINIA et al., 1963).

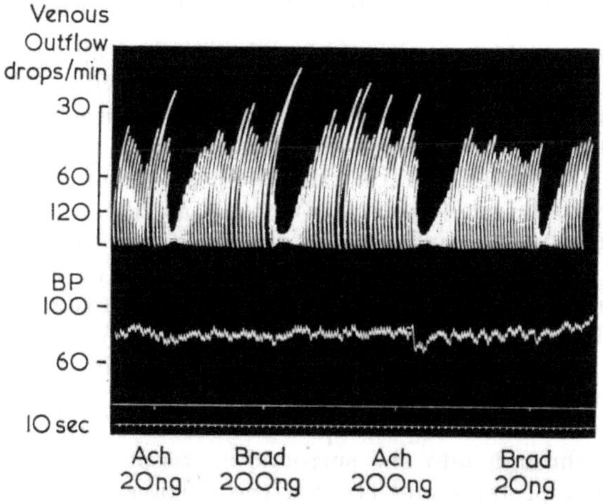

Fig. 4. Cat, 2.7 kg, anesthetized with sodium pentobarbital, 40 mg/kg. Upper record, venous outflow from hind limb (Gaddum drop-timer); lower record, arterial blood pressure. Response to intra-arterial injections of acetylcholine (Ach) and to bradykinin (Brad) 20 ng and 200 ng (LEWIS, 1963)

The same method was used by NICOLAIDES et al. (1965). WEBSTER et al. (1967) studied the effect of kinins on the muscle blood flow in the isolated perfused (constant flow) gracilis muscle of the dog.

These flow methods are based on the femoral *venous outflow technique*, according to GREEN et al. (1952). The procedure of LINDGREN (GREENBAUM and HOSODA, 1963) may also be used to study blood flow through the hind limb of the cat. Injections were made into the femoral artery, and the rate of blood flow was measured at the femoral vein by means of a photoelectric drop counter. In the cat 20 ng of bradykinin, which caused little change in the arterial blood pressure, showed a marked increase of the venous outflow (LEWIS, 1963) (Fig. 4).

ABE et al. (1968) described an improved bioassay method for kinins which utilizes the hindquarter of a rabbit. This procedure is about 20 times more sensitive for the assay of kinins than the dog hind limb preparation from BINIA et al. (1963) and allows the detection of less than 1 ng of bradykinin.

Albino rabbits of both sexes weighing 3–4 kg were anesthetized by i.v. urethane (1 g/kg). The carotid and femoral arteries were exposed and cannulated. Both vessels were connected and an extracorporeal circuit was established. Perfusion of the hindquarter of the rabbit was performed at a constant flow rate and the pressure in this system was recorded; 1 ng of bradykinin was easily detected in this preparation. Dose-response was linear in the range of 0.5–3 ng of bradykinin.

A very old pharmacological test object which allows the detection of vasoconstrictor and vasodilator substances is the isolated rabbit ear. It is perfused at room temperature through a cannula in the central artery. The ear is placed on a draining plate and the perfusate fluid (PAGE and GREEN, 1948) from the cut surface is led to a drop counter system (BOBBIN and GUTH, 1968).

To complete the blood flow methods I want to mention plethysmography for the measurement of the change of *in vivo* blood flow in single extremities (ERDÖS, 1966; MASHFORD and ZACEST, 1967; FREY et al., 1968) and the combined action of kinins on broncho- and vasoconstriction in the isolated perfused lung preparation in the guinea pig as semiquantitative bioassays (COLLIER, 1965; ERDÖS, 1966; GREEFF, 1968).

C. Increase of the Capillary Permeability as Bioassay

To study the possible physiological and pathological role of the kinins it is necessary to consider all biological activities of the kinins, especially the permeability-enhancing effect. This effect may be measured by the accumulation of an intravenously given vital dye at the intradermal injection site of the kinin (HOLDSTOCK et al., 1957; SCHACHTER, 1960). Pontamine blue or Evans blue (5–20 mg/kg) or India ink (1 ml/kg) was used as dye. The skin was dissected about 10–30 minutes after injection of the kinin and the diameter of the dye spots in the inner surface of the skin was examined (KONZETT and STÜRMER, 1960a; HABERMANN et al., 1966; DONALDSON and RATNOFF, 1967; WALDVOGEL and FRIMMER, 1967; OYVIN et al., 1967). CARR and WILHELM (1965) improved the method by extracting the dye from the excised skin with subsequent photometric estimation of the dye.

Even larger molecules may escape from the capillaries under the action of kinins and pass through into the surrounding tissue. WITTE et al. (1961) used fluorescent plasma proteins and studied the extravasation in the mesenterium with vital fluorescence microscopy. A loop of the jejunum of a rat was put into a perfusing chamber (2–3 ml) and 0.3 ml of a solution of 10 mg/ml brilliant sulfoflavine per 100 g animal body weight was injected intravenously. For the first 10 minutes after the local action of bradykinin the fluorescence was limited to the vessels and then spread into the perivascular tissue. FRIMMER (1961) took radioactive colloidal gold and ASCHEIM et al. (1963) I^{131}-labeled albumin as indicators.

D. Radioimmunoassay of Kinins

The availability of antisera to bradykinin and radioactive bradykinin now makes possible a quantitative immuno- or radioimmunoassay of the plasma kinins. This method is not quite so sensitive as the bioassay methods but the specificity of the assay is more reliable.

GOODFRIEND et al. (1964) were the first to describe the production of bradykinin antibody. They used as antigen a conjugate of bradykinin and rabbit serum albumin prepared by the carbodiimide method. The amount of bradykinin that could be detected by the complement fixation procedure was in the microgram range. SPRAGG et al. (1966) elicited the antibody with an antigen in which bradykinin was covalently bound to a nonimmunogenic carrier poly-L-lysine with the diisocyanate technique. Another carrier was rabbit serum albumin; 2–3 mg antigen was given with FREUND's adjuvant to rabbits three times with intermittent booster doses. The antiserum was collected after a six months' treatment. The antibody titer was determined by the microcomplement fixation procedure. The radioimmunoassay was performed with (H^3) acetyl bradykinin which was obtained by acetylation of bradykinin with (H^3) acetic anhydride.

To get a calibration curve, varying known concentrations of unlabeled bradykinin were incubated with 40 ng of labeled bradykinin and 50 μl of antiserum. The labeled antigen–antibody complex was separated from the bradykinin on Sephadex G-25 and the binding capacity plotted against the concentration of unlabeled bradykinin. Unknown samples of bradykinin can be detected in the nanogram range with a deviation of less than 5% from the mean value. The same good results were obtained by RINDERKNECHT et al. (1967). They used a bradykinin–hemocyanin conjugate as antigen. The lower specific activity of the C^{14}-acetyl bradykinin decreased somewhat the sensitivity of the immunoassay. In a further study TALAMO et al. (1968) tried different nonimmunogenic carriers for bradykinin and found that coupling bradykinin to ovalbumin via toluene diisocyanate gives an immunogen that reliably elicits bradykinin antibody of specificity and affinity appropriate for use in radioimmunoassay. The same group (SPRAGG et al., 1967) found that changes in amino acid side chains which altered charge or hydrophobic character of variants of bradykinin had little effect on binding to antibody. Change in length of the peptide chain, however, was of greater importance (see Chapter 6B, p. 531).

HABERMANN et al. (1968) combined the radioimmunoassay with the electrophoretic method, according to LAURELL (1966), and got an autoradiographic method by which nanograms of antigen may be determined.

E. Assay of Free Kinins in the Blood and Urine

I. Determination in Blood

Whether or not the kinins play a physiological role or are involved in pathological conditions can only be decided by the detection of free kinins *in vivo* or by the activation of kininogenases. This demands very sensitive assay methods for kinins, especially because of the very short half-life of the kinins *in vivo*.

Extraction Methods with Organic Solvents. The main problem is first to prevent destruction of kinins and activation of plasma kallikrein; then the purification and concentration of the kinins are carried out, together with the elimination of other biologically active substances that might impair the kinin bioassay. Glass contact should be avoided; the use of plastic material and siliconized glassware is recommended. The purified extracts from blood are subsequently submitted to bioassay as described above.

Methods which provide only deproteinization of the blood, concentration of the supernatant, and subsequent bioassay do not allow a reliable estimation of kinins. BINIA et al. (1963) treated the ethanol extract of dog blood after first evaporating the alcohol with ether in acidic solution; they then discarded the ether and extracted the kinins with n-butanol and re-extracted them into an aqueous solution. With this extraction method more than 95% of acetylcholine is eliminated and ATP is completely removed. The recovery of added bradykinin is $53.7 \pm 16\%$. With this method bradykinin levels of about 1.5 ng/ml of blood were detected in the dog. Ethanol denaturation with subsequent butanol treatment was also the principle of the method from BROCKLEHURST and ZEITLIN (1967). Butanol extraction at low pH eliminates all amines of high pK values, e.g. histamine, catecholamines, and serotonin. The recovery was $81.5 \pm 8\%$ and a level of 2.8 ng bradykinin/ml plasma was found in man. A similar butanol extraction was performed by ABE et al. (1966). They mixed the collected blood with cold EDTA solution and transferred it immediately into 0.8 N HCl before extraction. The recovery was $51.3 \pm 10.5\%$; 0–2 ng bradykinin/ml blood was found in healthy persons.

Deproteinization with ethanol and with thioglycolic acid as protector, ether extraction, and fractionation on Sephadex G-25 were the main steps of one of our own methods that gave a recovery of about 80%. Only traces of free kinin could be detected in normal venous human blood (Trautschold, 1965).

Methods Using Ion Exchange Chromatography. Speculation that the flushing episodes in the carcinoid syndrome are due to a kinin release stimulated the development of more accurate methods for the quantitative determination of human blood kinin.

Oates et al. (1964) applied the Amberlite IRC-50 chromatographic method, which had previously been used for the purification of kinins (Pierce and Webster, 1961; Werle and Trautschold, 1961), to the isolation of the blood kinins. Blood samples were collected from carcinoid patients at the beginning of the flush. The kinin peptides were isolated by rapid precipitation of the whole blood with ethanol followed by an ion exchange procedure and then assayed on the estrous rat uterus. Using this method Sardesai (1968) detected 1–4 ng of bradykinin/ml human blood.

In similar manner Webster and Gilmore (1965) stirred blood containing phosphoric acid (0.15 M) and 1 mg soybean inhibitor/10 ml with Amberlite IRC-50. Elution of the kinins from the resin was performed with ammonium formate, pH 8.2. Recovery was about 50%. With the same technique Melmon et al. (1968) found 2 ng bradykinin/ml in adult subjects and 12.8 ± 4.3 ng/ml in the cord blood of newborn infants. Zacest and Mashford (1967) first treated the ethanol extract with ether and then adsorbed the kinin onto Amberlite IRC-50. Recovery by this method was 97%. The average bradykinin level in brachial arterial blood of man was 0.25 ± 0.23 ng/ml.

II. Determination in Urine

The isolation of the urinary kinins was performed with the same techniques as those for blood. Yoshinaga et al. (1963) and Abe et al. (1964) used butanol extraction alone, whereas Jensen et al. (1965) and Webster and Gilmore (1965) applied the ion exchange method. Horton (1960) found a normal bradykinin excretion ranging from 10–30 µg per day; Abe et al. (1964) 5.3–36 µg (19.6 ± 9.1 µg) per day or 13.2 ± 6.3 ng bradykinin/min, ranging from 3.8–28 ng/min (Yoshinaga et al., 1964). Fractionation of the urinary kinin revealed the existence of two kinins. Total amount excreted in 24 hours is 34.2 ± 12 µg (16.6–55.7 µg) bradykinin equivalents. On the average 15.0 µg are bradykinin and 19.2 µg are identical with kallidin (Jensen et al., 1965) (see also p. 579).

Recently Miwa et al. (1968, 1969) detected in addition to bradykinin and kallidin the undecapeptide Met-Lys-bradykinin in human urine. They separated the three urinary kinins chromatographically and used the radioisotope dilution technique to identify urinary bradykinin.

Kininogen

The determination of the kinin precursor, kininogen, in plasma and other biological fluids is of obvious importance since it is the only parameter in the kinin system that might give information on the extent of activation of the kinin system and mobilization of free kinins. The facts known up to 1967 are reviewed in the monograph *The Kallikrein-Kinin-System and Its Inhibitors*, by Frey, Kraut, Werle, Vogel, Zickgraf-Rüdel, and Trautschold (Frey et al., 1968). The development of a simple method for the kininogen determination was essential for studying the whole kinin system.

Such a method had to meet the following requirements. (1) Kinin-destroying enzymes and factors that inhibit kinin release and impair the action of the kininogenase must be eliminated. (2) Only one kind of kininogenase should be active and only one kind of kinin released. (3) Activation of the endogen–kininogenase system must be prevented. (4) The kininogen must be suitably pretreated to get a 100% kinin release.

In the meantime there was great confusion since there are not only different kinin-releasing enzymes such as trypsin, kallikreins, acid-, glass-, or acetone-activated endogenous plasma kallikreins but also different kinds of kininogen. Two forms had been found (kininogen I and II) (HABERMANN, 1963; PIERCE and WEBSTER, 1966; NAGASAWA et al., 1966; VOGT et al., 1967) and an additional high molecular weight form (JACOBSEN and KRIZ, 1967; HENRIQUES et al., 1967; PIERCE, 1968; p. 42).

I. Pretreatment of the Plasma Kininogen

Blood samples must be collected in plastic tubes or siliconized glassware only. To prevent blood coagulation that might activate the endogenous kininogenases, heparinized blood is used. Oxalated or citrated plasma shows a significant decrease of bradykinin release. Storage of the plasma at 4° leads to a great loss of kininogen. Plasma stored at −20° does not change its kininogen content significantly for a week. WERLE (FREY et al., 1950) tried first to prevent the inactivation of kinin by kininases by adding cysteine or heating plasma for 3 hours at 56°. Other authors also prepared substrates for kininogen determination by heating with acid. VAN ARMAN (1955) added an equal volume of 0.3% acetic acid to plasma and heated it to 80–90° in a water bath. HAMBERG and ROCHA E SILVA (1957) used the same method. HORTON (1958) recommended the acidification to pH 2 and a 15-minute incubation at 37°. DINIZ and CARVALHO (1963) added 1.8 ml of 0.2% (v/v) acetic acid to 0.2 ml plasma and heated it at 100° for 30 minutes. RINVIK et al. (1966) heated the plasma at pH 2 for 30 minutes in a boiling water bath. Denaturation and enfolding of the kininogen molecule is an absolute requirement for an optimal bradykinin release by trypsin, whereas kallikrein gives the best yields of kallidin from an almost native kininogen. An untreated plasma that contained only kininase inhibitors without heating or acidification yielded 8 μg kallidin/ml after incubation with submaxillary kallikrein. Treatment of the same plasma for 15 minutes at pH 2 and 37° decreased the kallidin release to 4 μg/ml, and heating for 30 minutes in a boiling water bath at pH 2 lowered it to 0.4 μg/ml (TRAUTSCHOLD, 1965; p. 253).

II. Kinin Release with Trypsin

The best method for estimation of the total kininogen is the bioassay of the amount of bradykinin liberated from denatured plasma by an excess of trypsin. The acid–heat treatment destroys not only the kininogenases but also the α_1-trypsin inhibitor. Trypsin may be replaced by snake venom preparations as kininogenase (p. 193).

Original Method of DINIZ and CARVALHO (1963). Blood is collected by venipuncture in a 10-ml syringe moistened with a solution containing 20 U of heparin (Liquemine Roche), transferred to siliconized tubes, and immediately centrifuged; 0.2 ml of plasma is transferred with a siliconized pipette to an 18×50 tube containing 1.8 ml of 0.2% (v/v) of acetic acid and heated in a boiling water bath for 30 minutes. For the release of bradykinin the pH of denatured plasma is adjusted to 7.4–7.8 (Merck indicator paper) by addition of about 0.06 ml of N NaOH and the mixture buffered to pH 7.8 by addition of 0.5 ml of 0.2 M Tris buffer. The tubes are incubated with a solution containing 200 μg crystalline trypsin dissolved in 0.1 ml saline for 30 minutes at 37°. The reaction is stopped by addition of 5 ml absolute alcohol at boiling temperature. The tubes are heated for 10 minutes at 70° in a water bath and the suspension transferred to 125-ml round-bottom flasks and dried under reduced pressure. To facilitate the evaporation the flasks can be heated to a temperature not higher than 35°. Flasks can be kept in a desiccator under vacuum overnight without any loss of activity. The dried residue is suspended in 4 ml of saline and bradykinin is assayed in the bioassay (see p. 53).

Modifications of the Diniz Method. Numerous modifications of this method were published. The Diniz method was practised with little alteration by Aarsen (1968), Blümel et al. (1967), Greeff et al. (1966), Melmon et al. (1968), and Wiegershausen et al. (1967). A different pretreatment of the plasma was performed, for example, by Briseid et al. (1967), Brocklehurst and Mawer (1966), and Egorova and Paskhina (1967). A first real improvement of the method was proposed by Rinvik et al. (1966). They stopped the reaction by heating alone without alcohol. A 5-minute heating of the test solution at 100° before assay is not sufficient, however, to eliminate the trypsin effect on the smooth muscle preparation. Paskhina and Egorova (1966) stopped the reaction with trichloroacetic acid heating and subsequent neutralization. The best way to stop the enzymatic reaction is by the use of such trypsin inhibitors as soybean inhibitor or Trasylol (Greenbaum and Hosoda, 1963; Werle et al., 1964; Trautschold, 1965). Brocklehurst and Zeitlin (1967) described a method by which both the active kinin and the kininogen may be assayed in the same sample of blood. After denaturation of the blood with ethanol, the supernatant was used for the kinin determination, and the kininogen content was assayed in the washed precipitate.

III. Kinin Release with Kallikrein and by Glass Activation

The substrate for estimation of the kinin release by kallikrein must be free of kininase and kallikrein-inactivating factors, but in other respects it should be a native protein as far as possible (see p. 65). Kallikrein is not able to split all the kininogen. A subsequent incubation with trypsin gives an additional kinin release (Habermann and Blennemann, 1964; Garbe, 1967; see also p. 254). Care should be taken not to alter significantly the many factors involved in the release process. Briseid et al. (1967) proposed the use of a substrate which is prepared by adding 0.4 mg EDTA to 5 ml of citrated plasma with subsequent heating for 30 minutes at 37°. Other preparations of the substrate were performed by lowering the pH to 5.0 at 37° for 30 minutes or heating only for 10 minutes at 37° and pH 2.0. The first two substrates give good results with pancreas kallikrein as kininogenase and kinin release after addition of acetone which activates the plasma kallikrein. To 1 ml of substrate 4 ml of a mixture of acetone and saline (0.5 + 3.5) was added and incubated for several hours.

According to Garbe (1967) human plasma is acidified with 0.6 ml of 0.3 N HCl per ml of plasma to pH 2, incubated 30 minutes at 37° and again neutralized. One mg *o*-phenanthroline is added per ml of plasma (1% solution) and the pH is adjusted to 7.5; 2 KE/ml of plasma was added and incubated 45 minutes at 37° to release kallidin. The release of kallidin amounts to about 30% as compared to bradykinin (Trautschold, 1965). Acetone activates two kininogenases in human plasma. Seidel and Vogt (1969) called them kininogenase I and II. Kininogenase II is lost during longer incubation time. The remaining kininogenase I releases kinin only from kininogen I. Briseid et al. (1968b) examined the effect of different acetone concentrations on the kinin release in human citrated plasma stabilized with EDTA. About 10% acetone solution was required for effective inhibition of the kallikrein inhibitors. When a 20% concentration was used, a small amount of kinin was released because of a reversible acetone-dependent inhibition of factors in the releasing system. An acetone concentration of about 16.7% (V/V) in citrated plasma gave the highest yield of activity.

Glass activation was performed with glass ballotini, according to MARGOLIS (1963), or with silica powder (JACOBSEN, 1966a). Native plasma or plasma heated to 37° is used by adding such kininase inhibitors as EDTA or phenanthroline. In routine studies, 0.7 ml of a 0.2 M Tris buffer of pH 7.4 was added to a 0.5-ml citrated plasma and to 0.3 ml of 10^{-2} M 1,10-phenanthroline (ERDÖS et al., 1967b); 500 mg of washed glass beads were shaken in the incubation mixture. The activation of the kininogenase system in plasma by glass is completed in a few minutes by using glass ballotini (0.1 mm diameter) rotating at 37° (VOGT and WAWRETSCHEK, 1968).

Kininases

Cohn fraction IV-1 of human plasma contains kininogen and also inactivates kinins. This kininase resembles pancreatic carboxypeptidase B and was characterized by ERDÖS and SLOANE (1962) as carboxypeptidase N, which cleaves the Ph^8-Arg^9 bond of bradykinin. In 1967 YANG and ERDÖS described another kininase which inactivates the peptide by hydrolyzing the Pro^7-Phe^8 link. WEBSTER and PIERCE (1963) discussed the participation of aminopeptidases in the rapid destruction of the kinins. Kallidin is converted to bradykinin and Met-Lys-bradykinin is hydrolyzed by leucine aminopeptidase (see p. 314). ERDÖS (1966) found that bradykinin is resistant to leucine aminopeptidase but is destroyed by prolidase as the N-terminal arginine is hydrolyzed. The activity of kininases is much higher in tissues than in plasma. Cathepsins may also be involved in the overall kininase activity.

In the kinin assay the kininases are the greatest hindrance. Their existence is, however, essential to keep the kinin level low *in vivo*. Kininases could be of some help if an uncontrolled liberation of kinins is a mediator in hyperemia, shock, inflammation, or allergic disease. An application could efficiently diminish or even abolish the effects of locally formed kinins and kinins liberated in the blood by plasma kallikrein. An experimental blocking effect of kinin action *in vivo* was demonstrated by ERDÖS et al. (1963) who used carboxypeptidase B.

I. Determination of the Kininase Activity with Kinins as Substrate

The estimation of the kininase activity in blood or plasma samples is performed by incubating a given amount of kinin with the enzyme preparation for a known period of time, then halting the process and assaying the amount of residual kinin with smooth muscle preparations or on the blood pressure. This method records the sum of all kininases present. In most cases bradykinin is used as substrate in a buffered medium at pH 7.4, the optimum of the total kininase activity; 0.5–10 μg of bradykinin is incubated with Tris or other buffer (0.1–0.2 M, pH 7.4) in a total volume up to 2 ml, and various amounts of plasma, blood, or tissue extracts are added. The incubation is done at room temperature (exact control is necessary, best at 25°) or at 37° for a period ranging from a few seconds up to 30 minutes. The reaction is stopped by cooling, acidification with acetic acid or hydrochloric acid (sometimes with additional heating), or by denaturation with ethanol. In some methods the buffer is replaced by saline or Tyrode's solution. It is necessary to adjust the enzyme concentration to such a level that a 50% hydrolysis during incubation time is not exceeded, otherwise the saturation of the enzyme with the substrate is no longer guaranteed (ERDÖS and SLOANE, 1962; AARSEN and KEMP, 1963; ABE et al., 1965, 1966; AMUNDSEN and NUSTAD, 1965; RINVIK et al., 1966; RUGSTAD, 1966; WATANABE et al., 1966; ZACHARIAE et al., 1966; GREENBAUM and KIM, 1967; GARBE, 1967; MASHFORD and ZACEST, 1967; MELMON et al., 1968; WERLE et al., 1968).

II. Determination of the Kininase Activity with Synthetic Substrates

A major portion of the plasma kininase consists of a carboxypeptidase B-type enzyme which was called carboxypeptidase N. As the pancreatic carboxypeptidase B does, the plasma kininase also hydrolyzes substrates such as hippuryl-L-lysine, hippuryl-L-arginine, and hippuryl-L-ornithine (ERDÖS and WESTERMANN 1963; ERDÖS et al., 1964). The kininase also has an esterase activity and hydrolyzes the ester substrate hippuryl-L-argininic acid (ERDÖS et al., 1967b). These allow a spectrophotometric *determination of the carboxypeptidase* N according to the method of FOLK et al. (1960). The principle is based on the difference in spectra of hippuric acid and hippuryl-L-arginine. When the absorption of a 0.001 M solution of hippuric acid in 0.025 M Tris buffer, pH 7.65, containing 0.1 M NaCl, was measured against a blank consisting of a 0.001 M solution of hippuryl-L-lysine in the same buffered salt solution, a broad peak was observed in the ultraviolet region with a maximum at 254 nm. At this wavelength the difference in absorption in cells with 10-mm light path was 0.36. The assay was carried out in the following way: hippuryl-L-lysine, 0.001 M in the above buffered salt solution, was placed in 1-cm quartz cells in the spectrophotometer at 25° and the optical density was set to zero at 254 nm. The kininase-containing samples were introduced, the absorption again was reset to zero and the increase in o.d. was recorded as a function of time. A solution of hippuric acid, 0.001 M, was used as reference. Zero-order kinetics were observed up to about 40% hydrolysis. If greater amounts of sample are used, this volume must be compensated by less buffer to keep the total volume at 3.0 ml. The activity of the enzyme (μmoles hydrolysis/min) is calculated by the molar extinction coefficient or by a calibration curve or standard values. For optimal activity 1×10^{-4} M $CoCl_2$ is preincubated with the enzyme (ERDÖS et al., 1964, 1967b). The kininase activity of plasma from various species is given on p. 290.

The *second kininase* that splits the Pro^7-Phe^8 linkage does not hydrolyze hippuryl-L-lysine. This enzyme, which is very similar to the kininase found in the microsomal fraction of the kidney (ERDÖS and YANG, 1967) called peptidase P, was detected by using bradykinin as substrate (YANG and ERDÖS, 1967). For inhibitors of carboxypeptidase N and kininase II see Table 2.

Table 2. *Inhibition of the inactivation of bradykinin by kininase I and II of human plasma* (YANG and ERDÖS 1967)

Inhibitor	Concentration mmoles/liter)	Relative degree of inhibition	
		Kininase I	Kininase II
$CdSO_4$	1	++	0
$HgCl_2$	1	++	++
EDTA	3	++	++
1,10-Phenanthroline	1	++	++
ε-amino-n-caproic acid	3	+	0
H-Phe-Arg-OH	10	++	++
Arginine	3	++	0
Trasylol	125 KIU/ml	0/+	0

++ = Complete inhibition; + = partial inhibition; 0 = no inhibition.

For the *detection of amino peptidases* the β-naphthylamides of some amino acids may be used as substrates. These substrates are dissolved in a small amount of methyl alcohol and then diluted with water to a 1 mM solution containing about 10% alcohol. The assay mixture (1.0 ml Tris buffer, 0.1 M, pH 7.0, 0.5 ml substrate stock solution and 0.5 ml enzyme sample) is incubated at 37° for a given time (20–30 minutes). The naphthylamine liberated by the enzymatic activity is estimated colorimetrically after reacting with a diazonium salt dissolved in 1 M acetate–HCl buffer, pH 4.2, containing 10% Tween-20. The optical density was measured 15 minutes later at 525 nm against appropriate blanks (HOPSU-HAVU et al., 1966; HOPSU-HAVU and JANSEN, 1968).

The enzyme *prolidase* which can be found in blood and various tissues can be detected by hydrolysis of glycyl-L-proline at pH 7.5. The split products are determined by conventional methods.

III. Kininase Units

Most authors have defined their own units, expressed as percentage of hydrolysis of bradykinin in a given test method (ABE et al., 1965). Or, for example, one unit of kininase is defined as the amount of enzyme that will destroy 75% of 500 ng of synthetic bradykinin in 11 minutes (NILSEN and RUGSTAD, 1968). It is true that the kinin degradation is due to more than one enzyme; these attack the peptide at different sites and therefore the requirements for a definition of a unit are not met completely. But nevertheless it would be advisable, whatever the substrate used, to follow the recommendations of the IUB and define the kininase unit as that amount of activity that catalyzes a substrate turnover of 1 μmole per minute under optimal standard conditions. One milliunit (mU) of any kininase inactivates 1.06 μg of bradykinin or 1.19 μg of kallidin (respectively 1 nmole of kinin) per minute.

Kininogenases

Among the numerous identified kininogenases (kallikreins, trypsin, snake venoms, activation of plasma factors such as plasma kallikrein, plasmin, Hageman factor, permeability factor by glass contact, dilution, acid treatment, addition of casein or acetone) the kallikreins are the best known. The kallikreins are generally defined as a group of closely related enzymes which release kallidin from kininogen by a highly specific proteolytic activity and which have also an esterase activity. In a true sense of this definition the plasma kallikreins, which are only called kallikreins, because of a historical background, differ from the glandular kallikreins by having an unspecific proteolytic activity; they release bradykinin instead of kallidin. The relevant literature has been reviewed by ERDÖS (1966) and by FREY et al. (1968); see also Chapter 3, p. 82.

I. Estimation of Kininogenases by Bioassay

Action on Blood Pressure. Kallikrein has generally been estimated by comparing its depressor effect on dog blood pressure with that of a standard preparation (FREY et al., 1950, 1968). This hypotensive action drew attention first to the presence of kallikrein in the urine. Only a few facts have to be kept in mind for this method. The narcosis should be deep (butallylonal) to get a constant base line of blood pressure. Artificial respiration should be sufficient and constant. As reference substance for a quantitative assay it is advisable to take a kallikrein standard solution and not a solution of synthetic bradykinin, since the kinins cannot produce all the effects induced by kallikrein. Kallikrein has a longer-lasting effect on the circulation because it is not inactivated as quickly as the kinins are. As reference standard urinary kallikrein of a low degree of purity is recommended. Urine which is collected with toluene as preservative is treated with the same amount of acetone; the precipitate is discarded. To the supernatant the same amount of acetone is added again; the precipitate is then isolated, dried, and resolved in saline. Impurities are removed by centrifugation and the supernatant is standardized carefully against the action of standard kallikrein from the pig pancreas (Padutin) on the dog's blood pressure (WERLE and TRAUTSCHOLD, 1963). Another point that must be observed is to avoid too frequent injections of greater quantities of kallikrein in order not to exhaust the kinin precursor and lower the sensitivity of the assay, and the dog should not become tachyphylactic. The species specificity can influence the effect of kallikrein from various animals on dog blood pressure. Contamination of the crude kininogenase samples with kininases can be disregarded—it if is not extremely large—since the vascular system of the dog represents a great pool of kininases and the effect on blood pressure will be the result of kinin formation and degradation and of kininogenase inhibition in the test animal. Amounts of 0.05–0.1 KU are threshold doses that still give a good response in blood pressure. Other methods of kallikrein determination are based on the reduction of perfusion pressure in the perfused hind limb and the increase in capillary permeability (see pp. 59 and 62).

Estimation of Kininogenase Activity by Liberation of Kinins in vitro. The blood pressure assay method has several disadvantages. It is relatively insensitive, dose intervals are long, and the specificity is low since all vasoactive substances will give a response. In addition, dogs are expensive and are not always readily available. When smaller laboratory animals are used, only a few assays can be performed on one animal. Therefore HORTON (1959) developed a method in which dog plasma was treated to destroy the kininase and the kallikrein inactivators. After incubation of this substrate with kallikrein, the released kinin was assayed on the isolated smooth muscle preparation. Usually the kininogenases to be assayed are available as crude materials in various body fluids and tissue extracts. The assay by kinin liberation guarantees that no other enzymatic activity is recorded, provided the enzyme sample is free from substances which directly act on smooth muscle or contain kininase activity. The preparation of the substrate may be performed as described above for the assay of kininogen with kininogenases, particularly with kallikrein (see p. 66). It should not be denaturated, as far as possible, in order that it may be readily attacked by kallikrein, but it must be free from additional kininogenase and kininase activity. Kininase inhibitors, e.g., 1,10-phenanthroline, may be added to the incubation mixture. A spontaneous kinin formation caused by the pretreatment of the plasma must be taken into account. The standard and test curves were parallel in all assays. The activity of the kininogenase was calculated from standard preparations of the respective enzyme in various concentrations. The linearity of the reaction curve must be controlled and no more than 30% of the substrate should be hydrolyzed during the given reaction time. This determination of the kininogenase activity of kallikrein is about 100 times more sensitive than that of the dog blood pressure method and permits the detection of 0.001 KU (HORTON, 1959; AMUNDSEN et al., 1963; MIWA, 1965; MALOFIEJEW et al., 1966; BIELTVEDT and BRISEID, 1967; BRISEID et al., 1968a, b; ERDÖS et al., 1968; VOGT and WAWRETSCHEK, 1968; SEIDEL and VOGT, 1969).

II. Estimation of the Kininogenases with Synthetic Substrates

Kallikrein has an exceptionally high specificity of the proteolytic activity, but it is somewhat less specific as an esterase. The kallikreins are capable of cleaving only arginine esters such as α-N-benzoyl-L-arginine methyl ester (BzArgOMe or BAMe), α-N-benzoyl-L-arginine ethyl ester (BzArgOEt or BAEe), and α-N-*p*-tosyl-L-arginine methyl ester (TosArgOMe or TAMe) (HABERMANN, 1959; WERLE and KAUFMANN-BOETSCH, 1960; TRAUTSCHOLD and WERLE, 1961). Highly purified hog pancreatic kallikrein hydrolyzes also tyrosine and tryptophan esters (WEBSTER and PIERCE, 1961). This esterase activity of the kallikreins was used by TRAUTSCHOLD and WERLE (1961) to determine the activity of kallikrein by chemical assay. This method is easy to perform and has high reproducibility. The only disadvantage is the low specificity of the hydrolysis of arginine esters. This requires that the enzyme sample contain no other nonspecific esterase activity. But even this can be overcome by using specific kallikrein inhibitors. Such selective inhibitors for each kininogenase are now available (for a survey see the monograph of VOGEL, TRAUTSCHOLD, and WERLE, 1968). This will permit determination of any crude kininogenase preparation. BAEe was found to be the best substrate. Hydrolysis of the benzoyl-L-arginine ethyl ester to benzoyl-L-arginine and ethanol allows five different methods for assaying the esterolytic activity (1) recording the increase of absorbance at 253 nm due to the higher extinction of benzoyl arginine compared to the ester; (2) determination of the liberated ethanol enzymatically with an optical test; (3) titration of the liberated carboxyl group with an autotitrator; (4) volumetric determination of the acid carboxyl group by using the Warburg apparatus; (5) colorimetric determination of the decrease of the ester substrate concentration by using ROBERTS' modification of the Hestrin method (ROBERTS, 1958).

Spectrophotometric Determination of Kallikrein Activity (BAEe) by Direct Assay. (Method 1; TRAUTSCHOLD and WERLE, 1961, 1962.) The hydrolysis of BAEe has an optimum at pH 8.5. The molar extinction coefficient at 253 nm is 2.3×10^3 for BAEe and 3.45×10^3 for benzoyl arginine. The Michaelis constant at 25° and pH 8 varies according to the different kallikreins used from 2 to 8×10^{-4} M. The kallikrein samples should contain 0.1 KU/ml pancreatic kallikrein, 0.2 KU/ml submaxillary kallikrein, or 0.4 KU/ml urinary kallikrein.

Assay: wavelength 253 nm; 1 cm cells; total volume 3.0 ml; incubation temperature 25°; incubation time 15 minutes; 0.5 ml BAEe (3.10^{-3} M; 12.9 mg BAEe in 12.5 ml triethanol amine buffer; 0.067 M; pH 8.0) was mixed with 1.5–2.45 ml of the above buffer. The enzyme solution was introduced in a volume of 0.05–1.5 ml. One minute later the absorbance was checked and exactly 15 minutes later the increasing absorbance was recorded again. The reference contains buffered BAEe solution. Padutin is used as standard. The extinction difference during incubation time should not exceed 0.15 otherwise the enzyme sample will be diluted. The enzyme activity is calculated: (extinction of the sample) × (activity of standard) (in KU)/(extinction of the standard) × (volume of the sample). The result is given in KU per milliliter of sample. Since the molar extinction coefficient is known, the activity may be directly calculated in international units equivalent to the hydrolysis of 1 nmole of BAEe/min. One international milliunit (mU) of any BAEe-splitting enzyme is the amount that causes a change in absorbance at 253 nm of 0.000383 ΔE/min/3 ml test volume (TRAUTSCHOLD, 1965).

Spectrophotometric Determination of Kallikrein Activity (BAEe) by Enzymatic Ethanol Assay. (Method 2; TRAUTSCHOLD, 1965, TRAUTSCHOLD et al., 1961, 1969.) This method is preferable because there is no interference in the absorbance when protein-containing solutions at the test wavelength are used.

Assay: wavelength 366 nm; 1 cm cells; total volume 3.0 ml; temperature 25°; incubation time 5–10 minutes; 2.3 ml of pyrophosphate (0.2 M)–semicarbazide (0.2 M)–glycine (0.05 M) buffer was placed in the cell, 0.1 ml of nicotine amide adenine dinucleotide (NAD, 30 mM),

0.02 ml of alcohol dehydrogenase suspension (30 mg enzyme protein/ml) and 0.5 ml of BAEe-solution (6 mM) were added, mixed, and incubated for 5 minutes. The reaction was started by adding 0.1 ml of the kininogenase. The zero optical density is recorded against a blank containing 0.5 ml BAEe and 2.5 ml of buffer, and 5–10 minutes later the increased absorbance is registered again. The increase of absorbance per minute should not exceed 0.03. Without using a standard preparation, the activity of the enzyme may be calculated because a change of absorbance of 0.0011 ΔE/min/3 ml total test volume in every NAD-dependent reaction corresponds to an enzyme activity of 1 milliunit. This method permits the determination of about 5 mU or of an equivalent of about 0.1 KU of kallikrein.

Fluorometric Determination of Small Amounts of Kallikrein Activity with BAEe and the Enzymatic Ethanol Assay. Trautschold et al. (1969) used the principle of fluorometric determination of NAD, or its reduced form NADH according to Lowry et al. (1957), as a very sensitive determination of kallikrein activity. Ethanol which is released by the BAEe hydrolysis is enzymatically oxidized, and correspondingly the oxidized form of NAD is transferred in the reduced state. The reduced NAD is—after the surplus of oxidized NAD has been destroyed—transformed by alkali to a fluorescent product whose formation is referred to the time, the measure for the kallikrein activity. This method is about 500 times more sensitive than the spectrophotometric test; 0.01 mU of enzyme activity may be detected. For details of the method see Trautschold et al. (1969).

Automated Method for the Determination of Kallikrein and Prekallikrein Activity. Based on the foregoing principle of the enzymatic determination of ethanol which is released by the action of kallikrein on BAEe, Fiedler and Werle (1967) described a method for the determination of the kallikrein activity by means of the Technicon autoanalyzer (Trautschold et al., 1969). The solutions used for the assay are given in the legend to Fig. 5. A standard solution of 0.5–10 KU kallikrein/ml is necessary to get a calibration curve. The assay of kallikrein activity that uses other esters as substrate necessitates methods 3–5 (see p. 71), all of which are much more insensitive than the methods described here.

The activity of the other kininogenases or related enzymes (e.g. trypsin, plasmin, thrombin) is determined by conventional methods. The best substrate for trypsin is benzoyl arginine-*p*-nitroanilide (BANA) (Haverback et al., 1960; Nagel et al., 1965).

Assay: (Trautschold, 1965) wavelength 405 nm; 1 cm cells; total volume 3.0 ml; temperature 25°; incubation time 5 minutes; 1.0 ml BANA solution (1 mg/ml) is mixed with 1.9 ml triethanol amine buffer (0.1 M, pH 7.8, with 0.01 M $CaCl_2$) and 0.1 ml trypsin solution. The change in absorbance of 0.0032 ΔE/min/3 ml test volume corresponds to the hydrolysis of 1 nmole substrate/min and is equivalent to 1 mU of enzyme activity.

The use of proteins as substrates for the assay of the proteolytic kininogenases is not recommended. All methods known for the determination of proteolytic enzymes which are involved in the kinin system are compiled in the monograph by Vogel et al. (1968). In addition to the "recommendation for nomenclature and units" (see p. 659) and to the historical definition of the biological kallikrein unit (KU), there exist at least three alternatives for the definition of a chemical kininogenase unit. (1) Using synthetic substrates for the kininogenases one can select a substrate, which is *commonly* attacked by nearly all kininogenases like BAEe. The different kininogenase activities may be compared directly. Thus one milliunit of any BAEe-splitting kininogenase will give a change in extinction (253 nm) of 0.000383 ΔE/min/3 ml by the direct test method, or 0.0011 ΔE/min/3 ml by the ethanol dehydrogenase technique at 366 nm. (2) Selection of more or less specific synthetic substrates for each kininogenase. This will facilitate a differentiation of the kininogenases but will complicate a direct comparison since each enzyme has a different Michaelis constant for a specific substrate and a different turnover rate. With benzoyl-L-arginine-*p*-nitroanalide, a specific substrate for trypsin, one milliunit of enzyme activity will give a change of absorbance of 0.00332 ΔE/min/3 ml at 405 nm. (3) The third alternative is based on the common property of the kininogenases: kinin formation. One milliunit of kininogenase activity is the amount of enzyme that liberates a quantity of kinin per minute which is equivalent in its pharmacological activity (contracting smooth muscle or lowering blood pressure) to

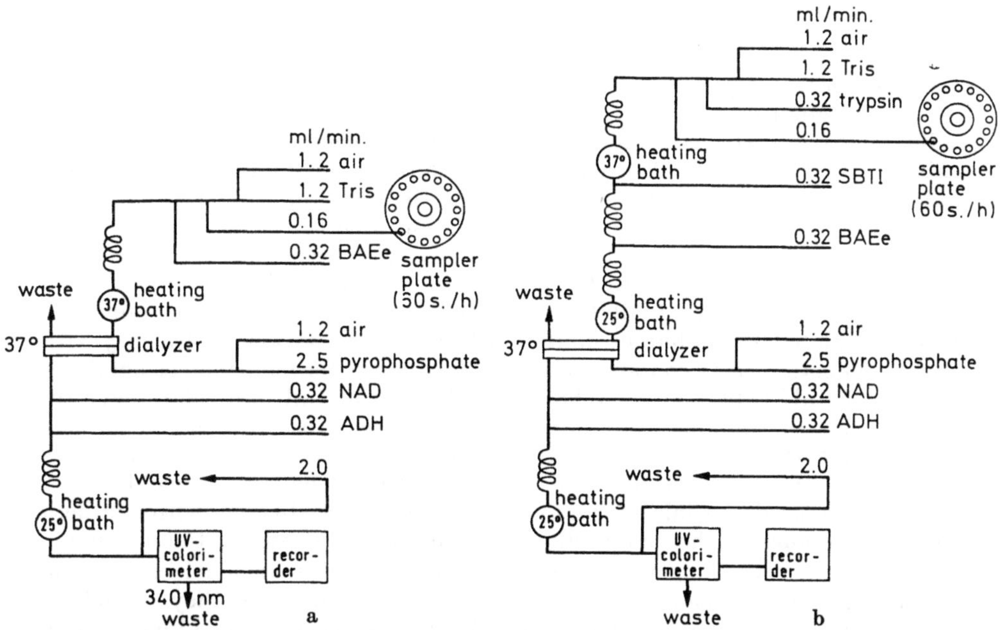

Fig. 5a and b. Automated method for determination of kallikrein and prekallikrein (FIEDLER and WERLE, 1967). a Determination of kallikrein. Tris: 0.05 Tris-HCl buffer, pH 7.8, with addition of 0.2 ml Triton X-100/liter. BAEe: 680 mg N-α-Benzoyl-L-arginine-ethyl-ester·HCl/100 ml water. Pyrophosphate: 30.4 g $Na_4P_2O_7 \cdot 10\,H_2O$, 8.2 g semicarbazide·HCl, 1.8 g glycine, 0.2 ml Triton-X 100/liter; adjust buffer with 2 N NaOH to pH 8.7. NAD: 150 mg nicotine amide adenine dinucleotide/100 ml water. ADH: 15 mg alcohol-dehydrogenase/100 ml water (ice bath). b Determination of prekallikrein. Trypsin: 50 mg/100 ml 0.001 N HCl (ice bath). SBTI: 500 mg soybean trypsin inhibitor/100 ml Tris buffer. Other reagents as in a

1.06 µg or 1 nmole bradykinin or to 1.19 µg or 1 nmole kallidin. Since the kinins differ in their quantitative pharmacological properties, the reference kinin must be identical with the kinin in the sample. This is not true for unknown kininogenases. It is recommended that only bradykinin be used as a reference substance for all kininogenases and that the biological parameter (e.g. rat uterus or dog blood pressure) of the assay method be specified.

Kininogenase Inhibitors

The natural inhibitors of proteolytic enzymes and kininogenases can be divided into a group of high molecular weight inhibitors (most inhibitors from plants, serum, egg white, urine) and a group of low molecular weight (inhibitor from bovine organs, pancreatic inhibitor, canine submandibulary inhibitor). For an extensive review see VOGEL et al. (1968) and FRITZ et al. (1969) (p. 213).

The mechanism of the enzyme inhibition is based on the formation of an enzyme inhibitor complex in which the enzymatic activity to natural and synthetic substrates is suppressed. In some cases the formation of the inhibitor complex with trypsin leads to a modified inhibitor molecule in which the peptide is split into two chains connected by an S–S bridge. The principle of the determination of the inhibitors is to preincubate the enzyme with the inhibitor (in absence of the substrate) and to measure subsequently, by any conventional test method, the remaining activity of the enzyme. A parallel assay without inhibitor serves as reference. Generally the complex formation is equilibrated in a few seconds, except the trypsin–kallikrein inhibitor from bovine organs (Trysalol) which needs a few minutes to complete the inhibition of kallikrein (Trautschold et al., 1966a). The pH optimum of inhibition ranges from 7 to 9, and the complex dissociates readily in acid and strong alkaline solutions. The dissociation constant at pH 7–9 is about 10^{-9} to 10^{-12} M. The detection of inhibitors in fluids and tissues containing simultaneously enzymes that may bind the inhibitor is done by extraction of the inhibitor in acidic solution or fractionation with the molecular sieve technique (Sephadex). On the other hand, if the activity of prekallikrein, prothrombin, or plasminogen in plasma is to be determined, a considerable amount of these enzymes is bound by the inhibitor after their activation. Glandular kallikreins are also inhibited by kallikrein inhibitors from plasma as well as by enzymatic activity. Human plasma contains an inhibitor capacity for pig pancreas kallikrein of 271 ± 72 ImU (Fritz et al., 1968) (for definition of ImU see below). For the determination of the inhibitors only small synthetic substrates should be used for measuring the remaining respective enzyme activity. Steric hindrance may influence the inhibition and substrate turnover when high molecular weight natural substrates are used. An inhibitor may sometimes be less effective with synthetic substrates because of the competitive effect of the substrate on the enzyme.

The system trypsin–benzoyl–arginine–*p*-nitroanilide is an ideal one for the detection and determination of kininogenase inhibitors since they all inhibit trypsin. BAEe is a universal substrate for the determination of the kininogenases, and trypsin–BANA is a universal system for the determination of the kininogenase inhibitors.

Assay: 0.2 ml of trypsin solution (50 μg/ml of 0.001 N HCl) was mixed with 1.7 ml buffer (triethanolamine 0.2 M, and $CaCl_2$ 0.02 M), 0.1 ml of the inhibitor solution, and incubated 5 minutes at room temperature. The subsequent procedure is identical with the trypsin assay (see p. 72). The reference assay contains 0.2 ml trypsin solution, 1.8 ml buffer, and 1.0 ml BANA solution (1 mg/ml). The calculation of the inhibitor content in inhibitor milliunits ImU (for definition see below) is carried out with the formula: (extinction reference-extinction sample)/0.00332.

Inhibitor Units. Several definitions of the inhibitor unit have been published by different authors. The basis of these definitions generally is the weight of enzyme that is inhibited or weight of the inhibitor used: (1) 100% or 50% inhibition of a definite quantity of enzyme by a tested quantity of inhibitor (also known as "enzyme ratio"). (2) Quantity of enzyme inhibited (100%) by a specified amount of inhibitor. (3) Kunitz's inhibitor unit (Kunitz, 1947) is defined as the quantity of inhibitor that causes a decrease in extinction of 1.0/min at 280 nm caused by the cleavage of a natural substrate in trichloroacetic acid filtrate. (4) According to Frey et al. (1950), 1 unit of kallikrein trypsin inhibitor (KIU) from bovine organs is the amount required for 50% inhibition of 2 units of kallikrein (KU).

These definitions require absolutely pure preparations of enzymes and inhibitors or need a standard preparation as reference. Trautschold proposed therefore to correlate the inhibitor unit with the international enzyme unit, thus with the decrease in the rate of substrate turnover (TRAUTSCHOLD, 1965; TRAUTSCHOLD et al., 1966a, b). According to this definition one inhibitor unit (IU) is that quantity of an inhibitor which inhibits completely the activity of one international enzyme unit (U), e.g. which causes a decrease in the rate of the substrate turnover of 1 micromole per minute.

Generally the inhibition of proteinases and kininogenases is related linearly to the inhibitor concentration only up to a certain degree of inhibition. In most cases the inhibition value must be calculated from 50% inhibition. This restriction is considered in the alternative formulation: one inhibitor unit (IU) is the quantity of inhibitor that inhibits the activity of two enzyme units (U) to 50%. The practical application of this definition to the inhibition of trypsin, with BANA as substrate, is: one inhibitor milliunit is that amount which causes a decrease in the absorbance at 405 nm of 0.00332 ΔE per min in a total test volume of 3 ml. The method of radioretention electrophoresis was applied by HABERMANN et al. (1968) to the detection of inhibitors in the nanogram range.

References

AARSEN, P. N.: Sensitization of guinea pig ileum to the action of bradykinin by trypsin hydrolysate of ox and rabbit plasma. Brit. J. Pharmacol. **32**, 453 (1968).
— KEMP, A.: Effect of pH and chloride ions on plasma kininase activity. Nature (Lond.) **198**, 687 (1963).
ABE, K., MOURI, T., SEKI, T., SUZUKI, M., TAKANO, T., YOSHINAGA, K.: An improved bioassay method for kinins. Experientia (Basel) **24**, 455 (1968).
— WATANABE, N., KUMAGAI, N., MIWA, I., MOURI, K., SEKI, T., OIKAWA, A., YOSHINAGA, K.: Assay of kininase activity in human blood. Tohoku J. exp. Med. **86**, 77 (1965).
— — — MOURI, T., SEKI, T., YOSHINAGA, K.: Estimation of kinin in peripheral blood in man. Tohoku J. exp. Med. **89**, 103 (1966).
— YOSHINAGA, K., MIWA, I., AIDA, M., MAEBASHI, M., WATANABE, N.: Excretion of urinary kinin in man. Tohoku J. exp. Med. **82**, 270 (1964).
ALLWOOD, M. J., LEWIS, G. P.: Bradykinin and forearm blood flow. J. Physiol. (Lond.) **170**, 571 (1964).
AMUNDSEN, E., NUSTAD, K.: Kinin-forming and destroying activities of cell homogenates. J. Physiol. (Lond.) **179**, 479 (1965).
— — WAALER, B.: A stable substrate for the assay of plasma kinin-forming enzymes. Brit. J. Pharmacol. **21**, 500 (1963).
ARMAN, C. G. VAN: Interrelationships among some peptide precursors. In: Polypeptides which stimulate plain muscle, p. 103, ed. by J. H. GADDUM. London: Livingstone 1955.
ASCHEIM, E., TSULUCA, V., COPLEY, A. L.: Quantitative relation between certain fibrinolysis factors and inflammation. Proc. Soc. exp. Biol. (N.Y.) **112**, 434 (1963).
BERGAMASCHI, M., GLÄSSER, A. H.: Effect of the undecapeptide eledoisin on the coronary blood flow. Comparison with nitroglycerin bradykinin and epinephrine. Circulat. Res. **13**, 329 (1963).
— — Peripheral vasodilator action of eledoisin, bradykinin and nitroglycerin in dog. Circulat. Res. **15**, 371 (1964).
BIELTVEDT, G., BRISEID, K.: An assay for Padutin (hog pancreas kallikrein). Based on the in vitro release of kinin in human plasma. Acta pharmacol. (Kbh.) **25**, 190 (1967).
BINIA, A., FASCIOLO, J. C., CARRETERO, O. A.: A method for the estimation of bradykinin in blood. Acta physiol. lat.-amer. **13**, 101 (1963).
BLÜMEL, G., FISCHER, M., LECHNER, K.: Plasmakininogen und Proteinasehemmkörper. Beobachtungen während der Substitutionstherapie bei Hämophilie A. Thrombos. diathes. haemorrh. (Stuttg.) **18**, 364 (1967).
BOBBIN, R. B., GUTH, P. S.: Venoconstrictive action of bradykinin. J. Pharmacol. exp. Ther. **160**, 11 (1968).
BRISEID, K., DYRUD, O. K., ARNTZEN, F. C.: Determination of prekallikrein in human plasma. Acta pharmacol. (Kbh.) **26**, 395 (1968a).
— — — Studies on the release of kinin by acetone and human plasma. Acta pharmacol. (Kbh.) **26**, 402 (1968b).
— — RINVIK, S. F.: In vitro estimation of the rate of release of kinin in human plasma. Acta pharmacol. (Kbh.) **25**, 201 (1967).

Brocklehurst, W. E., Mawer, G. E.: The purification of a kininogen from human plasma. Brit. J. Pharmacol. **27**, 256 (1966).
— Zeitlin, I. J.: Determination of plasma kinin and kininogen levels in man. J. Physiol. (Lond.) **191**, 417 (1967).
Carr, J., Wilhelm, D. L.: Interspecies differences in response to polypeptides as permeability factors. Nature (Lond.) **208**, 653 (1965).
Cleugh, J., Gaddum, J. H., Holton, P., Leach, E.: Assay of substance P on the fowl rectal caecum. Brit. J. Pharmacol. **17**, 144 (1961).
Collier, H. O. J.: Bronchoconstrictor action of bradykinin, kallidin and eledoisin. Nature (Lond.) **205**, 403 (1965).
Davies, G. E., Holman, G., Johnston, T. P., Lowe, J. S.: Studies on kallikrein. Failure of some anti-inflammatory drugs to affect release of kinin. Brit. J. Pharmacol. **28**, 212 (1966).
Diniz, C. R., Carvalho, I. V.: A micromethod for determination of bradykininogen under several conditions. In: Structure and function of biologically active peptides :bradykinin, kallidin and congeners, ed. by E. G. Erdös. Ann. N.Y. Acad. Sci. **104**, 77 (1963).
Donaldson, V. H., Ratnoff, O. D.: Effect of some analogues of bradykinin upon vascular permeability. Proc. Soc. exp. Biol. (N.Y.) **125**, 145 (1967).
Edery, H.: Potentiation of the action of bradykinin on smooth muscle by chymotrypsin, chymotrypsinogen and trypsin. Brit. J. Pharmacol. **22**, 371 (1964).
— New test for biological identification of bradykinin. Nature (Lond.) **217**, 70 (1968).
Egorova, T. P., Paskhina, T. S.: Purification of kininogen (bradykininogen) from rabbit blood plasma and study of its properties. Biokhimiya **32**, 354 (1967).
Elliott, D. F., Lewis, G. P.: Methionyl-lysyl-bradykinin, a new kinin from ox blood. Biochem. J. **95**, 437 (1965).
— — Smyth, D. G.: A new kinin from ox blood. Biochem. J. **87**, 21P (1963).
Erdös, E. G.: Hypotensive peptides. Bradykinin, kallidin and eledoisin. Advanc. Pharmacol. **4**, 1 (1966).
— Jackman, V., Barnes, U. C.: Instrument for recording isotonic contractions of smooth muscle. J. appl. Physiol. **17**, 367 (1962).
— Miwa, I., Graham, W. J.: Studies on the evolution of plasma kinins. Reptilian and avian blood. Life Sci. **22**, 2433 (1967a).
— Sloane, E. M.: An enzyme in human blood plasma that inactivates bradykinin and kallidin. Biochem. Pharmacol. **11**, 585 (1962).
— — Wohler, I. M.: Carboxypeptidase in blood and other fluids. I. Biochem. Pharmacol. **13**, 893 (1964).
— Tague, L. L., Miwa, I.: Kallikrein in granules of the submaxillary gland. Biochem. Pharmacol. **17**, 667 (1968).
— Westerman, M. P.: Properties of a carboxypeptidase in blood sera. Fed. Proc. **22**, 425 (1963).
— Wohler, J. R., Levine, M. I.: Blocking of the in vivo effects of bradykinin and kallidin with carboxypeptidase B. J. Pharmacol. exp. Ther. **142**, 327 (1963).
— Yang, H. Y. T.: An enzyme in microsomal fraction of kidney that inactivates bradykinin. Life Sci. **6**, 569 (1967).
— — Tague, L. L., Manning, N.: Carboxypeptidase in blood and other fluids. III. The esterase activity of the enzyme. Biochem. Pharmacol. **16**, 1287 (1967b).
Erspamer, V.: Active substances in the posterior salivary gland of octopoda. Acta pharmacol. (Kbh.) **4**, 213 (1948).
— Bioassay of indolealkylamines in 5-hydroxytryptamine and related indolealkylamines. In: Handbuch der experimentellen Pharmakologie, p. 113, ed. by O. Eichler and A. Farah. Berlin-Heidelberg-New York: Springer 1966.
— Bertaccini, G., Urakawa, N.: Biogenic amines and active polypeptides in the skin of ten Japanese amphibian species. Jap. J. Pharmacol. **14**, 468 (1964).
— Erspamer, F.: Pharmacological actions of eledoisin on extravascular smooth muscle. Brit. J. Pharmacol. **19**, 337 (1962).
— Glässer, A.: The action of eledoisin on the systemic arterial blood pressure of some experimental animals. Brit. J. Pharmacol. **20**, 516 (1963).
Fasciolo, J. C.: Bradykininogen, angiotensinogen and kallidinogen. Brit. J. Pharmacol. **21**, 250 (1963).
— Halvoresn, K. A., Itoiz, J. E., Paladini, A. C.: A vasodilator polypeptide present in purified hypertensin preparation. Acta physiol. lat.-amer. **8**, 133 (1958).
Feldberg, W., Schilf, E.: Histamin, seine Pharmakologie und Bedeutung für die Humoralphysiologie. Berlin 1930.

FERREIRA, S. H.: Bradykinin-potentiating factor (BPF) present in the venom of *Bothrops jararaca*. Brit. J. Pharmacol. **24**, 163 (1965).
— ROCHA E SILVA, M.: Potentation of bradykinin by dimercaptopropanol (BAL) and other inhibitors of its destroying enzyme in plasma. Biochem. Pharmacol. **11**, 1123 (1962).
— VANE, J. R.: The disappearance of bradykinin and eledoisin in the circulation and vascular beds of the cat. Brit. J. Pharmacol. **30**, 417 (1967).
FIEDLER, F., WERLE, E.: Vorkommen zweier Kallikreinogene im Schweinepankreas und Automation der Kallikrein- und Kininogenbestimmung. Hoppe-Seylers Z. physiol. Chem. **348**, 1087 (1967).
FISHLOCK, D. J.: Effect of bradykinin on the human isolated small and large intestine. Nature (Lond.) **212**, 1533 (1966).
FOLK, J. E., PIEZ, K. A., CARROLL, W., GLADNER, J. A.: Carboxypeptidase B. Purification and characterization of the porcine enzyme. J. biol. Chem. **235**, 2272 (1960).
FREY, E. K., KRAUT, H.: Ein neues Kreislaufhormon und seine Wirkung. Naunyn-Schmiedebergs Arch. exp. Path. Pharmak. **133**, 1 (1928).
— — WERLE, E.: Kallikrein (Padutin). Stuttgart: Enke 1950.
— — — VOGEL, R., ZICKGRAF-RÜDEL, G., TRAUTSCHOLD, I.: Das Kallikrein-Kinin-System und seine Inhibitoren. Stuttgart: Enke 1968.
FRIMMER, M.: Beeinflussung der Durchlässigkeit von Blut-Capillaren der Kaninchenhaut für Makromoleküle durch einige biogene, gefäßaktive Substanzen. Naunyn-Schmiedebergs Arch. exp. Path. Pharmak. **242**, 390 (1961).
FRITZ, H., TRAUTSCHOLD, I., HAENDLE, H., WERLE, E.: Chemistry and biochemistry of proteinase inhibitors from mammalian tissues. In: Chemistry, pharmacology and clinical applications of proteinase inhibitors, ed. by N. BACK. Ann. N.Y. Acad. Sci. **146**, 400 (1968).
— — WERLE, E.: Proteinaseinhibitoren. In: Methoden der enzymatischen Analyse, ed. by H.-U. BERGMEYER. Weinheim: Verlag Chemie 1969.
GADDUM, J. H.: Gefäßerweiternde Stoffe der Gewebe. Leipzig: Thieme 1936.
— The technique of superfusion. Brit. J. Pharmacol. **8**, 321 (1953).
— HAMEED, K. A.: Drugs which antagonize 5-hydroxytryptamine. Brit. J. Pharmacol. **9**, 240 (1954).
— LEMBECK, F.: Assay of substances from adrenal medulla. Brit. J. Pharmacol. **4**, 401 (1949).
GARBE, G.: Quantitative Kininogenbestimmung im menschlichen Plasma. Naunyn-Schmiedebergs Arch. exp. Path. Pharmak. **256**, 112 (1967).
— VOGT, W.: Zur Natur der im menschlichen Plasma durch PKE, Glaskontakt und Säurebehandlung gebildeten Kinine. Naunyn-Schmiedebergs Arch. exp. Path. Pharmak. **256**, 119 (1967).
GASCON, A. L.: Inhibition of eledoisin by morin on the isolated guinea pig ileum. Canad. J. Physiol. Pharmacol. **46**, 67 (1967).
GLADNER, J. A., MURTAUGH, P. A., FOLK, J. E., LAKI, K.: Nature of peptides released by thrombin. In: Structure and function of biologically active peptides. Bradykinin, kallidin and congeners, ed. by E. G. ERDÖS. Ann. N.Y. Acad. Sci. **104**, 47 (1963).
GOODFRIEND, T. L., LEVINE, L., FASMAN, D. G.: Antibodies to bradykinin and angiotensin; use of carbodiimides in immunology. Science **144**, 1344 (1964).
GREEFF, K.: Die Wirkung vasoaktiver Polypeptide auf Bronchien und Lungenkreislauf. Beitr. Klin. Erforsch. Tuberk. **138**, 306 (1968).
— SCHARNAGEL, K., LÜHR, R., STROHBACH, H.: Kininogengehalt des Plasmas beim Schock. Naunyn-Schmiedebergs Arch. exp. Path. Pharmak. **253**, 235 (1966).
GREEN, H. D., LITTLE, J. M., GADDY, C. G., FRANKLIN, L. T., WAYNE, H. H.: Vasodilator effects of a substance present in normal human urine in comparison with the effect of methacholine and sodium nitrite; statistical analysis of reliability of method of assay. Circulat. Res. **5**, 567 (1952).
GREENBAUM, L. M., HOSODA, T.: Studies on the isolation of bradykininogen. Biochem. Pharmacol. **12**, 325 (1963).
— KIM, K. S.: The kinin forming and kininase activity of rabbit polymorphonuclear leucocytes. Brit. J. Pharmacol. **29**, 238 (1967).
— YAMAFUJI, K., HOSODA, T.: Studies of the peptic degradation of bovine bradykininogen. Biochem. Pharmacol. **14**, 411 (1965).
HABERMANN, E.: Über Zusammenhänge zwischen esterolytischen und pharmakologischen Wirkungen von Jararacagift, Kallikrein und Thrombin. Naunyn-Schmiedebergs Arch. exp. Path. Pharmak. **236**, 492 (1959).
— Über pH-bedingte Modifikationen des kininliefernden α-Globulins (kininogen) aus Rinderserum und das Molekulargewicht von Kininogen I. Biochem. Z. **337**, 440 (1963).
— BLENNEMANN, G.: Über Substrate und Reaktionsprodukte der kininbildenden Enzyme Trypsin, Serum- und Pankreaskallikrein, sowie Crotalusgift. Naunyn-Schmiedebergs Arch. exp. Path. Pharmak. **249**, 357 (1964).

Habermann, E., Blennemann, G., Müller, B.: Charakterisierung und Reinigung peptischer kininliefernder Fragmente (PKF), sowie von Pepsitocin aus Rinderserum Kininogen. Naunyn-Schmiedebergs Arch. exp. Path. Pharmak. 253, 444 (1966).
— Klett, W., Rosenbusch, G.: Partielle Reinigung und Eigenschaften eines Kininogens aus Rinderblut. Hoppe-Seylers Z. physiol. Chem. 332, 121 (1963).
— Räker, K. O., Arndts, D.: Radio-Retentionselektrophorese; ein quantitatives und spezifisches Verfahren zur Bestimmung einzelner Proteine im Nanogrammbereich. Klin. Wschr. 46, 46 (1968).
Hamberg, U.: Structure and biological activity of bradykinin. Ann. Acad. Sci. fenn. A 106, 3 (1964).
— Rocha e Silva, M.: On the release of bradykinin by trypsin and snake venoms. Arch. int. Pharmacodyn. 110, 222 (1957).
Haverback, B. J., Dyce, B., Bundy, H., Edmondson, H. A.: Trypsin, trypsinogen and trypsin inhibitor in human pancreatic juice. Amer. J. Med. 29, 424 (1960).
Henriques, O. B., Kauritcheva, N., Kuznetsova, V., Astrakon, M.: Substrates of kinin releasing enzymes isolated from horse plasma. Nature (Lond.) 215, 1200 (1967).
Holdstock, D. J., Mathias, A. P., Schachter, M.: Comparative study of kinin, kallidin and bradykinin. Brit. J. Pharmacol. 12, 149 (1957).
Hopsu-Havu, V. K., Jansen, T.: Peptidase in the skin: I. Biochemical demonstration of an aminopeptidase in rat skin specific for N-terminal basic amino acids (aminopeptidase B). Arch. klin. exp. Derm. 233, 1 (1968).
— Mäkinen, K. K., Glenner, G. G.: 1. Purification of a mammalian peptidase selective for N-terminal arginine and lysine residue. 2. Characterization of aminopeptidase B: substrate specificity and affector studies. Arch. Biochem. 114, 557, 567 (1966).
Horton, E. W.: The assay of kallikrein in urine. J. Physiol. (Lond.) 142, 36P (1958).
— The estimation of urinary kallikrein. J. Physiol. (Lond.) 148, 267 (1959).
— Urinary kinin. In: Polypeptides which affect smooth muscle and blood vessels, p. 263, ed. by M. Schachter. Oxford: Pergamon 1960.
Jacobsen, S.: Substrates for plasma kinin forming enzymes in human, dog and rabbit plasma. Brit. J. Pharmacol. 26, 403 (1966a).
— Observations on the content of kininogen, kallikrein and kininase in lymph from limbs of dogs and rabbits. Brit. J. Pharmacol. 27, 213 (1966b).
— Kriz, M.: Some data on two purified kininogens from human plasma. Brit. J. Pharmacol. 29, 25 (1967).
Jensen, K. B., Venneröd, A. M., Rinvik, S. F.: Excretion of human urinary kinins. Acta pharmacol. (Kbh.) 22, 177 (1965).
Kellermeyer, R. W., Graham, R. C., Jr.: Kinins, possible physiologic and pathologic roles in man. New Engl. J. Med. 279, 754 (1968).
Khairallah, P. A., Page, I. H.: Mechanism of action of angiotensin and bradykinin on smooth muscle in situ. Amer. J. Physiol. 200, 51 (1961).
— — Effects of bradykinin and angiotensin on smooth muscle. In: Structure and function of biologically active peptides: bradykinin, kallidin and congeners, ed. by E. G. Erdös. Ann. N.Y. Acad. Sci. 104, 212 (1963).
Kobold, E. E., Thal, A. P.: Quantification and identification of vasoactive substances liberated during types of experimental intestinal ischemia. Surg. Gynec. Obstet. 117, 315 (1963).
Konzett, H., Stürmer, E.: Biological activity of synthetic polypeptides with bradykinin properties. Brit. J. Pharmacol. 15, 544 (1960a).
— — Synthetic bradykinin: its biological identity with natural pure trypsin bradykinin. Nature (Lond.) 188, 998 (1960b).
Kovalcik, V.: Effect of bradykinin on isolated coronary arteries. Nature (Lond.) 196, 174 (1962).
Kunitz, M.: Crystalline soybean trypsin inhibitor. II. General properties. J. gen. Physiol. 30, 291 (1947).
Laurell, C. B.: Quantitative estimation of proteins by electrophoresis in agarose gel containing antibodies. Analyt. Biochem. 15, 45 (1966).
Lecomte, J., Salmon, J.: Sur le role des kinines plasmatiqes dans la pathogenie du collapse anaphylactique du rat. Arch. int. Physiol. Biochem. 76, 273 (1968).
Lewis, G. P.: Active polypeptides derived from plasma proteins. Physiol. Rev. 40, 647 (1960).
— Pharmacological actions of bradykinin and its role in physiological and pathological reactions. In: Structure and function of biologically active peptides: bradykinin, kallidin and congeners, ed. by E. G. Erdös. Ann. N.Y. Acad. Sci. 104, 236 (1963).
Lowry, H. O., Roberts, N. R., Kupphahn, J. L.: The fluorometric measurement of pyridine nucleotides. J. biol. Chem. 224, 1047 (1957).
Malofiejew, M., Buluk, K., Czokalo, M.: A preparation of kininogen for the assay of kallikreins. Thromb. Diathes. haemorrh. (Stuttg.) 16, 723 (1966).

MARGOLIS, J.: The interrelationship of coagulation of plasma and release of peptides. In: Structure and function of biologically active peptides: bradykinin, kallidin and congeners, ed. by E. G. ERDÖS. Ann. N.Y. Acad. Sci. **104**, 133 (1963).
— BISHOP, E. A.: Studies on plasma kinins. 1. The composition of kininogen complex. Aust. J. exp. Biol. med. Sci. **41**, 293 (1963).
MASHFORD, M. L., ZACEST, R.: Physiological changes in blood bradykinin levels in man. Aust. J. exp. Biol. med. Sci. **45**, 661 (1967).
MCCARTHY, D. A., POTTER, D. E., NICOLAIDES, E. D.: Estimation of the potencies and half lives of synthetic bradykinin and kallidin. J. Pharmacol. exp. Ther. **148**, 117 (1965).
MELMON, K. L., CLINE, M. J., HUGHES, T., NIES, A. S.: Kinins: Possible mediators of neonatal circulatory changes in man. J. clin. Invest. **47**, 1295 (1968).
MIWA, I.: An incubation method for the estimation of urinary kallikrein. Tohoku J. exp. Med. **86**, 334 (1965).
— ERDÖS, E. G., SEKI, T.: Presence of three peptides in urinary kinin (substance Z) preparations. Life Sci. **7**, 1339 (1968).
— — — Separation of peptide components of urinary kinin (substance Z). Proc. Soc. exp. Biol. (N.Y.) **131**, 768 (1969).
NAGASAWA, S., MIZUSHIMA, Y., SATO, T., IWANAGA, S., SUZUKI, T.: Studies on the chemical nature of bovine bradykininogen: determination of amino acids, carbohydrate, amino and carboxyl terminals. J. Biochem. (Tokyo) **60**, 643 (1966).
NAGEL, W., WILLIG, F., PESCHKE, W., SCHMIDT, F. H.: Detection of trypsin and chymotrypsin with paranitroanilide derivates of amino acids. Hoppe-Seylers Z. physiol. Chem. **340**, 1 (1965).
NICOLAIDES, E. D., DEWALD, H. A., CRAFT, M. K.: The synthesis of kinin analogues. In: Structures and function of biologically active peptides: bradykinin, kallidin and congeners, ed. by E. G. ERDÖS. Ann. N.Y. Acad. Sci. **104**, 15 (1963).
— MCCARTHY, D. A., POTTER, D. E.: Bradykinin, configuration of the arginase moieties and biological activity. Biochemistry **4**, 190 (1965).
NILSEN, K. H., RUGSTAD, H. E.: Stability of kininase of microbiological origin in the blood of an isolated rat lung preparation. Life Sci. **7**, 921 (1968).
OATES, J. A., MELMON, K., SJOERDSMA, A., GILLESPIE, L., MASON, D. T.: Release of a kinin peptide in the carcinoid syndrome. Lancet **1964 I**, 514.
OLMSTED, F., PAGE, I. H.: Haemodynamic effects of eledoisin, kallidin and bradykinin on unanesthetized dogs. Amer. J. Physiol. **203**, 951 (1962).
OYVIN, I. A., GAPONIUK, P. Y., OYVIN, V. I.: The effect of bradykinin on permeability of skin blood vessels. Experientia (Basel) **23**, 925 (1967).
PAGE, I. H., GREEN, A. A.: Perfusion of rabbit's ear for study of vasoconstrictor substances. Meth. med. Res. **1**, 123 (1948).
PASKHINA, T. S., EGOROVA, T. P.: Purification and properties of kininogen (bradykininogen) from rabbit blood serum. Biokhimiya **31**, 468 (1966).
PEARSON, L., LANG, W. J.: A comparison in conscious and anesthetized dogs of the effect on blood pressure of bradykinin, kallidin, eledoisin and kallikrein. Europ. J. Pharmacol. **2**, 83 (1967).
PICARELLI, Z. P., HENRIQUES, O. B., OLIVEIRA, M. C. F.: Potentiation of bradykinin action on smooth muscle by cysteine. Experientia (Basel) **18**, 77 (1962).
PIERCE, J. V.: Structural features of plasma kinins and kininogens. Fed. Proc. **27**, 52 (1968).
— WEBSTER, M. E.: Human plasma kallidins: isolation and chemical studies. Biochem. biophys. Res. Commun. **5**, 353 (1961).
— — The purification and some properties of two different kallidinogens from human plasma. In: Hypotensive peptides, p. 130, ed. by E. G. ERDÖS, N. BACK and F. SICUTERI. Berlin-Heidelberg-New York: Springer 1966.
RINDERKNECHT, H., HAVERBACK, B. J., ALADJEM, F.: Radioimmunoassay of bradykinin. Nature (Lond.) **213**, 1130 (1967).
RINVIK, S. F., DYRUD, O. K., BRISEID, K.: Determination of plasma kininogen, plasma kininase and erythrocyte kininase. Acta pharmacol. (Kbh.) **24**, 169 (1966).
ROBERTS, P. S.: Measurement of the rate of plasmin action on synthetic substrates. J. biol. Chem. **232**, 285 (1958).
ROCHA E SILVA, M.: Method of assay of bradykinin upon guinea pig gut. Acta physiol. lat.-amer. **2**, 238 (1952).
— Bradykinin: occurrence and properties. In: Polypeptides which stimulate plain muscle, p. 45, ed. by J. H. GADDUM. Edinburgh and London: Livingstone Ltd. 1955.
— BERALDO, W. T., ROSENFELD, G.: Bradykinin, hypotensive and smooth muscle stimulation factor released from plasma globulin by snake venoms and by trypsin. Amer. J. Physiol. **156**, 261 (1949).
— LEME, J. G.: Antagonists of bradykinin. Med. exp. (Basel) **8**, 287 (1963).

Rugstad, H. E.: Kininase production by some microbes. Brit. J. Pharmacol. **28**, 315 (1966).
Sardesai, V. M.: Determination of bradykinin in blood and bradykininogen in tissues. Canad. J. Physiol. Pharmacol. **46**, 77 (1968).
Sarnoff, S. J., Case, R. B., Macruz, R.: Observation on the vasodilator properties of urine. Circulat. Res. **6**, 522 (1958).
Schachter, M.: Some properties of kallidin, bradykinin and wasp venom kinin. In: Polypeptides which affect smooth muscles and blood vessels, p. 232, ed. by M. Schachter. Oxford: Pergamon Press 1960.
Schröder, E., Hempel, R.: Bradykinin and kallidin and their synthetic analogues. Experientia (Basel) **20**, 529 (1964).
Seidel, G., Vogt, W.: Kininogenspezifität von acetonaktiviertem menschlichen Plasmakallikrein. Naunyn-Schmiedebergs Arch. exp. Path. Pharmak. **262**, 135 (1969).
Spragg, J., Austen, K. F., Haber, E.: Production of antibody against bradykinin. Demonstration of specificity by complement fixation and radio-immunoassay. J. Immunol. **96**, 865 (1966).
— Schröder, E., Stewart, J. M., Austen, K. F., Haber, E.: Structural requirements for binding to antibody of sequence variants of bradykinin. Biochemistry **6**, 3933 (1967).
Stopp, G., Jung, F.: Der Einfluß der Wasserstoffionenkonzentration, der Calziumkonzentration und der Temperatur auf die durch Eledoisin und Eledoisinpeptide hervorgerufene Kontraktion des Meerschweinchenileums. Acta biol. med. ger. **20**, 345 (1968).
Stürmer, E., Berde, B.: A pharmacological comparison between synthetic bradykinin and synthetic kallidin. J. Pharmacol. exp. Ther. **139**, 38 (1963a).
— — Pharmacological comparison between synthetic bradykinin and kallidin. Naunyn-Schmiedebergs Arch. exp. Path. Pharmak. **246**, 21 (1963b).
— — A comparative pharmacological study of synthetic eledoisin and synthetic bradykinin. J. Pharmacol. exp. Ther. **140**, 349 (1963c).
Talamo, R. C., Haber, E., Austen, K. F.: Antibody to bradykinin: effect of carrier and method of coupling on specificity and affinity. J. Immunol. **101**, 333 (1968).
Tella, A., Maegraith, B. G.: Studies on bradykinin and bradykininogen in malaria. Ann. trop. Med. Parasit. **60**, 304 (1966).
Trautschold, I.: Enzymes and inhibitors of the liberation and degradation of vasoactive polypeptides (kinins). Habil.-Schr. der Univ. München (1965).
— Fritz, H., Werle, E.: Kininogenases, kininases and their inhibitors. In: Hypotensive peptides, p. 221, ed. by E. G. Erdös, N. Back and F. Sicuteri. Berlin-Heidelberg-New York: Springer 1966b.
— Werle, E.: Spektrophotometrische Bestimmung des Kallikreins und seiner Inhibitoren. Hoppe-Seylers Z. physiol. Chem. **325**, 48 (1961).
— — Kallikrein. In: Methoden der enzymatischen Analyse, p. 880, ed. by H. U. Bergmeyer. Weinheim: Verlag Chemie 1962.
— — Fritz, H.: Zur Biochemie des Trasylols. In: Neue Aspekte der Trasylol-Therapie, ed. by R. Gross and G. Kroneberg. Stuttgart 1966a.
— — Schweitzer, G.: Kallikrein. In: Methoden der enzymatischen Analyse, 2nd ed., ed. by H. U. Bergmeyer. Weinheim: Verlag Chemie 1969.
Vane, J. R.: A sensitive method for the assay of 5-hydroxytryptamine. Brit. J. Pharmacol. **12**, 344 (1957).
— The blood-bathed isolated organ: a method of testing the circulating blood for active substances. J. Physiol. (Lond.) **143**, 75P (1958).
— The use of isolated organs for detecting active substances in the circulating blood. Brit. J. Pharmacol. **23**, 360 (1964).
— The release and fate of vaso-active hormones in the circulation. Brit. J. Pharmacol. **35**, 209 (1969).
Vogel, R., Trautschold, I., Werle, E.: Natural proteinase inhibitors. New York: Academic Press 1968.
Vogt, W., Garbe, G., Schmidt, G.: Untersuchung zur Existenz zweier verschiedener kininbildender Systeme im menschlichen Plasma. Naunyn-Schmiedebergs Arch. exp. Path. Pharmak. **256**, 127 (1967).
— Wawretschek, W.: Weitere Untersuchungen zur Existenz zweier kininbildender Systeme im menschlichen Plasma. Naunyn-Schmiedebergs Arch. exp. Path. Pharmak. **260**, 223 (1968).
Walaszek, E. J., Dyer, D. C., Gascon, A. L.: Polypeptide receptor mechanism. Fed. Proc. **27**, 67 (1968).
Waldvogel, G., Frimmer, M.: Untersuchungen zur Lokalisation von Änderungen der Gefäßpermeabilität. Naunyn-Schmiedebergs Arch. exp. Path. Pharmak. **258**, 321 (1967).
Watanabe, N., Abe, K., Kumagai, N., Mouri, T., Seki, T., Yoshinaga, K.: Kininase activity in human blood. Tohoku J. exp. Med. **89**, 383 (1966).

WEBSTER, M. E., GILMORE, J. P.: The estimation of the kallidins in blood and urine. Biochem. Pharmacol. **14**, 1161 (1965).
— PIERCE, J. V.: Action of the kallikreins on synthetic ester substrates. Proc. Soc. exp. Biol. (N.Y.) **107**, 186 (1961).
— — The nature of the kallidins released from human plasma by kallikreins and other enzymes. In: Structure and function of biologically active peptides: Bradykinin, kallidin and congeners, ed. by E. G. ERDÖS. Ann. N.Y. Acad. Sci. **104**, 91 (1963).
— SKINNER, N. S., POWELL, W. J.: Role of the kinins in vasodilatation of skeletal muscle of the dog. Amer. J. Physiol. **212**, 553 (1967).
WERLE, E., BEREK, U.: Zur Kenntnis des Kallikreins. Angew. Chem. **60** A, 53 (1948).
— GÖTZE, W., KEPPLER, A.: Wirkung des Kallikreins auf den isolierten Darm und eine neue darmkontrahierende Substanz. Biochem. Z. **289**, 217 (1937).
— HOCHSTRASSER, K., TRAUTSCHOLD, I.: Studies of bovine plasma, kininogen, ornitho-kallikrein and ornitho kinin. In: Hypotensive peptides, p. 105, ed. by E. G. ERDÖS, N. BACK and F. SICUTERI. Berlin-Heidelberg-New York: Springer 1966.
— — — LEYSATH, G.: Wirkung von Thioglykolsäure auf Kininogen und Kininase. Hoppe-Seylers Z. physiol. Chem. **337**, 286 (1964).
— KAUFMANN-BOETSCH, B.: Über esteratische Wirkungen von Kallikrein und Trypsin und ihre Hemmung durch Kallikrein und Trypsininhibitoren. Hoppe-Seylers Z. physiol. Chem. **319**, 52 (1960).
— LEYSATH, G.: Über das Molekulargewicht des Plasmakinins von Vögeln. Hoppe-Seylers Z. physiol. Chem. **348**, 352 (1967).
— — SCHMAL, A.: Behavior of the kininogen level after extirpation of rat kidneys and adrenal glands. Hoppe-Seylers Z. physiol. Chem. **349**, 107 (1968).
— TRAUTSCHOLD, I.: Isolierung und Struktur des Kallidins. Hoppe-Seylers Z. physiol. Chem. **326**, 174 (1961).
— — Kallikrein, kallidin, kallikrein inhibitors. In: Structure and function of biologically active peptides: Bradykinin, kallidin and congeners, ed. by E. G. ERDÖS. Ann. N.Y. Acad. Sci. **104**, 117 (1963).
WIEGERSHAUSEN, B., STOPP, G., EICHSTÄDT, M.: Zum Mechanismus der Bradykininwirkung am Meerschweinchendarm. Acta biol. med. germ. **12**, 443 (1964).
— PAEGELOW, J., NEUMAYER, E., WALTER, H.: Der Kininogengehalt in Plasma und Fruchtwasser. Acta biol. med. germ. **19**, 61 (1967).
WITTE, S., SCHRICKER, K. T., SCHMID, E.: Zur Wirkung von synthetischem Bradykinin auf die Gefäßpermeabilität. Arzneimittel-Forsch. **11**, 619 (1961).
YANG, H. Y. T., ERDÖS, E. G.: Second kininase in human blood plasma. Nature (Lond.) **215**, 1402 (1967).
YOSHINAGA, K., ABE, K., MIWA, I., AIDA, M., MAEBASHI, M., WADA, Y.: Assay of urinary kinin. Tohoku J. exp. Med. **81**, 246 (1963).
— — — FURUYAMA, T., SUZUKI, C.: Evidence for the renal origin of urinary kinin. Experientia (Basel) **20**, 396 (1964).
ZACEST, R., MASHFORD, M. L.: Blood bradykinin levels in the human. Aust. J. exp. Biol. med. Sci. **45**, 89 (1967).
ZACHARIAE, H., MALMQUIST, J., OATES, J. A.: Kininase in human polymorphonuclear leukocytes. Life Sci. **5**, 2347 (1966).

Plasma Kininogenases and Their Activators

V. Eisen and W. Vogt

With 4 Figures

A. Introduction

Plasma kinins can be released from the substrate globulins (kininogens) by enzymes which belong to the plasma proteins, and by enzymes derived from other tissues. We can therefore distinguish, by analogy with blood clotting, *intrinsic* and *extrinsic* plasma kinin formation.

Intrinsic plasma kinin formation must be viewed as part of an elaborate system of reactive mechanisms in which proteolytic enzymes play a dominant role. The most prominent of these mechanisms are blood clotting, fibrinolysis, complement, and plasma kinin formation (Fig. 1). Their function in pathological changes is often conspicuous. They are concerned with responses to a wide variety of noxious stimuli, ranging from trauma and other physical or chemical injury, to attack by microorganisms, immunological challenge, stress, and emotion. In most cases, the factors constituting the intrinsic systems collaborate with factors from cells and tissues to bring about hemostasis and removal of clotted blood, inflammation and other defense reactions, and repair of damaged structures. These are processes of utmost importance for survival. However, they may be mobilized at sites, at times, and with an intensity which are harmful to the organism. Such misplaced or excessive activity may then escape the normally controlling influence of the numerous inhibitors in tissues and body fluids. Occasionally this may happen because of primary defects among the inhibitors.

Very much less is known about the role, if any, of these plasma systems in undisturbed physiological conditions. It has been suggested that blood—circulating in a flexible, compliant vascular system of fluctuating calibre—remains fluid owing to a dynamic equilibrium between the continuous formation of fibrin along the endothelial surfaces of vessels and its equally continuous dissolution. Some types of physiological regional vasodilatation may be mediated by intrinsic plasma kinin formation. Complement assists phagocytosis and other activities which neutralize foreign particles and substances.

In recent years it has been recognized that these intrinsic plasma systems contain many instances of biological amplification by serial pre-enzyme–enzyme transformations. This concept was first evolved by Macfarlane (1964) and Davie and Ratnoff (1964) for blood clotting, and named *cascade* or *waterfall* sequence, respectively. According to this concept, most known clotting factors circulate as pre-enzymes; these can induce coagulation by activating each other in a definite sequence. Each pre-enzyme–enzyme transformation amplifies the reaction. The clotting process gathers speed as it progresses from the activation of less than 1 μg of factor XII in 1 ml of plasma, to the conversion of 3 mg of fibrinogen. This renders possible the rapid, almost explosive, formation of the hemostatic plug.

Such amplification also occurs in other triggered enzyme mechanisms in plasma. However, the systems contain several enzymes which act not only in sequence, as shown in Fig. 1, but also on other stages. This provides positive and negative feedback mechanisms, as well as possible shorter reaction chains. Other constituents, such as clotting factor V, may not act as enzymes but as cofactors or accelerators.

Of particular interest for the study of intrinsic plasma kinin formation are findings that several plasma proteases are active outside their own systems.

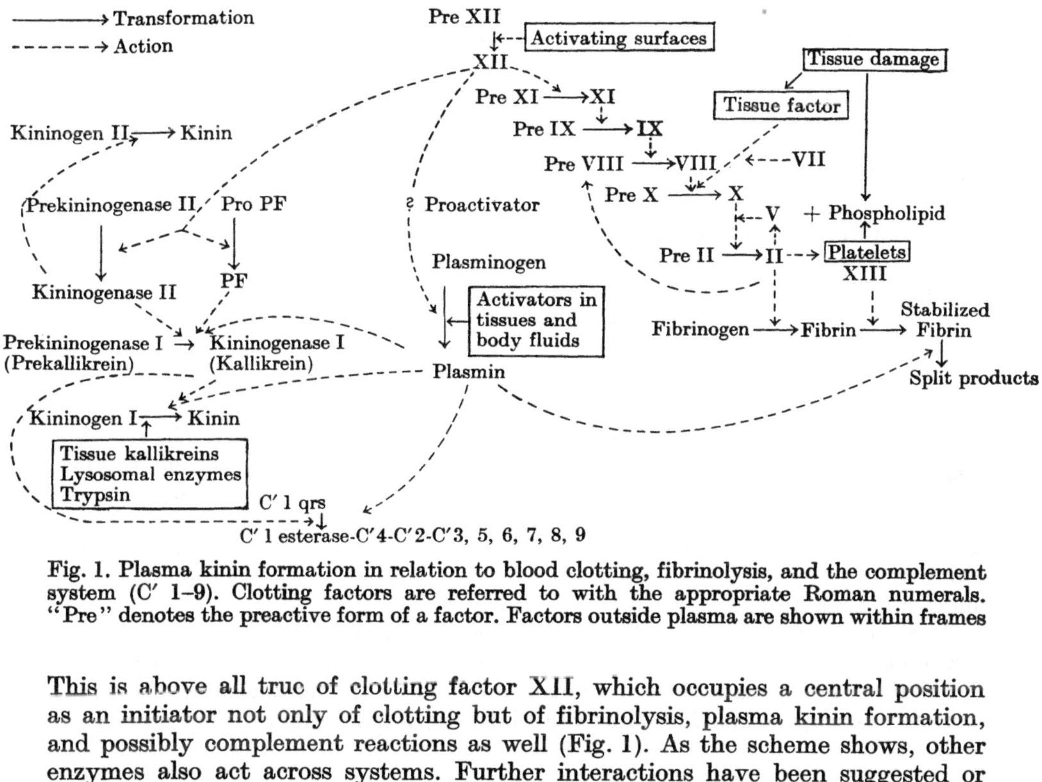

Fig. 1. Plasma kinin formation in relation to blood clotting, fibrinolysis, and the complement system (C′ 1–9). Clotting factors are referred to with the appropriate Roman numerals. "Pre" denotes the preactive form of a factor. Factors outside plasma are shown within frames

This is above all true of clotting factor XII, which occupies a central position as an initiator not only of clotting but of fibrinolysis, plasma kinin formation, and possibly complement reactions as well (Fig. 1). As the scheme shows, other enzymes also act across systems. Further interactions have been suggested or may be discovered; some of the currently postulated links may not be confirmed.

The fact that several of the enzymes can act out of sequence and in another system implies that their specificities for natural substrates often overlap. This is reflected by their bond specificities as determined with small-molecular synthetic weight substrates. These studies suggest that most enzymes of clotting, fibrinolytic, and kinin-forming cascades are endopeptidases which hydrolyze peptide bonds formed by a carboxyl group from the basic amino acids arginine or lysine, and situated in the amino acid chain. Only the complement system contains a proteolytic enzyme that more effectively attacks bonds formed by aromatic amino acids, in particular tyrosine. The cascade principle implies that the function of most of these enzymes is to activate another enzyme. It appears, therefore, that this activation is mostly achieved by the hydrolysis of an arginine or lysine bond, a fact which explains the numerous instances of autocatalysis.

A reaction engaging the complete cascade and passing through all stages of enzymatic amplification emerges therefore as the most efficient pathway, but not the only possible one. Intrinsic kinin formation in human plasma is generally regarded as a cascade consisting of three pre-enzyme–enzyme transformations. But so far, only the initial and the final links of this sequence are reasonably certain. In the light of recent reports that human plasma contains several activators of prekininogenases, the existence of further intermediate pre-enzyme–enzyme links cannot be excluded. On the other hand, shorter, less efficient sequences may also operate. As in the clotting system, this possibility is suggested by close similarities in the bond specificities of kininogenases and their activators. As the scheme shows, the kinin-forming cascade can both intervene in and be affected by other proteolytic processes.

Macfarlane (1965a) and Esnouf and Macfarlane (1968) have likened the amplification that occurs at each stage of an enzyme cascade to a photomultiplier in which the photoelectrons emitted from a photocathode elicit multiple electrons each time they strike one of a series of dynodes, until the greatly increased number of electrons is collected by the anode. If each of n dynodes emits m electrons for each incident electron, the overall gain will be m^n.

Several attempts have been made to formulate the immensely complicated kinetics of the cascade of intrinsic clotting factors. In most of these attempts, kinetic analysis has been simplified by assumptions that are justifiable for the clotting process but probably do not apply to the other proteolytic cascades. Thus, Kellerman (1964) considered the kinetics of a clotting cascade in which: (1) the reactants were present in very low molar concentrations, so that their rates of reaction were determined by the frequency of molecular collisions rather than by the resulting molecular rearrangements; (2) the consumption of the active enzymes by inhibitors could be neglected; (3) the end point of the reaction was reached with the formation of a fixed quantity of the final product. Levine (1966) analyzed the gain by enzymatic amplification in systems in a steady state. Hemker (1969) simplifies the analysis by regarding the clotting system as a "damped cascade" in which all activated enzymes have a short half-life owing to prompt inactivation. The kinetics of such a system mimic those of single-stage reactions.

It is not yet known whether in kinetic terms the intrinsic plasma kinin-forming cascade can be considered as damped, or in a steady state, or very dilute. The chain of reactions is certainly not terminated by the formation of a constant amount of end product. The kinetics of intrinsic plasma kinin formation remain to be explored.

B. Postulated Mechanisms of Intrinsic Plasma Kinin Formation

The plasma kininogenases circulate predominantly, in an inactive state, as pre-enzymes. This is evident from the following facts. (1) Plasma contains large amounts of kininogen, equivalent to 3–10 μg bradykinin/ml in most species; at the same time hardly any free kinin can be detected. (2) The potential capacity of plasma is such as to convert much of the kininogen present in the course of minutes once the enzymes have been activated in a suitable manner (e.g. by acetone).

In their early experiments Frey, Kraut, and Werle estimated the activation and activity of kallikrein directly, by measuring its hypotensive effect when injected intravenously into dogs (p. 115). Later, the amount of kinin formed on incubation with a substrate preparation was preferentially used as a measure of plasma kininogenase activity. The release of kinin is the most specific effect. Thus, experiments intended to elucidate mechanisms of kininogenase activation in plasma have rather been experiments measuring intrinsic kinin formation. This is not necessarily the same, as some procedure may have activated a kininogenase although no kinin formation was apparent. The reasons may be that: (1) the products were not sufficiently protected from destruction; (2) the kininogenase was blocked by an inhibitor; (3) it was destroyed in a secondary process activated simultaneously; (4) no susceptible substrate was present. These factors probably represent the main obstacles to the elucidation of plasma kininogenase activation, and one or the other of them may account for discrepancies among the results of various authors.

I. Early Views on the Origin and Activation of Serum Prekallikrein

Kraut and co-workers detected kallikrein in serum. Several experimental possibilities of activating it were found (Kraut et al., 1933; Werle et al., 1955) (see p. 110). Of these, two could possibly be of physiological or pathological significance—i.e. could occur as an endogenous kinin-forming process in vivo, namely the activation by lowering the pH or by trypsin. The first of these mechanisms was thought to be responsible for reactive hyperemia (Frey, 1930; Matthes and Gross, 1939).

At first it was assumed that activation of serum kallikrein was effected by the dissociation of an inhibitor from the otherwise active enzyme. This assumption stemmed from the idea that active glandular enzyme was secreted into the blood and there inactivated by combining with an inhibitor. It seemed to be supported by the finding of Schachter (1956) that dilution of plasma led to kinin formation, which could be plausibly attributed to the dissociation of an inhibitor from the plasma kininogenase. However, Werle (1936) recognized that plasma kallikrein is different from glandular kallikrein and, later, that its activation is the result of an enzymatic process which can be induced by plasma proteases or by trypsin (Werle et al., 1955). Treatment of plasma with acid, acetone, etc. has been assumed to trigger the same enzymatic activation. Detailed investigations into these endogenous activators, hypothetical at the time, were not performed by Werle and his co-workers.

II. The Fibrinolytic System

Plasmin (or fibrinolysin) is the endogenous proteolytic plasma enzyme that lyses fibrin clots. It circulates as the inactive precursor "plasminogen" (preplasmin) and can be activated by specific activators such as urokinase or tissue activators, or by exogenous substances like streptokinase.

Beraldo (1950) first observed that a plasmin preparation liberated kinin from dog plasma globulin *in vitro*, and that both plasmin activation and kinin formation accompanied the anaphylactic shock *in vivo*. He assumed that plasmin is the principal bradykinin-forming enzyme activated during shock. His findings have been extended to other species (Lewis and Work, 1956; Schachter, 1956; Lewis, 1958). According to Lewis (1958) there were two kinin-forming enzymes: plasmin was thought to be responsible mainly for slow kinin formation, whereas kallikreins released kinin from the same substrate much more quickly. This distinction was based on the observation that (depending on the conditions of activation) slow or fast formation of kinin was observed in dog pseudoglobulin. Also, two kinin-forming principles could be distinguished in urine: urinary kallikrein and urokinase. The former acted on substrate directly, the latter by activating plasminogen (Horton and Lewis, 1959). It was not known whether the two systems acted independently of each other or whether they were in some way connected.

The activation of plasminogen and subsequent kinin liberation were thought to be significant mainly in pathological conditions, where delayed reactions are known to occur. Thus tissue injury may liberate endogenous plasminogen activators, and these would—after the early increase in capillary permeability due to histamine liberation—come into contact with plasma-born plasminogen. The plasmin in turn would release kinin (Lewis, 1960). Other experimental procedures in which plasminogen was thought to be activated and to be responsible for the kinin formation observed were activation of serum by chloroform or by contact with glass and other surfaces (Lewis, 1958). Dilution of plasma which also leads to kinin formation (Schachter, 1956) was shown by Lewis (1958) to be independent of plasmin activation.

The suggestion that plasmin is a kininogenase has been challenged by various authors. The positive results have been attributed partly to contamination of the plasmin preparations with kallikrein, partly to activation by plasmin of prekallikrein present in the substrate preparations used (see p. 116). Activation of prekallikrein by plasmin has been demonstrated by various authors (e.g. Webster and Pierce, 1960; Back et al., 1963; Eisen, 1963b; Vogt, 1964). This seems to be a route by which activated plasmin may lead to kinin formation *in vivo*. The direct kinin-releasing effect requires high doses of plasmin even for slow formation and probably is possible only under special experimental conditions (Seidel et al., 1969). Still, in principle, plasmin is not only a prekallikreinase but also a kininogenase.

III. The Contact System

Kinin formation is only one of several proteolytic processes with which human blood responds to contact with foreign surfaces. The study of these reactions has revealed that the activation of the preactive proteases in blood, by surfaces differing in some way from the cell membranes of healthy blood cells and vascular endothelium, is not only an interesting artefact but a triggering mechanism of great biological importance. The first clue that a factor reacting to glass was involved in plasma kinin formation was obtained by Armstrong et al. (1954), who found that human plasma kept in glass containers developed a "pain-producing substance" (PPS) of polypeptide nature. Shortly afterward, Ratnoff and Colopy (1955) described a patient whose blood clotting system lacked a hitherto unrecognized clotting factor. The factor was named, after the patient, "Hageman factor," and later factor XII in accordance with the recommendations of an international committee (Koller, 1960).

In addition to glass, a large number of silicates and other surfaces activate factor XII, including some which may occur in the body. Most of the activating surfaces also adsorb factor XII. Once activated, it initiates the intrinsic enzymatic cascade of *blood clotting* by activating factor XI (Ratnoff and Davie, 1962; Macfarlane, 1964). The less effective activation of the *fibrinolytic system* by factor XII is also thought to be an enzymatic reaction. Margolis (1958) found that the kinin-forming response to glass required factor XII. When activated and adsorbed by a surface, this factor activated another enzyme *(component A)* which was thought to remain in the soluble phase where it released kinin from kininogen. Owing to the presence of plasma inhibitors, active factor XII and component A, like other plasma proteases, rapidly decayed in plasma.

The kinin-forming activity elicited by glass could not consume all kininogen in plasma. After prolonged exposure to glass, no more kinin was formed. This was demonstrated with plasma which had been exposed to glass powder (surface 20 cm^2/ml plasma) for 5–10 minutes, then separated from glass and left at room temperature for 3–4 hours until the generated kinin-forming activity (active component A) and kinin decayed. Renewed brief exposure (2–4 min) to glass induced in such plasma ample kinin-forming activity, but no kinin. The forming activity could be demonstrated immediately after separation from glass, non-contact plasma used as substrate ("two-stage test") (MARGOLIS, 1958). The failure to generate kinin was not due to lack of kininogen since trypsin and the tissue kallikreins could release large amounts of kinin from this plasma (KEELE, 1960). MARGOLIS (1960) therefore postulated that 10-minute exposure to glass depleted plasma of a "component B." Much longer treatment with glass was necessary to consume all of component A. Component B was first regarded as a cofactor required for the kinin-releasing action of active component A, but not of tissue kallikreins, trypsin, and other exogenous enzymes. Later, component B was described as that part of the plasma kininogen complex which interacts particularly readily with component A.

Recent studies of the intrinsic plasma kinin-forming system suggest that the main constituents of the contact system can be identified with enzymes or substrates described by other workers. MARGOLIS (1966) thought that component A was identical with plasma kallikrein. Similar views were expressed by WEBSTER and RATNOFF (1961) and EISEN (1963a). In the light of recent reports that factor XII activates prekallikrein not directly, but through the mediation of another protease such as permeability factor or kininogenase II, it may be more appropriate to equate component A with one of these intermediate enzymes, as suggested by VOGT (1966). The functional concept of component B is similar to that of VOGT's (1966) kininogen II (see pp. 89 and 117) and that of JACOBSEN's (1966a) kininogen I.

IV. The System of Globulin Permeability Factors

The name permeability factor (PF) was given to enzymatic plasma globulins that were initially detected and characterized by their ability to increase the permeability to proteins of venules and possibly capillaries (MILES and WILHELM, 1955). Globulins with this effect were demonstrated in the plasma of guinea pig, man, rat, and rabbit. Their biochemical and functional properties had been extensively studied before attempts were made to correlate them with the other plasma proteases discussed here.

In normal, quiescent conditions, permeability globulins were assumed to circulate as precursors (pro-PF). In guinea pig, man, and rat, activation of pro-PF was first induced by dilution of plasma (PF/dil; MACKAY et al., 1953). No PF developed in diluted rabbit plasma. PF/dil activity was transient owing to the presence in plasma of an inhibitor (IPF). Factors that increased vascular permeability also developed in plasma on aging. Their relationship to PF/dil is not certain.

Permeability factor has been differentiated from plasmin by several biochemical and functional criteria (ELDER and WILHELM, 1958; MILL et al., 1958). Findings that purified preparations of PF could induce kinin formation in human plasma (ARMSTRONG et al., 1957) and in dog pseudoglobulin (LEWIS, 1958) raised the question whether PF and plasma kallikrein were the same enzyme. This was also suggested by the finding that the development of measurable PF in diluted plasma was largely due to the glass surface of the containers (MILES, 1958/59), and that factor XII was an activator of pro-PF (RATNOFF and MILES, 1964). However, MASON and MILES (1962) were able to treat preparations of PF so that they activated only prekallikrein (prokininogenase) and no longer released kinin from kininogen. On the basis of this it was postulated that PF is activated by factor XII, and in turn activates prekallikrein (MILES, 1964; WEBSTER, 1966).

Further work will be necessary to differentiate fully PF from other activators of prekininogenases, in particular from factor XII. However, the most likely interpretation of the available evidence is that PF is an intermediate enzyme in the plasma kinin-forming cascade. When activated by factor XII, PF in turn activates prekallikrein (prekininogenase). The functional position postulated for PF thus resembles that of kininogenase II (Fig. 2). Their properties, however, are different, since PF is not regarded as a kininogenase. According to WEBSTER (1968), there may be further activators, but it is not known whether these are intercalated between factor XII and prekallikrein.

V. The Kininogenase I and Kininogenase II System

As outlined on p. 86, contact of plasma with glass activates "component A", a kininogenase that reacts with "component B" and eventually releases kinin (MARGOLIS, 1958, 1960). This process was originally not related to the kallikrein system. Later, however, a correlation was sought. The activated component A was identified tentatively (and then more or less definitely) with serum kallikrein (WEBSTER and RATNOFF, 1961; MARGOLIS and BISHOP, 1962, 1963; MARGOLIS, 1963). This made it difficult to define component B and to explain seemingly contradictory experimental findings (see VOGT, 1966). Thus MARGOLIS (1958, 1962, 1963) saw himself confronted with the paradoxical situation that plasma depleted of component B by glass activation still contained kininogen which would yield kinin on incubation with trypsin or glandular kallikreins, but was not converted by the activated component A also present in B-depleted plasma.

The active component A could be demonstrated by mixing the B-depleted plasma with noncontact plasma, which led to kinin formation. This effect is not due to the presence of Hageman factor, which might activate the prekallikrein or component A in the fresh plasma. It depends rather on the presence of a true kininogenase in the glass-activated sample, for this induces kinin formation also in heated substrate preparations which do not contain prekallikreins (EISEN, 1963a; VOGT, 1966).

On the basis of this paradox and additional experimental findings VOGT (1965, 1966; VOGT et al., 1967) has postulated that human plasma contains two kinin-forming systems (Fig. 2). The kininogenase and the kininogen demonstrable in human plasma after extensive activation by contact with glass are nonreactive with each other. The kininogenase active in such plasma (named kininogenase II) requires a different kininogen, which VOGT equates with MARGOLIS' component B. This kininogen (named kininogen II) is present in fresh plasma but is consumed during contact activation. Conversely, the kininogen left in plasma after contact activation (named kininogen I) can be utilized only by a plasma kininogenase (kininogenase I) which is absent from glass-treated plasma, hence different from the enzyme found therein. Trypsin digests kininogens I and II, pancreatic hog kallikrein only kininogen I.

The assumed reasons for the presence in plasma exposed to glass of kininogenase II and kininogen I and for the absence of kininogenase I and kininogen II are as follows: after activation by contact, kininogenase I is inactivated so rapidly that it has not sufficient time to consume kininogen I. In contrast, the activity of kininogenase II decays more slowly, allowing for total consumption of kininogen II and survival of sufficient enzyme activity to be demonstrable afterward. This is corroborated by earlier findings of MARGOLIS (1958) on active component A which is equated by VOGT with kininogenase II.

The activation of prekininogenase I prior to its disappearance in the course of glass treatment is indicated by the fact that a small proportion of kininogen is lost (GARBE and VOGT, 1967; VOGT and WAWRETSCHEK, 1968). The concept of a double kinin-forming system as presented in Fig. 2 requires that all kininogenase I be activated in a few minutes' exposure to glass and then be destroyed or blocked, because new glass contact does not give rise to any kinin formation. Kininogenase II is apparently less completely generated and inactivated, since further activity can be induced several times by repeated exposure of the same plasma to glass (MARGOLIS, 1960; VOGT et al., 1967).

It is surprising that kininogenase I should be activated so much more quickly and extensively. An alternative explanation of the experimental findings may be that an activator is activated and consumed during the first short period of glass contact, which is essentially involved in the activation of kininogenase I but not II. Then, glass-treated plasma would still contain prekininogenase I which, however, could not be activated by the mechanisms operating in normal plasma.

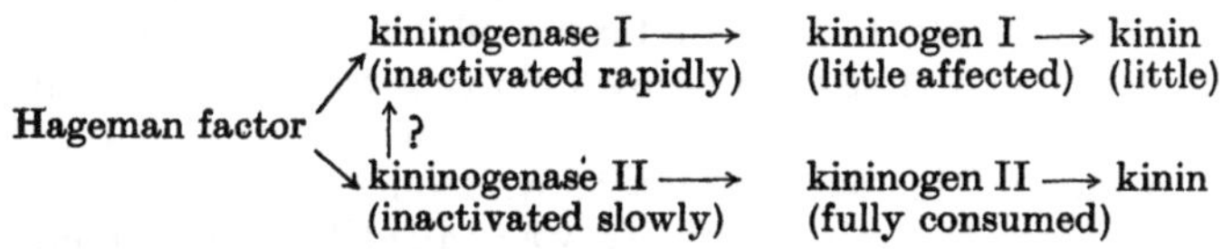

Fig. 2. Kininogenase I is the enzyme absent from glass-treated plasma; kininogenase II is the enzyme present in active form after glass contact. Kininogen I is the substrate largely left intact; kininogen II is the substrate consumed during glass activation of plasma

VOGT (1966) and VOGT et al. (1967) have assumed that kininogenase II itself activates kininogenase I, as it seems that kininogenase I cannot be activated by Hageman factor directly, e.g. in dog plasma which lacks prekininogenase II. However, the relation between the two kininogenases may be more complicated, and other activators may be intercalated in the activation of kininogenase I (see p. 110). The components of the proposed scheme have been related to factors defined earlier, as follows (VOGT, 1966): kininogenase I has been equated with serum kallikrein, as both act on the same substrate and are present in acid- or acetone-treated plasma. Kininogen I is identical, functionally, with the bovine kininogen preparation of HABERMANN et al. (1963). It seems reasonable to assume that it is also identical with bovine kininogen II prepared by YANO et al. (1967a) as well as with most other kininogen preparations described so far. As already stated, kininogenase II corresponds to activated component A and kininogen II to component B of MARGOLIS (1960).

The scheme of two kinin-forming systems reconciles various phenomena related to endogenous kinin formation in plasma which are difficult to explain on the basis of a single kininogenase (kallikrein) only (see p. 117). It is possibly corroborated by the description by ARMSTRONG and MILLS (1964) of a kinin-forming enzyme in human plasma which differs both from kallikrein and from plasmin, and certainly by results obtained by EISEN (1966a) with acetone-activated and glass-adsorbed kininogenases. Further, NAGASAWA et al. (1967) have prepared a glass-activated bovine serum kininogenase that corresponds to VOGT's kininogenase II (SEIDEL, 1969).

C. Activators

I. Hageman Factor

Clotting factor XII (Hageman factor, contact factor) initiates not only the intrinsic clotting reaction of blood to contact with certain abnormal or foreign surfaces, but also the kinin-forming, and possibly the fibrinolytic, response. Some of the proteases activated by factor XII may then mobilize enzymes and other components of the complement system (Donaldson, 1968). Factor XII thus appears to occupy a central position in the intrinsic triggering of proteolytic chain reactions in blood, all of which form part of defense mechanisms against various types of damage.

The existence of factor XII as a distinct molecular species is substantiated by a deficiency syndrome. This was first described by Ratnoff and Colopy (1955); they studied a patient with a greatly prolonged clotting time *in vitro*, who had no past or present bleeding tendency and no knowledge of a history of bleeding in his family. The abnormal laboratory findings could be corrected by small amounts of normal plasma, added either *in vivo* by transfusion or in the test tube. This indicated that the abnormalities were not caused by a circulating anticoagulant but by the lack of a clotting factor or factors responsive to glass. Having eliminated the possibility that a known clotting factor or an anticoagulant was responsible for the deficient blood coagulation, Ratnoff and Colopy (1955) concluded that an unknown clotting factor was missing. The clot-promoting effect of glass and certain other surfaces depended on the presence of this factor in blood. This asymptomatic syndrome was named Hageman trait after the first patient; the missing factor was called Hageman factor, and later factor XII (Koller, 1960). Subsequently, cases of Hageman trait with mild or moderate haemorrhagic tendencies were reported.

Mode of Inheritance. Ratnoff (1966) records that there are at least 89 cases of Hageman trait. Multiple cases have been found in 62 families. Detectable Hageman trait is now attributed to a homozygosis for an autosomal recessive gene (Margolius and Ratnoff, 1956; Ratnoff and Steinberg, 1962; Thompson et al., 1960). The concentration of factor XII was in these cases 1% or less of the normal plasma level, which was estimated to be about 10 μg/ml (Ratnoff, 1966). In a number of presumed heterozygous relatives of subjects with manifest Hageman trait, the levels of factor XII appeared to be lower than normal. Kasper et al. (1968) measured factor XII levels in 80 normal adults and in 39 members of an inbred kindred which included a girl whose factor XII concentration in plasma was 0.4% of the normal value. The results were compatible with the existence of two normal alleles of the gene governing factor XII synthesis: one associated with high levels, and one with low (Veltkamp et al., 1965). Two abnormal alleles of the same gene appear to be responsible for complete or partial deficiency of factor XII.

Occurrence in Species. Most mammalian species seem to possess a factor which in its reaction to surfaces corresponds to factor XII (Thompson et al., 1960; Ratnoff, 1966). Absence of such a plasma factor has been reported in the Peking duck (Ratnoff and Rosenblum, 1958), the chicken (Soulier and Prou-Wartelle, 1960), and in most other fowl (Ratnoff, 1966). Factor XII is low or absent in numerous species of reptiles, amphibians, and fishes (Ratnoff, 1966).

Chemistry and Purification of Factor XII. Factor XII as present in human plasma can be differentiated from most other clotting factors by simple means. It is not adsorbed by barium sulfate or aluminium hydroxide, and not destroyed by heating at 56° for 30 minutes; these procedures remove or inactivate all other known clotting factors except factor XI (Ratnoff and Rosenblum, 1958).

High degrees of purification have been reported by various groups of workers. RATNOFF and DAVIE (1962) adsorbed factor XII from human plasma with CM-cellulose and then eluted it with 0.6 M sodium acetate buffer at pH 5.2. The eluate was precipitated with 60% saturated ammonium sulfate, redissolved and dialyzed, and further purified by chromatography on CM- and DEAE-cellulose columns. A 3,000–5,000-fold purification was achieved; but, as later studies revealed (RATNOFF and MILES, 1964; RATNOFF and CRUM, 1964), the bulk of the purified factor had remained preactive, only 1–8% being present in active form. SPEER et al. (1965) prepared human factor XII by successive chromatography on diatomaceous earth, CM-cellulose, and phospho-cellulose. A million-fold purification and almost complete activation were reported. End-group analysis suggested that arginine was the only N-terminal amino acid, and methionine the only C-terminal amino acid. A molecular weight of 20,000 was calculated from ultracentrifugation data.

SCHIFFMAN et al. (1960) reported clear separation of human factors XII and XI by chromatography on DEAE-cellulose. SCHOENMAKERS et al. (1965) isolated bovine factor XII by adsorption onto glass powder, followed by elution at pH 9.6. Contaminating protein was then removed by cold ethanol. The purification was completed by precipitation with Zn and subsequent removal of Zn, and repeated ion-exchange chromatography on CM- and DEAE-Sephadex. The properties of the purified factor are summarized in Table 1.

Table 1. *Physical Properties and Chemical Composition of Bovine HF*

Properties	Values
Sedimentation coefficient S°_{20w}	7.08 S
Diffusion constant D°_{20w}	$7.14 \cdot 10^{-7}$ cm²/sec
Molecular weight (from D and S values)	82,000
Extinction coefficient, $E^{1\%}_{1\,cm}$ at 280 mμ	12.0
Polypeptide moiety (%)	86.3
Hexoses (%)	5.9
Galactose	3.6
Mannose	1.8
Fucose	0.5
Hexosamines (%) [a]	4.8
Glucosamine	3.2
Galactosamine	1.6
Sialic acid	4.4
Tyrosine/tryptophan ratio	0.45

[a] Value is expressed as the free base. When calculated as N-acetyl hexosamine the content would be 6.0%. (From SCHOENMAKERS et al., 1965).

Activation of Factor XII. The activation of factor XII from the preactive state in which it normally circulates appears to be generally due to contact with a surface. The bulk of the activated factor is usually found adsorbed onto this surface (RATNOFF and COLOPY, 1955; WAALER, 1959; MARGOLIS, 1957; SOULIER and PROU-WARTELLE, 1960; NOSSEL, 1964). HARDISTY and MARGOLIS (1959) even suggested that factor XII is active only in the adsorbed state, and that it reverts on elution to its preactive form. However, active factor XII in solution has been demonstrated by numerous workers (see *Chemistry and Purification*, above). At least one mode of activating factor XII by a soluble agent has been reported. RATNOFF and CRUM (1964) found that aged solutions of tannic acid, and certain *o*-dihydroxyl compounds related to it, activated human factor

XII. The most potent among them, ellagic acid (4.4′,5.5′,6.6′-hexahydroxydiphenic acid 2.6:2.6′dilactone) was effective in concentrations as low as 10^{-8} M. Nevertheless, there is little doubt that the biological importance of factor XII rests on its reaction to surfaces which in some way differ from the surfaces of normal blood cells, endothelium, and interstitial spaces. Macfarlane (1960)

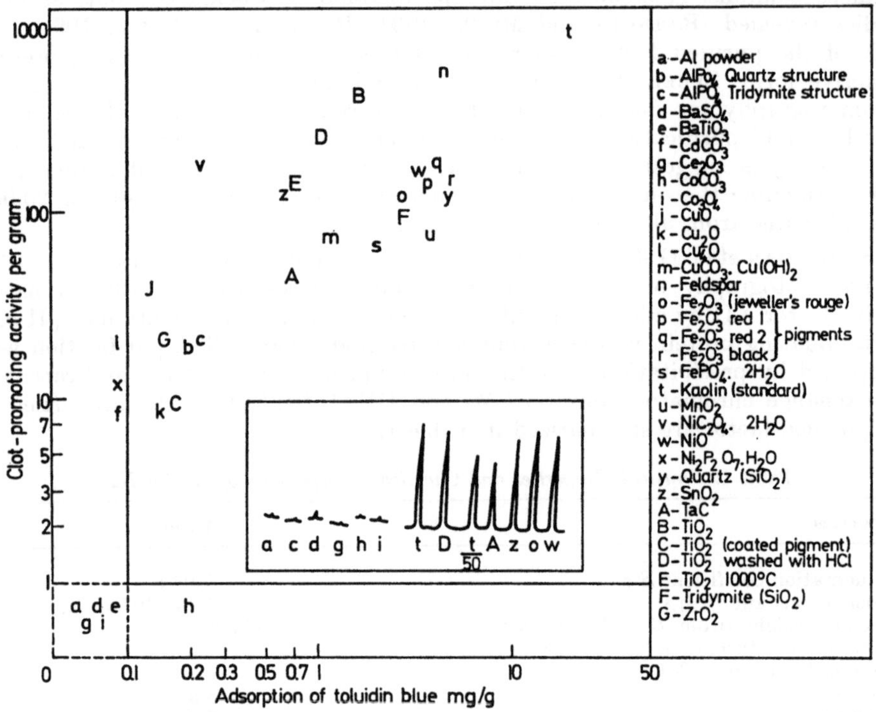

Fig. 3. Correlation between the affinity of various powders to toluidine blue and their ability to release kinin (inset) and promote clotting. Kaolin was used as reference and given an arbitrary value of 1,000. The values in the range $0 < x < 0.1$ and $0 < y < 1.0$ were too low for accurate representation and were grouped together. Uterus tracings were made after applications of 0.1 ml of plasma shaken for 2 minutes with 2 mg/ml of powders. Toluidine blue was adsorbed from 20 μg/ml solution at pH 7.0 for 10 minutes. The concentration in the supernatant was determined spectrophotometrically. (From Margolis, 1963)

thinks that the acute sensitivity of human blood to surfaces is phylogenetically descended from the surface precipitation reaction of monocellular organisms (Heilbrunn, 1961).

Surfaces of a large number of inorganic and organic materials activate factor XII (Margolis, 1963; Fig. 3). It may be assumed that activating surfaces are far more numerous than nonactivating "inert" ones. Indeed, the search for inert surfaces has assumed great practical importance in the technology of heart–lung machines, artificial kidneys, and the surgical replacement of body parts by artificial structures. Of obvious interest is the fact that several surfaces which may occur in the body, mostly as a result of injury or disease, are capable of activating factor XII (see p. 98).

The properties that enable a surface to activate factor XII have been the subject of considerable speculation but of comparatively little research. Lister (1863) noticed over a hundred years ago that glass and certain other foreign surfaces accelerated the coagulation of blood. Glass coated with nonwettable substances was less effective (FREUND, 1886; BORDET and GENGOU, 1901). However, early suggestions that the clot-promoting effect of a surface was due to its wettability by water, were contradicted by the finding that vessels lined with wettable collodion had no such effect (LAMPERT, 1931). Wettability and clot-promoting effects of a number of metal and plastic surfaces were not clearly correlated (ROSE and BROIDA, 1954). When in contact with electrolyte solutions whose pH is in the physiological range, most activating surfaces carry negative ionic charges (zeta potentials) and these are often regarded as responsible for the activation of factor XII. Some years before factor XII was recognized, WOOD et al. (1950) measured the zeta potentials of various particles by their mobility in an electrical field but found no correlation with their clot-promoting potency.

MARGOLIS (1963) thought that this lack of correlation could be explained by the nonhomogeneous nature of solid surfaces which are mostly composed of a mosaic of small areas with different ionic charges. Consequently, electronegative polar sites on a small proportion of the surface may suffice to adsorb and activate the positively charged molecules of factor XII without determining the mobility of the particle in an electrical field. A closer correlation was found between the adsorption of the basic dye toluidine blue by powders, and their clot-promoting and kinin-forming efficacy (Fig. 3). MARGOLIS (1961) reported that activating particles cease to be so when their size is reduced below a threshold value. The effectiveness of dispersions of colloidal silica diminished as the particle size fell below 150 Å, and became negligible at a particle diameter of 40–20 Å. Isolated areas with negative zeta potentials would thus have to be larger than 50 Å.

A different interpretation of the role of negative zeta polar sites was proposed by HUBBARD and LUCAS (1960). In their view these sites lead to an accumulation of blood Ca^{2+} at the solid-fluid interphase; the local high calcium concentration then accelerates clotting. Any role this mechanism may play is unlikely to involve activation or activity of factor XII which does not require calcium. Isolated negative polar sites may explain the activating power of particles with an overall positive charge, but not the inertness of negatively charged particles, such as the nonactivating $BaSO_4$ which carries a greater negative charge than does the activating $BaCO_3$ (Fig. 4). The activating properties of a surface are abolished when its negative potentials are neutralized or inverted by positively charged soluble compounds, like the antiheparin agents hexadimethrine bromide, protamine sulfate, or toluidine blue (HAANEN et al., 1961b; EISEN, 1964a, 1969b; Fig. 4).

Further positively charged inhibitors of factor XII activation were studied by NOSSEL et al. (1968). These included spermine tetrahydrochloride, cytochrome C, ribonuclease, and lysozyme. Protamine, hexadimethrine, *o*-toluidine blue, polylysine, polyornithine, and methyl blue inhibited also later stages of coagulation. Inhibition by polylysine increased with molecular weight ($4{,}000 < 40{,}000 < 400{,}000$). The available evidence thus suggests that negative polar sites are essential for the ability of a surface to activate factor XII. However, the potency of a surface is not determined solely by the magnitude of these negative zeta potentials; more specific properties of the surface seem to be involved.

The changes that the molecules of factor XII undergo during conversion from the preactive to the active state are not yet fully known. RATNOFF and ROSENBLUM (1958) suggested that surfaces act by adsorbing and sequestering from plasma an agent that opposes the activation of factor XII. Such an inhibitor had been found adsorbed onto glass after immersion in plasma lacking factor XII (Hageman trait or duck plasma). MARGOLIS (1957, 1958) at first expressed similar views, but later (MARGOLIS, 1963) thought that negatively charged surfaces lead to a partial, possibly reversible, unfolding of the tertiary structure of the adsorbed factor XII molecule, thus uncovering enzymatic sites. According to VROMAN (1964), adsorption onto polar solids such as glass exposes to the fluid phase a hydrophobic, relatively apolar region of the factor XII molecule which attracts and binds similar apolar sites of factor XI.

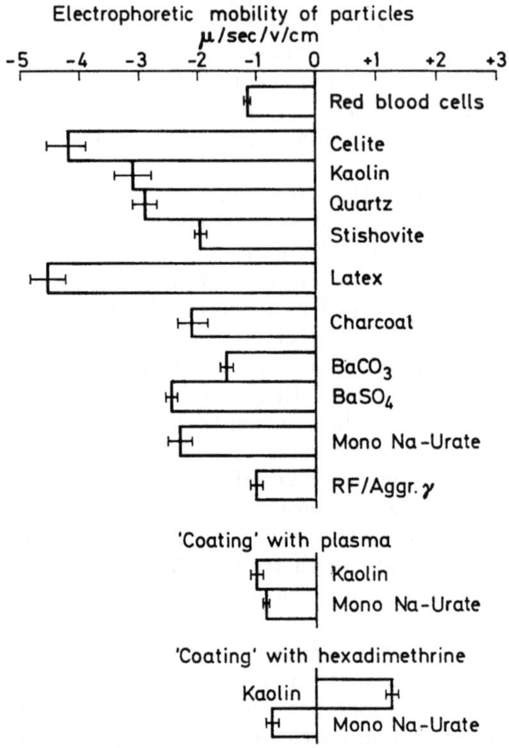

Fig. 4. Particles were suspended in 0.01 M phosphate buffer, pH 7.15, and their electrophoretic mobility measured in a Zeiss cytopherometer at 23° ($\pm$ 0.1). Columns to the left or right give the mean mobility of negatively or positively charged particles respectively. Brackets show the standard deviation of observations. RF/Aggr. γ = precipitated complexes of rheumatoid factor and heat-aggregated human γ-globulin. "Coating" of particles was carried out by mixing particles for 10 minutes with noncontact human plasma, or with a solution of hexadimethrine bromide (1 mg/ml), and then rinsing them thoroughly with buffer. Note the considerable negative charge on latex and $BaSO_4$ which activate factor XII little or not at all. Coating with hexadimethrine bromide, which renders particles nonactivating, reduces or even inverts negative charges. (From EISEN, 1969b)

DONALDSON and RATNOFF (1965) presented evidence for molecular changes of a different type. Ultracentrifugation in sucrose gradients showed that purified preactive factor XII had a sedimentation constant of 4.5–5.5 S. After activation with $BaCO_3$ or ellagic acid, followed by removal of these materials, the activated factor XII behaved in the ultracentrifuge and in a molecular filter gel (Sephadex G-200) like a large, possibly undissolved molecule; its sedimentation constant was now greater than 19 S. The increased sedimentation constant may have been due to lower solubility of active factor XII in aqueous solutions, since activation of factor XII in normal or factor XI-deficient plasma did not change the constant, which remained at 5.0–7.0 S.

Functions of Active Factor XII. Blood clotting. The initiation by active factor XII of the sequence of pre-enzyme–enzyme transformations which eventually leads to blood clotting, has been extensively reviewed in recent years (KLINE, 1965; RATNOFF, 1966; ESNOUF and MACFARLANE, 1968). Even the first step of this sequence, the activation of factor XI (BIGGS et al., 1958; RATNOFF et al., 1961) already has no connection with the intrinsic plasma kinin-forming process; accordingly, contact induces normal kinin formation in plasma deficient in factor XI (MARGOLIS, 1958). This is also true of kinin formation in plasma lacking most other clotting factors.

The suggested catalytic nature of the activation of factor XI by active factor XII (BIGGS et al., 1958; HARDISTY and MARGOLIS, 1959) was supported by kinetic studies with crude preparations (WAALER, 1959) and with more purified factors (RATNOFF et al., 1961). The last study showed that the *yield* of active factor XI was determined by the concentration of factor XI in the system, but not of factor XII. Conversely, the *rate* of activation of factor XI varied with the concentration of factor XII. This evidence for the catalytic nature of this process was strengthened by the inhibitory effect of diisopropyl-phosphofluoridate (DFP). Factor XII may promote blood clotting also by inducing viscous metamorphosis of platelets (BIGGS et al., 1958). This effect is probably due to factor XII which has been found by P. G. IATRIDIS et al. (1964) in the "plasmatic atmosphere" (ROSKAM, 1923) of platelets.

Fibrinolysis. Contact with surfaces that activate factor XII promotes fibrinolytic activity in plasma or plasma euglobulins (SOULIER and PROU-WARTELLE, 1959; IATRIDIS and FERGUSON, 1961, 1962; EISEN, 1961). The phenomenon does not occur in Hageman trait plasma. This has led to claims that factor XII triggers the intrinsic fibrinolytic system in plasma. IATRIDIS and FERGUSON (1961, 1962) concluded on the basis of extensive analyses, that factor XII does not activate plasminogen directly but by interacting with the precursor of plasminogen activator ("proactivator"). Factor XII would thus intervene in fibrinolysis in a manner similar to that of streptokinase. The view was based on differences between Hageman trait plasma and chicken plasma. The lysis of clots made of Hageman trait plasma was accelerated by streptokinase; the response to kaolin was deficient but could be corrected by crude factor XII adsorbed onto kaolin. Chicken plasma responded neither to streptokinase nor to kaolin, and the adsorbed factor XII did not promote fibrinolysis. This suggests that factor XII requires for its fibrinolytic function the same plasma constituent as does streptokinase. Streptokinase forms plasminogen activator not by a catalytic action but by combining stoichiometrically with a fibrinolytic precursor present in the plasma of man and some other species; factor XII may therefore also promote fibrinolysis *not* by acting catalytically but by forming a complex with the same fibrinolytic precursor. The increased factor XII activity induced *in vivo* by severe exercise (IATRIDIS and FERGUSON, 1963) or venous occlusion (HOLEMANS and ROBERTS, 1964) also leads to faster thrombolysis.

Tests with purified factor XII have not confirmed its activating effect on the fibrinolytic system (RATNOFF, 1966; SCHOENMAKERS et al., 1963). These contradictory findings may be due partly to different experimental conditions. The amounts of purified factor XII added to test systems were probably much lower than the large amounts that are activated when the plasma or euglobulin is in contact with silicates. Moreover, when the activating particles remain in the test system, most of the activated factor XII will be adsorbed onto them; and it is probable that, like plasmin, factor XII is less susceptible to its inhibitors when adsorbed than when in solution. RATNOFF (1966) thinks that both factor XII and factor XI may be required for the fibrinolytic response to contact.

Intrinsic Plasma Kinin Formation. The activation of the intrinsic plasma kinin-forming enzymes by glass was described by ARMSTRONG et al. (1954, 1957), who observed the reaction not only in plasma or serum but also in other extracellular fluids containing plasma proteins, for example blister fluid, synovial exudate, ascites, and other effusions. MARGOLIS (1957, 1958) established that this response was associated with the clotting system and depended on factor XII. This was evident from the failure of glass to induce kinin formation (or accelerate clotting) in Hageman trait plasma, although this plasma contained apparently normal levels of kininogen (MARGOLIS, 1960), and of plasma kininogenase (WEBSTER and RATNOFF, 1961; EISEN, 1961, 1963a). Moreover, factor XII was the only clotting factor concerned with the kinin-forming response to contact. The reaction was not detectably affected by the lack of clotting factors II (thrombin), IV (calcium), V, VII, VIII, IX, X, or XI (MARGOLIS, 1960; RATNOFF and MILES, 1964).

Other modes of inducing intrinsic plasma kinin formation also depended on factor XII. Thus, treatment of Hageman trait plasma with dilution, acetone, chloroform, euglobulin separation, acidification to pH 2, or incubation with kininase inhibitors did not lead to normal kinin formation (EISEN and KEELE, 1960; WEBSTER and RATNOFF, 1961; MARGOLIS and BISHOP, 1962). Activation by these chemical agents appeared to be independent of surfaces and could be carried out in silicone-coated vessels. However, later work (EISEN, 1964a) suggested that these procedures acted mainly by weakening the plasma constituents opposing kinin formation; the activation of factor XII seemed still determined by surfaces, even if these were as inert as silicone or polythene. It is generally assumed that factor XII initiates intrinsic plasma kinin formation by catalytically activating another enzyme. Kinetic evidence supporting this view was obtained by RATNOFF and MILES (1964) and is discussed on p. 103. Further support is provided by the action of numerous inhibitors (see p. 97).

The kinin-forming factor, presumably enzyme, with which active factor XII interacts is not yet definitely established. MARGOLIS (1958) at first thought that factor XII itself releases kinin from kininogen. Later he suggested that the adsorbed active factor XII converted a soluble prekininogenase (component A) into active kininogenase, which then attacked the substrate. EISEN (1961, 1963a) found that the distinction by adsorption was not complete, since the kininogenase was also adsorbed onto the activating surfaces. Factor XII proved, however, to be more resistant to 56° than the kininogenase.

More recent hypotheses proposing that factor XII initiates kinin formation by activating an intermediate enzyme such as PF/dil or plasma kininogenase II are discussed on pp. 103 and 117. A different view is put forward by ROCHA E SILVA et al. (1967). These workers think, on the basis of experiments with guinea pig plasma, that factor XII may possibly itself release kinin directly from kininogen.

The role of factor XII in plasma kinin formation was doubted by JOHNSTON and BARROW (1965), who found that euglobulin or protein eluate from glass powder, derived either from human normal or Hageman trait plasma, increased vascular permeability in rabbits equally well. Convincing support *for* such a role was provided by KELLERMEYER and RATNOFF (1967), who demonstrated that rabbit antiserum against purified human factor XII prevented the permeability-increasing effect of this factor XII preparation and the development of permeability factors in normal human plasma exposed to glass. No inhibition was seen when antiserum was added to human plasma *after* exposure to glass. Thus, the antiserum seemed directed against factor XII only, and not against the later stages of the kinin-forming process.

Activation of Complement by Factor XII. DONALDSON (1968) has reported that active factor XII may bring about the conversion of the first component of complement (C′1) to its active form C′1-esterase. In normal plasma, C′1-esterase is rapidly inactivated by its α-globulin inhibitor (PENSKY et al., 1961), and may therefore not be detected. In cases of an inherited deficiency of this inhibitor (hereditary angioneurotic edema), C′1-esterase persists and consumes the fourth and the second component of complement (C′4 and C′2); the esterolytic activity may be demonstrated with the substrate acetyl-tyrosine ethyl ester (ATEe). The activation, but not the activity, of C′1-esterase is inhibited by soybean trypsin inhibitor, heparin, and the proteolytic inhibitor from bovine lung. The results suggest that factor XII does not attack C′1 directly but through triggering the fibrinolytic and kinin-forming reactions in plasma. Plasmin is known to activate C′1 (RATNOFF and NAFF, 1967). If plasma kallikrein is indeed capable, as suggested, of the same activating function, C′1 will be the first natural kallikrein substrate to be found besides kininogen.

Action of Factor XII on Other Substrates. Attempts to confirm the enzymatic nature of factor XII with artificial substrates have not yet produced definite results. Casein, denatured hemoglobin, bovine albumin, egg albumen, β-lactoglobin were not attacked (RATNOFF, 1966). Reports that small-molecular trypsin substrates like tosyl- or benzoyl-arginine esters are hydrolyzed by isolated human factor XII (NIEWIAROWSKI et al. (1956) were not confirmed by RATNOFF et al. (1961) or SPEER et al. (1965). It is possible that the reported hydrolysis was due to contamination with enzymes activated by factor XII, such as factor XI, plasmin, or plasma kininogenases. These enzymes probably also account for the esterolysis observed in normal plasma exposed to silicates (EISEN, 1961, 1963b; SHERRY et al., 1966b).

Esters of substituted lysine are split by normal plasma (SHERRY et al., 1966b) and by purified, partly activated factor XII (RATNOFF, 1966), but the activity is not enhanced by further activation of factor XII. The ***esterolysis*** may therefore be due to another enzyme or to an enzymatic site of factor XII which is not concerned with the activation of factor XI. SCHOENMAKERS et al. (1965) found that their preparation of purified bovine factor XII hydrolyzed arginine esters; again, this activity could be dissociated from the clot-promoting function by inhibitors.

Inhibitors of Factor XII. The fluidity of circulating blood depends in part on the plasma constituent which ensures that factor XII remains preactive in normal conditions. In spite of this most important task, little is known about this factor. RATNOFF and ROSENBLUM (1958) suggested that surfaces activate by dissociating the factor XII–inhibitor complex and adsorbing the inhibitor. This hypothesis was based on findings that Hageman trait plasma inhibited the clotting (RATNOFF and ROSENBLUM, 1958) and kinin-forming (MARGOLIS, 1958) response to glass of normal plasma. The inhibiting protein could be removed from Hageman trait plasma by adsorption onto glass powder. The activating capacity of this glass was then reduced. LOELIGER and HENSEN (1960) and HAANEN et al. (1961a) thought the evidence showed that Hageman trait plasma contained factor XII, which occupied polar sites of surfaces but did not promote clotting. Surfaces also adsorb inhibiting protein from heated normal plasma (MARGOLIS, 1960). Since factor XII is also avidly adsorbed by activating surfaces, it appears that factor and inhibitor compete for binding sites.

Once activated, factor XII is destroyed by an enzyme in plasma (RATNOFF, 1958; MARGOLIS, 1957, 1958) although the adsorbed factor is relatively protected. The inhibitor is probably an α-globulin and an enzyme (RATNOFF and ROSENBLUM, 1958; NOSSEL and NIEMETZ, 1965). It is not removed from plasma by Celite or by procedures which extract lipids. The effects of artificial inhibitors require further study. The divergent results are often caused by difficulties of determining where in the chain of reactions the inhibitor acts.

DFP inhibited in a concentration of 5×10^{-4} M the activity but not the activation of crude human factor XII (RATNOFF et al., 1961). Purer preparations of factor XII were only little inhibited by 5×10^{-2} M DFP (RATNOFF and MILES, 1964). MASON (personal communication) could not detect inhibition of crude adsorbed or eluted guinea pig factor XII by DFP. Active factor XII is inhibited by cysteine, reduced glutathione, and poly-L-lysine, but not by soybean trypsin inhibitor (SBTI), EDTA-Na_3, ε-amino-n-caproic acid (EACA), or benzoyl-L-arginine methyl ester (BAMe) (RATNOFF et al., 1961; RATNOFF, 1966). The anticoagulants heparin (50 U/ml) and polyanetholsulfonate (4 μg/ml) inhibited both the activation and the activity of factor XII (RATNOFF and MILES, 1964), and similar effects were observed with the antiheparin agents toluidine blue, protamine sulfate (8 μg/ml) and hexadimethrine bromide (0.5–8 μg/ml) (HAANEN et al. 1961b; RATNOFF and MILES, 1964). According to EISEN (1964a), the heparin antagonists, in particular hexadimethrine, acted mainly by altering the activating surfaces, and not factor XII.

Activation of Factor XII in vivo. Little is known about the physiological role of factor XII. Hageman trait subjects are not manifestly handicapped by the failure of their blood to respond to abnormal or exogenous surfaces with clotting, fibrinolysis, and kinin formation. With the doubtful exception of slight bleeding, these patients react in seemingly normal, or at least adequate ways, to injury, microbial attacks, immunological challenge, or mechanical irritation.

On the other hand, factor XII seems to contribute to changes in clotting and in fibrinolytic factors which accompany certain physiological activities and stimuli. IATRIDIS and FERGUSON (1963) found that strenuous exercise increased in 30 subjects the factor XII level by 125 to 763% (average 318%); no increase was detected in one Hageman trait subject. Findings that venous occlusion promoted fibrinolysis much more in ten normal persons than in three subjects with Hageman trait, led HOLEMANS and ROBERTS (1964) to the conclusion that this procedure also increases the concentration of factor XII in circulating blood. Thus there is little evidence available that factor XII fulfills a useful function, and the question arises whether it is responsible for any untoward phenomena in pathological conditions. This possibility has stimulated investigations of whether surfaces or other stimuli produced by disease or injury may activate factor XII.

Damaged Tissues. KEELE and EISEN (EISEN, 1964b; see KEELE and ARMSTRONG, 1964) investigated whether contact between blood plasma and freshly damaged tissues might activate factor XII and thus induced kinin formation. Cantharidin blister bases on the forearm were damaged by rubbing them with moistened gauze, and used both as the source of tissue and as a means of detecting kinin formation by the algogenic effect. After the pain caused by the rubbing had subsided, application of fresh noncontact blood or cell-rich plasma caused considerable pain. Areas desensitized to 5-hydroxytryptamine (5-HT) responded with less pain; when these areas were covered with blood containing SBTI, no pain developed. This suggested that the pain was due partly to 5-HT released from platelets, and partly to plasma kallikrein and plasmin. Damaged tissues could activate these proteases by activating factor XII and/or by releasing plasminogen activator. Activation of factor XII seemed to be the more important mechanism, since even complete activation of the fibrinolytic system in blood produced only mild pain on the blister base.

Fatty Acid Salts. The postulated involvement of thrombotic changes in the pathogenesis of arteriosclerosis (DUGUID, 1946, 1948) has invited speculation that various types of lipids may activate factor XII. The acceleration of blood clotting by soaps of fatty acids with chains longer than 12 C-atoms, has been often described (STUBER and HEIM, 1914; POOLE, 1955; PILKINGTON, 1957; O'BRIEN, 1957), and may be produced by plasma concentrations occurring *in vivo* (CONNOR and POOLE, 1961; CONNOR, 1962). PILKINGTON (1957) and CONNOR and POOLE (1961) noticed that formation of thrombi was accelerated only by turbid solutions of fatty acids and thought that it was caused by negatively charged fatty acid ions aggregated into ionic micelles. Clear solutions had no effect. In dogs, intense thrombosis and death were caused by rapid infusions of salts of long-chain (C_{12}–C_{14}) saturated acids, but not by unsaturated acids of the same length, or by shorter saturated acids. The thrombotic effect was attributed to activation of factor XII (CONNOR et al., 1963). DIDISHEIM and MIBASHAN (1963) demonstrated the clot-promoting effect of 0.1 mM solutions of sodium stearate, and found by exclusion of other clotting factors that the salt activated factor XII; calcium was not required. MARGOLIS (1962) reported that the activation of factor XII by fatty acid soaps induced not only clotting but also kinin formation. The potency of the acids increased with chain length between C_8 and C_{22}. Hageman trait plasma did not respond and blocked the effect of the soaps on normal plasma. Calcium inactivated the sodium soaps, probably by converting them into calcium salts. BOTTI and RATNOFF (1963) claim that saturated fatty acid soaps promote clotting not through factor XII but by accelerating the activation of factor XI independently of factor XII. This hypothesis is difficult to reconcile with MARGOLIS' (1963) findings that fatty acid soaps also induce kinin formation, a process in which only clotting factor XII, but not factor XI, is involved.

Skin. Fatty acids in sebum, in particular stearic acid, may be partly responsible for the clot-promoting effect of healthy undamaged skin (NOSSEL, 1966). The effect is dependent on factor XII, and skin probably also activates by virtue of its surface properties.

Collagen. Activation of factor XII is one of several functions which have been attributed to collagen in the formation of the hemostatic plug (MACFARLANE, 1965b). NIEWIAROWSKI et al. (1964) found that collagen from bovine tendon adsorbed clotting factor XII extensively and selectively; factors XI, IX, VIII, VII + X, and V were only slightly adsorbed. High factor XII and some factor XI activity could be eluted from collagen, and the clotting effect demonstrated *in vitro* and *in vivo* in rabbits. DAVIES et al. (1967) found that collagen adsorbed from guinea pig serum a factor XII-like substance which activated partially purified guinea pig prekallikrein. Factor XII may also be activated by the mucopolysaccharides elastin (NIEWIAROWSKI et al., 1966) and chondroitin sulfate (EISEN, 1966b).

Urate Crystals. GARROD (1876) suggested that the urate crystals present in most gouty joint effusions contribute to the symptoms of the acute arthritis. This hypothesis was confirmed in recent years by dramatic experiments in healthy and gouty volunteers and in dogs. Intra-articular injections of suspended monosodium urate microcrystals produced intense acute arthritis (FAIRES and MCCARTY 1962; SEEGMILLER et al., 1962). The inflammatory changes were thought to be the result of the phagocytosis of urate crystals by the white blood cells in the synovial effusions, in the course of which the cells would release their lysosomal enzymes. Since some of these enzymes may induce kinin formation (GREENBAUM and YAMAFUJI, 1966; EISEN and KEELE, 1966), they could possibly account for the kinins detected in spontaneous and experimental gouty effusions (MELMON, et al., 1967). Another mode of promoting and maintaining inflammation was suggested by the finding that these crystals could activate factor XII in plasma (KELLERMEYER and BRECKENRIDGE, 1965) and in synovial exudates (EISEN, 1966b). Like other activating surfaces, monosodium urate crystals carried negative zeta potentials (KELLERMEYER and BRECKENRIDGE, 1965; cf. Fig. 4). The activated factor XII could be detected adsorbed onto the crystals; their activating properties were abolished by coating with hexadimethrine bromide (EISEN, 1966b). Rabbit antibody against human factor XII prevented the response of synovial fluids to crystals (KELLERMEYER, 1967). Compared with glass and other silicates, monosodium urate crystals were only weak activators of factor XII (EISEN, 1968); even so, biologically significant kinin concentrations can be generated. According to KELLERMEYER and BRECKENRIDGE (1965) amorphous particles of monosodium urate were less effective than crystals. This may have been partly due to the different size of particles. When microcrystals were broken up with ultrasound, their activating potency first increased and then decreased (KELLERMEYER, 1967).

Factor XII is present not only in joint effusions but also in normal synovial fluid, and could therefore conceivably *initiate* crystalline synovitis (KELLERMEYER and BRECKENRIDGE, 1966; KELLERMEYER, 1967). Synovial fluid from three healthy donors contained 21–50% of the plasma level of factor XII, and fluid from cadavers, 1–92%. The bulk of the synovial factor XII was in the preactive state and could be activated by ellagic acid or silicates. The precursors of uric acid, xanthine, and hypoxanthine also activate factor XII (EISEN, 1966b).

Crystals of Calcium Salts. Crystals of calcium pyrophosphate dihydrate are deposited in chondrocalcinosis, and when occurring in synovial tissues and spaces may produce the syndrome of pseudogout with episodes of acute arthritis. The pathogenetic mechanism of these attacks resembles acute gouty arthritis; it may involve factor XII, which is activated by these crystals (KELLERMEYER and BRECKENRIDGE, 1965). Arthritis attacks caused by calcium crystals in joints in patients with osteoarthritis and hyperparathyroidism (CURREY et al., 1966) possibly also result from activation of factor XII.

Precipitates Formed by Immune Reactions. DAVIES and LOWE (1960, 1962) reported that precipitated complexes of egg albumen and rabbit anti-egg albumen serum generated in guinea pig serum factors that increased vascular permeability. One part of this activity was inhibited by antihistamine drugs and could be attributed to components of the complement system. The other part was inhibited by SBTI; this could be attributed, in the light of later findings, to proteases mobilized by factor XII. These findings were extended by MOVAT (1967). Complexes of bovine serum albumin and rabbit antibovine serum albumin activated in guinea pig and rabbit serum permeability factors that could both be demonstrated in the supernatant and adsorbed onto the complexes. The activity developed in 5 minutes and persisted for 60 minutes. Its development in serum could be inhibited by a number of complement inhibitors, which was interpreted as evidence that complexes can activate factor XII only after they have fixed complement. Immune precipitates would in that case differ from other particles, most of which are known to activate factor XII in presence of the same complement and kininase inhibitors (ARMSTRONG et al., 1957;

MARGOLIS, 1966; ERDÖS and SLOANE, 1962). It is, however, possible that precipitated antigen–antibody complexes do not activate factor XII as a surface but by a catalytic mechanism for which enzymes of the complement system could well be responsible. The antigen–antibody complexes induced in serum clot-promoting activity and kinin formation confirmed that they activated factor XII.

Precipitates Formed by Aggregated γ-Globulin. Aggregation of 7S γ-globulin (γG or IGG) by heat, cross-linking with tetrazotized benzidine, or other means, results in molecular arrangements which are thought to resemble those occurring *in vivo* when 7S γ-globulins are combining with antigens. Such aggregated γ-globulins are capable of binding some 7S γ-globulin (TORRIGIANI and ROITT, 1967) and complement through the mediation of C′1q (11S component) (ISHIZAKA and ISHIZAKA, 1959; MÜLLER-EBERHARD and KUNKEL, 1961). In rheumatoid arthritis, plasma may contain *rheumatoid factor*, and a group of 19S and 7S globulins (IGM, IGG, and IGA), which form complexes, often precipitating, with aggregated γ-globulin.

EISEN (1969a) has demonstrated that the precipitated complexes formed by aggregated human γ-globulin in normal sera and in sera containing rheumatoid factor, induce kinin formation. The process appeared to involve adsorption and activation of factor XII and plasma kallikrein. Inactivation or inhibition of complement did not reduce the formation of complexes, or the kinin formation by formed complexes. In patients with rheumatoid factor, a soluble or precipitating 22S complex may be formed with the patient's own 7S γ-globulin (FRANKLIN et al., 1959). This complex is thought to play an important role in the pathogenesis of the disease (HOLLANDER et al., 1965). In particular, it may be partly responsible for the kinins found in rheumatoid joint effusions (MELMON et al., 1967; EISEN, 1969a) and these kinins, in turn, responsible for the pain.

Endotoxin Shock. ERDÖS and MIWA (1968) have described a type of activation of factor XII *in vivo*, which does not appear to be due to abnormal surfaces. *E. coli* endotoxin injected intravenously into rabbits activated and consumed factor XII. Glass powder induced the formation of about 95 ng of bradykinin in 1 ml of blood taken before the endotoxin shock. Only negligible amounts of kinin were formed in blood withdrawn 5 minutes after shock, but this blood formed about 60 ng/ml when mixed with glass powder which had adsorbed factor XII from pre-shock blood. Experiments using kinin-destroying carboxypeptidase B suggested that the released kinin was not responsible for the hypotensive effect of the endotoxin.

II. Permeability Factor (PF)

As outlined above, the current concept of the plasma globulins described in the preactive form as pro-PF, and in the active form as PF, is that of a pre-enzyme–enzyme link which occupies an intermediate position in the intrinsic plasma kinin-forming cascade (MILES, 1964). The term PF expressed the ability of these factors to increase the permeability of small vessel walls to proteins. This action was demonstrated by intravenous injection of dyes with a high affinity for plasma albumin (Evans blue, Pontamine sky blue or Trypan blue); the test solutions were then injected intradermally, and the effect on the local vascular permeability assessed by the size and intensity of the blue area of skin caused by leakage of stained plasma albumin (MILES and MILES, 1952). Since the extracellular fluid of the experimental animal or human volunteer contains precursors of all plasma kinin-forming factors, this method does not readily distinguish whether a kinin-forming agent acts as a kininogenase or as an activator of a pre-kininogenase. This is also the case when vascular permeability is studied on the cremaster muscle of the rat (MAJNO et al., 1961; MILES, 1964).

Occurrence of PF. The occurrence of PF in several mammalian species was studied before the present concepts of PF had evolved. As a result, the necessary differentiation of PF from factor XII and from plasma kininogenase has been attempted so far only in guinea pig and human plasma (MASON and MILES, 1962; KAGEN et al., 1963a, b; RATNOFF and MILES, 1964).

While searching for endogenous factors associated with the vascular changes of inflammation, MACKAY et al. (1953) observed that *guinea pig* serum, diluted in glass vessels 30 to 400 times with saline, generated within 10–12 minutes an agent which on intradermal injection increased the permeability of the local small vessels. The activity was described as PF by dilution (PF/dil). A PF/age, apparently distinct from PF/dil, developed when undiluted serum was allowed to age. A heat-labile, slow-acting inhibitor (IPF) was also found (MILES and WILHELM, 1955; WILHELM et al., 1955). In the *rat*, optimal activation of PF/dil was found in sera diluted up to 100 times. Rat serum contained a slow-acting IPF (SPECTOR, 1956; WILHELM et al., 1958). Dilution of *rabbit* serum generated little or no PF. However, the α- and β-globulins separated by cold ethyl ether contained a PF that acted slowly in rabbit skin, and quickly in rat and guinea pig skin. The serum contained a weak, slow-acting IPF (PASKHINA, 1956; WILHELM et al., 1958). *Human* serum, diluted 50 times in glass containers, developed a PF in 2–6 hours; 100–1,000-fold dilution of serum activated the PF after 1–4 days. The human PF was assayed in man by STEWART and BLISS (1957), and in the guinea pig by ELDER and WILHELM (1958).

Purification and Chemistry. Most of the attempts to isolate globulin PF from mammalian blood were based on the method developed by KEKWICK and MACKAY (1954) in which plasma is fractionated by cold ethyl ether at strictly controlled ionic strengths, pH, and temperature. It was soon established that pro-PF was activated in the course of this fractionation.

Fractionation of *guinea pig* plasma left the bulk of PF in the α-globulins. From these, PF could be further purified by repeated precipitation at pH 5 and low ionic strength, or by electrophoresis (WILHELM et al. 1955, 1957). Guinea pig PF proved to be an α_2-globulin, and IPF a heat labile α_1-globulin. The purest preparations of PF still contained kininogenase activity. However, MASON and MILES (1962) succeeded in removing this activity by exposure to pH 3.5 for 3 hours and then to 56° for 30 minutes. The resulting preparation still increased vascular permeability, and activated the prekininogenase in fresh noncontact plasma, but did not release kinin from kininogen. The PF in *rat* serum was also an α-globulin, while IPF was detected with α_1-globulin and albumin (WILHELM et al., 1958). *Rabbit* PF (activated by ether fractionation, but not by dilution) was associated with the α- and β-globulins; IPF was an albumin (PASKHINA, 1956; WILHELM et al., 1958). Exposure to 65° for 30 minutes reduced little or not at all the potency of isolated guinea pig, rat, and rabbit PF (WILHELM et al., 1957, 1958).

Human PF was found in a lipid-rich β_1-globulin fraction; the lipid could be removed without loss of potency (MILL et al., 1958). To obtain this PF, the plasma protein remaining after removal of fibrinogen was treated with 18.5% ethyl ether, at ionic strength 0.035, −3.5°, and pH 6.5. The precipitate was reprecipitated three times in water at pH 6.3 and 5.1, and ionic strength 0.006 and 0.01. This yielded a β-globulin which was virtually homogeneous on electrophoresis, and differed from plasmin by its lability at pH 2 or at 60°. However, heating mainly destroyed the contained kininogenase, and was therefore later exploited for abolishing this activity in PF preparations. The presence in human plasma of enzymes with the properties postulated for PF has in recent years been demonstrated by ion-exchange chromatography, electrophoresis, and gel filtration. Two peaks of permeability activity could be separated in human serum by starch block electrophoresis and by chromatography on DEAE-cellulose (KAGEN et al., 1963a, b). One, a γ-globulin with a sedimentation constant $S_{20w}=10.1–12.2$, was a kininogenase and resembled plasma kallikrein. The other, a β-globulin whose $S_{20w}=5.2–6.6$, activated plasma prekininogenase, but did not release kinin from kininogen (KAGEN, 1964); it was therefore identified with PF.

Activation of pro-PF. The early views that pro-PF is activated by dilution were modified when the important contribution of the glass surface of containers was recognized (MARGOLIS, 1958, 1959; MILES, 1958/59). SPECTOR (1957) was unable to detect PF in plasma diluted in silicone-coated vessels, a finding reflected in MILES' (1964) statement that "exposure to glass is the essence of the activation of PF/dil." However, this impression seems merely due to the fact that the enzymatic activities mobilized by dilution in siliconized or plastic vessels are too small to be detected by permeability tests; the kinin formation resulting from such dilution is easily measured on isolated organs (EISEN, 1963a, 1964a).

The postulated activation of pro-PF by activated factor XII was studied in detail by RATNOFF and MILES (1964). A mixture of preactive and active human factor XII, purified 3,000 to 5,000 times (RATNOFF and DAVIE, 1962), induced PF-like activity in human plasma and in a concentrate of human pro-PF. Pretreatment with ellagic acid increased the effectiveness of the partly activated factor XII. Its effect on pro-PF had the following characteristics of an enzymatic reaction: the *rate* of activation of pro-PF was at $0° < 25° < 37° < 45°$, and increased with higher concentrations of factor XII. The maximum final *yield* of PF was a function of the amount of pro-PF in the system, but not of active factor XII.

Functional Properties of PF. It is clear from the developments discussed earlier in this chapter that PF is now regarded as an enzyme whose natural substrate is a plasma prekininogenase. Although activation of plasma prekallikrein by PF is usually presented as an enzymatic process, definite kinetic proof is not yet available. The enzymatic nature of PF is, however, supported by evidence that it hydrolyzes synthetic esters of arginine acylated at the α-NH_2 group, and is protected by such ester substrates from inhibition by DFP (BECKER et al., 1959; KAGEN, 1964).

Inhibition of PF. PF generated in mammalian plasma or sera is inactivated by plasma inhibitors (IPF). The chemistry of the IPF in different species is discussed on p. 102. Their detailed mode of action is not yet known. IPF's seem to be closely related to the inhibitors of some other proteolytic enzymes in plasma. In some cases, inhibition of different proteases may be due to the same inhibitor. Thus, human IPF inhibits plasmin and trypsin (MILL et al., 1958). On the other hand, human PF (and to a lesser degree plasma kallikrein) is inhibited by the inhibitor of the activated first component of complement (C′1-esterase), which may be identical with IPF (BECKER and KAGEN, 1964; KAGEN, 1964). The inhibitor of C′1-esterase is a heat-labile α_2-globulin which acts by combining stoichiometrically with the enzyme (DONALDSON, 1966).

PF shares with plasmin, plasma kallikrein, and trypsin numerous exogenous and synthetic inhibitors, such as the trypsin inhibitors from soybeans and from the pancreas, and DFP (WILHELM et al., 1957, 1958). These inhibitors were studied in experimental conditions which did not always reveal whether PF, or later stages of the plasma kinin-forming process were inhibited. In a few instances, the site of inhibition could be more accurately determined, and PF differentiated in this way from other enzymes. Thus, protamine sulfate (8 μg/ml), sodium polyanetholsulfonate (4 μg/ml), hexadimethrine bromide (0.5–8 μg/ml), and heparin (50–200 units/ml) which inhibited the activity, and possibly activation of factor XII (see p. 98), did not inhibit PF (Elder and Wilhelm, 1958; Ratnoff and Miles, 1964). Higher concentrations of heparin were, however, effective against the later stages of plasma kinin formation. A heparin concentration of 320 units/ml inhibited PF by 50%; plasma kallikrein was inhibited to that degree only by 1,950 units/ml (McConnell et al., 1965). The different sensitivity to heparin was used as a further criterion of distinguishing PF from plasma kallikrein.

Biological Role of PF. Activation of pro-PF by factor XII is the only mode of generating PF so far described (Miles, 1964). Similarly, the actions of PF on the caliber and permeability of venules and capillaries are now entirely ascribed to the activation by PF of prekininogenase, and ultimate plasma kinin formation (Mason and Sparrow, 1965). The biological importance of active PF is therefore fully covered by the discussions of the activation and functions of factor XII, and of the effects of plasma kininogenases and kinins on living structures.

III. Plasmin (EC 3.4.4.14)

The fibrinolytic system has in the last three decades been the subject of extensive studies. The vast literature has been analyzed in numerous recent reviews in which the reader may obtain information on every aspect and constituent of this system (Macfarlane and Biggs, 1948; Sherry et al., 1959; v. Kaulla, 1963; Stafford, 1964; Fearnley, 1965; Pechet, 1965; Webster and Innerfield, 1965; Ambrus, 1966). Only features relevant to the role of the fibrinolytic system in plasma kinin formation will be briefly discussed here.

The main biological task of the fibrinolytic system is dissolution of unwanted clotted blood. Not only the fibrin strands in thrombi and emboli are digested but also the fibrin, which is believed to form continuously along the endothelial lining of vessels. In addition to these strictly fibrinolytic functions, the system is occasionally responsible for the consumption of clotting factors and the formation of clot-inhibiting substances, the digestion of hormones in blood, the mobilization of the complement system, the degradation of cartilage matrix and breakdown of protein–mucopolysaccharide complexes, and the formation of plasma kinins. The final operative agent in all these functions is the proteolytic enzyme *plasmin*. The fact that plasmin can assume such a diversity of roles in normal and morbid processes is a reflection of the complex and profound influences which environmental factors exert on this enzyme. Prominent among these factors is the avid adsorption of plasminogen and of its activator onto fibrin strands, where they are dissociated and/or protected from the potent inhibitors in plasma. The adsorbed plasmin then digests the fibrin, while the circulating plasmin is prevented by inhibitors from attacking its soluble protein substrates. In this way, the broad-spectrum protease plasmin functions as a relatively specific fibrinolytic agent.

Purification and Chemistry of Plasminogen. Plasminogen has been isolated by numerous methods. Several of these use as starting material the plasma fractions which contain α- and β-lipoprotein globulins. Such fractions are Cohn fraction III precipitated by 17% cold ethanol at pH 5.2 or fraction P precipitated by 10% cold ethyl ether at pH 5.3 (Kekwick et al., 1946; Kekwick and Mackay, 1954). Owing to its remarkable stability at acid pH values, it was possible to extract plasminogen from these fractions by dilute acids. Further purification was achieved by various combinations of heating, reprecipitation at pH 5.0–5.6 or at pH 8.5, or by ion-exchange chromatography and gel filtration. Plasminogen, which has in the course of preparation been exposed to an acid pH, is soluble and fairly stable at pH 2–3.5. Its instability and poor solubility in the neutral pH range can be impro ved by adding lysine to the solvent.

Plasminogen has also been isolated from plasma without exposure to acid pH's, by procedures involving chromatography on DEAE-cellulose and elution with lysine buffer (DERECHIN, 1962), or solubilization with ε-aminohexanoic acid (ALKJAERSIG, 1964). The resulting plasminogen is soluble at neutral pH and appears to have a lower SVEDBERG constant than acid-treated preparations.

Human plasminogen is a β-globulin whose molecular weight is about 143,000 (SHULMAN et al., 1958). Its molecule contains 5% hexose, 2.8% hexosamines, and 0.6% sialic acid (SLOTTA and GONZALEZ, 1964).

Activation of Plasminogen. Plasmin itself is a slow activator of plasminogen. Plasminogen solutions stabilized by 50% glycerol or by di- or triethylene glycol, are autocatalytically converted to plasmin in 3 to 4 days. Trypsin also activates plasminogen. Factors that promote the activation of plasminogen to plasmin are found in most tissues and body fluids (ASTRUP, 1966). ALI and LACK (1965) purified and studied a lysosomal enzyme from renal and other tissues which activated plasminogen. It was named cytokinase, and unlike most other lysosomal enzymes, it was active at neutral pH values. A very similar proteolytic enzyme is urokinase, which is found in urine and activates plasminogen by a direct catalytic action.

Most instances of raised fibrinolytic activity in plasma are due to higher blood levels of plasminogen activators, rather than of plasmin itself (SHERRY et al., 1959). These activators may be released into the blood stream from vessel walls and other tissues. The role of clotting factor XII as a plasminogen activator is discussed on p. 95. Factor XII probably contributes to the slow activation of plasminogen that occurs in human plasma whose plasmin inhibitors had been destroyed by chloroform.

Bacterial plasminogen activators are of great pathological importance; some of them are used clinically in the treatment of thromboembolic disease and for the clearance of other fibrin deposits. The cell-free filtrate or supernatant of cultures of growing streptococci belonging to LANCEFIELD's groups A, human C, and G contains *streptokinase* which activates human plasminogen very effectively; rabbit, monkey, dog, and cat plasminogen moderately or weakly; and bovine and pig plasminogen not at all. ASTRUP (1956) interpreted this difference in the response of various species as evidence that human and other activated plasmas contained a "proactivator," which was absent from unresponsive plasmas. Proactivator has not yet been unequivocally demonstrated. Most experimental findings can be adequately explained by assuming that streptokinase combines stoichiometrically with the plasminogen or plasmin of man and certain other species, but not with the ox or pig enzyme. The resulting complex is usually described as *plasminogen activator*, and its enzymatic properties differ from those of plasmin. The binding with streptokinase greatly enhances the ability of plasmin to activate plasminogen. Since most fibrinogen preparations contain plasminogen, the complex becomes a highly effective fibrinolytic agent. In contrast, the activity against protein substrates such as casein is progressively reduced as the concentration of streptokinase is increased (MARKUS and WERKHEISER, 1964). In this way, potent fibrinolytic preparations with negligible caseinolytic activity may be obtained. Staphylococci of several strains produce an enzyme *staphylokinase* which catalytically activates plasminogen of several species (LACK, 1948).

SHULMAN et al. (1958) reported that the molecular weight of human plasminogen was reduced on activation with glycerol, streptokinase, or urokinase by 24, 16, or 11% respectively. DAVIES and ENGLERT (1960) and ROBBINS et al. (1965) found no change in molecular weight on activation. ROBBINS et al. (1967) and SUMMARIA et al. (1967) think that only one arginyl-valine bond is split in the process. Several of these activators have been used for the preparation of plasmin. Highly purified preparations have been obtained by autocatalysis of plasminogen in the presence of glycerol, to stabilize the nascent plasmin. Alternatively, plasminogen is activated by streptokinase or urokinase which is later removed.

Chemistry of Plasmin. Plasmin has been prepared from plasminogen of several mammalian plasmas, but most studies have been conducted with human or bovine material. When subjected to electrophoresis, human plasmin migrates as a β-globulin. Plasmins activated by different methods appear to have different molecular weights; values in the range of 89,000 to 125,000 have been reported. Prominent among the chemical properties of plasmin is its remarkable stability at pH 2–3, where it withstands temperatures up to 100°. Its enzymatic activities proceed optimally at pH 7.4–8.4.

The substrate specificity of plasmin closely resembles that of trypsin, although quantitative differences have been reported. Numerous important proteins and polypeptides circulating in blood are attacked by plasmin. These include the clotting factors V, VIII, and IX; the hormones ACTH, growth hormone, and glucagon; components of the complement system; and constituents of the intrinsic plasma kinin-forming system. Plasmin also digests exogenous proteins such as denatured hemoglobin, gelatin, and casein. Some of these are used for measuring plasmin activity. The peptide bonds hydrolyzed by plasmin in these substrates appear to contain in all cases a carboxyl group supplied by an arginine or lysine residue. This has been deduced from the effects of plasmin on small-molecular synthetic esters of amino acids; only those of arginine and lysine are cleaved.

SHERRY et al. (1966a) reported that in contrast to trypsin and thrombin, human and bovine plasmin hydrolyzed lysine esters at higher rates than arginine esters. The MICHAELIS-MENTEN constant (K_m) at pH 7.6 was for a number of these esters of the order of 10^{-3} to 10^{-2} M, the lowest being 2.2×10^{-3} for BAMe. EISEN (1969c) found that human plasmin split BAEe at pH 8.0 with a K_m of 5×10^{-4} M and at pH 8.7 with a K_m of 3×10^{-4}. The hydrolysis of amides of acylated arginine has been denied (ABLONDI and HAGAN, 1960; KLINE, 1966).

Kinetic analyses of the esterolytic effects of plasmin (RONWIN, 1962a, b) according to DIXON (1953) and LAIDLER (1955) suggested that the active center of plasmin contained the sequence Gly-Asp-Ser-Gly, which has also been postulated for trypsin, chymotrypsin, thrombin, kallikreins, and other hydrolases.

Assays of Fibrinolytic Factors. Numerous methods for measuring every constituent of the fibrinolytic system have been developed. The very important and very difficult task of assaying the fibrinolytic activity in circulating blood can be attempted by observing the lysis of clots of *diluted plasma* (MACFARLANE, 1937) or *diluted blood* (FEARNLEY et al., 1957). These methods give an insight into the balance of factors promoting and opposing fibrinolysis. The lysis of plasma or serum *euglobulin clots* is an assay system largely free of inhibitors. All these methods measure both plasmin and plasminogen activator levels in plasma. This is also the case when fibrin plates or standard clots are used as substrate, since most fibrinogen preparations are contaminated with plasminogen. However, this plasminogen can be selectively destroyed by heating (ASTRUP and MÜLLERTZ, 1952). Also, fibrinogen essentially free of plasminogen has been prepared. The lysis of such heated or purified fibrin expresses plasmin activity only. The use of fibrinogen labeled with fluorescein or with I^{131} has been recommended for more accurate and sensitive assaying of fibrinolytic activity. The hydrolysis of both fibrinogen and fibrin may also be measured by the release of acid-soluble peptides.

Among various protein substrates, casein is the most widely used. Caseinolytic activity is often expressed in units based on the amount of tyrosine released. Such units were defined by KUNITZ (1947; 150 μg tyrosine/minute), REMMERT and COHEN (1949; 450 μg/hour), and ALKJAERSIG et al. (1959; 180 μg tyrosine/hour). The hydrolysis of synthetic arginine and lysine esters by plasmin is easily measured, and several methods suitable for continuous recording are available. The rates of hydrolysis are best expressed in international units (μmoles of substrate/minute).

Inhibitors of the Fibrinolytic System. A large number of natural and synthetic substances inhibit one or more phases of the fibrinolytic process. Blood itself contains a potent array of inhibiting factors, which are sometimes described as "antiplasmins." MACFARLANE and PILLING (1946) found that on precipitation of the plasma euglobulins, plasmin inhibitors remained in the supernatant. RATNOFF et al. (1954) distinguished three plasmin inhibitors, two of which were heat-stable. NORMAN (1958, 1966) described a heat-stable, immediately and reversibly inhibiting α_2-globulin, and a slowly and irreversibly acting α_1-globulin. The equilibrium between the inhibitors and the fibrinolytic potential in plasma is one of the most important factors controlling the functioning of the fibrinolytic system. Normally, the inhibitors have a considerably greater capacity than the enzymes. According to NORMAN (1958) this excess is 30-fold. SHERRY et al. (1959) reported that human plasma can inhibit a plasmin concentration releasing from casein about 0.9 mg of tyrosine/ml/hour; plasma in which the plasminogen had been fully activated by streptokinase released 0.7 mg/ml/hour. The inhibitory capacity of the plasma inhibitors was also evident from the finding that whole undiluted plasma activated by streptokinase released 0.07–0.45 mg/ml/hour, and the separated euglobulin fraction (essentially free of inhibitors) 0.7–1.4 mg/ml/hour (SGOURIS et al., 1960). Antiplasmins are thought to be distinct from the inhibitors of trypsin, plasma kallikreins, and C′1-esterase.

Mammalian tissues also contain several factors that inhibit fibrinolysis. Some of these, notably the inhibitor from bovine lung, are in clinical use. These and other proteolytic inhibitors have been recently reviewed by VOGEL et al. (1966). Many trypsin inhibitors, obtained from plants or synthetically, also inhibit plasmin. In some cases, considerable quantitative differences have been reported. Of clinical importance are inhibitors of plasminogen *activation*, such as EACA, 1-(aminomethyl)cyclohexane-4-carboxylic acid (AMCHA), and *p*-aminomethylbenzoic acid (PAMBA). EACA prevents the activation of plasminogen by streptokinase and urokinase (ALKJAERSIG et al., 1959), and by contact with surfaces (EISEN, 1963b), but not the activation occurring when plasma is incubated with chloroform (DONALDSON and RATNOFF, 1962).

Activation of Pre-Kallikrein by Plasmin. The overall contribution of the fibrinolytic system to intrinsic plasma kinin formation is discussed below. As outlined there, plasmin may act both as a kininogenase and as an activator of plasma prekallikreins. These two modes of inducing kinin formation were not distinguished in some of the early studies, which gave rise to divergent conclusions. Another source of disagreement was that the plasmin used was mostly obtained by activating plasminogen with high concentrations of streptokinase. As mentioned before, the stoichiometric complex of plasmin and streptokinase, usually termed plasminogen activator, has properties very different from those of plasmin itself (Markus and Werkheiser, 1964). When plasmin combines with streptokinase, its actions on prekallikreins and on kininogen are reduced as are the actions on casein (Eisen, 1963b). Indeed, streptokinase concentrations of 3,000–5,000 U-ml inhibit not only plasma kinin formation by plasmin but also by glass. This inhibition is evident long before a given sample of plasmin or plasma is fully saturated with streptokinase.

The possibility that plasmin is an activator of plasma prekallikrein was first considered by Webster and Pierce (1960). Their experiments led them to the conclusion that the fibrinolytic system plays a very small role in the generation of kallikrein in acetone-treated plasma, and after separation of the euglobulin fraction.

The dual role of plasmin in intrinsic plasma kinin formation emerged from comparisons of its effects on substrates containing prekininogenases, and on substrates from which prekininogenases had been removed. Eisen (1961, 1963b) found that mixtures of human plasmin and streptokinase (Thrombolysin; Merck, Sharf and Dohme) formed kinin at faster rates in fresh noncontact plasma than in plasma heated at 56° for 3 hours. The caseinolytic potency of the Thrombolysin concentrations used in these experiments was $^1/_3$ to $^1/_2$ of the caseinolytic potential in human plasma. Heating of Thrombolysin solutions at 100° and pH 2 for 20 minutes abolished their fibrinolytic effect but not the caseinolytic and kininogenase activities. The findings did not exclude the presence in Thrombolysin of other activators, such as clotting factor XII or PF/dil. However, the evidence that plasmin was both a kininogenase and an activator could be confirmed with highly purified glycerol-activated human plasmin. This was prepared by the method of Sgouris et al. (1960), which includes prolonged exposure to heat and acidity.

Vogt (1964) found that the kinin formation induced in dog pseudoglobulin by a mixture of human plasmin and streptokinase was largely due to activation of prekallikreins. When these had been destroyed by heating the pseudoglobulin at 56° for 2 hours, the fibrinolytic preparation did not induce kinin formation. Added to pseudoglobulin which had been activated by acidification to pH 2.1 for 15 minutes, the plasmin preparation accelerated only little the spontaneous generation of kinin. The activation of prekallikrein by plasmin was confirmed by inhibiting the formed kallikrein with DFP, and measuring the remaining prekallikrein. The activation of plasma prekallikrein by plasmin may be regarded as an instance of enzymatic amplification. It is therefore very likely that this mode of action is more efficient than the direct attack of plasmin on kininogen.

In certain pathological conditions, the extreme activation of the fibrinolytic factors in plasma will overwhelm the plasmin inhibitors, and free plasmin appears in blood. This has been observed in antepartum hemorrhage, abortion, retention of the dead fetus, abruptio placentae, and amniotic fluid embolism; cirrhosis of the liver and hepatic failure; cancer of the prostate; surgery of the lung, liver, or prostate; extracorporeal circulation; transfusions with incompatible blood; acute myeloblastic leukemia; shock etc. (Sharp, 1964; Back, 1966). In these conditions, the free circulating plasmin digests fibrinogen, clotting factors, and other plasma proteins and may rise sufficiently to act not only on prekallikreins but also on kininogens. Therapeutic infusions of human antihemophilic globulin concentrates have occasionally given rise to adverse circulatory effects. This has been attributed to their content of a plasminogen activator, inducing kinin formation, in the blood of the patient (Mackay et al., 1962). However, other proteases may contribute to the symptoms. The antihemophilic concentrates also contain an active kininogenase resembling kallikrein, preplasmin, and C′1-esterase (Eisen, 1965; Mackay et al., 1965; Eisen and Keele, 1966).

D. Kininogenases

I. Plasma Kallikrein (EC 3.4.4.21)

Definition. KRAUT et al. (1928, 1933) detected kallikrein in the blood. Originally, it was thought to be the same substance as pancreatic kallikrein. In fact the EC 3.4.4.21 refers to all kallikreins in tissues and body fluids. However, it is now established that serum kallikrein is different from glandular kallikreins. Further, even in serum itself more than one enzyme is capable of kinin formation. These have been distinguished by their mode of activation, by chemical differences, by their susceptibility to inhibitors, and by their substrate specificity.

In view of the existence of several serum kininogenases the term kallikrein will be used here for the kininogenase(s) which occur in plasma or serum of mammals as pre-enzyme and can be prepared in active form by treatment with acetone or acid, as first described by KRAUT et al. (1933). Kallikrein is synonymous with human serum kininogenase I (VOGT, 1966; VOGT et al., 1967). This definition is in accord with historical development as well as current use. It may not be unequivocal, because other kininogenases may also be activated by one or the other of the treatments mentioned. Serum kallikrein would then be better defined by its substrate specificity. It could possibly be described as the specific serum enzyme that reacts with the kininogen present in human, bovine, or dog serum and left there after the consumption of other kininogen(s) by glass contact (kininogen I of VOGT et al., 1967; kininogen II of YANO et al., 1967a).

Occurrence and Activation. Serum kallikrein has been found in all *mammalian* species investigated, in varying amounts. Hog serum has the highest, and bovine serum the lowest, content (Table 2). Kininogenases have also been detected in some *nonmammalian* plasmas. Fowl and other birds possess kininogenases ("ornithokallikreins") which release kinins ("ornithokinins") only from avian plasmas. WERLE and VOGEL (cf. FREY et al., 1968, p. 27) mention the presence

Table 2. *Serum kallikrein content after activation of sera from different species*[a]

Serum	Kallikrein content (units/ml)
Hog	10
Rat	5
Man	3—4
Dog	1—2
Ox	0,6

[a] From FREY et al. (1968), p. 25.

of an ornithokallikrein in hen serum. The Peking duck and domestic pigeon lack a plasma factor responsive to glass and other surfaces, which could correspond to factor XII. They possess however, according to ERDÖS et al. (1967) prekininogenases, since plasma kinin formation can be induced by acidification of plasma to pH 3 for 30 minutes, or by glass which had adsorbed factor XII from alligator plasma. Several reptile species, such as the common snapping turtle, the elegant slider turtle, and the alligator, possess a complete intrinsic plasma kinin-forming system responsive to contact (ERDÖS et al., 1967).

A kininogenase similar to plasma kallikrein has also been found outside the plasma, in guinea pig lung tissue. The enzyme is thought to have been adsorbed onto the lung vessel walls from plasma, or to have originated from lung tissue (JONASSON and BECKER, 1966).

As mentioned before, plasma kallikrein is normally present as an inactive pre-enzyme. This is not an enzyme–inhibitor complex as was assumed originally (WERLE, 1936). Rather, the prekallikrein is a single protein that can be converted to the active state by unknown molecular changes (WERLE et al., 1955). A purified prekallikrein preparation has not yet been prepared.

Experimental activation can be effected by various chemical treatments of serum, or by the addition of proteolytic enzymes. Among the latter, trypsin is most generally used (WERLE et al., 1955; WERLE and VOGEL, 1960). It gives a good yield of kallikrein activity. However, the fact must be considered that trypsin is itself a kininogenase and affects the blood pressure assay of kallikrein. WERLE et al. (1955) suggest the use of 1 mg trypsin/ml plasma. This concentration is high enough to overcome inactivation by serum inhibitors and, on the other hand, is thought to be sufficiently small not to interfere with the assay of kallikrein. Higher concentrations of trypsin may inactivate the kallikrein in whole serum (WERLE, 1960). A protease preparation from rice also activates serum prekallikrein (WERLE et al., 1955). Further, papain and plasmin have the same effect (KRAUT et al., 1928; WERLE and KORSTEN, 1938; BACK, 1960; BHOOLA et al., 1960; COPLEY, 1963; VOGT, 1964).

Treatment of serum or plasma with acetone, alcohol, or other organic solvents uncovers active kallikrein (KRAUT et al., 1933; WEBSTER and PIERCE, 1961; EISEN, 1963a; MORIYA et al., 1965). Dilution also leads to the appearance of kinin-forming activity, although in this case the identity with kallikrein has not been proved. Another mode of activating prekallikrein is acidification of plasma (KRAUT et al., 1933; WERLE, 1936; EISEN, 1963a). The yield is lower than that obtained by acetone treatment. This is probably due to the reported lability of serum kallikrein in an acid medium.

When a casein solution is added to serum and is precipitated by acidification of the mixture, the precipitate develops active kallikrein on redissolution in alkali (WERLE, 1936). JACOBSEN (1966a) and WEBSTER and PIERCE (1960) found active serum kallikrein mainly in the pseudoglobulin fraction, precipitated between 33 and 45% saturation with ammonium sulfate. Numerous other compounds induce kininogenase activity when added to plasma, particularly acidic polysaccharides (see e.g. ROTHSCHILD and GASCON, 1966). It is likely, however, that in these cases the activated enzyme is primarily kininogenase II. During contact with glass, serum kallikrein is also activated (besides kininogenase II); however, it does not become very effective, because of rapid inactivation (VOGT, 1966; VOGT et al., 1967).

The various chemical treatments of serum mentioned earlier probably do not convert the prekallikrein directly–e.g. by some kind of denaturation or physical dissociation from an inhibitor moiety. Rather, they activate one or more other endogenous serum enzymes which in turn act on prekallikrein. Thus, acetone and acid are ineffective in plasma from patients deficient in Hageman factor (EISEN and KEELE, 1960; WEBSTER and RATNOFF, 1961). The casein-precipitated preparations are not fully active immediately after redissolution, but their activity increases on standing (WERLE, 1936). With ammonium sulfate precipitation, a good yield of kallikrein activity is obtained only when it is repeated several times. WERLE (1936) assumes that the fractionation by casein or ammonium sulfate separates activating enzyme together with prekallikrein from their inhibitors. When ammonium sulfate is used, this separation is achieved only after several precipitations.

Little is known about the activating enzyme(s) contained in plasma except that in some cases at least Hageman factor is involved and probably PF/dil

(Miles, 1964; Webster, 1966). The active site of kallikrein is probably uncovered by a proteolytic process. Chemical treatments which activate prekallikrein are known to increase the proteolytic activity of plasma. The activation mechanism appears, therefore, to be similar to that induced by trypsin, plasmin, or papain. Activation by trypsin can proceed without the mediation of Hageman factor (Webster and Ratnoff, 1961). Plasmin, which is an endogenous plasma enzyme, may be involved in some of the activation procedures by chemical agents. However, acetone and acid activate serum kallikrein independently of plasmin (Webster and Pierce, 1960; Eisen, 1963b). Acid-treated human plasma does not exhibit fibrinolytic activity; inhibitors of plasminogen activation do not inhibit activation of the plasma kinin-forming system by contact and other means (Eisen, 1963b). In inflammatory reactions, plasma kallikrein is thought to be activated either by the lowering of the pH in the inflamed area (Lewis, 1964b), by unknown mechanisms accompanying tissue injury and leading to an increase in the proteolytic potential in plasma, or by a process similar to contact activation, taking place in the interstitial fluid of the injured tissue after the escape of prekallikrein from the vascular bed (Graham et al., 1965; Webster and Innerfield, 1965). These are, however, only hypothetical possibilities which have not yet been fully established. The participation of kinins in inflammatory reactions is still a matter of controversy. Even if the occurrence of kinins had been clearly demonstrated, this would not necessarily indicate increased activity of plasma kallikrein. A decrease of carboxypeptidase activity in plasma or tissue fluid—plausible because of decreased pH in the inflamed area—could cause a shift in the equilibrium between the formation and destruction of kinins toward higher kinin levels (Lewis, 1964a) (p. 516). On the other hand, the possibility of such a shift has been disputed by Trautschold et al. (cited from Frey et al., 1968, p. 223), who found with decreasing pH a parallel decrease in the kininase and the kallikrein activities in plasma.

Edery and Lewis (1963) observed an increase of active kininogenase in lymph coming from injured tissue. The activation seemed to depend on the previous liberation of histamine. Injection of histamine or of compound 48/80 led to the same increase of kinin-forming enzyme in lymph as that in injury caused by burning, freezing, mechanical pressure, or ischemia, though with a different time course. The permeability-increasing effect of histamine might explain an escape of plasma prekallikrein from the blood vessels and its penetration into the tissue spaces where it could be activated by injured structures. However, histamine apparently exerted a more specific effect, for mepyramine (pyrilamine) blocked the appearance of kinin-forming enzyme in the lymph, but not the increase in the protein content following local injury. Whether the enzyme observed was plasma kallikrein, is not known.

Jacobsen and Waaler (1965, 1966) and Jacobsen (1966b) interpreted the events in lymph from injured limbs in a different way. According to these workers, normal dog and rabbit lymph contained the same kininogens as plasma; their concentration was normally lower than in plasma but increased after scalding of the limb. Kinin-forming enzymes or free kinins were found neither before nor after scalding. Lowered plasma levels of kininogen have been found in various types of shock (see p. 279). This has been taken as evidence of an activation of plasma kallikrein. However, other kininogenases might also be responsible for the consumption of kininogen. Moreover, kininogen could disappear by nonspecific proteolysis, not involving kininogenases and not leading to kinin formation.

Changes in the Plasma Content of Prekallikrein. Like most other plasma proteins, plasma prekallikrein is synthesized in the liver. Extirpation of parts of this organ leads to a decrease of the concentration in plasma (WERLE and VORWALTER, cited from FREY et al., 1968). In hepatitis the prekallikrein level is also low (FORELL, 1957). Cortisone raises the plasma concentration of prekallikrein, which is also elevated in patients suffering from Cushing's disease. The level returns to normal after resection of the hypertrophic adrenals. Fever caused by bacterial endotoxin also causes the prekallikrein level in blood to rise (FORELL, 1957).

Purification. For the preparative purification of serum kallikrein, various sources and methods of activation have been used. WEBSTER and PIERCE (1960, 1961, 1963) start from acetone-activated human plasma. The acetone and salts are dialyzed off, and the bulk of inactive proteins is adsorbed onto DEAE-cellulose, leaving the active kallikrein together with other γ-globulins in the supernatant. Kallikrein is then adsorbed on the cation exchange resin Amberlite XE-64 (CM-cellulose in the earlier experiments). The resin is washed and eluted with solutions increasing stepwise in ionic strength and pH. The enzyme is recovered from the adsorbent with 0.2 M ammonium formate at pH 8.4–8.5. It is eventually stored as a powder, freeze-dried from a solution of pH 7.5.

In the method of MORIYA et al. (1965), acetone-activated human serum or plasma is precipitated by further addition of acetone, and the redissolved precipitate is fractionated with DEAE-cellulose, either in batches or on a column. Serum kallikrein remains unadsorbed, thus showing the properties of a γ-globulin. Further purification is achieved by ammonium sulfate fractionation, the main kallikrein activity being recovered from the precipitate obtained at 45% to 60% saturation. The preparation contains some esterase activity due to a thermolabile enzyme (60 min at 56°, pH 8.0), which is not or only partially inhibited by Trasylol. In a more analytical work KAGEN et al. (1963a, b) separated human serum kallikrein as a γ-globulin by chromatography of native serum on DEAE-cellulose, or by starch-block electrophoresis. The enzyme was also purified by these methods from ethanol fractions I+III-3 and III-1,2 (COHN et al., 1950).

HENRIQUES et al. (1966) activate human serum by acid. The pseudoglobulin fraction is then isolated by ammonium sulfate precipitation and subjected to DEAE-cellulose chromatography. Details of the elution have not been described. These authors have also prepared horse serum kallikrein after acid activation. Subsequently the serum was subjected to rather drastic treatment: it was heated at pH 2 to 90°. This raises some doubt about the nature of the enzyme, the more so as it does not attack horse serum kininogen.

ROCHA E SILVA et al. (1967) consider that these studies are in good agreement with their own work on kinin formation in guinea pig plasma, and suggest that plasmin may be the principal kininogenase in plasma. According to HAMBERG (1959) the kinin-forming activity that becomes apparent after heating rat plasma at low pH to the boiling point is due to plasmin.

HABERMANN and KLETT (1966) prepared kallikrein from casein-activated hog serum. The casein precipitate was redissolved at pH 7.5 and fractionated with ammonium sulfate. The fraction obtained between 30 and 60% saturation was then chromatographed on DEAE-Sephadex, Sephadex G-200, phospho-cellulose, and Sephadex G-100. A stable preparation was obtained which appeared homogeneous in the ultracentrifuge and in electrophoresis. It showed all functional properties of serum kallikrein: liberation of kinins (among other substrates also from a kininogen-I preparation VOGT et al., 1967), increase in vascular permeability, hypotensive effect, and esterase activity. A procedure similar in its early steps to HABERMANN and KLETT's (1966) method was used by TRAUTSCHOLD (cited from FREY et al., 1968; see also WERLE and TRAUTSCHOLD, 1963) for the preparation of hog serum kallikrein.

DAVIES and LOWE (1963a, b) obtained serum kallikrein from the γ-globulin fraction of guinea pig serum. The preparation seemed also to contain prekallikrein. Contact with glass beads, which had been coated with fresh guinea pig serum and washed afterward, markedly enhanced the esterase, kinin-forming, and permeability-increasing activities of the preparation. EISEN (1969b) fractionated whole human serum on DEAE-cellulose and obtained two kininogenase peaks; the first corresponded to γ-globulins, whereas the second contained a more anionic enzyme. In its functional properties it did not differ from the enzyme eluted first. Both showed properties of kallikrein, not of kininogenase II. They may be isoenzymes.

General Properties. Serum (pre)kallikrein is heat-labile. Heating of serum to 56° for 30 minutes leaves some activity, but after heating for 3 hours the activity is lost (WERLE, 1936; WERLE et al., 1937). Heating of plasma to 61° irreversibly destroys most of the kallikrein in 20 minutes (EISEN, 1963a). In contrast to plasmin, serum kallikrein is also labile at acid pH (WERLE and MAIER, 1952; EISEN, 1963a; HABERMANN and KLETT, 1966). In spite of this, acidification of serum is a means of activating prekallikrein. In view of the low resistance to acid, the finding of ROCHA E SILVA (1960) and of HENRIQUES et al. (1966) that rat plasma heated even to 90° at pH 2 shows kininogenase activity, is surprising. It is possible that the activity of these preparations was due not to kallikrein but to another kininogenase, possibly plasmin (HAMBERG, 1959). EISEN (1963a) found that human serum kallikrein preparations were not completely inactivated at acid pH. However, the hypotensive effect of the treated preparation was markedly reduced; the more stable kinin-forming activity, which was measured with unheated plasma as substrate, may have been due to an activator rather than kallikrein.

The serum kallikrein purified by HABERMANN and KLETT (1966) moves in electrophoresis between β- and γ-globulins. Its molecular weight is about 97,000 and its sedimentation constant 5.19. Other properties such as the failure to be adsorbed onto DEAE-cellulose suggest that it is a γ-globulin (WEBSTER and PIERCE, 1961; DAVIES and LOWE, 1963a, b; MORIYA et al., 1965).

Functional Properties. Like other kallikreins, serum kallikrein is a proteolytic hydrolase. The structural requirements for substrates are more specific than those of trypsin or plasmin. Kininogen denatured by heat is not or only poorly utilized by serum kallikrein (DINIZ and CARVALHO, 1963; HENRIQUES et al., 1966). On the other hand its specificity seems to be less marked than that of pancreatic kallikrein. In contrast to the latter, purified hog serum kallikrein has a weak but definite caseinolytic and fibrinolytic action (TRAUTSCHOLD, 1965; HABERMANN and KLETT, 1966). This proteolytic effect increases with higher purification, which implies that it is not (entirely) due to contamination with other enzymes.

Several amino acid amides or esters are cleaved, notably arginine derivatives like benzoyl-arginine-nitro-anilide, benzoyl-arginine-methyl-ester, the corresponding ethyl ester (BAEe) and tosyl-arginine-methyl-ester (TAMe) (TRAUTSCHOLD and WERLE, 1961; WEBSTER and PIERCE, 1961; HABERMANN and KLETT, 1966; HENRIQUES et al., 1966). Tyrosine esters are not attacked (WEBSTER and PIERCE, 1961). Of various kallikreins from other sources (hog) serum kallikrein is the most active on BAEe (TRAUTSCHOLD and WERLE, 1961). The esterase and hypotensive actions of serum kallikrein cannot be separated by fractionation procedures, which suggests that both are inherent properties of the same molecule.

The fact that kallikreins have esterase activities was regarded at one time as evidence that bradykinin is linked to the rest of kininogen by an ester bond (ROCHA E SILVA, 1960).

This view is not supported by recent investigations into the structure of bovine kininogen (HABERMANN, 1966b; HOCHSTRASSER and WERLE, 1967). The idea has, however, received new attention recently. There may exist some kininogens in which the bradykinin moiety is linked by a serine ester bond (PIERCE, 1968).

Serum kallikrein liberates kinin from a preparation of bovine kininogen (HABERMANN and BLENNEMANN, 1964) which shows exclusively properties of kininogen I as defined by VOGT (1966); kininogen II is not or is barely utilized. The main product released from kininogens of human and bovine sera is bradykinin (WEBSTER and PIERCE, 1963; HABERMANN and BLENNEMANN, 1964). Only a small amount of kallidin is formed. Since bradykinin is attached at its amino end to lysine, serum kallikrein splits a lysyl-arginyl-bond. This cleavage is possible only when the lysine is substituted on its α-amino group. Thus, serum kallikrein releases bradykinin from methionyl-lysyl-bradykinin (a peptide sequence that occurs in all known kininogen molecules) but not from lysyl-bradykinin (kallidin) (HABERMANN and BLENNEMANN, 1964). According to HABERMANN (1966b) bovine kininogen contains the sequence Ser-Val-Glu- next to the carboxyl end of the bradykinin moiety. It follows that serum kallikrein also cleaves an arginyl-seryl-bond. Whether the enzyme splits more readily the lysyl-arginyl-bond at the amino terminus, or the arginyl-seryl-bond at the carboxyl end of the bradykinin sequence in kininogen, depends on the nature of the substrate.

In intact kininogen the N-terminal end of bradykinin is liberated more easily. In contrast, the peptic fragment of kininogen, Met-Lys-bradykinin-Ser-Val-Glu, is attacked more easily at the carboxyl end of bradykinin, so that a considerable amount of the hendecapeptide, Met-Lys-bradykinin, is formed. HABERMANN and MÜLLER (1966) assume that the structural arrangement in these two substrates is different, resulting in different accessibilities of the two bonds to the enzyme. Under certain conditions, intact kininogen may acquire the tertiary structure of the peptic fragment, since ELLIOTT and LEWIS (1965) found that the hendecapeptide was formed "spontaneously" after neutralization of acid-treated bovine serum fractions (p. 260). Serum kallikrein does not split the bond between methionine and lysine, and therefore does not form kallidin (WEBSTER and PIERCE, 1963; HABERMANN and BLENNEMANN, 1964).

Inhibition and Inactivation. The inhibition and inactivation of plasma kininogenases is discussed in detail on p. 213 and will therefore be only briefly summarized here. Unless special precautions are taken, serum kallikrein is rapidly inactivated in serum or plasma. The inactivation appears to be irreversible, as neither treatment with acid nor acetone reactivates the enzyme (WERLE, 1936). This is different from the fate of pancreatic kallikrein, which is reversibly inactivated in plasma. The irreversible inhibition of serum kallikrein shows that inactivated serum kallikrein is different from prekallikrein. This does not mean, necessarily, that the active enzyme is destroyed, e.g. by proteolysis. Apparently irreversible inactivation may be caused by an inhibitor present in serum, which combines with the active site (protected in prekallikrein) with a high affinity. In acid- or acetone-treated plasma the kallikrein is stabilized, probably because of destruction of the inhibitor(s).

True enzymatic degradation of plasma kallikrein has recently been described in rat plasma (WERLE and SCHMAL, 1968). Unlike the inhibitors in other plasmas, this enzyme is capable of inactivating by digestion unlimited quantities of kallikrein. The process has an optimum at pH 6–8, and is dependent on the temperature and on the concentration of substrate (i.e. plasma kallikrein). It is inhibited by SBTI but not by other trypsin inhibitors, chelating agents, thioglycollate, or DFP.

Serum kallikrein also differs from glandular kallikreins in its reaction to exogenous inhibitors. In contrast to pancreatic and urinary kallikreins it is inhibited by SBTI (FREY et al., 1968). It is also said to be inhibited by lima bean inhibitor (EISEN, 1963a; MASON and SPARROW, 1965). However, the inhibition is weak (MASON and SPARROW, 1965) and BACK and STEGER (1968) recently found lima bean inhibitor quite ineffective. EACA at concentrations of 10^{-2} M does not inhibit serum kallikrein (EISEN, 1963b). Even at much higher doses its inhibitory effect is weak (BACK and STEGER, 1968). The kininogenolytic action of serum kallikrein is blocked by thiol compounds (WERLE, 1936; DAVIES and LOWE, 1966) whereas the esterase action is reported to remain unaffected (DAVIES and LOWE, 1966).

Serum kallikreins activated by different methods differ in their response to the ovomucoid inhibitor: papain-activated kallikrein is inhibited (WERLE and MAIER, 1952), whereas serum kallikrein preparations activated by acetone or chloroform are, like glandular kallikreins, resistant (WERLE and MAIER, 1952; WERLE et al., 1955; EISEN, 1963a; WEBSTER and PIERCE, 1963). Whether this is an indication that papain-activated serum kallikrein is a distinct enzyme (kininogenase II ?) is not known. The results with trypsin-activated human serum kallikrein seem to be divergent. WERLE et al. (1955) found that ovomucoid (2 mg/ml) did not inhibit the hypotensive effect of the enzyme. Later, WERLE and VOGEL (1960) mentioned that trypsin-activated serum kallikrein was inhibited by ovomucoid. The reaction with DFP blocks the action of serum kallikrein, indicating that its active center is similar to that of a wide variety of other hydrolases (trypsin, chymotrypsin, plasmin, cholinesterase, etc.) (HABERMANN, 1961, 1962, 1963).

Estimation of Serum Kallikrein. FREY et al. (1968) have devised a blood pressure assay for the quantitative estimation of glandular kallikreins, notably pancreatic kallikrein. One kallikrein unit (KU, also called FREY unit, FU) is the amount that produces the same hypotensive effect in dogs as 5 ml of pooled dialyzed human urine. As substandard, purified pancreatic kallikrein is mostly used. This assay has also been applied to serum kallikrein preparations. However, the activity ratio of two given samples of pancreatic and serum kallikrein may vary from one experimental animal to another and may even change after repeated injections in the same dog; furthermore, the time course of the circulatory effect is different (WEBSTER and PIERCE, 1961; HABERMANN and KLETT, 1966). These features have led to the preparation and use of individual standards in different laboratories. A general standard is lacking, and units declared for various preparations are probably only rough estimates of activity, and are not strictly comparable. Other possibilities for estimating serum kallikrein include kinin formation or the cleavage of amino acid esters (see p. 71).

II. Plasmin

There is no doubt that plasmin can induce kinin formation in plasma. Like certain other proteases it is able to activate serum kallikrein (see p. 107). Here the question will be discussed whether plasmin, in addition to being an activator, is also a kininogenase, capable of liberating kinin from kininogen directly, i.e. without the intervention of other enzymes. Apart from the earlier suggestion by BERALDO (1950), LEWIS (1958) was the first to investigate this possibility in detail. He was able to induce kinin formation in dog pseudoglobulin preparations with plasmin activated by streptokinase or chloroform. The formation was inhibited by antiplasmin. SCHACHTER (1956) needed rather high concentrations of bovine plasmin to develop kinin activity. He concluded that impurities (serum kallikrein) might have been responsible for the formation.

On i.v. injection into dogs, plasmin produces a hypotensive effect which is subject to tachyphylaxis and cross-tachyphylaxis with urinary kallikrein (Back, 1959, 1960, 1966). As neither the precursor, plasminogen, nor the activator, streptokinase, has a similar effect, intervention of contaminating enzymes was ruled out. The hypotensive effect of kallikreins can be attributed to the liberation of vasoactive kinins; the similar effect of plasmin has therefore also been interpreted as a kininogenase effect.

However, the fact that no cross-tachyphylaxis exists between plasmin preparations from different species (Back, 1959) indicates that the hypotensive action is not (entirely) due to kinin formation. There are other findings which suggest that plasmin may cause hypotension independently of kinin formation (Back et al., 1963). Conversely, Trautschold and Rüdel (1963) reported that highly purified plasmin does not cause hypotension.

These early observations do not yet prove a direct effect of plasmin on kininogen but could be explained by the activation of prekallikrein. Experiments by Bhoola et al. (1960), who were unable to generate kinin activity by incubating substrate preparations with plasmin, argue against a direct kinin-releasing activity. They further failed to produce a permeability-increasing effect in guinea pigs by injecting plasmin intradermally. The same negative result was also obtained by Copley (1963), who observed, however, a permeability-increasing action of plasminogen. This rather curious phenomenon indicates that increase in vascular permeability may not be taken as conclusive evidence for the presence of an active kinin-forming system.

There are further negative findings. In experiments by Vogt (1964), human plasmin did not release kinin from heated dog plasma globulins (2 hours, 56°) or from purified bovine kininogen. Haustein and Marquardt (1966) found that 3.6 casein units/ml plasmin did not release kinin from bovine kininogen purified by Habermann et al. (1963). According to Eisen (1963b), there is a considerable discrepancy between the development of fibrinolytic and of kinin-forming activities in plasma activated by various procedures. The fact that a high fibrinolytic potential may be accompanied by little kinin formation (and vice versa) indicates that plasmin may account for only a small fraction of the total kinin-forming capacity of blood.

The discrepancies between the findings by different authors seemed to be overcome when Vogt (1964) found that plasmin induces kinin formation in dog pseudoglobulin only if activatable plasma kallikrein is present (see also Lewis, 1960). This result was confirmed by Buluk and colleagues (Buluk and Malofiejew, 1965; Buluk et al., 1965), who used rabbit globulins as substrate, and by Haustein and Marquardt (1966) in human plasma. Accordingly, failure of plasmin to form kinin would be expected if no activatable kininogenase were present, and a demonstrable formation of kinin by plasmin would indicate the presence of a prekininogenase in the test system. However, there are indications that plasmin may also liberate kinins directly, in conditions under which activation of kallikrein is ruled out. Eisen (1963b) found a slight kinin formation in heated plasma. Back and Steger (1965) released kinin from bovine kininogen by incubating it with urokinase-activated human plasmin, in doses of 20 to 100 RPMI[1] units/ml. The reaction was slow and dependent on time and concentration.

1. The RPMI (Roswell Park Memorial Institute) unit is defined as that amount of plasmin which in 2 minutes will completely lyse 0.6 ml of a 0.3% purified human fibrin clot (formed with 1 NIH unit of purified thrombin) at 45° and pH 7.4 (Back et al., 1961). Human plasma contains from 3 to 15 RPMI units/ml after activation with streptokinase (Back, personal communication to W. V.)

Having been heated for 3 hours to 56° the substrate preparation was free from activatable prekallikrein. The possible participation of kallikrein, introduced as an impurity of the plasmin preparation, was excluded by demonstrating that antiplasmin blocked the reaction. Unfortunately, antiplasmin is not sufficiently well defined, and opinions about its specificity are not unanimous. LEWIS (1958) found that it did not inhibit kinin formation by dilution of plasma, and BACK and STEGER (1965) thought it was specific since it inhibited the hypotensive effect of plasmin but not of human urinary kallikrein. On the other hand the activation of plasma by contact with glass is also blocked by antiplasmin (LEWIS, 1958) although plasmin is probably not involved in this process to any significant extent (EISEN, 1963b). Further, WEBSTER and PIERCE (1960) found that antiplasmin inhibited human plasma kallikrein and plasmin equally strongly.

A clear demonstration of a kininogenase activity of plasmin at physiological concentrations has been given by HAMBERG (1959), who showed that rat or bovine plasma after heating at pH 1.5–1.8 in a boiling water bath acquired caseinolytic, fibrinolytic, and kinin-forming activities. In rat plasma treated this way, all these activities were demonstrable without further treatment but could be increased by addition of urokinase. In bovine plasma they were not (or weakly) present in direct assays, but they became apparent after treatment with the plasmin activator. In view of the acid and heat lability of serum kallikrein and of the specific plasmin activity demonstrated, these experiments strongly indicate that plasmin mainly, if not alone, was responsible for the kinin formation observed. HENRIQUES et al. (1966) prepared plasmin using RONWIN'S (1962a) method, which includes heating to 60° in acid solution. This preparation formed kinin from a heat-denatured substrate which was not utilized by kallikrein.

From these findings it seems obvious that plasmin is in fact able to cleave kininogen directly and to liberate kinin. It appears, however, that rather high concentrations are necessary, such as may not be attained *in vivo*; even these concentrations form kinin only at rather low rates. Much lower concentrations are sufficient to induce kinin formation indirectly by activating other kininogenases (VOGT, 1964; BACK and STEGER, 1965; HENRIQUES et al., 1966). Thus the direct kinin formation by plasmin is probably not very significant under physiological or pathological conditions (SEIDEL et al., 1969). It has even been suggested that the kallikrein and plasmin systems may act not as agonists but as antagonists in establishing an equilibrium of physiological importance (WEBSTER and INNERFIELD, 1965).

III. Kininogenase II

Definition. VOGT (1966) has defined (serum) kininogenase II as a kinin-forming enzyme present in human plasma as an inactive precursor, activated by contact with surfaces of glass etc. and distinct from serum kallikrein by its substrate specificity (see Fig. 2). It does not attack kininogen I, the substrate for pancreatic and serum kallikrein, but utilizes a different substrate—kininogen II—on which pancreatic kallikrein does not act and serum kallikrein acts only slightly. The enzyme is functionally identical with the "activated component A" of MARGOLIS (1958, 1960) (see p. 86) and with the glass-activated kinin-forming enzyme from bovine serum purified by NAGASAWA et al. (1967) (SEIDEL and VOGT, 1969a).

Activation in Plasma. Kininogenase II can be activated by contact with glass, quartz, or kaolin in human, rat, or bovine plasma. Since MARGOLIS (1958) found that any contact of human plasma with foreign surfaces leads to kinin formation only if Hageman factor is present and activated first (see p. 96), it follows that HF activates kininogenase II. Whether the permeability factor PF/dil is also an essential link in this sequence of reactions is not known. (PF/dil has been placed in the reaction sequence that leads to kallikrein activation, between HF and prekallikrein; see MILES, 1964; WEBSTER, 1966.) The amount of enzyme activated depends on the size of the surface available to contact, on time, and probably on temperature. Contact of 1 ml human plasma with 0.17 g glass beads of 0.1 mm ⌀ (350 cm^2 surface) for 5 min at 37° activates enough kininogenase II to consume all available kininogen II before the activated enzyme decays. Renewed contact with glass will again activate a considerable amount of kininogenase II. The generation of kininogenase activity on repeated exposure of plasma to glass is not due to a reactivation of enzyme, activated and inactivated before, but due to the fact that each time only a small proportion of pre-enzyme is activated. After sufficiently long or frequent exposure to glass surfaces, no further kininogenase activity can be generated by contact (MARGOLIS, 1958).

Evidence for the Existence of Kininogenase II as an Entity. As a result of the development of the kininogenase II concept, most data are concerned with the differentiation from serum kallikrein. Less is known about general properties, but some can be deduced from earlier results on component A. As mentioned above, human plasma which had been activated by contact with glass forms kinin and then ceases to do so well before the store of kininogen is exhausted. This occurs, even though the plasma still contains an active kininogenase (MARGOLIS, 1958, 1960; KEELE, 1960; EISEN, 1963a; VOGT, 1966) which is not plasmin, since plasmin is not activated significantly by glass contact (EISEN, 1963b; VOGT, 1964). Moreover, the inhibitor of plasminogen activation, EACA, does not inhibit prekininogenase activation during glass contact but even induces such activation itself. The enzyme present in contact-activated plasma can also be distinguished from plasma kallikrein by the following features: (1) various serum kallikrein preparations utilize the kininogen left in glass-activated plasma (kininogen I), although the kininogenase present therein (or activatable by renewed glass contact) does not. This is true of the purified hog serum kallikrein of HABERMANN (VOGT et al., 1967), of acid-treated human serum (VOGT et al., 1967; VOGT and WAWRETSCHEK, 1968) and for kallikrein obtained by acetone activation of human plasma (EISEN, 1966a; SEIDEL and VOGT, 1968).

MARGOLIS and BISHOP (1963) reported that acetone-activated human plasma did not release kinin from glass-treated plasma or only at a much slower rate. This has been regarded as evidence against the postulate of a specific kininogenase (WEBSTER and PIERCE, 1967). The negative finding may be explained by the exceedingly rapid inactivation of plasma kallikrein in glass-treated plasma (VOGT et al., 1967). If some time elapsed between glass treatment and incubation with the plasma kallikrein preparation, kinin formation has been regularly observed (SEIDEL and VOGT, 1969b). In the presence of acetone, MARGOLIS (1963) himself observed kinin formation in glass-treated plasma by acetone-activated plasma.

(2) The failure of the kininogenase in glass-treated plasma to utilize kininogen I is not due to an insufficient concentration of enzyme. The same concentration successfully forms kinin from kininogen II. Conversely, this substrate is not affected by concentrations of plasma kallikrein which effectively release kinin from kininogen I (VOGT and WAWRETSCHEK, 1968; SEIDEL and VOGT, 1968). Thus there is a qualitative difference in substrate specificity between plasma kallikrein (kininogenase I) as obtained by acid or acetone treatment of plasma and the enzyme (kininogenase II) in glass-activated plasma. It appears, therefore, that the two enzymes are different. (3) Kininogenase II is adsorbed by DEAE-cellulose in conditions under which plasma kallikrein is not (SEIDEL

and VOGT, 1969b). Kininogenase II releases kinin also from heated substrates (30 min, 61°) which do not form kinin on contact with glass or treatment with acetone and are regarded as being free of prekininogenases. It is thus not merely an activator but a true kininogenase.

Some Properties. With the possible exception of the preparation from bovine serum of NAGASAWA et al. (1967), kininogenase II has not yet been purified. Its properties are therefore mainly deduced from its apparent behavior in plasma, and the conclusions drawn may have to be revised as more is learned about purified material.

(Pre-)kininogenase II appears to be thermolabile, like plasma kallikrein. In human plasma heated for 3 hours to 56°, glass contact will not induce a kinin-forming enzyme although Hageman factor is still available (EISEN, 1963a). It seems also to be acid-labile, since practically no kininogenase II activity has been found in acid-treated human plasma (VOGT and WAWRETSCHEK, 1968). Once activated in whole plasma, the enzymatic activity decays rapidly. At room temperature, 90% of the activity disappears in 5 minutes (MARGOLIS, 1958). Still, kininogenase II is inactivated more slowly than serum kallikrein: in plasma treated with glass for several minutes, kininogenase II activity can be demonstrated at a time when kallikrein (kininogenase I) has already decayed (VOGT et al., 1967; VOGT and WAWRETSCHEK, 1968).

The inactivation proceeds more slowly in plasma heated for 20 minutes to 56° and in the pseudoglobulin fraction of human plasma (MARGOLIS, 1958). The process is irreversible. Once all the pre-enzyme available has been activated by prolonged contact of plasma with glass, and time has been allowed for decay, reactivation by renewed glass contact is no longer possible (MARGOLIS, 1958). After 5 minutes' contact with, e.g., 1 g of glass beads of 0.1 mm diameter and subsequent decay, fresh kinin-forming activity can be generated repeatedly by new contact (MARGOLIS, 1958). This indicates that each brief exposure to the glass surface activates only a small proportion of the pre-enzyme available, and that the activation is restricted to the actual period of contact and does not continue in solution after separation from the glass.

Prekininogenase II is precipitated from human and bovine plasma between 30 and 50% saturation with ammonium sulfate, i.e. with the pseudoglobulin fraction (NAGASAWA et al., 1967; SEIDEL and VOGT, in preparation). Unlike serum kallikrein, kininogenase II is presumably not a γ-globulin since it is adsorbed onto DEAE-cellulose from 0.01 M phosphate buffer at pH 8.0 (NAGASAWA et al., 1967; SEIDEL and VOGT, in preparation). Elution was done by passing 0.03 M buffer through the column.

Active kininogenase II is adsorbed onto glass surfaces (MARGOLIS, 1958, 1960; EISEN, 1963a; NAGASAWA et al., 1967). The pre-enzyme is probably not adsorbed since MARGOLIS (1958, 1960) was unable to coat glass beads with pre-enzyme from HF-deficient plasma. Kininogenase II is inhibited by SBTI and by Trasylol, but not by the ovomucoid trypsin inhibitor or lima bean trypsin inhibitor (MARGOLIS, 1958; NAGASAWA et al., 1967). Besides acting on kininogen II, it splits TAMe (NAGASAWA et al., 1967).

Purification. A stable preparation of what appears to be kininogenase II has been obtained so far only by NAGASAWA et al. (1967). These authors passed the pseudoglobulin fraction of bovine plasma through a glass powder column which adsorbed and simultaneously activated the enzyme. The active enzyme was then eluted with 1 M NaCl. Further purification was achieved by DEAE-cellulose chromatography. The results were confirmed and the functional identy with kininogenase II demonstrated by SEIDEL (1969).

IV. Kinin-Forming Substance

Armstrong and Mills (1963) found that in the incubated euglobulin fraction of human plasma, two plasma kinins, termed F and S, formed "spontaneously." They could be distinguished from bradykinin as well as from the lysyl- and methionyl-lysyl homologues (kallidin and Met-Lys-bradykinin). This and the fact that the forming enzyme was in the euglobulin rather than in the pseudoglobulin fraction, distinguished the enzyme from kallikrein. It was named "kinin-forming substance" (KFS) (Armstrong and Mills, 1964).

Purification. The euglobulins obtained by ammonium sulfate fractionation of human plasma were dialyzed at pH 6.3. This procedure precipitated the enzyme precursor, which was then activated with alcohol. The KFS was separated from γ-globulins on DEAE-cellulose. Further purification was achieved by electrophoresis (Armstrong and Mills, 1964).

Properties. The purified material liberated kinins from plasma of various species. It was active also in Hageman-factor-deficient plasma (Armstrong and Mills, 1964). KFS has been included among the kininogenases. However, a mere activator function has not been excluded. For example, the liberation of kinin has not been demonstrated in substrate preparations free of pre-enzymes. In view of the recently achieved separation of a series of kininogenase activators from human plasma by Webster (1968), it is not certain whether KFS is an activator or a kininogenase. (It released kinin from human plasma heated to 61° for 20 minutes but not from a kininogen I preparation. In this respect it was similar to kininogenase II; Vogt, unpublished observations.)

Depending on the degree of its purity and on the nature of the substrate (euglobulin fraction or whole plasma), KFS forms kinins F and S, only S, or another unknown kinin called E. This may be an indication that a complex sequence of reactions is induced, i.e. the participation of several enzymes. Besides kininogens, KFS hydrolyzes TAMe. The action is blocked by SBTI as well as by DFP. It is also blocked by hexadimethrine. This compound is known to inhibit the activation (by contact) of kinin-forming enzyme(s) in human plasma, but not their activity once induced (Eisen, 1964a). The effect of hexadimethrine, therefore, seems indicative of an activator function of KFS. In a semipurified state, KFS is unusually stable, resisting heating to 60° for more than an hour without significant loss of activity. Generally it is not possible to generate kinins in heated plasma by various methods of activation; this finding again suggests that KFS is an activator rather than a kininogenase. Unlike plasmin, KFS is acid-labile and has little fibrinolytic activity.

E. Differentiation of Kinin-Forming Enzymes and Activators of Plasma

Differences between the various kininogenases and their activators are apparent from the data given on pp. 90 and 109. Many of the individual properties are useful for practical purposes only when purified preparations are under investigation. In the case of unfractionated plasma or complex fractions, several active components of kinin-forming systems may be present, and identification may not be possible on the basis of properties which could well be used for pure factors. For example, the demonstration of casein-splitting and kinin-forming activities in plasma does not per se justify the conclusion that the casein-splitting enzyme, presumably plasmin, is responsible also for the kininogenolytic effect observed. Only those kinin-forming properties will be briefly summarized here which allow a rapid distinction even in mixtures. The distinction is based mainly on methods for selective elimination of one or the other substance, which permit a decision on the presence of that substance in the sample under investigation.

Kininogenases can be distinguished from their activators by comparing the result of incubation with normal (containing prekininogenases) and heat-denatured (e.g. 30, or better, 60 minutes at 62°, or 3 hours at 56°) plasma. Whereas an activator will induce kinin formation only in the fresh plasma specimen, a kininogenase will operate also (or even better, as inhibitors are likely to be destroyed) in the heated sample which is free of activatable enzyme. The finding that the "kinin-forming substance" (ARMSTRONG and MILLS, 1963, 1964) resists heating to 60° seems to contradict this statement. It may be, however, that it is not a kinin-forming enzyme per se, or that its precursor is less stable. MCCONNELL et al. (1965) distinguish serum kallikrein and PF/dil by their different sensitivities to inhibition by heparin. Among the activators, only Hageman factor and PF/dil can be distinguished, so far. HF can be eliminated by excessive contact with glass, kaolin, etc. (e.g. 2 m^2/ml human plasma), leaving PF/dil in solution (MARGOLIS, 1963; RATNOFF and MILES, 1964; B. MASON, personal communication).

Much work has been done on the differentiation between plasmin and plasma kallikrein. The dual nature of plasmin—being an activator as well as a kininogenase—and also the fact that both enzymes are often activated by the same initial process, have complicated these efforts. Unlike plasma kallikrein and kininogenase II, plasmin resists heating to 60° at pH 2 to 4. The persistence or loss of kinin-forming activity in plasma after treatment with acid and heat will therefore give an indication whether plasmin is or is not the actual kinin-forming enzyme. An inhibitor which effectively blocks plasmin but not plasma kallikrein is lima bean inhibitor (BACK and STEGER, 1968). Its effect on kininogenase II is not yet known. If one is dealing with the pre-enzymes and their activation, EACA will be useful for distinction. It blocks the activation of plasmin but not that of plasma kallikrein or kininogenase II.

Differences between plasma kallikrein (kininogenase I) and kininogenase II have been described in detail on p. 118. The distinction is based on the use of the two substrates, kininogen I and II (VOGT et al., 1967; VOGT and WAWRETSCHEK, 1968). The preparation of these substrates is also described in this handbook, in the chapters on kininogens by HABERMANN and by PIERCE.

Acknowledgment

One of us (V. E.) received generous financial help from the Medical Research Council and The Wellcome Trust.

References

ABLONDI, F. B., HAGAN, J. J.: Plasmin. In: The enzymes, vol. 4, p. 175, ed. by P. D. BOYER, H. LARDY and K. MYRBACK. New York: Academic Press 1960.

ALI, S. Y., LACK, C. H.: Studies on the tissue activator of plasminogen. Biochem. J. **96**, 63 (1965).

ALKJAERSIG, N.: The purification and properties of human plasminogen. Biochem. J. **93**, 171 (1964).

— FLETCHER, A. P., SHERRY, S.: ε-Amino caproic acid, an inhibitor of plasminogen activation. J. biol. Chem. **234**, 832 (1959).

AMBRUS, J. L.: The fibrinolysin system. Introduction. Fed. Proc. **25**, 28 (1966).

ARMSTRONG, D., JEPSON, J. B., KEELE, C. A., STEWART, J. W.: Pain-producing substance in human inflammatory exudates and plasma. J. Physiol. (Lond.) **135**, 350 (1957).

— KEELE, C. A., JEPSON, J. B., STEWART, J. W.: Development of pain-producing substance in human plasma. Nature (Lond.) **174**, 791 (1954).

Armstrong, D. A. J., Mills, G. L.: Chemical characterization of kinins of human plasma. Nature (Lond.) **197**, 490 (1963).
— — A highly purified kinin-forming enzyme from human plasma. Biochem. Pharmacol. **13**, 1393 (1964).
Astrup, T.: The biological significance of fibrinolysis. Lancet **1956 II**, 565.
— Tissue activators of plasminogen. Fed. Proc. **25**, 42 (1966).
— Müllertz, S.: The fibrin plate method for estimating fibrinolytic activity. Arch. Biochem. **40**, 346 (1952).
Back, N.: On the nature of plasmin-induced hypotension. Pharmacologist **1**, 56 (1959).
— In vivo formation of a vasodilator substance (plasma kinin) by plasmin. Fed. Proc. **19**, 55 (1960).
— Fibrinolysin system and vasoactive kinins. Fed. Proc. **25**, 77 (1966).
— Ambrus, J. L., Mink, I. B.: Distribution and fate of I^{131}-labeled components of the fibrinolysin system. Circulat. Res. **9**, 1208 (1961).
— Guth, P. S., Munson, A. E.: On the relationship beetween plasmin and kinin. Ann. N.Y. Acad. Sci. **104**, 53 (1963).
— Steger, R.: Activation of bovine bradykininogen by human plasmin. Life Sci. **4**, 153 (1965).
— — Effect of inhibitors on kinin-releasing activity of proteases. Fed. Proc. **27**, 96 (1968).
Becker, E. L., Kagen, L.: The permeability globulins of human serum and the biochemical mechanism of hereditary angioneurotic edema. Ann. N.Y. Acad. Sci. **116**, 866 (1964).
— Wilhelm, D. L., Miles, A. A.: Enzymic nature of the serum globulin permeability factor. (Nature (Lond.) **183**, 1264 (1959).
Beraldo, W. T.: Formation of bradykinin in anaphylactic and peptone shock. Amer. J. Physiol. **163**, 283 (1950).
Bhoola, K. D., Calle, J. D., Schachter, M.: The effect of bradykinin, serum kallikrein and other endogenous substances on capillary permeability in the guinea pig. J. Physiol. (Lond.) **152**, 75 (1960).
Biggs, R., Sharp, A. A., Margolis, J., Hardisty, R. M., Stewart, J., Davidson, W. M.: Defects in the early stages of blood coagulation: A report of 4 cases. Brit. J. Haemat. **4**, 177 (1958).
Bordet, J., Gengou, O.: Recherches sur la coagulation du sang et les serums anticoagulants. Ann. Inst. Pasteur **15**, 129 (1901).
Botti, R. E., Ratnoff, O. D.: The clot-promoting effect of soaps of long-chain saturated fatty acids. J. clin. Invest. **42**, 1569 (1963).
Buluk, K., Malofiejew, M.: Urokinase-induced activation of kallikreinogen and the release of plasma kinins in renal blood. Acta med. pol. **6**, 405 (1965).
— — Czokalo, M.: Activation of fibrinolysis and of plasma-kinin system during venostasis. Thromb. Diathes. haemorrh. (Stuttg.) **14**, 500 (1965).
Cohn, E. J., Gurd, F. R. N., Surgenor, D. M., Barnes, B. A., Brown, R. K., Derouaux, G., Gillespie, J. M., Kahnt, F. W., Lever, W. F., Liu, C. H., Mittelman, D., Mouton, R. F., Schmid, K., Uroma, E.: A system for the separation of the components of human blood: quantitative procedures for the separation of the protein components of human plasma. J. Amer. chem. Soc. **72**, 465 (1950).
Connor, W. E.: The acceleration of thrombus formation by certain fatty acids. J. clin. Invest. **41**, 1199 (1962).
— Hoak, J. C., Warner, E. D.: Massive thrombosis produced by fatty acid infusion. J. clin. Invest. **42**, 860 (1963).
— Poole, J. C. F.: The effect of fatty acids on the formation of thrombi. Quart. J. exp. Physiol. **46**, 1 (1961).
Copley, A. L.: Discussion. In: Ann. N.Y. Acad. Sci. **104**, 116 (1963).
Currey, H. L. F., Key, J. J., Mason, R. M., Swettenham, K. V.: Significance of radiological calcification of joint cartilage. Ann. rheum. Dis. **25**, 295 (1966).
Davie, E. W., Ratnoff, O. D.: Waterfall sequence for intrinsic blood clotting. Science **145**, 1310 (1964).
Davies, G. E., Holman, G., Lowe, J. S.: Role of Hageman factor in the activation of guinea-pig pre-kallikrein. Brit. J. Pharmacol. **29**, 55 (1967).
— Lowe, J. S.: A permeability factor released from guinea pig serum by antigen-antibody precipitates. Brit. J. exp. Path. **41**, 335 (1960).
— — Further studies on a permeability factor released from guinea-pig serum by antigen-antibody precipitates. Relationship to serum complement. Int. Arch. Allergy **20**, 235 (1962).
— — Guinea pig kallikrein system. Nature (Lond.) **198**, 94 (1963a).
— — Presence of kallikrein in the γ-globulin permeability factor of guinea-pig serum. Brit. J. Pharmacol. **21**, 491 (1963b).
— — Inhibitory effects of thiol compounds on kallikrein and on experimental burns in guinea pigs. Brit. J. Pharmacol. **27**, 107 (1966).

DAVIES, M. C., ENGLERT, M. E.: Physical properties of highly purified human plasminogen. J. biol. Chem. **235**, 1011 (1960).
DERECHIN, M.: Purification of human plasminogen. Biochem. J. **82**, 241 (1962).
DIDISHEIM, P., MIBASHAN, R. S.: Activation of Hageman factor (Factor XII) by long-chain saturated fatty acids. Thrombos. Diathes. haemorrh. (Stuttg.) **9**, 346 (1963).
DINIZ, C. R., CARVALHO, I. F.: A micromethod for determination of bradykininogen under several conditions. Ann. N.Y. Acad. Sci. **104**, 77 (1963).
DIXON, M.: The effects of pH on the affinities of enzymes for substrates and inhibitors. Biochem. J. **55**, 161 (1953).
DONALDSON, V. H.: Serum inhibitor of C'1-esterase in health and disease. J. Lab. clin. Med. **68**, 369 (1966).
— Mechanism of activation of C'1 esterase in hereditary angioneurotic edema plasma in vitro. J. exp. Med. **127**, 411 (1968).
— RATNOFF, O. D.: The enhancement of chloroform-induced plasma proteolytic activity by epsilon aminocaproic acid. J. exp. Med. **115**, 695 (1962).
— — Hageman factor: Alterations in physical properties during activation. Science **150**, 754 (1965).
DUGUID, J. B.: Thrombosis as a factor in the pathogenesis of coronary atherosclerosis. J. Path. Bact. **58**, 207 (1946).
— Thrombosis as a factor in the pathogenesis of aortic atherosclerosis. J. Path. Bact. **60**, 57 (1948).
EDERY, H., LEWIS, G. P.: Kinin-forming activity and histamine in lymph after tissue injury. J. Physiol. (Lond.) **169**, 568 (1963).
EISEN, V.: Modes of formation of human plasma kinin. Thesis for Ph.D. Degree, Univ. of London (1961).
— Observations on intrinsic kinin-forming factors in human plasma: the effect of acid, acetone, chloroform, heat and euglobulin separation on kinin formation. J. Physiol. (Lond.) **166**, 496 (1963a).
— Kinin formation and fibrinolysis in human plasma. J. Physiol. (Lond.) **166**, 514 (1963b).
— Effect of hexadimethrine bromide on plasma kinin formation, hydrolysis of *p*-tosyl-L-arginine methyl ester and fibrinolysis. Brit. J. Pharmacol. **22**, 87 (1964a).
— Fibrinolysis and formation of biologically active polypeptides. Brit. med. Bull. **20**, 205 (1964b).
— Studies on fibrinogen fractions isolated from human plasma by precipitation with cold ether. Brit. J. Haemat. **11**, 576 (1965).
— Kinin-forming enzymes and substrates in human plasma. J. Physiol. (Lond.) **186**, 133P (1966a).
— Urates and kinin formation in synovial fluid. Proc. roy. Soc. Med. **59**, 302 (1966b).
— Inflammation in gout. In: Rheumatic diseases, p. 255, ed. by J. J. R. DUTHIE and W. R. M. ALEXANDER). Edinburgh: University Press 1968.
— Kinin formation in human disease. Sci. Basis Med. ann. Rev. London, Athlone Press, p. 146 (1969a).
— Enzymic aspects of plasma kinin formation. Proc. roy. Soc. B **173**, 351 (1969b).
— Relation of the fibrinolytic mechanism to other proteolytic systems in plasma. Proc. roy. Soc. B **173**, 407 (1969c).
— KEELE, C. A.: Intrinsic plasma kinin forming factors in human plasma. J. Physiol. (Lond.) **154**, 20P (1960).
— — Possible modes of kinin formation in some pathological states in man. In: Hypotensive peptides, p. 551, ed. by E. G. ERDÖS, N. BACK and F. SICUTERI. Berlin-Heidelberg-New York: Springer 1966.
ELDER, J. M., WILHELM, D. L.: Enzyme-like globulins from serum reproducing the vascular. phenomena of inflammation. V. Activable permeability factor in human serum. Brit. J. exp. Path. **39**, 335 (1958).
ELLIOTT, D. F., LEWIS, G. P.: Methionyl-lysyl-bradykinin, a new kinin from ox blood. Biochem. J. **95**, 437 (1965).
ERDÖS, E. G., MIWA, I.: Effect of endotoxin shock on the plasma kallikrein-kinin system of the rabbit. Fed. Proc. **27**, 92 (1968).
— — GRAHAM, W. J.: Studies on the evolution of plasma kinins: reptilian and avian blood. Life Sci. **6**, 2433 (1967).
— SLOANE, E. M.: An enzyme in human blood plasma that inactivates bradykinin and kallidins. Biochem. Pharmacol. **11**, 585 (1962).
ESNOUF, M. P., MACFARLANE, R. G.: Enzymology and the blood clotting mechanism. Advanc. Enzymol. **30**, 255 (1968).
FAIRES, J. S., MCCARTY, D. J., JR.: Acute arthritis in man and dog after intrasynovial injection of sodium urate crystals Lancet **1962 II**, 682.

FEARNLEY, G. R.: Fibrinolysis. London: Arnold Ltd. 1965.
— BALMFORTH, G., FEARNLEY, E.: Evidence of a diurnal fibrinolytic rhythm; with a simple method of measuring natural fibrinolysis. Clin. Sci. 16, 645 (1957).
FORELL, M. M.: Untersuchungen über das Kallikreinogen im Serum des gesunden und kranken Menschen und seine Beeinflussung durch die Nebennierenrinde. Schweiz. med. Wschr. 87, 828 (1957).
FRANKLIN, E. C., EDELMAN, G., KUNKEL, H. G.: The rheumatoid factor. In: Immunity and virus infection, ed. by V. A. NAJJAR. New York: John Wiley & Sons, Inc. 1959.
FREUND, E.: Ein Beitrag zur Kenntnis der Blutgerinnung. Med. Jb. (Wien) 1, 46 (1886).
FREY, E. K.: Zur Deutung der reaktiven Hyperämie. Langenbecks Arch. klin. Chir. 162, 334 (1930).
— KRAUT, H., WERLE, E.: Das Kallikrein-Kinin-System und seine Inhibitoren. Stuttgart: F. Enke 1968.
GARBE, G., VOGT, W.: Zur Natur der in menschlichem Plasma durch Pankreaskallikrein, Glaskontakt und Säurebehandlung gebildeten Kinine. Naunyn-Schmiedebergs Arch. exp. Path. Pharmak. 256, 119 (1967).
GARROD, A. B.: A treatise on gout and rheumatic gout (rheumatoid arthritis). London: Longmans, Green & Co. 1876.
GRAHAM, R. C., EBERT, R. H., RATNOFF, O. D., MOSES, J. M.: Pathogenesis of inflammation. II. In vivo observations of the inflammatory effects of activated Hageman factor and bradykinin. J. exp. Med. 121, 807 (1965).
GREENBAUM, L. M., YAMAFUJI, K.: The in vitro inactivation and formation of plasma kinins by spleen cathepsins. Brit. J. Pharmacol. 27, 230 (1966).
HAANEN, C., HOMMES, F., BENRAAD, H., MORSELT, G.: A case of Hageman factor deficiency and a method to purify the factor. Thrombos. Diathes. haemorrh. (Stuttg.) 5, 201 (1961a).
— — MORSELT, G.: Some observations on the role of Hageman factor in blood coagulation. Thrombos. Diathes. haemorrh. (Stuttg.) 6, 261 (1961b).
HABERMANN, E.: Zur Reinigung und Wirkungsweise von Kallikrein. Naunyn-Schmiedebergs Arch. exp. Path. Pharmak. 241, 543 (1961).
— Unterscheidung von Kallikreinen und Kallikreinvorstufe mittels Antiseren und Diisopropylfluorophosphats. Hoppe-Seylers Z. physiol. Chem. 328, 24 (1962).
— Snake venoms, kallikreins and kininogen. Ann. N.Y. Acad. Sci. 104, 130 (1963).
— Enzymatic kinin release from kininogen and from low-molecular compounds. In: Hypotensive peptides, p. 116, ed. by E. G. ERDÖS, N. BACK, F. SICUTERI and A. F. WILDE. Berlin-Heidelberg-New York: Springer 1966a.
— Strukturaufklärung kininliefernder Peptide aus Rinderserum-Kininogen. Naunyn-Schmiedebergs Arch. exp. Path. Pharmak. 253, 474 (1966b).
— BLENNEMANN, G.: Über Substrate und Reaktionsprodukte der kininbildenden Enzyme Trypsin, Serum- und Pankreaskallikrein sowie von Crotalusgift. Naunyn-Schmiedebergs Arch. exp. Path. Pharmak. 249, 357 (1964).
— KLETT, W.: Reinigung und einige Eigenschaften eines Kallikreins aus Schweineserum. Biochem. Z. 346, 133 (1966).
— — ROSENBUSCH, G.: Partielle Reinigung und einige Eigenschaften eines Kininogens aus Rinderblut. Hoppe-Seylers Z. physiol. Chem. 332, 121 (1963).
— MÜLLER, B.: Zur enzymatischen Spaltung peptischer kininliefernder Fragmente (PKF) sowie von Rinderserum-Kininogen. Naunyn-Schmiedebergs Arch. exp. Path. Pharmak. 253, 464 (1966).
HAMBERG, U.: Fibrinolytic activation and bradykinin release. Biochim. biophys. Acta (Amst.) 36, 296 (1959).
HARDISTY, R. M., MARGOLIS, J.: The role of Hageman factor in the initiation of blood coagulation. Brit. J. Haemat. 5, 203 (1959).
HAUSTEIN, K. O., MARQUARDT, F.: Über den Einfluß von Fibrinolytica auf die Aktivierung des Kininsystems durch Fibrinolysevorgänge. Acta biol. med. germ. 16, 658 (1966).
HEILBRUNN, L. V.: The evolution of the haemostatic mechanism. In: Functions of the blood, ed. by R. G. MACFARLANE and A. H. T. ROBB-SMITH. Oxford: Blackwell 1961.
HEMKER, H. C., HEMKER, P. W.: General kinetics of enzyme cascades. Proc. roy. Soc. B 173, 411 (1969).
HENRIQUES, O. B., LAVRAS, A. A. C., FICHMAN, M., PICARELLI, Z. P.: Plasma enzymes that release kinins. Biochem. Pharmacol. 15, 31 (1966).
HOCHSTRASSER, K., WERLE, E.: Über kininliefernde Peptide aus pepsinverdauten Rinderplasmaproteinen. Hoppe-Seylers Z. physiol. Chem. 348, 177 (1967).
HOLEMANS, R., ROBERTS, H. R.: Hageman factor and *in vivo* activation of fibrinolysis. J. Lab. clin. Med. 64, 778 (1964).
HOLLANDER, J. L., MCCARTY, D. J., ASTORGA, G., CASTRO-MURILLO, E.: Studies on the pathogenesis of rheumatoid joint inflammation. Ann. intern. Med. 62, 271 (1965).

HORTON, E. W., LEWIS, G. P.: A comparison of the plasma kinin forming enzymes in urine. Kallikrein and urokinase. J. Physiol. (Lond.) **149**, 477 (1959).
HUBBARD, K., LUCAS, G. L.: Ionic charges of glass surfaces and other materials, and their possible role in the coagulation of blood. J. appl. Physiol. **15**, 265 (1960).
IATRIDIS, P. G., FERGUSON, J. H., IATRIDIS, S. G.: Surface factor mechanisms in relation to blood platelets; evidence that activated Hageman factor is present on the surface of platelets. Thrombos. Diathes. haemorrh. (Stuttg.) **11**, 355 (1964).
IATRIDIS, S. G., FERGUSON, J. H.: Effect of surface and Hageman factor on the endogenous or spontaneous activation of the fibrinolytic system. Thrombos. Diathes. haemorrh. (Stuttg.) **6**, 411 (1961).
— — Active Hageman factor: a plasma lysokinase of the human fibrinolytic system. J. clin. Invest. **41**, 1277 (1962).
— — Effect of physical exercise on blood clotting and fibrinolysis. J. appl. Physiol. **18**, 337 (1963).
ISHIZAKA, T., ISHIZAKA, K.: Biological activities of aggregated gamma globulin. I. Skin reactive and complement-fixing properties of heat denatured gamma globulin. Proc. Soc. exp. Biol. (N.Y.) **101**, 845 (1959).
JACOBSEN, S.: Substrates for plasmakinin-forming enzymes in human, dog and rabbit plasmas. Brit. J. Pharmacol. **26**, 403 (1966a).
— Observations on the content of kininogen, kallikrein and kininase in lymph from hind limbs of dogs and rabbits. Brit. J. Pharmacol. **27**, 213 (1966b).
— WAALER, B. A.: Lymph and plasma kinin formation. J. Physiol. (Lond.) **177**, 52P (1965).
— — The effect of scalding on the content of kininogen and kininase in limb lymph. Brit. J. Pharmacol. **27**, 222 (1966).
JOHNSTON, C. L., JR., BARROW, E. S.: A study of capillary permeability and its possible relationship to clotting factor XII. Scand. J. clin. Lab. Invest. **17**, Suppl., 84, 52 (1965).
JONASSON, O., BECKER, E. L.: Release of kallikrein from guinea pig lung during anaphylaxis. J. exp. Med. **123**, 509 (1966).
KAGEN, L. J.: Some biochemical and physical properties of the human permeability globulins. Brit. J. exp. Path. **45**, 604 (1964).
— LEDDY, J. S., BECKER, E.: Isolation of two permeability globulins from human serum. Nature (Lond.) **197**, 693 (1963a).
— — — The presence of two permeability globulins in human serum. J. clin. Invest. **42**, 1353 (1963b).
KASPER, C. K., WHISSELL BUECHY, D. Y. E., AGGELER, P. M.: Hageman factor (Factor XII) in an affected kindred and in normal adults. Brit. J. Haemat. **14**, 543 (1968).
KAULLA, K. N. v.: Chemistry of thrombolysis: Human fibrinolytic enzymes. Springfield, Ill.: Charles C. Thomas 1963.
KEELE, C. A.: Formation of pain-producing polypeptide (PPS) from plasma. In: Polypeptides which affect smooth muscles and blood vessels, p. 253, ed. by M. SCHACHTER. London: Pergamon Press 1960.
— ARMSTRONG, D.: Substances producing pain and itch. London: Arnold Ltd. 1964.
KEKWICK, R. A., MACKAY, M. E.: The separation of protein fractions from human plasma with ether. Spec. Rep. Ser. Med. Res. Coun., Lond., No. 286 (1954).
— — RECORD, B. R.: Fractionation of human plasma with ether. Nature (Lond.) **157**, 629 (1946).
KELLERMAN, G. M.: A simplified kinetic model of coagulation reactions. Brit. J. Haemat. **10**, 527 (1964).
KELLERMEYER, R. W.: Inflammatory process in acute gouty arthritis. III. Vascular permeability-enhancing activity in normal human synovial fluid; induction by Hageman factor activators; and inhibition by Hageman factor antiserum. J. Lab. clin. Med. **70**, 372 (1967).
— BRECKENRIDGE, R. T.: The inflammatory process in acute gouty arthritis. I. Activation of Hageman factor by sodium urate crystals. J. Lab. clin. Med. **65**, 307 (1965).
— — The inflammatory process in acute gouty arthritis. II. The presence of Hageman factor and plasma thromboplastin antecedent in synovial fluid. J. Lab. clin. Med. **67**, 455 (1966).
— RATNOFF, O. D.: Abolition of the permeability-enhancing properties of Hageman factor by specific antiserum. J. Lab. clin. Med. **70**, 365 (1967).
KLINE, D. L.: Blood coagulation; reactions leading to prothrombin activation. Ann. Rev. Physiol. **27**, 285 (1965).
— Chemistry and biochemistry of the fibrinolytic system. Fed. Proc. **25**, 31 (1966).
KOLLER, F.: New blood clotting factors. Thrombos. Diathes. haemorrh. (Stuttg.) Suppl. **4** (1960).

KRAUT, H., FREY, E. K., BAUER, E.: Über ein neues Kreislaufhormon. II. Mitt. Hoppe-Seylers Z. physiol. Chem. **175**, 97 (1928).
— — WERLE, E.: Über den Nachweis und das Vorkommen des Kallikreins im Blut. VIII. Mitt Über Kallikrein. Hoppe-Seylers Z. physiol. Chem. **222**, 73 (1933).
KUNITZ, M.: Crystalline soybean trypsin inhibitor. II. General properties. J. gen. Physiol. **30**, 291 (1947).
LACK, C. H.: Staphylokinase: an activator of plasma protease. Nature (Lond.) **161**, 559 (1948).
LAIDLER, K. J.: The physical chemistry of enzymes. Disc. Faraday Soc. No 20, 83 (1955).
LAMPERT, H.: Die physikalische Seite des Blutgerinnungsproblems. Leipzig: G. Thieme 1931.
LEVINE, S. N.: Enzyme amplifier kinetics. Science **152**, 651 (1966).
LEWIS, G. P.: Formation of plasma kinins by plasmin. J. Physiol. (Lond.) **140**, 285 (1958).
— Active polypeptides derived from plasma proteins. Physiol. Rev. **40**, 647 (1960).
— Plasma kinins and inflammation. Metabolism **13**, 1256 (1964a).
— Plasma kinins and other vasoactive compounds in acute inflammation. Ann. N.Y. Acad. Sci. **116**, 847 (1964b).
— WORK, T.: Formation of bradykinin or bradykinin-like substances by the action of plasmin on plasma proteins. J. Physiol. (Lond.) **135**, 7P (1956).
LISTER, J.: On the coagulation of the blood. Proc. roy. Soc. B **12**, 580 (1863).
LOELIGER, E. A., HENSEN, A.: Coagulation studies in a case of Hageman trait. Thrombos. Diathes. haemorrh. (Stuttg.) **5**, 187 (1960).
MACFARLANE, R. G.: Fibrinolysis following operation. Lancet **1937 I**, 10.
— The blood coagulation system. In: The plasma proteins, ed. by F. W. PUTNAM. New York and London: Acad. Press 1960.
— An enzyme cascade in the blood clotting mechanism and its function as a biochemical amplifier. Nature (Lond.) **202**, 498 (1964).
— The basis of the cascade hypothesis of blood clotting. Thrombos. Diathes. haemorrh. (Stuttg.) **15**, 591 (1965a).
— Hemostatic mechanisms in tissue injury. In: The inflammatory process, p. 465. New York and London: Acad. Press Inc. 1965b.
— BIGGS, R.: Fibrinolysis. Its mechanism and significance. Blood **3**, 1167 (1948).
— PILLING, J.: Observations on fibrinolysis: plasminogen, plasmin, and antiplasmin content of human blood. Lancet **1946 II**, 562.
MACKAY, M., MAYCOCK, W. D'A., COMBRIDGE, B. S.: Activation of endogenous plasma proteolytic enzymes with the consequent production of pharmacologically active polypeptides. Nature (Lond.) **195**, 1206 (1962).
— — SILK, E., COMBRIDGE, B. S.: Studies on fibrinogen fractions isolated from human plasma by precipitation with cold ether. I. Plasma kinin formation by the activation of contained plasminogen. Brit. J. Haemat. **11**, 563 (1965).
MACKAY, M. E., MILES, A. A., SCHACHTER, M., WILHELM, D. L.: Susceptibility of the guinea pig to pharmacological factors from its own serum. Nature (Lond.) **172**, 714 (1953).
MAJNO, G., PALADE, G. E., SCHOEFL, G. I.: Studies in inflammation. II. The site of action of histamine and serotonin along the vascular tree: A topographic study. J. biophys. biochem. Cytol. **11**, 607 (1961).
MARGOLIS, J.: Initiation of blood coagulation by glass and related surfaces. J. Physiol. (Lond.) **137**, 95 (1957).
— Activation of plasma by contact with glass. Evidence for a common reaction which releases plasma kinin and initiates coagulation. J. Physiol. (Lond.) **144**, 1 (1958).
— Hageman factor and capillary permeability. Aust. J. exp. Biol. med. Sci. **37**, 239 (1959).
— The mode of action of Hageman factor in the release of plasma kinin. J. Physiol. (Lond.) **151**, 238 (1960).
— The effect of colloidal silica on blood coagulation. Aust. J. exp. Biol. med. Sci. **39**, 249 (1961).
— Activation of Hageman factor by saturated fatty acids. Aust. J. exp. Biol. med. Sci. **40**, 505 (1962).
— The interrelationship of coagulation of plasma and release of peptides. Ann. N.Y. Acad. Sci. **104**, 133 (1963).
— Quantitative studies of kinin-releasing enzymes in plasma. In: Hypotensive peptides, p. 198, ed. by E. G. ERDÖS, N. BACK, F. SICUTERI and A. F. WILDE. Berlin-Heidelberg-New York: Springer 1966.
— BISHOP, E. A.: Interrelations between different mechanisms of release of biologically active peptides from blood plasma. Nature (Lond.) **194**, 749 (1962).
— — Studies on plasma kinins. I. The composition of kininogen complex. Aust. J. exp Biol. med. Sci. **41**, 293 (1963).
MARGOLIUS, A., RATNOFF, O. D.: Observations on the hereditary nature of Hageman trait. Blood **11**, 565 (1956).

MARKUS, G., WERKHEISER, W. C.: The interaction of streptokinase with plasminogen. I. Functional properties of the activated enzyme. J. biol. Chem. **239**, 2637 (1964).
MASON, B., MILES, A. A.: Globulin permeability factors without kininogenase activity. Nature (Lond.) **196**, 587 (1962).
— SPARROW, E. M.: The relationship between the permeability-increasing and the hypotensive proteases of plasma. Brit. J. Pharmacol. **25**, 257 (1965).
MATTHES, K., GROSS, F.: Zur Methode der fortlaufenden Registrierung der Farbe des menschlichen Blutes. Naunyn-Schmiedebergs Arch. exp. Path. Pharmak. **191**, 523 (1939).
McCONNELL, D. J., KAGEN, L. J., BECKER, E. L.: Use of heparin in distinguishing plasma kallikrein from Pf/dil. Proc. Soc. exp. Biol. (N.Y.) **119**, 652 (1965).
MELMON, K. L., WEBSTER, M. E., GOLDFINGER, S. E., SEEGMILLER, J. E.: The presence of a kinin in inflammatory synovial effusions from arthritides of varying etiologies. Arthr. and Rheum. **10**, 13 (1967).
MILES, A. A.: Mediators of the vascular phenomena of inflammation. Lect. sci. Basis Med. 8, 198 (1958/59).
— Large molecular substances as mediators of the inflammatory reaction. Ann. N.Y. Acad. Sci. **116**, 855 (1964).
— MILES, E. M.: Vascular reactions to histamine, histamine-liberator and leukotaxine in the skin of guinea-pigs. J. Physiol. (Lond.) **118**, 228 (1952).
— WILHELM, D. L.: Enzyme-like globulins from serum reproducing the vascular phenomena of inflammation. I. An activable permeability factor and its inhibitor in guinea-pig serum. Brit. J. exp. Path. **36**, 71 (1955).
MILL, P. J., ELDER, J. M., MILES, A. A., WILHELM, D. L.: Enzyme-like globulins from serum reproducing the vascular phenomena of inflammation. Brit. J. exp. Path. **39**, 343 (1958).
MORIYA, H., YAMAZAKI, K., FUKUSHIMA, H.: Biochemical studies on kallikreins. III. Preliminary experiment of studies on human plasma kallikrein. J. Biochem. **58**, 315 (1965).
MOVAT, H. Z.: Activation of the kinin system by antigen–antibody complexes. In: Internat. Symposium on Vasoactive Polypeptides: Bradykinin and Related Kinins, p. 177. São Paulo, 1967.
MÜLLER-EBERHARD, H. J., KUNKEL, H. G.: Isolation of thermolabile serum protein which precipitates γ-globulin aggregates and participates in immune hemolysis. Proc. Soc. exp. Biol. (N.Y.) **106**, 291 (1961).
NAGASAWA, S., HORIUCHI, K., YANO, M., SUZUKI, T.: Partial purification of bovine plasma kallikrein activated by contact with glass. J. Biochem. **62**, 398 (1967).
NIEWIAROWSKI, S., BANKOWSKI, E., FIEDORUK, T.: Adsorption of Hageman factor (Factor XII) on collagen. Experientia (Basel) **20**, 367 (1964).
— STACHURSKA, J., WEGRZYNOWICZ, Z.: Arginine esterase activity of the contact (Hageman) factor. Thrombos. Diathes. haemorrh. (Stuttg.) **7**, 514 (1956).
— STUART, R. K., THOMAS, D. P.: Activation of intravascular coagulation by collagen. Proc. Soc. exp. Biol. (N.Y.) **123**, 196 (1966).
NORMAN, P. S.: Inhibition of plasmin by serum or plasma. J. exp. Med. **108**, 53 (1958).
— Antiplasmins. Fed. Proc. **25**, 63 (1966).
NOSSEL, H. L.: The contact phase of blood coagulation. Oxford: Blackwell 1964.
— Activation of factors XII (Hageman) and XI (PTA) by skin contact. Proc. Soc. exp. Biol. (N.Y.) **122**, 16 (1966).
— NIEMETZ, J.: A normal inhibitor of the blood contact reaction product. Blood **25**, 712 (1965).
— RUBIN, H., DRILLINGS, M., HSIEH, R.: Inhibition of Hageman factor activation. J. clin. Invest. **47**, 1172 (1968).
O'BRIEN, J. R.: The effect of some fatty acids and phospholipids on blood coagulation. Brit. J. exp. Path. **38**, 529 (1957).
PASKHINA, T. S.: Homologous serum proteins and their role in phenomena of increased capillary permeability in inflammation. Clin. chim. Acta **1**, 24 (1956).
PECHET, L.: Fibrinolysis. New Engl. J. Med. **273**, 966 (1965).
PENSKY, J., LEVY, L. R., LEPOW, I. H.: Partial purification of a serum inhibitor of C'1 esterase. J. biol. Chem. **236**, 1674 (1961).
PIERCE, J. V.: Structural features of plasma kinins and kininogens. Fed. Proc. **27**, 52 (1968).
— WEBSTER, M. E.: The purification and some properties of two different kallidinogens from human plasma. In: Hypotensive peptides, p. 130, ed. by E. G. ERDÖS, N. BACK, F. SICUTERI and A. F. WILDE. Berlin-Heidelberg-New York: Springer 1966.
PILKINGTON, T. R. E.: The effect of fatty acids and detergents on the calcium clotting time of human plasma. Clin. Sci. **16**, 269 (1957).
POOLE, J. C. F.: Effect of certain fatty acids on the coagulation of plasma in vitro. Brit. J. exp. Path. **36**, 248 (1955).

Ratnoff, O. D.: An enzyme in plasma inactivating Hageman factor. J. clin. Invest. **37**, 923 (1958).
— The biology and pathology of the initial stages of blood coagulation. Progr. Hemat. **5**, 204 (1966).
— Colopy, J. E.: A familial hemorrhagic trait associated with a deficiency of a clot-promoting fraction of plasma. J. clin. Invest. **34**, 602 (1955).
— Crum, J. D.: Activation of Hageman factor by solutions of ellagic acid. J. Lab. clin. Med. **63**, 359 (1964).
— Davie, E. W.: The purification of activated Hageman factor (activated Factor XII). Biochemistry **1**, 967 (1962).
— — Mallet, D. L.: Studies on the action of Hageman factor. Evidence that activated Hageman factor in turn activates plasma thromboplastin antecedent. J. clin. Invest. **40**, 803 (1961).
— Lepow, I. H., Pillemer, L.: The multiplicity of plasmin inhibitors in human serum, demonstrated by the effect of primary amino compounds. Bull. Johns Hopk. Hosp. **94**, 169 (1954).
— Miles, A. A.: The induction of permeability-increasing activity in human plasma by activated Hageman factor. Brit. J. exp. Path. **45**, 328 (1964).
— Naff, G. B.: The conversion of C'1s to C'1 esterase by plasmin and trypsin. J. exp. Med. **125**, 337 (1967).
— Rosenblum, J. M.: Role of Hageman factor in the initiation of clotting by glass; evidence that glass frees Hageman factor from inhibition. Amer. J. Med. **25**, 160 (1958).
— Steinberg, A. G.: Further studies on the inheritance of Hageman trait. J. Lab. clin. Med. **59**, 980 (1962).
Remmert, L. F., Cohen, P.: Partial purification and properties of a proteolytic enzyme of human serum. J. biol. Chem. **181**, 431 (1949).
Robbins, K. C., Summaria, L., Elwyn, D., Barlow, G. H.: Further studies on the purification and characterization of human plasminogen and plasmin. J. biol. Chem. **240**, 541 (1965).
— — Hsieh, B., Shah, R. J.: The peptide chains of human plasmin. J. biol. Chem. **242**, 2333 (1967).
Rocha e Silva, M.: Biochemistry and pharmacology of bradykinin. In: Polypeptides which affect smooth muscles and blood vessels, p. 210, ed. by M. Schachter. London: Pergamon Press 1960.
— Reis, M. L., Ferreira, S. H.: Release of kinins from fresh plasma under varying experimental conditions. Biochem. Pharmacol. **16**, 1665 (1967).
Ronwin, E.: Properties of human plasmin. Canad. J. Biochem. **40**, 49 (1962a).
— The active center of human plasmin. Canad. J. Biochem. **40**, 57 (1962b).
Rose, J. C., Broida, H. P.: Effects of plastic and steel surfaces on clotting time of human blood. Proc. Soc. exp. Biol. (N.Y.) **86**, 384 (1954).
Roskam, J.: Contribution à l'étude de la physiologie normale et pathologique du globulin (plaquettes de Bizzozero). Arch. int. Physiol. **20**, 241 (1923).
Rothschild, A. M., Gascon, L.: Sulphuric esters of polysaccharides as activators of a bradykinin-forming system in plasma. Nature (Lond.) **212**, 1364 (1966).
Schachter, M.: A delayed slow contracting effect of serum and plasma due to the release of a substance resembling kallidin and bradykinin. Brit. J. Pharmacol. **11**, 111 (1956).
Schiffman, S., Rapaport, S. I., Ware, A. G., Mehl, J. W.: Separation of plasma thromboplastin antecedent (PTA) and Hageman factor (HF) from human plasma. Proc. Soc. exp. Biol. (N.Y.) **105**, 453 (1960).
Schoenmakers, J. G., Kurstjens, R. M., Haanen, C., Zilliken, F.: Purification of activated bovine Hageman factor. Thrombos. Diathes. haemorrh. (Stuttg.) **9**, 546 (1963).
— Matze, R., Haanen, C., Zilliken, F.: Hageman factor, a novel sialoglycoprotein with esterase activity. Biochim. biophys. Acta (Amst.) **101**, 166 (1965).
Seegmiller, J. E., Howell, R. R., Malawista, S. E.: The inflammatory reaction to sodium urate. J. Amer. med. Ass. **180**, 469 (1962).
Seidel, G.: Substrate specificity of glass-activated kininogenase from bovine plasma. Naunyn-Schmiedebergs Arch. Pharmak. **264**, 18–22 (1969).
— Stücker, H.-U., Vogt, W.: The role of plasmin for kinin formation in human plasma. Naunyn-Schmiedebergs Arch. Pharmak. **264**, 305–306 (1969).
— Vogt, W.: Kininogenspezifität von Aceton-aktiviertem menschlichem Plasma. Naunyn-Schmiedebergs Arch. exp. Path. Pharmak. **260**, 199 (1968).
— — Substratspezifität glasaktivierter Kininogenase aus Rinderplasma. Naunyn-Schmiedebergs Arch. Pharmak. **264**, 306–307 (1969a).
— — Kininogenspezifität von acetonaktiviertem menschlichem Plasmakallikrein. Naunyn-Schmiedebergs Arch. Pharmak. **262**, 135–138 (1969b).

SGOURIS, J. T., INMAN, J. K., McCALL, K. B., HYNDMAN, L. A., ANDERSON, H. D.: The preparation of plasminogen. Vox Sang 5, 357 (1960).
SHARP, A. A.: Pathological fibrinolysis. Brit. med. Bull. **20**, 240 (1964).
SHERRY, S., ALKJAERSIG, N., FLETCHER, A. P.: Activity of plasmin and streptokinase-activator on substituted arginine and lysine esters. Thromb. Diathes. haemorrh. (Stuttg.) **16**, 18 (1966a).
— — — Observations on the spontaneous arginine and lysine esterase activity of human plasma, and their relation to Hageman factor. Thrombos. Diathes. haemorrh. (Stuttg.) Suppl., **20**, 243 (1966b).
— FLETCHER, A. P., ALKJAERSIG, N.: Fibrinolysis and fibrinolytic activity in man. Physiol. Rev. **39**, 343 (1959).
SHULMAN, S., ALKJAERSIG, N., SHERRY, S.: Physicochemical studies on human plasminogen (profibrinolysin) and plasmin (fibrinolysin). J. biol. Chem. **233**, 91 (1958).
SLOTTA, K. H., GONZALEZ, J. D.: Native plasminogen. Biochemistry **3**, 285 (1964).
SOULIER, J. P., PROU-WARTELLE, O.: Nouvelles données sur les facteurs Hageman et P.T.A. et sur le «contact». Rev. franç. Étud. clin. biol. **4**, 932 (1959).
— — New data on Hageman factor and plasma thromboplastin antecedent: The role of "contact" in the initial phase of blood coagulation. Brit. J. Haemat. **6**, 88 (1960).
SPECTOR, W. G.: The mechanism of altered capillary permeability in acute inflammation. J. Path. Bact. **72**, 367 (1956).
— The activation of a globulin system controlling capillary permeability in inflammation. J. Path. Bact. **74**, 67 (1957).
SPEER, R. J., RIDGWAY, H., HILL, J. M.: Activated human Hageman factor (XII). Thrombos. Diathes. haemorrh. (Stuttg.) **14**, 1 (1965).
STAFFORD, J. L.: Fibrinolysis. Brit. med. Bull. **20**, 171 (1964).
STEWART, P. B., BLISS, J. Q.: The permeability-increasing factor in diluted human plasma. Brit. J. exp. Path. **38**, 462 (1957).
STUBER, B., HEIM, R.: Über Fettsäuren und Blutgerinnung, zugleich eine chemische Erklärung des Gerinnungsvorganges. Münch. med. Wschr. **61**, 1661 (1914).
SUMMARIA, L., HSIEH, B., ROBBINS, K. C.: The specific mechanism of activation of human plasminogen to plasmin. J. biol. Chem. **242**, 4279 (1967).
THOMPSON, J. H., JR., SPITTEL, J. A., JR., PASCUZZI, C. A., OWEN, C. A., JR.: Laboratory and genetic observations in another family with the Hageman trait. Proc. Mayo Clin. **35**, 421 (1960).
TORRIGIANI, G., ROITT, I. M.: Antiglobulin factors in sera from different patients with rheumatoid arthritis and normal subjects. Ann. rheum. Dis. **26**, 334 (1967).
TRAUTSCHOLD, I.: Habil.-Schrift, München 1965 (cit. from FREY, KRAUT and WERLE: Das Kallikrein-Kinin-System und seine Inhibitoren, 1968).
— RUDEL, G.: Neue Ergebnisse auf dem Gebiet der Plasmakinine. Klin. Wschr. **41**, 297 (1963).
— WERLE, E.: Spektrophotometrische Bestimmung des Kallikreins und seiner Aktivatoren. Hoppe-Seylers Z. physiol. Chem. **325**, 48 (1961).
VELTKAMP, J. J., HEMKER, H. C., LOELIGER, E. A.: Detection of heterozygotes for Factor VIII, IX and XII deficiency. Thrombos. Diathes. haemorrh. (Stuttg.) ,Suppl. **17**, 81 (1965).
VOGEL, R., TRAUTSCHOLD, I., WERLE, E.: Natürliche Proteinasen-Inhibitoren. Stuttgart: 1966.
VOGT, W.: Kinin formation by plasmin, an indirect process mediated by activation of kallikrein. J. Physiol. (Lond.) 170, 153 (1964).
— Ein komplettes zweites kininbildendes System in menschlichem Plasma. Naunyn-Schmiedebergs Arch. exp. Path. Pharmak. **251**, 186 (1965).
— Demonstration of the presence of two separate kinin-forming systems in human and other plasma. In: Hypotensive peptides, p. 185, ed. by E. G. ERDÖS, N. BACK and F. SICUTERI. Berlin-Heidelberg-New York: Springer 1966.
— GARBE, G., SCHMIDT, G.: Untersuchungen zur Existenz zweier verschiedener kininbildender Systeme in menschlichem Plasma. Naunyn-Schmiedebersg Arch. exp. Path. Pharmak. **256**, 127 (1967).
— WAWRETSCHEK, W.: Weitere Untersuchungen zur Existenz zweier kininbildender Systeme in menschlichem Plasma. Naunyn-Schmiedebergs Arch. exp. Path. Pharmak. **260**, 223 (1968).
VROMAN, L.: Effects of hydrophobic surfaces upon blood coagulation. Thrombos. Diathes. haemorrh. (Stuttg.) **10**, 455 (1964).
WAALER, B. A.: Contact activation in the intrinsic blood clotting system. Studies on a plasma product formed on contact with glass and similar surfaces. Scand. J. clin. Lab. Invest. Suppl. 37, **11**, 1 (1959).
WEBSTER, M. E.: The kallikrein-kininogen-kinin-system. Arthr. and Rheum. **9**, 473 (1966).
— Human plasma kallikrein, its activation and pathological role. Fed. Proc. **27**, 84 (1968).

WEBSTER, M. E., INNERFIELD, I.: Interrelationship of human plasma kallikrein and plasmin in inflammation. Enzym. biol. clin. **3**, 129 (1965).
— PIERCE, J. V.: Studies on plasma kallikrein and its relationship to plasmin. J. Pharmacol. exp. Ther. **130**, 484 (1960).
— — Action of the kallikreins on synthetic ester substrates. Proc. Soc. exp. Biol. (N.Y.) **107**, 186 (1961).
— — The nature of the kallidins released from human plasma by kallikreins and other enzymes. Ann. N.Y. Acad. Sci. **104**, 91 (1963).
— — Studies on the enzymes involved in the activation of human plasma kallikrein. In: M. ROCHA E SILVA and H. ROTHSCHILD, eds., Internat. Symposium on Vaso-active Polypeptides: Bradykinin and Related Kinins, p. 155, São Paulo, 1967.
— RATNOFF, O. D.: Role of Hageman Factor in the activation of vasodilator activity in human plasma. Nature (Lond.) **192**, 180 (1961).
WERLE, E.: Über Kallikrein aus Blut. Biochem. Z. **287**, 235 (1936).
— Kallikrein, kallidin and related substances. In: Polypeptides which affect smooth muscle, p. 199, ed. by M. SCHACHTER. London: Pergamon Press 1960.
— FORELL, M. M., MAIER, L.: Zur Kenntnis der blutdrucksenkenden Wirkung des Trypsins. Naunyn-Schmiedebergs Arch. exp. Path. Pharmak. **225**, 369 (1955).
— GÖTZE, W., KEPLER, A.: Über die Wirkung des Kallikreins auf den isolierten Darm und über eine neue darmkontrahierende Substanz. Biochem. Z. **289**, 217 (1937).
— KORSTEN, H.: Der Kallikreingehalt des Harns, des Speichels und des Blutes bei Gesunden und Kranken. Z. ges. exp. Med. **103**, 153 (1938).
— MAIER, L.: Über die chemische und pharmakologische Unterscheidung von Kallikreinen verschiedener Herkunft. Biochem. Z. **323**, 279 (1952).
— SCHMAL, A.: Über ein Kallikrein-abbauendes Enzym im Blutplasma der Ratte. Hoppe-Seylers Z. physiol. Chem. **349**, 521 (1968).
— TRAUTSCHOLD, I.: Kallikrein, kallidin, kallikrein inhibitors. Ann. N.Y. Acad. Sci. **104**, 117 (1963).
— VOGEL, R.: Über die Kallikreinausscheidung im Harn nach experimenteller Nierenschädigung. Arch. int. Pharmacodyn. **126**, 171 (1960).
WILHELM, D. L., MILES, A. A., MACKAY, M. E.: Enzyme-like globulins from serum reproducing the vascular phenomena of inflammation. II. Isolation and properties of the permeability factor and its inhibitor. Brit. J. exp. Path. **36**, 82 (1955).
— MILL, P. J., MILES, A. A.: Enzyme-like globulins from serum reproducing the vascular phenomena of inflammation. Brit. J. exp. Path. **38**, 446 (1957).
— — SPARROW, E. M., MACKAY, M. E., MILES, A. A.: Enzyme-like globulins from serum reproducing the vascular phenomena of inflammation. IV. Activable permeability factor and its inhibitor in the serum of the rat and the rabbit. Brit. J. exp. Path. **39**, 228 (1958).
WOOD, L. A., HORAN, F. E., SHEPPARD, E., WRIGHT, I. S.: Zetapotential measurements as a tool for studying certain aspects of blood coagulation. In: Blood clotting and allied problems, ed. by J. E. FLYNN. New York: J. Macy, Jr. Foundation 1950.
YANO, M., KATO, H., NAGASAWA, S., SUZUKI, T.: An improved method for the purification of kininogen II from bovine plasma. J. Biochem. **62**, 386 (1967a).
— NAGASAWA, S., HORIUCHI, K., SUZUKI, T.: Separation of a new substrate, kininogen-I, for plasma kallikrein in bovine plasma. J. Biochem. **62**, 504 (1967b).

Kallikreins in Glandular Tissues*

MARION E. WEBSTER

With the cooperation of MARCOS MARES-GUIA and CARLOS R. DINIZ

With 3 Figures

A. Introduction and History

The kallikreins have been defined as endogenous enzymes which rapidly and specifically liberate a kinin from plasma (Appendix on Nomenclature). Perhaps more comprehensively they might be defined as those proteolytic enzymes of animal origin which release a kinin from kininogen but, as far as is known, do not readily cleave peptide bonds in other proteins. The term kininogenase is a general one which has been applied to any enzyme that liberates a kinin from an inactive protein substrate. However, not all authors agree with this terminology, preferring to call all these enzymes kininogenins since to them the former expression implies the destruction of kininogen and the latter the formation (genesis) of active kinins (ROCHA E SILVA, 1962, 1963, 1965, and personal communication). For the purpose of this chapter the term kallikrein will be restricted to mammalian and avian kallikreins and will not include those enzymes found in snake venom, which may also be kallikreins (IWANAGA et al., 1965).

The kallikreins have been separated into two classes—those derived from glandular sources and those derived from plasma. All known plasma kallikreins are inhibited by soybean trypsin inhibitor (SBTI) (WERLE and MAIER, 1952; BHOOLA et al., 1960; WEBSTER and PIERCE, 1960, 1961; HABERMANN and KLETT, 1965, 1966; DAVIES et al., 1966; PASKHINA and EGOROVA, 1966; BRANDI et al., 1967; NAGASAWA et al., 1967), whereas the glandular kallikreins are not (WERLE and MAIER, 1952; WERLE and KAUFMANN-BOETSCH, 1960; WEBSTER and PIERCE, 1961; BRANDI et al., 1967; BACK and STEGER, 1968). Also, for those kallikreins that have been investigated, the plasma kallikreins release bradykinin from kininogens (WEBSTER and PIERCE, 1963; HABERMANN and BLENNEMANN, 1964; HABERMANN and KLETT, 1966; PASKHINA and EGOROVA, 1966) whereas the glandular kallikreins release kallidin (PIERCE and WEBSTER, 1961; WERLE et al., 1961; WEBSTER and PIERCE, 1963; HABERMANN and BLENNEMANN, 1964). In addition, the plasma kallikreins, in most species except the guinea pig, release a kinin only from the high molecular weight kininogens (JACOBSEN, 1966a, b, d; HENRIQUES et al., 1966, 1967; SUZUKI et al., 1967; YANO et al., 1967) and may be inactivated by different inhibitor(s) in plasma (WERLE, 1934; WERLE and MAIER, 1952) which do not inactivate the glandular kallikreins.

The first kallikreins to be discovered were the glandular kallikreins. ABELOUS and BARDIER, in a series of papers (1908–09) on the blood pressure effects of normal human urine, noted the presence of a hypotensive substance which they called urohypotensine. Similarly, PRIBRAM and HERRNHEISER (1920) and PETROFF

* Supported in part by Fundacao de Amparo a Pesquisa do Estado de Sao Paulo. Grant No. 68/638; National Institutes of Health, Special Fellowship, Grant No. 1 FO3 AM 42717–01.

and collaborators (MIGAY and PETROFF, 1923; PETROFF, 1925) noted the hypotensive effect of urine and pancreatic juice respectively. However, it was FREY (1926) and his associates, KRAUT and WERLE, who extensively studied the biologically active material and quickly showed that it was present in the urine (FREY and KRAUT, 1926, 1928; FREY, 1927; KRAUT et al., 1934), in the pancreas (FREY 1929; FREY et al., 1930; KRAUT et al., 1930), and in salivary glands (WERLE and VON RODEN, 1936, 1939) of many mammalian species. All exocrine fluids that were investigated, with the notable exception of the bile and gastric fluids, contained a kallikrein which was excreted by the gland. Thus saliva (WERLE and VON RODEN, 1936, 1939), pancreatic juice (PETROFF, 1925; WERLE, 1934), urine (FREY, 1926), feces (WERLE, 1934), but not bile or gastric juice (WERLE, 1934), contain a kallikrein that is excreted in a free active form except in pancreatic juice (MIGAY and PETROFF, 1923; WERLE, 1937) which contains mainly an inactive prekallikrein.

Whether these same glands also secrete the kallikreins under normal physiological conditions is less clearly established. Evidence for the internal secretion of pancreatic kallikrein was based originally on the observations (FREY et al., 1930) that ligation of all of the excretory ducts to the intestine does not alter the urinary excretion of kallikrein. These data, however, were based on the assumption that urinary kallikrein was derived from the pancreas, and they no longer seem applicable if it is concluded that the kallikrein found in urine is derived from the kidney (BERALDO et al., 1956; WEBSTER and PIERCE, 1960; WERLE, 1960; PRADO et al., 1962; MORIYA et al., 1963; CARVALHO and DINIZ, 1963, 1966; ABE, 1965). Also, no kallikrein could be detected in venous perfusates of the submaxillary gland when the gland was perfused with blood (HILTON and LEWIS, 1955). Further ligation of the ductus Whartoni in rats, mice, dogs, and cats (WERLE, 1960; WERLE et al., 1960; WERLE and FUCHS, 1965; BEILENSON et al., 1965) or of the pancreatic duct in rats (FORELL, 1960; FORELL et al., 1960) decreases the kallikrein content of the gland. These data suggest that the endocrine secretion of kallikrein is unlikely. Nevertheless, under pathological conditions evidence for the internal secretion of these kallikreins is being accumulated (Chapter 613, p. 552).

B. Subcellular Location and Activation of the Glandular Kallikreins

The subcellular localization of the glandular kallikreins has only recently been described. CARVALHO and DINIZ (1963, 1964, 1966) fractionated the kidney tissue of the rat in a manner similar to that described by DE DUVE et al. (1955) for the preparation of lysosomes from rat liver or to that reported by STRAUS (1954) for the preparation of "droplets" from rat kidney tissue. Both subcellular preparations contained a kallikrein which was inactive but could be activated either by dilution in hypotonic medium or by incubation in hypotonic medium at pH 5.0. It was suggested that this "activation" process reflects disruption of the subcellular particles and subsequent release of active kallikrein. These studies not only located a glandular kallikrein in a subcellular particle but for the first time demonstrated clearly that kidney tissue contains a kallikrein. Other investigators (WERLE, 1955) had mentioned that small amounts of kallikrein could be found in kidney tissue but no data were published.

In the submaxillary glands of the guinea pig (BHOOLA and OGLE, 1966; BHOOLA, 1968), the rat (ERDÖS et al., 1968), and the white mouse (CHIANG et al.,

1968) salivary kallikrein was also located in subcellular particles or granules. These granules were similar in appearance to those previously isolated from the pancreas, which had been shown to contain the digestive zymogens of this gland (Greene et al., 1963). The submaxillary granules were readily lysed by dilution in hypotonic (Bhoola and Ogle, 1966) or in isotonic (Erdös et al., 1968; Chiang et al., 1968) medium at 0° and released their kallikrein into the surrounding fluid.

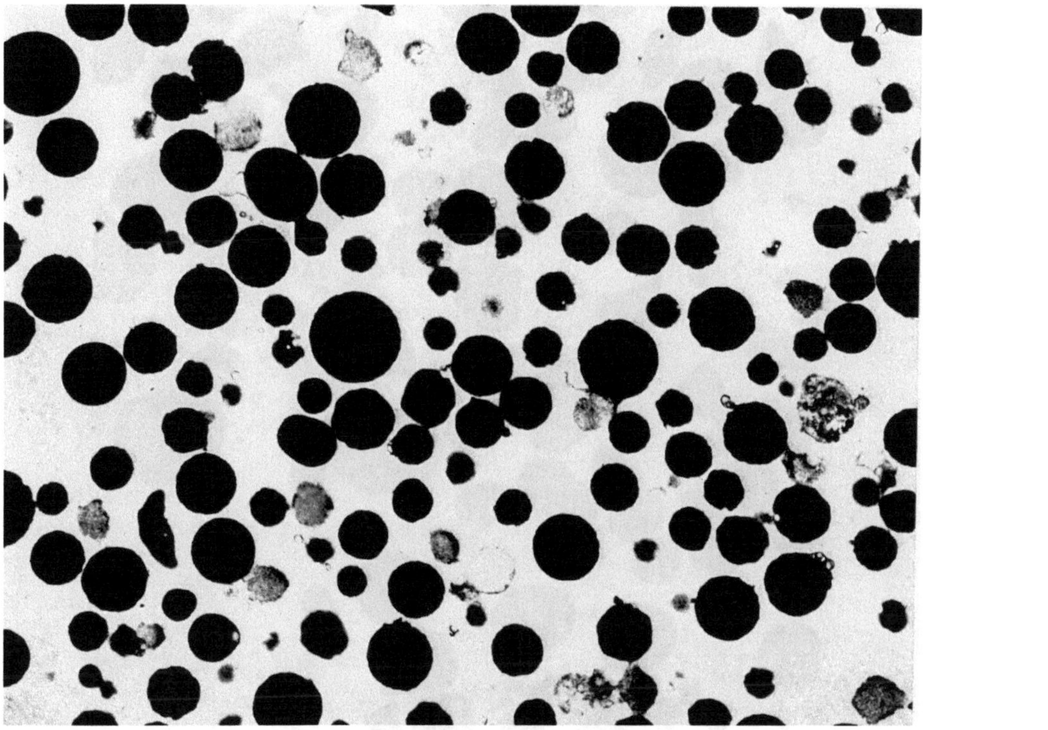

a

Fig. 1a and b. Electron photomicrographs of granules from submaxillary gland of the rat (a) and of the white mouse (b), that contain kallikrein, and kallikrein and renin, respectively. Magnification (a) 5,250 × and (b) 11,000 × (Erdös et al., 1968; Chiang et al., 1968) (reproduced with permission from Biochemical Pharmacology and Circulation Research)

Fig. 1 shows electron micrographs of the isolated granules obtained from the submaxillary glands of the rat and the white mouse. The granules from the rat were spherical bodies ranging in size up to 2 μ and were similar in appearance to the zymogen granules of the pancreas. Those from the white mouse, on the other hand, differed in size and shape. Some were spherical bodies resembling those from the rat gland while others were more elliptoid or amorphous. It has been known for some years that, in addition to kallikrein, renin is found in the submaxillary glands of the white mouse (Werle et al., 1957, 1963a; Turrian, 1960; Bing and Fårup, 1965; Oliver and Gross, 1967), and Carvalho and Diniz (1964) had suggested that, in the kidney, renin and kallikrein might be located in the same subcellular particle. The finding by Chiang and co-workers (1968) that the granular preparation from this submaxillary gland contains both renin and kallikrein suggested that the more amorphous granules might contain the renin and the round symmetrical ones the kallikrein. However, the authors, because of the similar distribution of the two activities during differential centrifugation, have mentioned the possibility that the same individual particles may contain both enzymes.

In both the kidney and the submaxillary gland no clear-cut evidence is available that the kallikrein is present as an inactive precursor. Although the kallikrein in the

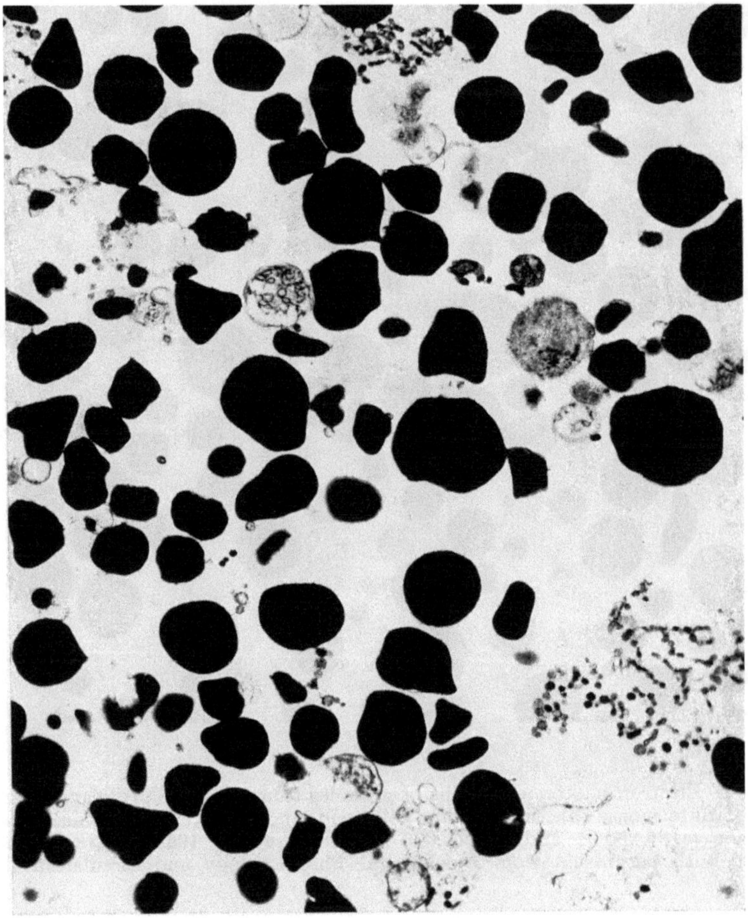

Fig. 1b

kidney particles required "activation," this process can be interpreted as simple disruption of the particle membrane and does not necessarily imply that an inactive enzyme precursor is present. In the pancreas, however, and in the internal secretion of this gland (Migay and Petroff, 1923; Werle, 1937), it has long been proposed that the kallikrein is present in an inactive form. Activation of the kallikrein in pancreatic juice can be accomplished by contact with gastric juice, and evidence was presented, in experiments using extracts from the pancreas (Werle and Urhahn, 1940), to suggest that the enterokinase in the gastric juice activates trypsin which in turn activates the kallikrein. Recently, however, the presence of an inactive enzyme precursor in pancreatic juice has been questioned (Hilton and JONES, 1968) and the apparent low concentration of kallikrein in this undiluted fluid has been attributed to the presence of kininases whose effect can be minimized by dilution. Nevertheless, it has been demonstrated clearly that the kallikrein in pancreas exists as inactive prekallikrein (FIEDLER and WERLE, 1967). Also, after several experimental procedures (FORELL, 1960; HILTON and JONES, 1968) a parallelism exists between the concentration of kallikrein and some of the digestive enzymes. These data would suggest that pancreatic kallikrein, like many of the digestive enzymes, is excreted as an inactive zymogen and may even be located in the same granules. Direct evidence for the location of pancreatic kallikrein in these granules is still lacking, although earlier studies (SIEBERT et al., 1955) have located hog pancreatic kallikrein in a mixed "microsomal-cytoplasmic" fraction and significant quantities in a "mitochondrial" fraction.

C. Tissue Concentrations of the Glandular Kallikreins

The content of the glandular kallikreins in various animal tissues and fluids is given in Table 1. Values are reported in terms of units per milliliter of fluid or per gram of fresh tissue. One unit (KU) was originally defined (FREY et al., 1950) as equal to the drop in the arterial blood pressure of the anesthetized dog, caused by the intravenous injection of 5.0 ml of dialyzed normal human urine which had been taken from a pool of 50 liters of urine. Pools of urine even of this magnitude, however, did not always contain 1.0 unit in 5.0 ml (F. SCHULTZ in FREY et al., 1950), and the unit has been maintained by exchanges of biologically active material between investigators. This unit of activity, although of great use to workers in this field, does not give the actual concentration of the kallikreins in the various tissues. Rather, it compares the ability of the various kallikreins to release kinins from dog kininogens. For example, for many years it was thought (FREY et al., 1950) that the horse had little kallikrein in its glands and fluids. However, ample amounts of kinins were formed *in vitro* if horse plasma, rather than dog plasma, was used as the substrate for the horse enzyme (PRADO and PRADO, 1961; PRADO et al., 1962). Therefore, the actual concentration of kallikrein cannot be determined by measuring the ability of these glandular extracts to depress dog blood pressure. If it is assumed, however, that the glandular kallikreins of a given species are equally potent in their ability to release kinins from dog blood, then values corresponding to their true concentrations may be obtained. On this assumption, the highest concentration of kallikrein is found in the pancreas in most animals except the rat and the mouse (Table 1). Of the various excretions tested, feces probably contain the highest concentration of kallikrein, followed by duodenal or pancreatic juice, saliva, and finally urine. In some species, such as the monkey, cow, hog and horse, however, no kallikrein could be detected in the feces, but this failure was thought to be due to bacterial decomposition (WERLE, 1934). The highest concentration of kallikrein as determined by this technique was found in the submaxillary gland of the rat, which contained 3,000 units per gram of wet tissue (WERLE, 1960).

The concentration of kallikrein within a given gland or fluid has been shown to vary 10-fold or more (Table 1). A partial explanation for this variation may be found in the following studies. It was noted that in man the daily excretion of urinary kallikrein varies more between individuals than in the same individual (KRAUT et al., 1930). The saliva secreted during or after eating in humans contains somewhat less kallikrein than in fasting saliva (WERLE and VON RODEN, 1939). In rats (WERLE, 1960; FORELL, 1960; VOGEL et al., 1962) and possibly in dogs, but not in man (Frey et al., 1950), a meat diet causes an increase in pancreatic and urinary kallikreins but no change in submaxillary kallikrein; an egg diet decreases the pancreatic kallikrein of the rat but increases the urinary kallikrein (Vogel et al., 1962), and a high-fat diet decreases both pancreatic and urinary kallikreins but does not alter submaxillary kallikrein. More kallikrein is found in human urine if it is collected during the day rather than at night (Elliot and Nuzum, 1934), and in that collected in summer rather than in winter (Kraut

Table 1. *Content of glandular kallikreins in various animal tissues and excretions*

Species	Glands				Excretions				
	Sub-maxillary	Sub-lingual	Parotid	Pancreas	Saliva	Pan-creatic	Dudoenal	Urine	Feces
Man	1–3	0.4–1	0.2–0.6	2–25	0–6		0.5–25	0.03–0.6	20
Monkey								0.2–1	<1
Whale				0.2–3					
Bovine	2–45	0.4–0.7	0.05–10	2–20	1–2			0.1–0.15	<1
Goat	0.5	0.5	0						
Hog	15–60	1	0.0–0.05	10–150				0.02–2	<1
Horse	<0.05–4	<0.05	<0.05–3	0.5–2	0.01–0.04			0.01	<1
Sheep	0.5	0.5	0	10					
Dog	2–40	0.07–7	0.1–4	10–100	1–7	9–25		0.4–1.5	1–60
Cat	15–110	2–3	4–5	20	5–10			2–4	
Rabbit					0.03			0.1–0.2	
Guinea pig					9			0.05–0.3	
Rat	3,000–4,000			70–80[a]	4			1.5	
Mouse	200			4	0.1				
Fox								2.5	
Lion								1.5	
Deer	7	4	0						

Content in units (KU) per gram fresh tissue or per milliliter fluid as measured by the fall in blood pressure of the dog (Frey et al., 1930, 1950, 1968; Kraut et al., 1930, 1934; Werle, 1934, 1937, 1960; Werle and Eckey, 1934; Werle and von Roden, 1936, 1939; Korányi et al., 1937; Webster et al., 1956; Kraut and Körbel, 1957; Moriya et al., 1958, 1963, 1965a, b; Habermann, 1962; Vogel et al., 1962; Werle and Trautschold, 1963).

[a] Values obtained with pancreas of albino rat. Pancreas of gray rat contained 5 KU/g fresh tissue.

et al., 1934), and prolonged bed rest may reduce the urinary excretion of kallikrein (Kraut et al., 1934; Werle and Korsten, 1938). During early and late stages of development in man the urinary excretion of kallikrein is lowered (Kraut et al., 1934; Elliot and Nuzum, 1936) and in the early development of a number of animal species the kallikrein concentration of the submaxillary gland and the pancreas is much lower than in the adult (Werle, 1960; Werle et al., 1960). More kallikrein is found in the submaxillary gland of the adult male rat than in the female (Erdös et al., 1968), but in the mouse no such difference was encountered (Trautschold et al., 1966b). These and other as yet unidentified factors may well influence the concentration of kallikrein in a given tissue.

In addition to the sources listed in Table 1, kinin-forming enzymes have been found in a number of other tissues and fluids. Thus a kininogenase has been found in perfusates of the glandular elements of the tongue (Hilton and Lewis, 1958), in sweat (Fox and Hilton, 1958), in accessory sex glands of the guinea pig (Bhoola et al., 1961, 1962), in lacrimal secretions (Lewis, 1959), and in milk and in rabbit bile (AMUNDSEN and NUSTAD, 1965). Similarly, small but distinct kinin-forming activity has been reported in acid-treated homogenates of squamous epithelial cells from the oral mucous membranes and in homogenates of cells from the gastric, duodenal, jejunal, ileal, and colonic mucosa of rats and rabbits (AMUNDSEN and NUSTAD, 1964, 1965). However, further studies are necessary on these kininogenases before they can be definitely classified as glandular kallikreins. For example, the enzyme which has been found in sweat still yields a kinin after the kininogen content of the serum has been depleted by a kallikrein (species and source not specified) (WERLE, 1960). Although a kallikrein has been reported to be present in milk (AMUNDSEN and NUSTAD, 1965), other investigators (GUTH, 1959; WERLE, 1960; WERLE and TRAUTSCHOLD, 1960; MORIYA et al., 1966) found only a substrate in bovine or human colostrum (p. 579). Also, the enzyme detected in rabbit bile (AMUNDSEN and NUSTAD, 1965) could not be found in liver homogenates and was not inhibited by Trasylol. This latter observation in itself does not preclude the existence of a kallikrein in bile since dog urinary kallikrein is not inhibited by Trasylol (FREY et al., 1950; WEBSTER et al., 1963). Nevertheless, the absence of a kallikrein in bile from other species (WERLE, 1934) suggests that further studies are necessary before the presence of a glandular kallikrein in rabbit bile can be established.

In addition, the small but distinct kinin-forming activity found in a number of acid-treated homogenates (AMUNDSEN and NUSTAD, 1964, 1965) might represent the activation of other endogenous proteases such as those found in lung extracts (WERLE and MAIER, 1955), in skin extracts (LEWIS, 1959), in cerebrospinal fluid CHAPMAN et al., 1960; HAMBERG, 1960; HILTON and SCHAIN, 1961; COPPEN and LEWIS, 1961; RAMOS et al., 1963), and those hypotensive substances found in water extracts of intestinal walls, lymph glands, milk, brain, and peripheral nervous tissue (WERLE, 1960; WERLE and VOGEL, 1961; WERLE et al., 1963b) which appear to be different from both plasma kallikrein and the glandular kallikreins. Attempts to detect glandular kallikreins in crude extracts of tissues and homogenates are fraught with difficulties. For example, the presence of appreciable amounts of kininases will interfere with their detection (WEBSTER and PIERCE, 1960; ERDÖS et al., 1962). The use of pseudoglobulin as a kininogen substrate which contains not only inactive kininogen but active plasma kallikrein may result in the identification of a kallikrein (EDERY and LEWIS, 1963) when actually a substrate is present (JACOBSEN, 1966c). Even the absence of blood in an organ does not ensure the absence of plasma kallikrein (JONASSON and BECKER, 1966). It is apparent, therefore, that the mere release of a kinin *in vitro* or of any hypotensive substance as measured in the dog does not necessarily identify the agent as a glandular kallikrein.

D. Purification and Some Properties of the Glandular Kallikreins

Attempts to purify the various glandular kallikreins were initiated as early as 1932 when KRAUT and co-workers reported the first partial purification of human urinary kallikrein. Table 2 enumerates the kallikreins which have been purified and the index of purification that was achieved by the various investigators. In addition to those listed, the purification of an immunologically homogenous kallikrein from the mucous of human bronchi and saliva (HAVEZ et al., 1965, 1966a, b) and a 30-fold purification of rat urinary kallikrein has been reported (MARES-GUIA and DINIZ, 1967). Four of the kallikreins—that is, those derived from human urine, human pancreas, hog pancreas, and horse urine—have been highly purified.

The first kallikrein to be so purified was that derived from hog pancreas and was reported by KRAUT and KÖRBEL (in WERLE, 1955) to have a molecular weight of 48,000. More recent studies of this same enzyme have resulted in the

Table 2. *Purification of glandular kallikreins from various animal tissues and fluids*

Species	Source	KU/mg or KU/E_{280}	Reference
Human	Urine	10	KRAUT et al. (1932)
		100–290	BISCHOFF and ELLIOT (1935)
		125–500	KRAUT and SCHWEITZER (1949)
		430	MORIYA et al. (1963)
	Pancreas	550	MORIYA et al. (1963)
	Saliva	365	MORIYA et al. (1965a, 1966)
Hog	Urine	200–500	WERLE and TRAUTSCHOLD (1963)
	Pancreas	30	WERLE and MARCUS (1938)
		500	FREY et al. (1950)
		100–200	KRAUT and KÖRBEL (1957)
		570	MORIYA and SCHIMAZAWA (1959a)
		800	HABERMANN (1962)
		100–588	WERLE and TRAUTSCHOLD (1963)
		320–450	MORIYA et al. (1965b)
		1,400	FRITZ et al. (1967)
		2,400	MORIYA et al. (1969)
	Submaxillary gland	900	FREY et al. (1950)
		200–510	WERLE and TRAUTSCHOLD (1963)
Bovine	Pancreas	70–100	WEBSTER et al. (1956)
Horse	Urine	820	PRADO et al. (1963)
Rat	Submaxillary	112	ERDÖS et al. (1968)

Units (KU) were determined by measuring the fall in blood pressure of the dog except for horse urinary kallikrein where one unit (KL) was defined as the activity per mg of a crude horse urinary kallikrein preparation and gives a calculated value of 0.25–0.75 KL units/ml horse urine (personal communication).

"The figure given by Moriya et al. for hog pancreatic kallikrein can be calculated to be 1,820. See p. 32, Table 6."

isolation of hog pancreatic kallikreins with a molecular weight of 33,000 (MORIYA, 1959e; MORIYA et al., 1963; FRITZ et al., 1967) and 24,000 (HABERMANN, 1962, 1963; MORIYA et al., 1969). Differences in the isoelectric point have also been reported: 4.2 for a partially purified preparation (WERLE and DÄUMER, 1940), 4.4 for the 24,000 molecular weight form (HABERMANN, 1962), and 2.4 for the 33,000 molecular weight form (MORIYA and SHIMAZAWA, 1959b). A partial explanation for these divergent results could be the presence of more than one form of this kallikrein in hog pancreas. HABERMANN (1962) was the first to separate two such forms by electrophoresis and suggested that their presence depended upon the degree of autolysis of the pancreas prior to its extraction. FRITZ et al. (1967) also noticed that their highly purified preparation contained multiple forms which differed in their content of sialic acid and suggested that these multiple forms could be due to contamination of the autolysates with neuraminidase-containing bacteria from the intestine. After removal of the sialic acid by treatment with neuraminidase, however, two forms of kallikrein (A and B) could still be separated by electrophoresis. Since chromatography of homogenates of hog pancreas on DEAE-cellulose columns (FIEDLER and WERLE, 1967) shows the presence of two prekallikreins, it is likely that this pancreas contains two distinct forms of kallikrein.

The amino acid composition has been determined on a number of highly purified hog pancreatic preparations (MORIYA, 1959c; TRAUTSCHOLD et al., 1966a; FRITZ et al., 1967) but no analyses have yet been done on the separated A and B forms. Both phenylalanine (MORIYA, 1959c) and alanine (TRAUTSCHOLD et al., 1966a) have been reported to be the amino terminal amino acid, and alanine is thought to occupy the carboxy terminus. However, the purity of these preparations makes these data questionable. Hog pancreatic kallikrein is a glycoprotein containing glucosamine, galactose, mannose, fucose, glucose, and sialic acid (MORIYA, 1959d; FRITZ et al., 1967). Phosphorus could not be detected (MORIYA, 1959d). Although lysine and arginine residues are present in these hog pancreatic kallikrein preparations, their biological activity is not altered after incubation with trypsin (WERLE and MAIER, 1952; MORIYA, 1959b). Similarly, incubation with papain only slightly reduced the biological activity of both hog pancreatic and human urinary kallikreins, although it completely destroyed the activity of hog submaxillary kallikrein. Pepsin only partially inactivated the three kallikreins. Like most enzymes the kallikreins are thermolabile (FREY et al., 1950) and inactivated by ultraviolet light (WERLE, 1936) even when combined with inhibitors.

Preparations of human urinary and human pancreatic kallikrein with molecular weights of 40,500 and 31,200 respectively (MORIYA et al., 1963), have been isolated. When these kallikreins were compared with hog pancreatic kallikrein for their electrophoretic mobility in polyacrylamide gel at pH 8.7, they migrated 3.2, 2.6, and 3.7 cm respectively. The biological potency of these three kallikreins as measured by their ability to produce vasodilatation in the dog was not markedly different. The two human glandular kallikreins had the same ratio of biological and esterase activity, whereas this ratio for hog pancreatic kallikrein was only one half.

Horse urinary kallikrein has also been purified to a state approaching homogeneity. This kallikrein is capable of hydrolyzing BAEe at a rate twice that of trypsin and is one third as active when TAMe is the substrate (PRADO et al., 1962, 1963). Loss of the kinin-forming activity of the enzyme was noted after exhaustive dialysis. Further investigation of this phenomena (PRADO et al., 1965) showed that Na^+, K^+, Li^+, Rb^+ or Cs^+ is required for the release of kinins from dialyzed horse plasma by this enzyme. Ca^{2+}, Mg^{2+}, and Al^{3+} did not alter this reaction, but preincubation of the kallikrein with Ag^+, Co^{2+}, Ni^{2+}, Cu^{2+}, Mg^{2+}, or Mn^{2+} strongly inhibits both the production of kinin and the hydrolysis of esters (KRAMER et al., 1966). FIEDLER and WERLE (1968) have also reported that the esterolytic activity of hog pancreatic kallikrein is inhibited by a number of heavy metal ions and is activated by sulfhydryl compounds or chelating agents. This latter activation has been interpreted as a reversal of heavy metal inhibition and this kallikrein is not thought to be either a "sulfhydryl" or a metal-dependent protease. Horse urinary kallikrein, like hog pancreatic kallikrein (CONTZEN et al., 1959) and human plasma kallikrein (WEBSTER and PIERCE, 1960), is incapable of digesting BAA amide or casein. It can, however, hydrolyze some of the arginyl peptide bonds in salmine (BRANDI et al., 1965, 1967) and the Arg-Arg bonds in poly-L-arginine peptides of four or more residues. It does not attack poly-L-lysine or dipeptides of arginine or lysine formed with other amino acids (PRADO et al., 1967). Similar studies with other glandular kallikreins have not yet been undertaken, although it has been demonstrated that hog and horse plasma kallikreins are also capable of hydrolyzing the arginyl bonds in salmine (BRANDI et al., 1967).

One or more of the glandular kallikreins, kinin-forming enzymes from snake venoms, or plasma kallikreins have been shown to hydrolyze the following substrates: BAMe (HAMBERG and ROCH E SILVA, 1957a, b; WEBSTER and PIERCE, 1961; HOLMAN et al., 1968); TAMe (CONTZEN et al., 1959; HABERMANN, 1959; WEBSTER and PIERCE, 1961; PRADO et al., 1962; DAVIES and LOWE, 1963; HABERMANN and KLETT, 1966); BAEe (WERLE and KAUFMANN-BOETSCH, 1960; WEBSTER and PIERCE, 1961; PRADO et al., 1962; DINIZ et al., 1965; HABERMANN and KLETT, 1966; ERDÖS et al., 1968; CHIANG et al., 1968); salmine (BRANDI et al., 1965, 1967); poly-L-arginine (PRADO et al., 1967); *p*-toluenesulfonyl-L-lysine methyl ester, acetylarginine methyl ester, acetyllysine methyl ester (SHERRY et al., 1965; HOLMAN et al., 1968); benzoyl-DL-arginine *p*-nitroanilide (HABERMANN and KLETT, 1966; MARES-GUIA and DINIZ, 1967; ERDÖS et al., 1968); benzoyl-L-lysine methyl ester (FIEDLER, 1968; HOLMAN et al., 1968); benzoyl-L-ornithine methyl ester, benzoyl-DL-methionine methyl ester (FIEDLER, 1968); *p*-toluenesulfonyl-L-arginine ethyl ester, *p*-toluenesulfonyl-L-lysine ethyl ester; a series of lysine methyl esters substituted in the N^{α}-position with *p*-methylbenzoyl, *p*-chlorobenzoyl, *p*-methoxybenzoyl, benzenesulfonyl, phenylacetyl, phenoxyacetyl, cyclohexylcarbonyl, 1-naphthoyl, 2-naphthoyl, 1-naphthylacetyl, and n-hexoyl; N^{α}-acetyl-O-(N^{α}-benzoyllysyl)-serine amide, N^{α}-acetyl-O-(N^{α}-acetyllysyl)-serine amide, N^{α}-acetyl-O-(N^{α}-benzoyllysyl)-tyrosine amide, and N^{α}-acetyl-O-(N^{α}-acetyllysyltyrosine) amide (HOLMAN et al., 1968).

There is little evidence that these enzymes digest casein (HAMBERG and ROCHA E SILVA, 1957a, b; MORIYA, 1959a; WEBSTER and PIERCE, 1960; HABERMANN, 1961a, b; PRADO et al., 1962; BAA (CONTZEN et al., 1959; HENRIQUES and FICHMAN, 1960; HABERMANN, 1961a; PRADO et al., 1963); hemoglobin, N-benzoyl-DL-arginine-β-naphthylamide, tributyrin, butyric acid methyl ester (WERLE and KAUFMANN-BOETSCH, 1960); benzoyl-DL-alanine methyl and ethyl ester, ATEe (WEBSTER and PIERCE, 1961); L-leucine ethyl ester, L-tyrosine methyl ester, N-acetyl-L-tryptophan ethyl ester (WEBSTER and PIERCE, 1961; DAVIES and LOWE, 1963); L-lysine methyl ester (WEBSTER and PIERCE, 1961; DAVIES and LOWE, 1963; SHERRY et al., 1965; HOLMAN et al., 1968); L-phenylalanine ethyl ester, DL-alanine ethyl ester, N-α-carboxybenzoxyaspartic acid methyl ester, N-α-carboxybenzoxyglutamic acid methyl ester (DAVIES and LOWE, 1963); arginine methyl ester (SHERRY et al., 1965); lysine ethyl ester (PRADO et al., 1967; HOLMAN et al., 1968); poly-L-lysine, arginylphenylalanine, arginylproline, arginylaspartic acid, arginylvaline, arginylisoleucine, arginylarginine, lysyl-L-phenylalanine, lysyl-L-valine, and lysyl-L-leucine (PRADO et al., 1967); N^{α}-acetyl-O-(N^{α}-acetyllysyl) threonine amide, and N^{α}-acetyl-O-(N^{α}-benzoyllysyl)$^{\alpha}$-threonine amide (HOLMAN et al., 1968).

During the above studies, some discrepancies have occurred which suggest the possibility that certain substrates are cleaved by only one of the kallikreins. Thus some preparations of hog pancreatic kallikrein have been reported to hydrolyze hemoglobin (WERLE and KAUFMANN-BOETSCH, 1960), tyrosine and tryptophan esters (WEBSTER and PIERCE, 1961), and even casein (JOLLÈS et al., 1963). However, the possibility that a contaminant was responsible for the observed effects has not been excluded. Also it has been reported (DINIZ et al., 1965, 1966) that certain partially purified preparations of human urinary kallikrein did not cleave BAEe. However, these results have not been confirmed with highly purified preparations. Acetyllysine methyl ester would appear to be a much better substrate for guinea pig plasma kallikrein (HOLMAN et al., 1968) than for human urinary kallikrein (SHERRY et al., 1965). Similarly, hog serum and rat urinary kallikreins hydrolyze BANA (HABERMANN and KLETT, 1966; MARES-GUIA and

DINIZ, 1967) while ornithokallikrein from the pancreas does not (WERLE et al., 1966). However, the ornithokallikreins might be quite different from the mammalian kallikreins since they do not appear to release bradykinin from their kininogens. Glandular kallikreins from different species and different sources can usually be distinguished by means of inhibitors (Chapter 3, p. 213) and hydrolyze synthetic substrates at different rates, but no clear-cut differences in their ability to cleave a particular substrate have yet been demonstrated.

Certain synthetic or isolated analogs of bradykinin have also been examined as possible substrates for some of the glandular kallikreins. PKFL and PKFS, kinin-yielding peptides isolated from pepsin digests of kininogen (HABERMANN and MÜLLER, 1966), contain methionyllysylbradykinin at the amino terminal end of the peptide (p. 262) and can act as substrates for some of the kallikreins. Hog pancreatic kallikrein forms methionyllysylbradykinin from these substrates while *Crotolus adamanteus* venom and hog serum kallikrein formed bradykinin. It has been reported that bradykinylserine is not a substrate for hog pancreatic kallikrein (HABERMANN, 1966), but it was cleaved at the Arg-Ser bond by horse urinary kallikrein (BABEL et al., 1968), hog serum kallikrein, *C. adamanteus* venom, and trypsin (HABERMANN, 1966). Horse urinary kallikrein slowly forms bradykinin from methionyllysylbradykinin and lysyllysylbradykinin, the latter being the more resistant substrate. In preliminary studies, liberation of a kinin-like material from 6-0-acetyl-Ser-bradykinyl-Gly-Val-Gln, bradykinyl-Gly and Gly-Gly-Lys-6-0-acetyl-Ser-bradykinin by hog pancreatic kallikrein and trypsin has also been reported (SUZUKI et al., 1966); the last substrate may be of use in distinguishing trypsin from hog pancreatic kallikrein. With most but not all of these substrates, relatively large amounts of the glandular kallikreins are required for hydrolysis. Further, it should be recalled that at least for hog pancreatic kallikrein the tertiary structure of bovine kininogen influences the rate of liberation of kinin (KATO et al., 1967).

E. The Active Center of the Kallikreins

(M. MARES-GUIA and C. R. DINIZ)

Attempts to determine the active center(s) of the glandular kallikreins are currently based on the use of competitive inhibitors or of specific labeling agents like DFP which bind to certain amino acids such as serine. In this discussion active center is defined as "that general region in the neighborhood of the catalytic residues identified with the binding and reaction of substrate" (KOSHLAND and NEET, 1968).

Competitive inhibition of purified rat urinary kallikreins by such compounds as benzamidine, β-naphthamidine, phenylguanidine, and cyclohexylguanidine has been demonstrated by MARES-GUIA and DINIZ (1967) (Fig. 2). Although this inhibition is qualitatively similar to that for trypsin (MARES-GUIA and SHAW, 1965), these compounds are less efficient inhibitors of this kallikrein, as shown in Table 3. Further, the Km value for the hydrolysis of BAEe by hog pancreatic kallikrein (Km 130 μM, Kcat 129 sec^{-1}) (FIEDLER and WERLE, 1968) is higher than that for trypsin (Km 4.3 μM, Kcat 14.6 sec^{-1}) (INAGAMI and STURTEVANT, 1960). Despite these quantitative differences, the data permit the inference that, as proposed for the active center of trypsin (MARES-GUIA and SHAW, 1965; MARES-GUIA, 1968), the active centers of the glandular kallikreins contain an anionic binding site and a hydrophobic site in addition to the catalytic site. FIEDLER and WERLE (1968) have also shown that, like trypsin (TROWBRIDGE et al., 1963), hog pancreatic kallikrein exhibits substrate activation with TAMe.

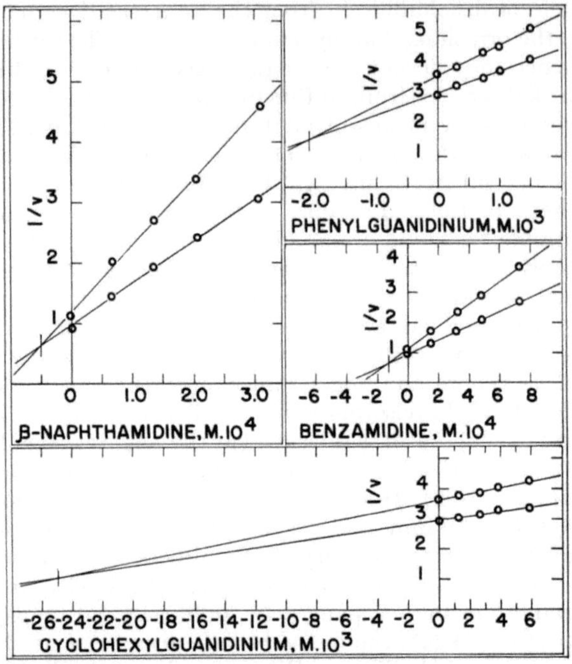

Fig. 2. Competitive inhibition of rat urinary kallikrein by amidines and guanidines. Ordinate: reciprocal of the rate in liters per mole $\times$ 10^{-7} per mintue. Abscissa: molar concentration of inhibitor multiplied by factor as given. Concentrations of DL-BANA: 5.05×10^{-4} M (lower lines) and 2.70×10^{-4} M (upper lines). Total volume was 2 ml; incubation was for 60 minutes at 37°; kallikrein concentration 0.3 mg/ml. Data for β-naphthamidine-HCl and benzamidine-HCl were obtained in 0.1 M Tris, pH 8.0; those for cyclohexylguanidine and phenylguanidine sulfates were obtained in 0.1 M phosphate (Na^+) buffer, pH 8.0. (Reproduced with permission from Archives of Biochemistry and Biophysics) (MARES-GUIA and DINIZ, 1967)

Table 3. *Comparison of the dissociation constants (Ki) for the competitive inhibition of trypsin and rat urinary kallikrein*

Inhibitor	Trypsin (Ki, μM[a])	Kallikrein (Ki, μM[a])
Benzamidine	16.6 ± 2[b]	125 ± 15[d]
β-Naphthamidine	14.6 ± 3[b]	50 ± 10[d]
Phenylguanidine	72.5[c]	2,130 ± 320[d]
Cyclohexylguanidine	1,540[c]	25,000 ± 5,000[d]

[a] Substrate used was DL-BANA and Ki values obtained from the following equations: EnI = En + I, Ki = (EN) (I)/(EnI).
[b] Measured at 15°, pH 8.15, in 0.1 M Tris (MARES-GUIA, 1968).
[c] Measured at 15°, pH 8.15, in 0.1 M Tris (MARES-GUIA and SHAW, 1965).
[d] Measured at 37°, pH 8.1 (MARES-GUIA and DINIZ, 1967).

This finding is probably best interpreted as a binding of the substrate to an auxiliary, perhaps adjacent, site. It is apparent that more studies with competitive models of the side chain are required to ascertain the contribution of the hydrophobic site to the overall binding in the active center of the kallikrein.

Many specific labeling agents have been tested for their ability to inhibit the glandular kallikreins. Thus DFP (p. 215) inhibits several of the glandular kallikreins, suggesting the presence of a reactive seryl residue in their active centers.

Indeed radioactive serine-phosphate was isolated by FIEDLER and co-workers (1968) from a hydrolysate of hog pancreatic kallikrein previously inactivated by ^{32}P-DFP. The authors found 1 mole of ^{32}P bound per mole of enzyme. This result adds the glandular kallikreins to the list of serine hydrolases (OOSTERBAAN and COHEN, 1964). Efforts, however, to demonstrate the presence of a histidyl residue in the active site by inactivation with 1-chloro-3-tosylamido-7-amino-2-heptanone (TLCK), as was done with trypsin (SHAW et al., 1965), have been unsuccessful. None of the kallikreins tested to date (i.e. those from rat urine, horse urine, human urine, hog pancreas, and human saliva (DINIZ et al., 1965; MARES-GUIA and DINIZ, 1967; FIEDLER and WERLE, 1968; PASKHINA et al., 1968) were inactivated by TLCK.

This lack of reactivity, however, does not exclude the participation of a histidyl residue in the catalytic mechanism. It could also be interpreted as an unfavorable fit between enzyme and TLCK which would render alkylation impossible (DINIZ et al., 1966). Indeed, several reports in the literature suggest the participation of a histidyl residue in the active center of a kallikrein. For example, WERLE and APPEL (1956) photochemically inactivated hog pancreatic kallikrein in the presence of methylene blue. MARES-GUIA and DINIZ (1967) proposed histidine participation in rat urinary kallikrein on the basis of the pH-dependent rate of BAEe and BANA hydrolysis. FIEDLER and WERLE (1968) analyzed the pH dependence of V_{max} and Km for hog pancreatic kallikrein and found a group with $pK = 5.7$ in the free enzyme and $pK = 6.9$ in the enzyme–substrate complex. A third reagent, TPCK (L-1-tosylamido-2-phenylethylchloromethyl ketone), which has been used in studies of the active center of chymotrypsin (SCHOELLMANN and SHAW, 1963), does not inactivate human urinary kallikrein. It was thought that if the reagent side chain was hydrophobic, like the methionyl residue in kininogen, some inactivation would occur. However, TPCK did not inhibit release of kinin by this kallikrein. Other new reagents such as ethyl *p*-guanidinobenzoate and *p*-nitrophenyl *p'*-guanidinobenzoate which inactivate trypsin (MARES-GUIA and SHAW, 1967; CHASE and SHAW, 1967) did not affect the rate of hydrolysis of BAEe and BANA by rat urinary kallikrein. In fact, rat urinary kallikrein at pH 8.3 slowly hydrolyzed the latter inhibitor, and at the end of the experiment no inhibition of BANA hydrolysis could be detected.

The ability of these guanidine esters to inactivate trypsin has been attributed to their rigid structure, which would bring the acyl enzyme into an unfavorable conformation so that the next step in the enzymatic catalysis, the hydrolysis of the acyl enzyme complex, was hindered. The failure of these esters to inhibit kallikreins would suggest that the active center of these kallikreins is less rigid than that of trypsin and possesses a higher degree of conformational adaptability. The bromoketones derived from *p*-guanidinobenzoic and *p*-amidinobenzoic acids have also been shown to inactivate trypsin by alkylation (SCHROEDER and SHAW, personal communication) the former alkylating trypsin faster than the latter compound. These results have been attributed to difference in accessibility and proximity of the site of alkylation in the active center. Both of these compounds inactivate rat urinary kallikrein, as shown in Fig. 3. Quantitative differences between the reactions of these reagents with trypsin and with rat urinary kallikrein were observed.

From these data it appears reasonable to propose (MARES-GUIA and DINIZ, 1967) that the active center of the glandular kallikreins includes the following sites:

1. *An anionic site* responsible for binding the substrate through electrostatic attraction for its positively charged nitrogen

2. *A hydrophobic site* that binds the carbon side chain of lysyl or arginyl residues
3. *A catalytic site* that most probably contains a seryl and a histidyl residue
4. *An auxiliary site* as evidenced by the activation of TAMe hydrolysis by TAMe itself

Other aspects of kininogen catalysis that might eventually enlarge or modify this view of the enzyme active center are:

i. Their pronounced protein specificity; kallikreins do not generally hydrolyze proteins other than kininogens and do not even hydrolyze reduced or otherwise denatured kininogens
ii. Their content of carbohydrate which might affect their tertiary structure and protein binding ability

In addition there are other curious aspects to their catalysis for which explanations must be found. For example, the glandular kallikreins, as far as is

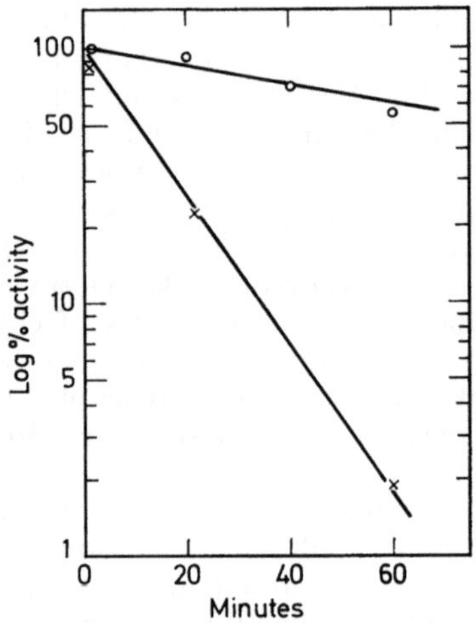

Fig. 3. Inactivation of rat urinary kallikrein by *p*-amidino and *p*-guanidinophenacyl bromides (APB and GPB). APB (x): 2 ml of 0.05 M phosphate (Na^+) buffer, pH 7.9 at 37°, containing 0.4 mg rat urinary kallikrein and 1.46 mM APB. GPB (○): 3 ml 0.1 M phosphate (Na^+) buffer, pH 7.9 at 37°, containing 0.6 mg rat urinary kallikrein and 0.65 mM GPB. Controls contained no APB or GPB. At suitable time intervals samples of 0.5 ml were removed and assayed with DL-BANA (MARES-GUIA and DINIZ, 1967)

known, form kallidin from kininogen, and current structural studies would suggest that this enzyme must preferentially split both a Met-Lys and an Arg-Ser peptide bond to release the decapeptide. This unusual specificity is further complicated by the observation that hog pancreatic kallikrein splits only the Arg-Ser bond in pepsin fragments of kininogen (PKFL) (p. 265) while leaving untouched the Met-Lys bond. These latter results, however, could be due to slowing of the rate of hydrolysis by the free amino group in the methionine, although studies with the tridecapeptides Gly-Arg-Met-Lys-bradykinin and Ser-Arg-Met-Lys-bradykinin (HOCHSTRASSER and WERLE, 1967) also indicate that only the Arg-Met bonds are cleaved by this enzyme. Nevertheless, FIEDLER (1968) has shown that the methyl ester of benzoyl-DL-methionine is weakly hydrolyzed by hog pancreatic kallikrein. Possible explanations for the specificity of the glandular kallikreins are that these enzymes have a site that recognizes both the Met- and Lys-residues of the Met-Lys bond. It would be possible to visualize the catalytic site as situated between these recognition sites, thus explaining the hydrolysis of this bond. A small molecule such as BAEe might fit this recognition site and be split by the enzyme. One substrate molecule might then bind two enzyme molecules—one splitting the Met-Lys bond and the other the Arg-Ser bond. Alternatively, there might be two catalytic subunits per enzyme molecule, each containing its own active site or two active sites in the same molecule. Further studies with purified kininogens might clarify this situation.

F. Species Differences Among the Glandular Kallikreins

The first observations of species differences among the kallikreins were made by (WERLE and HÜRTER (1936), who demonstrated that injection of large concentrations of human urinary kallikrein (80–100 KU) failed to affect the blood pressure of chickens or ducks. On the other hand, the pancreas from chicken or geese contained a kallikrein which lowered the blood pressure of birds but was inactive in mammals. They named this kallikrein ornithokallikrein. As in mammals, kallikreins could not be detected in chicken or goose liver or muscle (WERLE and HÜRTER, 1936) but were found in chicken, goose, and pigeon feces. These kallikreins could be inactivated either by bird serum or mammalian serum, although the inactivator from chicken and goose blood had little effect on the mammalian kallikreins. The above results were confirmed by LEHMANN and VAN WINKLE (1938), who found that pigeon urine raised the blood pressure in cats, dogs, and rabbits but reduced it in pigeons and chickens. More recent studies of ornithokallikrein from the pancreas (WERLE et al., 1966) have revealed that like the other glandular kallikreins it cleaves BAEe and is not inhibited by SBTI. This enzyme liberates ornithokinin from hen plasma, which contracts the hen ileum. Bovine trypsin can liberate an ornithokinin from hen plasma.

Species differences among the various mammalian kallikreins based on their different behaviour toward inhibitors has also been known for some time (WERLE and MAIER, 1952). Even as early as 1950 (FREY et al.), it was reported that the kallikrein of the dog (source not given but probably dog urinary kallikrein as mentioned by WEBSTER et al., 1963) could not be inactivated with Trasylol. (Other differences among the glandular kallikreins in their response to inhibitors have been detailed; see Chapter 3, p. 213.)

Species difference among the mammalian kallikreins based on their ability to release kinins from different sera or plasma has also been known for many years. In 1937 WERLE and co-workers noted that more human urinary kallikrein had to be added to bovine, dog, cat, rabbit, and sheep serum than to human serum in order to detect the release of a kinin *in vitro* and that no kinin was formed with this enzyme from hog, horse, or guinea pig serum. Kinin formation from plasma *in vitro* reflects not only the ability of an enzyme to release kinins from the kininogen under study but is also influenced by kallikrein inhibitors in the plasma and by the presence of kininases either in the partially purified enzyme preparation or in the plasma. Although the influence of kallikrein inhibitors on this reaction has not been clearly established, it has been known for some time that the kininases can effectively prevent the detection of kinin formation by rapidly destroying kinins. For example, the failure of a crude preparation of hog pancreatic kallikrein (containing 4 KU/mg when assayed in the dog) to release detectable levels of kinin when added to plasma directly in a tissue bath (WEBSTER and PIERCE, 1960) was probably due to the high content of carboxypeptidase B in this enzyme preparation (ERDÖS et al., 1962).

Table 4. *Species specificity of the mammalian glandular kallikreins*

Kallikreins derived from	Kinin formation from kininogens of different species										Reference
	Human	Bovine	Hog	Horse	Sheep	Dog	Cat	Rabbit	Guinea pig	Rat	
Human urine	+	+	−	−	+	+	+	+	−		Werle et al. (1937), Werle and Grunz (1939)
					+	+					
	+	−					−		−		Schachter (1956) Gaddum and Guth (1960)
Human saliva	+	+		−			+	+	−		Schachter (1956) Bhoola et al. (1965)
						+		+	−	−	Jacobsen (1966d)
Hog pancreas			+								Werle and Grunz (1939)
	−	±					−	−	+		Schachter (1956)
	+	+	+			+			−	−	Fasciolo and Halversen (1964)
	+					+		+	±[a]	−	Jacobsen (1966d)
Sheep urine					+	+					Gaddum and Guth (1960)
Horse urine	±	±		+		±				±	Prado and Prado (1961), Bhoola et al. (1965)
Horse saliva				+							
Dog urine		−				+					Beraldo (1955), Beraldo et al. (1956)
					+	+					Gaddum and Guth (1960)
Dog saliva	+					+		+	−	−	Jacobsen (1966d)
Cat saliva	+	+					+	+	−		Schachter (1956), Bhoola et al. (1965)
Rabbit saliva	+					+		+	−	−	Jacobsen (1966d)
Guinea pig urine	−	−					−	−	−		Schachter (1956)
Guinea pig saliva	+	+		−					−		Schachter (1960), Bhoola et al. (1965)
	+					+		+	+[a]	±	Jacobsen (1966d)
Rat urine										+	Beraldo et al. (1966, 1967), Jacobsen (1966d)
Rat saliva	+	+		−					−		Schachter (1960), Bhoola et al. (1965)
	+					+		+	−	+	Jacobsen (1966d), Erdös et al. (1968)
submaxillary	+										
Mouse submaxillary	+										Chiang et al. (1968)

+ Marked formation of kinin; ± small formation of kinin; — no detectable formation of kinin.
[a] Formation of kinin from low molecular weight substrate only.

The ability of several glandular kallikreins to form kinins from the plasma of different species as reported by a number of investigators is demonstrated in Table 4. As is shown, certain discrepancies exist in the literature concerning the release of kinins from the plasma of a particular species. Plausible explanations can be made for some of these divergent data. For example, the observations by SCHACHTER (1956) that no kinin was formed when human urinary kallikrein was added to bovine or cat serum could be due to the use of insufficient quantity of enzyme, since this investigator employed only 0.5 ml human urine (0.1 KU). Similar reasons may explain his failure to detect a kallikrein in guinea pig urine. An explanation, however, for the failure of hog pancreatic kallikrein to release a kinin from human, cat, and rabbit sera, although large amounts were formed with guinea pig sera, does not readily suggest itself; it may, however, simply reside in the particular enzyme preparation used by this investigator. Hog pancreatic kallikrein has been repeatedly shown to release a kinin from human plasma (WEBSTER and PIERCE, 1960, 1963; FASCIOLO and HALVORSEN, 1964; JACOBSEN, 1966d; VOGT et al., 1967). This same enzyme releases from guinea pig plasma only small amounts of kinin (JACOBSEN, 1966d) which were not detected by FASCIOLO and HALVORSEN (1964), who measured the decrease in kininogen rather than the generation of kinin—the former being a less sensitive method for the detection of kinin formation.

SCHACHTER (1960) was also unable to detect the release of a kinin when guinea pig saliva was added to guinea pig plasma and has used this observation to support the view that the glandular kallikreins do not play a role in functional vasodilatation of glands (SCHACHTER, 1960; BHOOLA et al., 1961, 1962, 1965; SCHACHTER, 1966). JACOBSEN (1966d), however, could detect the formation of kinin under these conditions provided an inhibitor of the kininases was present. This author noted that guinea pig salivary kallikrein and hog pancreatic kallikrein formed kinin only from the lower molecular weight kininogen of this species. The guinea pig, in this regard, is an unusual species in that the concentration of low molecular weight kininogen is slight, and the glandular kallikreins form kinin only from this substrate. In other mammalian species such as man, dog, rabbit, and rat the level of low molecular weight substrate is usually much higher and the glandular kallikreins will form kinins from both the low and high molecular weight kininogens. Plasma kallikrein, on the other hand, forms kinin from both the low and high molecular weight kininogens of the guinea pig but will form kinin only from the high molecular weight kininogen of other mammalian species. These unusual conditions, together with the high content of kininase in guinea pig plasma, make it difficult to detect the release of kinins by glandular kallikreins from this plasma. The use of *o*-phenanthroline or other chelating agents to inactivate the kininases is of particular importance when rat and guinea pig plasma are used as a source of substrate, since both of these plasma contain high concentrations of kininases (ERDÖS et al., 1963; FASCIOLO and HALVORSEN, 1964).

From the data currently available (Table 4), the hog, horse, guinea pig, and rat appear to have the most specific kininogens. In all these plasmas the greatest amounts of kinin are formed by the glandular kallikreins derived from the same species. To a lesser extent their glandular kallikreins may also show specificity. For example, horse urinary and salivary kallikreins are the only known glandular kallikreins that release kinins from horse plasma, but horse urinary kallikrein will release small quantities of kinin from the plasma of other mammalian species (PRADO and PRADO, 1961). The reason for this decreased kinin formation from heterologous plasma has not been established but very probably lies in differences in affinity of the enzyme for the substrate. Even human urinary kallikrein yields kinin best from human plasma (Werle et al., 1937) and must be used in higher concentrations to release kinins from other mammalian species. Further investigations, preferably with purified enzymes and substrates, are necessary.

G. Detection and Identification of a Glandular Kallikrein

Detection and identification of an enzyme as a glandular kallikrein, rather than some other proteolytic enzyme, is not an easy task and is particularly difficult when crude glandular extracts or fluids are examined. The following recommendations are based on our current knowledge of the properties of glandular kallikreins and may well have to be modified as further studies of these enzymes from other species are undertaken.

1. The glandular extract or fluid should be examined for its ability to inactivate bradykinin, since excessive amounts of kininases can destroy the formed kinin as rapidly as it is liberated. If the aliquot to be tested can inactivate one nanomole or more of bradykinin within one minute, methods for preventing this inactivation should be examined. Currently the use of various chelating agents is recommended (Chapter 2, p. 52). The concentration of chelating agent chosen should not alter the ability of bradykinin to contract the smooth muscle.

2. The extract can now be examined for its ability to release a kinin from plasma. Initially, citrated plasma taken from the same species in silicone-coated or otherwise protected containers should be used as substrate. It, too, should be preexamined for its ability to inactivate bradykinin, and chelating agents should be added if necessary. In order to ensure that substrate is present, the plasma should be tested whenever possible with a known glandular kallikrein which will form a kinin from the plasma of the species under investigation (see section on species differences, above). In these tests the plasma can be added directly to the isolated muscle in the tissue bath, followed in a minute or two by the enzyme preparation. Neither the plasma nor the enzyme preparation should cause contraction of the smooth muscle when added separately to the bath. Should the plasma and enzyme mixture cause contraction, the spasmogenic factor should be tentatively identified as a kinin by inactivation with carboxypeptidase B or the kininases of guinea pig plasma (Webster and Gilmore, 1965; Chapter 5, p. 304). Inactivation with chymotrypsin does not identify a kinin, since angiotensin is also destroyed by this enzyme. Other methods for identification of kinins which are based on the pharmacological properties of the kinins are given in Chapter 2, (p. 60).

3. If a kinin is formed, then the recommendations in No. 2 should be repeated, with plasma heated for 30 minutes at 60°. This procedure is thought to destroy prekallikrein and is thus useful in distinguishing between kallikreins and activators of prekallikreins.

4. The ability of inhibitors to prevent the formation of kinins should then be examined. SBTI is not known to inhibit any of the glandular kallikreins although it does block the formation of kinins by trypsin, plasmin, and plasma kallikrein (Chapter 3, p. 219). The response of the glandular kallikreins to other inhibitors is variable so that no single inhibitor (except possibly DFP) is known which will inhibit all the glandular kallikreins from the different species. Nevertheless, the action of the inhibitors on kinin formation provides useful information, and these same inhibitors can be used to inhibit the hydrolysis of substrates other than kininogen.

5. The glandular extracts or fluids can then be examined for their ability to hydrolyze synthetic arginine esters and other protein substrates such as casein, fibrinogen, hemoglobin, etc. Should the crude extracts cleave other protein substrates, purification of the kallikrein should be undertaken, and the separation of the kinin-forming activity from the proteolytic activity should be attempted. The kininogenase activity should correspond to at least a portion of the activity of the extract on synthetic arginine esters.

The substrate that is recommended above is plasma itself and not an isolated substrate. Difficulties have been encountered in the use of substrates which have been isolated by as simple a procedure as precipitation with ammonium sulfate. For example, this procedure when applied to plasma of humans, dogs, rabbits, guinea pigs, and rats caused the activation of endogenous plasma kallikrein and subsequent loss of the high molecular weight substrate (Jacobsen, 1966a, b, c, d). No satisfactory technique is as yet available which will rapidly isolate the kininogens from plasma free of kininases, prekallikrein, and plasma kallikrein. Further efforts in this direction should be undertaken.

References

ABE, K.: Urinary excretion of kinin in man with special reference to its origin. J. exp. Med. (Tohoku) 87, 175 (1965).

ABELOUS, J. E., BARDIER, E.: Action hypertensive de l'urine humaine normale. C. R. Soc. Biol. (Paris) 64, 848 (1908).

— — Les substances hypotensives de l'urine humaine normale. C. R. Soc. Biol. (Paris) 66, 511 (1909).

— — De l'action hypotensive et myotique de l'urine humaine normale. C. R. Soc. Biol. (Paris) 66, 876 (1909).

— — Effects physiologiques généraux de l'urohypotensine. C. R. Soc. Biol. (Paris) 67, 784 (1909).

— — L'Urohypotensine. J. Physiol. Path. gén. 11, 777 (1909).

— — Action de l'urohypotensine sur la pression artérielle. C. R. Acad. Sci. (Paris) 149, 142, 1395 (1909).

AMUNDSEN, E., NUSTAD, K.: Kinin-forming and -destroying activities of saliva. Brit. J. Pharmacol. 23, 440 (1964).

— — Kinin-forming and -destroying activity of cell homogenates. J. Physiol. (Lond.) 179, 479 (1965).

BABEL, I., STELLA, R. C. R., PRADO, E. S.: Action of horse urinary kallikrein on synthetic derivatives of bradykinin. Biochem. Pharmacol. 17, 2232 (1968).

BACK, N., STEGER, R.: Effect of inhibitors on kinin-releasing activity of proteases. Fed. Proc. 27, 96 (1968).

BEILENSON, S., SCHACHTER, M., SMAJE, L. H.: Kallikrein in the submaxillary gland of the cat. J. Physiol. (Lond.) 177, 61P (1965).

BERALDO, W. T.: Substance U and related substances from urine. In: Polypeptides which stimulate plain muscle, p. 58. Ed. by J. H. GADDUM. Edinburgh: Livingstone 1955.

— ARAUJO, R. L., MARES-GUIA, M.: Oxytocic esterases in rat urine. Amer. J. Physiol. 211, 976 (1966).

— — — On an esterasic activity of rat urine. In: International Symposium on vaso-active polypeptides: Bradykinin and related kinins, p. 229. Ed. by M. ROCHA E SILVA and H. A. ROTHSCHILD. São Paulo 1967.

— FELDBERG, W., HILTON, S. M.: Experiments on the factor in urine forming substance U. J. Physiol. (Lond.) 133, 558 (1956).

BHOOLA, K. D.: Intracellular distribution of submaxillary kallikrein. J. Physiol. (Lond.) 196, 431 (1968).

— CALLE, J. D., SCHACHTER, M.: The effect of bradykinin, serum kallikrein and other endogenous substances on capillary permeability in the guinea pig. J. Physiol. (Lond.) 152, 75 (1960).

— MAY YI, R., MORLEY, J., SCHACHTER, M.: Kinin releasing enzyme in the accessory sex glands of the guinea-pig. J. Physiol. (Lond.) 159, 34P (1961).

— — — — Release of kinin by an enzyme in the accessory sex glands of the guinea-pig. J. Physiol. (Lond.) 163, 269 (1962).

— MORLEY, J., SCHACHTER, M., SMAJE, L. H.: Vasodilatation in the submaxillary gland of the cat. J. Physiol. (Lond.) 179, 172 (1965).

— OGLE, C. W.: The subcellular localization of kallikrein, amylase and acetylcholine in the submaxillary gland of the guinea pig. J. Physiol. (Lond.) 184, 663 (1966).

BING, J., FÅRUP, P.: Location of renin (or a renin-like substance) in the submaxillary glands of albino mice. Acta path. microbiol. scand. 64, 203 (1965).

BISCHOFF, F., ELLIOT, A. H.: Purification of the depressor colloid of urine (callicrein). J. biol. Chem. 109, 419 (1935).

BRANDI, C. M. W., MENDES, J., PAIVA, A. C. M., PRADO, E. S.: Proteolysis of salmine by horse urinary kallikrein. Biochem. Pharmacol. 14, 1665 (1965).

— RONCADA, M. J., PRADO, E. S., PRADO, J. L.: Observations on the hydrolysis of salmine by kallikreins. In: Internat. Symposium on Vaso-active Polypeptides: Bradykinin and related kinins, p. 135. Ed. by M. ROCHA E SILVA and H. A. ROTHSCHILD. São Paulo 1967.

CARVALHO, I. F., DINIZ, C. R.: Kininogenin from renal tissue of the rat. Ciencia Cult. (São Paulo) 15, 286 (1963).

— — Cellular localization of renin and kininogenin. Ciencia Cult. (São Paulo) 16, 263 (1964).

— — Kinin-forming enzyme (kininogenin) in homogenates of rat kidney. Biochim. biophys. Acta (Amst.) 128, 136 (1966).

CHAPMAN, L. F., RAMNOS, A. O., GOODELL, H., SILVERMAN, G., WOLFF, H. G.: A humoral agent implicated in vascular headache of the migraine type. Arch. Neurol. (Chic.) 3, 223 (1960).

Chase, T., Jr., Shaw, E.: p-Nitrophenyl-p-guanidinobenzoate HCl: A new active site titrant for trypsin. Biochem. biophys. Res. Commun. **29**, 508 (1967).
Chiang, T. S., Erdös, E. G., Miwa, I., Tague, L. L., Coalson, J. J.: Isolation from a salivary gland of granules containing renin and kallikrein. Circulat. Res. **23**, 507 (1968).
Contzen, Ch., Holtz, P., Raudonat, H. W.: Über das bradykininbildende Prinzip des Bothrops-Giftes. Naturwissenschaften **46**, 402 (1959).
Coppen, A. J., Lewis, G. P.: An enzyme forming vasodilator polypeptides in human cerebrospinal fluid. J. Neurochem. **7**, 155 (1961).
Davies, G. E., Holman, G., Johnston, T. P., Lowe, J. S.: Studies on kallikrein. Failure of some anti-inflammatory drugs to affect release of kinin. Brit. J. Pharmacol. **28**, 212 (1966).
— Lowe, J. S.: Presence of kallikrein in the γ-globulin permeability factor of guinea-pig serum. Brit. J. Pharmacol. **21**, 491 (1963).
De Duve, C., Pressman, B. C., Gianetto, R., Wattiaux, R., Appelmans, F.: Tissue fractionation studies. 6. Intracellular distribution patterns of enzymes in rat-liver tissue. Biochem. J. **60**, 604 (1955).
Diniz, C. R., Pereira, A. A., Barroso, J., Mares-Guia, M.: On specificity of urinary kallikreins. Biochem. biophys. Res. Commun. **21**, 448 (1965).
— — — — Studies of the specificity of kinin-forming enzymes. The inhibition of the kininogenic activity of trypsin and kallikreins by model compounds. In: Hypotensive peptides, p. 175. Ed. by E. G. Erdös, N. Back and F. Sicuteri. Berlin-Heidelberg-New York: Springer 1966.
Edery, H., Lewis, G. P.: Kinin-forming activity and histamine in lymph after tissue injury. J. Physiol. (Lond.) **169**, 568 (1963).
Elliot, A. H., Nuzum, F. R.: The urinary excretion of a depressor substance (kallikrein of Frey and Kraut) in arterial hypertension. Endocrinology **18**, 462 (1934).
Erdös, E. G., McMennamin, M. A., Wohler, J. R.: Presence of carboxypeptidase B in crude kallikrein (Padutin) preparations. Life Sci. **2**, 765 (1962).
— Renfrew, A. G., Sloane, E. M., Wohler, J. R.: Enzymatic studies on bradykinin and similar peptides. Ann. N.Y. Acad. Sci. **104**, 222 (1963).
— Tague, L. L., Miwa, I.: Kallikrein in granules of the submaxillary gland. Biochem. Pharmacol. **17**, 667 (1968).
Fasciolo, J. C., Halvorsen, K.: Specificity of mammalian kallidinogen. Amer. J. Physiol. **207**, 901 (1964).
Fiedler, F.: Heterogenität und enzymatische Eigenschaften von Pankreaskallikrein. Hoppe-Seylers Z. physiol. Chem. **349**, 926 (1968).
— Müller, B., Werle, E.: Hemmung von Schweinepankreas-Kallikrein durch Diisopropylfluorophosphat. Hoppe-Seylers Z. physiol. Chem. **349**, 942 (1968).
— Werle, E.: Vorkommen zweier Kallikreinogene im Schweinepankreas und Automation der Kallikrein- und Kallikreinogenbestimmung. Hoppe-Seylers Z. physiol. Chem. **348**, 1087 (1967).
— — Activation, inhibition, and pH dependence of the hydrolysis of α-N-benzoyl-L-arginine ethyl ester catalyzed by kallikrein from porcine pancreas. Europ. J. Biochem. **7**, 27 (1968).
Forell, M. M.: Pancreatic kallikrein in physiological and pathological conditions. In: Polypeptides which affect smooth muscles and blood vessels, p. 247. Ed. by M. Schachter. New York: Pergamon 1960.
— Dobovicnik, W., Göldel, L.: Vergleichende Untersuchungen über Bildung und Verhalten des Kallikreins, der Diastase und Lipase im Pankreas, Blut und Harn nach Unterbindung der Pankreasausführungsgänge. Z. ges. exp. Med. **132**, 399 (1960).
Fox, R. H., Hilton, S. M.: Bradykinin formation in human skin as a factor in heat vasodilatation. J. Physiol. (Lond.) **142**, 219 (1958).
Frey, E. K.: Zusammenhänge zwischen Herzarbeit und Nierentätigkeit. Langenbecks Arch. klin. Chir. **142**, 663 (1926).
— Die Kreislaufwirkung eines neuen von der Niere ausgeschiedenen Stoffes. Langenbecks Arch. klin. Chir. **148**, 643 (1927).
— Kreislaufhormon und innere Sekretion. Münch. med. Wschr. **76**, 1951 (1929).
— Kraut, H.: Über einen von der Niere ausgeschiedenen, die Herztätigkeit anregenden Stoff. Hoppe-Seylers Z. physiol. Chem. **157**, 32 (1926).
— — Nachweis und Wirkung eines Kreislaufhormons. Münch. med. Wschr. **75**, 763 (1928).
— — Schultz, F.: Über eine neue innersekretorische Funktion des Pankreas. Naunyn-Schmiedebergs Arch. exp. Path. Pharmak. **158**, 334 (1930).
— — Werle, E.: Kallikrein (Padutin). Stuttgart: Enke 1950.
— — — Vogel, R., Zickgraf-Rüdel, G., Trautschold, I.: Das Kallikrein-Kinin-System und seine Inhibitoren. Stuttgart: Enke 1968.

FRITZ, H., ECKERT, I., WERLE, E.: Isolierung und Charakterisierung von sialinsäurehaltigem und sialinsäurefreiem Kallikrein aus Schweinepankreas. Hoppe-Seylers Z. physiol. Chem. **348**, 1120 (1967).

GADDUM, J. H., GUTH, P. S.: A comparison of the kallikrein-kinin system in sheep and dogs. Brit. J. Pharmacol. **15**, 181 (1960).

GREENE, L. J., HIRS, C. H. W., PALADE, G. E.: On the protein composition of bovine pancreatic zymogen granules. J. biol. Chem. **238**, 2054 (1963).

GUTH, P. S.: Kinins produced from bovine colostrum by kallikrein and saliva. Brit. J. Pharmacol. **14**, 549 (1959).

HABERMANN, E.: Über Zusammenhänge zwischen esterolytischen und pharmakologischen Wirkungen von Jararacagift, Kallikrein und Thrombin. Naunyn-Schmiedebergs Arch. exp. Path. Pharmak. **236**, 492 (1959).

— Zuordnung pharmakologischer und enzymatischer Wirkungen von Kallikrein und Schlangengiften mittels Diisopropylfluororphosphat und Elektrophorese. Naunyn-Schmiedebergs Arch. exp. Path. Pharmak. **240**, 552 (1961a).

— Über Beziehungen zwischen pharmakologischen und enzymatischen Wirkungen von Kallikrein und Viperidengiften. Naunyn-Schmiedebergs Arch. exp. Path. Pharmak. **241**, 202 (1961b).

— Trennung und Reinigung von Pankreaskallikrein. Hoppe-Seylers Z. physiol. Chem. **328**, 15 (1962).

— Snake venoms, kallikreins and kininogen. Ann. N.Y. Acad. Sci. **104**, 130 (1963).

— Enzymatic kinin release from kininogen and from low molecular compounds. In: Hypotensive Peptides, p. 116. Ed. by E. G. ERDÖS, N. BACK and F. SICUTERI. Berlin-Heidelberg-New York: Springer 1966.

— BLENNEMANN, G.: Über Substrate und Reaktionsprodukte der kininbildenden Enzyme Trypsin, Serum- und Pankreaskallikrein sowie von Crotalusgift. Naunyn-Schmiedebergs Arch. exp. Path. Pharmak. **249**, 357 (1964).

— KLETT, W.: Beiträge zur Biochemie und Pharmakologie eines Serumkallikreins. Naunyn-Schmiedebergs Arch. exp. Path. Pharmak. **250**, 253 (1965).

— — Reinigung und einige Eigenschaften eines Kallikreins aus Schweineserum. Biochem. Z. **346**, 133 (1966).

— MÜLLER, B.: Zur enzymatischen Spaltung peptischer kininliefernder Fragmente (PKF) sowie von Rinderserumkininogen. Naunyn-Schmiedebergs Arch. exp. Path. Pharmak. **253**, 464 (1966).

HAMBERG, U.: Cerebrospinal fluid and bradykinin release. Biochem. Pharmacol. **3**, 169 (1960).

— ROCHA E SILVA, M.: Release of bradykinin as related to the esterase activity of trypsin and of the venom of *Bothrops jararaca*. Experientia (Basel) **13**, 489 (1957a).

— — On the release of bradykinin by trypsin and snake venoms. Arch. int. Pharmacodyn. **110**, 222 (1957b).

HAVEZ, R., DEGAND, P., ROUSSEL, P., BISERTE, G.: Isolement et caractérization immunologique de la kallicréine bronchique humaine. C. R. Acad. Sci. (Paris) (D) **262**, 309 (1966a).

— — — VOISIN, C., BISERTE, G., GERNEZ-RIEUX, C.: Identification des γ-globulines, de la kallicréine et de la transferrine dans la muqueuse bronchique humaine. C. R. Acad. Sci. (Paris) (D) **262**, 1777 (1966b).

— ROUSSEL, P., MOSCHETTO, Y., DEGAND, P., BISERTE, G.: Caractérisation électrophorétique des composants du mucus bronchique. C. R. Acad. Sci. (Paris) **260**, 4853 (1965).

HENRIQUES, O. B., FICHMAN, M.: Bradykinin-releasing factor from *Bothrops jararaca* venom. Nature (Lond.) **187**, 414 (1960).

— KAURITCHEVA, N., KUZNETSOVA, V., ASTRAKAN, M.: Substrates of kinin-releasing enzymes isolated from horse plasma. Nature (Lond.) **215**, 1200 (1967).

— LAVRAS, A. A. C., FICHMAN, M., PICARELLI, Z. P.: Plasma enzymes that release kinins. Biochem. Pharmacol. **15**, 31 (1966).

HILTON, S. M., JONES, M.: The role of plasma kinin in functional vasodilatation in the pancreas. J. Physiol. (Lond.) **195**, 521 (1968).

— LEWIS, G. P.: The cause of the vasodilatation accompanying activity in the submandibular salivary gland. J. Physiol. (Lond.) **128**, 235 (1955).

— — Vasodilatation in the tongue and its relationship to plasma kinin formation. J. Physiol. (Lond.) **144**, 532 (1958).

— SCHAIN, R. J.: A search for pharmacologically active substances in fluid from the cerebral ventricles. J. Physiol. (Lond.) **157**, 46P (1961).

HOCHSTRASSER, K., WERLE, E.: Über kininliefernde Peptide aus pepsinverdauten Rinderplasmaproteinen. Hoppe-Seylers Z. physiol. Chem. **348**, 177 (1967).

HOLMAN, G., LOWE, J. S., MORLEY, J. S., SMITHERS, M. J.: The substrate specificity of guinea-pig plasma kallikrein. Biochem. biophys. Res. Commun. **33**, 140 (1968).

Inagami, T., Sturtevant, J. M.: Nonspecific catalyses by alpha-chymotrypsin and trypsin. J. biol. Chem. **235**, 1019 (1960).
Iwanaga, S., Sato, T., Mizushima, Y., Suzuki, T.: Studies on snake venoms. XVII. Properties of the bradykinin releasing enzyme in the venom of *Agkistrodon halys blomhoffii*. J. Biochem. (Tokyo) **58**, 123 (1965).
Jacobsen, S.: Separation of two different substrates for plasma kinin-forming enzymes. Nature (Lond.) **210**, 98 (1966a).
— Substrates for plasma kinin-forming enzymes in human, dog and rabbit plasmas. Brit. J. Pharmacol. **26**, 403 (1966b).
— Observations on the content of kininogen, kallikrein and kininase in lymph from hind limbs of dogs and rabbits. Brit. J. Pharmacol. **27**, 213 (1966c).
— Substrates for plasma kinin-forming enzymes in rat and guinea-pig plasma. Brit. J. Pharmacol. **28**, 64 (1966d).
Jollès, P., Alais, C., Jollès, J.: Action de la callicréine sur la caséine de vache. C. R. Acad. Sci. (Paris) **256**, 4308 (1963).
Jonasson, O., Becker, E. L.: Release of kallikrein from guinea pig lung during anaphylaxis. J. exp. Med. **123**, 509 (1966).
Kato, H., Nagasawa, S., Suzuki, T.: Relationship between tertiary structure and kinin yielding ability of bovine kininogen. Biochem. biophys. Res. Commun. **27**, 163 (1967).
Korányi, A., Szenes, T., Hatz, B. E.: Über das Vorkommen des Kallikreins im menschlichen Speichel und der tierischen Parotisdrüse. Kallikrein kein spezifisches Pankreashormon. Dtsch. med. Wschr. **63**, 55 (1937).
Koshland, D. E., Jr., Neet, K. E.: The catalytic and regulatory properties of enzymes. Ann. Rev. Biochem. **37**, 359 (1968).
Kramer, C., Prado, E. S., Prado, J. L.: Inhibition by ions of the esterolytic activity of horse urinary kallikrein. Med. Pharmacol. exp. **15**, 389 (1966).
Kraut, H., Frey, E. K., Bauer, E., Schultz, F.: Zur Kenntnis des Kallikreins. VII. Mitt. Hoppe-Seylers Z. physiol. Chem. **205**, 99 (1932).
— — Werle, E.: Der Nachweis eines Kreislaufhormons in der Pankreasdrüse. IV. Mitt. über dieses Kreislaufhormon. Hoppe-Seylers Z. physiol. Chem. **189**, 97 (1930).
— — — Schultz, F.: Nachweis und Vorkommen des Kallikreins im Harn. IX. Mitt über Kallikrein. Hoppe Seylers Z. physiol. Chem. **230**, 259 (1934).
— Körbel, W.: Versuche zur Isolierung des Kallikreins. III. Darstellung einer Kallikrein-Zink-Verbindung. Hoppe-Seylers Z. physiol. Chem. **309**, 248 (1957).
— Schweitzer, I.: Versuche zur Isolierung der Kallikreins. I. Hoppe-Seylers Z. physiol. Chem. **284**, 211 (1949).
Lehmann, A. J., Winkle, W. van, Jr.: Depressor effects from urine and tissue extracts: Comparison of different species, vasomotor changes, and related chemical agents. Arch. int. Pharmacodyn. **59**, 75 (1938).
Lewis, G. P.: Plasma-kinin-forming enzymes in body fluids and tissues. J. Physiol. (Lond.) **147**, 458 (1959).
Mares-Guia, M.: Hydrophobic interactions in the trypsin active center. The sensitivity of the hydrophobic binding site to side chain modifications in competitive inhibitors of the amidinium type. Arch. Biochem. **127**, 317 (1968).
— Diniz, C. R.: Studies on the mechanism of rat urinary kallikrein catalysis, and its relation to catalysis by trypsin. Arch. Biochem. **121**, 750 (1967).
— Shaw, E.: Studies on the active center of trypsin. The binding of amidines and guanidines as models of the substrate side chain. J. biol. Chem. **240**, 1579 (1965).
— — The specific inactivation of trypsin by ethyl p-guanidinobenzoate. J. biol. Chem. **242**, 5782 (1967).
Migay, T. I., Petroff, J. R.: Untersuchungen über die Wirkung des Pankreassaftes auf den Organismus bei parenteraler Einführung. Z. ges. exp. Med. **36**, 457 (1923).
Moriya, H.: Chemical studies on callicrein. II. Purification with acrinol. J. Pharm. Soc. (Japan) **79**, 32 (1959a).
— Chemical studies on callicrein. V. Stability of water solutions of callicrein. J. Pharm. Soc. (Japan) **79**, 1216 (1959b).
— Chemical studies on callicrein. VI. Amino acid composition and terminal amino acids. J. Pharm. Soc. (Japan) **79**, 1390 (1959c).
— Chemical studies on callicrein. VII. Structural sugar of callicrein. J. Pharm. Soc. (Japan) **79**, 1394 (1959d).
— Chemical studies on callicrein. VIII. Molecular weight of callicrein and the supplement. J. Pharm. Soc. (Japan) **79**, 1451 (1959e).
— Deguchi, M., Asano, H.: Chemical studies on callicrein. I. The amount of callicrein contained in various organs and its isolation and purification. J. Pharm. Soc. (Japan) **78**, 346 (1958).

MORIYA, H., KATO, A., FUKUSHIMA, H.: Further study on purification of hog pancreatic kallikrein. Biochem. Pharmacol. 18, 549 (1969).
— MORIWAKI, C., YAMAZAKI, K., AKIMOTO, S., FUKUSHIMA, H.: Human salivary kallikrein and liberation of colostrokinin. In: Hypotensive peptides, p. 161. Ed. by E. G. ERDÖS, N. BACK and F. SICUTERI. Berlin-Heidelberg-New York: Springer 1966.
— PIERCE, J. V., WEBSTER, M. E.: Purification and some properties of three kallikreins. N.Y. Acad. Sci. 104, 172 (1963).
— SHIMAZAWA, E.: Chemical studies on callicrein. III. Purification by zone electrophoresis. J. Pharm. Soc. (Japan) 79, 374 (1959a).
— — Chemical studies on callicrein. IV. The isoelectric point of callicrein. J. Pharm. Soc. (Japan) 79, 688 (1959b).
— YAMAZAKI, K., FUKUSHIMA, H.: Biochemical studies on kallikreins and their related substances. I. Isolation and purification of human saliva kallikrein. J. Biochem. (Tokyo) 58, 201 (1965a).
— — — MORIWAKI, C.: Biochemical studies on kallikreins and their related substances. II. An improved method of purification of hog pancreatic kallikrein and its some biological properties. J. Biochem. (Tokyo) 58, 208 (1965b).
NAGASAWA, S., HORIUCHI, K., YANO, M., SUZUKI, T.: Partial purification of bovine plasma kallikrein activated by contact with glass. J. Biochem. (Tokyo) 62, 398 (1967).
OLIVER, W. J., GROSS, F.: Effect of testosterone and duct ligation on submaxillary renin-like principle. Amer. J. Physiol. 213, 341 (1967).
OOSTERBAAN, R. A., COHEN, J. A.: The active site of esterases. In: Structure and activity of enzymes, p. 87. Ed. by T. W. GOODWIN, J. I. HARRIS and B. S. HARTLEY. New York: Academic Press 1964.
PASKHINA, T. S., EGOROVA, T. P.: Purification and some properties of kininogen (bradykininogen) of rabbit blood serum. Biokhimiya 31, 468 (1966). Chem. Abstr. 65, 10924h (1966).
— ZYKOVA, V. P., EGOROVA, T. P., NARTIKOVA, V. F., KARPOVA, A. V., GUZEVA, M. H.: Reaction of N-alpha-tosyl-L-lysylchloromethane with kallikrein from rabbit blood plasma and with kallikreins from human urine and saliva. Biokhimiya 33, 745 (1968). Chem. Abstr. 70, 420g (1969).
PETROFF, J. R.: Zur Kenntnis der Pankreassaftwirkung bei parenteraler Einführung. Z. ges. exp. Med. 44, 641 (1925).
PIERCE, J. V., WEBSTER, M. E.: Human plasma kallidins: Isolation and chemical studies. Biochem. biophys. Res. Commun. 5, 353 (1961).
PRADO, E. S., PRADO, J. L.: Partial purification of a plasma-kinin-forming enzyme from horse urine. Experientia (Basel) 17, 31 (1961).
— — BRANDI, C. M. W.: Further purification and some properties of horse urinary kallikrein. Arch. int. Pharmacodyn. 137, 358 (1962).
— STELLA, R. C. R., RONCADA, M. J., PRADO, J. L.: Action of horse urinary kallikrein on arginine and lysine-peptides. In: Internat. Symposium on Vaso-active Polypeptides: Bradykinin and Related Kinins, p. 141. Ed. by M. ROCHA E SILVA and H. A. ROTHSCHILD. São Paulo 1967.
PRADO, J. L., KATCHBURIAN, A. V., MENDES, J., PRADO, E. S.: Ions and the kininogenic activity of horse urinary kallikrein. Acta physiol. lat.-amer. 15, 386 (1965).
— PRADO, E. S., BRANDI, C. M. W., KATCHBURIAN, A. V.: Some properties of highly purified horse urinary kallikrein. Ann. N.Y. Acad. Sci. 104, 186 (1963).
PRIBRAM, H., HERRNHEISER, G.: Zur Kenntnis der adialysabeln Bestandteile des Menschenharnes. Biochem. Z. 111, 30 (1920).
RAMOS, A. D., CHAPMAN, L. F., RAMOS, L.: Neurokinin from cerebrospinal fluid. I. Some pharmacological properties. Arch. int. Pharmacodyn. 146, 501 (1963).
ROCHA E SILVA, M.: Definition of bradykinin and other kinins. Biochem. Pharmacol. 10, 3 (1962).
— The physiological significance of bradykinin. Ann. N.Y. Acad. Sci. 104, 190 (1963).
— Kinin-hormones. Proceedings, VI Pan-american Congress of Endocrinology, Mexico City. In: Excerpta Med. Int. Cong. Series 112, p. 47, 1965.
SCHACHTER, M.: A delayed slow contracting effect of serum and plasma due to the release of a substance resembling kallidin and bradykinin. Brit. J. Pharmacol. 11, 111 (1956).
— Some properties of kallidin, bradykinin and wasp venom kinin. In: Polypeptides which affect smooth muscles and blood vessels, p. 232. Ed. by M. SCHACHTER, New York: Pergamon 1960.
— Kallikrein and vasodilatation in the salivary gland. In: Hypotensive peptides, p. 275. Ed. by E. G. ERDÖS, N. BACK and F. SICUTERI. Berlin-Heidelberg-New York: Springer 1966.

SCHOELLMANN, G., SHAW, E.: Direct evidence for the presence of histidine in the active center of chymotrypsin. Biochemistry **2**, 252 (1963).
SHAW, E., MARES-GUIA, M., COHEN, W.: Evidence for an active-center histidine in trypsin through use of a specific reagent, 1-chloro-3-tosylamido-7-amino-2-heptanone, the chloromethyl ketone derived from N-tosyl-L-lysine. Biochemistry **4**, 2219 (1965).
SHERRY, S., ALKJAERSIG, N., FLETCHER, A. P.: Comparative activity of thrombin on substituted arginine and lysine esters. Amer. J. Physiol. **209**, 577 (1965).
SIEBERT, G., WERLE, E., JUNG, G., MAIER, L.: Intracelluläre Verteilung von Kallikrein und von Bradykininogen in Schweinepankreas. Biochem. Z. **326**, 420 (1955).
STRAUS, W.: Isolation and biochemical properties of droplets from the cells of rat kidney. J. biol. Chem. **207**, 745 (1954).
SUZUKI, K., SASAKI, K., KAMEYAMA, T., Interaction between kinin releasing enzymes and the synthesized bradykinin derivatives. Jap. J. Pharmacol. **16**, 486 (1966).
SUZUKI, T., IWANAGA, S., SATO, T., NAGASAWA, S., KATO, H., YANO, M., HORIUCHI, K.: Biochemical properties of kininogens and kinin releasing enzymes. In: International Symposium on Vaso-active Polypeptides: Bradykinin and Related Kinins, p. 27. Ed. by M. ROCHA E SILVA and H. A. ROTHSCHILD. São Paulo 1967.
TRAUTSCHOLD, I., FRITZ, H., WERLE, E.: Kininogenases, kininases and their inhibitors. In: Hypotensive peptides, p. 221. Ed. by E. G. ERDÖS, N. BACK and F. SICUTERI. Berlin-Heidelberg-New York: Springer 1966a.
— WERLE, E., SCHMAL, A., HENDRIKOFF, N. G.: Die hormonelle Beeinflussung des Isorenin-Spiegels der Submandibularisdrüse der weißen Maus und zur Lokalisierung des Enzyms in der Drüse. Hoppe-Seylers Z. physiol. Chem. **344**, 232 (1966b).
TROWBRIDGE, C. G., KREHBIEL, A., LASKOWSKI, M., JR.: Substrate activation of trypsin. Biochemistry **2**, 843 (1963).
TURRIAN, H.: Quelques caractéristiques du principe hypertensif contenu dans les glandes salivaires de la souris. Helv. physiol. pharmacol. Acta **18**, 259 (1960).
VOGEL, R. VON, RÜDEL, G., ZIEGESAR, L. VON: Die Beeinflussung der Kallikrein-Ausscheidung im Harn beim Menschen und bei der Ratte durch verschiedene Kostformen. Arzneimittel-Forsch. **12**, 881 (1962).
VOGT, W., GARBE, G., SCHMIDT, G.: Untersuchungen zur Existenz zweier verschiedener kininbildender Systeme in menschlichem Plasma. Naunyn-Schmiedebergs Arch. exp. Path. Pharmak. **256**, 127 (1967).
WEBSTER, M. E., CLARK, W. R., ANDERSON, P.: Purification of pancreatic and urinary callicrein. Proc. Soc. exp. Biol. (N.Y.) **93**, 181 (1956).
— EMMART, E. W., TURNER, W. A., MORIYA, H., PIERCE, J. V.: Immunological properties of the kallikreins. Biochem. Pharmacol. **12**, 511 (1963).
— GILMORE, J. P.: The estimation of the kallidins in blood and urine. Biochem. Pharmacol. **14**, 1161 (1965).
— PIERCE, J. V.: Studies on plasma kallikrein and its relationship to plasmin. J. Pharmacol. exp. Ther. **130**, 484 (1960).
— — Action of the kallikreins on synthetic ester substrates. Proc. Soc. exp. Biol. (N.Y.) **107**, 186 (1961).
— — The nature of the kallidins released from human plasma by kallikreins and other enzymes. Ann. N.Y. Acad. Sci. **104**, 91 (1963).
WERLE, E.: Zur Kenntnis des Haushalts des Kallikreins. Biochem. Z. **269**, 415 (1934).
— Über Kallikrein aus Blut. Biochem. Z. **287**, 235 (1936).
— Über den Aktivitätszustand des Kallikreins der Bauchspeicheldrüse und ihres äußeren Sekretes beim Hund. Biochem. Z. **290**, 129 (1937).
— The chemistry and pharmacology of kallikrein and kallidin. In: Polypeptides which stimulate plain muscle, p. 20. Ed. by J. H. GADDUM. London: Livingstone 1955.
— Kallikrein, kallidin and related substances. In: Polypeptides which affect smooth muscles and blood vessels, p. 199. Ed. by M. SCHACHTER. New York: Pergamon 1960.
— APPEL, W.: Photochemische Inaktivierung von Kallikrein durch Methylenblau. Z. Vitamin-, Hormon- u. Fermentforsch. 8, 24 (1956).
— DÄUMER, J.: Über das Verhalten des Kallikreins, des Inaktivators aus Lymphdrüsen, des Substance DK sowie der Histidin-decarboxylase bei der Kataphorese. Biochem. Z. **304**, 377 (1940).
— ECKEY, P.: Vergleichende Untersuchung über Kallikrein und Trypsinkonzentration im menschlichen Duodenalsaft. Biochem. Z. **269**, 435 (1934).
— FUCHS, P.: Verhalten des Transaminase-, Amylase- und Kallikreingehaltes von Unterkieferspeicheldrüsen von Ratten nach Unterbindung des Ductus Whartoni. Z. ges. exp. Med. **139**, 460 (1965).
— GÖTZE, W., KEPPLER, A.: Über die Wirkung des Kallikreins auf den isolierten Darm und über eine neue darmkontrahierende Substanz. Biochem. Z. **289**, 217 (1937).

WERLE, E., GRUNZ, M.: Zur Kenntnis der darmkontrahierenden uteruserregenden und blutdrucksenkenden Substanz DK. Biochem. Z. **301**, 429 (1939).
— HOCHSTRASSER, K., TRAUTSCHOLD, I.: Studies of bovine plasma kininogen, ornitho-kallikrein, and ornitho-kinin. In: Hypotensive peptides, p. 105. Ed. by E. G. ERDÖS, N. BACK and F. SICUTERI. Berlin-Heidelberg-New York: Springer 1966.
— HÜRTER, J.: Über Ornitho-Kallikrein. I. Mitt. Über kreislaufaktive Substanzen der Vögel. Biochem. Z. **285**, 175 (1936).
— KAUFMANN-BOETSCH, B.: Über esteratische Wirkungen von Kallikrein und Trypsin und ihre Hemmung durch Kallikrein- und Trypsininhibitoren. Hoppe-Seylers Z. physiol. Chem. **319**, 52 (1960).
— KORSTEN, H.: Der Kallikreingehalt des Harns, des Speichels und des Blutes bei Gesunden und Kranken. Z. Ges. exp. Med. **103**, 153 (1938).
— MAIER, L.: Über die chemische und pharmakologische Unterscheidung von Kallikreinen verschiedener Herkunft. Biochem. Z. **323**, 279 (1952).
— — Über das Vorkommen von Kallikrein in der Lunge. Klin. Wschr. **33**, 1103 (1955).
— MARCUS, A.: Die Anwendung der chromatographischen Adsorptionsmethode für die Reinigung des Kallikreins. Biochem. Z. **296**, 275 (1938).
— RODEN, P. VON: Über das Vorkommen von Kallikrein in den Speicheldrüsen und im Mundspeichel. Biochem. Z. **286**, 213 (1936).
— — Über das Vorkommen von Kallikrein in den Speicheldrüsen und im Mundspeichel und über eine blutdrucksteigernde Substanz in der Submaxillarisdrüse des Hundes. Biochem. Z. **301**, 328 (1939).
— TRAUTSCHOLD, I.: Colostrokinin und seine Bildung durch Kallikreine. Z. Biol. **112**, 169 (1960).
— — Kallikrein, kallidin, kallikrein inhibitors. N.Y. Acad. Sci. **104**, 117 (1963).
— — LEYSATH, G.: Isolierung und Struktur des Kallidins. Hoppe-Seylers Z. physiol. Chem. **326**, 174 (1961).
— — SCHMAL, A.: Über ein Iso-Enzym des Renins und über die Isolierung eines biologisch aktiven Spaltproduktes seines Substrates. Hoppe-Seylers Z. physiol. Chem. **332**, 79 (1963a).
— URHAHN, K.: Über den Aktivitätszustand des Kallikreins in der Bauchspeicheldrüse. Biochem. Z. **304**, 387 (1940).
— VOGEL, R.: Über die Freisetzung einer kallikreinartigen Substanz aus Extrakten verschiedener Organe. Arch. int. Pharmacodyn. **131**, 257 (1961).
— — GÖLDEL, L. F.: Über ein blutdrucksteigerndes Prinzip in Extrakten aus der Glandula submaxillaris der weißen Maus. Naunyn-Schmiedebergs Arch. exp. Path. Pharmak. **230**, 236 (1957).
— — KALIAMPETSOS, C.: Über das Kallikrein der Darmwand und seine Beziehung zum Blutkallikreingehalt bei Störungen des Darmfunktion. Proceedings, II World Congress of Gastroenterology (Munich 1962), vol. 2, p. 778. Basel: Karger 1963b.
— — LENTRODT, J.: Über den Kallikreingehalt der Glandula submandibularis während der Entwicklung einiger Säugerarten und nach Abbindung des Ductus Whartoni. Arch. int. Pharmacodyn. **126**, 187 (1960).
YANO, M., NAGASAWA, S., HORIUCHI, K., SUZUKI, T.: Separation of a new substrate, kininogen-I, for plasma kallikrein in bovine plasma. J. Biochem. (Tokyo) **62**, 504 (1967).

Proteolytic Enzymes as Kininogenases*

J. L. PRADO

With 2 Figures

A. Introduction

The discovery of enzymes, other than kallikreins, which release kinins from blood plasma was made by ROCHA E SILVA et al. (1949a) when they observed the formation of bradykinin by adding either trypsin or *Bothrops jararaca* venom to plasma globulins. One year later BERALDO (1950a, b) reported the kinin-liberating activity of fibrinolysin (plasmin), when it was incubated with plasma globulins precipitated by half saturation with ammonium sulfate. A cysteine-activated protease secreted by *Clostridium histolyticum* was next shown to release from fraction IV-4 of bovine plasma a bradykinin-like polypeptide (J. L. PRADO et al., 1956). This group of kinin-releasing enzymes, kininogenases, has been growing up to the present time and now includes several proteolytic enzymes.

I. Terminology

Names such as kinin-forming enzymes, kinin-releasing enzymes, and kinin liberators have also been used to designate the plasma kinin-forming enzymes. Since a shorter name would be more convenient, for this group of enzymes J. L. PRADO (1962, 1964) used the name kininogenase, and simultaneously and independently it was employed by BHOOLA et al. (1962) and by SCHACHTER (1963) to designate the kinin-releasing enzyme in accessory sex glands of the guinea pig. A similar term, kininogenins, was proposed by ROCHA E SILVA (1962, 1963) for the kinin releasers. The name kininogenase was recommended by the Committee on Nomenclature for Hypotensive Peptides (WEBSTER, 1966) as a general term including any enzyme that liberates a kinin from an inactive protein substrate. The corresponding adjectival term, kininogenic, for kinin-forming was not recommended by the Committee.

II. Kininogenases other than Kallikreins and Snake Venom Enzymes

Although, according to the definition used, the kininogenases include the kallikreins, some proteolytic enzymes found in snake venoms, plasmin (or fibrinolysin), and other kinin-releasing systems not well characterized (pp. 82 and 193), this chapter will be restricted mainly to the other known kininogenases: trypsin (EC 3.4.4.4), pepsin (EC 3.4.4.1), clostripain, subtilisin BPN′ (Nagarse), ficin (EC 3.4.4.12), papain (EC 3.4.4.10), *Streptomyces griseus* protease (Pronase), and chymotrypsin (EC 3.4.4.5).

* The financial support of this work by the National Institutes of Health (Grant No. HE 09267), Fundação de Amparo à Pesquisa do Estado de São Paulo and CAPES/BNDE/BID Project, is gratefully acknowledged.

B. Chemistry

I. Trypsin

Enzyme Preparations. Purity. Crystalline trypsin containing about 50% magnesium sulfate (commercial product of the Worthington Biochemical Laboratory, Freehold, N.J.) was the preparation first used by ROCHA E SILVA et al. (1949a). In a later paper ROCHA E SILVA (1951) used also a "new" trypsin preparation from the same laboratory, labeled TR 21, which, contrary to the first trypsin preparation (the "old" one), did not inactivate the liberated kinin; he then labeled the "old" trypsin preparation no. 483. WERLE et al. (1950a) used crystalline trypsin, supplied by Prof. M. KUNITZ, also containing about 50% $MgSO_4$ and observed that this preparation did not inactivate bradykinin and kallidin. Crystalline chymotrypsin (Prof. KUNITZ), on the other hand, quickly inactivated both polypeptides. The explanation offered by ROCHA E SILVA (1951) was that his old trypsin preparation was probably contaminated by chymotrypsin. He also showed that the pharmacologic effect of trypsin was not due to contamination of trypsin preparations with kallikrein, as suggested by WERLE et al. (1950a), but to trypsin itself. ELLIOTT et al. (1961), who first obtained pure bradykinin with crystalline trypsin, used a salt-free preparation (Armour Pharmaceutical Co. Ltd., Eastbourne) and confirmed that the biological activity of bradykinin was destroyed by chymotrypsin, but not by trypsin. WEBSTER and PIERCE (1963) used bovine pancreatic trypsin, salt-free, twice crystallized (Worthington Biochemical Corp.). The probable chymotrypsin impurity in a crystalline trypsin preparation (C. F. Boehringer & Soehne, Mannheim) was inactivated by incubation with N/20 HCl for 14 hours at 37° by HABERMANN and BLENNEMANN (1964) and HABERMANN and MÜLLER (1966).

Assay. Trypsin (Worthington) is assayed[1] by the method of SCHWERT and TAKENAKA (1955), which measures the absorbancy difference at 253 mμ between N-benzoyl-L-arginine and its ethyl ester (BAEe). One unit is equal to an increase in absorbancy of 0.001/min under the defined conditions at 25°. Trypsin, once or twice crystallized, maximum 50% $MgSO_4$, minimum activity 8,000 units/mg.

II. Pepsin

Enzyme Preparations. CROXATTO et al. (1950, 1951, 1953) used crystalline pepsin, without mentioning its source. TURBA and HETZEL (1954) used Merck pepsin. GREENBAUM et al. (1965) employed twice-crystallized pepsin (Worthington), and HABERMANN et al. (1966), thrice-crystallized pepsin (Serva, Heidelberg).

Assay. The Worthington crystalline enzyme is assayed by measuring the rate of hydrolysis of denatured hemoglobin (ANSON, 1938). One unit is equal to an increase in absorbancy of the TCA-soluble hydrolysis products of 0.001/min under standard conditions at 280 mμ. Worthington crystalline pepsin is a lyophilized preparation, twice crystallized, containing approximately 2,500 units/mg.

III. Clostripain

Enzyme Preparations. When first used by J. L. PRADO et al. (1956) a pure enzyme had not yet been obtained. It was known as the cysteine-activated protease secreted by *Clostridium histolyticum* and it was prepared by the method of MONIER et al. (1955). A strain of *Cl. histolyticum* from the Pasteur Institute, Paris, was cultivated in anaerobiosis in a medium with peptone and salts. The

1. Worthington Enzymes, Worthington Biochemical Corp., Freehold, N.J. (1963).

filtered and dialyzed culture medium was fractionated with salt solutions (ammonium sulfate and barbital/HCl buffer containing calcium) at −3 to −5°. Two fractions, A and B, were finally obtained, Fraction A contained 57% of the cysteine-activated protease and 31% of the collagenase activity and was contaminated by small amounts of other proteases. It was further purified by passage through a column of silica gel which completely eliminates the collagenase and the cysteine-inhibited proteases. At this stage it was 150 times purer than the dialyzed culture medium. The second time that clostripain was used as kininogenase (J. L. and E. S. PRADO, 1962) it was supplied by Dr. B. LABOUESSE, Paris, who had obtained a pure component on ultracentrifugation. The steps of the purification procedure (LABOUESSE and GROSS, 1960) were: (1) ammonium sulfate fractionation between 40 and 70% saturation; (2) incubation in the presence of 5×10^{-2} M cysteine and 1×10^{-2} M calcium chloride for 4 to 6 hours; (3) chromatography on DEAE-cellulose; (4) chromatrography on hydroxylapatite. The final purification was 530-fold, and the specific activity was 48 coagulating units/mg. The name clostripain was given to the enzyme (LABOUESSE and GROSS, 1960).

Assay. The proteolytic activity is assayed routinely at 35°, pH 7.4, by the milk coagulation test of GORINI and LANZAVECCHIA (LABOUESSE and GROSS, 1960). To 5 ml of "synthetic" milk (1% defatted milk in 0.3 M cacodylic acid triethanolamine buffer, containing 0.03 M calcium chloride) are added 0.5 ml of 0.3 M cysteine and 0.5 ml of enzyme solution. When this enzymatic solution contains 0.1 coagulating unit/ml, coagulation occurs in 500 seconds.

IV. Subtilisin BPN' (Nagarse)

Enzyme Preparations. J. L. PRADO et al. (1964) used two samples of the crystalline bacterial proteinase (Nagase and Co. Ltd., Osaka, Japan). It was prepared (HAGIHARA et al., 1958a) from submerged culture solutions of *Bacillus subtilis* N′ by using a cation exchange resin, Duolite C-10. The enzyme crystallized as needles or plates from acetone solution. The material was shown to be homogeneous by ultracentrifugal analysis (MATSUBARA et al., 1958). HUGGINS et al. (1964) used a lyophilized crystalline bacterial proteinase (Nagarse) from *B. subtilis* N′ (Enzyme Development Corp., New York) and later HUGGINS and THAMPI (1967) seem to have used the same enzyme preparation.

Assay. The assay of proteinase activity is based on the digestion of casein at 30°, pH 7.5. The optical density of the filtrates was read at 275 mμ. One unit liberates digestion products equivalent to 1 μg of tyrosine in 1 minute. The crystalline enzyme assayed by the casein-275 mμ method, by reagent B (HAGIHARA et al., 1958a, b) had 12.4 units/mg protein nitrogen.

Similarity to Subtilisin. A similarity between NAGARSE and CARLSBERG subtilisin had been detected by HUNT and OTTENSEN (1961). The complete amino acid sequence of the single BPN′ subtilisin polypeptide chain was determined by SMITH et al. (1966) and MARKLAND and SMITH (1967), who found that it differed from CARLSBERG subtilisin.

V. Ficin

Ficin Preparations. J. L. PRADO et al. (1965b) used two ficin preparations: crude ficin (C grade, lot 105662, California Corp. for Biochemical Research, Los Angeles) from fig latex; and crystalline ficin, which is a twice-crystallized product from fig latex (Worthington Biochemical Corp., Freehold, N.J.). The sample used was a suspension in 0.001 M EDTA, 19 mg/ml, batch Fi 688 A, assaying 3.8 units/mg.

Assay. The Worthington enzyme is assayed by potentiometric titration of acid produced during enzymatic hydrolysis of BAEe. One unit will hydrolyze 1 μmole of benzoyl-L-arginine ethyl ester/min. at 25°, pH 6.2. The crystallized product contains approximately 4 units/mg.

Ficin Components. The proteolytic ficin components B, C, D, E, F, G, H, and I, separated from *Ficus glabrata* latex by SGARBIERI et al. (1964), were used by J. L. PRADO et al. (1965b). Dr. J. R. WHITAKER, University of California, determined the activity of the components by the KUNITZ (1947) method (1% casein; 1.25×10^{-2} M each of EDTA and cysteine; 0.15 M, pH 7.0, phosphate buffer at 35° for 20 minutes) and supplied the *F. glabrata* components. According to SGARBIERI et al., twice-crystallized ficin (Nutritional Biochemicals Corp., Cleveland, Ohio) contained 70% of its activity as component G; components B, C, E, F, H, and I accounted for the other 30% of activity. Both this crystalline ficin and the Worthington crystalline enzyme used by PRADO et al. (1965b) were obtained by the same crystallization method.

VI. Papain

Enzyme Preparations. KRAUT et al. (1928) used *Succus caricae papayae* Merck as their papain source, and WERLE and KORSTEN (1938) used Merck papain. Even this last preparation must have been a crude one because papain was not crystallized until 1939. WERLE and BEREK (1950) used Merck papain. Unpublished results cited by WERLE (1963) were obtained with a papain whose source and degree of purity are not mentioned. MOSS et al. (1963) did not mention the source of papain and ficin used in their experiments. J. L. PRADO et al. (1965b) used twice-crystallized papain (Worthington Biochemical Corp.), batch PAP 5542, specific activity 7.2. It was supplied as a suspension in 0.05 M sodium acetate, pH 4.5. Crystallized from dried papaya latex by the method of KIMMEL and SMITH (1954), it is electrophoretically and ultracentrifugally homogeneous.

Assay. Potentiometric determination of the acid produced by hydrolysis of benzoylarginine ethyl ester: one unit will hydrolyze 1 μmole of BAEe/min at 25°. The twice-crystallized Worthington papain has a specific activity of approximately 10 units/mg.

VII. Streptomyces griseus Protease (Pronase)

Enzyme Preparations. REIS et al. (1966) did not mention the preparation used. J. L. PRADO and MENDES (1965) used Pronase, B grade, lot 502117, with 45,000 proteolytic units/g (California Corp. for Biochemical Research, Los Angeles).

Assay. One unit of proteolytic activity liberates from casein (pH 7.4, 40°) 25 microequivalents tyrosine/min.

Purity. The proteolytic enzyme of *St. griseus* was purified by NOMOTO and NARAHASHI (1958) and its homogeneity confirmed by ultracentrifugal and electrophoretic analyses and enzymological methods.

VIII. Carboxypeptidase A

Enzyme Preparations. The carboxypeptidase A preparation used by HABERMANN and MÜLLER (1966) was a five-times crystallized enzyme (Serva, Heidelberg) free of trypsin and chymotrypsin.

Assay. The recrystallized enzyme (Worthington Biochemical Corp.) is assayed by measuring the hydrolysis rate of 0.025 M carbobenzoxyglycyl-L-phenylalanine. Calculated from first-order reaction kinetics, its proteolytic coefficient is approximately 20.

IX. Chymotrypsin

Enzyme Preparations. Rocha e Silva et al. (1967) used α, β, γ and δ chymotrypsins from Mann Research Laboratories (personal communication). The chymotrypsin preparations from this company are as follows: α-ChT, 3× cryst., salt-free; β, γ, and δ ChT are 2× cryst., salt-free preparations.

Assay. The Mann enzymes are all assayed by the method of Schwert and Takenaka (1955) and their activities are[2]: 9,000 units/mg for α-ChT and 13,000 units/mg for δ-ChT; the activities for β and γ-ChT are not given.

C. Kinin Formation

I. Demonstration of Kinin-Forming Activity

Trypsin; Bradykinin. Before 1941 several workers attempted to identify substances liberated from tissues by trypsin which could account for the pharmacological effects of trypsin *in vitro* and *in vivo*. Heparin and histamine had been identified (cf. Rocha e Silva, 1941a, b), and a "slow-reacting substance" was mentioned as a possibility (cf. Rocha e Silva, 1941a). As the trypsin effects had been confirmed with a preparation of the enzyme crystallized by Prof. J. Northrop (Rocha e Silva, 1939a, b) and as they were inhibited by the crystallized Kunitz and Northrop trypsin inhibitor (Rocha e Silva, 1941a), the pharmacological effects of trypsin were considered to be dependent on its proteolytic activity. They were independent, however, of a digestive effect of trypsin on the smooth muscle (Rocha e Silva, 1939a, b). To demonstrate the liberation by trypsin of a "slow-reacting substance" whose action on the smooth muscle was resistant to atropine, and yet was not histamine, remained as a challenge (Rocha e Silva, 1939a). The existence of such a "slow-reacting muscle-stimulant substance" was also envisaged as a possibility by Trethewie (1942), who recorded its effect on smooth muscle. He observed that when 40 mg of (Difco) trypsin, 1:250, was perfused through the isolated rabbit liver, an adenyl compound and its inactivating enzyme, as well as the "slow-reacting muscle stimulant" (guinea pig jejunum) were liberated in the perfusate. When Wells et al. (1946) found that diphenhydramine (Benadryl), a potent antagonist to either injected or liberated histamine, did not alter the lethal action of trypsin in the guinea pig and dog and, even more, that the hypotension caused by the intravenous injection of nonlethal doses of trypsin (0.05 to 1 mg/kg) in the dog was reduced only 8% by diphenhydramine while the histamine hypotension was reduced 65%, the pressure to find a new chemical mediator for trypsin kept rising steadily.

The work of Rocha e Silva et al. (1949a) thus came as a relief for all workers in this field. In effect these investigators were the first to *isolate* and to *characterize* a substance which was liberated by crystalline trypsin and had chemical and pharmacological properties that explained several facts previously observed and new ones described in their paper. It was known (Rocha e Silva, 1939a) that the addition of 250–500 µg of crystalline trypsin to the isolated guinea pig ileum bath produced a strong and slow contraction. On successive enzyme additions the smooth muscle was finally desensitized to trypsin. Using this refractory guinea pig gut, Rocha e Silva et al. (1949a) demonstrated several facts. (1) Aliquots of defibrinated or oxalated plasma of several species (dog, ox, cat) may be added to the trypsin resistant guinea pig ileum bath without eliciting any response. If, however, 0.2 ml of plasma is added to the bath, followed by small

2. Reference Guide and Price List no. 134 of Biochemicals for Research (1967), Mann Research Laboratories, Inc., New York, N.Y.

amounts of trypsin (about 250 μg), a powerful contraction occurs after a short latency. (2) A mixture of the plasma globulin fraction (precipitated at 30 to 45% saturation with ammonium sulfate) and trypsin generates an active substance, the maximum effect being observed between 1 and 3 minutes of incubation. If incubation is prolonged (15–30 min) the active principle disappears. If a large enough dose of trypsin is added to a fresh sample of globulin solution, the active principle is liberated, inactivated, and the generating potency of the globulin solution is exhausted. This was interpreted as exhaustion of the precursor of the active principle. The names bradykinin and bradykininogen were given to the active principle and to its precursor. (3) A crude bradykinin was released from ox plasma or serum globulins with *Bothrops jararaca* venom (which liberated a principle similar to bradykinin). From each liter of globulin solution (approximately the original plasma volume), about 450 mg of the crude bradykinin was obtained with alcohol extraction. Crude bradykinin was redissolved in 80 to 90% ethyl alcohol and the filtrate dried *in vacuo*, yielding purified bradykinin 8 to 12 times more active than crude bradykinin. (4) The chemical and pharmacological observations permitted bradykinin to be defined as a smooth-muscle-stimulating and hypotensive principle, released from its plasma precursor (bradykininogen) by proteolytic and coagulating venoms of the *Bothrops* genus and by trypsin. Its pharmacological actions were not blocked by antihistamines and atropine. The evidence available showed that it was a polypeptide (Rocha e Silva et al., 1949b).

Two aspects of the characterization of bradykinin were not dealt with in that classic paper: (1) the possible identification of bradykinin with kallidin and (2) the identity, which was admitted by the authors, of the principle liberated by trypsin with that released by *B. jararaca* venom. Kallidin was rather well characterized by that time (Werle et al., 1937; Werle and Grunz, 1939; Werle and Däumer, 1940; Werle, 1948) but these results were not discussed by the discoverers of bradykinin (Rocha e Silva et al., 1949a). Although Werle and Berek (1950) and Werle et al. (1950a) immediately claimed that bradykinin might be identical with kallidin, much of the scientific world remained unaware of this possibility for some further years. In the words of the late Prof. J. H. Gaddum (1960), then at the Institute of Animal Physiology, Cambridge, England, the discovery of bradykinin proved to be a "very potent stimulus to research. People who had not really been attracted to this field took up work on this substance because Rocha's results were so clear-cut and simple." Werle himself (1962) expressed the opinion that the discovery of bradykinin strongly stimulated the research on kallidin[3]. Thus, in spite of having missed the contribution of the German researchers at the time of the discovery of bradykinin, Rocha e Silva et al. (1949a) rendered a fundamental service to this area of knowledge.

The second aspect mentioned, which was settled much later, was discussed by Werle et al. (1950b), who thought incorrectly at this time that the hypotensive effect of crystalline trypsin on dogs was produced by traces of kallikrein impurities in their trypsin. They were led to this opinion by two observations: a short boiling of a trypsin solution would leave its proteolytic effect practically unaltered, but the hypotensive and kinin-liberating activities were lost; the kallikrein inactivator of parotid glands would inhibit partially (75%) the pharmacological properties of trypsin. Rocha e Silva (1951) reacted immediately to this opinion. Using a sample of a commercial kallikrein preparation (Bayer

3. This opinion is missing in a later publication of this symposium article: E. Werle, Über Plasmakinine [Naunyn-Schmiedebergs Arch. exp. Path. Pharmak. **245**, 254 (1963)], but appears in the publication (Werle, 1962) mentioned above.

Padutin, supplied by Quimica Bayer Ltd., São Paulo; 1-ml ampoules containing 4 units) he observed that Padutin did not liberate a smooth-muscle contracting factor (guinea pig ileum) either from a sample of dried lyophilized human plasma (ELI LILLY) or from beef plasma globulin solution, but released it from dog plasma, a release which was not inhibited by soybean trypsin inhibitor. Crystalline trypsin, on the other hand, liberated the active principle from the three substrates, and the liberation was inhibited by SBTI. Although his interpretations about the inability of Padutin to release an active principle from human and beef plasma were open to criticism, ROCHA E SILVA (1951) concluded correctly that the kinin-liberating activity of crystalline trypsin was not due to contaminating kallikrein.

Several laboratories confirmed the formation of bradykinin by crystalline trypsin. VAN ARMAN (1952, 1955) gave the important information that serum or partly purified globulins of several species, even denatured by 10 to 30 minutes' boiling with an equal volume of N/20 acetic acid, were as good substrates as the native materials. These include fraction IV–6 (Cohn's method). J. L. PRADO et al. (1956) used bovine globulins (1.25–1.70 M ammonium sulfate) and crystalline trypsin (Delta Chemical Works). Fraction IV–4 of bovine plasma globulins (lot BP-45, Armour Research Division, Chicago, Ill.) was also used as substrate. HOLDSTOCK et al. (1957) used crystalline trypsin and ox serum or its globulins heated to 56–58° (WERLE et al., 1937). Finally, in 1959, at a meeting of the Biochemical Society, ELLIOTT et al. (1959b) reported the isolation of pure bradykinin, obtained by the action of pure trypsin on ox serum proteins separated by ammonium sulfate fractionation between 33 and 45% of saturation. At the same time ELLIOTT et al. (1959a), at a meeting of the Physiological Society, described the biological properties of pure bradykinin on several pharmacological preparations and concluded that pure bradykinin probably was responsible for most of the biological activity found in the crude mixture. These results were also published later (ELLIOTT et al., 1960a). The isolation of pure bradykinin, produced by pure trypsin and ox serum globulins was published in detail (ELLIOTT et al., 1961). ANDRADE and ROCHA E SILVA (1956) obtained a highly purified bradykinin which may have been pure (ROCHA E SILVA, 1963), but this bradykinin was obtained from ox plasma globulins and *B. jararaca* venom, and at that time (1956) it was not yet known whether it was identical with bradykinin formed by trypsin. This information became available later (HAMBERG et al., 1961).

Direct and indirect Actions. Besides the bradykinin-releasing effect of trypsin on plasma, WERLE et al. (1955) showed that a second hypotensive substance is formed when fresh plasma and crystalline trypsin are incubated. While the liberated bradykinin was inactivated within minutes, the second hypotensive factor remained active for a much longer time, was not dialyzable, and had chemical and pharmacological properties similar to those of pancreatic and urinary kallikreins and identical with serum kallikrein. These results were interpreted by them as due to the transformation of serum prekallikrein into serum kallikrein by trypsin. The activation of a kinin-forming factor in fresh plasma by trypsin was recently investigated by ROCHA E SILVA et al. (1967). They observed that when trypsin is added to fresh guinea pig plasma (50 μg to 1 mg/ml), proportional amounts of kinins are released, but the maximal liberation (as indicated by using denatured plasma substrate) is not reached. If the fresh plasma was previously treated with glass powder, trypsin released no kinin activity. The total and residual kininogen contents were also determined and were consistent with the interpretation that trypsin activates a kinin-releasing system in plasma which, when removed by glass powder, can no longer be activated.

The nature of the systems activated by trypsin is open to discussion at the present time (see Chapter 1, p. 3).

Kallidin. When WEBSTER and PIERCE (1963) incubated human plasma with crystalline trypsin (200 μg/ml) they recovered 2.5% of the total pharmacological activity as kallidin and the remainder as bradykinin. The finding of kallidin was confirmed by HABERMANN and BLENNEMANN (1964) when they incubated purified beef kininogen (from fraction IV–6) with crystalline trypsin (50 μg-ml) and found that about 8% of the total activity was caused by kallidin. Because their trypsin was contamined with chymotrypsin (inactivated by special treatment), they thought that possible traces of pancreatic kallikrein might explain the presence of kallidin. Later, however, HABERMANN and MÜLLER (1966) used a lower trypsin concentration (1.25 μg/ml) and were still able to detect traces of kallidin in their incubates. It may thus be concluded that kallidin is released from kininogen by trypsin.

Methionyllysyl-Bradykinin (MLBr). It was shown by HABERMANN and MÜLLER (1966) that crystalline trypsin (12.5 μg/ml) liberates from PKFL (a kinin-yielding peptide from bovine kininogen; structure under C II below, p. 171) about 31% of MLBr and 68% bradykinin.

Glycine[1]*-Kallidin* (Glycyl-Bradykinin). This peptide was identified (see references under C II, p. 173) as the main active peptide formed by trypsin digestion of the major kinin fraction of wasp (*Polistes*) venom. The proposed structure for this wasp kinin (PISANO, 1967) contains glycyl-bradykinin in its C-terminus.

Pepsin; Pepsitocin. CROXATTO et al. (1950) showed that prolonged digestion of the plasma globulin fraction which contains angiotensinogen (hypertensinogen), or of pepsitensin solutions with crystalline pepsin, is accompanied by a decrease or disappearance of the pressor activity and the formation of an oxytocic substance. Pressor activity was measured on cat blood pressure and the oxytocic activity mainly on isolated guinea pig uterus. As substrates the following were used: human and horse plasmas and some of their fractions such as angiotensinogen (precipitated at 30% with ammonium sulfate), fibrinogen and albumin fraction, and purified angiotensinogen. Solutions of these substrates were digested twice with crystalline pepsin. In a few cases the digestion was repeated a third time to obtain sufficient inactivation of the pressor action. During the second digestion the pressor effect (pepsitensin) was totally or partially inactivated, while the oxytocic effect remained unaltered or increased. Digests obtained from the globulin fractions (angiotensinogen) had larger pressor and oxytocic effects when compared to digests from the other plasma fractions which had very weak actions. According to the authors, digestion of pepsitensin by pepsin might produce a similar peptide with oxytocic properties which was resistant to peptic digestion. This characteristic and its solubility in ethyl alcohol, stability in acid medium, and the resistance of the uterotonic effect to atropine were similar to those described for oxytocin.

In a paper describing the antidiuretic factor formed by pepsin, CROXATTO et al. (1951) mention that hypertensinogen, especially after the second digestion with pepsin, releases the most potent uterotonic (guinea pig uterus) substance. Human or horse plasma globulin fractions (1:6 to 1:2 saturation with ammonium sulfate, adjusted to pH 3.5 or 2.5), were digested with crystalline pepsin at 38° for 4 to 24 hours and extracted with alcohol. This solution was tested for its pressor effect and antidiuretic and oxytocic activities. A second digestion with pepsin, under identical conditions, was carried out, and the final concentrated solution was assayed again as after the first digestion. In some instances the procedure was repeated a third time. Table 1 shows some of the results. The authors concluded that more than one substance is involved because it is clear that, although the pressor action decreases, the other two activities remain practically unaltered or increase. There is no indication in this paper, however, that the oxytocic principle might be different from the antidiuretic factor. In 1953, however, CROXATTO et al. claimed that the oxytocic substance, formed by digestion of human, ox, and horse plasma or hypertensinogen (α_2-globulins) by crystalline pepsin was different from the antidiuretic substance; it resisted crystalline trypsin and pepsin but was inactivated by chymotrypsin. Further physical and chemical characteristics of the oxytocic principle, now called pepsitocin, are given

Table 1. *Antidiuretic, pressor, and oxytocic actions of the products obtained from plasma globulin fractions by successive digestions with crystalline pepsin and from the first pepsin digestion of albumin fraction.* (From CROXATTO et al., 1951)

Digestion	Pepsin (mg/100 ml)	Incubation time (hrs)	Water excretion in 90 min (%)	Pressor units (per ml)	Oxytocic units (per ml)
		Human hypertensinogen, pH 3.5			
I	20	4	61	1.8	0.005
II	120	24	23	1.2	0.005
III	400	24	6	0.0	0.005
		Horse hypertensinogen, pH 3.0			
I	15	5	50	6	0.003
II	60	19	5	2	0.015
		Albumin fraction, pH 3.0			
I	10	14	66	0	0.001

Antidiuretic activity measured on groups of rats according to H. J. BURN, Quart. J. Pharmacol. 4, 517 (1931); the pressor action was tested on cats and rats, recording the effect from the carotid arteries, and the oxytocic action was assayed on the isolated guinea pig uterus.

by CROXATTO (1955). From 1 ml of horse plasma digested twice with pepsin, pepsitocin equivalent to 2 to 4 mU of oxytocin was obtained. It remained to be demonstrated whether pepsitocin was different from pepsanurin, the antidiuretic factor. Starting from 100 liters of ox serum, TURBA and HETZEL (1954) digested the globulin fraction separated between 40 and 65% of ammonium sulfate saturation, with Merck pepsin (50 mg/liter), pH 2.5, 37° for 4–6 hours[4]. From 100 liters of serum, 1,000 g of an oxytocic preparation was obtained. The oxytocic activity was measured on rat uterus and expressed as Voegtlin units per gram. The purification procedure consisted of: (1) extraction with 96% ethyl alcohol and with pyridine; (2) chromatography on paper pulp column, where two oxytocic peaks were found; (3) submission of the sharper peak to paper electrophoresis (50 V/cm; pH 6.4); (4) migration of the oxytocic material cathodically and its further purification by paper chromatography. The oxytocic activity increases from 0.06 to 2,500 units/g; 0.8 mg of a pure peptide was obtained and its only N-terminal amino acid (phenylisothiocyanate method) was asparagine. The other amino acids found were: glycine, alanine, valine, leucine (isoleucine), serine, threonine, glutamic acid, arginine, lysine, histidine. No mention of antidiuretic activity determination was made and doubt remained that pepsitocin would be different from pepsanurin. DENGLER (1957) reported finding

4. Digestion of 24-hr duration and six times higher pepsin concentration did not increase the yield of active substance.

a paper chromatogram fraction, obtained by peptic digestion from ox serum globulin, which was pressor and acted on smooth muscles but without anti-diuretic activity.

Hypotensive Action of Pepsitensin and Relationship with Kinins. When WEBER et al. (1942) confirmed the production of pepsitensin, they also reported that, in incubations between pH 5 and 3, the resulting solution was in some instances strongly depressor. BRAUN-MENENDEZ et al. (1943) showed that when dog angiotensinogen was hydrolyzed by swine renin, the resulting angiotensin dialyzed,

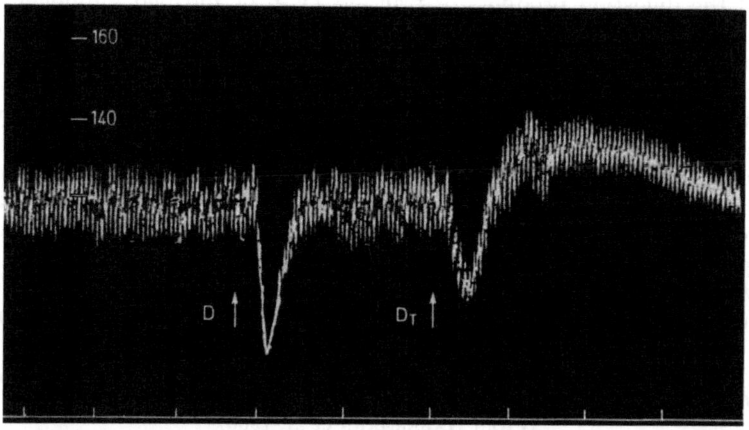

Fig. 1. Blood pressure responses in dog produced by: *D* extract from plasma treated with renin, dialyzed, and treated with pepsin; *DT* extract from dialyzed plasma treated with pepsin. (From BRAUN-MENENDEZ et al., 1943)

and the residual plasma incubated with pepsin, only a depressor material was formed. In contrast, the control plasma had a biphasic response (depressor and pressor) on dog blood pressure after digestion with pepsin (Fig. 1). Actually, they showed also that when dog plasma (1 vol.) was treated with renin and its proteins precipitated with cold alcohol (3 vol.), resuspended in water (1.3 vol.), and incubated with pepsin at pH 3.5, only a depressor response was detected, which is a variation of the first observation. Zeal to study the hypertensive substance, owing to its obvious relationship with angiotensin and human hypertension, delayed for several years further studies on the depressor substance formed by pepsin digestion. PAIVA (1954) obtained from pepsitensin paper chromatograms a fraction which was hypotensive in the cat, distinct from the pressor and smooth-muscle-stimulating factor (pepsitensin). As a consequence of more recent studies of kininogen, several other findings were made. WERLE and HOCHSTRASSER (1963) found that when bovine plasma globulins are digested with crystalline pepsin (pH 2.0, 37°, 40 hr.), kininogen may be degraded to dialyzable products which keep their kinin-forming activity when treated with trypsin. HABERMANN and SCHUCK (1964) made similar observations and reported also that the pepsitocin activity could not be completely separated from the kinin-producing kininogen fragments by paper and column chromatography. GREENBAUM et al. (1965) obtained by peptic degradation of partially purified bovine kininogen a hypotensive basic peptide fraction, which served as substrate for the kinin-forming activity of trypsin. Its spasmogenic (guinea pig ileum) and hypotensive (rabbit blood pressure) activities increased 9- and 4-fold after trypsin digestion.

HABERMANN et al. (1966) finally identified the polypeptides by studying the digestion products of purified beef serum kininogen or plasma fractions such as IV–6 (which contains kininogen) with thrice-crystallized pepsin. They showed that the pepsitocic fractions (direct activity) and the kinin-releasing fractions (indirect activity by incubation with kininogenases) could not be separated during purification. Pepsin liberates from kininogen 0.5 to 2% of spasmogenic activity (guinea pig ileum) as compared with that liberated by trypsin or *Crotalus adamanteus* venom (indirect activity). Then, having determined the optimum conditions for these digestions (pH 1.8, 4 hr., 37°, enzyme 20 to 100 μg/ml) they separated the digestion products of fraction IV–6 or purified kininogen on CM-cellulose microcolumns. In both cases two peaks with direct (guinea pig ileum and rabbit blood pressure) and indirect (*Crotalus* venom and kallikrein) activities were partially separated. The peak, eluted at 0.27 M ammonium formate buffer, was about 100 times more active than the starting material as a kinin-yielding substance, and was the only one to be further purified. Paper chromatography gave two zones of kinin-yielding fractions (*peptische kininliefernde Fragmente*), called PKFS (faster, Rf about 0.34) and PKFL (slower, Rf about 0.25) and only two, which had pepsitocin activity and released kinins with *Crotalus* venom, pancreas kallikrein, or carboxypeptidase A. These fragments (PKFS and PKFL) were purified by rechromatography on microcolumns of either CM-cellulose or P-cellulose, and the final yield is shown in Table 2. The purity of these fragments

Table 2. *Yield of kinin-releasing peptides (PFKS and PKFL*[a]*) obtained by chromatography on CM-cellulose, paper chromatography, and chromatography on phosphorylated cellulose*
(From HABERMANN et al. 1966)

	(mg)	Total activity as bradykinin	Yield (%)	Bradykinin/ Material (μg/mg)
Starting material	465	5,110	100	11
CM-cellulose	25	5,280	103	211
Paper chrom. and P-cellulose				
PFKS	1.4	385	8	275
PKFL	6.4	2,240	44	350
Total	7.8	2,625	52	

[a] PKFS and PKFL = *peptische kininliefernde Fragmente*, "*schneller*" or "*langsamer*" in paper chromatography.

was tested in high-voltage paper electrophoresis and paper chromatography and their amino acid compositions determined. PKFL: Lys (1.16), Arg (1.96), Ser (1.91), Glu (1.07), Pro (2.71), Gly (1.10), Val (1.16), Met (0.97), Phe (1.94). PKFS: Lys (1.14), Arg (2.00), Ser (1.96), Glu (1.07), Pro (3.06), Gly (1.03), Val (2.07), Met (1.67), Phe (1.89). PKFL contains all of the amino acids of Met-Lys-bradykinin plus Val, Ser, and Glu (one mole of each). Both kinin-yielding fragments can be called pepsitocin. The direct activity on the ileum of PKFL and PKFS (expressed as micrograms of bradykinin per milligram) were 2.0 and 2.6 as compared with 350 and 275 (Table 2) when treated with trypsin or *Crotalus* venom. The direct uterotonic (rat) actions (as micrograms bradykinin per milligram) were 2 (PKFL) and 0.7 (PKFS). They were both hypotensive (rabbit blood pressure). They increase vascular permeability (rabbit skin) approximately to the same extent.

Although the kinin activities of PKFL and PKFS are rather low when compared with bradykinin and kallidin, they may be classified as kinins and thus pepsin could be classified as a kininogenase. There is no doubt, however, that pepsin cannot be compared with kininogenases such as trypsin, clostripain, and others. Kininogen fragments produced by pepsin (the pepsitocins) are similar to the major kinin in wasp venom described by J. L. PRADO et al. (1966), because this wasp kinin, although much more potent as a kinin, serves as substrate for trypsin as well as for horse urinary kallikrein (PISANO, 1967), giving rise to glycylbradykinin.

The pepsitocin purified by TURBA and HETZEL (1954), although obtained from beef serum and claimed by them to be pure, had a qualitative amino acid composition different from PKFL and PKFS. Pepsanurin was not studied by HABERMANN et al. (1966); its possible identity with the pepsitocins remains an open question.

Clostripain; Kinin Formation. The kinin-forming activity of clostripain was found by J. L. PRADO et al. (1956) when they demonstrated that by incubating bovine plasma globulins (precipitated between 0.30 and 0.41% saturation with ammonium sulfate) or Cohn fraction IV–4 from bovine plasma (lot BP–45, Armour Research Division, Chicago) with the cysteine-activated enzyme, a substance that contracted the isolated guinea pig ileum accumulated in the incubation mixture. The slowly contracting substance, named clostridin for convenience, was prepared either from bovine globulins or fraction IV–4 and exhibited the following main characteristics: (1) it was readily adsorbed on animal charcoal and eluted by glacial acetic acid; (2) it was purified by extracting it from saturated NaCl solution, pH 1.0, with butanol (GOMES, 1955); (3) it was dialyzable, resisted boiling for 1 hour in water or 0.1 N HCl but was partially destroyed in 0.07 N NaOH solution at 100°; (4) clostridin was inactivated by chymotrypsin but resisted trypsin (1 hr.) and pepsin (4 hr.) digestion; (5) in diferent paper chromatograms there was about 30% recovery of clostridin and its Rf varied from 0.30 to 0.42; (6) in paper electrophoresis (pH 4.0 and 7.4) it migrated cathodically, with 10 to 20% recovery. All these properties were compared, in simultaneous experiments, with those shown by bradykinin prepared and purified from bovine globulins with crystalline trypsin. Mixtures of both active substances could not be resolved by paper chromatography or paper electrophoresis. The slow contraction of guinea pig ileum produced by clostridin was not abolished by atropine and pyrilamine (Neoantergan); its effect on rat blood pressure was biphasic, a transitory fall followed by a transient blood pressure rise, identical with that observed with the bradykinin preparation. Indices of discrimination (rat uterus, guinea pig ileum, hen rectal caecum, rat blood pressure) could not differentiate between the preparations of clostridin and bradykinin. J. L. PRADO et al. (1956) concluded that clostridin was similar to, if not identical with, bradykinin.

Direct Action. Although it had been suggested (LEWIS, 1960) that kinin formation by clostripain might be indirect, through plasmin activation, this possibility was disproved by the experiments of J. L. and E. S. PRADO (1962), who showed that by incubating heat-treated horse plasma (6 hr., 56–58°) with highly purified clostripain, the fast kinin formation was not inhibited by soybean trypsin inhibitor, which is known (LEWIS, 1958) to abolish kinin formation by plasmin. They have also shown that addition of 1 mg urokinase (18,000 units/mg, Leo Pharmaceutical Products) to heat-treated horse plasma (0.4 ml) in the guinea pig ileum bath liberated negligible amounts of kinin, while doses as low as 25 μg cysteine-activated clostripain were followed by an immediate kinin formation in the muscle bath.

As prekallikrein does not resist the heat treatment of plasma (Werle et al., 1955; Fasciolo, 1964) and is inhibited by SBTI, activation of prekallikrein in plasma by clostripain is also ruled out. Thus although never proven directly, the site of action of clostripain must be on kininogen.

Subtilisin BPN' (Nagarse); Kinin Formation. When a crystalline preparation of the proteinase from *Bacillus subtilis* N', commercially available as Nagarse, was incubated for 10 min at 37° with heat-treated horse plasma (3 hr., 56–58°, pH c. 7.4), in the proportion of 200–400 μg enzyme/ml plasma. a pharmacologically active substance, provisionally called substance N, accumulated in the incubation mixture (J. L. Prado et al., 1964). Interrupting the incubation by adding boiling ethyl alcohol and purifying the substance N formed by extracting it from NaCl-saturated solution at pH 1.5 with butanol, then with glacial acetic acid and precipitating it with eight volumes of ethyl ether, a small-scale preparation of the liberated substance was obtained. Substance N was inactivated by chymotrypsin but resisted trypsin digestion, being inactivated slowly by Nagarse itself. In paper electrophoresis it could not be separated from authentic bradykinin. In the dog, substance N produced a transitory hypotension which, like bradykinin hypotension, was potentiated by BAL. Although not mentioned in the text of the above paper (J. L. Prado et al., 1964) the transitory hypotension was followed by a less marked and transitory hypertension. In the rat, substance N had a pressor effect. Indices of discrimination with synthetic bradykinin varied from 2 to 50. Like bradykinin, substance N relaxed rat duodenum. Since intravenously injected Nagarse produced shock in both rat and dog the above results, as a whole, led the authors to accept Nagarse as a kininogenase, because they thought that a material similar to bradykinin had been liberated by the enzyme.

Vasopressor Principle. Huggins et al. (1964) incubated human plasma fraction IV–4 with Nagarse and found a vasopressor substance in the cat, dog, and rat. The principle contracted the isolated guinea pig ileum and rat uterus. Chymotrypsin, trypsin, and Nagarse inactivated the material, while pepsin (500 μg-ml) inactivated only 40% in 30-minute and 80% in 1-hour incubation. In chromatography on a CM-cellulose column its behavior was identical with Val^5-angiotensin II. These properties led the authors to conclude that the pressor principle was similar to Val^5-angiotensin II and identical with or similar to a pressor substance of Walaszek and Huggins (1959), formed on incubation of plasma fraction IV–4 and some α-amylase preparations. These amylase preparations were found later (Huggins et al., 1964) to possess high proteolytic activity on hemoglobin. One of these amylase preparations (NBC-7942) was obtained from *B. subtilis*. This pressor principle, named substance A, had been characterized by Walaszek et al. (1962) as closely related to the octapeptides Val^5-angiotensin II and Ile^5-angiotensin II. They also reported in this paper the complete inactivation of purified substance A (Huggins and Walaszek, 1962) by pepsin and the transformation of two angiotensins (I) probably into the corresponding octapeptides by the α-amylase preparation used.[5] Huggins et al. (1964) finally suggested that Nagarse was the contaminating enzyme in their α-amylase preparations responsible for the formation of the vasopressor principle. Taking into consideration the findings described by J. L. Prado et al. (1964), the formation of a vasoactive principle liberated by Nagarse from heat-treated horse plasma was reinvestigated by Huggins and Thampi (1967); they concluded that the vasoactive material was vasopressor and very similar to a standard preparation of substance A (Huggins and Walaszek, 1962).

5. Based on observations showing that the octapeptides are several times more uterotonic than the decapeptides (Carlini et al., 1958; Carlini and Huggins, 1962).

There is no doubt, however, that Nagarse also forms a bradykinin-like material when incubated with plasma globulin. When substance A was prepared in large scale from fraction IV–4 of human plasma and α-amylase (NBC-7942), HUGGINS and WALASZEK (1962) found that approximately 10% of the total biological activity on the guinea pig ileum was separated on a CM-cellulose column from the main vasopressor material, it relaxed rat duodenum and was recognized as bradykinin-like. HUGGINS and THAMPI (1967) observed a biphasic response of rat duodenum with the active powder obtained from heat-treated horse plasma; the relaxation would be explained by the formation of a bradykinin-like material. Their substance A from heat-treated plasma was resistant to pepsin and partially resistant to trypsin which would, again, point to the presence of a kinin-like principle in their preparation. The observations of J. L. PRADO et al. (1964) called attention specifically to this bradykinin-like substance. In deep shock in dogs, produced by Nagarse, large amounts of kinin are found in the blood stream, and bradykininogen disappears entirely from the circulating blood (CORRADO et al., 1966).

It seems in conclusion that Nagarse liberates from blood plasma globulins both a vasopressor peptide, similar to the angiotensin octapeptides, and a vasodepressor polypeptide of kinin nature. This situation is analogous to that found with pepsin and may be common to other proteolytic enzymes, the amount of each vasoactive peptide formed depending on enzyme and substrates used and on incubating conditions. It should also be pointed out that Val^5-angiotensin II amide is inactivated within 20 seconds by Nagarse in concentrations of 0.5 and 5.0 μg/ml (ENDO et al., 1966) and that HUGGINS and THAMPI (1967) used in heat-treated horse plasma around 200 μg/ml, a situation that would not favor an accumulation of angiotensin II. Synthetic bradykinin, on the contrary, is destroyed slowly by 50 μg Nagarse/ml (J. L. PRADO et. al., 1964).

Ficin; Kinin Formation. J. L. PRADO et al. (1965b, 1967) also proved that crystalline ficin liberates a kinin-like substance or substances from heat-treated horse plasma (3 hr, 56–58°). They demonstrated the formation of a smooth-muscle (guinea pig ileum) stimulating agent by adding the crystalline enzyme (down to 38 μg), neutralized cysteine hydrochloride (5×10^{-3} M final concentration), and 0.4 ml horse plasma to the muscle bath (7–8 ml). The kinin liberation by ficin is not affected by 1 mg SBTI. The slow contraction is not affected by atropine and antihistamine (not mentioned in their paper). The active agent was prepared by incubating dialyzed fresh horse plasma and crude ficin (880 μg/ml plasma plus 1×10^{-2} M cysteine·HCl) for 4 minutes at 37°. The kinin was extracted as described (p. 168). The activity of this partially purified active material was destroyed by chymotrypsin and resisted trypsin and pepsin digestion. When assayed on guinea pig ileum, rat uterus, and rat duodenum, it could not be distinguished from authentic bradykinin. Both bradykinin and the active agent are rapidly destroyed by crystalline ficin. Dialyzed crude ficin (132 mg) produced in an 11 kg dog, anesthetized with morphine and pretreated with atropine sulfate (1 mg) and diphenhydramine (1 mg), a marked hypotension which lasted more than 20 minutes. All these findings were interpreted as the result of liberation of a kinin-like peptide by ficin from plasma, either *in vitro* or *in vivo*. In the whole animal, of course, other hypotensive agents and effects might also be responsible for the marked drop in blood pressure.

Ficin Components. The approximate kinin-forming activity of the ficin components separated by SGARBIERI et al. (1964) was estimated by the method of E. S. PRADO et al. (1962). This consisted in adding excess heat-treated horse plasma to the guinea pig ileum chamber, pipetting in the respective ficin component (equi-caseinolytic amounts), and recording the muscle contraction for a fixed period of time (60–90 sec). The results (J. L. PRADO et al., 1965b) showed that components B, C, and F were the most active; D and G were intermediate; and E, H, and I had no kinin-forming activity. No correlation was found between kinin-forming and caseinolytic activities.

Papain. When studying the kinin-forming activity of ficin, J. L. PRADO et al. (1965b) observed that crystalline papain, in the presence of 5×10^{-3} M cysteine, liberates rapidly from heat-treated horse plasma large amounts of a smooth-muscle-contracting principle. The liberation is not inhibited by SBTI, and both the active principle and bradykinin were rapidly inactivated by activated papain itself. As with ficin, crystalline-activated papain (3.7 mg/kg) produced a marked hypotension in the dog, which lasted more than 20 minutes. These observations were interpreted as caused by either *in vitro* or *in vivo* liberation of a kinin-like principle or principles.

WERLE and KORSTEN (1938) developed a procedure to estimate serum kallikrein by incubating 10 ml serum (pH 5.0) with Merck papain (2 mg/ml serum) at room temperature for 48 hours, with simultaneous dialysis against running water. The activated serum kallikrein was precipitated with uranyl acetate and finally assayed in the dog. Any kinin thus formed would be removed by dialysis. These results appear also in book of (FREY et al. (1950). WERLE and BEREK (1950) were unable to find any guinea pig ileum-contracting activity on incubation of blood serum with Merck papain. Much later (WERLE, 1963), the claim was made of unpublished results showing the kinin-forming activity (not prekallikrein activation) of papain. Therefore, when J. L. PRADO et al. (1965b) made their observations with crystalline papain, they were still uncertain about the direct kinin-liberating activity of papain.

Streptomyces griseus protease (Pronase). HUGGINS et al. (1964) were unable to demonstrate that Pronase had a kininogenase activity on human plasma fraction IV–4. J. L. PRADO and MENDES (1965) made the following unpublished observations. In a mixture (2 ml) containing 20 μg synthetic bradykinin and 2 μg Pronase, 80% of the peptide activity disappeared within 4 minutes. When trying to demonstrate the kinin-releasing activity of Pronase directly in the smooth-muscle chamber, they found that a minimum of 50 μg Pronase induced a contraction in guinea pig ileum when added to 0.4 ml of heat-treated horse plasma. When the dose was increased to 100 μg, the contraction appeared but the muscle relaxed before the Pronase was washed out. Even 50 μg of the substance, when present in the muscle chamber, reduced the response to 0.1 or 0.2 μg bradykinin by about 50%. Although the release of a smooth-muscle stimulant was evident, the apparently fast inactivation of the released agent by Pronase led them to abandon the experiments. REIS et al. (1966) studied the kinin-releasing action of Pronase on denatured bradykininogen and were unable to detect the release of any activity by adding Pronase to kininogen in the isolated guinea pig ileum bath. They found, however, that among several fractions separated from the Pronase preparation by paper electrophoresis (barbital buffer, pH 8.6) the most basic one released bradykinin-like material and also split ATEe and BAEe. The bradykinin-like peptide relaxed rat duodenum, contracted guinea pig ileum and rat uterus, and was inactivated by chymotrypsin. The other fractions, slower in paper electrophoresis, had only a kinin-inactivating activity. When they were added to the kinin-releasing fraction, the mixture seemed inactive as a kininogenase. The Pronase preparation used may have been impure. NOMOTO and NARAHASHI (1958) have proved the electrophoretic homogeneity of pure Pronase.

Pronase, like Nagarse, probably liberates from blood plasma both pressor and depressor polypeptides. The inactivation of angiotensin-like polypeptides by Pronase has not been reported, although the broad proteolytic specificity of this enzyme (NOMOTO et al., 1959), would suggest that the pressor polypeptides would also be quickly inactivated.

Carboxypeptidase A. Although they were unable to liberate a kinin from beef kininogen, carboxypeptidase A was shown by HABERMANN and MÜLLER (1966) to release methionyllysyl-bradykinin from PKFL. Carboxypeptidase A should not be classified as a true kininogenase as its kinin-releasing activity can be demonstrated only on fragments of kininogen.

Chymotrypsin. A liberation of a kinin-like activity from fresh guinea pig plasma by chymotrypsin (α, β, γ, and δ) was recently reported by ROCHA E SILVA et al. (1967) when they inhibited the kinin inactivation with 8-hydroxyquinoline. As an example, chymotrypsin (80 μg/ml plasma in 9 min) released the equivalent of 2.0 μg synthetic bradykinin, as compared to 2.4 liberated by trypsin (1 mg/ml plasma in 10 min) from 1 ml plasma. This corresponds to about 20% of the total kininogen content. From other fresh plasmas tried (dog, hamster, rabbit, and man) there was no kinin released by chymotrypsin *in vitro*. The kinin release was accompanied by a demonstrable kininogen consumption of guinea pig plasma. From denatured as well as from fresh guinea pig plasma treated with glass powder (30-min shaking with 0.2 g glass powder/3 ml plasma), chymotrypsin released no kinin. This situation is similar to the liberation of kinin by trypsin from fresh guinea pig plasma. Trypsin, however, liberates kinin from denatured guinea pig plasma kininogen, but chymotrypsin does not. Thus, liberation by chymotrypsin in this species is only indirect, probably through activation of a plasma kinin-releasing system. The enzyme should not be classified as a true kininogenase. When acting *in vivo* on kininogen it seems that chymotrypsin may even attack it without liberating a kinin. ROCHA E SILVA et al. (1967) observed, indeed, a drastic reduction of circulating kininogen in dogs without any effect on the blood pressure.

II. Nature of Kinin Liberated

Table 3 shows the nature and chemical structure of kinins released from blood plasma globulins or from other natural substrates by the kininogenases reviewed in this chapter. These include trypsin, pepsin, clostripain, Nagarse, ficin, papain, and Pronase. Structures of kinins liberated only by trypsin and pepsin have been determined. Bradykinin represents more than 90% of the total peptide activity released from kininogen by trypsin. Relatively small amounts of kallidin were also found by WEBSTER and PIERCE (1963) and HABERMANN and BLENNEMANN (1964). The crystalline trypsin preparation used by the last authors was contaminated with chymotrypsin, which was previously inactivated. The contamination of crystalline trypsin with pancreatic kallikrein would explain the formation of kallidin (about 8% of total activity, HABERMANN and BLENNEMANN, 1964; 2.5% of recovered activity, WEBSTER and PIERCE, 1963). However, it does not seem to be the correct explanation, because trypsin itself seems to liberate kallidin from kininogen, although in a much smaller percentage than bradykinin. Even at the concentration of 1.25 μg/ml, trypsin still releases trace amounts of kallidin from beef kininogen (HABERMANN and MÜLLER, 1966).

The structures of kinin-yielding peptides formed by pepsin from bovine kininogen were determined by HABERMANN (1966a, b). PKFL corresponds to Met^1-Lys^2-Arg^3-Pro^4-Pro^5-Gly^6-Phe^7-Ser^8-Pro^9-Phe^{10}-Arg^{11}-Ser^{12}-Val^{13}-Gln^{14}; PKFS

Table 3. *Kinins formed by several kininogenases* [a]

Kininogenase	Kinin found	Kinin structure	References
Trypsin (C)	Bradykinin	Not determined	Rocha e Silva et al. (1949a)
Trypsin (C)	Bradykinin	Not determined	Van Arman (1955)
Trypsin (C)	Bradykinin	Not determined	J. L. Prado et al. (1956)
Trypsin (C)	Bradykinin	Not determined	Holdstock et al. (1957)
Trypsin (C)	Bradykinin	Not determined	Elliot et al. (1959b)
Trypsin (C)	Bradykinin	Not determined	Elliot et al. (1959a, 1960c, 1961)
Trypsin (C)	Bradykinin	Octapeptide	Elliot et al. (1960a)
Trypsin (C)	Bradykinin	Nonapeptide	Elliot et al. (1960b)
Trypsin (C)	Bradykinin, kallidin	Nona and decapeptide	Webster and Pierce (1963)
Trypsin (C)	Bradykinin, kallidin	Nona and decapeptide	Habermann and Blennemann (1964)
Trypsin (C)	Bradykinin, methionyllysyl-bradykinin	Nona and hendecapeptide	Habermann and Müller (1966)
Trypsin (C)	Glycine[1]-kallidin (glycyl-bradykinin)	Decapeptide	Pisano et al. (1965); J. L. Prado et al. (1965c, 1966)
Pepsin (C)	PKFL PKFS	Tetradecapeptide Hexadecapeptide	Habermann et al. (1966; Habermann and Müller (1966); Habermann (1966a, b)
Clostripain	Bradykinin-like	Not determined	J. L. Prado et al. (1956)
Nagarse (C)	Bradykinin-like	Not determined	Huggins and Walaszek (1962); J. L. Prado et al. (1964); Corrado et al. (1966)
Ficin	Bradykinin-like	Not determined	J. L. Prado et al. (1965b, 1967)
Papain (C)	Uncharacterized kinin	Not determined	J. L. Prado et al. (1965b)
Pronase	Bradykinin-like	Not determined	Reis et al. (1966)

[a] Kallikreins and snake venoms are not included. (C) = crystalline enzyme preparations.

has one valine and probably one methionine residue attached to the C-terminus of PKFL. Their first eleven amino acid residues correspond to the structure of methionyl-lysyl-bradykinin.

From the major kinin found in wasp venom, PISANO et al. (1965) and J. L. PRADO et al. (1965c, 1966) liberated by trypsin digestion glycine[1]-kallidin (glycyl-bradykinin) which had previously been synthesized by SCHRÖDER and HEMPEL (1964).

Clostripain, Nagarse, and ficin release bradykinin-like peptides, but no chemical studies were made of the structures. The kinin-like principles released by papain and Pronase were even less well characterized.

III. Action on the Substrate

Kinin-Forming Substrates. From the work with the renal vasopressor system (e.g. BRAUN-MENENDEZ et al., 1946), it became evident that blood plasma globulins contained the precursors of pressor and depressor substances liberated by incubation with renin and pepsin. When bradykinin was discovered, trypsin was shown to act on the plasma globulin fraction precipitated by a 30–45% saturation with ammonium sulfate. Forty-five per cent saturation precipitated completely the bradykinin precursor named bradykininogen (ROCHA E SILVA et al., 1949a). The work which followed or preceded this observation will be reviewed under *kininogen* (see Chapter 4, p. 250), a name now used for the main natural substrate of the kininogenases. It was only in recent years, however, that it became tenable that the kinin-liberating action of trypsin is dependent on the proteolytic action of this enzyme on kininogen. The structure of kinin-releasing peptides obtained from bovine kininogen was clarified (HABERMANN, 1966b) and it was shown that the releasing of bradykinin by the action of trypsin on this substrate was a proteolytic action (HABERMANN and MÜLLER, 1966). The idea that bradykinin may be released from kininogen by breaking an ester linkage (ROCHA E SILVA, 1960; ELLIOTT, 1963) is, however, not yet abandoned (PIERCE, 1968); this author still believes that the carboxyl end of bradykinin may be linked by an ester linkage to a serine residue in kininogen. Only future results will provide a final answer.

Besides plasma kininogen or its fragments, the major kinin in wasp venom is also a kininogen substrate of trypsin (PISANO et al., 1965; J. L. PRADO et al., 1965c, 1966). The kinin-releasing activity of trypsin has been tested with success (Table 4) on natural and denatured serum globulins, plasma globulins heated at 56–58°, Cohn fractions IV–4 and the narrower IV–6, purified kininogens from human plasma and from several animal species, polypeptides resulting from digestion of kininogen by pepsin, and a natural polypeptide with kinin-like activity found in wasp venom. Table 4 shows also the substrates which were tried with other kininogenases. When it was found that plasma kininogen may be resolved into two components it was also observed that trypsin released kinin activity from both kininogens (JACOBSEN, 1966a, b; HENRIQUES et al., 1966, 1967; PIERCE and WEBSTER, 1966).

Direct and Indirect Actions. It was mentioned on pages 162 and 170 that trypsin and papain possess besides their direct kininogenase action an indirect kininogenase activity with plasma because they activate a plasma system (pre-kallikrein and/or plasminogen) which has a kinin-forming activity in itself. A direct kinin-releasing action was demonstrated for the following kininogenases: trypsin, pepsin, clostripain, Nagarse, ficin, papain, and Pronase. While the direct action of trypsin and pepsin was demonstrated with purified kininogen, for the

Table 4. *Kinin-forming substrates*

Kininogenase	Substrate	References
Trypsin (C)[a]	Bovine plasma globulin fraction (30—45% am. sulf.)	ROCHA E SILVA et al. (1949a)
Trypsin (C)	Denatured serum globulins	VAN ARMAN (1955)
Trypsin (C)	Beef serum or globulins (50% am. sulf.) heated 3 hr 56—58°	HOLDSTOCK et al. (1957)
Trypsin (C)	COHN's fractions IV-4 and IV-6	VAN ARMAN (1952, 1955); J. L. PRADO et al. (1956); HABERMANN et al. (1966)
Trypsin (C)	Purified horse kininogen	HENRIQUES et al. (1962)
Trypsin (C)	Purified bovine kininogen	GREENBAUM and HOSODA (1963)
Trypsin (C)	Purified beef kininogen from fraction IV-6	HABERMANN et al. (1963); HABERMANN and BLENNEMANN (1964)
Trypsin (C)	Purified bovine kininogen	SUZUKI et al. (1965)
Trypsin (C)	Purified human kininogen	BROCKLEHURST and MAWER (1966)
Trypsin (C)	Fragments from plasma globulins by pepsin digestion	WERLE and HOCHSTRASSER (1963); HABERMANN and SCHUCK (1964); GREENBAUM et al. (1965)
Trypsin (C)	Wasp kinin 3	PISANO et al. (1965); J.L. PRADO et al. (1965c, 1966).
Trypsin (C)	Fragments of peptic digestion from purified beef serum kininogen or from plasma fraction IV-6	HABERMANN et al. (1966); HABERMANN and MÜLLER (1966); HABERMANN (1966a, b)
Pepsin (C)	Plasma globulin fraction (30% am. sulf.)	CROXATTO et al. (1950)
Pepsin (C)	Purified beef kininogen and fraction IV-6	HABERMANN et al. (1966)
Clostripain	Beef plasma globulin (0.30-0.41%) (am sulf.) and	J. L. PRADO et al. (1956)
Clostripain	Horse plasma heated twice, 3 hr 56—58°	J. L. and E. S. PRADO (1962)
Nagarse (C)	Horse plasma heated 3 hr 56—58°	J. L. PRADO et al. (1964)
Nagarse (C)	Human fraction IV-4	HUGGINS and WALASZEK (1962)
Ficin (C) and Papain (C)	Horse plasma heated 3 hr 56—58°	J. L. PRADO et al. (1965b)
Pronase	Horse plasma heated 3 hr 56—58°	J. L. PRADO and MENDES (1965)
Pronase	Plasma denatured by boiling with N/20 acetic acid	REIS et al. (1966)
Carboxy-peptidase A (C)	PKFL	HABERMANN and MÜLLER (1966)

[a] C = crystalline.

other kininogenases the substrates were not pure (Table 4). Clostripain, Nagarse, ficin, papain, and Pronase released a kinin from horse plasma heated for 3 hours at 56–58°. This substrate, as shown by J. L. and E. S. PRADO (1962), liberates only a small amount of kinin on addition of urokinase, in contrast to fresh horse plasma. This is an indication of a low plasminogen content. Further, the kinin liberation by clostripain, Nagarse, ficin, and papain is not inhibited by SBTI, which inhibits plasmin and plasma kallikrein. Plasma prekallikrein is also inactivated by the heat treatment of horse plasma, which is even more drastic in the VAN ARMAN (1955) denaturation procedure. A direct hydrolysis of kininogen is thus common to all kininogenases mentioned. The indirect mechanism which was demonstrated for trypsin and papain has not been investigated for the other kininogenases.

IV. Relative Kinin-Forming Activity

It is impossible at the present time to compare the specific kinin-releasing activities of the kininogenases reviewed in this chapter. The enzymatic activities of trypsin, pepsin, clostripain, Nagarse, ficin, papain, and Pronase preparations used by several authors were measured with different substrates (BAEe, denatured hemoglobin, casein, milk, and probably others) but the kinin-releasing activities of these enzymes were never determined under comparable conditions.

For crystalline trypsin SUZUKI et al. (1965) published the time curve of kinin release from purified bovine kininogen under conditions of zero-order kinetics. Recalculating from their graph and data, I have found that 1 mg trypsin/ml liberated the equivalent of 9 μg bradykinin in 1 minute (0.05 M ammonium

Table 5. *Esterase and kininogenase activities of trypsin and three kallikrein preparations*[a]. *(Initial rates in mμmoles/min/mg enzyme; pH 8.0, 37°)*

Enzymes[b]	BAEe hydrolysis	Bradykinin released
Trypsin	69	8.5
Ho UK	11.3	26.7
RUK	4.7	0.72
Hu UK	0.028	0.83

[a] Data recalculated and rearranged from DINIZ et al. (1965).

[b] Trypsin, twice crystallized (Worthington Biochem. Corp.); Ho UK, RUK, and Hu UK are urinary kallikrein preparations from horse, rat, and man, with different degrees of purity.

Table 6. *Comparative determinations of esterase and bradykinin-releasing activities* (From IWANAGA et al., 1965). *(Rates expressed as mμmole/min/mg enzyme; esterase activity measured at pH 8.5, 37°; kinin release determined at pH 8.0; temperature not given)*

Enzymes[a]	TAMe hydrolysis	Bradykinin released
Trypsin	43	4.7[b]
"Mamushi"	1.65	4.4
Hg PK	10	53.8

[a] Trypsin, crystalline (Sigma Chemical Co.); *Mamushi*, partially purified bradykinin-releasing enzyme from the venom of *Agkistrodon halys blomhoffii*; Hg PK, partially purified hog pancreatic kallikrein.

[b] It is uncertain whether this value corresponds to initial rate because according to my calculations from their time-course curves, SUZUKI et al. (1965) found 8.5 mμmoles/min/mg trypsin (38°, pH 8).

formate buffer, pH 8, 37°). Since the molecular weights of kininogen and bradykinin are approximately 48,000 and 1,000 respectively and assuming that each mole of kininogen releases 1 mole of bradykinin, 1 mg trypsin transforms 9 mμmoles kininogen/min (432 μg kininogen). The specific kinin-releasing activity of trypsin would thus be 9 mU. Results reported by DINIZ et al. (1965) were probably obtained with crude kininogen. Recalculating, however, from their time-course curve the same value of 9 mU for the specific kinin-releasing activity of trypsin (Tris 0.2 M, pH 8.0, 37°) was also found. This approximate calculation could not be done with the other results utilizing trypsin which were reported in the literature, because the measurements were not made under conditions of zero-order kinetics. For the other kininogenases even the approximate value found for trypsin could not be calculated, because pertinent data were not disclosed. Unless determinations can be obtained with excess purified kininogen (zero-order kinetics) comparative observations among several enzymes will be subject to false interpretations.

When the arginine esters are used as substrates, no correlation is found between initial rates of esterase and kinin-releasing activities of trypsin and kallikreins (Table 5). Data in Table 6 confirm this statement, including results with the bradykinin-releasing enzyme from the Japanese snake *Mamushi*. This does not, however, mean that there exists no correlation between esterase and kinin-releasing activities of a single enzyme. At present there is no substrate to substitute for kininogen.

V. Specificity

Substrates. HAMBERG and ROCHA E SILVA (1957a, b) showed a relationship between the esterase activity with BAEe and BAMe and the kininogenase activities of trypsin and snake venom enzymes. They reported their results before two scientific meetings (HAMBERG and ROCHA E SILVA, 1956 and ROCHA E SILVA and HAMBERG, 1956). Their main findings, which came from comparing the kinin-releasing activities of trypsin and *B. jararaca* and *Agkistrodon mokasen* venoms on several substrates were the following. Heating venom for 3–5 minutes in a boiling water bath abolished its proteolytic action on casein and diminished its esterolytic action on BAMe, but its kinin-releasing activity remained unaltered. Solutions of trypsin and heated venom, with equipotent esterolytic activities on BAMe, were also equally potent in their kinin-releasing activites on denatured plasma, but their proteolytic actions on casein were completely different. While caseinolytic action of trypsin roughly paralleled its kinin-releasing activity, practically no caseinolytic action was found in the heated venom. Although these results will be dealt with in more detail in other chapters it should be emphasized that the finding that trypsin is a kinin-releasing enzyme (ROCHA E SILVA et al., 1949a) affected also, in an important way, studies of the enzymatic specificities of kininogenases in general. As a consequence of the results mentioned above, ROCHA E SILVA (1960) reached two main conclusions: the bradykinin molecule would be in a terminal position in kininogen; and it would probably be linked to this protein molecule by an ester linkage next to a basic amino acid (lysine or arginine). The importance of the esterolytic activity (on BAEe and TAMe) of kinin-releasing enzymes received support from independent findings showing a parallel between these two activities in hog pancreatic and submaxillary kallikreins (HABERMANN, 1959, 1960; WERLE and KAUFMANN-BOETSCH, 1960) and horse urinary kallikrein (E. S. and J. L. PRADO, 1961; E. S. PRADO et al., 1962). When we found, however, (J. L. PRADO et al., 1962), that subtilisin BPN′ (Nagarse) did not cleave TAMe while comparable doses would liberate the maximum amount of a kinin-like activity from plasma, we concluded (J. L. PRADO et al., 1964) that the two activities were not necessarily linked to each other.

This finding led us finally to formulate the following working hypothesis (J. L. PRADO, 1962, 1964): kininogenases are serine proteinases (HARTLEY, 1960) which hydrolyze peptide bonds involving the carboxyl side of arginine residues in the middle of the kininogen molecule. This was based on a review of some properties and effects of three inhibitors (DFP, OMTI, and SBTI) on six kininogenases: clostripain, hog pancreatic and horse urinary kallikreins, Nagarse, plasmin, and trypsin. Among the properties considered were casein hydrolysis; esterase activity with BAEe, BAMe, and TAMe substrates; and BAA hydrolysis and splitting of a peptide bond involving the carboxyl side of arginine. Because of experimental and theoretical considerations, the last one was proposed as the common and fundamental property of every kininogenase. This hypothesis was used by our group to demonstrate that the proteolytic activity of purified horse urinary kallikrein on salmine parallels its kinin-releasing activity (BRANDI et al., 1965, 1967) and to show that this kallikrein hydrolyzes Arg-Arg bonds in poly-L-arginine of four or more residues, while poly-L-lysine was not split (E. S. PRADO et al., 1967). It is also compatible with the type of action of horse urinary kallikrein on methionyllysyl-bradykinin (MLBr), lysyllysyl-bradykinin (LLBr), bradykinyl-serine (BrSer) (BABEL et al., 1967), and *Polistes* kinin 3 (PISANO, 1967). In fact, this kallikrein liberated small amounts of lysyl-bradykinin from MLBr but even less when the substrate was LLBr, as compared to complete hydrolysis of BrSer through splitting of an arginyl-serine bond in the last substrate. These results show that the peptide bond on the carboxyl side of arginine is split more easily than on its amino side. The splitting of wasp kinin by kallikrein occurred probably at the arginyl side of an arginine-glycine bond with the formation of glycyl-bradykinin.

In the last few years, results of other investigators, however, have stemmed from different considerations, but they may be grouped into two main types of findings: 1. those that derived from studies of the purification and structure of kininogen and its fragments as well as their use or that of synthetic peptides as substrates for kininogenases (WEBSTER and PIERCE, 1963; PIERCE and WEBSTER, 1966; HABERMANN and BLENNEMANN, 1964; HABERMANN, 1965, 1966a, b; HABERMANN and MÜLLER, 1966; SUZUKI et al., 1966, 1967); 2. those that related to the use of new trypsin inhibitors on the kininogenase activity of kallikreins (DINIZ et al., 1965, 1966; MARES-GUIA and DINIZ, 1967). All these studies were done with the kallikreins, snake venom kininogenases, and trypsin. It also became evident, from section C of this chapter, that the proteolytic specificities of ficin, papain, and Pronase should be considered if a common enzymatic specificity is to be found to explain the kinin-releasing activity of the whole group of kininogenases.

Table 7 summarizes the specificities of proteolytic enzymes which are kininogenases. Trypsin splits the bond that links the carboxyl group of a basic amino acid (arginine or lysine) to the amino group of another amino acid or to the hydroxyl group of an alcohol. Although this is highly specific, trypsin does not split all basic bonds at the same rate. Papain has a specificity similar to trypsin but not nearly so limited. The most sensitive substrate found is BAA, which is also a substrate for trypsin. Papain, however, hydrolyzes typical substrates of pepsin, carboxypeptidase, and peptidases. The proteolytic specificity of ficin closely resembles papain; this is true also regarding its esterase action. Its best substrate is also BAA or the corresponding ester (BAEe). It should be mentioned that the specific BAA hydrolytic activities found by KRAMER and WHITAKER

Table 7. *Specificity of some proteases with kininogenase activity*

Protease	Substrates attacked[a]	References
Trypsin	-Arg↓-, Lys↓-, BAA, BAMe, BAEe, TAMe	[1]
Clostripain	Narrower specificity than trypsin; -Arg↓-, -Lys↓-, BAA, BAEe, TAMe	[2]
Subtilisin BPN′	Very wide specificity; N- and C-sides of neutral and acidic residues; ↓-Arg↓-, ↓-Lys↓-; BAMe	[1, 3, 4]
Ficin	Wider specificity than trypsin; -Arg↓-, Lys↓-, BAA, BAEe	[1]
Papain	Specificity similar to trypsin but not nearly so	[1]
	limited; -Arg↓-, -Lys↓-, BAA, TAMe	[1]
St. griseus protease	Exceptionally wide specificity; ↓-Arg↓-, BAA, BAMe	[1]

[a] Arrows show peptide bonds cleaved.

References: Data taken from 1. *The Enzymes*, ed. by P. D. BOYER, H. LARDY and K. MYRBÄCK, vol 4 (Part A), Academic Press, 1960. 2. GROSS and LABOUESSE (1960). 3. OKUNUKI et al. (1956). 4. CORRADO et al. (1966) (BAMe).

(1964) for eight ficin components varied from a minimum 0.048 (component A) to a maximum 1.881 (component D), bearing no relation to the kinin-releasing activities determined approximately by J. L. PRADO et al. (1965b). Subtilisin BPN′ (Nagarse) shows a very wide specificity. OKUNUKI et al. (1956) concluded that it hydrolyzes bonds of neutral and acidic amino acid residues at the amino and carboxyl end generally and aromatic and basic amino acid residues partially in proteins. J. L. PRADO et al. (1964) found no esterase activity with TAMe and a weak one with BAEe and were unable to detect any amidase activity with BAA. CORRADO et al. (1966) have found that BPN′ has an esterase activity (1.2 μmoles/mg/min) with BAMe which is less than the esterolytic activity (16.0 μmoles/mg/min) of trypsin. GLAZER (1967) studied the kinetics of BAEe and ATEe hydrolysis by subtilisin BPN′, finding that the profile of the pH velocity curve was very similar to those obtained with trypsin and BAEe or chymotrypsin and ATEe. BAA and acetyl-L-tyrosinamide were not hydrolyzed. The *St. griseus* protease has an exceptionally wide proteolytic specificity, hydrolyzing 75% of the peptide bonds in casein, while trypsin hydrolyzes one fourth and BPN′ half of that. The use of synthetic substrates indicated that it splits dipeptides at the N- and C-sides of arginine, BAA, and BAMe (cf. HAGIHARA, 1960). Clostripain specificity, contrary to the other proteases mentioned above, is narrower than the trypsin specificity.

GROSS and LABOUESSE (1960) have shown that in the β-chain of insulin the ratio of initial velocities of hydrolysis for the bonds Arg-Gly and Lys-Ala is 500. Using synthetic esters of arginine and lysine, they found clostripain is about ten times more effective with the arginine derivatives. Clostripain hydrolyzes BAEe about ten times faster than trypsin. The preference of clostripain for the carboxyl group of arginine was confirmed with glucagon. The relative initial velocities for splitting the bonds Arg-Arg, Arg-Ala, and Lys-Tyr were 1, 1/7, and 1/300 respectively (LABOUESSE, 1960). Considering that clostripain attacks glucagon more actively than trypsin and that its molecular weight is larger, LABOUESSE (1960) calculated that at equivalent molecular concentrations clostripain would be 400 to 1,000 times more active than trypsin in splitting the Arg-Arg bond of glucagon. No unusual cleavages, such as occur with trypsin, were observed on prolonged digestion with clostripain. All these observations point to clostripain as the kinin-releasing protease with the highest proteolytic specificity at present and would leave the splitting at the carboxyl group of arginine as the main common proteolytic specificity found in kininogenases.

For comparative purposes Fig. 2 includes results with the kallikreins, although their specificity will be dealt with in detail in Chapter 3, p. 131. The figure

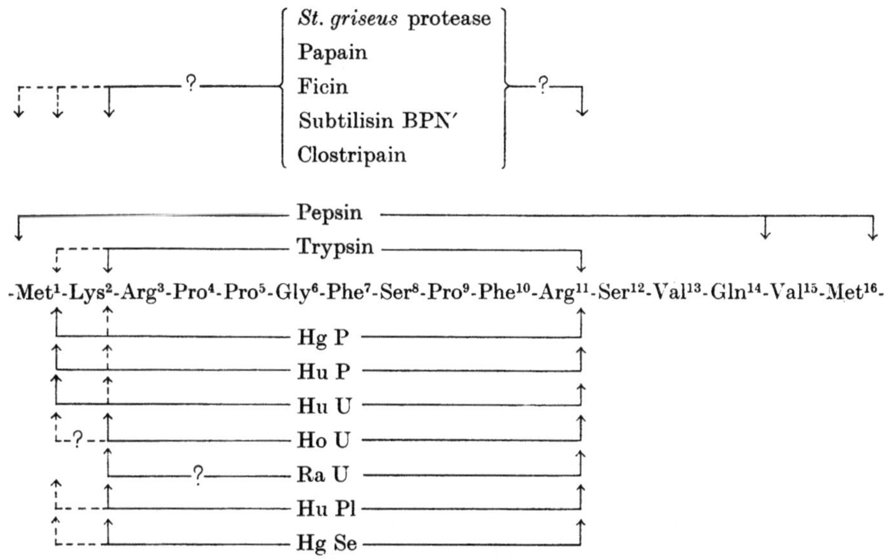

Fig. 2. Action of several kininogenases on the kinin-containing fragment of kininogen. *Lower part:* the action of kallikreins. *Hg P* hog pancreatic (Habermann, 1966a); *Hu P* human pancreatic (Webster and Pierce, 1963); *Hu U* human urinary (Webster and Pierce, 1963; Pierce and Webster, 1966); *Ho U* horse urinary (Stella et al., 1968); *Ra U* rat urinary (Diniz et al., 1966); *Hu Pl* human plasma (Webster and Pierce, 1963); *Hg Se* hog serum (Habermann and Blennemann, 1964). *Upper part:* the effect of kinin-releasing proteases. Solid arrows, main cleavages; interrupted arrows, secondary splits. Question marks mean probable but not proven splits

shows the polypeptide sequence that contains bradykinin in the middle of the kininogen molecule. It may be seen that all kallikreins studied cleave the Arg^{11}-Ser^{12} bond. To release a kinin, a second[6] bond has to be split in this substrate, and in general the kallikreins split either a Met^{1}-Lys^{2} or a Lys^{2}-Arg^{3} bond.

Stella et al. (1968) incubated partially purified horse urinary kallikrein (specific activity 160) with fresh horse plasma in the presence of 3×10^{-3} M *o*-phenanthroline. The active material was adsorbed on Amberlite (XE-64); the eluted kinin was purified on Sephadex G-15 and finally chromatographed on microcolumns of CM-cellulose. Only one peak was found, which behaved on the microcolumn as bradykinin. This suggests only a Lys^{2}-Arg^{3} split. These results are somewhat doubtful because fresh plasma contains an aminopeptidase that transforms kallidin into bradykinin (Webster and Pierce, 1963; Erdös et al., 1963). A B-aminopeptidase from rat liver, which is able to liberate lysine from kallidin to form bradykinin (Hopsu-Havu et al., 1966) was strongly inhibited by

6. Actually it is not known whether the bonds are split simultaneously or not; no kinetic studies have been made.

o-phenanthroline when L-Arg-β-naphthylamide was the substrate (Hopsu et al., 1966), but it has not yet been shown whether plasma aminopeptidase would also be blocked by *o*-phenanthroline. Diniz et al. (1966), on the basis of their observation that rat urinary kallikrein is inhibited by benzamidine and not by TLCK (which is a specific trypsin inhibitor), suggested that this kallikrein would liberate bradykinin and not kallidin from kininogen, since this would require hydrolysis of the Met^1-Lys^2 bond; evidence in favor of this suggestion is still lacking. Thus it seems that either of the two links on the N- and C-sides of Lys^2 in kininogen may be cleaved by kallikreins as well as the carboxyl side of Arg^{11} already mentioned.

Returning now to the proteases, we may observe (Fig. 2) that trypsin was shown by Habermann and Blennemann (1964) to split the Arg^{11}-Ser^{12} as well as the Lys^2-Arg^3 bonds in purified beef kininogen; secondarily, however, the Met^1-Lys^2 link may also be cleaved, even by low (1:800,000 w/v) trypsin concentrations (Habermann and Müller, 1966). Methionyllysyl-bradykinin (MLBr) was also found (31%) when they used PKFL as substrate, showing that in this substrate the link between Met^1 and the amino acid which precedes it in kininogen was also split. With this substrate, however, both pancreatic (50 μg/ml) and hog serum (250 μg/ml) kallikreins also formed MLBr. Suzuki et al. (1967) showed that when the methionine residues of pure bovine kininogen are oxidized to methionine sulfoxide, trypsin and pancreatic kallikrein no longer liberate kinin activity. It may thus be said that trypsin mimics the kinin-releasing activities of kallikreins very closely. Contrary to what was observed for pancreatic kallikrein, the conformation of bovine kininogen is not necessary for kinin release by trypsin (Kato et al., 1967). The four proteases with specificity wider than trypsin (*St. griseus* protease, papain, ficin, and subtilisin BPN′) probably split kininogen at the indicated places (Fig. 2). Clostripain would cleave the Arg^{11}-Ser^{12} bond very easily but would probably be a poor enzyme for the bonds Met^1-Lys^2 or Lys^2-Arg^3. Both J. L. Prado (1964) and Diniz et al. (1966) have expressed their difficulty in reconciling the knowledge about proteolytic specificities of several kininogenases and the fact that several types of peptide bonds have to be split in kininogen to explain the formation of bradykinin, lysyl-bradykinin, and methionyllysyl-bradykinin. J. L. Prado (1964) suggested the presence of an arginyl residue on the N-side of the kinin sequence in kininogen, and Mares-Guia and Diniz (1967) predicted two types of kallikreins in an attempt to understand the specificity of all kinin-releasing enzymes. The recent finding by Hochstrasser and Werle (1967) would lend support to Prado's suggestion; these authors have indeed found the sequence Ser-Arg-Met^1-Lys^2 ... or Gly-Arg-Met^1-Lys^2 ... in kinin-yielding fragments obtained from bovine kininogen by pepsin digestion. This finding would explain, for instance, the kinin-releasing activity of clostripain. Only future research on kinin-releasing activity of kininogenases, on structure determination of kinins actually liberated by different enzymes, and on sequential and conformational studies of kininogens might permit a general interpretation of kininogenase specificity.

It seems clear that pepsin should not be classified as a true kininogenase, because it has entirely different (Fig. 2) proteolytic specificities.

As ficin and papain are "thiol proteinases" (Hartley, 1960), the idea that all kinin-releasing enzymes belong to the group of "serine proteinases" (J. L. Prado, 1964), must be discarded.

Inhibitors. Enzyme inhibitors have been used by several authors in attempts to characterize the kinin-releasing activity of proteases at least qualitatively. Table 8 lists results obtained with five inhibitors of proteases (I to VI) and,

Table 8. *Action*[a] *of some inhibitors and activators*[b] *on release of kinin by kininogenases*

Kininogenase		SBTI	Trasylol	OMTI	Bzd	TLCK	Activators
I	Trypsin	+[1]	+[8]; +[cf. 9]	+[8]; +[3]	+[14]	+[14]	
II	Clostripain	−[2]; −[6]	0	0	0	0	Cysteine [2,6]
III	Subtilisin BPN′	−[3]; −[13]	0	+[3]; −[13], pressor peptide	0	−[13], pressor peptide	
IV	Ficin	−[4]	0	0	0	0	Cysteine [4]
V	Papain	−[4]	0	0	0	0	Cysteine [4]
VI	*St. griseus* protease	0	0	0	0	0	
VII	Hg P	−[1]	+[cf. 9]	0	+[15]	−[15]	
VIII	Hu P	−[cf. 19]	+[cf. 9, 19]	−[cf. 19]	0	0	
IX	Hu U	−[10]; [cf. 19]	+[cf. 9, 19]	−[cf. 19]	−[14]; −[15]	−[15]	
X	Ho U	−[5]; [−7]	+[cf. 9]	−[5]; −[7]	+[14]	−[14]	Some monov. cations [11, 18]
XI	Ra U	0	0	0	+[14]	−[14]	
XII	Hu Pl	+[10]; +[12]; +[cf. 9, 19]	+[cf. 9]	−[cf. 19]	0	0	
XIII	Hg Se	+[17]; +[cf. 9]	+[cf. 9]; +[17]	0	+[16]	0	
XIV	Ho Pl	+[cf. 16]	+[cf. 16]	−[cf. 16]	0	−[20]	

[a] Inhibition, +; no inhibition, −; data not found, 0; references in parentheses.

[b] Only those that were found indispensable for kinin release.

Abbreviations: SBTI = soybean trypsin inhibitor; OMTI = ovomucoid trypsin inhibitor; Bzd = benzamidine HCl; TLCK = 1 chloro-3-tosylamide-7-amino-2-heptanone. The kallikreins are: Hg P = hog pancreas; Hu P = human pancreas; Hu U = human urinary; Ho U = horse urinary; Ra U = rat urinary; Hu Pl = human plasma; Hg Se = hog serum; Ho Pl = horse plasma.

References: 1. Rocha e Silva, 1951. 2. J. L. Prado et al. 1956. 3. J. L. Prado et al., 1964. 4. J. L. Prado et al., 1965b. 5. E. S. and J. L. Prado, 1961. 6. J. L. and E. S. Prado, 1962. 7. E. S. Prado et al., 1962. 8. Werle et al., 1952. 9. Trautschold et al., 1967. 10. Werle and Maier, 1952. 11. J. L. Prado et al., 1963. 12. Webster and Pierce, 1960. 13. Huggins and Thampi, 1967. 14. Diniz et al., 1965, 1966. 15. Mares-Guia and Diniz, 1967. 16. Brandi et al., 1967. 17. Habermann and Klett, 1965. 18. J. L. Prado et al., 1965a. 19. Webster and Pierce, 1963. 20. Stella, 1968.

for comparative purposes, includes data obtained with eight kallikreins (VII to XIV). This table is incomplete because many experiments have not yet been done, which makes it difficult to establish the inhibition characteristics of kinin-releasing proteases. One generalization possible for these proteases is that the kinin-releasing activity of only trypsin is inhibited by SBTI. The other four inhibitors also block the kinin-releasing activity of trypsin. With the exclusion of subtilisin BPN′, however, no data were found with the other proteases. J. L. PRADO et al. (1964) found that OMTI was at least ten times less effective in inhibiting subtilisin BPN′ than trypsin, but they found around 50% inhibition when 100 μg enzyme/ml was preincubated 5 minutes at 37° with 0.4 mg inhibitor/ml. HUGGINS and THAMPI (1967) did not observe inhibition (20-min preincubation; 33 μg enzyme, and 0.4 mg of inhibitor/ml) with OMTI, but it should be noted that they were measuring the formation of a pressor polypeptide. They were also unable to inhibit this subtilisin with TLCK.

Among the kinin-forming proteases, the inhibition of the kinin-releasing action of trypsin in thus the one best characterized. ROCHA E SILVA (1941a) already knew that the soybean inhibitor-trypsin complex was pharmacologically inactive, and consequently his demonstration (1951) that the kinin-releasing activity of trypsin was inhibited by SBTI was a logical consequence of his previous findings. WERLE et al. (1952) showed that the kallikrein inhibitor from bovine lymph nodes and parotid gland inhibits also trypsin and chymotrypsin. Recently, two new synthetic inhibitors of trypsin, benzamidine (competitive) and TLCK (a specific trypsin active-center reagent), were shown to be effective inhibitors of the kinin-releasing activity of trypsin (DINIZ et al., 1965). These results are important because this was the first occasion on which the effect of inhibitors on the kinin-releasing activity of trypsin was quantitatively determined. In addition, of the kininogenases so far tested, the chloroketone TLCK seems to be specific for the kinin-releasing activity of trypsin. Benzamidine (8.0×10^{-4} M) and TLCK (1×10^{-3} M) inhibited about 90% of the initial rate of kinin release by crystalline trypsin.

Results with kallikreins are much more abundant and will be presented in detail in p. 213, but those included in Table 8 permit a few comparisons. Trasylol and benzamidine are the least specific among the five inhibitors under consideration. OMTI inhibits trypsin and, less effectively, subtilisin BPN′, but has not affected the kallikreins studied. Among the natural trypsin inhibitors OMTI seems to be the most specific one. The inhibition of plasma kallikreins by SBTI would make these kallikreins look similar to trypsin, but the failure of OMTI to inhibit plasma kallikreins reveals a difference between these kininogenases. And finally the mode of action of TLCK on plasma kallikreins is still unknown (MARES-GUIA and DINIZ, 1967). It would be interesting to learn whether this inhibitor would behave like OMTI or SBTI toward plasma kallikreins. It was demonstrated recently (STELLA, 1968) in this department that preincubation of TLCK (pH 7.5; 7×10^{-4} to 5×10^{-3} M) for 50–60 minutes with a partially purified horse plasma kallikrein had no effect on its kininogenase action on fresh horse plasma containing *o*-phenanthroline (3×10^{-3} M). In a test run, the kinin release by crystalline trypsin was completely blocked.

In a recent symposium on vasoactive peptides, BACK and STEGER (1968) reviewed the effect of inhibitors on the release of kinin by proteases and presented semiquantitative results on the effect of several synthetic and natural inhibitors. They observed that OMTI inhibited only trypsin strongly, and not at all or just slightly some other kininogenases, including plasma kallikrein. BHOOLA et al. (1960) observed that the permeability-increasing ability of serum (species not given) kallikrein was unaffected by 30-min preincubation with concentrations up to 500 μg/ml crystalline OMTI.

One important point in future studies would be to compare the effect of inhibitors on several of the activities of the kininogenases such as the kinin-releasing, proteolytic, and esterolytic actions to make sure that extrapolations which have been based on assays of only one activity are really acceptable.

Activators. As shown in Table 8, cysteine is necessary for the kinin release by clostripain, ficin, and papain. Observations with clostripain (J. L. and E. S. PRADO, 1962) showed that when heat-treated horse plasma was incubated with cysteine or clostripain alone, no kinin was formed for about 30 minutes, while in the complete mixture about half the amount of the activity was formed within 5 minutes of incubation. The concentration of cysteine in the incubation mixture was 1.3×10^{-3} M. The amount of cysteine contained in the aliquots tested was sufficient to potentiate the guinea pig ileum response (PICARELLI et al., 1962) to the kinin formed. This may have introduced an error into the observations. However, when the kinins liberated either by clostripain (J. L. PRADO et al., 1956) or by ficin (J. L. PRADO et al., 1965b) were isolated and partially purified, this source of error was, of course, absent in the final assays of the active factors.

With the exception of horse urinary kallikrein, no activators seem to be necessary for the release of kinin by kallikreins (Table 8). This exception is intriguing and should be examined in other laboratories and with other kallikreins. It has been shown (KRAMER et al., 1966) that the inhibition of the kinin-releasing activity of horse urinary kallikrein by Co^{++}, Hg^{++}, Cu^{+}, Ni^{++}, and Mn^{++} (1×10^{-3} to 1×10^{-2} M) runs parallel with the inhibition of its esterolytic activity on TAMe.

D. Kininase Activity

Trypsin. Trypsin will be discussed in the chapter dealing with kininases (p. 289).

Trypsin can slowly convert kallidin to bradykinin (WEBSTER and PIERCE, 1963; ERDÖS et al., 1963; cf. ERDÖS, 1966); and it transforms methionyllysyl-bradykinin more easily into methionyl-lysine and bradykinin (ELLIOTT et al., 1963; ELLIOTT and LEWIS, 1965; SCHRÖDER, 1964; HABERMANN and BLENNEMANN, 1964). As there is no inactivation of the original substrates because the end product is active, these hydrolytic actions of trypsin do not conform to the definition of kininase adopted by the committee on nomenclature (WEBSTER, 1966).

Pepsin. When pepsitocin was discovered by CROXATTO et al. (1950) they observed that the uterotonic action was very resistant to pepsin digestion. This was confirmed by HABERMANN et al. (1966) when they studied the yield of kinin from kinin-releasing peptides, although they found some loss of activity during the 23-hour digestion period. Crude bradykinin and clostridin activities were not inactivated during incubation for 4 hours with pepsin (500 μg/ml) (J. L. PRADO et al., 1956).

Clostripain. The peptide liberated by clostripain was stable in the incubation mixture for 3 hours (J. L. PRADO et al., 1956), indicating that clostripain has no kininase activity. This was confirmed later (J. L. and E. S. PRADO, 1962) when heat-treated horse plasma was incubated for 40 minutes with purified clostripain (83 μg/ml) and the active peptide formed was not inactivated. These observations are compatible with the similarity of the kinin formed with bradykinin and with the proteolytic specificities of clostripain.

Subtilisin BPN' (Nagarse). J. L. PRADO et al. (1964) incubated synthetic bradykinin with subtilisin BPN' (enzyme:substrate molar ratio, 1.6:1.0; pH 7.1; 37°; BPN' conc. 1.6 mμmoles/ml) and found that 1 mμmole of bradykinin was inactivated in 60 minutes, corresponding to about 50% inactivation of the peptide present. This enzyme is, therefore, a very poor kininase, particularly when the wide proteolytic specificity of subtilisin BPN' is considered. Carboxypeptidase B (enzyme:substrate molar ratio higher than 1:10,000) inactivated more than 1.6 mμmoles of bradykinin (3.2 mμmoles/ml) within half-an-hour, and chymotrypsin was roughly 50 to 100 times less active than carboxypeptidase B in a similar experiment (ERDÖS et al., 1963). These two enzymes are thus much more active than subtilisin BPN'.

Ficin and Papain. Cysteine-activated crystalline ficin inactivates synthetic bradykinin quickly (enzyme:substrate molar ratio 1:23, pH 7.4, 37°; ficin conc. 0.2 mμmole/ml); 5.7 mμmoles corresponding to 60% of total activity of the peptide (J. L. PRADO et al., 1965b) were inactivated in 3 minutes. This kininase activity would be roughly 15 times weaker than the bradykinin-inactivating activity of carboxypeptidase B cited above. The kinin-inactivating activity of ficin components was estimated from the time in minutes necessary to inactivate approximately 50% of 1 μg synthetic bradykinin/ml in Tyrode's solution at 37°. These times were different for the several components tried by J. L. PRADO et al. (1965b) and did not parallel their kinin-forming activities. It was mentioned in this paper that cysteine-activated crystalline papain also has marked kininase activity. Reviewing their original results, which were not published in their paper, I found that at an enzyme concentration of 0.12 mμmole/ml (enzyme: substrate ratio 1:80, pH 7.4, 37°) papain inactivated 4 mμmoles/bradykinin/min (90% inactivation). This rough estimation shows that in this respect papain is several times more active than ficin and would probably approach the bradykinin-inactivating potency of carboxypeptidase B.

St. griseus protease (Pronase). From the unpublished results of PRADO and MENDES (1965) a similar rough estimation shows that this protease is about twice as active a kininase as papain.

Final Remarks. Evidently, a careful analysis of the kinin-inactivating action of these kininogenases is still lacking. The kininase action of chymotrypsin was mentioned only briefly, since this enzyme shows only an indirect kinin-releasing activity in guinea pig plasma.

E. Other Pharmacological Effects

I. Stimulating Effect on Smooth Muscles

Trypsin. The study of the pharmacological action of trypsin on smooth muscles was important in the discovery of bradykinin; this aspect was reviewed in Section C I of the present article and in the summary of the Spanish and Portuguese literature (p. 634). A detailed paper by ROCHA E SILVA (1940a) on this subject may be summarized as follows. 1. With one exception (mouse jejunum), crystalline trypsin contracted all smooth muscles studied (guinea pig, cat, dog, rat, and rabbit ilia; guinea pig, rabbit, and virgin rat uteri). 2. Repetition of the same trypsin dose evoked smaller responses and longer latent periods, a phenomenon which was named trypsin desensitization and which occurred in all smooth muscles studied. 3. The trypsin contraction was not blocked by atropine, was independent of the enzyme digestive action on muscle fibrils, and was thought to be due to liberation of a pharmacologically active substance.

Under certain conditions (concentration 2×10^{-5}, cycles of 8 min, time of contact 20 sec) trypsin may stimulate repeatedly isolated rat uterus without inducing desensitization. Other enzymes tried (chymotrypsin, papain, carboxypeptidase, lysozyme, and several others) had no action on rat uterus up to concentrations 2×10^{-5} to 1×10^{-4} (20–50 µg/ml). This trypsin contraction of rat uterus is inhibited by SBTI, OMTI, and also by drugs (isopropyl-norepinephrine) which do not affect the trypsin proteolytic activity (JAQUES and SCHÄR, 1957). They believe that it is a direct effect of trypsin on the rat uterus, independent of the liberation of bradykinin.

Since the discovery of bradykinin (ROCHA E SILVA et al. 1949a), no other mediator of trypsin action on muscle has been described. The significance of kinins in other areas has occupied the attention of researchers in this field, but only future investigation will determine whether any new substance or substances are actually liberated.

Other Proteases. Phenomena identical with trypsin desensitization were observed on guinea pig ileum with clostripain (J. L. and E. S. PRADO, 1962), and subtilisin BPN′ (J. L. PRADO et al., 1964); they are not so conspicuous as with trypsin, because the initial contractions are not so marked. Rat submaxillary gland kallikrein is oxytocic on the isolated rat uterus (ERDÖS et al., 1968).

Potentiation of Kinins. See Chapter 6, p. 425.

II. Shock

Trypsin. When the pharmacology of crystalline trypsin was studied by ROCHA E SILVA (1939a, b, 1940b), its marked circulatory effects on cat, rabbit, and dog were described. Intravenous injection of trypsin to cats (0.1–0.5 mg/kg) produced a steep fall in carotid blood pressure and even (1.0–2.0 mg/kg) fatal circulatory collapse within a few minutes. Repeated small doses produced a desensitization, similar to that observed on smooth muscles. There was a concomitant rise in the pulmonary blood pressure. Results in the rabbit and dog confirmed these observations in the cat. In the dog, which is very sensitive, a conspicuous hypotensive action was found with trypsin doses from 0.05 to 0.1 mg/kg. Injection into the portal vein produced stronger systemic hypotension than injection into the femoral vein. Atropinization did not alter the hypotension. The significance of these observations for the finding of bradykinin was emphasized in Section C I. The similarity of symptomatology produced by trypsin injections and those produced by the antigen on sensitized isolated organs or on intact animals (cats, rabbits, dogs) led ROCHA E SILVA (1941a, b) to call this complex condition tryptic shock. From the beginning he tried to understand its mechanism; at that time, however, histamine liberation seemed to be its most important cause.

Studies by ROSENFELD (1950) showed that in shocks produced in dogs by crystalline trypsin, histamine, or partially purified bradykinin, a constant feature was hemoconcentration. Part (10 to 67%) of the plasma fluid lost during induced shock is absorbed into the red blood cells. In some cases this absorption may be larger than the total plasma loss. The increase in mean corpuscular volume leads to increased fragility and detectable hemolysis. In shock produced by *Bothrops* venom the same changes were noticed. In this case a direct effect of venom on red cells was also produced *in vitro*. The other shocking agents had no direct effect on red blood cells.

Other Proteases. Nagarse (BPN′) was found by J. L. PRADO et al. (1964) to produce lethal hypotension in the rat and dog when injected intravenously. Similar observations were made with ficin and papain (MOSS et al., 1963; J. L. PRADO et al., 1965b).

Participation of Kinins. The cardiovascular shock produced by trypsin and Nagarse was studied by CORRADO et al. (1966), who measured several biochemical and hematological parameters in dogs. Smaller enzyme doses (3 mg trypsin/kg and 1.5 mg Nagarse/kg) produced transient blood pressure drops; when intermediate doses were given repeatedly or with larger doses (24 mg trypsin or 6 mg Nagarse/kg) a rapid and irreversible fall in blood pressure killed the animals in 15 to 20 minutes. Changes in blood were studied after repeated and after single enzyme injections. The results were similar but of different intensity. They were compared with the effect of a crude hog pancreas kallikrein preparation (Padutin Bayer, 10 units/mg). These enzymes produce a remarkably similar pattern—depletion of kininogen stores and kinin liberation—but they also have separate distinctive characteristics. Thus, trypsin liberates also histamine, while Nagarse and kallikrein do not. When the initial kininogen concentrations drop to about half the value, hypotension is invariably irreversible. The large amount of kinin liberated was suggested as the triggering mechanism for this irreversible fall in blood pressure. Most of these results are included in a thesis (CORRADO, 1964), which was reviewed on p. 643. Independent observations made by FASCIOLO and HALVORSEN (1964) showed that lethal shock by trypsin in rats exhausted plasma kininogen. In the dog they used only enough trypsin (5–10 mg per dog) to provoke a severe and long-lasting hypotension but permitting a tendency to recover, and then found no reduction of kininogen.

III. Pruritus

ARTHUR and SHELLEY (1955) introduced 48 different enzyme preparations into the epidermis of man; they observed that only endopeptidases of animal or vegetable sources produce a sustained pruritus, in the absence of any visible cutaneous changes. Only proteinases active at pH 7 to 8 were effective: bacterial proteinase, bromelain, ficin, fungal proteinase, mucunain (from *Mucuna pruriens*), and twice-crystallized papain (vegetal enzymes); chymotrypsin, pancreatin, plasmin, and twice-crystallized trypsin (animal source). Intradermal injection of 20 μg enzyme in 0.02 ml of 0.9% sodium chloride solution (1:1,000 dilution) was one of the administration methods used. Papain, which proved to be the most effective enzyme, was ineffective when diluted beyond a concentration of 1:10,000 and the other proteases showed critical dilutions below this level. It was postulated that release or activation of proteinases in the epidermis plays a significant role in itching. CORMIA et al. (1957) confirmed this observation with crystallized trypsin, fibrinolysin, ficin, and papain. ARTHUR and SHELLEY (1958) used crystallized trypsin as a clinical test to measure itch sensitivity of skin areas. CORMIA and DOUGHERTY (1960) observed that the intradermal injection of as little as 200 ng proteolytic enzymes (trypsin, ficin, papain) provokes itching. Kallikrein (purity and species not given) and crude bradykinin were also very active in doses of 2–20 ng. Bradykinin produced burning pain (42 times out of 56) and itch (36 out of 56). YAMURA and CORMIA (1961) found in human epidermis a proteolytic enzyme activity which hydrolyzes BAMe and TAMe.

References

ANDRADE, S. O., ROCHA E SILVA, M.: Purification of bradykinin by ion-exchange chromatography. Biochem. J. **64**, 701 (1956).

ANSON, M. L.: The extinction of pepsin, trypsin, papain and cathepsin with hemoglobin. J. gen. Physiol. **22**, 79 (1938).

ARMAN, C. G. VAN: Origin of bradykinin. Proc. Soc. exp. Biol. (N.Y.) **79**, 356 (1952). Chem. Abstr. **46**, 5625f (1952).

ARMAN, C. G. VAN: Interrelationship among some peptide precursors. In: Polypeptides which stimulate plain muscle, p. 103, ed. by J. H. GADDUM. London 1955.
ARTHUR, R. P., SHELLEY, W. B.: The role of proteolytic enzymes in the production of pruritus in man. J. invest. Derm. 25, 341 (1955).
— — The nature of itching in dermatitic skin. Ann. intern. Med. 49, 900 (1958).
BABEL, I., STELLA, R. C. R., PRADO, E. S.: Action of horse urinary kallikrein on synthetic derivatives of bradykinin. Ciencia Cult. (S. Paulo) 19, 395 (1967).
BACK, N., STEGER, R.: Effect of inhibitors on kinin-releasing activity of proteases. Fed. Proc. 27, 96 (1968).
BERALDO, W. T.: Formation of bradykinin in anaphylactic and peptone shock. Amer. J. Physiol. 163, 283 (1950a).
— Bradykinin formation by the action of peptone and fibrinolysin on plasma globulins *in vitro*. Ciencia Cult. (S. Paulo) 2, 300 (1950b).
BHOOLA, K. D., CALLE, J. D., SCHACHTER, M.: The effect of bradykinin, serum kallikrein and other endogenous substances on capillary permeability in the guinea pig. J. Physiol. (Lond.) 152, 75 (1960).
— YI, R. M. M., MORLEY, J., SCHACHTER, M.: Release of kinin by an enzyme in the accessory sex glands of the guinea pig. J. Physiol. (Lond.) 163, 269 (1962).
BRANDI, C. M. W., MENDES, J., PAIVA, A. C. M., PRADO, E. S.: Proteolysis of salmine by horse urinary kallikrein. Biochem. Pharmacol. 14, 1665 (1965).
— RONCADA, M. J., PRADO, E. S., PRADO, J. L.: Observations on the hydrolysis of salmine by kallikreins. In: Internat. Symposium on Vasoactive Polypeptides: Bradykinin and Related Kinins, p. 135, ed. by M. ROCHA E SILVA and H. A. ROTHSCHILD. São Paulo 1967.
BRAUN-MENENDEZ, E., FASCIOLO, J. C., LELOIR, L. F., MUÑOZ, J. M., TAQUINI, A. C.: Relationship between hypertensin and pepsitensin. Rev. Soc. argent. Biol. 19, 304 (1943).
— — — — — Renal hypertension. Springfield, Ill. 1946.
BROCKLEHURST, W. E., MAWER, G. E.: The purification of a kininogen from human plasma. Brit. J. Pharmacol. 27, 256 (1966).
CARLINI, E. A., HUGGINS, C. G.: Enzymic conversion of valine[5]-angiotensin-I into an oxytocic principle by impure preparations of alpha-amylase. Biochem. Pharmacol. 11, 171 (1962).
— PICARELLI, Z. P., PRADO, J. L.: Pharmacological activity of hypertensin I and its conversion into hypertensin II. Bull. Soc. Chim. biol. (Paris) 40, 1825 (1958).
CORMIA, F. E., DOUGHERTY, J. W.: Proteolytic activity in development of pain and itching: Cutaneous reactions to bradykinin and kallikrein. J. invest. Derm. 35, 21 (1960).
— — UNRAU, S. A.: Proteolytic activity in dermatoses. J. invest. Derm. 28, 425 (1957).
CORRADO, A. P.: Considerations upon the participation of bradykinin and analogous peptides on the hemodynamic effects produced by proteolytic enzymes. Thesis, Faculdade de Medicina, Ribeirão Preto (1964).
— REIS, M. L., CARVALHO, I. F., DINIZ, C. R.: Bradykininogen and bradykinin in the cardiovascular shock produced by proteolytic enzymes. Biochem. Pharmacol. 15, 959 (1966).
CROXATTO, H.: Active polypeptides formed by pepsin. In: Polypeptides which stimulate plain muscle, p. 92, ed. by J. H. GADDUM. Edinburgh and London 1955.
— BARNAFI, L., ROJAS, G., REYES, A., INFANTE, A.: Antidiuretic and oxytocic substances liberated by the digestion of plasmatic proteins with pepsin. Nature (Lond.) 171, 82 (1953).
— ROJAS, G., BARNAFI, L.: Separable oxytocic and pressor actions of pepsitensin. Bol. Soc. Biol. Santiago 8, 84 (1950).
— — — The liberation of an antidiuretic factor by the hypertensinogen pepsin reaction. Acta physiol. lat.-amer. 1, 178 (1951).
DENGLER, H.: Untersuchungen über Pepsitensin. Z. ges. exp. Med. 127, 153 (1956). Biol. Abstr. 31, 31581 (1957).
DINIZ, C. R., PEREIRA, A. A., BARROSO, J., MARES-GUIA, M.: On the specificity of urinary kallikreins. Biochem. biophys. Res. Commun. 21, 448 (1965).
— — — — Studies of the specificity of kinin-forming enzymes: The inhibition of the kininogenic activity of trypsin and kallikreins by model compounds. In: Hypotensive peptides, p. 175, ed. by E. G. ERDÖS, N. BACK and F. SICUTERI. Berlin-Heidelberg-New York: Springer 1966.
ELLIOTT, D. F.: Bradykinin and its mode of release. Ann. N.Y. Acad. Sci. 104, 35 (1963).
— HORTON, E. W., LEWIS, G. P.: Biological activity of pure bradykinin. J. Physiol. (Lond.) 150, 6P (1959a).
— — — Actions of pure bradykinin. J. Physiol. (Lond.) 153, 473 (1960c).
— LEWIS, G. P.: Methionyl-lysyl-bradykinin, a new kinin from ox blood. Biochem. J. 95, 437 (1965).
— — HORTON, E. W.: The isolation of bradykinin: A plasma kinin from ox blood. Biochem. J. 74, 15P (1959b).

Elliott, D. F., Lewis, G. P., Horton, E. W., The structure of bradykinin. Biochem. J. **76**, 16P (1960a).
— — — The structure of bradykinin: A plasma kinin from ox blood. Biochem. biophys. Res. Commun. **3**, 87 (1960b).
— — — The isolation of bradykinin, a plasma kinin from ox blood. Biochem. J. **78**, 60 (1961).
— — Smyth, D. C.: A new kinin from ox blood. Biochem. J. **87**, 21P (1963).
Endo, R. M., Santos, M., Carlini, E. A.: Effects of a crystalline proteinase from *Bacillus subtilis* (Nagarse) on angiotensins I and II. Experientia (Basel) **22**, 757 (1966).
Erdös, E. G.: Hypotensive peptides: Bradykinin, kallidin and eledoisin. Advanc. Pharmacol. **4**, 1 (1966).
— Renfrew, A. G., Sloane, E. M., Wohler, J. R.: Enzymatic studies on bradykinin and similar peptides. Ann. N.Y. Acad. Sci. **104**, 222 (1963).
— Tague, L. L., Miwa, I.: Kallikrein in granules of the submaxillary gland. Biochem. Pharmacol. **17**, 667 (1968).
Fasciolo, J. C.: Formation and destruction of plasma kinins. Acta physiol. lat.-amer. **14**, 170 (1964).
— Halvorsen, K.: Specificity of mammalian kallidinogen. Amer. J. Physiol. **207**, 901 (1964).
Frey, E. K., Kraut, H., Werle, E.: Kallikrein (Padutin), p. 107. Sutttgart 1950.
Gaddum, J. H.: Summary of meeting. In: Polypeptides which affect smooth muscles and blood vessels, p. 329, ed. by M. Schachter. Edinburgh and London 1960.
Glazer, A. N.: Esteratic reactions catalyzed by subtilisins. J. biol. Chem. **242**, 433 (1967).
Gomes, F. P.: A slow contracting substance in normal human urine. Brit. J. Pharmacol. **10**, 200 (1955).
Greenbaum, L. M., Hosoda, T.: Studies on the isolation of bradykininogen. Biochem. Pharmacol. **12**, 325 (1963).
— Yamafuji, K., Hosoda, T.: Studies on the peptic degradation of bovine bradykininogen. Biochem. Pharmacol. **14**, 411 (1965).
Gross, P., Labouesse, B.: La clostripaine, protéase de *Clostridium histolyticum*. II. Specificité. Bull. Soc. Chim. biol. (Paris) **42**, 559 (1960).
Habermann, E.: Über Zusammenhänge zwischen esterolytischen und pharmakologischen Wirkungen von Jararacagift, Kallikrein und Thrombin. Naunyn-Schmiedebergs Arch. exp. Path. Pharmak. **236**, 492 (1959).
— Diisopropylfluorophosphat-Hemmung esterolytischer und pharmakologischer Wirkungen von Kallikrein und Schlangengiften. Naturwissenschaften **47**, 111 (1960).
— Enzymatic kinin release from purified kininogen and from low molecular compounds. Biochem. Pharmacol. **14**, 1393 (1965).
— Enzymatic kinin release from kininogen and from low molecular compounds. In: Hypotensive peptides, p. 116, ed. by E. G. Erdös, N. Back and F. Sicuteri. Berlin-Heidelberg-New York: Springer 1966a.
— Strukturaufklärung kininliefernder Peptide aus Rinderserum-Kininogen. Naunyn-Schmiedebergs Arch. exp. Path. Pharmak. **253**, 474 (1966b).
— Blennemann, G.: Über Substrate und Reaktionsprodukte der kininbildenden Enzyme Trypsin, Serum und Pankreaskallikrein sowie von Crotalusgift. Naunyn-Schmiedebergs Arch. exp. Path. Pharmak. **249**, 357 (1964).
— — Müller, B.: Charakterisierung und Reinigung peptischer kininliefernder Fragmente (PKF) sowie von „Pepsitocin“ aus Rinderserum-Kininogen. Naunyn-Schmiedebergs Arch. exp. Path. Pharmak. **253**, 444 (1966).
— Klett, W.: Beiträge zur Biochemie und Pharmakologie eines Serumkallikreins. Naunyn-Schmiedebergs Arch. exp. Path. Pharmak. **250**, 253 (1965).
— — Rosenbusch, G.: Partielle Reinigung und einige Eigenschaften eines Kininogens aus Rinderblut. Hoppe-Seylers Z. physiol. Chem. **332**, 121 (1963).
— Müller, B.: Zur enzymatischen Spaltung peptischer kininliefernder Fragmente (PKF) sowie von Rinderserumkininogen. Naunyn-Schmiedebergs Arch. exp. Path. Pharmak. **253**, 464 (1966).
— Schuck, S.: Einige Beziehungen zwischen „Pepsitocin“ und Plasmakininen. Naturwissenschaften **51**, 61 (1964).
Hagihara, B.: Bacterial and mold proteases. In: The enzymes, 2nd ed., vol. 4, pt. A, p. 193, ed. by P. D. Boyer, H. Lardy, and K. Myrbäck. New York and London 1960.
— Matsubara, H., Nakai, M., Okunuki, K.: Crystalline bacterial proteinase. I. Preparation of crystalline proteinase of *Bacillus subtilis*. J. Biochem. (Tokyo) **45**, 185 (1958a).
— Nakai, M., Matsubara, H., Komaki, T., Yonetani, T., Okunuki, K.: Crystalline bacterial proteinase. III. Comparison of crystalline proteinase of *Bacillus subtilis* with crystalline trypsin. J. Biochem. (Tokyo) **45**, 305 (1958b).

HAMBERG, U., BUMPUS, F. M., PAGE, I. H.: Isolation and amino acid composition of bradykinin released by venom of *Bothrops jararaca* from bovine plasma. Biochim. biophys. Acta (Amst.) **52**, 533 (1961).

— ROCHA E SILVA, M.: On the nature of the bond split by agents releasing bradykinin from plasma proteins. Proc. XX. Internat. Physiol. Congr., p. 390. Brussels 1956.

— — Release of bradykinin as related to the esterase activity of trypsin and of the venom of *Bothrops jararaca*. Experientia (Basel) **13**, 489 (1957a).

— — On the release of bradykinin by trypsin and snake venoms. Arch. int. Pharmacodyn. **110**, 222 (1957b).

HARTLEY, B. S.: Proteolytic enzymes. Ann. Rev. Biochem. **29**, 45 (1960).

HENRIQUES, O. B., KAURITCHEVA, N., KUZNETSOVA, V., ASTRAKAN, M.: Substrates of kinin-releasing enzymes isolated from horse plasma. Nature (Lond.) **215**, 1200 (1967).

— LAVRAS, A. A. C., FICHMAN, M., PICARELLI, Z. P.: Plasma enzymes that release kinins. Biochem. Pharmacol. **15**, 31 (1966).

— PICARELLI, Z. P., FERRAZ DE OLIVEIRA, M. C.: Partial purification of the plasma substrate for the bradykinin-releasing enzyme from the venom of *Bothrops jararaca*. Biochem. Pharmacol. **11**, 707 (1962).

HOCHSTRASSER, K., WERLE, E.: Über kininliefernde Peptide aus pepsinverdauten Rinderplasmaproteinen. Hoppe-Seylers Z. physiol. Chem. **348**, 177 (1967).

HOLDSTOCK, D. J., MATHIAS, A. P., SCHACHTER, M.: A comparative study of kinin, kallidin and bradykinin. Brit. J. Pharmacol. **12**, 149 (1957).

HOPSU, V. K., MÄKINEN, K. K., GLENNER, G. G.: Characterization of aminopeptidase B: substrate specificity and affector studies. Arch. Biochem. **114**, 567 (1966).

HOPSU-HAVU, V. K., MÄKINEN, K. K., GLENNER, G. G.: Formation of bradykinin from kallidin-10 by aminopeptidase B. Nature (Lond.) **212**, 1271 (1966).

HUGGINS, C. G., PAVESI, L., ARIAS, F.: The enzymatic formation of the vasopressor polypeptide substance A by a crystalline enzyme of *Bacillus subtilis*. Biochem. Pharmacol. **13**, 697 (1964).

— THAMPI, S. N.: Vasopressor principle liberated by a crystalline enzyme of "Bacillus subtilis" (Nagarse) from heat treated horse plasma. In: Internat. Symposium on Vasoactive Polypeptides: Bradykinin and Related Kinins, p. 127, ed. by M. ROCHA E SILVA and H. A. ROTHSCHILD. São Paulo 1967.

— WALASZEK, E. J.: Large scale preparation and purification of the vasopressor polypeptide, substance A. J. med. pharm. Chem. **5**, 183 (1962).

HUNT, J. A., OTTENSEN, M.: A comparison of three proteinases from various strains of *Bacillus subtilis*. Biochim. biophys. Acta (Amst.) **48**, 412 (1961).

IWANAGA, S., SATO, T., MIZUSHIMA, Y., SUZUKI, T.: Studies on snake venoms. XVII. Properties of the bradykinin releasing enzyme in the venom of *Agkistrodon halys blomhoffii*. J. Biochem. (Tokyo) **58**, 123 (1965).

JACOBSEN, S.: Substrates for plasma kinin-forming enzymes in human, dog and rabbit plasmas. Brit. J. Pharmacol. **26**, 403 (1966a).

— Separation of two different substrates for plasma kinin-forming enzymes. Nature (Lond.) **210**, 98 (1966b).

JAQUES, R., SCHÄR, B.: Fermentwirkungen an isolierten glattmuskulären Organen und Zellen, unter besonderer Berücksichtigung proteolytischer Fermente. Helv. physiol. pharmacol. Acta **15**, 134 (1957).

KATO, H., NAGASAWA, S., SUZUKI, T.: Relationship between tertiary structure and kinin yielding ability of bovine kininogen. Biochem. biophys. Res. Commun. **27**, 163 (1967).

KIMMEL, J. R., SMITH, E. L.: Crystalline papain. I. Preparation. specificity and activation. J. biol. Chem. **207**, 515 (1954).

KRAMER, C., PRADO, E. S., PRADO, J. L.: Inhibition by ions of the esterolytic activity of horse urinary kallikrein. Med. Pharmacol. exp. (Basel) **15**, 389 (1966).

— WHITAKER, J. R.: *Ficus* enzymes. II. Properties of the proteolytic enzymes from the latex of *Ficus carica* variety *Kadota*. J. biol. Chem. **239**, 2178 (1964).

KRAUT, H., FREY, E. K., BAUER, E.: Über ein neues Kreislaufhormon. II. Mitt. Hoppe-Seylers Z. physiol. Chem. **175**, 97 (1928).

KUNITZ, M.: Crystalline soybean trypsin inhibitor. II. General properties. J. gen. Physiol. **30**, 291 (1947).

LABOUESSE, B.: L'hydrolyse du glucagon par la clostripaïne. Bull. Soc. Chim. Biol. (Paris) **42**, 1293 (1960).

— GROSS, P.: La clostripaïne, protéase de *Clostridium histolyticum*. I. Purification et activation par les thiols. Bull. Soc. Chim. biol. (Paris) **42**, 543 (1960).

LEWIS, J. P.: Formation of plasma kinins by plasmin. J. Physiol. (Lond.) **140**, 285 (1959).

— Active polypeptides derived from plasma proteins. Physiol. Rev. **40**, 647, cf. p. 657 (1960).

Mares-Guia, M., Diniz, C. R.: The specificity of kallikreins, as studied with model compounds. In: Internat. Symposium on Vasoactive Polypeptides: Bradykinin and Related Kinins, p. 149, ed. by M. Rocha e Silva and H. A. Rothschild. São Paulo 1967.

Markland, F. S., Smith, E. L.: Subtilisin BPN'. VII. Isolation of cyanogen bromide peptides and the complete amino acid sequence. J. biol. Chem. **242**, 5198 (1967).

Matsubara, H., Hagihara, B., Nakai, M., Komaki, T., Yonetani, T., Okunuki, K.: Crystalline bacterial proteinase. II. General properties of crystalline proteinase of *Bacillus subtilis* N'. J. Biochem. (Tokyo) **45**, 251 (1958).

Monier, R., Litwack, G., Somlo, M., Labouesse, B.: Les enzymes protéolytiques de *Clostridium histolyticum*. Influence de la complexone III et du calcium sur la stabilité de deux de ces enzymes. Biochim. biophys. Acta (Amst.) **18**, 71 (1955).

Moss, J. N., Frazier, C. V., Martin, G. J.: Bromelains: The pharmacology of the enzymes. Arch. int. Pharmacodyn. **145**, 166 (1963).

Nomoto, M., Narahashi, Y.: Proteolytic enzyme of *Streptomyces griseus*. I. Purification of protease of *Streptomyces griseus*. Rikagaku Kenkyusho Hokoku **34**, 381 (1958). III. Homogeneity of highly purified enzyme. Rikagaku Kenkyusho Hokoku **34**, 393 (1958). Cf. Chem. Abstr. **54**, 688d (1960).

— — Murakami, M.: A proteolytic enzyme of *Streptomyces griseus*. VII. Hydrolysis of synthetic substrate by *St. griseus* protease (specificity of *St. griseus* protease). Rikagaku Kenkyusho Hokoku **35**, 261 (1959). Cf. Chem. Abstr. **54**, 21269i (1960).

Okunuki, K., Matsubara, H., Nishimura, S., Hagihara, B.: Specificity of crystalline bacterial proteinase. J. Biochem. (Tokyo) **43**, 857 (1956).

Paiva, A. C. M.: Comparative study of pepsitensin and hypertensin, p. 30. Thesis, Escola Paulista de Medicina, São Paulo (1954).

Picarelli, Z. P., Henriques, O. B., Oliveira, M. C. F.: Potentiation of bradykinin action on smooth muscle by cysteine. Experientia (Basel) **18**, 77 (1962).

Pierce, J. V.: Structural features of plasma kinins and kininogens. Fed. Proc. **27**, 52 (1968).

— Webster, M. E.: The purification and some properties of two different kallidinogens from human plasma. In: Hypotensive peptides, p. 130, ed. by E. G. Erdös, N. Back, and F. Sicuteri. Berlin-Heidelberg-New York: Springer 1966.

Pisano, J. J.: Studies on the structure of the major kinin in wasp venom. In: Internat. Symposium on Vasoactive Polypeptides: Bradykinin and Related Kinins, p. 35, ed. by M. Rocha e Silva and H. A. Rothschild. São Paulo 1967.

— Tamura, Z., Furano, E., Udenfriend, S.: Vasoactive peptides in wasp venom. Fed. Proc. **24**, 488 (1965).

Prado, E. S., Prado, J. L.: Partial purification of a plasma kinin-forming enzyme from horse urine. Experientia (Basel) **17**, 31 (1961).

— — Brandi, C. M. W.: Further purification and some properties of horse urinary kallikrein. Arch. int. Pharmacodyn. **137**, 358 (1962).

— Stella, R. C. R., Roncada, M. J., Prado, J. L.: Action of horse urinary kallikrein on arginine and lysine-peptides. In: Internat. Symposium on Vasoactive Polypeptides: Bradykinin and Related Kinins, p. 141, ed. by M. Rocha e Silva and H. A. Rothschild. São Paulo 1967.

Prado, J. L.: Kininogenases, plasmakinin-liberating enzymes. Ciencia Cult. (S. Paulo) **14**, 231 (1962).

— Considerations upon the enzymic specificities of kininogenases. Acta physiol. lat.-amer. **14**, 215 (1964).

— Katchburian, A. V., Mendes, J., Prado, E. S.: Ions and the kininogenic activity of horse urinary kallikrein. Acta physiol. lat.-amer. **15**, 386 (1965 a).

— Mendes, J.: Unpublished observations (1965).

— — Rosa, R. C.: On the kininogenic activity of ficin, with a note on papain. An. Acad. bras. Cien. **37**, 295 (1965b).

— — Stella, R. C. R.: Crystalline ficin and papain as kinin-forming enzymes. In: Internat. Symposium on Vasoactive Polypeptides: Bradykinin and Related Kinins, p. 192, ed. by M. Rocha e Silva and H. A. Rothschild. São Paulo 1967.

— Monier, R., Prado, E. S., Fromageot, C.: Pharmacologically active polypeptide formed from blood globulin by a cysteine-activated protease from *Clostridium histolyticum*. Biochim. biophys. Acta (Amst.) **22**, 87 (1956).

— Prado, E. S.: Plasmakinin liberation by clostripaine. An. Acad. bras. Cien. **34**, 51 (1962).

— — Brandi, C. M. W., Katchburian, A. V.: Some properties of highly purified horse urinary kallikrein. Ann. N.Y. Acad. Sci. **104**, 186 (1963).

— — Jurkiewicz, A.: On the liberation of plasmakinin/s by a crystalline protease from *B. subtilis* (Nagarse). Ciencia Cult. (S. Paulo) **14**, 223 (1962).

— — — Crystalline bacterial proteinase from *B. subtilis* (Nagarse) as a new kininogenase. Arch. int. Pharmacodyn. **147**, 53 (1964).

PRADO, J. L., TAMURA, Z., FURANO, E., PISANO, J. J., UDENFRIEND, S.: Characterization of kinins in wasp venom. Biochem. Pharmacol. **14**, 1397 (1965 c).

— — — — — Characterization of kinins in wasp venom. In: Hypotensive peptides, p. 93, ed. by E. G. ERDÖS, N. BACK, and F. SICUTERI. Berlin-Heidelberg-New York: Springer 1966.

REIS, M. L. DOS, MEDEIROS, M. C., ROCHA E SILVA, M.: Release and destruction of kinins by a proteolytic enzyme (Pronase) derived from a fungus *Streptomyces griseus*. Abstracts of III. Internat. Pharmacol. Congr., No 485. São Paulo 1966.

ROCHA E SILVA, M.: Pharmacology of trypsin. Action on mammalian smooth muscles and isolated heart. Circulatory effects of trypsin. Experiments with a crystalline material. Arch. Inst. biol. (S. Paulo) **10**, 93 (1939 a).

— Pharmacology of trypsin. Toxicity and circulatory effects on cat and rabbit. Folia clín. biol. (S. Paulo) **11**, 70 (1939 b).

— Beiträge zur Pharmakolgie des Trypsins. I. Wirkung des Trypsins auf die glatten Muskeln des Dünndarms und die Gebärmutter von Säugetieren. Die Freisetzung von Histamin nach Durchströmung der Meerschweinchenlunge mit Trypsin. Naunyn-Schmiedebergs Arch. exp. Path. Pharmak. **194**, 335 (1940 a).

— Beiträge zur Pharmakologie des Trypsins. II. Wirkung des Trypsins auf den Blutkreislauf bei Katze, Kaninchen und Hund. Naunyn-Schmiedebergs Arch. exp. Path. Pharmak. **194**, 351 (1940b).

— Tryptic shock. Arch. Inst. biol. (S. Paulo) **12**, 155 (1941a).

— Concerning the mechanism of anaphylactic and tryptic shock. J. Immunol. **40**, 399 (1941b).

— Bradykinin: Mechanisms of its release by trypsin and kallikrein. Arch. int. Pharmacodyn. **88**, 271 (1951).

— Biochemistry and pharmacology of bradykinin. In: Polypeptides which affect smooth muscles and blood vessels, p. 210, ed. by M. SCHACHTER. Oxford 1960.

— Definition of bradykinin and other kinins. Biochem. Pharmacol. **10**, 3 (1962).

— The physiological significance of bradykinin. Ann. N.Y. Acad. Sci. **104**, 190 (1963).

— BERALDO, W. T., ANDRADE, S. O.: On a new hypotensive and smooth muscle stimulating factor (bradykinin) liberated from plasma globulin by snake venom and by trypsin. Proc. First Internat. Congr. of Biochemistry, p. 119. Cambridge 1949 b.

— — ROSENFELD, G.: Bradykinin, a hypotensive and smooth muscle stimulating factor released from plasma globulin by snake venoms and by trypsin. Amer. J. Physiol. **156**, 261 (1949 a).

— HAMBERG, U.: On the nature of the bond split by bradykinin releasing agents. Ciencia Cult. (S. Paulo) **8**, 177 (1956).

— REIS, M. L., FERREIRA, S. H.: Release of kinins from fresh plasma under varying experimental conditions. Biochem. Pharmacol. **16**, 1665 (1967).

ROSENFELD, G.: Hematimetric studies in shock produced by animal venoms. Trypsin, histamine and snake venom. Absorption of fluid by the red blood cells. Proc. Internat. Soc. of Hematology, p. 84. 1950.

SCHACHTER, M.: Kinins of different origins. Ann. N.Y. Acad. Sci. **104**, 108 (1963).

SCHRÖDER, E.: Über Peptidsynthesen. Synthese von Methionyl-Lysyl-Bradykinin, eines Kinin aus Rinderblut. Experientia (Basel) **20**, 39 (1964).

— HEMPEL, R.: Bradykinin, kallidin and their synthetic analogues. Experientia (Basel) **20**, 529 (1964).

SCHWERT, G. W., TAKENAKA, Y.: Spectrophotometric determination of trypsin and chymotrypsin. Biochim. biophys. Acta (Amst.) **16**, 570 (1955).

SGARBIERI, V. C., GUPTE, S. M., KRAMER, D. E., WHITAKER, J. R.: *Ficus* enzymes. I. Separation of the proteolytic enzymes of *Ficus carica* and *Ficus glabrata* latices. J. biol. Chem. **239**, 2170 (1964).

SMITH, E. L., MARKLAND, F. S., KASPER, C. B., DELANGE, R. J., LONDON, M., EVANS, W. H.: The complete amino acid sequence of two types of subtilisin, BPN' and Carlsberg. J. biol. Chem. **241**, 5974 (1966).

STELLA, R. C. R.: Study on the liberation of kinins in horse plasma by acid activation or by horse urinary kallikrein. Thesis, Escola Paulista de Medicina, São Paulo (1968).

— MENDES, J., PRADO, J. L.: Identification of kinins liberated from equine plasma by acidification and by addition of horse urinary kallikrein. Ciencia Cult. (S. Paulo) **20**, 422 (1968).

SUZUKI, T., IWANAGA, S., NAGASAWA, S., SATO, T.: Purification and properties of bradykininogen and of the bradykinin-releasing and destroying enzymes in snake venom. In: Hypotensive peptides, p. 149, ed. by E. G. ERDÖS, N. BACK, and F. SICUTERI. Berlin-Heidelberg-New York: Springer 1966.

SUZUKI, T., IWANAGA, S., SATO, T., NAGASAWA, S., KATO, H., YANO, M., HORIUCHI, K.: Biochemical properties of kininogens and kinin releasing enzymes. In: Internat. Symposium on Vasoactive Polypeptides: Bradykinin and Related Kinins, p. 27, ed. by M. ROCHA E SILVA and H. A. ROTHSCHILD. São Paulo 1967.
— MIZUSHIMA, Y., SATO, T., IWANAGA, S.: Purification of bovine bradykininogen. J. Biochem. (Tokyo) 57, 180 (1965).
TRAUTSCHOLD, I., WERLE, E., ZICKGRAF-RÜDEL, G.: Trasylol. Biochem. Pharmacol. 16, 59 (1967).
TRETHEWIE, E. R.: Tissue injury by trypsin. Aust. J. exp. Biol. med. Sci. 20, 49 (1942).
TURBA, F., HETZEL, H.: Über ein oxytocisch wirkendes Peptid aus Serumprotein. Biochem. Z. 325, 524 (1954).
WALASZEK, E. J., BUÑAG, R. D., HUGGINS, C. G.: The characterization of the hypertensive polypeptide substance A. J. Pharmacol. exp. Ther. 138, 139 (1962).
— HUGGINS, C. G.: Substance A: A hypotensive polypeptide from fraction IV-4 of plasma protein. J. Pharmacol. exp. Ther. 126, 258 (1959).
WEBER, C. J., MAJOR, R. H., LOBB, D.: The production of a pressor substance from serum globulin by action of pepsin. Science 96, 44 (1942).
WEBSTER, M. E.: Report of the committee on nomenclature for hypotensive peptides. In: Hypotensive peptides, p. 648, ed. by E. G. ERDÖS, N. BACK, and F. SICUTERI. Berlin-Heidelberg-New York: Springer 1966.
— PIERCE, J. V.: Studies on plasma kallikrein and its relationship to plasmin. J. Pharmacol. exp. Ther. 130, 484 (1960).
— — The nature of the kallidins released from human plasma by kallikreins and other enzymes. Ann. N.Y. Acad. Sci. 104, 91 (1963).
WELLS, J. A., MORRIS, H. C., DRAGSTEDT, C. A.: Significance of histamine in trypsin shock as determined by Benadryl. Proc. Soc. exp. Biol. (N.Y.) 62, 209 (1946).
WERLE, E.: Zur Kenntnis des Kallikreins. Angew. Chem. 60, 53 (1948).
— Über Plasmakinine. In: Symposium Biologisch aktive Polypeptide, p. 57. Vienna 1962.
— Plasma-Kinine. Münch. med. Wschr. 50, 2846 (1963).
— BEREK, U.: Über Kallidin. Biochem. Z. 320, 136 (1950).
— DÄUMER, J.: Über das Verhalten des Kallikreins, des Inaktivators aus Lymphdrüsen, der Substanz DK, sowie der Histidindecarboxylase bei der Kataphorese. Biochem. Z. 304, 377 (1940).
— FORELL, M. M., MAIER, L.: Zur Kenntnis der blutdrucksenkenden Wirkung des Trypsins. Naunyn-Schmiedebergs Arch. exp. Path. Pharmak. 225, 369 (1955).
— GÖTZE, W., KEPPLER, A.: Über die Wirkung des Kallikreins auf den isolierten Darm und über eine neue darmkontrahierende Substanz. Biochem. Z. 289, 217 (1937).
— GRUNZ, M.: Zur Kenntnis der darmkontrahierenden, uteruserregenden und blutdrucksenkenden Substanz DK. Biochem. Z. 301, 429 (1939).
— HOCHSTRASSER, K.: Versuche zur Isolierung eines niedermolekulären Kininogens. Hoppe-Seylers Z. physiol. Chem. 332, 322 (1963).
— KAUFMANN-BOETSCH, B.: Über esteratische Wirkungen von Kallikrein und Trypsin und ihre Hemmung durch Kallikrein und Trypsininhibitoren. Hoppe-Seylers Z. physiol. Chem. 319, 52 (1960).
— KEHL, R., KOEBKE, K.: Über Bradykinin, Kallidin und Hypertensin. Biochem. Z. 320, 372 (1950a).
— — — Über Trypsin, Chymotrypsin, Kallidin und Bradykinin. Biochem. Z. 321, 213 (1950b).
— KORSTEN, A.: Der Kallikreingehalt des Harns, des Speichels und des Blutes bei Gesunden und Kranken. Z. ges. exp. Med. 103, 153 (1938).
— MAIER, L.: Über die chemische und pharmakologische Unterscheidung von Kallikreinen verschiedener Herkunft. Biochem. Z. 323, 279 (1952).
— — RINGELMANN, E.: Hemmung von Proteinasen durch Kallikrein-Inaktivatoren. Naturwissenschaften 39, 328 (1952).
YAMURA, T., CORMIA, F. E.: Studies on human skin protease. J. invest. Derm. 37, 121 (1961).

Snake Venoms

TOMOJI SUZUKI and SADAAKI IWANAGA

With 14 Figures

A. Bradykinin-Releasing Enzyme in Snake Venom

For many years pharmacologists have been interested in biologically active proteins in snake venoms (KAISER and MICHEL, 1958). Highly specific methods are often necessary in enzymatic studies, and enzymes from snake venoms are used in some of these methods. These enzymes include phospholipase A (EC 3.1.1.4), L-amino-acid oxidase (EC 1.4.3.2), phosphodiesterase (EC 3.1.4.1), and 5′-nucleotidase (EC 3.1.3.5). Much of the literature on these has been reviewed (ZELLER, 1948, 1951; VAN HEYNINGEN, 1954; SLOTTA, 1955; SARKER and DEVI, 1968). The availability of highly purified enzyme proteins has enabled rapid progress in the characterization of many enzymes and of their biological activity, so more up-to-date reviews are constantly required. Proteinase and arginine ester hydrolase activity have been found in the venoms of Crotalidae (*Agkistrodon*, *Bothrops*, *Crotalus*, *Lachesis*, and *Trimeresurus* species) and some venoms of Viperidae. The venoms of Elapidae usually do not contain proteinase or arginine ester hydrolase activity and thus they do not digest proteins, but they react strongly toward peptides of rather small molecular weight (MURATA et al., 1963).

Proteinases and arginine esterases are related to the toxic and physiological actions of the venoms of the Crotalidae family. EAGLE (1937) studied the mechanism of blood coagulation by various snake venoms and found that nine of seventeen venoms tested could coagulate citrated blood or plasma. Trypsin may replace Ca^{2+} and platelets in activation of prothrombin to thrombin, and this thrombin is itself a proteolytic enzyme, reacting with fibrinogen to form fibrin. Most coagulant and proteolytic snake venoms also react with fibrinogen to form fibrin. Therefore, the proteinase in snake venom was formerly considered to be a thrombin-like enzyme. Moreover, trypsin hydrolyzes benzoylarginine methyl ester (BAMe) (SCHWER et al., 1948) and, since Crotalidae venom also hydrolyzes this synthetic substrate (DEUTSCH and DINIZ, 1955), venom proteinase seemed to be a trypsin-like enzyme. However, trypsin and venom proteinase can be distinguished from each other by means of trypsin inhibitors (DEUTSCH and DINIZ, 1955).

The most characteristic physiological symptoms resulting from injection of Crotalidae venoms into an animal are hemorrhage and lowering of the blood pressure. Around 1940 ROCHA E SILVA (1939a, b, 1940a, b) observed that a pure preparation of trypsin had strong spasmogenic effects on smooth muscles of the isolated guinea pig ileum and uterus, rabbit intestine and rat uterus and liberated a small amount of histamine from guinea pig lung. A few years previously, FELDBERG and KELLAWAY (1937a, b) had reported the release of histamine when guinea pig or cat lung was perfused with the venoms of some snakes, such as *Crotalus atrox*, *Denisonea superba* (Australian copperhead) and *Naja naja* (Indian cobra). At first the role of histamine in the resulting toxic and traumatic conditions seemed to be the central theme of their studies. However, it became evident that the effect of histamine alone could not explain the physiological actions of these snake venoms. Thus a search for mediators other than histamine to explain the effects of venoms upon living tissues was started by FELDBERG et al. (1937d). One of the active principles they found caused a slow contraction of guinea pig ileum (FELDBERG and KELLAWAY, 1937c).

ROCHA E SILVA et al. studied the pharmacological actions of the strongly proteolytic *Bothrops jararaca* venom upon the intestine and uterus of guinea pig, uterus and intestine of rat, intestine of rabbit, and smooth muscle of dog. They

Table 1. *Liberation of bradykinin from bovine serum*

Time of incubation (min)	Maximal activity (%)
0	10
1	60
2	80
3	100
4	50
10	15
30	0

Five ml serum and 0.5 mg venom were incubated. After the indicated times, liberation of bradykinin was assayed on guinea pig ileum. (From ROCHA E SILVA et al. 1949).

observed that venom acted like trypsin on these tissues and that an active principle was released even when the venom of *B. jararaca* was added directly to bovine serum or oxalated plasma, and especially to the pseudoglobulin fraction (ROCHA E SILVA et al., 1949). The active principle could not be histamine or acetylcholine, because it affected guinea pig ileum even in the presence of atropine or antihistamines. The guinea pig ileum responded to the active principle slowly, compared to the quick response to histamine or acetylcholine, and the active principle was named bradykinin. Bradykinin, liberated by the action of the venom of *B. jararaca*, was rapidly destroyed by an enzyme in the crude venom (Table 1), and bradykinin was considered to be a polypeptide. When bradykinin was discovered, there was no indication that any hypotensive or smooth-muscle-stimulating principle was liberated from the globulin fraction of normal plasma by incubation with venom enzymes, even though lowered blood pressure after snakebite had been noted before 1920. MITCHELL (1861) and MITCHELL and REICHERT (1886) demonstrated the hypotensive action of *Crotalus horridus* and *C. atrox* venoms on mammals, and ARTHUS (1921) called attention to the similarity of symptoms caused by *C. adamanteus*, *Vipera russelli*, and *V. aspis* venoms. The venoms of Crotalidae have proteolytic activity, unlike the venoms of Elapidae. Bradykinin is a polypeptide; thus the bradykinin-releasing effect of the venom is believed to be due to a proteinase with the specificity of trypsin. This seemed reasonable, because trypsin had the same effects as *B. jararaca* venom upon guinea pig ileum and uterus and blood pressure of the cat. These physiological actions were also seen from a crude bradykinin preparation isolated from a mixture of bovine pseudoglobulin and venom by boiling it and adding alcohol.

Moreover, ROCHA E SILVA and ANDRADE (1945) observed a trypsin-like activity of the venoms of *C. terrificus terrificus*, *B. jararaca*, and *B. atrox* related to the hydrolysis of benzoyl-L-arginine amide (BAA). In 1955, in a study of proteinases in snake venoms, DEUTSCH and DINIZ (1955) could find no definite relationship between the proteolytic and bradykinin-releasing activities. They also observed that the venoms of Crotalidae species hydrolyze benzoyl-L-arginine ethyl ester (BAEe). Although the venom of *B. neuweidii* has little BAA hydrolyzing and kininogenase activities (MARSANO et al., 1945), both exist in the venom of *B. jararaca* (HENRIQUES et al., 1966). However, *Agkistrodon halys blomhoffii* venom, which releases bradykinin, does not hydrolyze BAA (SATAKE et al., 1965). Thus it is concluded that the enzyme in the Crotalidae venom which liberates bradykinin may hydrolyze BAEe but not proteins or BAA. HOLTZ and RAUDONAT (1956) reported that the proteinase fraction of *B. jararaca* venom precipitated at 40% saturation with ammonium sulfate does not release bradykinin, whereas the fraction precipitated at 60% saturation with ammonium sulfate had kininogenase, a slight proteinase, and clotting activities. Subsequently, HAMBERG and ROCHA E SILVA (1957a) reported that on heat treatment the kininogenase and esterase activities of snake venom remained, although the caseinolytic activity was quickly destroyed. They indicated that the common mediator of bradykinin release in both trypsin and snake venom may be the esterase activity. The esterase activity of venom is also effective in clotting blood.

Table 2. *Hemorrhagic, lethal, and various enzymatic activities of A. halys blomhoffii venom after treatment with DFP and EDTA*

Toxic and enzymatic activities	Untreated	DFP treated	EDTA treated	DFP and EDTA treated
Hemorrhage	100	89	0	0
Lethality (LD_{50})	1.20 mg	1.04 mg	none[a]	none[a]
Proteinase	100	150	8	18
BAEe-esterase	100	0	100	0
Bradykinin-releasing enzyme	100	0	100	0
Phospholipase A	100	115	[b]	128
Hyaluronidase	100	60	[b]	60
L-Amino acid oxidase	100	88	[b]	191
Phosphodiesterase	100	110	[b]	130
5′-Nucleotidase	100	123	[b]	129

Values are expressed as specific activities relative to that of the untreated crude venom. LD_{50} = Mg/kg of mouse.
[a] No lethality was observed at doses up to 15 mg/kg.
[b] Not examined.
(From OMORI et al., 1964).

When venom was treated with EDTA, proteinase was completely lost while esterase remained unchanged (DEUTSCH and DINIZ, 1955; OMORI et al., 1964). Conversely, on treatment with diisopropyl phosphorofluoridate (DFP), both esterase and kininogenase actions were completely lost (OMORI et al., 1964; HABERMANN, 1960) while proteinase activity and toxicity remained unchanged (Table 2). Recent experiments with purified enzyme have showed that venom proteinases and venom arginine ester hydrolases are quite distinct enzymes, and that venom proteinases are almost inactive against arginine esters in general (SATAKE et al., 1965).

It was also shown that Crotalidae venoms usually contain three or more proteinases (SATAKE et al., 1965; PFLEIDERER and SUMYK, 1961), one being a main principle of the kininases and also one of the two hemorrhagic proteins with lethal toxicity (SUZUKI et al., 1966a; IWANAGA et al., 1965a). Therefore, immersion of the venom in a boiling water bath for a few minutes raises the release of bradykinin from fresh plasma by the venom to a maximum (HAMBERG and ROCHA E SILVA, 1957a), owing to heat denaturation of the proteinase with bradykinin-destroying activity (Fig. 1). Enzymes which release and destroy bradykinin are widely distributed in the venom of snakes such as *B. jararaca* (fer-de-lance), *C. adamanteus* (rattlesnake), *C. atrox*, *A. contortrix* (copperhead), *A. piscivorus* (water moccasin), and *A. halys blomhoffii* (Japanese trivial name "mamushi"). The distribution of proteinases, BAEe esterases, and kininogenases

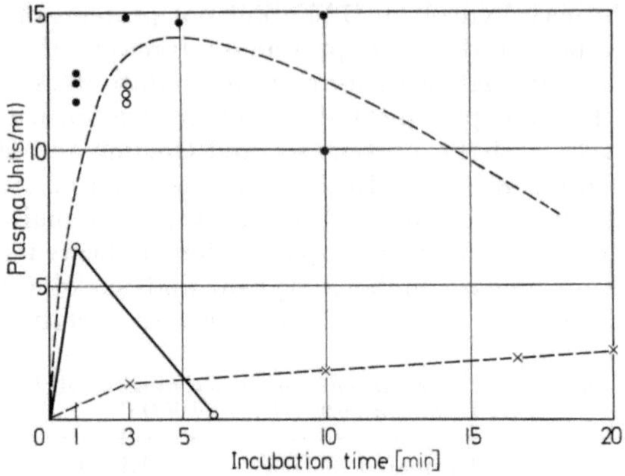

Fig. 1. Release of bradykinin by *B. jararaca* venom. Fresh plasma with untreated dry venom (o), heat-denatured venom from fresh (•) and denatured (×) plasma. Concentration of venom, 1 mg/ml plasma. (From HAMBERG and ROCHA E SILVA, 1957a)

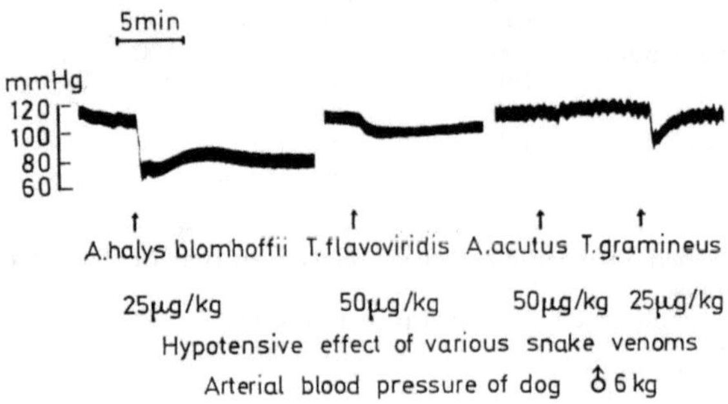

Fig. 2. Hypotensive effects of some snake venoms. (From OSHIMA et al., 1969)

in the venoms of various species are shown in Tables 3 (DEUTSCH and DINIZ, 1955) and 4 (OSHIMA et al., 1969). Venoms of some snakes such as *Trimeresurus flavoviridis* (Japanese trivial name "habu") and *A. acutus* (Formosan trivial name "hyapoda") did not show appreciable bradykinin-releasing activity, although they contained considerable amounts of BAEe hydrolytic activity. When these two venoms are injected into the dog, there is little or no hypotensive effect (Fig. 2), unlike the venoms of *A. halys blomhoffii* and *T. gramineus* (OSHIMA et al., 1969).

SATO et al., (1965) reported the separation of arginine ester hydrolase of *A. halys blomhoffii* venom into three enzymatic entities, "bradykinin releasing," "clotting," and "permeability increasing," and that the last two enzymes were purified to physicochemically homogeneous states. It is interesting that the venom secreted from the salivary gland of the snake is similar to mammalian plasma in that it contains clotting, kinin-releasing, and permeability-increasing

Table 3. *Proteolytic, BAEe esterase, and bradykinin-releasing activities of venoms of various common snakes in Brazil and North America*

Venom[a]	Activity[b]							Clotting Hb ratio
	Hb	Hb + EDTA[c]		BAEe	Clotting[d]	Bradykinin		
						Formation	Destruction	
Trypsin	610	610	(0.02)	56	none	5.2	0.14	
Chymotrypsin						0	94.1	
A. piscivorus piscivorus	30	17	(0.25)	8.0	none	13.5	0.0	
L. muta	29	18	(0.75)	8.3	12	41.1	0.10	0.41
C. atrox	21	3.2	(0.3)	2.8	none	46.2	5.60	
C. horridus	17	2.7	(0.4)	5.9	2	31.2	0.44	0.12
A. contortrix	13	9	(0.4)	11.6	none	53.0	0.0	
B. neuweidii	7.9	3	(1.0)	2.2	1.6	0.9	0.04	0.2
B. jararacaussu	4.4	0.8	(1.5)	3.8	3		0.15	0.68
B. jararaca	3.1	0.8	(2.0)	3.7	11	17.2	0.72	3.5
B. insularis	2.5	0.8	(4.0)	2.9	3.6	1.4	0.50	3.4
B. cotiara	2.1	0.6	(1.5)	7.9	2.3	2.5	0.93	1.1
B. alternatus	1.5	0.3	(12)	0.4	0.25	0.5	0.35	0.17
B. atrox	1.5	0.7	(3.0)	3.8	7.8	3.7	0.49	5.2
C. adamanteus	1.0	0.3	(10)	2.3	7	36.3	0.07	7
C. terrificus terrificus (yellow)	0.01	0.01	(20)	0.7	3	1.7	0.30	300
C. terrificus terrificus (white)	0.005	0.005	(20)	1.4	2	2.5	0.23	400

[a] *A.* = *Agkistrodon*; *C.* = *Crotalus*; *B.* = *Bothrops*; *L.* = *Lachesis*.

[b] For hemoglobin, milliequivalents of tyrosine $\times 10^4$ per mg/15 min liberated at 37°, pH 7.4; for (BAEe), moles hydrolyzed $\times 10^6$ per mg/min at 22°. For bradykinin, units formed or destroyed per mg venom/min at 37° are shown.

[c] Concentration of EDTA 5.6×10^{-4}M. The figures in parentheses indicate milligrams of venom used in each test.

[d] Clotting activity is expressed as the reciprocal of the amount in milligrams venom required to clot 1 ml of 300 mg% solution of fibrinogen at pH 7.4 in 30 sec at 25°.

(From Deutsch and Diniz, 1955.)

(in mammalian plasma this is the permeability globulin) enzymes with arginine esterase activity. These enzymes are in an active state in venom, unlike those in plasma which exist as inactive pre-enzymes.

Pharmacological investigations of snake venoms are complicated by the fact that these venoms can be called solutions of toxins in saliva and contain many components with physiological activities. To elucidate the physiological actions of snake venoms it is important to purify each component from each venom. Although we are as yet far from this goal, we have several techniques for this purpose. Chromatography on ion-exchange cellulose and gel filtration are excellent methods for the purification of proteins; they have limitations, but fortunately they are not the same for each material. Recently, the bradykinin-releasing and inactivating enzymes (kininogenases and kininases) from snake venom and their substrates (kininogens and bradykinin and its analogs) have been well purified or synthesized. Investigations of the liberation and destruction of bradykinin by snake venoms, with these highly purified materials, are some of the most comprehensive ever conducted.

Table 4. *Enzyme activities of various snake venoms treated with EDTA*

Venom[a]	TAMe hydrolysis (μmole/min/mg)	Bradykinin release (μg equivalent of synth. BK/min/mg)
A. halys blomhoffii	1.8	25.2
A. piscivorus piscivorus	4.6	28.0
A. contortrix contortrix	11.1	72.6
A. contortrix mokasen	10.2	38.6
A. acutus	2.9	0.5
B. jararaca	2.3	10.4
B. atrox	3.8	5.0
Bi. javonica	2.7	215.0
Bi. arietans	1.0	6.57
C. adamanteus	16.8	20.4
C. atrox	4.2	124.3
C. durissus terrificus	8.9	56.5
C. viridis viridis	9.1	233.5
C. basiliscus	4.0	24.5
Causus rhombeatus	1.8	6.6
Echis carinatus	1.1	9.6
T. flavoviridis	1.5	3.0
T. okinavensis	2.2	4.3
T. macrosquamatus	34.1	28.6
T. gramineus	8.0	54.4
V. russellii	0.4	1.3
V. palestinae	5.0	40.0
V. ammodytes	1.1	107.8

[a] *A.* = *Agkistrodon*; *B.* = *Bothrops*; *Bi.* = *Bitis*; *C.* = *Crotalus*; *T.* = *Trimeresurus*; *V.* = *Vipera*.

Each 2 mg of venoms was treated with 2 μmoles EDTA at 37° for 1 hr. The *p*-toluenesulfonyl-L-arginine methyl ester hydrolysis in each 0.1 ml aliquot was assayed by using 10 μmoles substrate. The bradykinin release by the crude venoms was assayed on guinea pig ileum with the method of ROCHA E SILVA. (From OSHIMA et al., 1969).

B. Purification of Bradykinin-Releasing Enzyme (Kininogenase) from Snake Venom

ROCHA E SILVA et al. (1949) found that if appropriate doses of trypsin or *B. jararaca* venom were incubated with bovine pseudoglobulin, maximum release of bradykinin was observed after 2 to 3 minutes. When the incubation was prolonged for 20 to 30 minutes, the liberated bradykinin was completely inactivated (Table 1).

Table 3 shows that some crude venoms, such as that of *A. contortrix* which is a potent kininogenase, have no kininase activity. Some other crude venoms which are kininogenases do not clot blood.

HAMBERG and ROCHA E SILVA (1957a) found that bradykinin-releasing and clotting activities remained even after *B. jararaca* venom had been heated at 100° for 3 to 5 minutes. Heat treatment destroyed the proteolytic activity of the venom. On prolonged heating the kininogenase, BAEe esterase, and coagulating activities decreased in parallel. It therefore seemed that the clotting and bradykinin-releasing activities might be due to the same principle in the venom of *B. jararaca*. Subsequently, HAMBERG and DEUTSCH (1958) attempted large-scale preparation of bradykinin from bovine serum globulin and reported that the kininase, but not the kininogenase, was inhibited by the addition of cysteine during incubation of whole plasma with *B. jararaca* venom. These facts suggest that the release of bradykinin and the inactivation of bradykinin are caused by different enzymes. In addition, HABERMANN found (1959) that the TAMe hydrolytic activity in the venom of *B. jararaca* can be partially separated by electrophoresis and that the peak of bradykinin-releasing activity did not coincide with the peak of clotting activity. Moreover, the fraction with clotting activity also had strong permeability-increasing activity.

It is now known that snake venom contains considerable amounts of permeability-increasing and clotting enzymes other than bradykinin-releasing enzyme (SATO et al., 1965). HOLTZ et al. (1960) observed that addition of alcohol

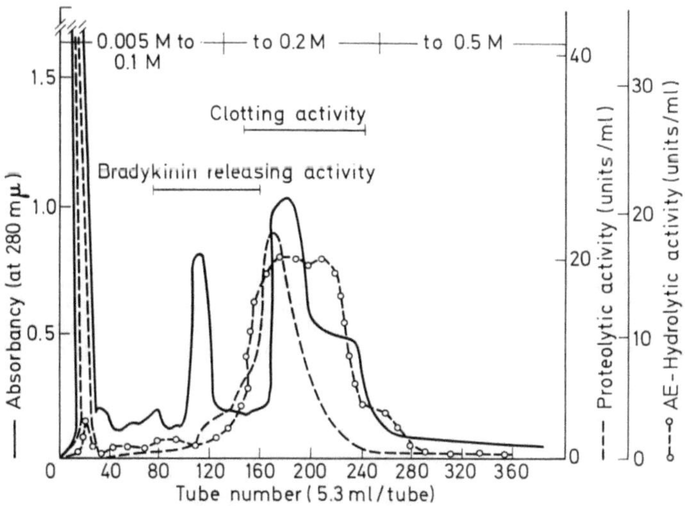

Fig. 3. Chromatographic separation of kininogenase and clotting enzyme of *C. adamanteus* venom on a DEAE-cellulose column. The lyophilized venom (500 mg) was applied to a column (2.5×26.5 cm) of DEAE-cellulose. Gradient elution was performed with 400 ml of 0.005 M sodium acetate (pH 7.0) in the mixing vessel and 0.1, 0.2, and 0.5 M sodium acetate (pH 7.0) in the reservoir. The flow rate was 65 ml/hr at 4°. (From SATO, 1968)

to a solution of heat-treated *B. jararaca* venom precipitated the clotting and bradykinin-releasing enzymes and on further addition of ether to the supernatant, bradykinin-releasing activity, but not clotting activity, was found in the precipitate. They also reported that about 10% of the kininogenases in *B. jararaca* and *C. atrox* venoms can be dialyzed through cellophane tubing (HOLTZ et al., 1960), or an Lsg *60* Göttingen membrane filter (CONTZEN et al., 1959) and that no proteolytic activity is detectable in the dialysate. The presence of a low molecular weight kininogenase in snake venom was also observed in the venom of *C. adamanteus* (SATO ,1965, 1968). The kininogenase and clotting enzyme of the venom are capable of being separated from each other by column chromatography on DEAE-cellulose (Fig. 3). When the kininogenase fraction in Fig. 3 was filtered through a Sephadex G-25 column in order to remove sodium acetate, it was found that the bradykinin-releasing activity was separated into two fractions, as shown in Fig. 4. The kininogenase activity, which appeared in the later fraction of the Sephadex column, corresponded to about 30% of the total activities of the venom used. This enzyme molecule could be smaller than that of the kininogenase eluted in the void volume fraction of the column. Therefore, it seems that *C. adamanteus* venom contains two different kininogenases with respect to their molecular weights.

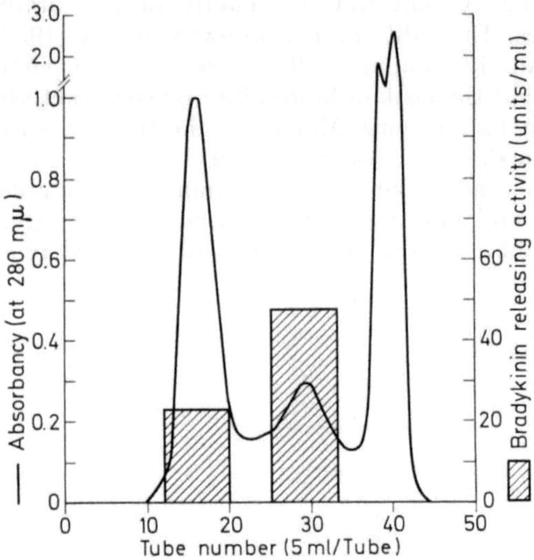

Fig. 4. Gel filtration of kininogenase fraction of *C. adamanteus* venom on a Sephadex G-25 column. The kininogenase fraction obtained from DEAE-cellulose column was gel filtered through a column (3.0×41 cm) of Sephadex G-25 (Fine) and eluted with distilled water adjusted to pH 8.0 with ammonia. The flow rate was 40 ml/hr at 4°. (From SATO, 1965)

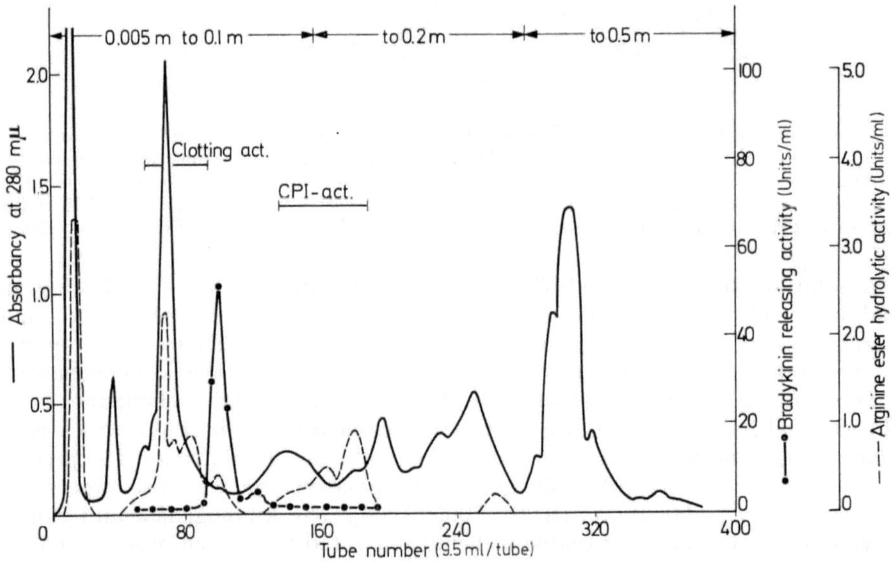

Fig. 5. Chromatographic behavior of arginine esterase of *A. halys blomhoffii* venom. One gram of lyophilized venom was applied to a column (3×40 cm) of DEAE-cellulose (0.68 meq/g), and subjected to gradient elution. Esterase was assayed with BAEe as substrate. One unit of esterase was defined as the amount of enzyme needed to hydrolyze 1 μmole BAEe per minute. (From SATO et al., 1965)

HAMBERG and ROCHA E SILVA (1957b) and HENRIQUES et al. (1960) also partially separated the bradykinin-releasing and clotting enzymes by starch-column electrophoresis and reported that both enzymes cleave arginine ester.

RAUDONAT and ROCHA E SILVA (1962) partially separated clotting and bradykinin-releasing enzymes by paper electrophoresis, and found that BAEe esterase is present in both fractions. Thus, until recently, venom kininogenase completely free from clotting activity had not been obtained in good yield, and it has not been proven that kininogenase action of the venom depends directly on its activity to split N-substituted arginine esters.

On chromatography of *A. halys blomhoffii* venom on DEAE-cellulose, SATO et al. in 1965 found that the kininogenase can easily be separated from the main

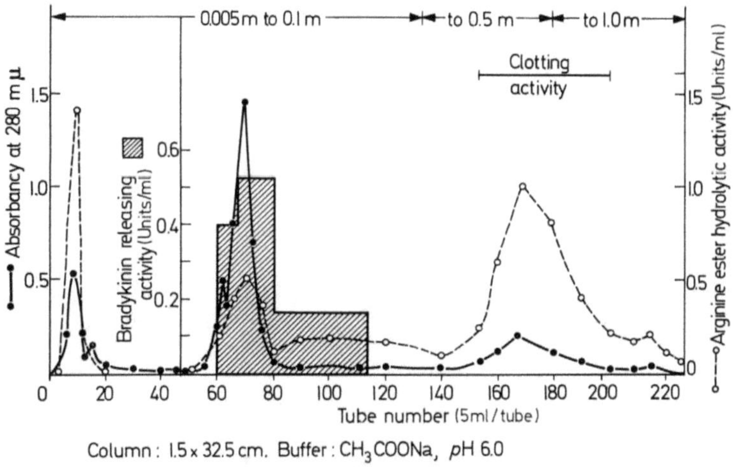

Fig. 6. Purification of kininogenase on a CM-cellulose column. The partially purified kininogenase, almost free of clotting enzyme, was applied to a CM-cellulose column. One mg of the applied sample hydrolyzed 1.65 μmoles of TAMe per minute, and released from kininogen bradykinin corresponding to 4.7 μg synthetic bradykinin per minute. (From SUZUKI et al., 1966b)

principle with kininase activity, namely proteinase b. By this means the kininogenase is partially purified and separated from the clotting and permeability-increasing enzymes (Fig. 5).

Purified kininogenase, completely free of kininase and clotting enzymes, is prepared by successive rechromatography on DEAE-cellulose and chromatography on a CM-cellulose column (SUZUKI et al., 1966b) (Fig. 6). Chromatography on a CM-cellulose column completely removes the kininase which contaminates the partially purified preparation.

The arginine esterase activity in the kininogenase accounts for less than 10% of the total esterase present in the venom. A physicochemically homogeneous enzyme, unlike the clotting and permeability-increasing enzymes, has not yet been obtained. The unexpectedly low level of arginine esterase in the kininogenase preparation raises the question of whether the release of bradykinin is directly related to the hydrolysis of its arginine ester. Moreover, the venom of *B. jararaca* released more bradykinin from purified kininogen than did trypsin, although the crude venom hydrolyzed arginine ester more slowly than trypsin does (HENRIQUES et al., 1962). However, the inseparability of the arginine esterase and the kininogenase activities was demonstrated in the experiments described below.

C. Dependency of the Kininogenase on the Arginine Esterase in the Venom

As mentioned elsewhere (p. 198) prolonged heat treatment decreased the clotting and the kininogenase and esterase activities in parallel manner. HABERMANN (1960) observed that the bradykinin release, clotting, and TAMe cleavage

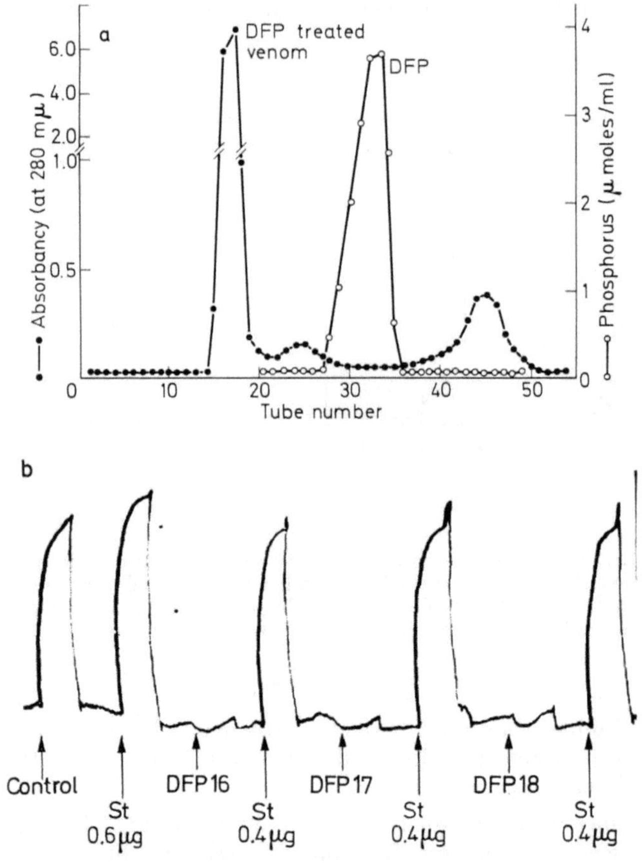

Fig. 7a and b. Inhibition of kininogenase of venom by DFP. Top: Gel filtration; a solution of DFP-treated venom was applied to a column (2.4 × 40 cm) of Sephadex G-25, and fractions of about 5 ml were collected at a flow rate of 20 ml/hr. Bottom: Bradykinin release by the protein fraction of DFP-treated venom. Samples from the Sephadex G-25 column (above) were assayed on the guinea pig ileum. Control, untreated venom; *St* = synthetic bradykinin. DFP 16, DFP 17, and DFP 18 are samples of DFP-treated venom, the numbers corresponding to the tube numbers above. (From IWANAGA et al., 1965b)

by *B. jararaca* venom were inhibited by DFP. The treatment also destroyed the permeability-increasing factor of the venom (Evans blue test). The esterase and the hypotensive and permeability-increasing effects of pancreatic kallikrein also disappeared on treatment with DFP. Subsequently, HABERMANN (1961) also observed the same effects of DFP on the venoms of *Vipera ammodytes*, *C. adamanteus*, and *B. jararaca*. α-N-Substituted arginine esters, but not argininamide, also inhibited the kininogenase in these venoms.

In 1965 IWANAGA et al. (1965b), using purified bradykinin-releasing enzyme of *A. halys blomhoffii*, clearly demonstrated that the kininogenase completely depends upon the arginine esterase activity of the enzyme. After incubation with DFP, both the kininogenase and the esterase were inhibited (Fig. 7). On heat

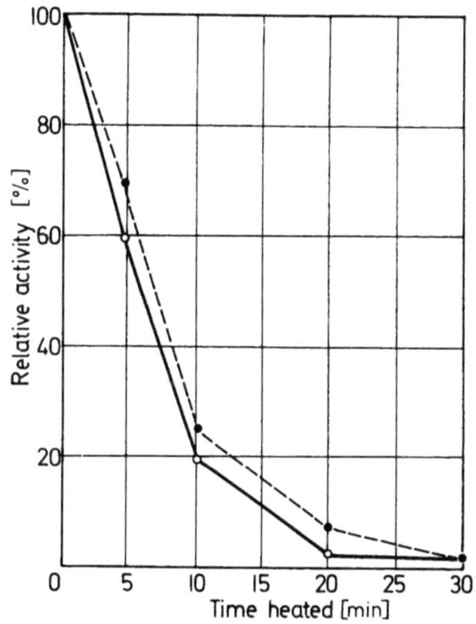

Fig. 8. Effect of heat treatment on bradykinin release by venom of *A. halys blomhoffii*. Purified kininogenase was diluted with 0.1 M sodium acetate (pH 7.0) to give a 0.012% solution. After heating in a boiling water bath, the solutions were cooled in an ice bath, and the residual kininogenase and esterase activities were estimated; —o—: bradykinin release; — —•— —: BAEe hydrolysis. (From IWANAGA et al., 1965b)

Table 5. *Effect of BAEe on Kininogenase*

Synthetic substrate added	Final concentration of substrate (M)	Maximal bradykinin release (%)
Benzoyl-L-arginine ethyl ester	none	100
	2.5×10^{-7}	100
	2.5×10^{-6}	68
	2.5×10^{-5}	40
	2.5×10^{-4}	10
	2.5×10^{-3}	0
L-Lysine ethyl ester	2.5×10^{-3}	100
Benzoyl-L-arginine amide	2.5×10^{-3}	100

To a mixture containing 1.0 ml kininogen and 25 μg purified kininogenase, various amounts of BAEe were added in a total volume of 1.4 ml. After incubation for 3 minutes at 37°, the bradykinin liberated was estimated on the guinea pig ileum. (From IWANAGA et al., 1965b).

treatment, kininogenase and the esterase actions decreased simultaneously; both activities are almost completely lost by heating the preparation in a boiling water bath (Fig. 8).

Also, when the synthetic substrate, BAEe, was added to a mixture of kininogen and kininogenase, the inhibition of liberation of bradykinin by BAEe depended on the concentration of the latter. At high enough concentration, the release of bradykinin was completely inhibited. L-Lysine ethyl ester and BAA which are not hydrolyzed by kininogenase, do not inhibit the liberation of bradykinin (Table 5).

D. The Kinin Liberated by Venom Enzymes and the Properties of Kininogenase in Venoms

ZUBER and JAQUES (1960) and MEIER (1960) found no difference between the kinin liberated from plasma by *B. jararaca* venom and that liberated by trypsin. HAMBERG (1962) observed the release of kinin from human plasma by *B. jararaca* venom and identified it as bradykinin. HABERMANN isolated bradykinin after incubating partially purified bovine kininogen with *C. adamanteus* venom (HABERMANN and BLENNEMANN, 1964). With purified kininogen (SUZUKI

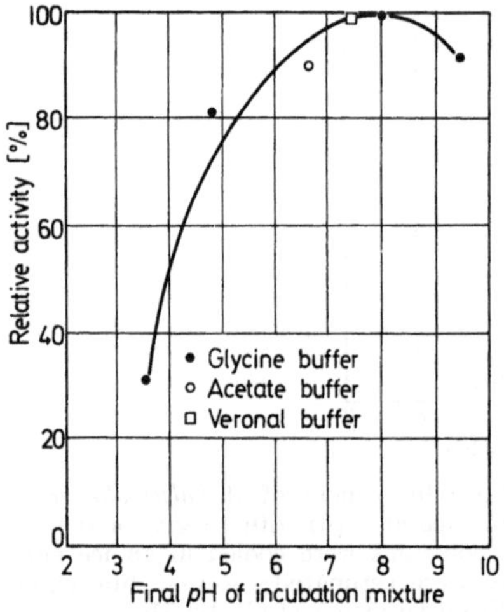

Fig. 9

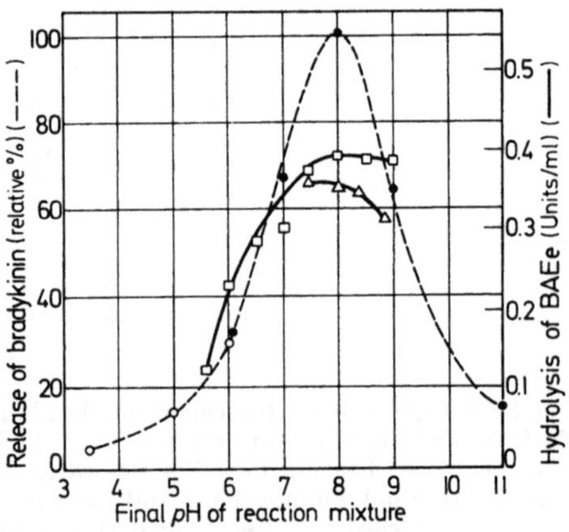

Fig. 10

Fig. 9. Stability of purified kininogenase (*A. halys blomhoffii*) at various pH values. Thirty-four μg of purified kininogenase was dissolved in 0.2 ml of 0.05 M buffer. The mixture was heated for 3 minutes at 85°, and the residual enzyme activity was assayed with guinea pig ileum. (From IWANAGA et al., 1965b)

Fig. 10. Optimum pH of the purified kininogenase of *A. halys blomhoffii*. The reaction mixture contained 0.1 ml (about 200 μg) kininogen, 4.2 μg purified kininogenase, and 0.5 ml of 0.1 M buffer, in a total volume of 2.0 ml. After incubation for 3 minutes at 37°, the bradykinin released was assayed on the guinea pig ileum. The reaction mixture for assay of esterase contained 5 μmoles BAEe, 156 μg purified enzyme, and 0.5 ml of 0.1 M buffer, in a total volume of 1.0 ml; —●—: phosphate–NaOH buffer; —○—:acetate buffer; --□--: barbital–acetate buffer; —△—: Tris buffer. (From IWANAGA et al., 1965b)

et al., 1965) and purified venom kininogenase of *A. halys blomhoffii*, and converting the kinin liberated to the 1-dimethyl-aminonaphthylsulfonyl derivative (KATO and SUZUKI, 1968a) by the so-called dansyl method (GRAY and HARTLEY, 1963), it was found that the venom enzyme liberated bradykinin directly from the kininogen molecule. On the other hand, WEBSTER and PIERCE (1963) found evidence that the venom of *A. contortrix* might liberate kallidin in addition to bradykinin.

The kininogenase isolated from the venom of *A. halys blomhoffii* (IWANAGA et al., 1965b) is stable in the frozen state for at least six months, and there is no loss of activity after freezing–thawing or lyophilization. It is most stable at pH 7–8 during heating (Fig. 9).

Cations such as Ca^{2+}, Mg^{2+}, Mn^{2+}, Zn^{2+}, Cd^{2+}, Fe^{3+}, K^{+}, and Na^{+} have no effect in tests using dialyzed kininogen and kininogenase of *A. halys blomhoffii* venom. The pH optimum of the enzyme is about 8.5 in various buffers, and its activity is highest in phosphate buffer (Fig. 10). The same pH was optimal for the hydrolysis of BAEe and liberation of bradykinin from kininogen. Two kinds of kininogen have been found in mammalian plasma (SUZUKI et al., 1966b; MARGOLIS and BISHOP, 1963; PIERCE and WEBSTER, 1966; JOHN and VOGT, 1965; VOGT, 1965, 1967), and the kininogenase of *A. halys blomhoffii* venom liberates bradykinin from both bovine kininogens (SUZUKI et al., 1966b). In one of the kininogens, the kinin moiety is located approximately at the central part of the kininogen molecule (SUZUKI et al., 1966a; HABERMANN, 1966; NAGASAWA

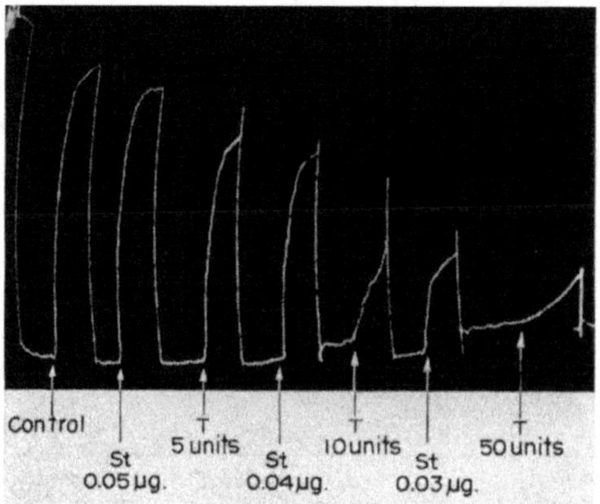

Fig. 11. Inhibition of purified kininogenase (*A. halys blomhoffii*) by Trasylol. The incubation mixture contained 58 µg enzyme, 0.5 ml of 0.0066 M phosphate buffer (pH 8.0), and 0.1 ml Trasylol (T) solution, in a total volume of 0.7 ml. After incubation for 5 minutes at 37°, 0.3 ml kininogen was added to the mixture and after 3 minutes, 0.8 ml of the reaction mixture was used for assay. Control, without T; St., synthetic bradykinin. (From IWANAGA et al., 1965b)

et al., 1966; KATO and SUZUKI, 1968b). Even after the conformation of the kininogen is changed by reducing all the disulfide bridges of the kininogen with β-mercaptoethanol and then converting them to carboxymethyl derivatives with monoiodoacetic acid, bradykinin is released from them by snake venom enzymes and by trypsin (KATO et al., 1967). In contrast, hog pancreatic kallikrein does not release kinin from these modified kininogens.

By the cyanogen bromide treatment of human kininogen, a fragment yielding kinin was released from the kininogen molecule (AXÉN et al., 1966). Subsequently, KATO and SUZUKI (1968b) isolated a peptide yielding kinin by applying the cyanogen bromide method of WITKOP (GROSS and WITKOP, 1962) to the bovine kininogen, and its amino acid sequence was identified as: Lys-Arg-Pro-Pro-Gly-Phe-Ser-Pro-Phe-Arg-Ser-Val-Gln-Val-Homoser.

Snake venom kininogenase, trypsin, or pancreatic kallikrein could release kallidin from this peptide by cleaving only the arginyl-seryl linkage in the fragment. Human thrombin did not liberate kinin from this peptide. HABERMANN (1966) also obtained pepsitocin, a peptide yielding kinin, by digesting bovine kininogen with pepsin. In this peptide, the methionyl residue is attached to the N-terminal lysine of the peptide obtained by the cyanogen bromide treatment. Kininogenase of venom liberated bradykinin from this peptide by cleaving the arginyl-serine and lysyl-arginine bonds. So it seems that the tertiary structure of the kininogen is not essential for the liberation of bradykinin by snake venom enzyme or by trypsin. However, the tertiary structure of native kininogen around the methionyl-lysyl linkage seems to be essential for the cleavage of the methionyl-lysine bond in the kininogen molecule by pancreatic kallikrein.

----Met-Lys-Arg-Pro-Pro-Gly-Phe-Ser-Pro-Phe-Arg----
↑ ↑——trypsin, snake venom enzyme——↑
└——pancreatic kallikrein——┘

Trasylol, a potent inhibitor of purified urinary (PRADO et al., 1963) and purified pancreatic (IWANAGA et al., 1965b; WEBSTER and PIERCE, 1961) kallikreins, markedly inhibits the bradykinin release by the venom kininogenase (Fig. 11). The decrease in bradykinin release is proportional to the amount of Trasylol added. Although the kininogenase activities of trypsin and kallikrein are completely inhibited by Trasylol, the release of bradykinin is only partially but not completely inhibited, even when a high concentration of Trasylol is added to the venom (Table 6).

Table 6. *Trasylol inhibits the contraction of the ileum induced by A. halys blomhoffii venom kininogenase, pancreatic kallikrein, or trypsin*

Trasylol (KIU)	Relative activity (%)		
	Bradykinin-releasing enzyme	Kallikrein	Trypsin
none	100	100	100
5	80	20	0
10	40	0	0
50	13	—	—
100	10	—	—

The assay conditions were the same as for bradykinin-releasing enzyme in Figure 11; 58 μg kininogenase, 5.8 μg kallikrein, or 10 μg trypsin was used. The values in the column for kininogenase were calculated from contractions shown in Figure 11. (From IWANAGA et al., 1965b).

Table 7. *Absence of inhibition by Trasylol of the "capillary permeability-increasing" (CPI)-enzyme and "clotting" (clot)-enzyme of the venom of A. halys blomhoffii*

Inhibitor (KIU)	Relative activity (%)	
	CPI-enzyme	Clot-enzyme
none	100	100
10	104	—
100	92	—
200	104	—
300	100	100

The activities of the CPI-enzyme (26 μg) and clot-enzyme (38 μg) were estimated by assaying the hydrolysis of TAMe. (From IWANAGA et al., 1965b).

Trasylol, on the other hand, does not inhibit the hydrolysis of arginine ester by the "clotting" and "capillary permeability-increasing" enzymes of the venom (Table 7). This is interesting because these two enzymes have the same specificity toward synthetic substrates that the kininogenase has. It is now assumed that the kininogenase in venom is the salivary kallikrein of the snake. SBTI (WEBSTER and PIERCE, 1960, 1961; NAGASAWA et al., 1967), which inhibits plasma kallikreins, does not affect the venom kininogenase (HABERMANN, 1959).

E. Kininases and Bradykinin Potentiators in Snake Venoms

When ROCHA E SILVA observed liberation of bradykinin from pseudoglobulin by *B. jararaca* venom (Table 1), the bradykinin-destroying activity in the venom was also seen on prolonged incubation (ROCHA E SILVA et al., 1949).

DEUTSCH and DINIZ (1955) found that none of the snake venoms which release bradykinin hydrolyzes acetyl-L-tyrosine ethyl ester, a synthetic substrate

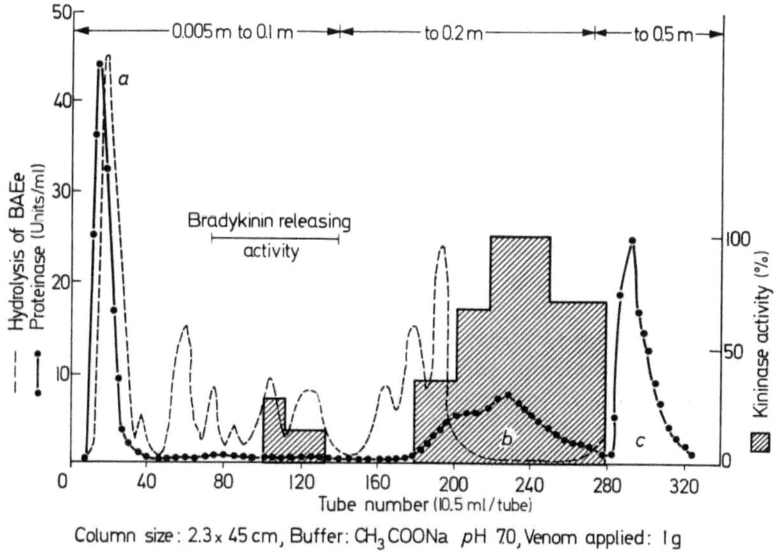

Fig. 12. Chromatography of the venom of *A. halys blomhoffii* on a DEAE-cellulose column. Distribution of the bradykinin-releasing and -destroying activities in the eluate. (From SUZUKI et al., 1966a)

for chymotrypsin. Thus these venoms do not contain a proteinase with the characteristics of chymotrypsin.

The enzymes that liberate or inactivate bradykinin migrated together in paper electrophoresis (DEUTSCH and DINIZ, 1955). However, cysteine inhibited the kininase but not the kininogenase in *B. jararaca* venom (HAMBERG and DEUTSCH, 1958). Moreover, kininase but not the kininogenase activity was destroyed by heat treatment (HAMBERG and ROCHA E SILVA, 1957a). The kininogenase and the main principle with bradykininase activity in the venom of *A. halys blomhoffii* were separated in chromatography on DEAE-cellulose (SUZUKI et al., 1966a, b), and were highly purified (Fig. 12).

Proteinase of the venom of *A. halys blomhoffii* was separated by chromatography into three entities, proteinase a, b, and c. The activities of all three were inhibited by cysteine (SATAKE et al., 1965). Of the three, only proteinase b has bradykininase activity. This proteinase can easily be purified to a physicochemically homogeneous state by rechromatography on DEAE-cellulose and by gel filtration on a Sephadex G-100 column (OSHIMA et al., 1968a). Of the three, proteinase b was present in largest quantity, amounting to approximately 10% of the lyophilized venom. It is interesting that proteinase b produces petechiae when injected intravenously into albino rabbits (IWANAGA et al., 1965a), and purified proteinase c causes more marked edema than other proteinases of plant and animal origin when injected subcutaneously into depilated albino rabbit (OSHIMA et al., 1968b). When purified proteinase b was incubated with synthetic bradykinin, the glycyl-phenylalanine bond was hydrolyzed.

On the other hand, when synthetic bradykinin was incubated with kininogenase of *A. halys blomhoffii* venom which had been partially purified by chromatography on DEAE-cellulose (Fig. 12), bradykinin was slowly inactivated.

Bradykinin was hydrolyzed at its phenylalanyl-seryl linkage by the enzyme contaminating the partially purified kininogenase preparation (SUZUKI et al., 1966a) (Fig. 13).

Enzymes with weak kininase activity
↓
H-Arg-Pro-Pro-Gly-Phe-Ser-Pro-Phe-Arg-OH
↑
Proteinase b

Fig. 13. Peptide bonds in bradykinin cleaved by kininase from *A. halys blomhoffii* venom

The distribution of kininases in various Crotalidae venoms can be seen in Table 8. The venoms of *C. atrox*, *C. adamanteus*, and *Trimeresurus flavoviridis* split the two peptide bonds of the bradykinin molecule, whereas the venoms of *A. contortrix contortrix*, *B. jararaca*, and *Vipera russellii* split only one peptide bond. All these venoms hydrolyzed the glycyl-phenylalanine bond of bradykinin.

Table 8. *Distribution of the bradykinin-releasing, inactivating and hemorrhage-causing activities in snake venoms*

Venom	Bond hydrolyzed in bradykinin		Hemorrhage	Bradykinin release (U/mg)
	Gly-Phe	Phe-Ser		
A. halys blomhoffii	++	+	++	27.3
C. atrox	++	+	+	42.0
C. adamanteus	++	+	+++	63.0
T. flavoviridis	++	+	+	0
A. contortrix contortrix	+	−	−	52.5
B. jararaca	+	−	±	52.3
V. russelli	+	−	−	0

One μmole bradykinin and 300 μg venom were incubated for 3 hours. (From SUZUKI et al., 1966a).

The glycyl-phenylalanine bond of bradykinin was hydrolyzed by proteinase b with hemorrhagic activity of *A. halys blomhoffii* venom. The venom of *A. contortrix contortrix* had no hemorrhagic activity, and the venom of *B. jararaca* and *V. russellii* had very little, although all three hydrolyzed the same peptide bond of bradykinin as *A. halys blomhoffii* venom. These results indicate that different enzyme proteins in the venoms of poisonous snakes may hydrolyze the same peptide bond of bradykinin.

FERREIRA and ROCHA E SILVA (1965), and FERREIRA (1966) reported the existence of a substance in the venom of *B. jararaca* which potentiates bradykinin activity. Potentiation of the effect of bradykinin by bovine fibrinopeptide B (GLADNER et al., 1963) or human fibrinopeptide A-β (OSBAHR et al., 1964) was also observed. The contraction of ileum by synthetic bradykinin was also markedly potentiated by addition of heat-treated venom of *A. halys blomhoffii* (SUZUKI et al., 1966b).

KATO and SUZUKI (1968a), isolated a bradykinin potentiator from the lyophilized venom of *A. halys blomhoffii*, using the procedures as follows: 2 g of the venom was gel-filtered through a column (4.5 × 90 cm) of Sephadex G-100. Bradykinin potentiating activity was found in a low molecular weight fraction. This fraction was subjected twice to gel filtration on a column (3 × 90 cm) of Sephadex G-25, and contaminating protein and salt were removed. To purify

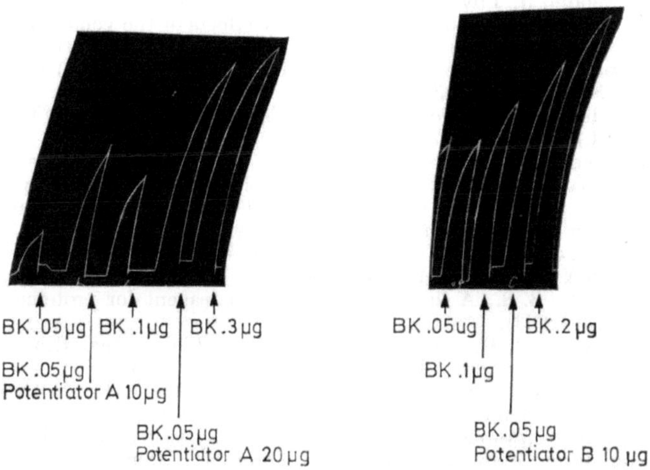

Fig. 14. Effect of snake venom potentiators A and B on the bradykinin-induced contraction of guinea pig ileum. Before the addition of synthetic bradykinin (BK), the potentiator was in contact for 5 to 10 seconds with the guinea pig ileum suspended in 5 ml Tyrode's solution. (From KATO and SUZUKI, 1968a)

the principles further, the desalted fraction was applied to a column (1.5 × 92 cm) of CM-Sephadex C-50, equilibrated with 0.005 M sodium acetate (pH 5.0), and exponential gradient elution was performed by increasing ionic strength with 1 M sodium acetate (pH 5.0) at room temperature. By this procedure, five potentiators, A, B, C, D, and E were separated. Each (5 to 20 µg) of the peptides had a potentiating effect in two or three trials upon the bradykinin-induced contraction of isolated guinea pig ileum.

Each peptide gave a single spot in high-voltage paper electrophoresis at pH 3.5. In the peptides, potentiators A, C, and D were unreactive to ninhydrin reagent, indicating no free amino groups at their N-terminal ends. Their amino acid compositions, however, were quite analogous to that of potentiator B. Potentiator B was composed of ten amino acid residues as follows: Lys_1, Arg_1, Glu_1, Pro_4, Gly_1, Ile_1, Leu_1. All other potentiators except E-peptide showed almost the same amino acid composition as potentiator B, and they seem to have a molecular weight of about 1,000 to 1,500. It is very interesting that all these potentiators in *A. halys blomhoffii* venom have a characteristically high proline content. If the structure of the potentiator is similar to bradykinin this may afford us interesting information on the mechanism of the pharmacological actions of bradykinin while studies of the amino acid sequence of the potentiators are in progress (KATO and SUZUKI, 1969; GREENE et al., 1969).

References

Arthus, M.: De l'Anaphyloxie à l'Immunité. Paris 1921.

Axén, R., Gross, R., Witkop, B., Pierce, J. V., Webster, M. E.: Release of kinin activity from human kininogens and fresh plasma. Biochem. biophys. Res. Commun. **23**, 92 (1966).

Contzen, C., Holtz, P., Raudonat, H. W.: Über das Bradykinin bildende Prinzip des Bothrops-Giftes. Naturwissenschaften **46**, 402 (1959).

Deutsch, H. F., Diniz, C. R.: Some proteolytic activities of snake venoms. J. biol. Chem. **216**, 17 (1955).

Eagle, H.: The coagulation of blood by snake venoms and its physiologic significance. J. exp. Med. **65**, 613 (1937).

Feldberg, W., Holden, H. F., Kellaway, C. H.: Liberation of histamine from the perfused lung by snake venom. J. Physiol. (Lond.) **90**, 257 (1937d).

— Kellaway, C. H.: The circulatory and pulmonary effects of the venom of the Australian copperhead (*Denisonia superba*). Aust. J. exp. Biol. med. Sci. **15**, 81 (1937a).

— — Circulatory effects of the venom of the Indian cobra (*Naja naja*) in dogs. Aust. J. exp. Biol. med. Sci. **15**, 441 (1937b).

— — Liberation of histamine and formation of lysolecithin-like substances by cobra venom. J. Physiol. (Lond.) **94**, 187 (1937c).

Ferreira, S. H.: Bradykinin-potentiating factor. In: Hypotensive peptides, p. 356, ed. by E. G. Erdös, N. Back and F. Sicuteri. Berlin-Heidelberg-New York: Springer 1966.

— Rocha e Silva, M.: Potentiation of bradykinin and eledoisin by BPF (bradykinin potentiating factor) from *Bothrops jararaca* venom. Experientia (Basel) **21**, 347 (1965).

Gladner, J. A., Murtagh, P. M., Folk, J. E., Laki, K.: Nature of peptides released by thrombin. Ann. N.Y. Acad. Sci. **104**, 47 (1963).

Gray, W. R., Hartley, B. S.: A fluorescent end-group reagent for proteins and peptides. Biochem. J. **89**, 59 (1963).

Greene, L. J., Stewart, J. M., Ferreira, S. H.: Bradykinin-potentiating peptides from the venom of *Bothrops jararaca*. Pharmacol. Res. Comm. **1**, 159 (1969).

Gross, E., Witkop, B.: Nonenzymatic cleavage of peptide bonds: The methionine residues in bovine pancreatic ribonuclease. J. biol. Chem. **237**, 1856 (1962).

Habermann, E.: Über Zusammenhänge zwischen esterolytischen und pharmakologischen Wirkungen von Jararacagift, Kallikrein und Thrombin. Naunyn-Schmiedebergs Arch. exp. Path. Pharmak. **236**, 492 (1959).

— Diisopropylfluorophosphat-Hemmung esterolytischer und pharmakologischer Wirkungen von Kallikrein und Schlangengiften. Naturwissenschaften **47**, 111 (1960).

— Zuordnung pharmakologischer und enzymatischer Wirkungen von Kallikrein und Schlangengiften mittels Diisopropylfluorophosphat und Elektrophorese. Naunyn-Schmiedebergs Arch. exp. Path. Pharmak. **240**, 552 (1961).

— Strukturaufklärung kininliefernder Peptide aus Rinderserum-Kininogen. Naunyn-Schmiedebergs Arch. exp. Path. Pharmak. **253**, 474 (1966).

— Blennemann, G.: Über Substrate und Reaktionsprodukte der kininbildenden Enzyme Trypsin, Serum- und Pankreas-Kallikrein sowie von Crotalusgift. Naunyn-Schmiedebergs Arch. exp. Path. Pharmak. **249**, 357 (1964).

Hamberg, U.: Isolation and molar activity of human bradykinin. Biochem. biophys. Res. Commun. **7**, 95 (1962).

— Deutsch, H. F.: A large scale preparation of bradykinin. Arch. Biochem. **76**, 262 (1958).

— Rocha e Silva, M.: Release of bradykinin as related to the esterase activity of trypsin and of the venom of *Bothrops jararaca*. Experientia (Basel) **13**, 489 (1957a).

— — On the release of bradykinin by trypsin snake venoms. Arch. int. Pharmacodyn. **110**, 222 (1957b).

Henriques, O. B., Fichman, M., Beraldo, W. T.: Bradykinin-releasing factor from *Bothrops jararaca* venom. Nature (Lond.) **187**, 414 (1960).

— Mandelbaum, F. R., Henriques, S. B.: Proteolytic enzymes of Bothrops venom. Mem. Inst. Butantan Simp. Internac. **33**, 359 (1966).

— Picarelli, Z. P., Ferrase de Oliveira, M. C.: Partial purification of the plasma substrate for the bradykinin-releasing enzyme from the venom of *Bothrops jararaca*. Biochem. Pharmacol. **11**, 707 (1962).

Heyningen, W. E. van: Toxic proteins. In: The proteins, 1st ed., vol. 2, p. 345, ed. by H. Neurath. New York 1954.

Holtz, P., Raudonat, H. W.: Über Beziehungen zwischen proteolytischer Aktivität und blutcoagulierender sowie bradykinin-freisetzender Wirkung von Schlangengiften. Naunyn-Schmiedebergs Arch. exp. Path. Pharmak. **229**, 113 (1956).

— — Contzen, C.: Über das bradykininbildende Prinzip des Schlangengiftes. Naunyn-Schmiedebergs Arch. exp. Path. Pharmak. **239**, 54 (1960).

IWANAGA, S., OMORI, T., OSHIMA, G., SUZUKI, T.: Studies on snake venoms. XVI. Demonstration of a proteinase with hemorrhagic activity in the venom of *Agkistrodon halys blomhoffii*. J. Biochem. **57**, 392 (1965a).
— SATO, T., MIZUSHIMA, Y., SUZUKI, T.: Studies on snake venoms. XVII. Properties of the bradykinin releasing enzyme in the venom of *Agkistrodon halys blomhoffii*. J. Biochem. **58**, 123 (1965b).
JAQUES, R., MEIER, R.: Pharmacological characteristics of bradykinin B. Experientia (Basel) **16**, 371 (1960).
JOHN, G., VOGT, W.: Kininbildung in frischem und glasaktiviertem menschlichem Plasma. Naunyn-Schmiedebergs Arch. exp. Path. Pharmak. **251**, 186 (1965).
KAISER, E., MICHEL, H.: Die Biochemie der tierischen Gifte. Vienna 1958.
KATO, H., NAGASAWA, S., SUZUKI, T.: Relationship between tertiary structure and kinin yielding ability of bovine kininogen. Biochem. biophys. Res. Commun. **27**, 163 (1967).
— SUZUKI, T.: Structures of bradykinin potentiators isolated from snake venoms. (In Japanese.) J. Jap. Biochem. Soc. **40**, 574 (1968a).
— — The location and nature of the linkage of kinin moiety in bovine kininogen-II. Biochem. biophys. Res. Commun. **32**, 800 (1968b).
— — Isolation and identification of bradykinin potentiators in snake venoms. Pharmacol. Res. Comm. **1**, 166 (1969).
MARGOLIS, J., BISHOP, E. A.: Studies on plasma kinins. I. The composition of kininogen complex. Aust. J. exp. Biol. med. Sci. **41**, 293 (1963).
MARSANO, A., CROXATTO, R., CROXATTO, H.: Proteolytic action of the venom of *Lachesis neuwiedii*. Bol. Soc. Biol. Santiago **2**, 350 (1945).
MITCHELL, S. W.: Physiology and toxicology of the venom of the rattlesnake. Smithson. Contrib. **12**, 1 (1861).
— REICHERT, E. T.: Researches upon the venoms of poisonous serpents. Smithson. Contrib. **26**, 1 (1886).
MURATA, Y., SATAKE, M., SUZUKI, T.: Studies on snake venom. XII. Distribution of proteinase activities among Japanese and Formosan snake venoms. J. Biochem. **53**, 431 (1963).
NAGASAWA, S., HORIUCHI, K., YANO, M., SUZUKI, T.: Partial purification of bovine plasma kallikrein activated by contact with glass. J. Biochem. **62**, 398 (1967).
— SATO, T., MIZUSHIMA, Y., IWANAGA, S., SUZUKI, T.: Studies on the chemical nature of bovine bradykininogen: Determinations of amino acid, carbohydrate, amino and carboxyl terminal residues. J. Biochem. **60**, 643 (1966).
OMORI, T., IWANAGA, S., SUZUKI, T.: The relationship between the hemorrhagic and lethal activities of Japanese mamushi (*Agkistrodon halys blomhoffii*) venom. Toxicon **2**, 1 (1964).
OSBAHR, A. J., GLADNER, J. A., LAKI, K.: Studies on the physiological activity of the peptide released during the fibrinogen-fibrin conversion. Biochim. biophys. Acta (Amst.) **86**, 535 (1964).
OSHIMA, G., IWANAGA, S., SUZUKI, T.: Studies on snake venoms. XVIII. An improved method for purification of the proteinase b from the venom of *Agkistrodon halys blomhoffii* and its physicochemical properties. J. Biochem. **64**, 215 (1968a).
— MATSUO, Y., IWANAGA, S., SUZUKI, T.: Studies on snake venoms. XIX. Purification and some physicochemical properties of proteinase a and c from the venom of *Agkistrodon halys blomhoffii*. J. Biochem. **64**, 227 (1968b).
— SATO-OMORI, T., SUZUKI, T.: Distribution of proteinase, arginine-ester hydrolase and kinin releasing enzyme in various kinds of snake venoms. Toxicon **7**, 229 (1969).
PFLEIDERER, T., SUMYK, G.: Investigation of snake venoms enzyme. I. Separation of rattlesnake venom proteinases by cellulose ion-exchange chromatography. Biochim. biophys. Acta **51**, 482 (1961).
PIERCE, J. V., WEBSTER, M. E.: The purification and some properties of two different kallidinogens from human plasma. In: Hypotensive peptides, p. 130, ed. by E. G. ERDÖS, N. BACK and F. SICUTERI. Berlin-Heidelberg-New York: Springer 1966.
PRADO, J. L., PRADO, E. S., CATHARINA, M., BRANDI, W., KATCHBURIAN, A. V.: Some properties of highly purified horse urinary kallikrein. Ann. N.Y. Acad. Sci. **104**, 186 (1963).
RAUDONAT, H. W., ROCHA E SILVA, M.: Separation of the bradykinin releasing enzyme from the clotting factor in venom from *Bothrops jararaca*. Naunyn-Schmiedebergs Arch. exp. Path. Pharmak. **243**, 232 (1962).
ROCHA E SILVA, M.: Action de la trypsin sur l'utérus de cobaye. C. R. Soc. Biol. (Paris) **130**, 184 (1939a).
— Liberation de l'histamine par la perfusion du poumon de cobaye au moyen de la trypsine. C. R. Soc. Biol. (Paris) **130**, 186 (1939b).
— Beiträge zur Pharmakologie des Trypsins. I. Wirkung des Trypsins auf die glatten Muskeln des Dünndarms und die Gebärmutter von Säugetieren. Die Freisetzung von Histamin nach Durchströmung der Meerschweinchenlunge mit Trypsin. Naunyn-Schmiedebergs Arch. exp. Path. Pharmak. **194**, 335 (1940a).

Rocha e Silva, M.: Beiträge zur Pharmakologie des Trypsins. II. Wirkung des Trypsins auf den Blutkreislauf bei Katze, Kaninchen und Hund. Naunyn-Schmiedebergs Arch. exp. Path. Pharmak. **194**, 351 (1940b).
— Andrade, S.: Studies on dicoumarin-3,3′-methylene-*bis*-(4-hydroxycoumarin). II. Coagulant effect of snake venoms (from Bothrops and Crotalus) upon oxalated plasmas from normal and dicoumarin treated animals. Arch. Inst. Biol. **16**, 115 (1945).
— Beraldo, W. T., Rosenfeld, G.: Bradykinin, a hypotensive and smooth muscle stimulating factor released from plasma globulin by snake venoms and by trypsin. Amer. J. Physiol. **156**, 261 (1949).
Sarker, N. K., Devi, A.: Enzymes in snake venoms. In: Venomous animals and their venoms, p. 167, ed. by W. Bucherl, E. Buckley and V. Dirlofeu. New York 1968.
Satake, M., Murata, Y., Suzuki, T.: Studies on snake venoms. XIII. Chromatographic separation and properties of three proteinases from *Agkistrodon halys blomhoffii* venom. J. Biochem. **53**, 438 (1965).
Sato, T.: Unpublished observation (1965).
— Thesis, Faculty of Pharmaceutical Sciences, Kyoto Univ. (1968).
— Iwanaga, S., Mizushima, Y., Suzuki, T.: Studies on snake venoms. XV. Separation of arginine ester hydrolase of *Agkistrodon halys blomhoffii* venom into three enzymatic entities; "bradykinin releasing," "clotting" and "permeability increasing." J. Biochem. **57**, 151 (1965).
Schwer, G. H., Neurath, H., Kaufman, S., Snolke, J.: The specific esterase activity of trypsin. J. biol. Chem. **172**, 221 (1948).
Slotta, K.: Chemistry and biochemistry of snake venoms. Progr. Chem. Org. Nat. Prod. **12**, 406 (1955).
Suzuki, T., Iwanaga, S., Nagasawa, S., Sato, T.: Purification and properties of bradykininogen and of the bradykinin-releasing and -destroying enzymes in snake venom. In: Hypotensive peptides, p. 149, ed. by E. G. Erdös, N. Back and F. Sicuteri. Berlin-Heidelberg-New York: Springer 1966a.
— — Sato, T., Nagasawa, S., Kato, H., Yano, M.: Biochemical properties of kininogen and kinin releasing enzymes. In: Internat. Symposium on Vasoactive Polypeptides: Bradykinin and Related Kinins, p. 27, ed. by M. Rocha e Silva and H. A. Rothschild. São Paulo 1966b.
— Mizushima, Y., Sato, T., Iwanaga, S.: Purification of bovine bradykininogen. J. Biochem. **57**, 14 (1965).
Vogt, W.: Ein komplettes zweites kininbildendes System in menschlichem Plasma. Naunyn-Schmiedebergs Arch. exp. Path. Pharmak. **251**, 186 (1965).
— Untersuchungen zur Existenz zweier verschiedener kininbildender Systeme in menschlichem Plasma. Naunyn-Schmiedebergs Arch. exp. Path. Pharmak. **256**, 127 (1967).
Webster, M. E., Pierce, J. V.: Studies on plasma kallikrein and its relationship to plasmin. J. Pharmacol. exp. Ther. **130**, 484 (1960).
— — Action of the kallikreins on synthetic ester substrates. Proc. Soc. exp. Biol. (N.Y.) **107**, 186 (1961).
— — The nature of the kallidins released from human plasma by kallikreins and other enzymes. Ann. N.Y. Acad. Sci. **104**, 91 (1963).
Zeller, E. A.: Enzymes of snake venoms and their biological significance. Advanc. Enzymol. 8, 459 (1948).
— Enzymes as essential components of toxins. In: The proteins, 1st ed., vol. 1, p. 986, ed. by H. Neurath. New York 1951.
Zuber, H., Jaques, R.: Isolierung von Bradykinin aus Rinderplasma nach Einwirkung von Schlangengift (*Bothrops jararaca*). Helv. chim. Acta **43**, 1128 (1960).

Kallikrein Inhibitors

ROSMARIE VOGEL and EUGEN WERLE

With 3 Figures

A. Introduction

A system in the body having as potent a biological activity as the kininogenase-kinin system requires a regulating mechanism that limits the concentration of the active principles. The activity of kininogenases can be controlled either by blocking with inhibitors or by degradation with enzymes. Under normal conditions the system is regulated with remarkable precision; in pathological states the mechanism may be overwhelmed.

The inhibition of proteolytic enzymes by extracts of plants or animal tissues was first reported at the turn of the century. Around 1930 attempts were made to isolate and characterize the inhibitors. Kallikrein studies were already successful in these early years.

WERLE described the first experiments (p. 2 and 4) with the "inactivators" of kallikrein (FREY, 1927; KRAUT et al., 1928). At that time kallikrein was called a hormone. Since 1936, when WERLE found the enzymatic effect of kallikrein (WERLE et al., 1937), it has become obvious that the reversible "inactivation" of kallikrein could be compared to the actions of proteinase inhibitors, which were known at that time.

The general characteristics of the reactions of the proteinase inhibitors with the enzymes are: pH-dependent forming of an enzymatically inactive complex with the enzyme at a definite (frequently at a 1:1) molar ratio, rapid equilibrium of the reaction, and finally complete recovery of activity of the enzyme after splitting of the complex. The inhibitors block the active centers of the susceptible enzymes, thus preventing the degradation of the substrates, especially those of high molecular weight.

In most cases crude organ extracts were tested as potential kallikrein inhibitors. After thirty years of investigation it is obvious that the early selection of the inhibitor of bovine origin for intensive studies was the right approach.

Twenty years after the detection of the kallikrein inhibitors in plasma and bovine organs WERLE and co-workers tested all known trypsin inhibitors for their kallikrein-inhibiting capacity. At that time they used soybean (SBTI) and ovomucoid inhibitors (OMTI) and found that they inhibited plasma kallikrein selectively, thus enabling differentiation of plasma kallikrein from other kallikreins.

The therapeutic evaluation of proteinase inhibitors led to intensive attempts to study the occurrence, physiological importance, and similarities of mammalian and human inhibitors. One of the most important findings was the difference between the specific trypsin inhibitor of mammalian and human pancreas and the polyvalent inhibitor of bovine pancreas and other bovine organs (called Trasylol or Kunitz inhibitor). The difficulties in distinguishing the inhibitors isolated by different investigators were discussed in detail by VOGEL et al. (1966, 1968). Many proteinase inhibitors are very specific, especially as kallikrein

Table 1. *Inhibition spectra of the most important natural proteinase inhibitors*

Inhibitor Source	Trypsin	Chymo-trypsin	Kallikrein			Plasmin
			Plasma	Organ	Urine	
Soybean and lima bean	+	+	+	—	—	+
Ovomucoid	+	—	+	—	—	—
Urine, human	+	+	—	—	—	+
Serum, human						
α_1	+	+	—	—	—	—
Inter-α	+	—	—	—	—	—
α_2	+	+	—	—	—	+
Postalbumin	—	+	—	—	—	—
$\alpha+\beta$	—	—	+	+	+	—
Bovine organs						
Pancreas (Kunitz)	+	+	+	+	+	+
Parotid gland	+	+	+	+	+	+
Lung	+	+	+	+	+	+
Pancreas, mammalian	+	—	—	—	—	[illegible]
Submandibular gland, canine	+	+	—	—	—	—
Seminal vesicles						
Guinea pig	+	—	—	—	—	+
Bull I	+	—	—	—	—	+
Bull II	+	+	+	+	+	+

inhibitors. Therefore availability of a variety of pure inhibitors is a great help for the differentiation of the closely related kininogenases (Table 1).

Another possibility for regulation is offered by kallikrein-degrading enzymes. These "kallikreinases" are differentiated from natural inhibitors only by kinetic studies of the inactivation.

Antibodies to kallikrein are unknown in the native state. If natural inhibitors and immune bodies are compared with respect to the nature of the synthesizing system in the organism, there is a distinct difference: natural inhibitors are built up in accordance with a species-specific code; the antibodies are synthesized after repeated application of kallikrein. When the relatively high molecular weight of the kallikreins and the differences between several kallikreins became known, interesting studies of the immunological properties of the kallikreins developed.

Finally, because of the position of kallikrein among the peptide peptido-hydrolases, synthetic proteinase blockers were tested *in vitro* for inhibition of kallikreins. Many substances are called inhibitors of kallikrein, but a number first became known as inhibitors of trypsin or chymotrypsin. Among them are blocking agents for specific amino acids of the kallikrein molecule or blockers of the active center, and also substances which compete with the substrates of the enzyme and inhibit competitively. Although tested mainly *in vitro*, these blockers are of great interest in studying the pharmacological properties of the kininogenases, especially kallikrein.

B. Kallikrein Blocking Agents

Many inorganic and organic compounds of relatively low molecular weight block kallikreins. In most cases these substances were known first as blockers of some of the peptide-peptidohydrolases. Proteolytic and/or esterase activity is inhibited. So far as is known, the reactions are mostly irreversible, causing partial destruction. *In vivo* inhibition by some drugs may be a competitive inhibition of the receptors of the tissue, i.e. the receptors for the kinin effect.

1. Amino group blocking agents: ninhydrin, formaldehyde, benzaldehyde, phenylisocyanate, benzoylchloride, and ketene (BISCHOFF and ELLIOTT, 1937; WERLE and FLOSSDORF, 1938).

2. Amino- and hydroxyl-group reagents: benzoylchloride, ketene, acetic acid anhydride, diazomethane, dimethyl sulfate (WERLE and FLOSSDORF, 1938).

3. Serine blocking agents: diisopropylfluorphosphate (DFP) (HABERMANN, 1960, 1961a, b, 1962; WERLE and TRAUTSCHOLD, 1960; WEBSTER and PIERCE, 1961; HABERMANN and KLETT, 1966)[1]. It may be mentioned that prekallikrein is not inactivated by DFP (HABERMANN, 1962; KAGEN, 1964), the OH-group being masked as found with trypsinogen. Also kallikrein bound in the inhibitor complex cannot be blocked by DFP (HABERMANN, 1962).

4. Oxidizers: iodine, permanganate, hydrogen peroxide, methylene blue (WERLE, 1936; WERLE and APPEL, 1956).

5. Histidine-destroying reaction: treatment with ultraviolet rays (WERLE, 1936). Because of the finding that kallikrein bound in complex with bovine inhibitor is not destroyed, the inhibitor presumably masks this amino acid (WERLE and APPEL, 1956).

6. Sulfhydryl-group reagents: a) Low molecular weight thiols: cysteine, glutathione, and β-mercaptoethanol are inactivators only for plasma kallikrein (WERLE, 1936; WERLE et al., 1950b), but not for kallikrein from urine or tissues (WERLE, 1936). Plasma kallikrein also is blocked by thioglycolic acid (WERLE, unpublished). According to DAVIES and LOWE (1966) the kinin-liberating activity of plasma kallikrein is blocked whereas the esterase capacity is still active. The esterase activity of pancreas kallikrein is enhanced in presence of cysteine or thioglycolic acid (FIEDLER, 1968) or chelating agents (FIEDLER and WERLE, 1968) and in contrast blocked by

b) heavy metals (PRADO et al., 1965; FIEDLER, 1968; FIEDLER and WERLE, 1968).

7. Competitive inhibitors of natural substrates (kininogen) are used: synthetic substrates of kallikreins (WERLE and KAUFMANN-BOETSCH, 1959; TRAUTSCHOLD and WERLE, 1961; WEBSTER and PIERCE, 1961); benzamidine (DINIZ et al., 1965, 1966; BRANDI et al., 1966); benzoyl-L-arginine amide (WEBSTER and PIERCE, 1961).

8. Macroionic inhibition: heparin (MCCONNELL et al., 1965).

9. Various synthetic substances: ε-aminocaproic acid (EACA) (BACK and STEGER, 1968), 0,0-bis-(2-chloroethyl)-0-(2-dichlorovinyl) phosphate (WEBSTER and PIERCE, 1960); 1-chloro-3-tosylamido-7-amino-2-heptanone (TLCK) (BRANDI and PRADO, 1966) for inhibition of salmine splitting by hog plasma kallikrein, ineffective with pancreas kallikrein (FIEDLER, 1968) and rat urine kallikrein (MARES-GUIA et al., 1966; MARES-GUIA and DINIZ, 1967).

10. Anti-inflammatory drugs: salicylate, aspirin, indomethacin (probably acting as kinin receptor blockers) (GUTH, 1960; NORTHOVER and SUBRAMANIAN, 1961; SPECTOR and WILLOUGHBY, 1962, 1963; WALTER and WILLOUGHBY, 1965). Negative results also are reported (HEBBORN and SHAW, 1963; BERTELLI et al., 1965; DAVIES et al., 1966; ERDÖS et al., 1967) (see LEWIS, p. 516).

1. Bimolecular velocity constant of the inhibition at pH 7.2 = 7 ($1 \cdot mole^{-1} \cdot min^{-1}$). Analysis of [^{32}P] DFP-treated hog pancreas kallikrein identified one serine (of 17 found in the molecule) as phosphorylated (FIEDLER et al., 1968).

Table 2. *Immunochemical differentiation of kallikreins*[a]

Kallikrein antigen	Immune bodies against kallikrein from								
	Pancreas (pig)		Submandibular gland (pig)	Pancreas (man)		Urine (man)		Bronchial mucosa (man)	*Vipera amydotes* toxin
	[1]	[2]	[2]	[3]	[4]	[3]	[4]	[5]	[6]
Pancreas, pig	+++	+++	+	0		0			
Submandibular, pig		+	+++						
Plasma, pig	0								
Pancreas, man				+++	+++	+	0		
Urine, man				+	0	+++	+++		+
Urine, dog				0		0			
Bronchial mucosa, man								+++	
Submandibular, man								+++	

[a] 0 = no inactivation; + = inactivation; +++ = strong inactivation.

References: 1. HABERMANN, 1961a, 1963a, b; 2. VOGEL, 1968; 3. WEBSTER et al., 1963; 4. AUNGST et al., 1966; 5. HAVEZ et al., 1966a, b; 6. WERLE et al., 1951a.

C. Immune Bodies against Kallikreins

In 1961 HABERMANN reported that after repeated application of pig pancreas kallikrein, rabbits produce antibodies against this kallikrein. One ml serum inhibits 5–8 KU; after a longer period of immunization, up to 40 KU (HABERMANN, 1961a, 1962, 1963a, b). According to other authors (WEBSTER et al., 1963; AUNGST et al., 1966) immune bodies are also produced by rabbits against human kallikrein from urine and pancreas.

With kallikrein from pig pancreas and submandibular gland in the purest state available VOGEL (in FREY et al., 1968) immunized rabbits and achieved antibody serum levels equivalent to 2.5–10 KIU.

Also, kallikrein from bronchial mucosa evokes antibodies (HAVEZ et al., 1966a, b). According to VOGEL (in FREY et al., 1968) normal rabbit serum has a titer for kallikrein inhibition in the range of 0.2–1 KIU/ml. This inactivating capacity is due to the natural serum kallikrein inhibitor (see p. 225). Real kallikrein immune bodies may be distinguished from the serum kallikrein inhibitor by their stability against acetone, the inhibitor being precipitated and denatured by this procedure (WEBSTER et al., 1963).

The findings of these research groups result in the conclusion that the kallikreins are immunologically strongly specific. From the combined results (Table 2) it is obvious that immunological differentiation is not only reported among the kallikreins of different organs or body fluids but also that more distinct differentiation takes place in the mammalian species, i.e. at least in mammalian orders.

Various kallikreins from one species have lower titer values in the cross-over immunochemical reaction than are found with kallikreins from the same source in different species. The studies support the thesis that kallikreins are species-specific (VOGEL, 1968).

Inactivation of the kallikreins by DFP does not influence their antigenic properties (HABERMANN, 1961a, 1962). Probably the active center is not identical with the immunochemically important part of the kallikreins.

D. Natural Kallikrein Inhibitors

I. Units

1. KIU. On the basis of kallikrein inhibition the kallikrein inhibitor unit is defined as follows: one unit of the kallikrein-trypsin inhibitor of bovine origin (1 KIU) is the amount that inhibits 2 KU (pig pancreas kallikrein) by 50%, biologically determined under standard conditions (incubation for 15 minutes, pH 8, 37°) (WERLE and KAUFMANN-BOETSCH, 1960).

2. eIU. The enzymatic inhibitor unit (1 eIU) is the quantity of any natural inhibitor which inhibits the enzymatic activity of 2 KU by 50% under standard conditions (15-minute preincubation at optimal pH of enzyme reaction and 25°); i.e. that reduces the rate of splitting the substrate of kallikrein or other proteolytic-esterase enzymes by 1 μmole per minute under standard conditions (TRAUTSCHOLD, 1965; TRAUTSCHOLD et al., 1966a, b; VOGEL et al., 1966; FRITZ et al., 1968).

As most of the kallikrein inhibitors also inhibit trypsin, the definition of the enzymatic unit is important for comparative studies, not only in respect to the different inhibitors but especially for comparison of observations of different authors, most of whom use trypsin for the estimation of the inhibiting capacity. It is important to refer to the nature of the substrate used because of kinetic differences in presence of natural or synthetic substrates: rate and degree of inhibition (competitive or noncompetitive inhibition).

Other definitions of inhibitor units (especially for the polyvalent inhibitor of bovine origin) (GREEN, LASKOWSKI, and others) are given in Table 3. Most of the proposed definitions for the inhibitor capacity are based on the ratio of the weight of enzyme and inhibitor at which the inhibition is just 100%. However, the complex binding ratio is strictly proportional to the quantity of inhibitor only up to a certain degree of inhibition. Therefore the quantity of inhibitor required for 50% inhibition cannot be deduced from 100% inhibition.

Table 3. *Definitions of inhibitor units with special reference to the polyvalent proteinase inhibitor of bovine origin*

1 KIU	Amount of kallikrein-trypsin inhibitor of bovine origin which inhibits the biological activity of 2 U of kallikrein by 50% under specified conditions (references, p. 000)
1 eIU	Amount of any natural inhibitor for 50% inhibition of the enzymatic activity of 2 KU under standard conditions or for the 50% reduction of the rate of substrate splitting by kallikrein or other proteinases (1 μmole/minute under standard conditions) (references p. 217)
Specific activity	Quantity of enzyme inhibited 100% or approximately 100% by a specified quantity of inhibitor (e.g. 1 μg or 1 ml of a specified solution) (LASKOWSKI, JR. et al. 1952; LASKOWSKI et al., 1957; PEANASKY and LASKOWSKI, 1960; WU and LASKOWSKI, 1960; LEBOWITZ and LASKOWSKI, JR., 1962; KASSELL et al., 1963a; KASSELL 1964; KRESS and LASKOWSKI, 1967; see also review by VOGEL et al., 1966, 1968)
Enzyme ratio or inhibition quotient	Inhibition of a definite quantity of enzyme (e.g. 1 μg) to 100% or approximately 100% by a tested quantity of inhibitor (GREEN, 1957), for 50% inhibition (see TRAUTSCHOLD et al., 1963, 1964)
Kunitz inhibitor unit	Defined as the quantity of inhibitor that causes a decrease in extinction of 0.1/minute at 280 mμ during the cleavage of a natural substrate in trichloroacetic acid filtrate (KUNITZ, 1947a)

II. Methods of Determination

Principle. 1. The amount of inhibitor is indicated by the decrease of the enzyme activity (kallikrein or other kininogenases) in the presence of the inhibitor[2]. 2. In 1967 methods were published for direct immunochemical determination of the inhibitors independent of any enzyme.

For review of methods for estimation of proteinases (kininogenases) see VOGEL et al. (1966, 1968). For references to specific kallikrein inhibitor determination see Table 4.

2. Method for estimation of the polyvalent inhibitor from bovine organs and blood (TRAUTSCHOLD and WERLE, 1962): 5 ml of blood or supernatant of homogenized organs is mixed with the same volume of cold 6% (w/w) perchloric acid. After centrifugation a sample of the supernatant is adjusted to pH 7 with 2 N KOH. Within 10 minutes at 0° potassium perchlorate precipitates. After decantation, a sample of the supernatant is incubated with a definite amount of enzyme, and the remaining activity of the enzyme is tested. With BAEe as substrate for kallikrein, 1 inhibitor-milli-U causes the reduction of the change in extinction of $\Delta E_{253} = 0.000383$ at 50% inhibition (TRAUTSCHOLD, 1965).

Table 4. *Determination of naturally occurring kallikrein inhibitors*

Source of Inhibitors	Biological Method	Splitting of Synthetic Esters	Radio-immuno-chemical Method
Plant inhibitors, particularly Leguminosae	WERLE and MAIER (1952a, b) WERLE et al. (1951b) WERLE et al. (1959) WEBSTER and PIERCE (1963)	WEBSTER and PIERCE (1961)	
Inhibitors from blood serum	WERLE and MAIER (1952b) WEBSTER and PIERCE (1963)		
Inhibitor from colostrum	WERLE and TRAUT-SCHOLD (1960)		
Inhibitors from egg white	WERLE and MAIER (1952a) WEBSTER and PIERCE (1963)		
Inhibitor from bovine organs	WERLE and MAIER (1952b) WERLE et al. (1958) WERLE and APPEL (1958) APPEL and WERLE (1959) WEBSTER and PIERCE (1963)	WEBSTER and PIERCE (1961) WERLE et al. (1964) WERLE and KAUFMANN-BOETSCH (1960) WERLE and TRAUTSCHOLD (1961, 1963), TRAUT-SCHOLD and WERLE (1961, 1962)	HABERMANN et al. (1968)

III. Plant Inhibitors

In 1951 WERLE found an inhibitor for kallikrein in potatoes (WERLE et al., 1951b; WERLE and MAIER, 1952a). In 1952 WERLE reported that crystalline SBTI also inhibits plasma kallikrein (WERLE and MAIER, 1952b). These initial investigations already showed a specific inhibitor capacity for different kallikreins, a property characteristic of all kallikrein inhibitors except bovine inhibitor.

Leguminosae

Investigations of the last ten years suggest that all the leguminosae contain proteinase inhibitors, only some of them known also as inhibitors of kallikrein.

Inhibitor from Soybean (SBTI). As shown in Table 5, the commercial crystalline salt-free inhibitor is not homogeneous when tested after using modern purification methods. Different charges also contain different impurities (OZAWA and LASKOWSKI, JR., 1966). Therefore the physicochemical constants obtained by various authors differ over a relatively wide range. (For physicochemical properties and constants of SBTI see reviews by VOGEL et al., 1966, 1968.) SBTI is the only inhibitor of a relatively high molecular weight (mean value 22,000) without a carbohydrate component. The inhibitor is sensitive against extreme pH values and is heat unstable: both reactions of denaturation are reversible in a wide range if pH is changed at normal temperature or temperature is elevated in neutral media. SBTI is rapidly degraded by pepsin (KASSELL and LASKOWSKI, 1956) but is not destroyed by trypsin and chymotrypsin.

The amino acid composition of pure SBTI preparations is shown in Table 6. The N-terminal amino acid is aspartic acid (NEURATH and DAVIE, 1954; DAVIE

Table 5. *Isolation of soybean inhibitor*

Methods	Fractions	Reference
Marketed salt-free product: extraction with aqueous acid; adsorption on bentonite; elution with pyridine; fractional precipitation with acid; recrystallization from water and dilute ethanol		KUNITZ (1946, 1947a, b), LASKOWSKI (1955)
Electrophoresis, paper chromatography	5	STRÄSSLE (1960), WINTERSTEIN and STRÄSSLE (1962)
Physicochemical analysis	1	JIRGENSONS et al., (1960)
Electrophoresis in polyacrylamidgel	3—4	STEINER (1966), FRATTALI and STEINER (1968)
Chromatography on Sephadex	2	OZAWA and LASKOWSKI, JR. (1966)
Electrophoresis in polyacrylamidgel	6	ELDRIDGE et al. (1966)
Chromatography on DEAE-cellulose and rechromatography	4	RACKIS et al., (1959, 1962), RACKIS (1963), RACKIS and ANDERSON (1964)

Table 6. *Amino acid composition of plant inhibitors*[a]

Amino Acid	Soybean Inhibitor		Lima Bean Inhibitor		
	[1]	[2]	[3]	[4]	[5]
Lys	10.7	11	6.1	4.0— 4.6	4
His	2.0	2	5.4	4.1— 5.4	3—6
Arg	9.3	10	4.1	2.3	2
Asp	28.9	28	16.0	12.4—15.1	12—14
Thr	8.3	8	5.3	4.2— 4.8	3—5
Ser	13.3	12	13.5	12.0—13.4	12—15
Glu	21.2	21	8.7	5.8— 6.5	5—7
Pro	10.2	10	8.5	6.7—11.4	6—7
Gly	18.4	18	0.4	0.87— 0.98	0—1
Ala	9.2	9	1.9	2.7— 4.0	3—4
Cys $^1/_2$	4.0	4	16.5	13.0—13.8	12—16
Val	11.6	15	1.5	0.81—1.7	1
Met	2.6	2	—	—	—
Ile	13.8	15	7.0	3.6— 4.1	4—5
Leu	15.6	16	4.9	3.5— 3.7	3
Tyr	4.1	4	1.7	1.2— 1.5	1—2
Phe	9.0	9	3.1	1.2— 2.2	1—2
Try	1.7	8	—	0.16— 0.41	—
Amid N	13.6	—	0.92	3.5— 6.5	4—5
Amin N	25.8	—	0.83	—	—
Total N	251.1	—	16.2	15.65—15.78	—

[a] Numbers in parentheses at top of columns refer to the following units and sources: 1. Moles/21,500 gm protein (WU and SCHERAGA, 1962a). 2. Moles/mole inhibitor (OZAWA and LASKOWSKI, JR., 1966). 3. Per cent (FRAENKEL-CONRAT et al., 1952). 4. Moles/10,000 gm (JIRGENSONS et al., 1960). 5. Moles/mole inhibitor (JONES et al., 1963).

and NEURATH, 1955; RACKIS and ANDERSON, 1964); the C-terminal residue is leucine (NEURATH and DAVIE, 1954; DAVIE and NEURATH, 1955). Partial sequences of the molecule are known (see reviews by VOGEL et al., 1966, 1968), especially the sequence around the two disulfide bridges, the possible active center (BROWN et al., 1966) (Fig. 1). From physicochemical studies it is concluded that the molecule has a random coil structure occasionally interrupted by an organized structure consisting of helices (Wu and Scheraga, 1962b). A partial α-helical formation was found in high-percentage propanol solution (Jirgensons, 1967).

Inhibition of kallikrein. SBTI inhibits only the bradykinin liberation by plasma kallikrein activated by acetone or enzymes, whereas the liberation of kallidin by kallikreins from organs and urine is unaffected. This observation, first published by Werle and Maier (1952b) is confirmed by all later publications. The only exceptions are the partial inhibition of the kallikreins of sweat glands (Werle, 1964b), of the intestinal wall and brain of mammals (Werle and Vogel, 1961), and of carcinoid tumors (Melmon et al., 1965; Oates and Melmon, 1966). SBTI inhibits the hypotensive effect of plasma kallikrein (Werle

H$_2$N-Glu-Arg-Cys-Pro-Leu-Thr-COOH
|
H$_2$N-(Try)-Leu-Cys-Val-Gly-Ile-Pro-Thr-Glu-COOH

(I)

H$_2$N-Val-Phe-Cys-Pro-Gln-Gln-Ala
| |
HOOC-Gly-Ile-Asp-Gly-Cys-Lys-Asp-Asp-Glu

(II)

Fig. 1. Possible active center of soybean trypsin inhibitor. (After Brown et al., 1966)

and Maier, 1952a; Werle et al., 1952; Werle and Kaufmann-Boetsch, 1960; Werle and Vogel, 1960; Werle, 1960, 1962; Webster and Pierce, 1961; Werle and Trautschold, 1963).

According to Werle and Kaufmann-Boetsch (1959, 1960), Habermann (1959), Webster and Pierce (1961), and Chambers et al. (1963), the esterase activity of plasma kallikrein also is inhibited, although four times as much SBTI is required as for inhibition of proteolytic cleavage (Webster and Pierce, 1961). The kininogenase of plasma is affected *in vitro* and *in vivo* (Rocha e Silva, 1951; Schachter, 1956; Bhoola et al., 1960; Werle and Trautschold, 1960; Prado and Prado, 1961; Prado et al., 1963; Back and Steger, 1968) and *in vivo* according to Werle and Vogel (1961) by pretreatment of the animals with SBTI.

Table 7 shows the origin of all kallikreins tested with SBTI and the specific references. It should be noted that all the investigations are made with commercial SBTI preparations. Only one of the homogeneous fractions referred to in Table 5 was tested for kallikrein inhibition (the inhibitor fraction of Birk), though differences in inhibition spectrum could be shown. The activity of SBTI fraction from Birk resembles that of lima bean inhibitor (Back and Steger, 1968).

Relatively early Beraldo found, without any knowledge of the nature of the kininogenase, that SBTI inhibits the liberation of kinins in peptone shock, and improves the pathologic state (Beraldo, 1950). The importance and expansion of these early experiments are discussed later (see p. 559).

Inhibition of other enzymes (kininogenases) of the kinin system. Soybean inhibitor is primarily known as trypsin inhibitor. The inhibition of trypsin affects the proteolytic, esterase, and kininogenase (Rocha e Silva, 1951) activities of trypsin. Studies of the formation of the trypsin–SBTI complex have been made over a wide range, and many kinetic facts about this reaction and the inhibitor complex are known (for references, see reviews by Vogel et al., 1966, 1968).

Table 7. *Kallikrein inhibition spectrum of plant inhibitors*

Inhibitors	Source of Kallikrein												
	Serum			Pancreas			GI Tract	Submandibular Gland			Urine		
	man	bov.	pig	man	bov.	pig	dog	man	bov.	pig	man	pig	horse
Soybean	+ [1]	± [2]	+ [3]	− [1,4]	− [1]	− [5]	+ [6]	− [2]	− [1]	− [5]	− [11]		− [7]
Lima bean	+ [8, 9]			(−) [9]							+ [9]	− [10]	
Potato, crude extract	+ [1]				+ [1]	+ [11]			+ [1]		+ [1]		
Potato, trypsin inhibitor	− [8]												
Beet			+ [12]			+ [12]				− [13]	− [13]		

References: 1. Werle and Maier, 1952b; 2. Schachter, 1956; 3. Bhoola and Schachter, 1959; 4. Webster and Pierce, 1961; 5. Werle et al., 1952; 6. Werle and Vogel, 1961; 7. Brandi et al., 1966; 8. Mason and Sparrow, 1965; 9. Back and Steger, 1968; 10. Chambers et al., 1963; 11. Werle and Trautschold, 1963; 12. Vogel, in Vogel et al., 1966; 13. Werle et al., 1951b.

Only the most important study is referred to here: the trypsin-binding reaction consisting of the cleavage of a special "susceptible bond" of the inhibitor by the enzyme with subsequent formation of a covalent bond between enzyme and inhibitor. If the complex is split, the inhibitor structure is partially modified as the active center proved by LASKOWSKI is cleaved (FINKENSTADT and LASKOWSKI JR., 1965, 1967; FINKENSTADT et al., 1965; OZAWA and LASKOWSKI JR., 1966; HIXSON JR., et al., 1967). With benzoyl-L-arginine-ethyl ester as substrate, 1 µg SBTI inhibits 1.3 µg trypsin (mean value; the values referred to are between 0.5 and 2.3 µg trypsin inhibited, depending on the purity of the enzyme and inhibitor preparations).

Inhibition of the other factors see Table 8. Administration of SBTI (i.p.) protects rabbits against lethal doses of trypsin (BOWMAN, 1954; JAQUES, 1957).

Table 8. *Inhibition of kininogenases (except kallikrein and trypsin) by soybean inhibitor*

Enzyme or Activator	Inhibition of Activity		References
Plasmin	protease	+	KLINE and FISHMAN (1961)
	esterase	+	MARKUS and WERKHEISER (1962)
	[kininogenase	+]	SCHACHTER (1956), EISEN and KEELE (1960)
Hageman factor	esterase	—	SCHOENMAKERS et al. (1964)
Snake venom	kininogenase	—	HAMBERG and ROCHA E SILVA (1957)
	esterase	—	HABERMANN (1959), SUZUKI et al. (1966), TU et al. (1966)
C'1-Esterase	esterase	—	RATNOFF and LEPOW (1957)
PF/dil	esterase	+	MILES and WILHELM (1960)
Cellulose sulfate	kininogenase	+	ROTHSCHILD (1966)
Spontaneous (dilution of plasma)	kininogenase	+	SCHACHTER (1956, 1960)

+ = Inhibition; — = no inhibition.

Inhibitor from Lima Beans (Phaseolus lunatus). Besides SBTI, the lima bean inhibitor is the only other Leguminosa inhibitor that has been investigated for kallikrein inhibition. It is unknown whether other isolated Leguminosae inhibitors (e.g. beans, peas, lucerne, lentils, peanuts) inhibit kallikrein.

Lima bean inhibitor is marketed as an amorphous preparation (method of FRAENKEL-CONRAT et al., 1952). Like SBTI it is not homogeneous and can be fractionated chromatographically into four to six active fractions (JIRGENSONS et al., 1960; JONES et al., 1963; HAYNES and FEENEY, 1967). The amino acid composition of different fractions is similar (Table 6), particularly with regard to the high cystine content. The stability toward proteolytic enzymes including pepsin, acids, and heat, is characteristic for proteins with the low molecular weight of 9,000 from lima bean inhibitor; for constants see VOGEL et al. (1966, 1968).

The inhibition spectrum of this substance, so far as is known, is similar to that of SBTI. According to MASON and SPARROW (1965), acetone activated plasma kallikrein is inhibited. BACK and STEGER (1968) were unable to confirm this. Also, NAGASAWA et al. (1967) report no inhibitory effect for glass-activated kallikrein. A permeability factor is inhibited (MASON and SPARROW, 1965), whereas pig urinary kallikrein (CHAMBERS et al., 1963), human pancreatic kallikrein, and human urinary kallikrein (BACK and STEGER, 1968) are not affected.

Inhibition spectrum for other kininogenases. The molar inhibition quotient of lima bean inhibitor for trypsin is approximately 1:1(RYAN et al., 1965). Inhibition of plasmin is described by MAXWELL et al. (1964).

Proteinase Inhibitors from Potatoes (Solanum tuberosum)

According to WERLE (WERLE et al., 1951b, 1955; WERLE and MAIER, 1952a; WERLE, 1962; TRAUTSCHOLD et al., 1964) crude potato extracts inhibit all kallikreins. The kallikrein inhibitor has been partially purified by fractional precipitation with ammonium sulfate. This inhibitor is not dialyzable and is stable to acid (WERLE et al., 1951b), but is unstable to heat (WERLE and MAIER, 1952a). The optimal pH for inhibition covers a wide range (between 5 and 9). In a more acid medium the complex dissociates quickly (WERLE et al., 1959). Depending on the type and the season, potatoes contain 10 to 40 KIU/g fresh weight (WERLE et al., 1951b, 1959).

Besides the kallikrein inhibitor, the existence of a distinct inhibitor for trypsin was postulated by WERLE and described by MANSFELD, who separated chromatographically three fractions with different inhibitory capacities for trypsin, chymotrypsin, and plasmin (RÁBEK and MANSFELD, 1963). The fraction with the highest trypsin–chymotrypsin inhibitory capacity also inhibits kallikrein, though, like SBTI, it inhibits only acetone-activated plasma kallikrein (MASON and SPARROW, 1965; LOGAN and WILHELM, 1966).

Inhibitor from Beet (Beta vulgaris)

Another proteinase inhibitor, with the highest concentration in the root, was found by VOGEL in beetroot and sugarbeet (VOGEL et al., 1966). The inhibitor was purified by precipitation with ammonium sulfate and column chromatography. The inhibitor is stable to acid, unstable to heat. It is precipitated by trichloroacetic acid, degraded by pepsin, and not dialyzable. From these properties, it is concluded that the substance has a high molecular weight (like SBTI); it inhibits kallikreins from pancreas and serum, and also trypsin. Kallikreins from urine and submandibular gland are not inhibited.

Physiological Importance

While the occurrence of proteinase inhibitors in animal organisms can be explained by their regulatory function, especially of the kininogenase–kinin system, their occurrence in plants is a matter of speculation. MANSFELD et al. (1959) suggest their importance lies in maintaining the latent life of the plant by suppressing the proteolytic autolysis.

We consider the plant inhibitors in combination with the specific features of Leguminosae, potatoes, and beets. They exist in symbiosis with *Bacterium radicicola* or *Azotobacter*. The inhibitors may be present for protection against proteolytic attack by the symbionts, or in general they may prevent the plant from being overrun by the symbionts (VOGEL et al., 1966).

In other species, inhibitor activity is found only in the seeds; it disappears during germination. Therefore the proteolytic processes are probably halted in the resting state of the seed. No function explains the inhibition of kallikrein, an enzyme not found in plants. We suppose that the inhibition of kallikrein is an accidental property due to the polyvalent inhibition capacity of the plant inhibitors. It may be based, e.g., on the similarities of the active centers of the proteolytic-esterase enzymes of plants and animals.

IV. Inhibitors of Animal and Human Origin

Inhibitors from Blood Serum

Kallikrein Inhibitors. Kallikrein administered *in vivo* causes a quickly transient decrease in systemic blood pressure. For the fast normalization of the blood pressure five reasons may be important: sympathetic contra-regulation, degradation of the pharmacologically active kinins, enzymatic destruction and inhibition of kallikrein by natural serum inhibitor(s), and escape of kinins into the interstitial space. With the knowledge of the importance of the kinins, studies of all parts of this reaction were intensified, and it was finally confirmed that the reactions together give the pharmacological result.

All serums studied so far (of cold-blooded and warm-blooded animals) inhibit kallikreins from any origin (KRAUT et al., 1928; WERLE et al., 1952; WERLE and APPEL, 1958, 1959), though quantitative differences have been observed (WERLE and MAIER, 1952b; WEBSTER and PIERCE, 1960, 1961; BACK et al., 1963; MORIYA et al., 1965; VOGEL et al., 1966). Hemolymph of snails and celom fluid of Ascaris also have inhibitory capacity for kallikrein (APPEL, 1957; WERLE et al., 1958; WERLE and APPEL, 1959); 1 ml serum contains 1–5 KIU dependent on the species (WERLE and APPEL, 1958). For inhibition see Table 9.

It is obvious that at least some sera contain two inhibitory principles for kallikrein. Horse serum contains two kallikrein inhibitors, one with optimal pH$>$7, the other $<$7. The latter is one of the rare serum inhibitors that inhibit only distinct kallikreins (WERLE, in FREY et al., 1968). According to PASKHINA and SHIMONAEVA (1967) rabbit serum also contains two kallikrein inhibitors. A kallikrein inhibitor of bovine serum isolated chromatographically inhibits serum kallikrein but not pancreas kallikrein (HABERMANN and KLETT, 1966; HABERMANN, 1968). According to HABERMANN, this inhibitor may be identical with the inhibitor isolated and crystallized by WU and LASKOWSKI (1960) that inhibits kallikrein in addition to other proteinases (WEBSTER and PIERCE, 1960; BACK et al., 1963).

In human serum two inhibitory principles were postulated (WERLE, 1955) and confirmed by kinetic studies of kallikrein inhibition (TRAUTSCHOLD et al., 1966a; TRAUTSCHOLD et al., in VOGEL et al., 1966). One inhibitor causes instantaneous inhibition of 2–3 KU/ml serum after 10-minute incubation; the other inhibitory substance inactivates 3–4 KU/ml serum during 5 hours. The latter principle is destroyed when heated for 1 hour at 56°. The separation and identification of both these principles are difficult because of their low concentration in serum, their minimal polar properties, and their high lability (FRITZ et al., 1968); fractionation on DEAE-Sephadex results in separation of α_1-fraction with immediate inhibition and a slow reacting α_2-fraction.

According to the kinetic studies, the slow-reacting factor may be a kallikreinase, i.e. a kallikrein-destroying enzyme; also kallikrein cannot be reactivated completely after splitting the complex (see p. 239). According to WERLE and VOGEL (1960), trypsin does not displace kallikrein from the complex with kallikrein serum inhibitor even after hours of incubation.

The kallikrein inhibitors are not identical with any of the numerous specific proteinase inhibitors isolated from human serum; e.g. the serum trypsin inhibitors obtained by SCHULTZE et al. (1962) in highly purified state do not inhibit kallikrein even in large excess (WERLE et al., 1964; TRAUTSCHOLD et al., in VOGEL et al., 1966; see Table 1).

According to KAGEN and BECKER (1963), BECKER and KAGEN (1964), and KAGEN (1964), a factor concentrated from human serum by LEVY and LEPOW

Table 9. *Kallikrein inhibition spectrum of colostrum and human and animal blood*

Inhibitors	Source of Kallikrein												
	Serum		Pancreas				Submandibular Gland			Urine			
	man	pig	man	pig	dog	bird	pig	dog	cat	man	pig	dog	rat
Colostrum		+ [1]					+ [1]			+ [1]			
Serum													
Man, unfractionated	A + [2] B + [3]		+ [3]	+ [4]	+ [5]	+ [16]	+ [4]	+ [2]	+ [2]	+ [6]			+ [9]
Trypsin inhibitors	— [7]			— [8]			— [8]				— [8]		
Cattle	B + [3]	+ [10]		— [10]						+ [11]			
Horse				+ [16]			+ [16]						
Rabbit			+ [12]	+ [13]						+ [12]		+ [12]	
Rat				+ [14]						+ [9]			
Bird						+ [16]				— [16]			
Cold-blooded animals				+ [15]			+ [15]			+ [15]			

A = enzymatically activated; B = acetone activated.

References: 1. WERLE and TRAUTSCHOLD, 1960; 2. WERLE, 1936; 3. WEBSTER and PIERCE, 1960; 4. WERLE and TRAUTSCHOLD, 1963; 5. WERLE, 1934; 6. WERLE and TRAUTSCHOLD, 1966; 7. VOGEL et al., 1966; 8. WERLE et al., 1964; 9. WERLE and VOGEL, 1960; 10. HABERMANN and KLETT, 1966; 11. HORTON and LEWIS, 1959; 12. WEBSTER et al., 1963; 13. STEVENS and FEENEY 1963; 14. MORIYA et al., 1965; 15. WERLE et al., 1952; 16. WERLE and HÜRTER, 1936.

(1959) and PENSKY et al. (1961), especially inhibiting C′1-esterase, also inhibits kallikrein. BECKER and KAGEN discuss the identity with one of the kallikrein inhibitors and with the inhibitor of the permeability factor PF/dil from MILES and WILHELM (1955). Colostrum contains an inhibitor for kallikrein that resembles the serum kallikrein inhibitor (WERLE and TRAUTSCHOLD, 1960; see Table 9).

Inhibition of other Kininogenases and Plasmin. Especially in human serum great numbers of proteinase inhibitors are well known, isolated in high purity, and characterized in detail. Some inhibitors are polyvalent, others strongly specific for a single proteinase (Table 1). Ninety per cent of the trypsin inhibiting capacity is characterized as α_1-globulin (JAKOBSSON, 1955; SCHULTZE et al., 1955; DYCE and HAVERBACK, 1960); 1 ml serum inhibits 0.4–1.9 mg trypsin by 100% (for literature see VOGEL et al., 1968).

Many methods are published for the isolation of the different inhibitors and are referred to by VOGEL et al. (1968). One method mentioned here is useful for the simultaneous separation of four inhibitors (SCHWICK et al., 1966): α_1-trypsin inhibitor, α_2-macroglobulin plasmin-trypsin inhibitor, the inter-α-trypsin inhibitor, and the α_1-chymotrypsin inhibitor. After fractionating serum with ammonium sulfate and rivanol, the inhibitors are resolved by zone electrophoresis, column chromatography, and ultracentrifugation. At the end of this purification process the inhibitors are in an immunologically and ultracentrifugally pure state. For constants see reviews by VOGEL et al. (1966, 1968). Serum of cold-blooded and warm-blooded animals also inhibits trypsin (review of LASKOWSKI and LASKOWSKI, JR., 1954; NAKAMURA and WAKEYAMA, 1961), but only the inhibitors of cattle and sheep serum are partly purified. Kininogenase from snake venom is not inhibited by human serum (WERLE et al., 1950a).

Physiological Importance. As mentioned earlier, intravenous administration of kallikrein causes a transient fall in blood pressure. According to WERLE (1953) trypsin acts on the dog circulation in concentrations several orders of magnitude higher than kallikrein. *In vivo* injections of trypsin lead to liberation of bradykinin and to activation of kallikrein; the latter liberates bradykinin. So bradykinin is the pharmacologically active agent after trypsin injection (WERLE et al., 1955; WERLE, 1963). The quantitative difference between the pharmacological actions elicited by kallikrein and trypsin is caused by the different quantities of inhibitors circulating in blood. The concentration of trypsin inhibitor is 860–1,260 ImU/ml, of kallikrein inhibitor 0.5–3 ImU/ml (VOGEL et al., 1966). The role of inhibitors in physiological regulation of kinin liberation is obvious from these experimental findings. Local, minimal activation of kininogenases is blocked instantaneously.

It should be mentioned again that plasma kallikrein is pharmacologically inactive in the native form (see WERLE, p. 3), this state being a precursor of the enzyme and not a kallikrein serum inhibitor complex. Securing the circulation against uncontrolled kinin liberation is of such great importance that for each kininogenase several independent natural inhibitors are present in the circulating blood. Still it is impossible to prevent overproduction of kinins. Here the therapeutic use of the polyvalent inhibitor is indicated.

Pathophysiology. According to WERLE and VOGEL (1960) experimental injury of the kidney tubules is followed by excretion of the serum inhibitor in urine; 1 ml urine inhibits about 0.5 U kallikrein. In the normal state, urine contains no inhibitor of kallikrein, only inhibitor of trypsin, this inhibition being due to the main serum trypsin inhibitor (FAARVANG and LAURITSEN, 1962, 1963, 1964). A change in the kallikrein inhibitor level of the serum is reported during surgical intervention (VOGEL and KALIAMPETSOS, 1959; WERLE et al., 1962).

According to Donaldson (1966), the level of C′1-inhibitor that also inhibits kallikrein is decreased in the last weeks of pregnancy, increased in hypertension and uremia.

Confirmation that the synthesis of serum proteinase inhibitors is controlled by genes is provided by the genetic absence of serum proteinase inhibitors. In hereditary angioneurotic edema the kallikrein-inhibiting capacity is decreased (Landermann et al., 1962; Becker and Kagen, 1964; Webster and Innerfield, 1965); also the inhibiting capacity for C′1-esterase (Donaldson and Evans, 1963; Donaldson and Rosen, 1964; Charache et al., 1964; Burdon et al., 1965). It is obvious that gene mutation causes the partial loss of inhibitor synthesis (see also the section on Pathophysiology above).

Egg White Inhibitors

Whole Egg White. It has been known for many years that native egg white possesses inhibitory capacity against a great number of proteinases. Egg white from chicken and duck eggs reversibly inhibits human urinary kallikrein (Werle et al., 1954) and enzymatically activated plasma kallikrein (Werle and Maier, 1952b), but pancreas kallikrein from man (Webster and Pierce, 1963) or pig (Werle et al., 1954) is not inhibited. It is not known how ornitho-kallikrein reacts to egg white inhibitor. One ml egg white inhibits 10–60 KIU. The inhibitor which has not been concentrated is unstable to heat and to acids (Werle et al., 1954).

Table 10. *Amino acid composition of mammalian inhibitor*[a]

Amino Acid	Ovomucoid Chicken		Bovine Organs Pancreas (Kunitz)	Parotid gland	Lung		Liver
	1	2	3	4	4	5	6
Lys	4.1	4.10	4	8	8	4.00	4
His	1.38	1.56	—	—	—	—	—
Arg	2.1	1.92	6	9	9	6.01	6
Asp	9.8	9.52	5	8	8	4.99	5
Thr	4.6	4.53	3	5	5	2.98	3
Ser	4.0	3.55	1	3	2	1.03	1
Glu	4.4	4.71	3	5	5	3.00	3
Pro	2.36	2.03	4	9	8	3.90	4
Gly	5.1	4.94	6	10	10	6.08	6
Ala	2.6	3.56	6	10	11	5.87	6
Cys $^1/_2$	5.5	5.84	6	8	8	5.81	6
Val	5.1	5.00	1	2	2	1.00	1
Met	1.76	1.51	1	2	2	0.90	1
Ile	1.1	1.07	2	2	3	1.76	2
Leu	3.9	3.66	2	3	3	1.97	2
Tyr	1.76	1.90	4	4	5	3.63	4
Phe	1.76	1.51	4	6	7	3.74	4
Try	<0.15	<0.15	—	—	—	—	—
Amino-N			—	13	11	4.92	—

[a] The numbers above the columns indicate units and references as follows: 1. Moles/10,000 gm protein (Lewis et al., 1950). 2. Moles/10,000 gm protein (Stevens and Feeney, 1963). 3. Moles/mole inhibitor (Kassell et al., 1963a). 4. Moles/mole inhibitor (Kraut and Bhargava, 1964). 5. Moles/mole inhibitor (Anderer and Hörnle, 1965). 6. Moles/mole inhibitor (Fritz et al., 1967).

Table 11. *Kallikrein inhibition spectrum of egg white inhibitors*

Inhibitors	Source of Kallikrein											
	Serum		Pancreas			Submandibular Gland			Urine			
	man	pig	man	bov.	pig	man	bov.	pig	man	pig	horse	rat
Egg white	A+ [4] B− [4]		− [2]		− [5]				+ [5]			
Ovomucoid	A+ [1] B− [2]	A+ [3] B− [4]	− [4]	− [4]	− [5]	− [6]	− [4]	− [7]	− [4]	− [8]	− [9]	− [10]

A = enzymatically activated; B = acetone activated.

References: 1. Werle and Vogel, 1958; 2. Webster and Pierce, 1963; 3. Trautschold et al., 1964; 4. Werle and Maier, 1952b; 5. Werle et al., 1954; 6. Schachter, 1956; 7. Werle et al., 1952; 8. Chambers et al., 1963; 9. Prado and Prado, 1961; 10. Werle and Vogel, 1960.

Ovomucoid. One fraction of egg white, the so-called ovomucoid (OMTI), has been well known for a long time as an inhibitor. Isolation methods for an amorphous product were referred to by LINEWEAVER and MURRAY in 1947 and FREDERICQ and DEUTSCH in 1949, and a variant of these methods yields the marketed product. For other inhibitors the technical product can be separated electrophoretically and chromatographically into three active fractions (for methods of isolation and fractionation and for physicochemical constants see reviews by VOGEL et al., 1966, 1968).

For amino acid composition of ovomucoid, see Table 10. Ovomucoid is a mucoprotein with 10–20% average carbohydrate content (for review see ADAM-CHOSSON and MONTREUIL, 1965). LASKOWSKI postulates for ovomucoid as for other inhibitors a Lys-X bridge in the active center (OZAWA and LASKOWSKI, JR., 1966). Ovomucoid is degraded by pepsin (KASSELL and LASKOWSKI, 1956).

WERLE and MAIER (1952b) observed that commercially produced ovomucoid inhibited only the enzymatically activated plasma kallikrein. WERLE and co-authors tested the inhibition of the plasma kallikreins from man and cattle. Many authors acknowledged the lack of inhibition of all other kallikreins (see Table 11). The separated ovomucoid fractions have not yet been tested for plasma kallikrein inhibition. The trypsin-kallikrein inhibitor ovomucoid is heat stable (to 56°) and acid stable (2 hours at pH 1.5) (JIRGENSONS et al., 1960). By these means the specific kallikrein inhibitor of egg white and ovomucoid can be differentiated, the kallikrein inhibitor being destroyed as is the serum kallikrein inhibitor.

Inhibition of other kininogenases. One μg of ovomucoid inhibits 0.25 or 0.36 μg trypsin by 50% (JUSTISZ et al., 1957; BANGA and MAYLATH-PALAGYI, 1963). Ovomucoid inhibits trypsin from mammals and birds (VITHAYATHIL et al., 1961; RYAN et al., 1965), but human trypsin is not inhibited even by a large excess of inhibitor (BUCK et al., 1962a). No inhibitory effect is observed against plasmin (CLEMENTE, 1957; SCHULTZ, 1959; MANSFELD et al., 1960; BHOOLA et al., 1960) or against the permeability factor (MASON and SPARROW, 1965).

Physiological Importance. The similarity between the egg white and the serum inhibitors is remarkable. It may be that the similarity is caused by excretion of the serum inhibitor in the egg as a protective mechanism against unspecific proteolytic reactions during the hatching process. During brooding the concentration of the egg white inhibitor remains unchanged (COHEN and BALLS, 1955).

The Polyvalent Inhibitor in Bovine Organs and Body Fluids

The polyvalent bovine inhibitor is the most important of the discussed kallikrein inhibitors because of its possible therapeutic use. In 1929 WERLE and co-workers FREY and KRAUT found a kallikrein-inhibiting substance in lymph nodes, parotid gland, spleen, liver, and spinal marrow of cattle (BAUER et al., 1929; KRAUT et al., 1930). Lung and pancreas contain the inhibitor in the highest concentration of the whole organism (WERLE and APPEL, 1959). The inhibitor is also found in the vesicular glands and semen of the bull (HAENDLE et al., 1965a, b). In other species of bovines and the goat family the inhibitor is found mainly in the spleen. So far as determined, the occurrence in ruminants is shown in Table 12.

In 1936 KUNITZ and NORTHROP isolated an inhibitor for trypsin from bovine pancreas. For the next thirty years the substance of FREY, KRAUT, and WERLE and the substance of KUNITZ were studied along parallel lines by different research teams. A plasmin inhibitor from bovine lung described first by ASTRUP (1950) also belongs here.

Table 12. *Occurrrence of the kallikrein trypsin inhibitor in ruminants (KIE/gm)* [a]

	Liver	Spleen	Lung	Mucosa Trachea	Mucosa Esophagus Stomach	Intestinal Tract	Seminal Vesicle [b]
Cattle	200—400	40—100	1,500	+	80—120	200—250	120—180
Sheep	0	50—160	70			120—160	
Goat	100	10—90	0				
Chamois	0						
Stag		75—100					
Roe		0—50	0				
Reindeer	0		0				
Elk	0						

	Pancreas	Parotis	Kidney	Lymph Nodes	Thyroid	Colostrum
Cattle	200—600	400	80—200	80—800	400—800	2—7
Sheep	0	10—50			15	
Goat				10		
Chamois						
Stag		0—10		10		
Roe						
Reindeer						
Elk						

[a] Werle and Appel, 1959; Werle, 1964a.
[b] Haendle, unpublished.

In 1967 it was concluded that the three substances are identical because of findings that the inhibitor for kallikrein also inhibits trypsin and chymotrypsin (Werle et al., 1952) and plasmin (Marx et al., 1959). Astrup (1952a, b) and Astrup and Albrechtsen (1957) referred to the trypsin and chymotrypsin inhibiting capacity of the plasmin inhibitor. On the other side Trautschold and Werle (Trautschold, 1960; Trautschold and Werle, 1961) and Webster and Pierce (1961) reported that the Kunitz inhibitor also inhibits kallikrein.

Besides having identical spectra, the inhibitors were finally proven identical by crystallization, ultraviolet absorption spectra, and by structure (Kraut et al., 1963; Kraut and Bhargava, 1964; Anderer, 1965a, b; Anderer and Hörnle, 1966, 1968; Nissen and Astrup, 1966; Werle et al., 1967).

The discovery of the trypsin inhibitor by Kunitz provided the incentive for many experimental studies of its physiological role since it was assumed that this inhibitor occurs in all mammals including man. It should be pointed out that the uncritical acceplance of many authors of the occurrence of the Kunitz inhibitor in the pancreas of all mammals resulted in erroneous theories of its physiological function and in the discussion of its possible therapeutic use.

Isolation. The various research groups independently developed methods for isolation of the polyvalent inhibitor (for review see Table 13). The process of Kunitz formed the basis for the isolation of the commercial preparation. According to Scevola et al. (1962) and Avineri et al. (1963) Kunitz preparations can be resolved into two inhibitor fractions, whose purity at the same time is doubled. Jeanteur and Fournier (1965) reported that the commercial product can be resolved chromatographically into one active and three inactive fractions. In the crystalline state, also after chromatographic purification, the activity of 1 KIU corresponds to 0.14–0.15 μg of organic substance (Schultz et al., 1963; Kraut et al., 1963; Schultz, 1967; Werle et al., 1967).

Table 13. *Isolation methods for the polyvalent inhibitor of bovine organs*

Material of bovine organism	Isolation method	Specific activity U/mg protein	References
Lymph nodes; parotid gland crude material	Extraction with acetic acid; fractionation with ethanol or acetone; precipitation with picrolonic acid	500—1,000 KIU	KRAUT et al. (1930), WERLE, in FREY et al. (1950)
Lymph nodes, spleen crude material	Deproteinization with trichloroacetic acid		GARDNER et al. (1944)
Parotis crude material	Deproteinization with alcohol; fractionation by preparative high volt electrophoresis	5,000 KIU	KRAUT and KOERBEL-ENKHARDT (1957, 1958)
Parotis commercial product	Spontaneous crystallization of the free base	7,100 KIU	SCHULTZ (1967)
Liver crude material	Deproteinization with trichloroacetic acid; fractionation with ammonium sulfate; precipitation with picric acid; chromatography with Amberlite IRC-50; purification on kieselguhr, paper chromatography; paper electrophoresis	2,000 KIU	WERLE and APPEL (1959)
Liver crude material	Cation exchange-chromatography with P-cellulose; fractionation on Sephadex G-50 bound in trypsin complex; splitting of the complex (6% perchloric acid); desalination	6,450 KIU	WERLE et al. (1967)
Liver crude material	Trypsin resin column chromatography	3.28 TIU	WERLE et al. (1967), FRITZ et al. (1967)
Lung crude material	Thiocyanate extract; deproteinization (thiosalicylic acid); precipitation with tungstic acid; fractionation with ethanol		ASTRUP and STAGE (1956)
Lung or liver crude material	Deproteinization with methanol and calcium chloride; adsorption on kieselguhr; precipitation with acetone; elution, fractionation, and gradient elution on CM-and SE-cellulose	7,500—10,000 KIU	TRAUTSCHOLD (1965), TRAUTSCHOLD et al. (1966a)
Pancreas crude material	Complex binding with trypsin; cleavage with trichloroacetic acid; crystallization with magnesium sulfate	180 Kunitz U	KUNITZ and NORTHROP (1936) see review LASKOWSKI (1955)
Pancreas crude material	Trypsin inhibitor complex; column chromatography on Dowex 1-X 2; splitting by dialysis against HCl; fractionation on Sephadex G-50, Amberlite XE-64	3.3—3.7 TIU	KASSELL et al. (1963a, b)
Pancreas; fraction from insulin isolation	Deproteinization with trichloroacetic acid at 80°	220 Kunitz U	GREEN and WORK (1953)
Pancreas commercial product	Chromatography on CM-cellulose	192.8 U (F.I.P.)	SACH et al. (1965)
Pancreas crude material	Deproteinization with perchloric acid; chromatography on chymotrypsin-maleic acid ethylene copolymer		FRITZ et al. (1966)

The commercial products of the polyvalent inhibitor of bovine origin are Trasylol, Zymofren, Iniprol, and Contrycal. Many patents have been obtained for their isolation on an industrial scale.

Properties. The polyvalent inhibitor is characterized by a high stability against acid and heat (KUNITZ and NORTHROP, 1936). Only 50% of its activity is lost on heating for one hour at 100° (TRAUTSCHOLD, 1965). If a suspension of crystallized inhibitor (pH 10) is heated to 60°, the crystals dissolve; above 63° irreversible coagulation takes place (SCHULTZ, 1967). The stability decreases with increasing alkalinity. The inactivation is reversible up to pH 11 (TRAUTSCHOLD et al., 1966b). In solution with higher pH the inhibitor is destroyed irreversibly. Modification of the molecule is seen in a change of the absorption spectrum (TRAUTSCHOLD, 1965). The inhibitor is stable against proteolytic enzymes (KUNITZ and NORTHROP, 1936; KRAUT and KOERBEL-ENKHARDT, 1958; DLOUHÁ et al., 1966; KRAUT and BHARGAVA, 1967a). No enzyme is known to degrade the native inhibitor (AUHAGEN, 1967). The inhibitor can be degraded by proteinases only after oxidation with performic acid (CHAUVET et al., 1964; DLOUHÁ et al., 1965b) or reduction and carboxymethylation (KASSELL et al., 1965; KASSELL and LASKOWSKI, 1966). For constants see Table 14.

Table 14. *Constants of the bovine inhibitor*

Constant	Value	Reference
Isoelectric point	pH 10 10.5	GREEN and WORK (1953) CHAUVET et al. (1964), TRAUTSCHOLD (1965)
Molecular weight	Osmotic pressure 6,500; inhibitor-trypsin relation 6,500; amino acid composition 6,511; sedimentation and diffusion constant 11,600—11,700	KUNITZ and NORTHROP (1936) GREEN and WORK (1953) (see Table 6) KRAUT et al. (1960)
	Sephadex G-25 molecular sieve 6,700 ± 200	ANDERER and HÖRNLE (1965), TRAUTSCHOLD (1965), FRITZ et al. (1965), SCHOLTAN and LIE (1966)
	Native inhibitor: sedimentation and diffusion constant 10,300—11,800	ANDERER and HÖRNLE (1965)
Sedimentation constant, pH 7	$s_{20w} = 1.28$—1.32 S 1.0 S	KRAUT et al. (1960) BUCK et al. (1962b)
Diffusion constant	15.2—11.0 $cm^2\ sec^{-1}$	KRAUT et al. (1960)
Specific rotation	$[\alpha]_{578}$ pH 7.4 = 116	SCHOLTAN and ROSENKRANZ (1966)
Dispersion constant	$\lambda_c = 234$	SCHOLTAN and ROSENKRANZ (1966)
Ultraviolet absorption spectrum, pH 5.9	maximum: 280 mμ minimum: 250 mμ	TRAUTSCHOLD (1965)

The molecular form of the native inhibitor has not yet been fully elucidated. If the molecular weight 6,511 from the amino acid composition is taken as basis, the inhibitor must be present largely as a dimeric aggregate, the mean molecular weight of 10,300 to 11,800 being attributed to the presence of a small amount of the monomeric compound. Already fractionation on Sephadex results in dissociation to the monomer (TRAUTSCHOLD, 1965; FRITZ et al., 1965). At the isoelectric point (pH 10.5) the higher molecular weight decreases to the value of 6,500, found also in 8 M urea. The high molecular weight is not changed by the addition of small amounts of urea, mercaptoethanol, or formic acid (ANDERER and HÖRNLE, 1965). ANDERER suggested cross-linking by an agent of low molecular weight which is not yet identified (ANDERER and HÖRNLE, 1965). In the complex with enzyme the inhibitor is bound in the monomeric state.

From SCHOLTAN's investigation of the sedimentation, diffusion, and viscosity, it can be seen that the molecule is not at all globular (SCHOLTAN and LIE, 1966). From the optical rotatory dispersion and values for circular dichroism it follows that there is no α-helix structure although the inhibitor has a partly organized structure (tested by Cotton effect) (SCHOLTAN and ROSENKRANZ, 1966). The

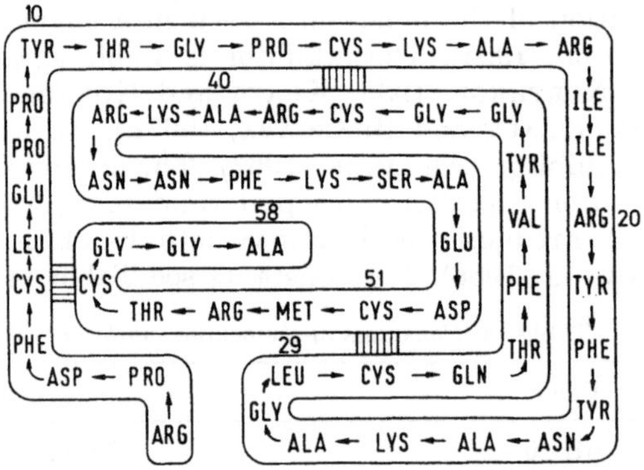

Fig. 2. A schematic representation of the structure of the kallikrein-trypsin inhibitor. (After KASSELL and CHOW, 1966)

covalent structure is postulated to be a compact molecule because of the high stability against proteolytic enzymes and degradation (CHAUVET and ACHER, 1967c).

Structural Analysis. The amino acid composition of the Kunitz inhibitor was determined by GREEN and WORK (1953) and KASSELL et al. (1963a). The inhibitor preparations isolated from lung and parotis were analyzed by KRAUT and BHARGAVA (1964), the inhibitor from liver by FRITZ et al. (1967). The results agree qualitatively, although it must be assumed that the Kunitz preparation still contains impurities. For amino acid composition see Table 10. The inhibitor contains no histidine or tryptophan.

The amino acid sequence of the inhibitors of parotid gland and lung of cattle is the same as that for the pancreas trypsin inhibitor (KUNITZ). Sequence analyses were published first by CHAUVET et al. (1964) for the Kunitz inhibitor (CHAUVET et al., 1966a, b; CHAUVET and ACHER, 1966a). ŠORM and co-workers reported the same amino acid sequence, yet constructed from 57 amino acids, the isoleucine in position 19 being absent (DLOUHÁ et al., 1965a, b). KASSELL et al. (1965b), ANDERER (1965b), and ANDERER and HÖRNLE (1966) gave identical analyses for the sequence of the commercial preparations from WORTHINGTON and BAYER (see Fig. 2). (For discussion of the results see the review of VOGEL et al., 1968.)

The positions of the S-S bridges have also been established. LASKOWSKI and ANDERER agree in the conclusion the three S-S bridges join the half cystine residues in positions 5 and 55, 14 and 38, and 30 and 51 (see Fig. 2) (KASSELL and LASKOWSKI, 1965b, 1966; KASSELL and CHOW, 1966; ANDERER and HÖRNLE, 1966; DLOUHÁ et al., 1966; CHAUVET and ACHER, 1967c; ACHER and CHAUVET, 1967).

Many investigations examine the active center. Changes in the molecule concerning methionine (KASSELL, 1964), tyrosine (SHERMAN and KASSELL, 1967), serine (KASSELL and LASKOWSKI, 1965a) and four lysines (KASSELL and CHOW, 1966; CHAUVET and ACHER, 1967b) are without effect on the inhibitor activity. Lys^{15} participates in the complex binding (CHAUVET and ACHER, 1967a). Acetylation and methylation of the inhibitor lead to almost complete loss of inhibiting activity, for the carboxyl and primary amino groups are involved in binding of the enzyme. Reduction in acidic solution leads to loss of the inhibiting capacity, pointing to the role of cysteine residues (GREEN and NEURATH, 1954).

Remarkable results are reported by ANDERER and LASKOWSKI: after reduction of the S-S bridges and slow reoxidation with atmospheric oxygen, the inhibitory activity lost by reduction is reacquired, the S-S bridges being in the same position as before (ANDERER and HÖRNLE, 1965). The degree of reactivation depends on the nature of the reducing agent (ANDERER and HÖRNLE, 1966). Selective reduction of the S-S bridge linking the half cystines 14 and 38 results in no loss of the activity. The reduction of more than one disulfide bond results in a loss of the activity (KRESS and LASKOWSKI, 1967). Complex binding of trypsin with the partially reduced inhibitor and the following oxidation result in a missing reoxidation of the inhibitor.

According to CHAUVET and ACHER (1967a) and ACHER et al. (1968) the amino end-group of the inhibitor is not involved in the active center but several of the lysine ε-NH_2 groups. Shortening of the chain (modified method according to the Edman technique) results in the loss of one arginine and a modified inhibitor with 92% activity of the intact guanidinated inhibitor. The elongation at the N-terminal end of the inhibitor chain results in a product with 88% of the inhibitor capacity of the native inhibitor. Blockade of the α-amino group leads to the reduction of the inhibitory activity to 7%. It is therefore concluded that the inhibitor capacity will not be changed if the fixed alanine chain has two residues, but the inhibiting capacity is lost if the chain is elongated by 12 or 13 residues (CHAUVET and ACHER, 1967; ACHER et al., 1968). The activity is also lost by blocking the end groups (ANDERER, personal communication). From the conclusions drawn in the case of SBTI and OMTI, LASKOWSKI JR. postulated a Lys-X bridge in the active center of the bovine inhibitor (OZAWA and LASKOWSKI JR., 1966).

Inhibition of Kallikrein. The inhibitor affects the hypotensive, esterase, and kininogenase activities of most of the kallikreins. The inhibition spectrum is shown in Table 15. The complex formation is a reversible reaction (FREY et al., 1950; WERLE et al., 1951b; WERLE and MAIER, 1952b). On the basis of the definition, 1 KIU inhibits 2 KU by 50%; i.e. 0.17 μg inhibitor inhibits 1.6 μg kallikrein by 50%. The molecular weight of the kallikrein inhibitor complex determined by gel filtration on Sephadex is 39,500 (calculated 49,500) (FRITZ et al., 1965).

A remarkable specificity exists with respect to the mammalian species, though it should be emphasized that these observations cannot be generalized for all kallikrein activities. The studies of esterase activity and reaction on isolated organs (of plasma kallikrein) are not completed.

Changes in the active center of the kallikreins (e.g. destruction by acid or alkaline solution, ultraviolet irradiation, oxidation, or phosphorylation with DFP) leads to hindrance of complex binding. Complex binding in turn protects the enzyme against inactivation by irradiation and by DFP (WERLE and APPEL, 1956; WERLE and TRAUTSCHOLD, 1963). Plasma kallikrein is inhibited three

Table 15. *Kallikrein inhibition spectrum of the polyvalent bovine inhibitor*

Source of Kallikrein	Inhibition	Reference
Man		
Serum	+	WERLE et al. (1955)
Pancreas	+	WEBSTER and PIERCE (1961)
Submandibular	+	VOGEL (1968)
Urine	+	WERLE et al. (1937)
Ox		
Serum	+	VOGEL (1968)
Pancreas	+	WEBSTER and PIERCE (1961)
Submandibular	+	WERLE and MAIER (1952b)
Urine	+	VOGEL (1968)
Pig		
Serum	+	BRANDI et al. (1966)
Pancreas	+	WERLE et al. (1937)
Submandibular	+	VOGEL (1968)
Urine	+	WERLE et al. (1937)
Horse		
Serum	+	BRANDI et al. (1966)
Urine	+	PRADO et al. (1963)
Dog		
Serum	(+)	VOGEL (1968)
Pancreas	—	WERLE (1934)
Submandibular	—	WERLE (1936)
Urine	—	KRAUT et al. (1934)
Gastrointestinal Tract	+	WERLE and VOGEL (1961)
Cat		
Submandibular	—	WERLE (1936)
Urine	—	KRAUT et al. (1934)
Rat		
Serum	(+)	VOGEL (1968)
Pancreas	—	WERLE and TRAUTSCHOLD (1966)
Submandibular	— Kininogenase	VOGEL (1968)
	+ Esterase	ERDÖS et al. (1968)
Urine	—	VOGEL (1968)
Mouse		
Serum	(+)	VOGEL (1968)
Pancreas	—	VOGEL (1968)
Submandibular	—	VOGEL (1968)
Urine	—	VOGEL (1968)
Guinea Pig		
Serum	(+)	VOGEL (1968)
Pancreas	—	VOGEL (1968)
Submandibular	—	VOGEL (1968)
Urine	—	VOGEL (1968)
Bird		
Pancreas	+	WERLE, in FREY et al. (1950)

times more by the borine inhibitor than by SBTI (WEBSTER and PIERCE, 1961). The inhibition is greater with synthetic ester substrates than with natural substrates (WERLE and KAUFMANN-BOETSCH, 1960). The complex binding reaction is characterized by the fact that total inhibition cannot be achieved even with a large excess of inhibitor (TRAUTSCHOLD and WERLE, 1961). This incomplete inhibition (maximum 95% at an inhibitor–enzyme ratio of 6 KIU/1 KU) is explained by the relatively high dissociation constant of the kallikrein inhibitor complex. (At pH 7.8 $K_i = 1.2 \times 10^{-8}$ mole/liter; at pH 4.0 the complex is completely dissociated; TRAUTSCHOLD, 1965).

The equilibrium of the reaction depends on the pH of the medium. The maximal velocity of the reaction lies in the range of pH 8, the velocity falling quickly as the pH becomes acid. The pH optimum of the reaction indicates that the inhibitor combines with the enzyme only as the free base. The degree of inhibition increases linearly up to 80% with increasing inhibitor concentration. The inhibition of kallikrein is not instantaneous: at 33% inhibition the reaction reaches equilibrium after 2 minutes, for 55% inhibition after 3 minutes (TRAUTSCHOLD, 1965). The reaction is noncompetitive and proceeds independently of the nature of the substrate.

A solution of the kallikrein inhibitor complex obtained from the pure components contains up to 5% of the kallikrein in unbound form. Such a preparation represents a depot of kallikrein from which active kallikrein is split off after intravenous administration. The splitting of the complex has been demonstrated *in vivo* by pharmacological methods, especially by observing a prolonged depressor effect (GOLENHOFEN et al., 1958; KRONEBERG, personal communication). This observation is the basis of the application of Complex-Padutin.

Inhibition Spectrum of Other Kininogenases and Plasmin. The inhibition of trypsin, chymotrypsin, and plasmin led to the name of *polyvalent inhibitor* for the bovine inhibitor.

Trypsin-inhibiting capacity: the Kunitz-Green preparation inhibits 1 mg trypsin per 0.242 ± 0.005 mg inhibitor (GREEN, 1957). A preparation of LASKOWSKI inhibits 3.3 to 3.7 parts by weight of trypsin (KASSELL et al., 1963a). The inhibition is competitive (JEANTEUR and FOURNIER, 1965). As in the reaction with kallikrein, equilibrium is reached only after 20 minutes (GREEN, 1957). For reaction constants see the review of VOGEL et al. (1968). As with kallikrein, the activity of trypsin toward the natural substrate kininogen is inhibited (WERLE and TRAUTSCHOLD, 1960; BANASZKIEWICZ and CHODERA, 1963). Porcine and bovine trypsin are bound in equal ratios (KRAUT and BHARGAVA, 1967b).

For comparing the various units used, the following values on the basis of trypsin inhibition in TIU (trypsin inhibitor units) and ImU (inhibitor milliunits) are given: 1 KIU = 0.56 ImU, 1 TIU = 0.75 KIU, or 1 KIU = 1.33 TIU (VOGEL et al., 1966).

The reaction with trypsin is stoichiometric, i.e. the molar ratio is 1:1. The reaction is linear up to 90–95% with increasing inhibitor concentration (TRAUTSCHOLD et al., 1966b; SCHOLTAN, 1967). The inhibition is competitive if inhibitor and substrate are added to the enzyme at the same time, but it is noncompetitive if the complex formation takes place without the addition of the synthetic substrate (TRAUTSCHOLD, 1965). On the basis of a molecular radius of 20 Å for trypsin and 13 Å for the inhibitor, AUHAGEN proposed a contact zone having a radius of 7 Å, corresponding to five amino acids (AUHAGEN, 1967). The molecular weight of the complex determined by gel filtration on Sephadex is 26,000 (calculated 30,300) (FRITZ et al., 1965) with sedimentation analysis $30{,}500 \pm 1{,}000$ (SCHOLTAN, 1967).

In a mixture of kallikrein and trypsin the complex binding of kallikrein occurs first (KRAUT and KOERBEL-ENKHARDT, 1958; SINGH and HOWARD, 1965). However, after incubation for 24–48 hours, more trypsin than kallikrein is bound (TRAUTSCHOLD, 1965). This deviation is a result of the different dissociation contants of the complexes formed. For the binding of trypsin, chymotrypsin, and kallikrein the same active center of the inhibitor is responsible (KRAUT and BHARGAVA, 1967c).

Other kininogenases: the bovine inhibitor also inhibits the kinin-liberating activity of snake venom (Iwanaga et al., 1965; Sugino, 1965) and the permeability factor (Burke et al., 1964).

Plasmin: According to the observation of Astrup, the extracts of bovine lung inhibit fibrinolysis (Astrup, 1950). The inhibition of pure plasmin by the substance from Astrup was referred to in 1966 by Egeblad and Astrup. The different commercial preparations inhibit the fibrinolytic, caseinolytic, and esterase action of streptokinase-activated plasmin (Hladovec et al., 1958;

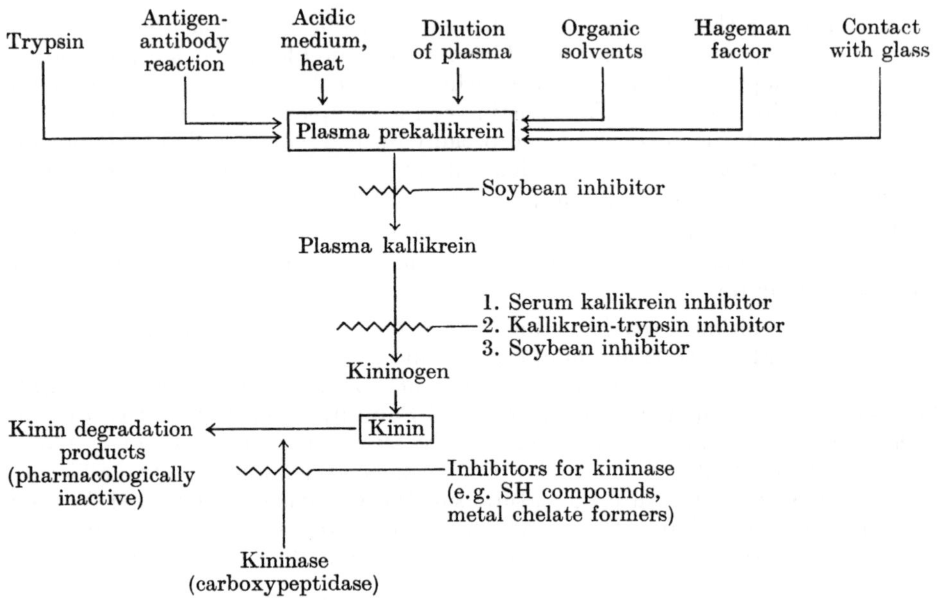

Fig. 3. Mechanism of the liberation and inactivation of kinins in plasma. (From Vogel et al., 1966)

Marx et al., 1959; Soulier, 1959, 1962; Benzer et al., 1960; Mansfeld et al., 1960; Soulier et al., 1960; Marx and Henning, 1962; Schmutzler and Beck, 1962; Berghoff and Glatzel, 1963; de Barbieri et al., 1964; Godal and Theodor, 1965; Maxwell et al., 1965; Beller, 1966; Maki and Beller, 1966). 1 μg bovine inhibitor inhibits 38.4 μg plasmin Novo; i.e. 1 KIU inhibits 6 μg plasmin (1.7 μg enzyme protein corresponds to 1 mU). The inhibition was measured by the splitting of synthetic substrate (Vogel et al., 1966). The effect on streptokinase and the related activator system has not been studied in detail (for review see Gross and Kroneberg, 1966).

Fibrinolysis is inhibited not only *in vitro* but also *in vivo* (Marx et al., 1959; Marggraf, 1961; Steichele and Herschlein, 1961, 1962; Marx, 1962; Gibelli et al., 1964; Schulz, 1965; Ferrauto et al., 1965a, b; Verstraete et al., 1965; Encke et al., 1966; Mann, 1966; Markwardt et al., 1966; Larsen et al., 1966; Mammen, 1968; Ambrus, et al. 1968). The inhibition of clotting is also observed by an inhibitor preparation from liver (Marx et al., 1959, 1963).

Physiological Importance: The polyvalent inhibitor is not secreted into pancreatic juice, saliva, or semen. This is in contrast to other inhibitors from pancreas, submandibular gland, and seminal vesicles. The inhibitor is not detectable in blood (Frey et al., 1950; Werle, 1964a). Therefore it is concluded that the function of the inhibitor must be endocellular. The unknown function probably is not connected with the fundamental biochemical processes of cells since the inhibitor appears only in bovines, and in bovine organs only after birth (WERLE, 1964a). We assume that the function of the inhibitor is related to the specificities of the ruminant species. It may be thought that the inhibitor plays some role in the more complicated digestion system of ruminants and the special growth of bacteria and protozoa in their gastrointestinal tract (VOGEL et al., 1966). According to LASKOWSKI (1968), all tissues containing the inhibitor must contain proteolytic systems, the equilibrium with the inhibitor contributing to the function of these systems. But since the inhibitor also occurs in tissues which possess no enzymes accessible to the inhibitor action (WERLE, 1964b), we discuss defense against the free motile protozoa of the rumen and their metabolites. ASTRUP proposes that the absence of certain diseases of the respiratory tract among cattle is attributable to the presence of the inhibitor (ASTRUP, 1968).

Pharmacology and Therapeutical Purposes. The pharmacological properties of the polyvalent bovine inhibitor and its application in therapy of pathological states connected with the kinin system are discussed later, see p. 550. Fig. 3 gives a scheme for the liberation of kinins and shows the points of attack of various inhibitors.

D. Kallikrein-destroying Enzymes

In mammalian serum, enzymes exist for kallikrein inactivation or destruction — the so-called kallikreinases. Years ago they were postulated by WERLE and co-workers from kinetic data differentiating real inhibitors and possible kallikrein-destroying enzymes in horse serum or human serum. These factors are described as "slow-reacting" inhibitors (see p. 225). The "complex-binding" reaction is temperature dependent, and so far as is known, is irreversible. Kinetic measurements indicate that it could involve enzymatic degradation of kallikrein.

In 1968 WERLE and SCHMAL found that 1 ml of rat serum is able to degrade hundreds of kallikrein units. Repeated addition of kallikrein invokes a repeated turnover. The range of kallikrein degradation by rat serum is not seen in other mammalian serums and cannot be attributed to a real kallikrein inhibitor. Most likely the kallikrein-destroying principle is an enzyme, which could be enriched to some degree by conventional methods.

Only kallikrein from plasma is destroyed by trypsin, pepsin, papain, and proteinases from mould fungus. The other kallikreins are resistant to proteolytic degradation, with the exception of pancreas kallikrein which is destroyed by pepsin (WERLE and MAIER, 1952b; WERLE, in FREY et al., 1968).

References[3]

ACHER, R., CHAUVET, J.: La structure covalente d'un polypeptide pancréatique inhibiteur de la trypsine. Bull. Soc. Chim. Fr. 3954 (1967).

— — ARMAN, R., SELA, M.: Préparation et propriétés de dérivés poly-DL-alanylés d'un inhibiteur de la trypsine (inhibiteur de Kunitz et Northrop). Europ. J. Biochem. **3**, 476 (1968).

ADAM-CHOSSON, A., MONTREUIL, J.: Glycoproteins. X. Structure of oligosides isolated from ovomucoid partial hydrolysates. Bull. Soc. Chim. biol. (Paris) **47**, 1881 (1965).

AMBRUS, C. M., AMBRUS, J. L., LASSMAN, H. B., MINK, I. B.: Studies on the mechanism of action of inhibitors of the fibrinolysin system. Ann. N.Y. Acad. Sci. **146**, 430 (1968).

3. Literature references included up to Spring of 1968.

ANDERER, F. A.: Zur Identität des Kallikrein-Inaktivators aus Rinderlunge und Rinderparotis. Z. Naturforsch. **20b**, 499 (1965a).
— Strukturuntersuchungen am Kallikrein-Inaktivator aus Rinderlunge. II. Bestimmung der Aminosäuresequenz. Z. Naturforsch. **20b**, 462 (1965b).
— HÖRNLE, S.: Strukturuntersuchungen am Kallikrein-Inaktivator aus Rinderlunge. I. Molekulargewicht, Endgruppenanalyse und Aminosäure-Zusammensetzung. Z. Naturforsch. **20b**, 457 (1965).
— — The disulfide linkages in kallikrein inactivator of bovine lung. J. biol. Chem. **241**, 1568 (1966).
— — Chemical studies on kallikrein inactivator from bovine lung and parotid gland. Ann. N.Y. Acad. Sci. **146**, 381 (1968).
APPEL, W.: Darstellung und Charakterisierung eines einheitlichen, kristallinen, natürlich vorkommenden bifunktionellen Hemmkörpers für Trypsin und das Kreislaufhormon Kallikrein. Diss. Naturwiss. Fakultät, Techn. Hochschule, München, 1957.
— WERLE, E.: Über einen Hemmkörper für Kallikrein und verschiedene Proteinasen aus Rinderleber. III. Z. Naturforsch. **14b**, 648 (1959).
ASTRUP, T.: A proteolytic inhibitor in lung tissue. 18th Int. Physiol. Congr. Copenhagen, Abstr. p. 81, 1950.
— Ox lung tissue as a proteolytic inhibitor. Acta physiol. scand. **26**, 243 (1952a).
— Fibrinolysis. Acta haemat. (Basel) **7**, 271 (1952b).
— Comparative studies of some antifibrinolytic agents and proteinase inhibitors. Ann. N.Y. Acad. Sci. **146**, 601 (1968).
— ALBRECHTSEN, O. K.: Estimation of the plasminogen activator and the trypsin inhibitor in animal and human tissue. Scand. J. clin. Lab. Invest. **9**, 233 (1957).
— STAGE, A.: A protease inhibitor in ox lung tissue. Acta chem. scand. **10**, 617 (1956).
AUHAGEN, E.: Chimica e biochimica del Trasylol. In: Drugs of animal origin, p. 69, ed. by A. LEONARDI and J. WALSH. Milan 1967.
AUNGST, C. W., BACK, N., BARLOW, B., TSUKADA, G. A.: Immunologic studies of components of the kallikrein-kinin system. In: Hypotensive Peptides, ed. by E. G. ERDÖS, N. BACK, and F. SICUTERI. Berlin-Heidelberg-New York: Springer 1966.
AVINERI, R., BLAUER, G., RIGBI, M.: Studies on the pancreatic trypsin inhibitor and its interaction with trypsin. Israel J. Chem. **1**, 199 (1963).
AVINERI-GOLDMAN, R., SNIR, I., BLAUER, G., RIGBI, M.: Studies on the basic trypsin inhibitor of bovine pancreas and its interaction with trypsin. Arch. Biochem. **121**, 107 (1967).
BACK, N., GUTH, P. S., MUNSON, A. E.: On the relationship between plasmin and kinin. Ann. N.Y. Acad. Sci. **104**, 53 (1963).
— STEGER, R.: Effects of inhibitors on kinin releasing activity of proteases. Fed. Proc. **27**, 96 (1968).
BANASZKIEWICZ, W., CHODERA, A.: Effect of Trasylol on the vascular reaction to kallikrein. Acta physiol. pol. **14**, 431 (1963).
BANGA, I., MAYLATH-PALÁGYI, J.: Effect of inhibitors on the activity of trypsin and collagen mucoproteinase. Acta physiol. Acad. Sci. hung. **24**, 151 (1963).
BARBIERI, A. DE, SCEVOLA, M. E., FRANCHINI, M.: Antiplasmin activity of pancreatic trypsin inhibitor and ε-aminocaproic acid. Boll. chim. farm. **103**, 37 (1964).
BAUER, E., FREY, E. K., KRAUT, H., SCHULTZ, F., WERLE, E.: Über neue Funktionen von Pankreas und Lymphdrüsen. Naturwissenschaften **17**, 672 (1929).
BECKER, E. L., KAGEN, L. J.: The permeability globulins of human serum and the biochemical mechanism of hereditary angioneurotic edema. Ann. N.Y. Acad. Sci. **116**, 866 (1964).
BELLER, F. K., GÖSSWALD, R. K.: Zur Inhibitionswirkung von Proteinaseninhibitoren auf Plasmin und Urokinase. In: Neue Aspekte der Trasyloltherapie, p. 161, ed. by R. GROSS and G. KRONEBERG. Stuttgart 1966.
BENZER, H., BLÜMEL, G., PIZA, F.: Einflüsse von Trypsininhibitoren auf die Blutgerinnung. Wien. med. Wschr. **110**, 609 (1960).
BERALDO, W. T.: Formation of bradykinin in anaphylactic and peptone shock. Amer. J. Physiol. **163**, 283 (1950).
BERGHOFF, A., GLATZEL, H.: Über die Hemmung des fibrinolytischen Potentials durch Trasylol. Med. Klin. **58**, 476 (1963).
BERTELLI, A., CERRATI, A., DONATI, L., ROSSANO, M. A.: Attivitá antipeptidasica di farmaci entireazionali. Atti Accad. med. lombarda **20**, 442 (1965).
BHOOLA, K. D., CALLE, J. D., SCHACHTER, M.: The effect of bradykinin, serum kallikrein and other endogenous substances on capillary permeability in the guinea-pig. J. Physiol. (Lond.) **152**, 75 (1960).
— SCHACHTER, M.: A comparison of serum kallikrein, bradykinin and histamine on capillary permeability in the guinea-pig. J. Physiol. (Lond.) **149**, 80P (1959).
BISCHOFF, F., ELLIOTT, A. H.: Chemical studies of callicrein. J. biol. Chem. **117**, 7 (1937).

BOWMAN, E.: Influence of bean trypsin inhibitors on thromboplastic properties of trypsin. Proc. Soc. exp. Biol. (N.Y.) **86**, 491 (1954).
BRANDI, C. M. W., MENDES, J., PAIVA, A. C. M., PRADO, E. S.: Proteolysis of salmine by horse urinary kallikrein. Biochem. Pharmacol. **14**, 1665 (1965).
— PRADO, E. S.: Proteolysis of salmine by three kallikreins and the effect of some inhibitors. III. Internat. Symposium on Vasoactive Polypeptides. Sao Paulo 1966.
— RONCADA, M. J., PRADO, E. S., PRADO, J. L.: Observations on the hydrolysis of salmine by kallikreins. III. Internat. Symposium on Vasoactive Polypeptides. Sao Paulo 1966.
BROWN, J. R., LERMAN, N., BOHAK, Z.: The amino acid sequence around the disulfide bonds of soybean trypsin inhibitor. Biochem. biophys. Res. Commun. **23**, 561 (1966).
BUCK, F. F., BIER, M., NORD, F. F.: Some properties of human trypsin. Arch. Biochem. **98**, 528 (1962a).
— VITHAYATHIL, A. J., BIER, M., NORD, F. F.: On the mechanism of enzyme action. LXXIII. Studies on trypsin from beef, sheep and pig pancreas. Arch. Biochem. **97**, 417 (1962b).
BURDON, K. L., QUENG, J. T., THOMAS, O. C., MCGOVERN, J. P.: Observations on biochemical abnormalities in hereditary angioneurotic edema. J. Allergy **36**, 546 (1965).
BURKE, J. S., URIUHARA, T., MACMORINE, D. R. L., MOVAT, H. Z.: A permeability factor released from phagocytosing PMN-leukocytes and its inhibition by protease inhibitors. Life Sci. **3**, 1505 (1964).
CHAMBERS, D. A., GREEP, J. M., BOSSER, C., NARDI, G. L.: Enzymatic studies on partially purified hog kallikrein. Fed. Proc. **23**, 542 (1963).
CHARACHE, P., DONALDSON, V., PENSKY, J., FIREMAN, P., ROSEN, F. S., JANEWAY, C. A.: Genetic abnormalities in hereditary angioneurotic edema. J. clin. Invest. **43**, 1250 (1964).
CHAUVET, J., ACHER, R.: Séquence des acides aminés d'un polypeptide pancréatique inhibiteur de la trypsine (inhibiteur de Kunitz et Northrop). Bull. Soc. Chim. Fr. 1280 (1966a).
— — Inactivation et réactivation d'un inhibiteur pancréatique de la trypsine (inhibiteur de Kunitz et Northrop) par réduction réversible des ponts disulfures. Bull. Soc. Chim. biol. (Paris) **48**, 1284 (1966b).
— — The reactive site of the basic trypsin inhibitor of pancreas. J. biol. Chem. **242**, 4274 (1967a).
— — Active derivatives of a polypeptide inhibitor of trypsin (Kunitz and Northrop inhibitor). Biochem. biophys. Res. Commun. **27**, 230 (1967b).
— — La structure covalente d'un inhibiteur polypeptidique de la trypsine (inhibiteur de Kunitz et de Northrop). Bull. Soc. Chim. biol. (Paris) **49**, 985 (1967c).
— NOUVEL, G., ACHER, R.: Structure primaire d'un inhibiteur pancréatique de la trypsine (inhibiteur de Kunitz et Northrop). Biochim. biophys. Acta (Amst.) **92**, 200 (1964).
— — — Structure primaire d'un inhibiteur pancréatique de la trypsine (inhibiteur de Kunitz et Northrop). I. Enchaînements N- et C-terminaux. Biochim. biophys. Acta (Amst.) **115**, 121 (1966a).
— — — Structure primaire d'un inhibiteur pancréatique de la trypsine (inhibiteur de Kunitz et Northrop). II. Caractérisation des peptides résultant de l'hydrolyse trypsique. Biochim. biophys. Acta (Amst.) **115**, 130 (1966b).
CLEMENTE, P.: Methodenkritische Arbeit über quantitative und qualitative Bestimmung fibrinolytisch und antifibrinolytisch wirksamer Substanzen. Diss. Med. Fakultät Univ. München, 1957.
COHEN, W., BALLS, A. K.: Behaviour of antitrypsin in egg white during storage and brooding. Poultry Sci. **34**, 290 (1955).
DAVIE, E. W., NEURATH, H.: The terminal groups of the soybean trypsin inhibitor. J. biol. Chem. **212**, 507 (1955).
DAVIES, G. E., HOLMAN, G., JOHNSTON, T. P., LOWE, J. S.: Studies on kallikrein: Failure of some antiinflammatory drugs to affect release of kinin. Brit. J. Pharmacol. **28**, 212 (1966).
— LOWE, J. S.: Inhibitory effects of thiol compounds on kallikrein and on experimental burns in guinea-pigs. Brit. J. Pharmacol. **27**, 107 (1966).
DINIZ, C. R., PEREIRA, A. A., BARROSO, J., MARES-GUIA, M.: On the specifity of urinary kallikreins. Biochem. biophys. Res. Commun. **21**, 448 (1965).
— — — — Studies on the specificity of kinin-forming enzymes. The inhibition of the kininogenic activity of trypsin and kallikreins by model compounds. In: Hypotensive Peptides, p. 175, ed. by E. G. ERDÖS, N. BACK and F. SICUTERI. Berlin-Heidelberg-New York: Springer 1966.
DLOUHÁ, V., NEUWIRTHOVÁ, J., MELOUN, B., ŠORM, F.: On proteins. XCV. Preparation of pancreatic trypsin inhibitor. Coll. czech. chem. Commun. **30**, 1705 (1965a).
— POSPÍŠILOVÁ, D., MELOUN, B., ŠORM, F.: On proteins. XCIV. Primary structure of basic trypsin inhibitor from beef pancreas. Coll. czech. chem. Commun. **30**, 1311 (1965b).
— — — — On proteins. C. Disulfide bonds of basic trypsin inhibitor from beef pancreas. Coll. czech. chem. Commun. **31**, 346 (1966).

DONALDSON, V. H.: Serum inhibitor of C′1-esterase in health and disease. J. Lab. clin. Med. **68**, 369 (1966).
— EVANS, R. R.: A biochemical abnormality in hereditary angioneurotic edema, absence of serum inhibitor of C′1-esterase. Amer. J. Med. **35**, 37 (1963).
— ROSEN, F. S.: Action of complement in hereditary angioneurotic edema: The role of C′1-esterase. J. clin. Invest. **43**, 2204 (1964).
DYCE, B., HAVERBACK, B. J.: Serum trypsin inhibitors in the normal and in patients with acute pancreatitis. Amer. J. Gastroent. **34**, 481 (1960).
EGEBLAD, K., ASTRUP, T.: Fibrinolysis and the bovine lung trypsin inhibitor ("Pulmin"). Scand. J. clin. Lab. Invest. **18**, 567 (1966).
EISEN, V., KEELE, C. A.: The formation of plasma kinin by the action of human plasmin on human plasma. J. Physiol. (Lond.) **150**, 21P (1960).
ELDRIDGE, A. C., ANDERSON, R. L., WOLF, W. J.: Polyacrylamide-gel electrophoresis of soybean whey proteins and trypsin inhibitors. Arch. Biochem. **115**, 495 (1966).
ENCKE, A., SCHIMPF, K., KOMMERELL, B., GRÖZINGER, K. H., GILSDORF, H., WANKE, M., LASCH, H. G.: Veränderungen der Blutgerinnung bei der akuten experimentellen Pankreatitis des Hundes. Klin. Wschr. **44**, 90 (1966).
ERDÖS, E. G., HINSHAW, L. B., GILL, C. C.: Effect of indomethacin in endotoxin shock in the dog. Proc. Soc. exp. Biol. (N.Y.) **125**, 916 (1967).
— TAGUE, L. L., MIWA, I.: Kallikrein in granules of the submaxillary gland. Biochem. Pharmacol. **17**, 667 (1968).
FAARVANG, H. J., LAURITSEN, O. S.: Relationship between serum concentration and urinary output of trypsin inhibitor during operative stress. Enzymol. Biol. Clin. **1**, 189 (1962).
— — Increase of trypsin inhibitor in serum during pregnancy. Nature (Lond.) **199**, 290 (1963).
— — Relationship between serum concentration and urinary output of trypsin inhibitor after cortisone administration. Scand. J. clin. Lab. Invest. **15**, 483 (1964).
FERRAUTO, A., CRISTALDI, R., GUISTOLISI, R.: Azione di un inhibitore triptico sulla fibrinogenolisi e fibrinolisi plasmatiche. Ricerche in vitro. Boll. Soc. ital. Biol. sper. **41**, 1281 (1965a).
— — TERRANOVA, R., GIUFFRIDA, G.: Il comportamento dell'attività fibrinogenolitica plasmatica dopo attivazione con streptokinasi ed urokinasi in presenza di acido epsilon amino-capronico e dell'inhibitore parotideo della tripsina. Boll. Soc. ital. Biol. sper. **41**, 1486 (1965b).
FIEDLER, F.: Heterogenität und enzymatische Eigenschaften von Pankreaskallikrein. Hoppe-Seylers Z. physiol. Chem. **349**, 926 (1968).
— MÜLLER, B., WERLE, E.: Hemmung von Schweinepankreas-Kallikrein durch Diisopropylfluorphosphat. Hoppe-Seylers Z. physiol. Chem. **349**, 942 (1968).
— WERLE, E.: Activation, inhibition and pH-dependence of the hydrolysis of BAEE catalyzed by kallikrein from porcine pancreas. Europ. J. Biochem. **7**, 27 (1968).
FINKENSTADT, W. R., LASKOWSKI, M., JR.: Peptide bond cleavage on trypsin-trypsin inhibitor complex formation. J. biol. Chem. **240**, PC 962 (1965).
— — Resynthesis by trypsin of the cleaved peptide bond in modified soybean trypsin inhibitor. J. biol. Chem. **242**, 771 (1967).
— OZAWA, K., LASKOWSKI, M.: The active center of trypsin inhibitors. Fed. Proc. **24**, 593 (1965).
FRAENKEL-CONRAT, H., BEAN, R. C., DUCEY, E. D., OLCOTT, H. S.: Isolation and characterization of a trypsin inhibitor from lima beans. Arch. Biochem. **37**, 393 (1952).
FRATTALI, V., STEINER, R. F.: Soybean inhibitors. I. Separation and some properties of three inhibitors from commercial crude soybean trypsin inhibitor. Biochemistry **7**, 521 (1968).
FREDERICQ, E., DEUTSCH, H. F.: Studies on ovomucoid. J. biol. Chem. **181**, 499 (1949).
FREY, E. K.: Die Kreislaufwirkung eines neuen von der Niere ausgeschiedenen Stoffes. Langenbecks Arch. klin. Chir. **148**, 643 (1927).
— KRAUT, H., WERLE, E.: Kallikrein (Padutin). Stuttgart 1950.
— — — VOGEL, R., ZICKGRAF, G., TRAUTSCHOLD, I.: Das Kallikrein-Kinin-System und seine Inhibitoren. Stuttgart 1968.
FRITZ, H., HUTZEL, M., WERLE, E.: Über Proteaseninhibitoren. VI. Zur Identität des Proteaseninhibitors aus Rinderleber mit dem Trypsin-Kallikrein-Inhibitor (Trasylol). Hoppe-Seylers Z. physiol. Chem. **348**, 950 (1967).
— SCHULT, H., NEUDECKER, M., WERLE, E.: Isolierung von Protease-Inhibitoren. Angew. Chem. **78**, 775 (1966).
— TRAUTSCHOLD, I., HAENDLE, H., WERLE, E.: Chemistry and biochemistry of proteinase inhibitors from mammalian tissues. Ann. N.Y. Acad. Sci. **146**, 400 (1968).
— — WERLE, E.: Bestimmung der Molekulargewichte von neuen Trypsin-Inhibitoren mit Hilfe der Sephadex-Gelfiltration. Hoppe-Seylers Z. physiol. Chem. **342**, 253 (1965).

GARDNER, L. I., WESTERFIELD, W. W., WEISIGER, J. R.: Callicrein inactivators. Amer. J. Physiol. **142**, 541 (1944).

GIBELLI, A., CIPOLLI, P. L., MOREO, G. C., BOLANDRINA, E., MAINIERI, L.: The antifibrinolytic action of the parotid inhibitor. Minerva med. **55**, 488 (1964).

GODAL, H. C., THEODOR, I.: In vitro inhibition of streptokinase-induced proteolysis by Trasylol and by epsilon-amino caproic acid (EACA). Scand. J. clin. Lab. Invest. **17**, Suppl. 84, 199 (1965).

GOLENHOFEN, G., HENSEL, H., PAPENBERG, I.: Über die Wirkung von aktivem und inaktiviertem Kallikrein auf die Muskel- und Hautdurchblutung des Menschen. In: Leistungen und Ergebnisse der neuzeitlichen Chirurgie, p. 49. Stuttgart 1958.

GREEN, N. M.: Kinetics of the reaction between trypsin and the pancreatic trypsin inhibitor. Biochem. J. **66**, 407 (1957).

— NEURATH, H.: Proteolytic enzymes. In: The Proteins, vol. IIB, ed. by H. NEURATH. New York 1954.

— WORK, E.: Pancreatic trypsin inhibitor. I. Preparation and properties. Biochem. J. **54**, 257 (1953).

GROSS, R., KRONEBERG, G.: Neue Aspekte der Trasylol-Therapie. Stuttgart 1966.

GUTH, P. S.: Discussion. In: Polypeptides Which Affect Smooth Muscles and Blood Vessels, p. 322, ed. by M. SCHACHTER. Oxford 1960.

HABERMANN, E.: Über Zusammenhänge zwischen esterolytischen und pharmakologischen Wirkungen von Jararacagift, Kallikrein und Thrombin. Naunyn-Schmiedebergs Arch. exp. Path. Pharmak. **236**, 492 (1959).

— Diisopropylfluorophosphat-Hemmung esterolytischer und pharmakologischer Wirkungen von Kallikrein und Schlangengift. Naturwissenschaften **47**, 111 (1960).

— Zur Reinigung und Wirkungsweise von Kallikreinen. Naunyn-Schmiedebergs Arch. exp. Path. Pharmak. **241**, 543 (1961a).

— Über Beziehungen zwischen pharmakologischen und enzymatischen Wirkungen von Kallikrein und Viperidengiften. Naunyn-Schmiedebergs Arch. exp. Path. Pharmak. **241**, 202 (1961b).

— Unterscheidung von Kallikreinen und Kallikreinvorstufe mittels Antiseren und Diisopropylfluorophosphat. Hoppe-Seylers Z. physiol. Chem. **328**, 24 (1962).

— Fortschritte auf dem Gebiet der Plasmakinine. Naunyn-Schmiedebergs Arch. exp. Path. Pharmak. **245**, 230 (1963a).

— Snake venoms, kallikreins, and kininogen. Ann. N.Y. Acad. Sci. **104**, 130 (1963b).

— Inhibitors of kallikrein and other proteinases from animal blood. Ann. N.Y. Acad. Sci. **146**, 479 (1968).

— KLETT, W.: Reinigung und einige Eigenschaften eines Kallikreins. Biochem. Z. **346**, 133 (1966).

— RÄKER, K. O., ARNDTS, D.: Radio-Retentionselektrophorese: Ein quantitatives und spezifisches Verfahren zur Bestimmung einzelner Proteine im Nanogrammbereich. Klin. Wschr. **46**, 46 (1968).

HAENDLE, H., FRITZ, H., TRAUTSCHOLD, I., WERLE, E.: Über einen hormonabhängigen Inhibitor für proteolytische Enzyme in männlichen accessorischen Geschlechtsdrüsen und im Sperma. Hoppe-Seylers Z. physiol. Chem. **343**, 185 (1965a).

— TRAUTSCHOLD, I., FRITZ, H., WERLE, E.: Über einen neuen Trypsin-Inhibitor. Herbsttg. Dtsch. Ges. Physiol. Chem. Berlin, 1965b.

HAMBERG, U., ROCHA E SILVA, M.: On the release of bradykinin by trypsin and snake venoms. Arch. int. Pharmacodyn. **110**, 222 (1957).

HAVEZ, R., DEGAND, P., ROUSSEL, P., BISERTE, G.: Isolement et caractérisation immunologique de la kallicréine bronchique humaine. C. R. Acad. Sci. (Paris) **262**, 309 (1966a).

— — — VOISIN, C., BISERTE, G., GERNEZ-RIEUX, C.: Identification des γA-globulines, de la kallicréine et de la transferrine dans la muqueuse bronchique humaine. C. R. Acad. Sci. (Paris) **262**, 1777 (1966b).

HAYNES, R., FEENEY, R. E.: Fractionation and properties of trypsin and chymotrypsin inhibitors from lima beans. J. biol. Chem. **242**, 5378 (1967).

HEBBORN, P., SHAW, B.: The action of sodium salicylate and aspirin on some kallikrein systems. Brit. J. Pharmacol. **20**, 254 (1963).

HIXSON, H. F., JR., FINKENSTADT, W. R., LASKOWSKI, M., JR.: Kinetics of the reaction between trypsin and soybean trypsin inhibitor. Fed. Proc. **26**, 276 (1967).

HLADOVEC, J., MANSFELD, V., HORÁKOVÁ, Z.: Antifibrinolytische Aktivität einiger Trypsin-Inhibitoren. Naturwissenschaften **45**, 575 (1958).

HORTON, E. W., LEWIS, G. P.: A comparison of the plasma kinin forming enzymes in urine, kallikrein and urokinase. J. Physiol. (Lond.) **149**, 477 (1959).

IWANAGA, S., SATO, T., MIZUSHIMA, Y., SUZUKI, T.: Studies on snake venoms. XVII. Properties of the bradykinin releasing enzyme in the venom of *Agkistrodon halys blomhoffii*. J. Biochem. **58**, 123 (1965).
JAKOBSSON, K.: Studies on fibrinogen. II. Studies on the trypsin and plasmin inhibitors in human blood serum. Scand. J. clin. Lab. Invest. **7**, Suppl. 14 (1955).
JAQUES, R.: Schutz gegenüber letalem Trypsinschock am Meerschweinchen. Helv. physiol. pharmacol. Acta **15**, C 69 (1957).
JEANTEUR, P., FOURNIER, E.: Etude sur la nature de l'inhibition de l'activité endopeptidasique de la trypsine par un inhibiteur extrait de la parotide de bœuf. C. R. Acad. Sci. (Paris) **260**, 722 (1965).
JIRGENSONS, B.: Effects of n-propyl alcohol and detergents on the optical rotatory dispersion of α-chymotrypsinogen, β-casein, histone, fraction F1, and soybean trypsin inhibitor. J. biol. Chem. **242**, 912 (1967).
— IKENAKA, T., GORGURAKI, V.: A study of trypsin inhibitors. Makromolekul. Chem. **39**, 149 (1960).
JONES, G., MOORE, S., STEIN, W. H.: Properties of chromatographically purified trypsin inhibitors from lima beans. Biochemistry **2**, 66 (1963).
JUSTISZ, M., KAMINSKI, M., LEGAULT-DÉMARE, J.: Purification de l'ovomucoide par électrophorèse de zone. Biochim. biophys. Acta (Amst.) **23**, 173 (1957).
KAGEN, L. J.: Some biochemical and physical properties of the human permeability globulins. Brit. J. exp. Path. **45**, 604 (1964).
— BECKER, E. L.: Inhibition of permeability globulins by C'1-esterase inhibitor. Fed. Proc. **22**, 613 (1963).
KASSELL, B.: The basic trypsin inhibitor of bovine pancreas. II. Alteration of the methionine residue. Biochemistry **3**, 152 (1964).
— CHOW, R. B.: Modification of the basic trypsin inhibitor of bovine pancreas. The ε-amino-groups of lysine and the amino-terminal sequence. Biochemistry **5**, 3449 (1966).
— LASKOWSKI, M.: The comparative resistance to pepsin of six naturally occurring trypsin inhibitors. J. biol. Chem. **219**, 203 (1956).
— — Further experiments on the basic pancreatic trypsin inhibitor. Fed. Proc. **24**, 593 (1965a).
— — The basic trypsin inhibitor of bovine pancreas. V. The disulfide linkages. Biochem. biophys. Res. Commun. **20**, 463 (1965b).
— — The basic trypsin inhibitor of bovine pancreas. VI. Sequence studies and disulphide linkages. Acta biochim. pol. 18, 287 (1966).
— RADICEVIC, M., ANSFIELD, M. J., LASKOWSKI, M.: The basic trypsin inhibitor of bovine pancreas. IV. The linear sequence of the 58 amino acids. Biochem. biophys. Res. Commun. 18, 255 (1965).
— — BERLOW, S., PEANASKY, R. J., LASKOWSKI, M.: The basic trypsin inhibitor of bovine pancreas. I. An improved method of preparation and amino acid composition. J. biol. Chem. **238**, 3274 (1963a).
— — LASKOWSKI, M.: A new method of preparation of pancreatic trypsin inhibitor. Fed. Proc. **22**, 529 (1963b).
KLINE, D. L., FISHMAN, J. B.: Proactivator function of human plasmin as shown by lysine esterase assay. J. biol. Chem. **236**, 2807 (1961).
KRAUT, H., BHARGAVA, N.: Versuche zur Isolierung des Kallikrein-Inaktivators. V. Isolierung eines Kallikrein-Inaktivators aus Rinderlunge und seine Identifizierung mit dem Inaktivator aus Rinderparotis. Hoppe-Seylers Z. physiol. Chem. **338**, 231 (1964).
— — Das Verhalten des Kallikrein-Inhibitors gegenüber Fermenten. III. Verhalten des Kallikrein-Inhibitors gegenüber Proteinasen. Hoppe-Seylers Z. Physiol. Chem. **348**, 1498 (1967a).
— — Das Verhalten des Kallikrein-Inhibitors gegenüber Fermenten. IV. Verhalten des Kallikrein-Inhibitors gegenüber Trypsin und Chymotrypsin. Hoppe-Seylers Z. physiol. Chem. **348**, 1500 (1967b).
— — Über Symplexbildung des Kallikrein-Inhibitors aus Rinderorganen mit Heparin. Hoppe-Seylers Z. physiol. Chem. **348**, 1502 (1967c).
— — SCHULTZ, F., ZIMMERMANN, H.: Versuche zur Isolierung des Kallikrein-Inaktivators. IV. Kristallisation und Aminosäurezusammensetzung, Vergleich mit dem Trypsin-Inhibitor von Kunitz und Northrop. Hoppe-Seylers Z. physiol. Chem. **334**, 230 (1963).
— FREY, E. K., BAUER, E.: Über ein neues Kreislaufhormon. II. Mitt. Hoppe-Seylers Z. physiol. Chem. **175**, 97 (1928).
— — WERLE, E.: Über die Inaktivierung des Kallikreins. Hoppe-Seylers Z. physiol. Chem. **192**, 1 (1930).
— — — SCHULTZ, F.: Nachweis und Vorkommen des Kallikreins im Harn. Hoppe-Seylers Z. physiol. Chem. **230**, 259 (1934).

KRAUT, H., KÖRBEL, W., SCHOLTAN, W., SCHULTZ, F.: Versuche zur Isolierung des Kallikrein-Inaktivators. II. Elektrophoretische Reinigung und Molekulargewichtsbestimmung in der Ultrazentrifuge. Hoppe-Seylers Z. physiol. Chem. **321**, 90 (1960).
— KOERBEL-ENKHARDT, R.: Versuche zur Isolierung des Kallikrein-Inaktivators. I. Hoppe-Seylers Z. physiol. Chem. **309**, 243 (1957).
— — Das Verhalten des Kallikrein-Inaktivators aus Rinderparotis gegenüber proteolytischen Fermenten. In: Leistungen und Ergebnisse der neuzeitlichen Chirurgie, p. 62. Stuttgart 1958.
KRESS, L. F., LASKOWSKI, M.: The basic trypsin inhibitor of bovine pancreas. VII. Reduction with borohydride of disulfide bond linking half-cystine residues. J. biol. Chem. **242**, 4925 (1967).
KUNITZ, M.: Crystalline soybean trypsin inhibitor. J. gen. Physiol. **29**, 149 (1946).
— Crystalline soybean trypsin inhibitor. II. General properties. J. gen. Physiol. **30**, 291 (1947a).
— Isolation of a crystalline protein compound of trypsin and of soybean trypsin and of soybean trypsin inhibitor. J. gen. Physiol. **30**, 311 (1947b).
— NORTHROP, J. H.: Isolation from beef pancreas of crystalline trypsinogen, trypsin, trypsin inhibitor, and an inhibitor-trypsin compound. J. gen. Physiol. **19**, 991 (1936).
LANDERMAN, N. S., WEBSTER, M. E., BECKER, E. L., RATCLIFFE, H. E.: Hereditary angioneurotic edema. Deficiency of inhibitor for serum-globulin-permeability factor and/or plasma kallikrein. J. Allergy **33**, 330 (1962).
LARSEN, V., AMRIS, C. J., BRØCKNER, J., STORM, O.: Fibrinolytic treatment with activator-free porcine plasmin. Scand. J. clin. Lab. Invest. 18, Suppl. 89, 34 (1966).
LASKOWSKI, M.: Naturally occurring trypsin inhibitors. In: Methods in Enzymology, vol. II, p. 36, ed. by S. P. COLOWICK and N. O. KAPLAN. New York 1955.
— The mechanism of formation of a trypsin-trypsin inhibitor complex. Ann. N.Y. Acad. Sci. **146**, 364 (1968).
— KASSELL, B., HAGERTY, G.: A crystalline trypsin inhibitor from swine colostrum. Biochim. biophys. Acta (Amst.) **24**, 300 (1957).
— LASKOWSKI, M., JR.: Naturally occurring trypsin inhibitors. In: Advances in Protein Chemistry, vol. IX, p. 203, ed. by M. L. ANSON, K. BAILEY, and J. T. EDSALL. New York 1954.
LASKOWSKI, M., JR., MARS, P. H., LASKOWSKI, M.: Comparison of trypsin inhibitor from colostrum with other crystalline trypsin inhibitors. J. biol. Chem. **198**, 745 (1952).
LEBOWITZ, J., LASKOWSKI, M., JR.: Potentiometric measurement of protein-protein association constants. Soybean trypsin inhibitor-trypsin association. Biochemistry **1**, 1044 (1962).
LEVY, L. R., LEPOW, J. G.: Assay and properties of serum inhibition of C′1 esterase. Proc. Soc. exp. Biol. (N.Y.) **101**, 608 (1959).
LEWIS, J. C., SNELL, N. S., HIRSCHMANN, D. J., FRAENKEL-CONRAT, H.: Amino acid composition of egg proteins. J. biol. Chem. **186**, 23 (1950).
LINEWEAVER, H., MURRAY, C. W.: Identification of the trypsin inhibitor of the egg white with ovomucoid. J. biol. Chem. **171**, 565 (1947).
LOGAN, G., WILHELM, D. L.: Vascular permeability changes in inflammation. I. The role of endogenous permeability factors in ultraviolet injury. Brit. J. exp. Path. **47**, 300 (1966).
MAKI, M., BELLER, F. K.: Comparative studies of fibrinolytic inhibitors in vitro. Thrombos. Diathes. haemorrh. (Stuttg.) **16**, 668 (1966).
MAMMEN, E. F.: Natural proteinase inhibitors in extracorporeal circulation. Ann. N.Y. Acad. Sci. **146**, 754 (1968).
MANN, R. D.: Method of estimating the inhibitory effect of plasma or serum upon urokinase-activated fibrinolysis. J. clin. Path. **19**, 233 (1966).
MANSFELD, V., RYBÁK, M., HORÁKOVÁ, Z., HLADOVEC, J.: Die antitryptische, antifibrinolytische und antiphlogistische Aktivität natürlicher Proteinasen-Inhibitoren. Hoppe-Seylers Z. physiol. Chem. **318**, 6 (1960).
— ZIEGELHÖFFER, A., HORÁKOVÁ, Z., HLADOVEC, J.: Isolierung der Trypsin-Inhibitoren aus einigen Hülsenfrüchten. Naturwissenschaften **46**, 172 (1959).
MARES-GUIA, M., DINIZ, C. R.: Studies on the mechanism of rat urinary kallikrein catalysis, and its relation to catalysis by trypsin. Arch. Biochem. **121**, 750 (1967).
— PEREIRA, A. A., BARROSE, I., DINIZ, C. R.: The inhibition of kallikreins by model compounds. II. In: Internat. Symposium on Vasoactive Polypeptides. Sao Paulo 1966.
MARGGRAF, W.: Die posttraumatische intravasale Proteolyse und ihre Behandlung. Verhandl. Dtsch. Ges. Unfallheilk. 1961, p. 238.
MARKUS, G., WERKHEISER, W. C.: Distinction between esterase and protease activities derived from plasminogen. Fed. Proc. **21**, 65 (1962).
MARKWARDT, F., KLÖCKING, H. P., HAUSTEIN, K. O., PERLEWITZ, J.: Tierexperimentelle Untersuchungen über die Wirkung eines Proteaseninhibitors aus Rinderlunge. Acta biol. med. germ. **16**, 15 (1966).

MARX, R.: Wirkungsweise der Fibrinolytika und Antifibrinolytika. 5. Hamburger Symp. über Blutgerinnung, 1962.
— CLEMENTE, P., WERLE, E., APPEL, W.: Zum Problem eines Antidotes in der internen Thrombotherapie mit Fibrinolytika. Blut 5, 367 (1959).
— — — — Über die Wirkung von Proteinaseinhibitor-Präparaten (Leber- und Parotis-inhibitor) auf die extravasale Fibrinolyse, Fibrinogenolyse und Blutgerinnungskonstanten im Menschenblut. Blut 9, 164 (1963).
— HENNIG, K.: Über Verstärkersubstanzen der Antifibrinolysewirkung der Epsilon-Aminocapronsäure im Organismus. Verhandl. VIII. Congr. Europ. Soc. Haematol., p. 454. Basel, 1962.
MASON, B., SPARROW, E. M.: The relationship between the permeability-increasing and the hypotensive proteases of plasma. Brit. J. Pharmacol. 25, 257 (1965).
MAXWELL, R. E., LEWANDOWSKI, V., NICKEL, V. S.: Enhancement of fibrinolysis and antagonism of antiplasmin by reversible plasmin inhibitors. Life Sci. 4, 45 (1965).
MCCONNELL, D. J., KAGEN, L. J., BECKER, E. L.: Use of heparin in distinguishing plasma kallikrein from PF/dil. Proc. Soc. exp. Biol. (N.Y.) 119, 652 (1965).
MELMON, K. L., LOVENBERG, W., SJOERDSMA, A.: Characteristics of carcinoid tumor kallikrein. Identification of lysyl-bradykinin as a peptide it produces in vitro. Clin. chim. Acta 12, 292 (1965).
MILES, A. A., WILHELM, D. L.: Enzyme-like globulins from serum producing the vascular phenomena of inflammation. I. An activable permeability factor and its inhibitor in guinea pig serum. Brit. J. exp. Path. 36, 71 (1955).
— — Globulins affecting capillary permeability. In: Polypeptides Which Affect Smooth Muscles and Blood Vessels, p. 309, ed. by M. SCHACHTER. Oxford 1960.
MORIYA, H., YAMAZAKI, K., FUKUSHIMA, H., MORIWAKI, C.: Biochemical studies on kallikreins and their related substances. II. An improved method of purification of hog pancreatic kallikrein and its some biological properties. J. Biochem. 58, 208 (1965).
NAGASAWA, S., HORIUCHI, K., YANO, M., SUZUKI, T.: Partial purification of bovine plasma kallikrein activated by contact with glass. J. Biochem. 62, 398 (1967).
NAKAMURA, S., WAKEYAMA, T.: Distribution of trypsin inhibitors in the sera of various animals. Nature (Lond.) 192, 1077 (1961).
NEURATH, H., DAVIE, E. W.: Terminal groups of components of the trypsin system. Fed. Proc. 13, 268 (1954).
NISSEN, U., ASTRUP, T.: Purity and specific activity of plasmin preparations determined with inhibitors. Fed. Proc. 25, 193 (1966).
NORTHOVER, B. J., SUBRAMANIAN, G.: Analgesic-antipyretic drugs as inhibitors of kallikrein. Brit. J. Pharmacol. 17, 107 (1961).
OATES, J. A., MELMON, K. L.: Biochemical and physiological studies of the kinins in carcinoid syndrome. In: Hypotensive Peptides, p. 565, ed. by E. G. ERDÖS, N. BACK, and F. SICUTERI. Berlin-Heidelberg-New York: Springer 1966.
OZAWA, K., LASKOWSKI, M., JR.: The reactive site of trypsin inhibitors. J. biol. Chem. 241, 3955 (1966).
PASKHINA, T. S., SHIMONAEVA, E. E.: Some properties of thermolabile trypsin, plasmin and kallikrein inhibitor from rabbit blood serum. Vopr. med. Khim. 13, 464 (1967).
PEANASKY, R. J., LASKOWSKI, M.: Chymotrypsin inhibitor from *Ascaris*. Biochim. biophys. Acta (Amst.) 37, 167 (1960).
PENSKY, J., LEVY, L. R., LEPOW, J. H.: Partial purification of a serum inhibitor of C′1-esterase. J. biol. Chem. 236, 1674 (1961).
PRADO, E. S., PRADO, J. L.: Partial purification of a plasma-kinin-forming enzyme from horse urine. Experientia (Basel) 17, 31 (1961).
PRADO, J. L., PRADO, E. S., BRANDI, C. M. W., KATCHBURIAN, A. V.: Some properties of highly purified horse urinary kallikrein. Ann. N.Y. Acad. Sci. 104, 186 (1963).
— KATCHBURIAN, A. V., MENDES, J., PRADO, E. S.: Ions and the kininogenic activity of horse urinary kallikrein. Acta physiol. lat.-amer. 15, 386 (1965).
RÁBEK, V., MANSFELD, V.: Gel filtration of protease inhibitors from potatoes. Experientia (Basel) 19, 151 (1963).
RACKIS, J. J.: Isolation and characterization of soybean trypsin inhibitors. Proc. Seed Protein Conf., p. 98. New Orleans 1963.
— ANDERSON, R. L.: Isolation of four soybean trypsin inhibitors by DEAE-cellulose chromatography. Biochem. biophys. Res. Commun. 15, 230 (1964).
— SASAME, H. A., ANDERSON, R. L., SMITH, A. K.: Chromatography of soybean proteins. I. Fractionating of whey proteins on diethyl-aminoethyl-cellulose. J. Amer. chem. Soc. 81, 6265 (1959).
— — MANN, R. K., ANDERSON, R. L., SMITH, A. K.: Soybean trypsin inhibitors: Isolation, purification and physical properties. Arch. Biochem. 98, 471 (1962).

Ratnoff, O. D., Lepow, I. H.: Some properties of an esterase derived from preparations of the first component of complement. J. exp. Med. **106**, 327 (1952).
Rocha e Silva, M.: Bradykinin — mechanism of its release by trypsin and kallikrein. Arch. int. Pharmacodyn. **88**, 271 (1951).
Rothschild, A. M.: Pharmacodynamic properties of cellulose sulfate and related polysaccharides. — A group of bradykinin-releasing compounds. In: Internat. Symposium on Vaso-Active Polypeptides, III, p. 197. Sao Paulo 1966.
Ryan, C. A., Clary, J. J., Tomimatsu, Y.: Chicken chymotrpysin and turkey trypsin. Arch. Biochem. **110**, 175 (1965).
Sach, E., Thély, M., Choay, J.: Données supplémentaires sur l'inhibiteur de trypsine de pancréas du bœuf. C. R. Acad. Sci. (Paris) **260**, 3491 (1965).
Scevola, M. E., Franchini, M., Barbieri, A. D. de: Purification of the tryptic inhibitor of Kunitz and its isolation from two fractions endowed with different specific inhibitory activity. Boll. Soc. ital. Biol. sper. **38**, 1771 (1962).
Schachter, M.: A delayed slow contracting effect of serum and plasma due to the release of a substance resembling kallidin and bradykinin. Brit. J. Pharmacol. **11**, 111 (1956).
— Some properties of kallidin, bradykinin and wasp venom kinin. In: Polypeptides Which Affect Smooth Muscles and Blood Vessels, p. 232, ed. by M. Schachter. Oxford 1960.
Schmutzler, R., Beck, E.: Effect of ε-aminocaproic acid and of Trasylol by fibrinolysis. Schweiz. med. Wschr. **92**, 1368 (1962).
Schoenmakers, J., Matze, R., Haanen, C., Zilliken, F.: Proteolytic activity of purified bovine Hageman factor. Biochim. biophys. Acta (Amst.) **93**, 433 (1964).
Scholtan, W.: Bestimmung der Wechselwirkung zwischen Trypsin und dem Kallikrein-Inaktivator mittels der Ultrazentrifuge. Hoppe-Seylers Z. physiol. Chem. **348**, 1193 (1967).
— Lie, S. Y.: Molekulargewichtsbestimmung des Kallikrein-Inaktivators mittels der Ultrazentrifuge. Makromolek. Chem. **98**, 204 (1966).
— Rosenkranz, H.: Optisches Drehungsvermögen, Circulardichroismus und Ultraviolett-Spektrum des Kallikrein-Inaktivators. Makromolek. Chem. **99**, 254 (1966).
Schultz, F.: Verfahren zur Herstellung von reinen Lösungen des Kallikrein-Inaktivators. DBP 1084433 (1959).
— Kristallisation des Kallikrein-Trypsin-Inhibitors als freies basisches Polypeptid. Naturwissenschaften **54**, 338 (1967).
— Kraut, H., Bhargava, N.: Darstellung von kristallisiertem Kallikrein-Inaktivator und kristallisiertem Inaktivator-Trypsin-Komplex. Naturwissenschaften **50**, 375 (1963).
Schultze, H. E., Göllner, I., Heide, K., Schönenberger, M., Schwick, H. G.: Zur Kenntnis der α-Globuline des menschlichen Normalserums. Z. Naturforsch. **10**b, 463 (1955).
— Heide, K., Haupt, H.: α_1-Antitrypsin aus Humanserum. Klin. Wschr. **40**, 427 (1962).
Schulz, K.: Antifibrinolyse durch einen neuen Proteaseinhibitor. Z. ges. inn. Med. **20**, 325 (1965).
Schwick, H. G., Heimburger, N., Haupt, H.: Antiproteinasen des Humanserums. Z. ges. inn. Med. **21**, 1 (1966).
Sherman, M. P., Kassell, B.: Modification of the tyrosine residues of the basic trypsin inhibitor of bovine pancreas. Fed. Proc. **26**, 825 (1967).
Singh, L. M., Howard, J. M.: Studies of Trasylol. Arch. Surg. **91**, 635 (1965).
Soulier, J. P.: Les inhibiteurs naturelles de la coagulation. Sang **30**, 262 (1959).
— Progress in Coagulation. Stuttgart 1962.
— Prou-Wartelle, O., Dormont, J.: Etude de divers inhibiteurs d'enzymes protéolytiques sur la coagulation et la fibrinolyse. Rev. Hémat. **15**, 431 (1960).
Spector, W. G., Willoughby, D. A.: Salicylate and increased vascular permeability. Nature (Lond.) **196**, 1104 (1962).
— — The antagonism of substances that increase vascular permeability. J. Path. Bact. **86**, 487 (1963).
Steichele, D. F., Herschlein, H. J.: Zur antifibrinolytischen Wirkung des Trypsin-Kallikrein-Inaktivators. Med. Welt 2170 (1961).
— — Klinik und Therapie der durch Fibrinolyse und Fibrinogenolyse hervorgerufenen Blutungen. Med. Welt 141 (1962).
Steiner, R. F.: Accessibility and structural function of particular amino acid residues of soybean trypsin inhibition. Arch. Biochem. **115**, 257 (1966).
Stevens, F. C., Feeney, R. E.: Chemical modification of avian ovomucoids. Biochemistry **2**, 1346 (1963).
Strässle, R.: Antifibrinolyse. Schweiz. med. Wschr. **90**, 1249 (1960).
Sugino, R.: The dynamic equilibrium of the fibrinolytic system, especially the tissue activator and inhibitor of the dog. Nagoya Shirutsu Daigaku Igakkai Zasshi **16**, 535 (1965).

SUZUKI, T., IWANAGA, S., NAGASAWA, S., SATO, T.: Purification and properties of bradykininogen and of the bradykinin-releasing and -destroying enzymes in snake venom. In: Hypotensive Peptides, p. 149, ed. by E. G. ERDÖS, N. BACK, and F. SICUTERI. Berlin-Heidelberg-New York: Springer 1966.
TRAUTSCHOLD, I.: Zur Bestimmung der Enzymaktivität von Kallikreinen. Gemeinsame Tagung der deutschen, französischen und schweizer Biochemiker. Zürich, 1960.
— Enzyme und Inhibitoren der Bildung und des Abbaues gefäßaktiver Polypeptide (Kinine). Habil.-Schr. Med. Fakultät, Univ. München, 1965.
— FRITZ, H., WERLE, E.: Kininogenases, kininases, and their inhibitors. In: Hypotensive Peptides, p. 221, ed. by E. G. ERDÖS, N. BACK, and F. SICUTERI. Berlin-Heidelberg-New York: Springer 1966a.
— WERLE, E.: Spektrophotometrische Bestimmung des Kallikreins und seiner Inaktivatoren. Hoppe-Seylers Z. physiol. Chem. **325**, 48 (1961).
— — Kallikrein. In: Methoden der enzymatischen Analyse, p. 880, ed. by H. U. BERGMEYER. Weinheim 1962.
— — FRITZ, H.: Zur Biochemie des Trasylol. In: Neue Aspekte der Trasylol-Therapie, p. 3, ed. by R. GROSS u. G. KRONEBERG. Stuttgart 1966b.
— — HAENDLE, H., SEBENING, H.: Über einen neuen Trypsin-Chymotrypsin-Inhibitor. Hoppe-Seylers Z. physiol. Chem. **332**, 328 (1963).
— — — — Neuere experimentelle Ergebnisse über Proteaseinhibitoren. In: Pathogenese, Diagnostik, Klinik und Therapie der Erkrankungen des exokrinen Pankreas, p. 289, ed. by N. HENNING, K. HEINKEL u. H. SCHÖN. Stuttgart 1964.
TU, A. T., CHUA, A., JAMES, G. P.: Proteolytic enzyme activities in a variety of snake venoms. Toxicol. appl. Pharmacol. 8, 218 (1966).
VERSTRAETE, M., VERMYLEN, J., VERMYLEN, C., VREKER, R. A. DE: On the combined administration of streptokinase and pancreatic trypsin inhibitor. Thrombos. Diathes. haemorrh. (Stuttg.) **12**, 391 (1964).
VITHAYATHIL, A. J., BUCK, F., BIER, M., NORD, F. F.: On the mechanism of enzyme action. LXXII. Comparative studies on trypsin of various origins. Arch. Biochem. **92**, 532 (1961).
VOGEL, R.: Differenzierung der Kallikreine untereinander und Abgrenzung gegen andere vasoaktive Substanzen. Hoppe-Seylers Z. physiol. Chem. **349**, 926 (1968).
— KALIAMPETSOS, G.: Über den Blut-Kallikreinspiegel beim postoperativen Verlauf. Langenbecks Arch. klin. Chir. **292**, 894 (1959).
— TRAUTSCHOLD, I., WERLE, E.: Natürliche Proteinasen-Inhibitoren. Stuttgart 1966.
— — — Natural Proteinase Inhibitors. New York 1968.
WALTER, M. N. I., WILLOUGHBY, D. A.: Indomethacin, a new anti-inflammatory drug: Its potential use as a laboratory tool. J. Path. Bact. **90**, 641 (1965).
WEBSTER, M. E., EMMART, E. W., TURNER, W. A., MORIYA, H., PIERCE, J. C.: Immunological properties of the kallikreins. Biochem. Pharmacol. **12**, 511 (1963).
— INNERFIELD, I.: Interrelationship of human plasma kallikrein and plasmin in inflammation. Enzymol. Biol. Clin. **5**, 129 (1965).
— PIERCE, J. C.: Studies on plasma kallikrein and its relationship to plasmin. J. Pharmacol. exp. Ther. **130**, 484 (1960).
— — Action of kallikreins on synthetic ester substrates. Proc. Soc. exp. Biol. (N.Y.) **107**, 186 (1961).
— — The nature of the kallikreins released from human plasma by kallikreins and other enzymes. Ann. N.Y. Acad. Sci. **104**, 91 (1963).
WERLE, E.: Zur Kenntnis des Haushaltes des Kallikreins. Biochem. Z. **269**, 415 (1934).
— Über Kallikrein aus Blut. III. Biochem. Z. **287**, 235 (1936).
— Über Kallidin und Bradykinin. Arch. int. Pharmacodyn. **92**, 427 (1953).
— The chemistry and pharmacology of kallikrein and kallidin. In: Polypeptides Which Stimulate Pain Muscle, p. 20, ed. by J. H. GADDUM. Edinburgh and London 1955.
— Kallikrein, kallidin and related substances. In: Polypeptides Which Affect Smooth Muscles and Blood Vessels, p. 199, ed. by M. SCHACHTER. Oxford 1960.
— Über Plasmakinine. 27. Tagg. Dtsch. Pharmakol. Ges., Wien, 1962.
— Über Plasmakinine. Naunyn-Schmiedebergs Arch. exp. Path. Pharmak. **245**, 254 (1963).
— Über einen Hemmkörper für Kallikrein und Trypsin in der Rinderlunge. Hoppe-Seylers Z. physiol. Chem. **338**, 228 (1964a).
— Biochemische Betrachtungen zur Regulierung der Gewebsdurchblutung. Ärztl. Forsch. 18, 281 (1964b).
— APPEL, W.: Photochemische Inaktivierung von Kallikrein durch Methylenblau. Z. Vitamin-, Hormon- u. Fermentforsch. 8, 24 (1956).
— — Isolierung eines natürlichen Inaktivators für Kallikrein und einige Proteinasen aus Rinderleber. Naturwissenschaften **45**, 60 (1958).

WERLE, E., APPEL, W.: Über einen Hemmkörper für Kallikrein und verschiedene Proteinasen aus Rinderleber. II. Z. Naturforsch. **14b**, 385 (1959).

— — HAPP, E.: Über Hemmkörper für Trypsin und Kallikrein im Blut der Weinbergschnecke (*Helix pomatia*) und über eine Kreislauf-Schockwirkung des Schneckenblutes. Naunyn-Schmiedebergs Arch. exp. Path. Pharmak. **234**, 364 (1958).

— — — Über den Kallikrein-Inaktivator aus Kartoffeln und seine Abgrenzung gegen Proteinase-Inhibitoren. Z. Vitamin-, Hormon- u. Fermentforsch. **10**, 127 (1959).

— FLOSSDORF, K.: Zur Kenntnis der Chemie und Pharmakologie des Kallikreins. Biochem. Z. **296**, 282 (1938).

— FORELL, M. M., MAIER, L.: Über einen neuen Inaktivator des Kallikreins in Eiklar. Naturwissenschaften **41**, 89 (1954).

— — — Zur Kenntnis der blutdrucksenkenden Wirkung des Trypsins. Naunyn-Schmiedebergs Arch. exp. Path. Pharmak. **225**, 369 (1955).

— GÖTZE, W., KEPPLER, A.: Über die Wirkung des Kallikreins auf den isolierten Darm und über eine neue darmkontrahierende Substanz. Biochem. Z. **289**, 217 (1937).

— HÜRTER, J.: Über Ornitho-Kallikrein. I. Mitteilung über kreislaufaktive Substanzen der Vögel. Biochem. Z. **285**, 176 (1936).

— KAUFMANN-BOETSCH, B.: Über eine esterspaltende Wirkung von Kallikrein. Naturwissenschaften **46**, 559 (1959).

— — Über esteratische Wirkungen von Kallikrein und Trypsin und ihre Hemmung durch Kallikrein- und Trypsininhibitoren. Hoppe-Seylers Z. physiol. Chem. **319**, 52 (1960).

— KEHL, R., KOEBKE, K.: Über Bradykinin, Kallidin und Hypertensin. Biochem. Z. **320**, 372 (1950a).

— — — Über Trypsin, Chymotrypsin, Kallidin und Bradykinin. Biochem. Z. **321**, 213 (1950b).

— — — Über die Freilegung von Bradykinin und Kallidin aus Immunserum. Biochem. Z. **321**, 348 (1951a).

— MAIER, L.: Zur Kenntnis des Kallikrein-Inaktivators aus Kartoffeln. Biochem. Z. **322**, 414 (1952a).

— — Über die chemische und pharmakologische Unterscheidung von Kallikreinen verschiedener Herkunft. Biochem. Z. **323**, 279 (1952b).

— — LÖFFLER, F.: Über einen Kallikrein-Inaktivator aus pflanzlichem Material. Biochem. Z. **321**, 372 (1951b).

— — RINGELMANN, E.: Hemmung von Proteinasen durch Kallikrein-Inaktivatoren. Naturwissenschaften **39**, 328 (1952).

— MARX, R., TRAUTSCHOLD, I., REICHENBACH-KLINKE, K. E.: Vergleich der Proteinasen-Inhibitoren aus Lunge und Leber vom Rind mit besonderer Berücksichtigung ihres Einflusses auf Fibrinolyse und Blutgerinnung. Blut **14**, 206 (1967).

— SCHMAL, A.: Über ein Kallikrein-abbauendes Enzym im Blutplasma der Ratte. Hoppe-Seylers Z. physiol. Chem. **349**, 521 (1968).

— TRAUTSCHOLD, I.: Colostrokinin und seine Bildung durch Kallikrein. Z. Biol. **112**, 169 (1960).

— — Bestimmung des Kallikrein-Inaktivators „Trasylol“ im Blut und in Organen und seine Verteilung nach Injektionen. Münch. med. Wschr. **103**, 773 (1961).

— — Kallikrein, kallidin, kallikrein inhibitors. Ann. N.Y. Acad. Sci. **104**, 117 (1963).

— — Physiology, pharmacology and pathology of exocrine pancreas enzymes with special reference to proteolytic enzymes. Paper read: 6th Ann. Meeting Anglo-German Medical Society, Manchester 1965. Anglo-Germ. med. Rev. **3**, 212 (1966).

— — SEBENING, H., FRITZ, H., HUTZEL, M.: Enzym-Inhibitoren des exokrinen Pankreas. Verh. dtsch. Ges. inn. Med. **70**, 801 (1964).

— VOGEL, R.: Vorkommen von Kallikreinogen im Urin von Nierenkranken. In: Leistungen und Ergebnisse der neuzeitlichen Chirurgie, p. 59. Stuttgart 1958.

— — Über die Kallikreinausscheidung im Harn nach experimenteller Nierenschädigung. Arch. int. Pharmacodyn. **126**, 171 (1960).

— — Über die Freisetzung einer kallikreinartigen Substanz aus Extrakten verschiedener Organe. Arch. int. Pharmacodyn. **131**, 257 (1961).

— — KALIAMPETSOS, G.: Über das Kallikrein der Darmwand und seine Beziehung zum Blutkallikreingehalt bei Störungen der Darmfunktion. In: Proceedings, II. Weltkongr. Gastroenterologie, München, vol. 2, p. 778, 1962.

WINTERSTEIN, A., STRÄSSLE, R.: Antifibrinolytic effect of soybean trypsin inhibitor. In: Proceedings, 8th Internat. Congr. of Hematology, Tokyo, 1960, vol. 3, p. 1708, 1962.

WU, F. C., LASKOWSKI, M.: Crystalline acid-labile trypsin inhibitor from bovine blood plasma. J. biol. Chem. **235**, 1680 (1960).

WU, Y. V., SCHERAGA, H. A.: Studies of soybean trypsin inhibitor. I. Physicochemical properties. Biochemistry **1**, 698 (1962a).

— — Studies of soybean trypsin inhibitor. II. Conformational properties. Biochemistry **1**, 905 (1962b).

Kininogens

E. HABERMANN

With 3 Figures

A. History and Definition

The discovery of kininogen dates back to the observation made by WERLE et al. in 1937 that kallikrein by itself fails to contract isolated smooth muscular organs; addition of serum was necessary. WERLE had already excluded a possible "cofactor" function of serum—the relationship between kallikrein and serum resembled that between enzyme and substrate. The second observation was made by ROCHA E SILVA et al. (1949) a decade later: they described a gut-stimulating principle in blood after application of snake venom *in vivo* or *in vitro*. From the historical point of view it is remarkable that both independent groups detected kinin activity only in combination with the kinin precursor. This applies to all the progress made in exploring the kinin system. Better knowledge of biochemistry and pharmacology of kinins contributed to our understanding of kininogen and vice versa. The definition of the term kininogen is unambiguous. It covers every protein that yields kinin(s) on incubation with suitable enzymes.

It is not recommended that the precursor be designated "kallidinogen" or "bradykininogen". Although historically well founded, these terms are not useful, since no protein is known which yields exclusively bradykinin or kallidin. It was preferred, therefore, to name the highly purified protein *kininogen* (HABERMANN and ROSENBUSCH, 1962). Later it was confirmed that it contains indeed the sequences of all three mammalian kinins known. The terms bradykininogen and kallidinogen should be reserved exclusively for proteins still to be detected which yield solely the nonapeptide (bradykinin) or the decapeptide (kallidin).

It is also not recommended that low molecular substances, e.g. enzymatic (peptic) or synthetic kininogen fragments, also be called kininogen; otherwise, one would be compelled to list Met-Lys-bradykinin (kinin-11) among the kininogens since it yields another kinin, namely bradykinin with trypsin or snake venoms. They should be labeled kinin-yielding peptides, a term that cannot be misunderstood.

No evidence indicates that kininogen is a single substance. There are species differences, as well as indications for the simultaneous occurrence of more than one kininogen in the blood of the same animal.

The terms "kininogen I" and "kininogen II" have been introduced by various authors, but with quite different meanings (Table 1).

HABERMANN (1963) referred to the monomer of bovine kininogen as I, the polymer as II. VOGT (1966) described a second "functional" kininogen in human plasma which he called kininogen II. Its substrate function distinguishes that kininogen II from human kininogen I which is apparently similar to HABERMANN's kininogen I (see p. 254). In contrast, the latter was called kininogen II by SUZUKI et al. (1967); a fraction sensitive to plasma kallikrein was named kininogen I. JACOBSEN's (1966a, b) "substrate I" is distinguished from "substrate II" by its higher molecular weight. PIERCE and WEBSTER (1966) differentiate kininogen I from kininogen II by the electrophoretic behavior and by the position of the kinin-yielding group.

Table 1. *Discrimination of kininogens*

Source	Degree of purity	Distinctive properties	Reference
Bovine serum	high	Substrate of kinin-9 and kinin-10 enzymes	HABERMANN and BLENNEMANN (1964b)
Bovine serum	good	Molecular weight (gel filtration)	HABERMANN et al. (1963)
Bovine serum	high[a] low[b]	Substrates of serum kallikrein and other enzymes	SUZUKI et al. (1967)
Human plasma	moderate	Molecular weight (gel filtration)	BROCKLEHURST and MAWER (1966)
Human plasma	good	Sensitivity to carboxypeptidase B and BrCN Electrophoretic and chromatographic behavior	PIERCE and WEBSTER (1966); AXÉN et al. (1966); PIERCE (1968)
Equine serum	good	Sensitivity to serum kallikrein and other enzymes	HENRIQUES et al. (1967)
Various sera	low	Molecular weight, electrophoretic behavior; sensitivity to different kininogenases[c]	JACOBSEN (1966a, b); MARGOLIS and BISHOP (1963); VOGT (1966); EISEN (1966); GAUTVIK (1969)

[a] LMW kininogen. [b] HMW kininogen. [c] See also Table 5, 10, 13.

It would therefore be premature to recommend any of these classifications for general use; more information should be collected. The nomenclature used in this paper follows mainly the suggestions of the individual authors. Discrepancies among them will be noted. As will be shown, highly purified kininogens of various species have in common the relatively low molecular weight of about 50,000. They apparently form a group and will therefore be named LMW kininogens in contrast to, in our view either hypothetical or artificial, kininogens of higher molecular weight (HMW).

B. Estimation

I. Important Factors

An ideal method for determination of kininogens should fulfill the following criteria: the kinin-yielding sequence of kininogen should be converted completely into one kinin; the kinin released should be preserved from hydrolysis by enzymes added or present in the substrate; the kinin should be assayed quantitatively on a stable organ against a stable test solution. The simple addition of enzyme to the substrate with subsequent testing of the reaction products is only possible when highly purified proteins are used. As a rule, however, kininogen is determined in the presence of other plasma proteins. Often kinin is released with the aid of enzyme preparations which are themselves not homogeneous. At least seven factors can interfere with the evaluation.

Inhibitors present in the test system may antagonize the releasing enzyme. Kinin release is not possible except by proteolysis. If trypsin is used, various (at least four) trypsin inhibitors of human blood plasma (SCHWICK et al., 1966) may interfere. The same is true when snake venoms or pancreatic or serum kallikrein are applied instead of trypsin. The main trypsin inhibitor of bovine plasma is identical with the serum kallikrein inhibitor (HABERMANN, 1968b). Heating at an acidic pH destroys the inhibitory capacity.

This procedure, however, introduces another difficulty. Heated and reneutralized whole serum becomes turbid. Crude serum fractions can form coarse sediments coprecipitating kininogen. In such cases, only trypsin is a suitable reagent because it digests the clot, thus exposing the kinin-yielding sequence. The more specific the enzyme is, the more the kinin release depends upon the *physical state of the substrate*. Pancreatic kallikrein, for example, is practically devoid of nonspecific proteolytic potency and therefore gains only limited access to the kinin-yielding sequence of denatured substrates (Habermann et al., 1963; Suzuki et al., 1967; see Table 2). To a lesser degree this also applies to certain snake venom enzymes (see Table 13).

Table 2. *Kinin release from native and chemically modified bovine LMW kininogen.* (Suzuki et al., 1967)

Kininogen	Enzyme		
	Snake venom enzyme	Trypsin	Pancreatic kallikrein
Native	100	100	100
Reduced	50	100	<4
Reduced and carboxymethylated	10	100	<4

Release from native kininogen = 100.

The *kininogenases* should be added *in sufficient amount and purity*. It is tempting to use a high excess to be sure that all the substrate will be converted to kinin. Many enzyme preparations, however, contain trace impurities that can destroy the released kinin and/or the kinin-yielding sequence. This is true for trypsin, even when recrystallized several times. Since in this case the kininase activity is due to chymotrypsin, the trypsin preparations should be pretreated with diluted hydrochloric acid which preferentially inactivates chymotrypsin (Northrop and Kunitz, 1936). Among the snake venoms we found a batch of *Crotalus adamanteus* venom which was devoid of kininase activity. Pancreatic kallikrein must be prepurified *in extenso*. Commercial preparations (e.g. Padutin) contain a series of proteolytic enzymes, including kininases. Use of saliva, pseudoglobulin, and other crude preparations should be avoided. For example, we found human pseudoglobulin *not* to be a suitable enzyme preparation to distinguish between Jacobsen's substrate I and II, since it contains — in contrast to what is stated by other authors — kininogen susceptible to trypsin and to Hageman-factor activated serum kallikrein (Jahrreiss and Habermann, unpublished).

As Werle et al. (1937) found many years ago, blood plasma inactivates kinins (see p. 5). Because of the lability of *kininases* they are inactivated by the procedure to eliminate the kallikrein and trypsin inhibitors. The rather drastic treatment (see p. 254) can interfere occasionally with the experiments. Then, addition of kininase inhibitors is indicated, especially of sequestering agents such as *o*-phenanthroline, 2,2′-dipyridyl, or EDTA (Erdös and Sloane, 1962; Erdös et al., 1963). Experiments with relatively intact plasma show the quantitative turnover of kininogen less accurately because without heating the plasma inhibitors are still active.

A technical source of error in testing the released kinins stems from the considerable *lability of highly purified kinin solutions*. Crude extracts or incubation mixtures are relatively stable because of the large amounts of impurities present. Very dilute test solutions, e.g. 0.01 to 1 μg/ml bradykinin, are subject to aging. They should be preserved in carefully cleaned plastic vessels in an ice bath and checked every hour for stability with a freshly diluted solution, since the process of aging proceeds rather irregularly (Habermann et al., 1963). Loss of activity on standing is not a peculiarity of kinins: histamine (Bosse and Wassermann, 1967) and lysophospholipids (Arnold and Weltzien, 1968) for example are also adsorbed on to glass.

Incubation mixtures may contain several factors that *sensitized* the guinea pig ileum to the action of bradykinin. Some snake venoms, especially that of *Bothrops jararaca*, contain a "bradykinin-potentiating factor", probably a kininase inhibitor (Ferreira, 1966). Such venoms must not be used for estimation of kininogen. Pretreatment with trypsin, as with other proteolytic enzymes, increases the sensitivity of the ileum for kinins in a relatively specific manner. This "doping" of isolated organs has been adopted by us as a routine procedure for many years. Edery (1964) has described the phenomenon in detail. To avoid any interference, either the organ should be sensitized maximally by trypsin or snake venom, or the incubation mixture should be boiled (5 min/98°) after kinin release. Pretreatment of the test organ with the kininogenase used is indispensable. Many of these enzymes are known to cause contractions, of the guinea pig ileum for example, with subsequent tachyphylaxis. The test organs should be sensitized maximally for kinins and desensitized against kininogenases. AARSEN (1968) has emphasized an additional source of error. Tryptic hydrolysates of ox and rabbit plasma contain sensitizing, probably acidic peptides, deriving from various plasma proteins, among them bovine serum albumin. Since the slope of the dose–effect curves is significantly steeper for tryptic hydrolysates than for solutions of synthetic bradykinin, comparison between the two kinin sources seems to be inaccurate. According to various authors (LEWIS, 1960; CÎRSTEA, 1965), cysteine and other sulfhydryl compounds sensitize the rat uterus and guinea pig ileum to bradykinin. Such substances may be present in tryptic hydrolysates of plasma.

Finally, native plasma contains *aminopeptidase activity* that can convert some of the available kallidin into bradykinin (WEBSTER and PIERCE, 1963; ERDÖS et al., 1963). Such a process leads to about a threefold increase in kinin activity when tested on the guinea pig ileum. Therefore the action on that organ by kallikrein incubates may be more than calculated on the basis of kallidin release alone (see Table 13).

The different susceptibility of normal and heated plasma to kininogenases results from a combination of the variables mentioned (Table 13). Bradykinin equivalents obtained from unheated plasma with kininogenases decrease in the order Crotalus venom > pancreatic kallikrein > trypsin > glass contact; for heated plasma, the order is trypsin > Crotalus venom >> pancreatic kallikrein.

Consequently, methods to differentiate various kinds of kininogens in whole plasma are subject to severe errors. For example, MOURI (1969) tried to distinguish two human kininogens by successive treatment with casein-activated plasma kallikrein and trypsin. Even if we pass over the erroneous assumption that casein-activated kallikrein would attack a special substrate (see p. 258), such an approach ignores the very different reaction conditions required by the two enzymes. Perhaps various functional states of kininogen can be distinguished in that manner but not various kininogens.

II. Typical Procedures for Kinin Release

Three typical procedures suitable for determination of kinin-yielding groups used by the author will be described. Contact activation (see p. 86) of the kinin system should be avoided during preparation of the plasma.

Kinin Release from Purified Kininogen. Neither kininogenase nor kininase should be present in the substrate.

0.1 ml substrate solution (equivalent to about 1 μg kinin) in water or saline +0.3 ml 0.05 M phosphate buffer (pH 7.8) +0.1 ml crystallized trypsin (acid-treated) 1:2,000, or *Crotalus adamanteus* venom 1:2,000, or pancreatic kallikrein, 1:100,000 (w/v). Incubate for 15 minutes at 37°, cool to 0°, test on the guinea pig ileum (previously desensitized against the kinin-releasing enzyme used) in the presence of atropine and an antihistamine (HABERMANN et al., 1963). Modification using volatile buffers, useful for subsequent chromatography and electrophoresis (HABERMANN and BLENNEMANN, 1964b): 0.5 ml kininogen solution in 0.05 N HCOOH are kept for 10 minutes at 37° (for destruction of traces of kininase; can be omitted otherwise); add 0.25 ml 0.125 M (gives pH 8.6) or 0.1 M (gives pH 7.8–8.2) $(NH_4)_2CO_3$ and 0.25 ml enzyme solution in water. Incubate for the desired time (usually 15–30 min) at 37°, cool to room temperature, add 0.2 ml 1 N HCOOH. The mixture can be either freed from salt by repeated lyophilization or tested directly.

Kinin Release from Intact or Partially Denaturated Plasma. Enzyme inhibitors in plasma must be overcome. Plasma kininogenases should be neither present nor activated during incubation.

0.05 ml of enzyme solution +0.05 ml 0.04 M Na_2–EDTA +0.2 ml intact substrate plasma are incubated for 1–5 min (usually 2 min) at room temperature, then tested on the rat uterus (MARGOLIS, 1966). A modification excludes, at least partially, kininogenase inhibitors and kininases by acid treatment (HORTON's substrate, 1958) and addition of *o*-phenanthroline (GARBE, 1967). According to ERDÖS et al. (1963), EDTA inhibits human kininases well, but not the enzymes in animal plasma. Therefore, *o*-phenanthroline is preferred.

Kinin Release from Denaturated Plasma. Protease inhibitors, kininogenases and their precursors, and kininases are destroyed by acid treatment. A drawback, however, is the simultaneous denaturation of kininogen which renders it less susceptible for certain kininogenases, e.g. pancreatic kallikrein (HABERMANN et al., 1963).

A frequently used procedure was described by DINIZ and CARVALHO (1963) (p. 65). We modified and simplified this technique the following way. To 0.05–0.5 ml solution containing substrate, we add 0.2% acetic acid up to 1.7 ml; after heating for 10 min at 98° in a sealed vessel, the cooled solution is mixed with 0.1 ml 1 M sodium phosphate buffer (pH 7.8), 0.05 ml of 1 N $NaHCO_3$, and 0.2 ml *Crotalus adamanteus* venom or acid-treated trypsin solution 1:1,000 (w/v). Depending on protein content, the mixture is incubated for 15–30 min at 37°, then cooled to 0° and tested as soon as possible (HABERMANN et al., 1963).

To compensate for sensitization by the incubation mixture, a tryptic hydrolysate of pooled plasma is used as internal standard. The standard has been tested repeatedly and very cautiously against synthetic bradykinin. This is possible since some intestinal strips are not sensitized by plasma hydrolysate (HABERMANN, et al., 1969).

BROCKLEHURST and ZEITLIN (1967) developed another procedure which permits the simultaneous determination of free kinin and of kininogen. Immediately after withdrawal, the blood is diluted by 15 ml ethanol. The sediment is washed with dilute alcohol, denatured with heat, washed with water, homogenized, and digested by trypsin.

Each of the methods proposed has its advantages and limitations; an ideal procedure is not yet available. Therefore, for each problem the least unsatisfactory one should be selected (see TRAUTSCHOLD, p. 66).

C. Isolation and Biochemical Properties

ROCHA E SILVA et al. observed in 1949 that plasma bradykininogen precipitates at 50% saturation with $(NH_4)_2SO_4$. Later, the bulk of kinin-yielding globulin was localized in the fraction sedimenting between 33 and 45% saturation. It did not precipitate on dialysis and was therefore called a pseudoglobulin (ROCHA E SILVA et al., 1949; ELLIOTT, 1963). In our unpublished experiments, the precipitation of kininogen from serum of man, rabbit, or cattle was similar. VAN ARMAN (1955) found that the substrate for the *Bothrops jararaca* enzyme and for trypsin and kallikrein is concentrated in COHN's fraction IV-4 (subfraction IV-6). WERLE (1955) localized the substrate for trypsin and kallikrein in the α_2 globulin fraction of human plasma. Bovine kininogen, either purified (HABERMANN et al., 1963) or in whole serum (unpublished experiments), moved like an α_1 globulin. Since kininogen(s) contain neuraminic acid (see below), slight migration differences may be due to variations in the content of this strongly electronegative residue.

I. Bovine Kininogens

LMW Bovine Kininogen[1] *as a "Model" for the Class of Kininogens.* Highly purified bovine kininogen has been obtained by combining various procedures of protein fractionation. HABERMANN and ROSENBUSCH (1962), and later HABERMANN et al. (1963), started with fraction IV-6 which had been prepared by a simplified COHN method 6. The precipitate was adsorbed first on a calcium hydroxylapatite column at pH 5.3 and eluted with acetate-phosphate buffers of low ionic strength. The final step consists of a chromatography on a DEAE-Sephadex column. High ionic strength is necessary to elute the protein from this basic ionic exchanger, indicating a relatively low isoelectric point (HABERMANN, 1963). Initially, two acidic proteins were found which had different molecular weight and could be separated by gel filtration. The HMW kininogen was later characterized as an

1. II according to SUZUKI's nomenclature; I according to VOGT's nomenclature.

artifact, very probably a dimer, originating during preparation. It does not appear when the temperature is kept low and the pH above 5.0 (HABERMANN, 1963). Angiotensinogen, serum kallikrein, and inhibitor of pancreatic kallikrein are removed during purification. Traces of serum kininases are still present but can be inactivated by mild acid treatment.

During purification, some physical parameters of the molecule are altered. Whereas kininogen coprecipitates with the bulk of serum proteins on treatment with heat, perchloric acid, or ethanol, purified kininogen is relatively resistant against heat, soluble in dilute perchloric acid, and less easily precipitated by ethanol. Electrophoretic movement in starch gel and behavior in gel filtration, are, however, not changed.

The kinin content by weight of various kininogen preparations showed some variations, probably as a result of degradation by serum enzymes activated during purification. At least 12 μg kinin/mg kininogen were obtained (incubation with Crotalus venom) (HABERMANN et al., 1963); the best fractions contained 20 ± 2 μg/mg (HABERMANN, 1963).

Crude mixtures, e.g. serum, especially when denatured, are relatively insensitive to pancreatic kallikrein when compared with trypsin or snake venom. With increasing purity, the sensitivity to pancreatic kallikrein also increases. About 10–20% of the kininogen molecules remain, however, resistant to pancreatic kallikrein (see below). No evidence indicates that the kinin-yielding substrates would dissociate into different fractions which would be sensitive exclusively to trypsin, Crotalus venom, or pancreatic kallikrein.

In addition to physicochemical experiments, pharmacological studies can be used for the determination of molecular weight of kininogens. If production of 1 mole of kinin per mole of kininogen is assumed, a molecular weight of $53{,}000 \pm 5{,}000$ can be calculated. This is, however, a maximum value since, as mentioned above, some degradation during purification cannot be ruled out. Sedimentation and diffusion measurements in the analytical ultracentrifuge confirmed the biological data. A molecular weight $\overline{SD} = 48{,}000$ results from $S_{0,20°} = 3.58 \times 10^{-13}$, $D_{0,20°} = 6.15 \times 10^{-7}$ and an assumed partial specific volume $\bar{v} = 0.70$ (HABERMANN and ROSENBUSCH, 1962; HABERMANN et al., 1963; HABERMANN, 1963). Kininogen may be the first protein whose molecular weight has been evaluated from biological data.

Bovine LMW kininogen is an acidic glycoprotein. We (HABERMANN, 1963) found 6.1% N-acetyl-neuraminic acid (calculated from BIAL'S reaction), 8.5% hexosamine (calculated as glucosamine HCl), and 5.5% hexoses (calculated as galactose). This composition, especially the rich content in neuraminic acid or in its derivates, explains the low (pH 3.3–3.6) isoelectric point. The glycoprotein character may also be responsible for a relatively expanded molecular size. During gel filtration of whole bovine serum, its kininogen moiety appears in the eluate shortly before the albumin peak, at about the same position as purified kininogen. This would indicate a molecular weight higher than that of albumin ($> 68{,}000$), not in accordance with the values obtained by biological and physicochemical means (see above). Therefore, other glycoproteins of known molecular weight, such as orosomucoid (human, molecular weight 44,100), β_2-mucoid (human, molecular weight 40,000), and α_2HS-glycoprotein (molecular weight 49,000) have been applied to the same column. All three glycoproteins behaved as if they possessed a higher molecular weight than albumin (HABERMANN, unpublished). Ample evidence has been accumulated for atypical behavior of many glycoproteins during gel filtration (ANDREWS, 1965). Their folding may be less compact when compared with true globular proteins consisting of amino acid residues only. The hydrophilic carbohydrate moieties may attract a water layer which restricts diffusion into the gel grana.

On immunoelectrophoresis, serum of rabbits immunized with purified kininogen yields a single precipitation line with kininogen as well as with bovine serum. The migration velocity of the antigen is independent of the degree of purity. At least 90% of the kininogen contained in bovine serum is precipitated by the specific immunoglobulin; this indicates close antigenic relationship of the kinin-yielding protein(s) with the isolated material (p. 255). The kinin-yielding group is, however, not the only antigenic determinant of that protein, since kinin-free kininogen still precipitates with antiserum. Two very close lines appear when (normal or kinin-free) antigen diffuses in the Ouchterlony plate against antiserum (HABERMANN, unpublished).

SUZUKI's group (SUZUKI et al., 1966; NAGASAWA et al., 1966) succeeded in another way in isolating a bovine kininogen indistinguishable from the protein described above. They combined fractionation with ammonium sulfate, heat

Table 3. *Amino acid composition of LMW human kininogens and bovine LMW kininogen before and after treatment with cyanogen bromide*

	Moles of amino acid/mole kininogen (assumed MW = 50,000)				
	bovine kininogen (Germany)		bovine kininogen (Japan)[b]	human kininogen[c]	
	before BrCN[a]	after BrCN[a]		I	II
Asp	31	31	36	30	24
Thr	20	20	23	22	17
Ser	24	24	28	21	18
Hoser	0	3			
Glu	39	39	43	38	33
Pro	20	19	25	14	13
Gly	16	17	19	16	15
Ala	21	22	27	16	16
Val	21	21	30	15	15
$^1/_2$ Cys	12	10	13[d]	12	6
Met	3	$\leq$0,3	3	2	2
Ile	12	11	15	13	11
Leu	19	20	26	16	14
Tyr	11	11	11	9	8
Phe	12	12	13	12	10
Lys	21	21	22	20	
His	6	7	8	4	
Arg	8	10	10	10	
Try			4		

[a] Hydrolysis, 22 hours (HABERMANN, unpublished).
[b] Accumulated values from 24, 48, and 72 hours of hydrolysis (NAGASAWA et al., 1966).
[c] PIERCE, 1968.
[d] Six or seven cystine residues in the native molecule (KATO et al., 1967a).

treatment, pH treatment (pH 4.9), and column chromatography on DEAE-cellulose and CM-cellulose. Additional purification was accomplished by chromatography on DEAE-Sephadex A-50 and gel filtration on Sephadex G-100 or G-200 columns. Later on they changed the working procedure, replacing heat treatment with zinc acetate precipitation (YANO et al., 1967a). As in our experiments, a HMW compound was separated during gel filtration on Sephadex G-200. It exhibited the same amino terminal (serine) and carboxyl terminal ends (leucine) as the main fraction. The kinin yield per weight was the same for the heavier and the lighter compound. Therefore, the heavier compound may be a dimer of the natural protein. The carboxyl terminal leucine is deduced from experiments with carboxypeptidase A. The same amino acid has been found by the German group (HABERMANN and HELBIG, 1966). From quantitative amino acid analysis, a molecular weight of 49,500 has been calculated. The amino acid compositions of the two preparations are not very different. Certain discrepancies may be due to differences in conditions during hydrolysis. With respect to kinin-yielding peptides, the low methionine content is important; BrCN treatment converts this amino acid nearly completely into the homoserine derivative (Table 3).

The sulfhydryl groups of the cysteine residues are connected to disulfide linkages since ^{14}C-monoiodoacetic acid is not incorporated into the molecule. When purified kininogen is incubated with pancreatic kallikrein or with the purified kininogenase

Table 4. *Comparison of data on LMW bovine kininogen prepared by the Japanese and German groups*

	NAGASAWA et al. (1966); KATO et al. (1967b)	HABERMANN (1963); HABERMANN et al. (1963)
Origin	plasma	serum
Kinin content (μg/mg)	17	18—20
N-Terminal end	Ser	?
C-Terminal end	-Leu	-Ala-Leu
Kinin-yielding group:		
Resistant to carboxypeptidase A and B	yes	yes
Released by BrCN treatment	yes	yes
Sedimentation coefficient ($S^0_{20,w}$)	3.66	3.58
Diffusion coefficient ($D^0_{20,w}$)	6.16	6.15
Partial specific volume $\bar{v}$ (ml/g)	0.688	0.700[a]
Isoelectric point (*pI*)	3.3	3.3–3.6
Intrinsic viscosity (η)	0.063	
Electrophoretic mobility (*u*)	−8.21 (pH 8.20)	
Frictional rate (f/f_{min})	1.48	
Extinction coefficient $E^{1\%}_{1cm}$	6.7	
Molecular weight:		
From kinin content		53,000 ± 10%
From sediment. and diffus.	46,000	48,000
From sediment. and intrinsic viscosity	47,600	
From Archibald method	47,000	
Galactose (%)	4.9	5,5 (Galactose + Mannose)
Mannose (%)	2.5	
Glucosamine (%)	6.7	7.0
Sialic acid (%)	5.7	6.1
Total carbohydrate (%)	19.8	18.6
Nitrogen (%)	13.1	13.4

[a] Assumed.

from *Agkistrodon halys blomhoffii* venom, the kinin-free protein behaves as a single substance. Since the kinin-yielding sequence is neither in the C-terminal nor in the N-terminal position, it must be bridged by at least one disulfide bond (SUZUKI et al., 1967; Table 9; see also p. 268).

KATO et al. (1967b) measured the optical rotatory dispersion, the circular dichroism, and spectral changes of that kininogen. The results argue for a low α-helical content; some parts of the molecule may possess β-structure. With enzymatic kinin release, the α-helix or β-structure content of the residual protein increases. Reduction and carboxymethylation alter the conformation considerably. This is evident also from loss of reactivity with antibodies against native kininogen and from loss of susceptibility against a "specific" kininogenase (pancreatic kallikrein) (Kato et al., 1967a).

Considering the different analytical procedures used, the reports of the carbohydrate contents of kininogen prepared by the two groups are in good agreement. The relation between galactose and mannose was reported to be 2:1 (Nagasawa et al., 1966). All the sialic acid located in the kininogen molecule could be removed by bacterial neuraminidase, thus changing the electrophoretic mobility (Nagasawa et al., 1966; Habermann, unpublished). A comparison between the chemical and physicochemical values obtained by the two laboratories demonstrates beyond doubt that they are dealing with the same protein (Table 4).

Bovine LMW kininogen is so far the best characterized kininogen; it is the only protein that yields the theoretical amount of kinin. Its parameters are checked by two independent groups.

HMW Bovine Kininogen[2]. Like other proteins, purified bovine kininogen tends to aggregate into high molecular forms (Habermann, 1963; Nagasawa et al., 1966). — Suzuki's group suggested that the pseudoglobulin fraction of bovine plasma contains a kininogen which in contrast to LMW kininogen is said to be sensitive to a glass-activated kallikrein (Nagasawa et al., 1967) from bovine plasma. It is the substrate of all enzymes that attack LMW kininogen. More detailed information about this compound is still lacking; as deduced from its behavior on gel filtration and on DEAE-Sephadex, HMW kininogen molecules seemed to be more extended and more acidic than those of LMW kininogen (Yano et al., 1967b). Jahrreiss and Habermann (unpublished), however, failed to find any HMW kininogen in native, contact-free bovine plasma. In contrast, Habermann's LMW kininogen was converted quantitatively into kinin by a purified preparation of F XII-activated kallikrein (Jahrreiss and Habermann, 1969b). It is also the substrate for porcine serum kallikrein activated by casein (Habermann and Klett, 1966). I hesitate, therefore, to distinguish various kininogens in bovine plasma. Differences in enzymatic susceptibility are a question of circumstances (see B I), rather than a question of the actual biochemistry of kininogen.

II. LMW Human Kininogens

Pierce and Webster (1966) purified human plasma kininogens. Repeated column chromatography (first with stepwise, then with linearly increased molarity of the eluant) on DEAE-cellulose and on calcium hydroxylapatite yielded two peaks of activity; the first had 32%, the second 68% of the kinin-yielding groups. Human urinary kallikrein was the source of kininogenase. The first peak consisted of relatively impure material which could be resolved further by gel filtration (Sephadex G-200) into probably dimeric and monomeric forms. The second fraction recovered from hydroxylapatite contained only traces of polymeric material; subsequent to gel filtration, it was rechromatographed on hydroxylpatite in the presence of 1 M sodium chloride. Two peaks appeared which were called kininogen I and kininogen II. The ratio of distribution of kinin-yielding groups was 2:1 between the two peaks. The overall recovery was about 2.2%. The kininogen fraction obtained by gel filtration had an average molecular weight of 50,000 ± 5,000 on equilibrium centrifugation (assumed $\bar{v} = 0.70$). Gel filtration on a cali-

2. I According to Suzuki's nomenclature; II according to Vogt's nomenclature.

brated Bio-Gel P-200 column suggested a molecular weight of 52,000 ± 5,000. Both kininogen I and II were acidic glycoproteins. They contained 5.4 and 5.0% hexose (16 and 15 moles/mole), 1.8 and 1.2% of hexosamine (5 and 3 moles/mole), as well as neuraminic acid. Like LMW bovine kininogen (Table 3), they were rich in glutamic and aspartic acid, contained considerable amounts of cystine, but only two methionine residues per mole. Sheep antiserum obtained with the product of gel filtration revealed a single line of identity for kininogen I and II and for kinin-free kininogen. This would indicate a close antigenic similarity between the two kininogens that does not depend entirely on the kinin-yielding group.

Another approach to human kininogen has been tried by BROCKLEHURST and MAWER (1966). They used contact-free plasma which they desalted first with Sephadex G-50, then fractionated by chromatography on DEAE-Sephadex and finally by gel filtration on Sephadex G-200 columns. The bradykinin content was 5.2 μg/mg protein. Some evidence argued for traces of a higher molecular compound (dimer ?) also yielding kinins. The relationship between HMW and LMW kininogen is, however, much lower than has been reported by JACOBSEN (1966a, b, c) (see below). From gel filtration experiments, these authors estimated a molecular weight of about 100,000 for the LMW kininogen. This value is, however, subject to corrections since the glycoprotein kininogen has been compared with the globular proteins, rabbit gamma globulin and bovine albumin. However, in the light of the above discussions (see p. 255), this is not feasible. In our hands (JAHRREISS and HABERMANN, unpublished), fresh, contact-free human plasma proved to be devoid of HMW kininogen on gel filtration. The peak containing LMW kininogen served as substrate not only for trypsin but also for bovine serum kallikrein activated by Hageman factor.

III. Horse Kininogens

Horse kininogen has been prepared by acidification of plasma to pH 2.0 and heating to 38°, followed by fractional precipitation with ammonium sulfate between 33 and 50% and chromatography on DEAE-cellulose; 5.0 μg bradykinin/mg protein was released by the enzyme from *Bothrops jararaca* venom. As with bovine kininogen (HABERMANN et al., 1963) there was an inverse relationship between sensitivity to trypsin or snake venom enzyme and degree of purification: the purer the preparation, the higher the relative sensitivity to snake venom enzyme. As judged from its behavior on ion-exchange chromatography, horse kininogen is quite acid. At least in this respect, the protein resembles the kininogens described above (HENRIQUES et al., 1962).

More recently, HENRIQUES et al. (1967) succeeded in separating two kininogens from horse plasma. The 20–35% ammonium sulfate fraction from fresh, heat-treated horse plasma was chromatographed on DEAE-Sephadex. One kinin-yielding peak (kininogen I) appeared at lower, the other (kininogen II) at higher ionic strength. Kininogen I released kinin when incubated with snake venom enzyme, trypsin, or plasma kallikrein; kininogen II with snake venom enzyme, trypsin, plasmin, and urinary kallikrein, but not with plasma kallikrein. Kinin released from substrate II by purified human plasmin behaves like Met-Lys-bradykinin on peptide mapping (HENRIQUES et al., 1969).

IV. LMW Rabbit Kininogen

EGOROVA and PASKHINA (1968) purified and characterized this kininogen. The glycoprotein (15.2% carbohydrate), obtained by precipitation and chromatographic procedures, contains about 22 μg bradykinin/mg protein. This value, together with the physicochemical data ($S_{20,w} = 3.3$ S) indicates a molecular weight of about 48,000. The native molecule serves as substrate for every kininogenase tested (trypsin, rabbit plasma kallikrein, and human salivary and urinary kallikrein) and can be exhausted by each one of these enzymes. The kallikreins mentioned do not release kinin when the substrate has been heated at pH 7 or 8. From substrate heated at pH 2 or 4, plasma (but not salivary or urinary) kallikrein releases kinin. As with LMW bovine kininogen (see p. 258), the tertiary structure seems to be important for the attack by kallikreins.

The kinin-yielding sequence is probably not at the carboxyl-terminal end of rabbit kininogen since it is resistant against carboxypeptidases A and B (PASHKINA, personal communication).

D. Kinin Release and Its Relationship to the Structure of Kininogens

The kininogen molecules can be regarded, by analogy with enzymes, as proteins composed of two parts. The activable center yields the kinins; this is fitted into the much bigger core serving as a high molecular weight carrier. This view can raise some questions. (a) What is the composition of the kinin-yielding group? (b) How is it attached to the remainder of the molecule? (c) Where is the position of the activable center?

The composition of the kinin-yielding group follows from the structure of the kinins. Three kinins are identified (see p. 265): the nonapeptide (kinin-9) bradykinin from bovine serum, the decapeptide (kinin-10 = Lys-bradykinin) kallidin, and the hendecapeptide (kinin-11) Met-Lys-bradykinin. The triplicity of the kinins might be explained in two different ways. All three may originate from a single sequence; the nature of kinin produced would then depend mainly on the enzyme used. The second hypothesis would imply that more than one kininogen exists—each possessing an individual kinin-yielding group. Both hypotheses seem to be inadequate. Ample evidence has been accumulated that some sera contain more than one kininogen. There is, however, at present no evidence for the existence of different kinin-yielding groups. Only the kinins mentioned have been identified in incubated mammalian blood, despite species specificity, molecular heterogeneity, and different enzymatic actions on kininogens. Ornithokinin, however, a kinin from the blood of birds, seems to be a different kinin (p. 593).

I. Bovine LMW Kininogen

Most experiments relevant in this context are performed with bovine LMW kininogen. This material is available in the greatest amount and purity. Therefore experiments with this kininogen will serve as a model, followed by discussion of other kininogens. The following facts argue for the "unitarian" theory of the kinin-yielding group of bovine LMW kininogen(s).

Proteins that release either bradykinin or kallidin only with various kininogenases (K-9 enzymes or K-10 enzymes) cannot be separated during purification. Quantitative differences in recovery can be attributed to other factors (HABERMANN et al., 1963, 1966).

The purified bovine LMW kininogen is substrate for both kinin-9 and kinin-10 enzymes: trypsin, *Crotalus adamanteus* venom, and pig serum kallikrein release exclusively or nearly exclusively bradykinin; pig pancreatic kallikrein liberates kallidin. Kallidin is not an intermediate in the production of bradykinin since the lysyl-bradykinin bond is relatively stable against the kinin-9 enzymes mentioned. This is probably due to the free α-amino group at the lysyl residue (HABERMANN and BLENNEMANN, 1964a, b).

One experiment does not appear to support the unitarian hypothesis. When purified bovine kininogen is incubated first with a kinin-9 enzyme, then with a kinin-10 enzyme, only bradykinin is formed. This means that kallidin originates from a group that also yields bradykinin. When, however, a kinin-10 enzyme (pancreatic kallikrein) is allowed to act first, a kinin-9 enzyme applied subsequently still releases some (10–20%) bradykinin in addition to the kallidin already present (HABERMANN and BLENNEMANN, 1964a, b). Discrepancies between susceptibility to trypsin and pancreatic kallikrein also occur in other plasmas. Rat and guinea pig kininogens seem to be completely resistant to swine pancreatic kallikrein (Padutin); swine plasma is also relatively resistant (FASCIOLO and HALVORSEN, 1964). Here again two explanations can be offered. Two kininogens may exist with different primary structures. Both could be sensitive to kinin-9 enzymes but only one of them to kinin-10 enzymes as well. A second working hypothesis seems to be more feasible. This correlates the properties of bovine kininogen as substrate with its tertiary structure (KATO et al., 1967a, b). According to SUZUKI's group, bovine kininogen contains six or seven disulfide bridges but not free sulfhydryl groups. Destruction of disulfide linkages by oxidation with performic acid, or reduction with subsequent conversion to carboxymethyl derivatives, renders at least one linkage resistant to pancreatic kallikrein. Kinin is no longer released by this enzyme. Reoxidation in absence of cupric ions restores the sensitivity to pancreatic kallikrein to about 50%; in the presence of cupric ions, no substrate function is regained. Kininogen treated with urea was still fully sensitive to pancreatic kallikrein. The authors mention that trypsin and snake venom enzyme still released kinin from reduced and carboxymethylated kininogen. Splitting by pancreatic kallikrein depends, therefore, on a rigid conformation of kininogen, which is not necessary for susceptibility to kinin-9 enzymes. The structural changes that follow the modification of the disulfide groups are accompanied by loss of antigenic properties. Despite the identical kinin-yielding sequence, difference in tertiary structure may therefore offer another explanation for the partial resistance of purified bovine kininogen to pancreatic kallikrein (Table 2).

According to a third explanation pancreatic kallikrein first releases Met-Lys-bradykinin. Then trypsin is added as the second enzyme and it splits the intermediary kinin into methionyl-lysine and bradykinin. The first hypothesis is contradicted by the identification of kallidin (Lys-bradykinin) as the main product of kallikrein action. (The transformation Met-Lys-bradykinin → Met + Lys-bradykinin could be achieved, however, by an aminopeptidase accompanying the usual kallikrein preparations.)

For a better understanding of the mechanism of kinin release, the amino acid sequences around the kinin moiety of the precursor molecule should be known. This goal has been achieved in two ways. The first started with the observation that, on peptic degradation, the kinin-yielding part of the kininogen remained intact (GREENBAUM and HOSODA, 1963a; GREENBAUM et al., 1965; WERLE and HOCHSTRASSER, 1963; HABERMANN and BLENNEMANN, 1964a; HABERMANN and SCHUCK, 1964). Pepsin releases a small amount of "direct" kinin-like pharmacological activity which may be called "pepsitocic". In CM-cellulose chromatography, "pepsitocin" is distributed into various fractions that do not always coincide with the kinin-yielding peptides. The single components have not been characterized further. By far the major part of the kinin-yielding group is in a pharmacologically inactive state due to attachment of a few additional amino acids. It can be purified by combined CM-cellulose and paper chromatography. By the latter procedure, two kinin-yielding peptides have been separated which were brought to electrophoretic and chromatographic purity by ion-exchange chromatography on phosphorylated cellulose. Combination of quantitative amino acid analysis, enzymatic breakdown, and Edman degradation revealed the following structure:

(a) Met-Lys-Bradykinin-Ser-Val-Gln-Val-Met (?)
(b) Met-Lys-Bradykinin-Ser-Val-Gln

(HABERMANN, 1965, 1966a, b; HABERMANN et al., 1966; HABERMANN and MÜLLER, 1966).

Sequence (b) has been synthesized by E. SCHRÖDER (unpublished). Its identity with the isolated fragment has been shown by enzymatic analysis, in electrophoresis and in chromatography (HABERMANN, 1966a). There is no evidence for the existence of an ester bond between the bradykinin sequence and the rest of the molecule as repeatedly postulated (see ROCHA E SILVA in SCHACHTER, 1960b; ELLIOTT, 1963; HOLMAN et al., 1968) on the basis of the esterase activity of pancreatic kallikrein (HABERMANN, 1959). Pancreatic kallikrein belongs, like the other kallikreins, to the esterolytic proteases. Splitting of N-substituted amino acid esters is merely an aid for grouping these enzymes—it is not a model for their action on natural substrates. Otherwise, one could also assume that trypsin splits ester bonds in its natural substrates because it hydrolyzes synthetic esters. Kallikreins are highly specific proteolytic enzymes.

HOLMAN et al. (1968) were able to split N_α-acetyl-O-(N_α-acetyl-lysyl)-serine amide and the corresponding tyrosine derivative, but not the threonine derivative, by guinea pig plasma kallikrein. They conclude that a similar binding may connect the kinin with the remainder of the kininogen molecule. The peptidic -Arg-Ser- linkage at the carboxylic side of the kinin-yielding peptides (see above) is said to be an artifact due to O→N shift. Irrespective of the acceptance of these conclusions, kallikreins cannot be classified as pure esterases. At least the N-terminal linkage of the kinin-yielding group with the core is peptidic. But also the O→N shift poses some logical difficulties. MORLEY (1968), apologizing for his hypothesis, states that O-(N_α-acetyl-l-lysyl)-l-serine is rearranged to the corresponding peptide during a few seconds at pH 8. Why should the rearrangement not occur at pH 7.3–7.4, in the physiological range? Why should the hypothesis be restricted to the kinin-yielding sequence? Every -x-Ser-linkage in peptides and proteins could be regarded as primarily esteratic. An exceptional mechanism in protein synthesis should then be postulated.

The second, not less important result is the location of the bradykinin sequence inside the kininogen molecule. This explains why kininogen is resistant to carboxypeptidase N present in plasma (p. 290) and why purified kininogen is resistant to added carboxypeptidase B (NAGASAWA et al., 1966; HABERMANN and HELBIG, 1967). The C-terminal methionine of the kinin-yielding fragment (Table 9) represents, however, not the C-terminal end of the intact kininogen which is -Ala-Leu. Neither does the N-terminal methionine occupy the N-terminal end of kininogen which is serine (see Table 4).

The correctness of the sequences of the peptic kinin-yielding peptides has been checked by nonenzymatic cleavage of kininogen. As described above, bovine LMW kininogen contains only three methionine residues per molecule. Formula (a) above shows that the peptic sequence starts and ends with this amino acid.

Application of cyanogen bromide here was obvious; this reagent is, according to GROSS and WITKOP (1961) selective for cleavage of methionyl peptide bonds. On treatment with BrCN, purified bovine LMW kininogen yielded, as with pepsin, only negligible "direct" activity. More than 50% of the kinin-yielding group was eluted from a Sephadex G-50 column together with short fragments. This was subfractionated on CM-cellulose. Two peaks were obtained which represented homogeneous substances. As expected from the structure of the peptic peptides and the mechanism of action of cyanogen bromide, the amino acid analysis of both BrCN-peptides corresponded to that of kallidin plus 1 serine, 2 valine, and 1 glutamic acid residues and, in addition, homoserine or homoserine lactone. The difference between the two BrCN-peptides obtained rests only on the C-terminal end. The more basic peptide ends with homoserine lactone, the less basic with free homoserine. The amino acid sequence, established in a manner similar to that of the peptic kinin-yielding peptides, is

(kallidin)-Ser-Val-Gln-Val-hoSer or -hoSer lactone

(hoSer = homoserine). The high molecular weight moiety of the BrCN-treated kininogen, which releases relatively little kinin, has not been investigated further. It is not clear whether it is the product of incomplete splitting of a single kininogen or the manifestation of a distinct kininogen which is partially or totally resistant to cyanogen bromide (HABERMANN and HELBIG, 1966, 1967).

KATO and SUZUKI (1968) confirmed and extended these observations. Kinin-free bovine LMW kininogen, prepared by incubation with pancreatic kallikrein or snake venom enzyme, has the same sedimentation constant (3.3 S) as native kininogen. Reduction and carboxymethylation of kinin-free kininogen yields two proteins (1.32 S) differing only slightly in molecular weight. This is in favor of the structure proposed in Table 9. Treatment with cyanogen bromide, followed by combined enzymatic and chemical analysis, confirmed the sequence (kallidin)-Ser-Val-Gln-Val-homoserine.

By using these small kinin-yielding peptides as substrates, some of the reaction mechanisms of kininogenases can be established. Each of these enzymes splits preferentially at the arginyl bond (HABERMANN and MÜLLER, 1966; HABERMANN and HELBIG, 1967); the Arg-Ser linkage seems to be unusually susceptible. The points of attack at the N-terminal end of the peptides depend on the length of the adjacent sequence to be cleaved. In the intact kininogen molecule, the N-terminal end is very long: kinin-9 enzymes split the Lys-Arg bond, kinin-10 enzymes probably the Met-Lys bond. When, after peptic cleavage, methionine occupies the N-terminal position, the Met-Lys bond is stable against the kinin-10 enzyme pancreatic kallikrein; this enzyme now releases Met-Lys-bradykinin instead of kallidin. However, the resistance of the Lys-Arg bond against kinin-9 enzymes is also increased. They now release Met-Lys-bradykinin besides bradykinin, since transformation of Met-Lys-bradykinin into bradykinin is a relatively slow process with kinin-releasing enzymes. The Lys-Arg-bond of BrCN-peptides, like that of kallidin, is resistant to each of the enzymes mentioned. Therefore it is paradoxical only with respect to the nomenclature that kallidin is formed from BrCN-peptides, regardless of whether the enzyme is of the kinin-9 or of the kinin-10 type. Carboxypeptidase A releases kinin from peptic kinin-yielding peptides and from certain BrCN-peptides (homoserine terminal), of course not from intact kininogen (Table 5).

HOCHSTRASSER and WERLE (1967) tried to isolate the kinin-yielding sequence after peptic degradation of crude substrate. They started with fraction IV-6 and fractionated the hydrolysate by ion exchange on Dowex and CM-Sephadex

Table 5. *Dependence of kinin formation on enzymes and substrates (compiled by* HABERMANN, *1966a; results of* HABERMANN *and* HELBIG, *1967, added)*

Enzyme		Substrates				
Type[a]	Name	Bovine kininogen	Kinin-yielding peptic peptide	Kinin-yielding BrCN-peptide	Met-Lys-bradykinin	Bradykinyl serine
k-9	Trypsin	Bradykinin Kallidin (little)	Bradykinin Met-Lys-bradykinin	Kallidin	Bradykinin	Bradykinin
k-9	*Cr. adamanteus* venom	Bradykinin	Bradykinin Met-Lys-bradykinin	Kallidin	Bradykinin	Bradykinin (little)
k-9	Pig serum kallikrein	Bradykinin	Bradykinin Met-Lys-bradykinin	Not investigated	Bradykinin	Bradykinin
k-10	Pig pancreatic kallikrein	Kallidin	Met-Lys-bradykinin	Kallidin	No degradation	No degradation
	Carboxypeptidase A	No kinin	Met-Lys-bradykinin	Kallidin	No degradation	Bradykinin

[a] For nomenclature see HABERMANN and BLENNEMANN, 1964b.

and by chromatography on Sephadex G-25, silica gel, and paper. Although a homogeneous product was not obtained, indirect evidence was given for the existence of two peptides:

Ser-Arg-(Met-Lys-bradykinin)
Gly-Arg-(Met-Lys-bradykinin)

The structure of WERLE's peptides and ours is in agreement in the crucial part, the sequence Met-Lys-(bradykinin). We found, as well as NAGASAWA et al. (1966) and KATO and SUZUKI (1968), a prolongation at the C-terminal end; WERLE et al. found it at the N-terminal end. There are three possible explanations for these discrepancies. (1) NAGASAWA et al. and KATO and SUZUKI, like ourselves, worked with highly purified kininogen, HOCHSTRASSER and WERLE with a crude fraction treated with perchloric acid. Perhaps the attack on kininogen by pepsin is modified by inert materials and/or pretreatment. (2) Preparation of substrate could lead to activation of kininogenases present in plasma. If we assume that they open the Arg-Ser linkage, which is especially susceptible, then the kinin sequences would have an artificial C-terminal end. (3) Finally, the possible existence of more than one kininogen in crude fractions should not be ruled out. We have already mentioned the different sensitivity of bovine kininogen preparations to pancreatic kallikrein or trypsin (KATO et al., 1967a, b). Kininogens could also be grouped according to their susceptibility to carboxypeptidase B preparations. Bovine serum and human plasma both are partially sensitive; about 20% of the kinin-yielding group of bovine plasma and about 40% of human plasma are lost. Unfortunately, however, the usual commercial enzyme preparations contain, besides carboxypeptidase B, still other enzymes. Therefore they are relatively unreliable analytical tools (HABERMANN and HELBIG, 1967).

The evidence for the structure of the activable center of bovine LMW kininogen is summarized in Table 6, the general structure of kininogens in Table 9.

Table 6. *Sequences around the kinin-yielding group of bovine kininogen.* (From HABERMANN and HELBIG, 1967)

Designation[a]	Sequence	Origin	Technique of preparation	Reference
PKFS	-Met-(kallidin)-Ser-Val-Gln-Val-Met(?)-	Purified LMW kininogen	Peptic	HABERMANN (1965, 1966b)
PKFL	-Met-(kallidin)-Ser-Val-Gln-	Purified LMW kininogen; whole serum	Peptic	HABERMANN (1965, 1966b); JAHRREISS and HABERMANN (1969a)
BrCN-carboxyl	-(kallidin)-Ser-Val-Gln-Val-hoSer	Purified LMW kininogen	BrCN	HABERMANN and HELBIG (1967); KATO and SUZUKI (1968)
BrCN lactone	-(kallidin)-Ser-Val-Gln-Val-hoSer lactone	Purified LMW kininogen	BrCN	HABERMANN and HELBIG (1967)
Werle's peptide (1)	Gly-Arg-Met-(kallidin)	Fraction IV-6	Peptic	HOCHSTRASSER and WERLE (1967)
Werle's peptide (2)	Ser-Arg-Met-(kallidin)	Fraction IV-6	Peptic	HOCHSTRASSER and WERLE (1967)

[a] PKFS = peptic kinin-yielding fragment S; PKFL = peptic kinin-yielding fragment L.

Experiments with purified kininogen are not quite satisfactory since some distinct kinin-yielding proteins could have been lost during preparation. We therefore tried to hydrolyze whole bovine serum with BrCN or with pepsin in order to isolate kinin-yielding peptides. At least four kinin-yielding fractions appeared after BrCN treatment, but purity and recovery were disappointing (Table 7). Nevertheless, some conclusions can be drawn from the following results.

Table 7. *Separation of kinin-yielding BrCN fractions* (HELBIG, 1968)

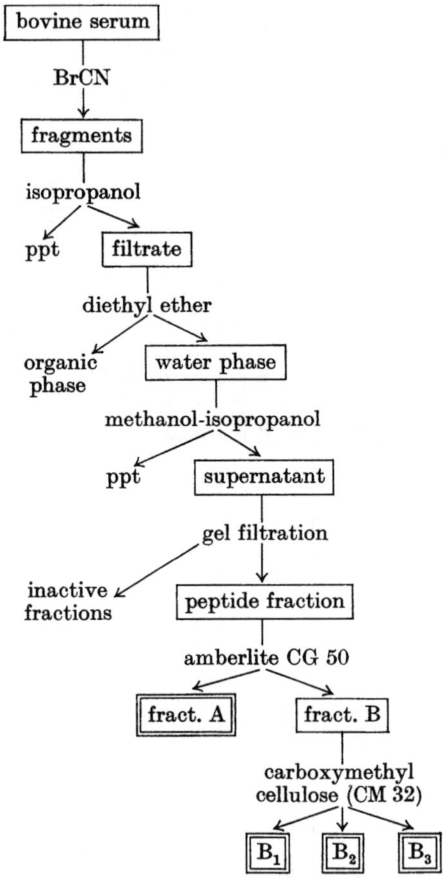

(1) BrCN treatment of whole bovine or human serum yields very low "direct" kinin activity, which means that only a small percentage of kininogen(s) ends with -Met-Lys-bradykinin. One of the peptide fractions (B_3) finally obtained possesses, however, mainly "direct" kinin activity; therefore it may be a kinin that previously occupied the C-terminal end of a kininogen. (2) One of the kinin-yielding fractions (A) yielded, when treated with pancreatic kallikrein, a kinin which behaved like bradykinin on CM-cellulose chromatography but corresponded to the longer kinins with respect to its index of discrimination. It was relatively more active on the rabbit blood pressure than on the guinea pig ileum. (3) BrCN treatment seems to produce more kinin-yielding peptides than there are kinin-yielding sequences. This is secured at least for purified bovine kininogen from which two identical sequences with different physicochemical behavior are released:

one, the more acidic and hydrophilic, ends with homoserine; the other ends with homoserine lactone (see p. 263). The reaction products of whole plasma may be still more complicated (HELBIG, 1968).

In contrast, purification of peptic peptides from bovine serum resulted in the isolation of two components which yielded kinins and were homogeneous on peptide mapping (Table 8). Amino acid analysis of the main peptide proved that the composition is identical with that from purified bovine kininogen (see p. 262). Methionine was the only N-terminal amino acid, followed by the kallidin sequence, as disclosed by Edman degradation. Both peptic peptides are resistant to carboxypeptidase B; they can be activated by carboxypeptidase A. The

Table 8. *Isolation of peptic kinin-yielding fragments from whole bovine serum (*JAHRREISS *and* HABERMANN, *1969a)*

	Activity equivalents (μg bradykinin)	
	per mg protein or peptide	total
Serum (4.7 l)	0.08	17,400
Treatment with isopropanol-ether		15,779
Treatment with isopropanol-petrol ether	1.25	11,364
Gel filtration on Sephadex G-25	1.17	10,000
Chromatography on CM-cellulose	26.0	8,860
Chromatography on P-cellulose	75	5,200
Paper chromatography (main peptide)	139	2,100
Paper chromatography (additional peptide)	63	420
High voltage electrophoresis (main peptide)	530	1,668

pharmacologically active hydrolysis products obtained with various kininogenases correspond to those given in Table 5 for peptic kinin-yielding peptides (JAHRREISS and HABERMANN, 1969a). In summary, the results with whole serum confirm those with purified kininogen. They suggest the overall structure x-bradykinin-y, where y is constituted by neutral and/or acidic amino acids. Nevertheless, the possible existence of more than one kinin-yielding sequence in whole bovine plasma is not excluded by these findings. Minor peptides differing by primary structure could have been lost during preparation, although there is no evidence in favor of such considerations.

II. Human Kininogens

Ample evidence is available for the existence of at least two human kininogens. Like bovine kininogen and crude substrates of other origin (see p. 252), partially purified human kininogen (GREENBAUM and HOSODA, 1963b) yields quantitatively different activities when incubated with various kininogenases. BACK and STEGER (1968) propounded the following series: trypsin>plasmin, plasma kallikrein> urinary kallikrein, pancreatic kallikrein. According to unpublished experiments of these authors, kininogen or human plasma completely activated by plasmin or "kallikrein" yields additional kinin when incubated with trypsin. Such experiments, for reasons given on p. 252, are not very conclusive. Nevertheless they are strengthened by preparative separation of various kininogens.

PIERCE and WEBSTER (1966) distinguished, as mentioned above, two proteins by chromatography on hydroxylapatite which are, according to their molecular weight of around 50,000, classified as LMW kininogens. The proteins differed in that only one of them was inactivated by carboxypeptidase B treatment, thus suggesting that the bradykinin sequence is in the C-terminal position. Their different behavior with BrCN indicated the same. The carboxypeptidase B-sensitive kininogen I yielded "direct" activity corresponding to 2.5 μg kallidin/mg of protein (kallikrein treatment revealed 8 μg/mg); the carboxypeptidase B-resistant kininogen II released only 0.8 μg kallidin (from a total of 6 μg) on incubation with cyanogen bromide. The cleavage by cyanogen bromide indicates that methionine precedes the kallidin in the human kininogens as in bovine kininogen. Until now, however, Met-Lys-bradykinin has not been identified directly in human plasma or in its proteins. A small amount of kinin activity (about 10% of that released by urinary kallikrein) can be detected after BrCN

Table 9. *Structural models proposed for LMW bovine kininogen and LMW human kininogen I and II (summarized by* Pierce, *1968)*

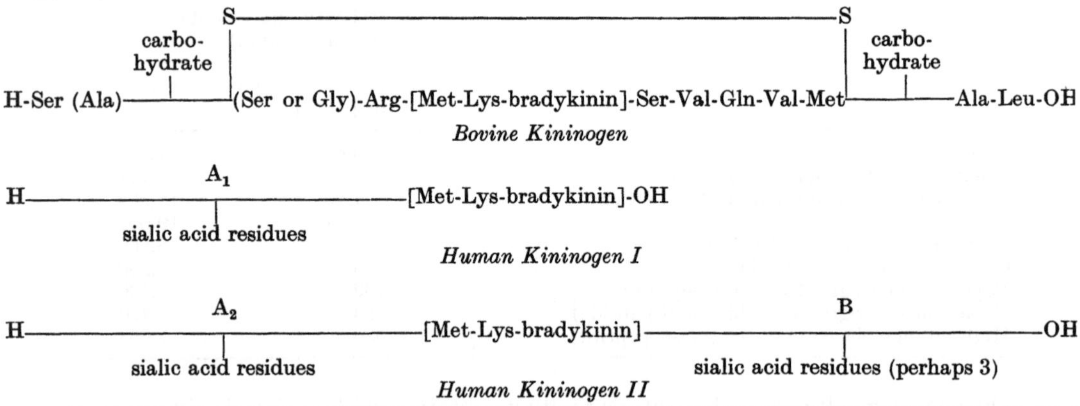

A_1 and A_2 are high molecular, B is probably low molecular.

treatment of whole human plasma. Since the release of kinin from whole human plasma by kallikreins is incomplete (see Table 13), only a small percentage of the total kinin-yielding group of human plasma fulfills the requirements of BrCN activation: C-terminal position and methionine being located near the kallidin sequence (Axén et al., 1966). For the first view, this argues against a significant role of Pierce and Webster's kininogen I in human plasma. BrCN treatment of whole plasma or serum is, however, both inefficient and not very specific when compared with enzymatic (e.g. peptic) hydrolysis (see p. 266).

A second difficulty is the simultaneous occurrence in plasma of a kininogen with free C-terminal bradykinin residue and of carboxypeptidase N which hydrolyzes the C-terminal arginine from bradykinin and related peptides. It must be assumed that the C-terminus of Pierce and Webster's kininogen I is, perhaps for steric reasons, susceptible to carboxypeptidase B from pancreas but not to carboxypeptidase N from plasma. Kininogen I (but not II) elicits and binds antibodies against bradykinin (Pierce, 1968); this argues for C-terminal position of bradykinin residue in kininogen I. The particular antibody against bradykinin used binds chiefly if not exclusively the C-terminus of that peptide and requires that -Arg^9 be free (Pierce, personal communication). The proposed structures of human kininogens, and that of bovine kininogen, are given in Table 9.

The existence of functional differences among various human kininogens is beyond doubt. According to Margolis and Bishop (1963), intact human plasma exposed to glass or treated with a preparation of plasma kallikrein loses about

20—40% of its kininogen which appears to be specifically susceptible to plasma kallikrein and probably corresponds to component B. B-depleted plasma still reacts with trypsin, venoms, and glandular kallikrein but not with plasma kallikrein. VOGT (1966) extended these observations (see p. 117) in pointing out that human plasma contains two kininogens, one (kininogen II)[3] being sensitive to the plasma enzyme activated by glass (kininogenase II), but not to pancreatic kallikrein. The other (kininogen I, which can be replaced by bovine LMW kininogen), is said to be the substrate not of the glass enzyme but of trypsin, pancreatic kallikrein, and serum kallikrein. The last enzyme has been called kininogenase I. The mode of activation of serum kallikrein (e.g. by casein, acid, or acetone) is irrelevant (SEIDEL and VOGT, 1968; VOGT and WAWRETSCHEK, 1968). Kininogen II is synonymous with component B. EISEN (1966) also found a glass-activated kininogenase attacking a kininogen from which acetone-activated plasma kallikrein, pancreatic kallikrein, plasmin, or trypsin released very little kinin. In the schema given by EISEN, Hageman factor or trypsin activates kininogenaseII which then activates plasma kallikrein (kininogenase I).

Other criteria for differentiation of various kininogens are used by JACOBSEN and co-workers. Separation by gel filtration and sensitivity to various enzyme preparations led him to the following classification (Table 10; JACOBSEN, 1966a, b, c; JACOBSEN and KRIZ, 1967).

Table 10. *Differentiation of various kininogens by gel filtration and in vitro sensitivity to enzymes (JACOBSEN, 1966b)*

Enzyme preparation	Rat plasma		Guinea pig plasma		Human, rabbit, dog plasma	
	substrate 1	substrate 2	substrate 1	substrate 2	substrate 1	substrate 2
Rat saliva	+	+	0	0	+	+
Guinea pig saliva	(+)	(+)	0	+	+	+
Saliva from man, dog, rabbit	0[a]	0[a]	0	0	+	+
Padutin[b]	0[a]	0[a]	0	(+)	+	+
Human pseudoglobulin	+	0	+	+	+	0

[a] Nevertheless, rat blood pressure is lowered by human saliva and by Padutin (LECOMTE, 1968a).
[b] Hog pancreatic kallikrein.

From gel filtration and ultracentrifugation measurements a molecular weight of 197,000 has been deduced for human substrate 1 (HMW kininogen) and a molecular weight of 57,000 for human substrate 2 (LMW kininogen). The molecular weight calculated for substrate 2 may be somewhat too high, to judge from findings given above. On disk electrophoresis, substrate 1 moved with the β-globulins, substrate 2 with the α_2-globulins. Since PIERCE and WEBSTER (1966) found two human kininogens possessing a molecular weight around 50,000, JACOBSEN'S "substrate 1" may be a third kinin-yielding protein to be added to the already known human kininogens; it seems to account for about 20% of the total kinin-yielding sequence present in human plasma. The close similarity of the three human kininogens becomes apparent from immunological tests: they give a

3. It should be stressed again that VOGT'S nomenclature is the opposite of SUZUKI'S.

single line of identity when tested with sheep antiserum elicited against kininogen I or II on Ouchterlony plates. Disk electrophoresis of the kininogens, isolated from fresh human serum by means of their specific precipitation with antibody to kininogen I, gave bands for I and II and a third kininogen having an electrophoretic mobility similar to Jacobsen's substrate 1. Gel filtration of human HMW kininogen in 8 M urea on Bio-Gel P-200 revealed a kinin-yielding protein which appeared at about the same retention volume as LMW kininogen I or II (Pierce, 1968).

The apparent correlations between the chemical approach to the kininogen problem and the enzymatic approach must be further substantiated. The experiments with whole plasma (Margolis, Vogt, Jacobsen, Eisen) are beset by many sources of error: activation of enzymes present in plasma, presence of inhibitors which may inhibit or stabilize (e.g. macroglobulins) the action of proteolytic enzymes including kininogenases. Work with crude enzyme preparations, e.g. saliva, Padutin, bulk fractions of plasma, carries the possibility of error by multiplicity of enzymes. The various criteria for discriminating between kininogens are set out in Table 1.

In the author's laboratory, considerable effort has been devoted to demonstrating HMW kininogen, but without success (Jahrreiss and Habermann, unpublished). He is now convinced that HMW kininogen is non-existent in native human plasma, for the following reasons: a) Gel filtration of fresh, contact-free human plasma revealed no HMW kininogen activable by trypsin or HF-activated serum kallikrein. Conversely, the LMW-fractions of the same plasma were substrates for both enzymes. b) The susceptibility of human plasma for the two enzymes depended on its physical pretreatment. c) Human pseudoglobulin, prepared scrupulously according to Gautvik (1969) or Jacobsen (1966a, b) contained large amounts of substrate for both enzymes. It is, therefore, not a suitable analytical tool.

E. Kininogen Level *in vivo*

I. General Considerations

It is very difficult to measure reliably the degree of activation of the kinin system *in vivo*. It is tacitly assumed that the system—like that of the coagulation—is in a state of "latent activation", the degree of which depends on physiological or pathological processes. The activity should be reflected by the kinin or kallikrein content of body fluids. Unfortunately, these factors are unstable. They can be demonstrated under highly artificial conditions only. The kinin level of blood is kept low by the kininases (see p. 289); any circulating kallikrein would be inactivated by inhibitors present in blood or tissues. It is tempting to correlate the loss of kininogen with the activation of the kinin system. The correctness of this approach rests, however, upon two premises.

First, the decrease in plasma kininogen and the formation of kinin are not necessarily linked. The measured disappearance of kininogen yields valid data when typical kininogenases are injected, e.g. trypsin, snake venoms, kallikrein, or Nagarse (see Fig. 2), but the assumption is incorrect when enzymes are used that split the kinin-yielding sequence without kinin release. Chymotrypsin belongs to those enzymes that depress the kininogen level *in vivo* and *in vitro* (Habermann, 1968a) although it is not a kinin-releasing kininogenase (Fig. 1). Chymotrypsin-like enzymes are probably activated during pathophysiological conditions, e.g. mast cell degranulation (Mongar and Perera, 1962). Therefore, in most cases the loss of kininogen does not allow any conclusions about its cause.

The second assumption implies that the kininogen level is changed only by enzymatic breakdown of the circulating protein. It does not make allowance for formation and redistribution of kininogen. Sometimes an increase of kininogen level has been found under conditions that should favor kininogen depletion. This is true for the anaphylactic shock (p. 280) of the rat (DAWSON et al., 1966),

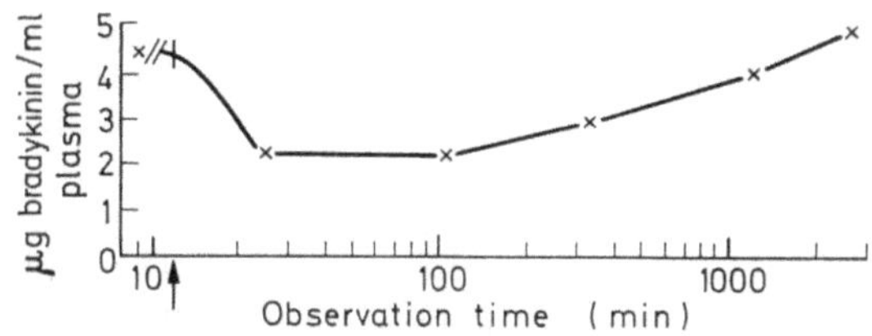

Fig. 1. Loss of kininogen without concomitant kinin release by intravenous injection of 20 mg/kg chymotrypsin (at arrow) to a rabbit. (HABERMANN, 1968a)

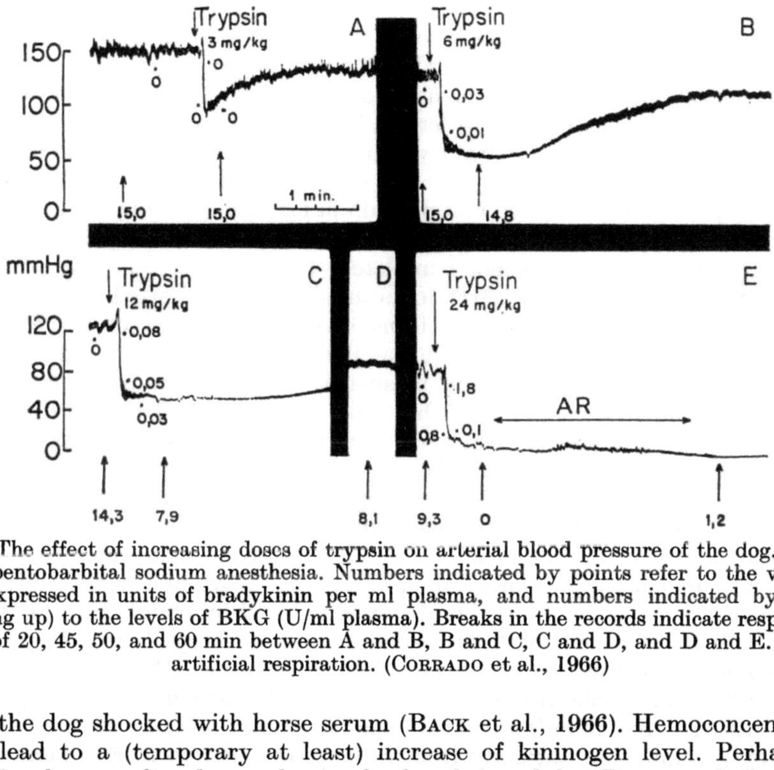

Fig. 2. The effect of increasing doses of trypsin on arterial blood pressure of the dog. Animal under pentobarbital sodium anesthesia. Numbers indicated by points refer to the values of kinin expressed in units of bradykinin per ml plasma, and numbers indicated by arrows (pointing up) to the levels of BKG (U/ml plasma). Breaks in the records indicate respectively lapses of 20, 45, 50, and 60 min between A and B, B and C, C and D, and D and E. At *AR*, artificial respiration. (CORRADO et al., 1966)

or for the dog shocked with horse serum (BACK et al., 1966). Hemoconcentration could lead to a (temporary at least) increase of kininogen level. Perhaps the biphasic change after hemorrhagic shock, observed by DINIZ and CARVALHO (1963) in dogs, may be explained this way: the initial hemoconcentration raises the kininogen concentration, the secondary hemodilution decreases it below normal levels. We noticed a close parallel between decrease of kininogen and plasma protein in rabbits during shock elicited by hemorrhage, trauma, or burning (URBANITZ et al., 1969b; HABERMANN et al., 1969).

A difficulty arises from the supposed existence of more than one kinin-forming system in blood plasma. It is not clear whether one is more easily activated than the other. In human plasma, for example, glass activates only a fraction (in our hands about 10%) of the total kinin-yielding material. Incubation of tested plasma with trypsin releases the whole kinin (see Table 13). Usual estimation of bradykinin has a confidence limit of at least ± 5 to 10%. Therefore, a selective drop of glass-activable kininogen could escape detection unless specialized procedures are applied. An elimination of the glass-activated kininogen without affecting the second system seems to be possible in rats given ellagic acid; the experimental design was, however, unsatisfactory in my view (GAUTVIK and RUGSTAD, 1967). According to LECOMTE and DAMAS (1968), the desensitization of rats to a given kallikrein, for example hog pancreatic kallikrein, includes the resistance against ellagic acid and vice versa. Homologous rat salivary kallikrein is said to attack still another substrate. Such *in vivo* experiments do not allow the differentiation of substrates since other factors of the kinin system may be involved. The potency of activation by glass is lost not only by kininogen depletion but also by consumption of contact factors (factor XII). For instance, the apparent depletion of the kinin system in rabbits shocked by endotoxin can be corrected by adding glass beads rotated in normal plasma (ERDÖS and MIWA, 1968), thus adding fresh contact factor.

It would be of considerable interest to employ animals with completely depleted plasma kininogen. They could be useful for evaluating the importance of the kinin system under experimental conditions. As mentioned above, ellagic acid seems to remove completely a certain kininogen fraction, but total depletion does not seem feasible in laboratory animals by present methods unless the animal is simultaneously damaged to a severe degree by general proteolysis. We tried chymotrypsin, papain, and plasmin in rats and/or rabbits; only a partial depletion was possible without toxic effects. CORRADO et al. (1966) also were unable to deplete dog kininogen completely by sublethal amounts of trypsin (Fig. 2), Nagarse, or Padutin. MARGOLIS et al. (1965) reported the exhaustion of sheep kininogen by continuous infusion of 2 μg/min/kg of *Crotalus atrox* venom for 30–60 minutes and even by a single dose of 20 μg/kg. In our hands, it was not possible to deplete rabbit plasma *in vivo*, not even by excessive doses of *C. atrox* venom. WERLE reported the complete desensitization of a dog against the hypotensive effects of trypsin and kallikrein after infusion of 200 kallikrein units (see FREY et al., 1968). A complete depletion has, however, not been achieved (WERLE, personal communication). Every desensitization experiment should include controls of the kininogen levels attained.

Partial depletion of kininogen by cellulose sulfuric acid ester reduces the severity of some pathophysiological processes. In dogs, moderate reduction of the kininogen level prevents further decrease induced by endotoxin in untreated animals. Hypotension and death due to endotoxin were delayed; especially striking was the absence of the immediate fall of blood pressure (ROTHSCHILD and CASTANIA, 1968; see Table 15). Another example also has been given by ROTHSCHILD (1968b): the manifestation of passive cutaneous anaphylaxis, induced in rats by precipitating antibody from rabbits, is much weaker in animals pretreated with cellulose sulfate than in controls. Of course, such experiments indicate a role of bradykinin in those processes but do not prove it. Cellulose sulfate may change other body functions besides kininogen level. For example, activation of the fibrinolytic system has been established by ROTHSCHILD (1968a). Cellulose sulfate fails to release histamine or to change blood platelet, plasma protein, or hematocrit values (Fig. 3). Kininogen depletion is accompanied, however, by short-lasting increase of esterolytic (BAEe substrate) activity of blood, by marked fibrinolytic activity, and by moderate leukocytosis. Soybean inhibitor prevents the drop of blood pressure, which argues strongly for

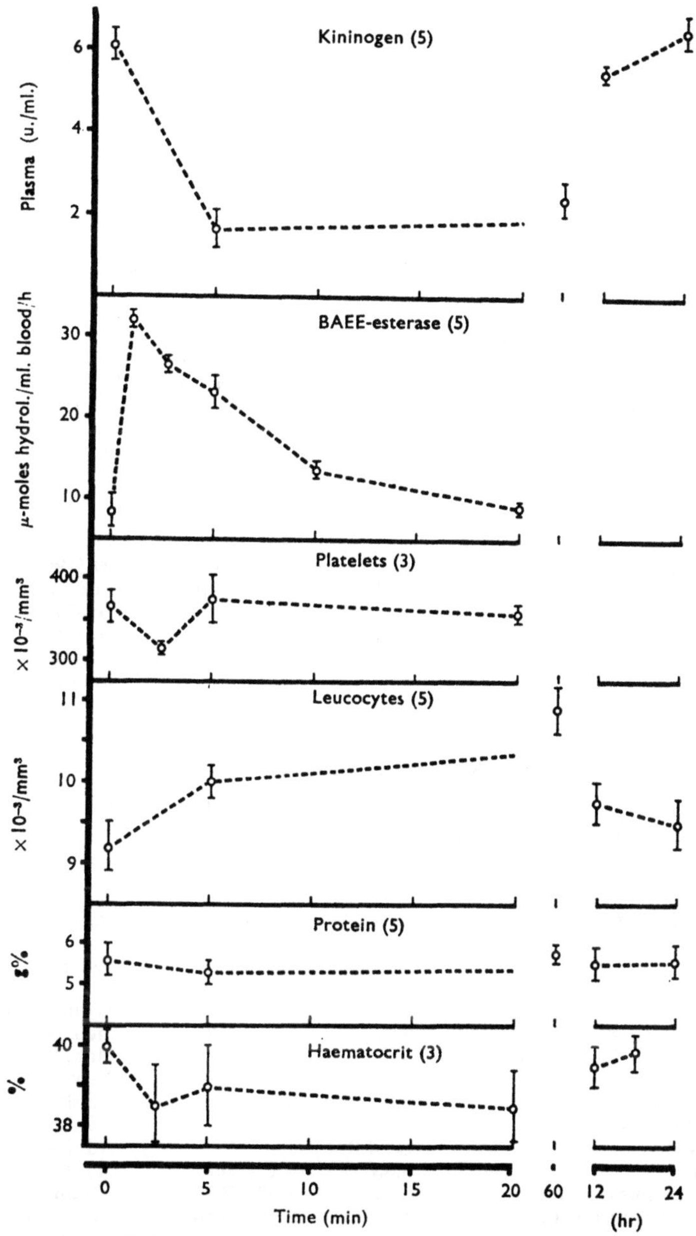

Fig. 3. Effect of the intravenous administration of cellulose sulfate on blood components of the rat. Figures in parentheses refer to the number of experiments performed. One unit of kininogen is equivalent to 0.44 μg of synthetic bradykinin. (ROTHSCHILD, 1968a)

participation of enzymes similar to trypsin or serum kallikrein. The mechanism of their activation is still obscure. Hageman factor may be involved since kinin release *in vitro* by cellulose sulfate is greatly retarded in human plasma deficient in factor XII. The activation of the fibrinolytic system also seems to be mediated by a plasminogen activator (ROTHSCHILD et al., 1969). It is remarkable that even the maximum possible kininogen depletion (about $^2/_3$ of original value) is not followed by severe or lethal shock or related symptoms. The decrease of blood pressure in rats is massive but always reversible and lasts only a few minutes (ROTHSCHILD, 1968a).

LECOMTE (1968a) tried to differentiate the substrates S_1 and S_2 *in vivo* by alternate application of ellagic acid (I), heterologous kallikreins (Padutin; human saliva) (II), and extracts of rat salivary glands (III). S_1 proved to be substrate for I and II, S_2 for III. Rabbits were nearly resistant against I but reacted well to Padutin. For depleting rats of kininogen, the author recommends combined application of I and III. He did not release data on the kininogen content of plasma withdrawn from treated animals.

On the basis of those experiments, LECOMTE (1968b, d) treated rabbits sensitized against egg white with ellagic acid, trypsin, chymotrypsin, exogenous kallikreins, a mixture of streptokinase and streptodornase, or a combination of ellagic acid (20 mg/kg) and Padutin. Such animals died, like the controls, on subsequent application of egg white. By a similar technique, DAMAS and LECOMTE (1968; see also LECOMTE and DAMAS, 1968) tried to evaluate the role of kinin release during the hypotensive response to dextran of the rat. Although dextran application reduced the subsequent response to ellagic acid, previous intravenous injection of that acid did not prevent the hypotension and edema due to dextran. The protective action of intraperitoneal ellagic acid could not be explained. It can be concluded that kininogen is not essential for the reactions due to dextran.

In a further short communication, LECOMTE (1968c) deals with the role of kininogens in the anaphylactic (ovalbumin) shock of rats. In contrast to his earlier report (1968a), the author succeeded in desensitizing against ellagic acid by repeated application of extracts from rat salivary glands. Such animals invariably were shocked by intravenous ovalbumin.

Intravenous injection of bromelain (10 mg/kg), but not of papain, in rats prevents glass activation of plasma obtained 10 minutes later. A reduction of kininogen by 40–50% has been found. Bromelain also initiated kinin formation *in vitro* which was inhibited by soybean inhibitor (KATORI and SHIGEI, 1968).

II. Normal Kininogen Values

Blood Kininogen. Despite the similarity of methods used, the kininogen values given by various authors are hardly comparable. Possible causes of deviation are compiled above (see p. 251). Tables 11 and 12 demonstrate the differences

Table 11. *Normal values for venous kininogen in man (μg bradykinin equivalents/ml plasma)*

Reference	Mean	Range	Remarks
BROCKLEHURST and ZEITLIN (1967)	7.1	6.0 – 8.2	Women, 61–85 years
BROCKLEHURST and ZEITLIN (1967)	6.2	5.1 – 7.3	Men, 49–61 years
BROCKLEHURST and ZEITLIN (1967)	5.1	3.9 – 6.3	Men, 20–30 years
DINIZ et al. (1967)	0.97	0.66– 1.64	Newborn
DINIZ et al. (1967)	9.3	6.5 –12.6	Adults
HABERMANN (unpublished)		3 – 5	Adults
MARGOLIS (1966)	ca. 4.0		Adults
MOURI (1969)	5.63	4.1 – 6.9	Adults
PERITI and GASPARRI (1966)	2.77	1.67– 3.87	Nonpregnant women
PERITI and GASPARRI (1966)	4.55	2.95– 6.15	Pregnant women

between various laboratories and various animals. The general trend is the same but the absolute values differ widely. The same is true for the maximum kinin activities obtained by various releasing agents, e.g. glass, various kinds of organ or plasma kallikreins, or venoms. Whereas trypsin releases a defined product—bradykinin—other enzymes may produce, when applied to whole plasma, any of the three known kinins with varying potency on the guinea pig ileum. For the sake of comparison, we incubated human and bovine plasma with trypsin,

Table 12. *Kininogen content in the blood of various animals*

Mean values after tryptic digestion according to DINIZ and CARVALHO (1963) or DINIZ et al. (1967) (I) and HABERMANN (unpublished) (II) in μg/ml plasma or serum.

	I	II		I	II
Mouse	13.2–22.2		Sheep	5.3–6.1	
Cattle	10.5–14.9	5–10	Dog	5.3–5.7	
Rabbit	7.7–10.0	6– 8	Frog	2.2–2.3	
Horse	7.8– 8.7		Rat	1.1–2.2	1–2
Guinea pig	7.0– 8.8	2– 4	Toad	1.1–2.2	
Cat	5.9– 8.4		Pigeon	0.9–1.1	
Pig	2.4– 5.1		Hen	traces[a]	

[a] Ornithokinin; probably different from mammalian kinins (see WERLE et al., 1966).

Table 13. *Kinin release from human and bovine blood by trypsin, pancreatic kallikrein, and Crotalus adamanteus venom as well as by glass (*HABERMANN*, unpublished)*

Conditions: (a) Glass activation: 0.5 ml plasma (heparinized) + 0.05 ml 1% phenanthroline + 10 mg Bio-glass; rotate for 30 min.

(b) Experiments with unheated plasma: 0.1 ml plasma + 0.1 ml 0.5% phenanthroline + 0.7 ml 0.05 M phosphate buffer (pH 7.8) + 0.1 ml enzyme solution.

(c) Experiments with heated plasma: slightly modified procedure of DINIZ and CARVALHO (1963); see p. 254.

Enzyme (μg added to 0.1 ml plasma)	Bovine plasma		Human plasma	
	heated	unheated	heated	unheated
Trypsin (200)		1.5		
Trypsin (100)	10.0	1.5	3.0	0.5
Trypsin (10)	6.0	≪0.5	0.7	0.5
Venom (100)	6.7	6.0	2.0	2.0
Venom (10)	5.0	1.0	1.4	1.5
Kallikrein (10)	≪0.5	4.0	0.15	1.25
Kallikrein (1)	<0.5	0.75	0.15	1.25
Kallikrein (0.1)	<0.25	<0.5	0.15	0.5
Control	<0.25	≪0.5		<0.25
Glass		1.00		0.44
Control		≪0.055		<0.055

Kinin values are given as bradykinin equivalents (μg/ml plasma) tested on guinea pig ileum.

pancreatic kallikrein, *Crotalus adamanteus* venom or glass (Table 13). It is evident that heating decreases the sensitivity against pancreatic kallikrein but increases it against trypsin. For explanation see p. 251 and 261.

Nonmammalian animals contain kininogens too. Alligator and turtle plasma yield, when activated with glass, a kinin indistinguishable from bradykinin (1.4 or 2.0 μg/ml plasma). Low amounts (equivalent to 0.1 or 0.034 μg/ml) also have been found in pigeon and duck plasma. Since the plasma of these animals is free from contact factor, glass-adsorbed activator from mammalian or reptilian plasma is necessary for contact activation (ERDÖS et al., 1967). In addition, plasma of birds seems to contain another kininogen which is part of the ornithokinin system. There is considerable evidence that the kinin-yielding group is different from that of mammalian kininogen (WERLE et al., 1966; and p. 593).

Localization and control of kininogen synthesis have not yet been subjected to intensive investigation. The liver seems to be involved. After partial hepatectomy or treatment with CCl_4, the blood kininogen content decreases considerably.

Liver cirrhosis and steatosis in humans are said to be accompanied by a drop in blood kininogen (DINIZ and CARVALHO, 1963). Elimination of kininogen is perhaps effected—at least partially—by the kidneys. After nephrectomy, the kininogen level in rats increases from 5 μg bradykinin equivalents/ml to 17 μg/ml during about 24 hours. A comparable elevation after adrenalectomy has been explained by diminished kallikrein synthesis in the kidneys. Serum kallikreinogen and kininase level have not been changed by those procedures (WERLE et al., 1968).

Some reports describe arteriovenous differences in human kininogen levels, in some cases as large as 200 or even 1,000 ng bradykinin equivalents/ml (SICUTERI et al., 1966). After induced ischemia, the venous blood is said to lose about 60% of kininogen (discussion of SICUTERI et al., 1966). SCHARNAGEL and GREEFF (1966) described normal arteriovenous differences in dogs ($12.4 \pm 0.7/11.3 \pm 0.1$) which were sharply increased by electrically induced muscular activity and ischemia. PERITI and GASPARRI (1966) found an arteriovenous quotient of 2.91/2.68 for nonpregnant women, 4.84/3.87 for pregnant women.

It is quite improbable that arteriovenous differences in resting, undamaged organs are in the measurable range. When a circulation time of 20 seconds and a mean arteriovenous difference of only 5% (the methodological limit of discrimination) is assumed, the kininogen level of blood would be exhausted in a few minutes unless the protein were quickly synthesized *de novo*. One ml human plasma (4 μg bradykinin equivalents/ml) contains about 0.2 mg kininogen, if we accept a molecular weight of 50,000 (see p. 257). The blood of one person contains roughly 0.6 g of kininogen. This amount should then be replaced several times every hour—a task that is beyond the possibilities of the protein-synthetizing apparatus. If an arteriovenous difference does exist, it must be either circumscribed and/or short-lived or not measurable by present methods. In some cases it may be an artifact due to the method of withdrawal used. This could be especially true of the extreme difference between venous (ca. 3 μg/ml) and pulmonary capillary (ca. 1.3 μg/ml) kininogen reported in man (discussion of the communication of SICUTERI et al., 1966).

The measurements and calculations of the kininogen turnover furnish weighty arguments against a dominant role of kinins in prolonged shock. Only short and/or local actions are debatable, since the kininogen pool is quickly exhausted and the supply is slow. Rats tolerate "explosive" kinin release from most of their kininogen (ROTHSCHILD, 1968a); therefore, the comparatively slow and moderate release of kinins in several acute pathophysiological conditions may not contribute very much to the lethal outcome. URBANITZ et al. (1969b) and HABERMANN et al. (1969) questioned whether the release of total kinin available in blood would generate a shock syndrome. For that purpose, kinin solutions containing more than the amount of plasma precursor (calculated from kininogen level) have been infused into the arterial output of the heart via a catheter introduced into the ascending aorta of rabbits and rats. This way has been chosen since most of circulating bradykinin is eliminated during passage through the lungs (see p. 308). Although the blood pressure dropped rapidly during infusion, recovery started promptly after the end of the infusion, None of the animals died. Intravenous challenge yielded the same result.

Turnover studies have been performed with ^{125}I-labeled, highly purified bovine kininogen in rabbits. The elimination rate is similar to that of labeled albumin. Radioactivity decays in the usual exponential manner. The half-life is at least one day. This is a minimum value since it is well known that iodinated proteins have a shorter half-life than the corresponding native ones. It could be objected that the radioactive label is attached not to the bradykinin moiety but to the remainder of the kininogen. Although kinin release cannot be recorded by the method used, the long sojourn of kininogen in the circulation precludes the assumption of quick turnover. Otherwise, a lot of kininogen free of kinin should be found in the blood; but this is not so (HABERMANN et al., 1969). Resynthesis of kininogen lost by single injections of chymotrypsin in rabbits (HABERMANN, 1968a), ellagic acid in rats (GAUTVIK and RUGSTAD, 1967), or cellulose sulfate in guinea pigs (ROTHSCHILD, 1967) needs about 24 hours. This is in accordance with the half-life time calculated from radioactivity measurements. The slow restoration of the kininogen level lowered by ellagic acid is not due to persistence of this agent in blood; it disappears quickly (<15 min; GAUTVIK and RUGSTAD, 1967).

Kininogen in Other Body Fluids. Like the other plasma proteins, the high molecular weight members of the kinin system are continuously exchanged between the intravasal and the extravasal space. Increase in permeability will be followed by accelerated exchange. Therefore, normal lymph contains substrate for kinin-forming enzymes, e.g. lymph of the thoracic duct (SCHACHTER, 1960a), of hind limbs of dogs or rabbits (JACOBSEN, 1966c; JACOBSEN and WAALER, 1966). The increase in lymphatic kininogen on scalding probably reflects the increased escape of plasma proteins from blood vessels into tissue spaces. The migration of ^{125}I-labeled bovine kininogen into the interstitial fluid of the heated (46.5°) rat paw parallels that of ^{131}I-labeled human albumin. The higher apparent molecular weight of kininogen on gel filtration may be recalled here (see p. 255) (URBANITZ et al., 1969a). The fluids of human cantharides blister (HABERMANN, unpublished) and human ascites contain substrates of kininogenases. Kininogen content of human cerebrospinal fluid has not yet been demonstrated beyond doubt (see FREY et al., 1968). Peritoneal exudate resulting from experimental pancreatitis in dogs may exhibit kininogen concentrations just below plasma (1.08 vs. 1.44 µg bradykinin equivalents/ml). Simple shift of kininogen into exudate may account for the kininogen lost from plasma (NUGENT et al., 1969).

Cow colostrum kininogen yields a kinin (colostrokinin; p. 582) on incubation with trypsin, urinary, pancreatic, or submaxillary kallikreins but not with pepsin, papain, plasmin, or serum kallikrein (casein-activated). Pepsin and chymotrypsin both inactivate colostrokinin; the latter enzyme seems to possess some kinin-releasing activity also. The kininogen content is highest post partum and decreases eightfold during the first four days of the postpartum period. Acid treatment, followed by fractionation with methanol and acetone, yields a 15–20-fold enrichment of kininogen. Human, goat, and dog colostrums also contain kininogen (WERLE and TRAUTSCHOLD, 1960).

For the sake of completeness, two low molecular kinin precursors may be mentioned which bear some similarity to peptic, low molecular kinin-yielding peptides. The major wasp kinin corresponds to the general structure of x-kinin, whereas phyllokinin has the structure of kinin-y (see Chapter 8). Trypsin releases the kinin sequence from both precursor molecules.

III. Variations of Kininogen Level

In Chapter 6, changes that occur in the kinin system under physiological and pathophysiological conditions are described. Therefore and because of the wide variations in quantitative and qualitative results reported by various workers, Tables 14–18 will be presented without special comment. The data should be interpreted very cautiously because of the reasons summarized again below.

Table 14. *Kininogen depletion by enzymes*[b]

References	Animal	Agent	Dosage	Decrease of kininogen[a]
WEBSTER and CLARK (1959)	Dog	Human urinary kallikrein	14–600 FU	40–90% loss of kallidinogen
		Bovine pancreatic kallikrein	300–1800FU	68–88% loss of kallidinogen
DINIZ and CARVALHO (1963)	Dog	"Kallikrein"	300 FU	about 60% loss of kininogen
FASCIOLO and HALVORSEN (1964)	Dog	Hog pancreatic kallikrein	2–10 FU	no decrease but hypotension
	Rat	Hog pancreatic kallikrein	20 FU	no effect
CORRADO et al. (1966)	Dog	Hog pancreatic kallikrein (Padutin)	12 mg/kg	15 μg/ml → 0
WERLE (1967; cf. FREY et al., 1968)	Dog	200 kallikrein units	infusion	6.3 μg/ml → 0; desensitization against trypsin and kallikrein
DINIZ and CARVALHO (1963)	Dog	*Bothrops jararaca* venom	?	about 70% loss of kininogen
MARGOLIS et al. (1965)	Sheep	*Crotalus atrox* venom	1.5–2.0 μg/min/kg for 30–60 min	2.5 μg/ml → 0
FASCIOLO and HALVORSEN (1964)	Rat	Trypsin	5 mg	nearly total loss of kininogen
CORRADO et al. (1966)	Dog	Nagarse Trypsin Padutin	1.5–6 mg/kg 6–25 mg/kg 3–12 mg/kg	depending on dose, decrease from 9.3–16.3 μg/ml to or nearly to 0
DINIZ et al. (1967)	Dog	Trypsin Padutin Nagarse	12 mg/kg 6 mg/kg 3 mg/kg	45–55% loss of kininogen
KATORI and SHIGEI (1968)	Rat	Bromelain	10 mg/kg	40–50% loss of kininogen

[a] Given in percent or μg bradykinin equivalent/ml plasma or serum.
[b] Intravenous application.

Table 15. *Kininogen depletion by substances activating the kinin system in vivo and in vitro*[b]

Reference	Animal	Agent	Dosage	Decrease of kininogen[a]
ROTHSCHILD and GASCON (1965)	Rat	Hydrolyzed agar	0.5 g/kg	5.16 ± 0.61 μg/ml → 0.85 ± 0.08 μg/ml
GAUTVIK and RUGSTAD (1967)	Rat	Ellagic acid	0.3 μmole	Total loss of "substrate 1"
LEME et al. (1967)	Rat	Cellulose sulfate	treatment (12-hour interval) with 2 × 10 mg/kg and 2 × 12 mg/kg	about 40% loss
	Rat	Carrageenin	same	about 10% loss
ROTHSCHILD (1967)	Rat	Cellulose sulfate	0 mg/kg 0.3 mg/kg 1.0 mg/kg 3.0 mg/kg	4.5 ± 0.35 μg/ml 2.7 ± 0.22 μg/ml 1.3 ± 0.09 μg/ml 0.9 ± 0.09 μg/ml
	Guinea pig	Cellulose sulfate	0 mg/kg 0.3 mg/kg 1.0 mg/kg 3.0 mg/kg	7.5 ± 0.6 μg/ml 7.8 ± 0.8 μg/ml 4.0 ± 0.4 μg/ml 1.6 ± 0.2 μg/ml

Table 15 (continued)

Reference	Animal	Agent	Dosage	Decrease of kininogen
ROTHSCHILD (1968b)	Rat	Cellulose sulfate	0.1 mg/kg 0.3 mg/kg 1.0 mg/kg	25% loss (5 min after challenge) 62% loss 85% loss
ROTHSCHILD and CASTANIA (1968)	Dog	Cellulose sulfate	0 mg/kg 20 mg/kg	7.9 ± 0.4 μg/ml → 5.3 ± 0.26 μg/ml; no further loss of kininogen on subsequent endotoxin injection; hypotension and death due to endotoxin delayed, but not abolished

[a] Given in percent or μg bradykinin equivalent/ml plasma or serum.
[b] Intravenous application.

Table 16. *Kininogen depletion during shock-like syndromes*

Reference	Animal	Agent	Dosage	Decrease of kininogen
		a) Endotoxin application		
WEBSTER and CLARK (1959)	Dog	*Salm. typhosa*	50 mg	no decrease
GREEFF et al. (1966)	Dog	Endotoxin Flexner	10 mg/kg i.v.	10.8 ± 0.6 → 1.1 ± 0.5 μg/ml
MEYER (1966)	Dog	Coli or proteus endotoxin	0.2–5 mg/kg i.v.	decrease
DINIZ et al. (1967)	Dog	Endotoxin from *Serratia marcescens* or *E. coli*	5 mg/kg	31.3% (10–49%) loss of kininogen
ROTHSCHILD and CASTANIA (1968)	Dog	*E. coli* endotoxin	5 mg/kg	8.4 ± 0.4 → 5.7 ± 0.3 μg/ml; no further decrease after previous application of cellulose sulfate
SARDESAI and WALT (1969)	Rat	*E. coli* endotoxin	10 mg/kg i.p.	significant decrease of plasma kininogen
ERDÖS and MIWA (1968)	Rabbit	*E. coli* endotoxin	2 mg/kg	no decrease of kininogen activable by pancreatic kallikrein; some loss of glass-activable kininogen[a]
NIES et al. (1968)	Monkey (*Macaca mulatta*)	*E. coli* endotoxin or *P. pseudomallei* endotoxin	9.0–12.5 mg/kg 0.2– 0.3 mg/kg i.v. infusion	decrease (100 → 50–60%); depending on severity of intoxication
URBANITZ et al. (1969b)	Dog	*E. coli* endotoxin	1 mg/kg i.v.	not significant
HABERMANN et al. (1969)	Rabbit	*E. coli* endotoxin	1 mg/kg i.v.	not exceeding the (small) decrease of plasma protein concentration
	Cat	*E. coli* endotoxin	1 mg/kg i.v.	not exceeding the (small) changes of plasma protein concentration
		b) Anaphylactic and anaphylactoid reactions		
LECOMTE (1961)	Rabbit	Egg white Human erythrocytes	? ?	kininogen content (hydrolysis by saliva) decreased
DINIZ and CARVALHO (1963)	Rabbit	Egg albumin	?	about 50% loss of kininogen

Table 16 (continued)

Reference	Animal	Agent	Dosage	Decrease of kininogen
CÎRSTEA et al. (1966)	Dog	Horse serum	?	decrease less than 20%
DINIZ et al. (1967)	Dog	Horse serum	1 ml/kg i.v.	depending on severity of shock; up to 25–55% loss
CÎRSTEA et al. (1966)	Rabbit	Egg albumin	?	significant decrease (22–61%)
	Guinea pig	Egg albumin	?	not significant
GREEFF et al. (1966)	Guinea pig	Egg white	0.2 ml $^1/_{10}$ i.v.	10.6 ± 0.9 µg/ml→ 4.5 ± 1.2 µg/ml plasma
	Dog	Polyvinylpyrrolidon	50 mg/kg i.v.	11.1 ± 0.7 µg/ml→ 3.4 ± 0.6 µg/ml plasma
	Rat	Dextran	40 mg/kg i.p.	12.3 ± 0.9 µg/ml→ 3.0 ± 0.3 µg/ml plasma
			40 mg/kg i.p. following cortisone	13.5 ± 0.9 µg/ml plasma
URBANITZ et al. (1969b); HABERMANN et al. (1969)	Dog	Polyvinyl-pyrrolidone	50 mg/kg i.v.	not significant
STARR and WEST (1969)	Rat	Horse serum + Pertussis vaccine	0.5 ml i.p., 2.5×10^7 organisms i.p.	increase of plasma kininogen[b], decrease of liver kininogen[b]
BACK et al. (1966)	Dog	Horse serum	10 ml i.v.	ca. 7 µg/ml→ca. 8.5 µg/ml
ANKIER and STARR (1967)	Rat	Dextran	40–240 mg/kg	ca. 5 µg/ml→ca. 7 µg/ml during 30 min; then return to normal values
BRISEID et al. (1968)	Man	Specific, exogenous allergies		no differences against healthy subjects
		c) Other Agents		
WERLE (1966b)	Dog	Coelomic fluid from *Ascaris lumbricoides*	0.1 ml i.v.	40→0 µg/ml
GREEFF et al. (1966)	Rat	Compound 48/80	2 mg/kg	$12.3 \pm 0.9 \rightarrow 4.4 \pm 0.4$ µg/ml

[a] Probably not responsible for the sudden drop of blood pressure since carboxypeptidase B (3.9 mg/kg) fails to prevent it.
[b] When challenged 10 days after sensitization. No change on 20th day.

Table 17. *Kininogen level in other physiological and pathological conditions*

Reference	Animal	Condition	Changes in kininogen content
WEBSTER and CLARK (1959)	Dog	Hemorrhagic shock	1 of 4 dogs showed decrease of kininogen level which was normalized after reinfusion
DINIZ and CARVALHO (1963)	Dog	Hemorrhagic shock	first rise (to 160%) then fall (to about 60%)
MEYER (1966)	Dog	Hemorrhagic shock	14 µg/ml→5 µg/ml
URBANITZ et al. (1969b), HABERMANN et al. (1969)	Rabbit, dog	Hemorrhagic shock	Simultaneous decrease of kininogen and total protein

Table 17 (continued)

Reference	Animal	Condition	Changes in kininogen content
URBANITZ et al. (1969b), HABERMANN et al. (1969)	Rabbit	Traumatic shock	Simultaneous decrease of kininogen and total protein
WERLE (1966a)	Man	Traumatic shock	15–20 μg/ml → 2.0–7.8 μg/ml
URBANITZ et al. (1969b), HABERMANN et al. (1969)	Rabbit	Burning	No significant deviations between changes of kininogen and total protein level
RYAN et al. (1964, 1965)	Dog	Acute hemorrhag. pancreatitis	47% kininogen lost without Trasylol, 25% kininogen lost with Trasylol
NUGENT et al. (1969)	Dog	Acute pancreatitis (taurocholate + trypsin)	No decrease of concen. of plasma kininogen (1.49 μg/ml → 1.44 μg/ml); loss of total kininogen equal with loss of plasma volume
GREEFF (1966)	Man	Cholecystitis; pancreatitis; ulcus duodeni	14 μg/ml → 5 μg/ml 14 μg/ml → 7 μg/ml 14 μg/ml → 8 μg/ml
DINIZ et al. (1967)	Dog	Acute pancreatitis (bile injection)	35% decrease without Trasylol, no significant decrease with Trasylol
NAGEL et al. (1968)	Dog	Perforation peritonitis	18.0 μg/ml → 10.9 μg/ml (mean values from 6 dogs)
GREEFF (1966)	Rat	Environmental temperature (30 min) 35° 45° 52°	 13 μg/ml → 12 μg/ml 13 μg/ml → 5 μg/ml 13 μg/ml → 6 μg/ml
GREEFF and SCHARNAGEL (1966)	Rat	Environmental temperature: normal 35° 45° 52°	 11.4 ± 0.2 μg/ml 6.2 ± 0.6 μg/ml 3.7 ± 1.0 μg/ml 4.3 ± 0.6 μg/ml
CUSCHIERI et al. (1969)	Man	Cold vasodilatation in the finger	0.30 ± 0.03 μg/ml → 0.23 ± 0.03 μg/ml
WIEGERSHAUSEN et al. (1969b)	Man	Myocardial infarction	No change on first day; decrease 2nd to 6th day
SICUTERI et al. (1966)	Man	Myocardial infarction	ca. 3.0 μg/ml → 0.5 μg/ml
DINIZ and CARVALHO (1963)	Man	Liver cirrhosis; liver metastases	3.85—6.3 μg/ml instead of 7.4–14.3 μg/ml
DINIZ and CARVALHO (1963)	Rabbit	CCl_4 poisoning	decrease with severity of liver damage, maximally 50%
SCHARNAGEL and GREEFF (1966)	Dog	Oxygen deficiency 3–6 min	11.2 ± 1.5 μg/ml → 6.0 ± 0.9 μg/ml
EIGLER and HABERMANN (unpublished)	Dog	Tourniquet shock (aorta abdominalis)	No significant deviations between changes of kininogen and plasma protein level
EIGLER and HABERMANN (unpublished)	Dog	Tourniquet shock (aorta mesenterica)	
BOREHAM and GOODWIN (1969)	Man	Trypanosomiasis	6 μg/ml → 2.4 μg/ml during parasitaemic wave

Table 17 (continued)

Reference	Animal	Condition	Changes in kininogen content
GAUTVIK et al. (1968)	Cat	Stimulation of chorda tympani	No effect on concentration of "substrate 1"; reduction (from 20–60%) of "substrate 2"
PERITI and GASPARRI (1969)	Man	Cancer chemotherapy with trisethylene-iminoquinone	3.05 ± 1.14 μg/ml→ 0.72 ± 0.31 μg/ml
WERLE et al. (1968)	Rat	Nephrectomy (bilateral)	5 μg/ml→17 μg/ml after 24 hours
	Rat	Adrenalectomy (bilateral)	5 μg/ml→13 μg/ml after 24 hours

Table 18. *Kininogen level during birth*

Reference	Stage of birth	Animal	Venous plasma (μg/ml)
PERITI and GASPARRI (1966)	Beginning of labor	Man	4.81 ± 1.30
	Full dilatation and expulsion		3.74 ± 1.20
	Few hours post partum		3.68 ± 1.30
	During puerperium		normal values
DINIZ and CARVALHO (1963)	During delivery	Man	25% loss of kininogen
	During puerperium	Man	normal values
ARMSTRONG and MILLS (1966)	During puerperium (?)	Man	loss of glass-activable kininogen[a]
WIEGERSHAUSEN et al. (1967, 1969a)	During mens IX/X	Man	up to threefold normal values
	During birth		decrease to a value still higher than normal
	In amniotic fluid		0.2–0.5
DELHAYE et al. (1967)	In amniotic fluid	Man	present
WIEGERSHAUSEN et al. (1968a, b, 1969a)	End of pregnancy	Rabbits, rats	increase
	Birth		small, not significant decrease to nearly normal values
	Puerperium		temporary increase

[a] At least partially due to "cold activation".

Kininogen values may change concomitantly with total plasma protein, for instance by hemodilution or hemoconcentration (see p. 271). Only a few investigators communicated the changes of both kininogen and total protein levels. In our hands, no dissociation of those values occurred in rabbits shocked by trauma, hemorrhage, burn or endotoxin. The same was true for dogs shocked by hemorrhage, endotoxin or polyvinylpyrrolidone and for cats shocked with endotoxin (see Tables 16 and 17).

The kinin-yielding sequence of kininogen can be degraded without kinin release (see p. 270).

If only one of the plasma kininogens is affected by a pathophysiological process (see p. 271), and if it constitutes a small fraction of that group, its decrease will not be detected; the global determinations currently used are not precise enough.

Measurable arteriovenous differences of the kininogen content due to kinin release cannot be maintained for longer than a few minutes except in a very small vascular area; otherwise the supply of kininogen would be exhausted (see p. 276).

Because of the quick elimination of bradykinin by blood and tissues, concentrations of more than a few nanograms bradykinin/ml circulating blood can be maintained for only a few minutes if the kinin-releasing process is a local one. Otherwise the kininogen reserves would be exhausted within a few minutes.

Decrease of kininogen may be involved in a given pathophysiological process as its cause or its consequence. This must be ascertained by other criteria.

References

AARSEN, P. N.: Sensitization of guinea pig ileum to the action of bradykinin by trypsin hydrolyzate of ox and rabbit plasma. Brit. J. Pharmacol. **32**, 453 (1968).

ANDREWS, P.: The gel-filtration behaviour of proteins related to their molecular weights over a wide range. Biochem. J. **96**, 595 (1965).

ANKIER, S. I., STARR, M. S.: The importance of plasma kinins in the anaphylactoid reaction in rats. Brit. J. Pharmacol. **31**, 331 (1967).

ARMAN, C. G. VAN: Interrelationship among some peptide precursors. In: Polypeptides which stimulate plain muscle, p. 103, ed. by J. H. GADDUM. Edinburgh 1955.

ARMSTRONG, D., MILLS, G. L.: Physiological influence on the liberation of human plasma kinin at low temperatures. In: Hypotensive peptides, p. 139, ed. by E. G. ERDÖS, N. BACK and F. SICUTERI. Berlin-Heidelberg-New York: Springer 1966.

ARNOLD, D., WELTZIEN, H. V.: Über die strukturabhängige hämolytische Aktivität einiger Cholin-Phosphatide. Z. Naturforsch. **23**b, 675 (1968).

AXÉN, R., GROSS, E., WITKOP, B., PIERCE, J. V., WEBSTER, M. E.: Release of kinin activity from human kininogens and fresh plasma by cyanogen bromide. Biochem. biophys. Res. Commun. **23**, 92 (1966).

BACK, N., STEGER, R.: Effect of inhibitors on kinin-releasing activity of proteases. Fed. Proc. **27**, 96 (1968).

— WILKENS, H., STEGER, R.: Fibrinolysis and vasoactive peptides in anaphylaxis. In: Hypotensive peptides, p. 485, ed. by E. G. ERDÖS, N. BACK and F. SICUTERI. Berlin-Heidelberg-New York: Springer 1966.

BOREHAM, P. F. L., GOODWIN, L. G.: The release of kinins as a result of an antigen-antibody reaction in trypanosomiasis. Symposium on cardiovascular actions of kinins. Fiesole 1969 (in press).

BOSSE, J.-A., WASSERMANN, O.: Über eine Adsorption von Histamin an Glas. Med. Pharmacol. exp. **16**, 459 (1967).

BRISEID, K., DYRUD, O. K., LANGE-NIELSEN, F.: Determination of factors of the plasma kinin system in plasma substrate specimens from patients with specific, exogenous allergies. Acta allerg. (Kbh.) **23**, 413 (1968).

BROCKLEHURST, W. E., MAWER, G. E.: The purification of a kininogen from human plasma. Brit. J. Pharmacol. **27**, 256 (1966).

— ZEITLIN, I. J.: Determination of plasma kinin and kininogen levels in man. J. Physiol. (Lond.) **191**, 417 (1967).

CÎRSTEA, M.: Potentiation of some bradykinin effects by thiol-compounds. Brit. J. Pharmacol. **25**, 405 (1965).

— SUHACIU, G., BUTCULESCU, I.: Evaluation du rôle de la bradykinine dans le choc anaphylactique. Arch. Int. Pharmacodyn. **159**, 18 (1966).

CORRADO, A. P., REIS, M. L., CARVALHO, I. F., DINIZ, C. R.: Bradykininogen and bradykinin in the cardiovascular shock produced by proteolytic enzymes. Biochem. Pharmacol. **15**, 959 (1966).

CUSCHIERI, A., ONABANJO, O. A., JAMES, P. B.: Kinin release during cold vasodilatation. Symposium on cardiovascular actions of kinins. Fiesole 1969 (in press).

DAMAS, J., LECOMTE, J.: Kininogènes plasmatiques et réactions vasomotrices provoquées chez le rat, par le dextran. C. R. Soc. Biol. (Paris) **162**, 809 (1968).

DAWSON, W., STARR, M. S., WEST, G. B.: Inhibition of anaphylactic shock in the rat by antihistamines and ascorbic acid. Brit. J. Pharmacol. **27**, 249 (1966).

Delhaye, C., Reuse, J.-J., Vanden Driessche, B.: Studies on smooth muscle active substances in human amniotic fluid. In: Bradykinin and related kinins, p. 113, ed. by M. Rocha e Silva and H. Rothschild. São Paulo 1967.
Diniz, C. R., Carvalho, I. F.: A micromethod for determination of bradykininogen under several conditions. Ann. N.Y. Acad. Sci. **104**, 77 (1963).
— — Reis, M. L., Corrado, A. P.: Bradykininogen in some experimental conditions. In: Bradykinin and related kinins, p. 15, ed. by M. Rocha e Silva and H. Rothschild. São Paulo 1967.
Edery, H.: Potentiation of the action of bradykinin on smooth muscle by chymotrypsin, chymotrypsinogen and trypsin. Brit. J. Pharmacol. **22**, 371 (1964).
Egorova, T. P., Paskhina, T. S.: The liberation of kinins from rabbit kininogen by different kallikreins, p. 180. Abstracts, 5th FEBS Meeting. Prague 1968.
Eisen, V.: Kinin-forming enzymes and substrates in human plasma. J. Physiol. (Lond.) **186**, 133P (1966).
Elliott, D. F.: Bradykinin and its mode of release. Ann. N.Y. Acad. Sci. **104**, 35 (1963).
Erdös, E. G., Miwa, I.: Effect of endotoxin shock on the plasma kallikrein-kinin system of the rabbit. Fed. Proc. **27**, 92 (1968).
— — Graham, W. J.: Studies on the evolution of plasma kinins; reptilian and avian blood. Life Sci. **6**, 2433 (1967).
— Renfrew, A. G., Sloane, E. M., Wohler, J. R.: Enzymatic studies on bradykinin and similar peptides. Ann. N.Y. Acad. Sci. **104**, 222 (1963).
— Sloane, E. M.: An enzyme in human blood plasma that inactivates bradykinin and kallidins. Biochem. Pharmacol. **11**, 585 (1962).
Fasciolo, J. C., Halvorsen, K.: Specificity of mammalian kallidinogen. Amer. J. Physiol. **207**, 901 (1964).
Ferreira, S. H.: Bradykinin-potentiating factor. In: Hypotensive peptides, p. 356, ed. by E. G. Erdös, N. Back and F. Sicuteri. Berlin-Heidelberg-New York: Springer 1966.
Frey, E. K., Kraut, H., Werle, E., Vogel, R., Zickgraf, G., Trautschold, I.: Das Kallikrein-Kinin-System und seine Inhibitoren. Stuttgart: Ferdinand Enke 1968.
Garbe, G.: Quantitative Kininogenbestimmung in menschlichem Plasma. Naunyn-Schmiedebergs Arch. Pharmak. exp. Path. **256**, 112 (1967).
Gautvik, K. M.: Kininogen in plasma from cat, hamster and guinea pig. Acta physiol. scand. **76**, 191 (1969).
— Hilton, S. M., Torres, S. H.: Consumption of the plasma substrate for glandular kallikrein on activation of the submandibulary salivary gland. J. Physiol. (Lond.) **197**, 22P (1968).
— Rugstad, H. E.: Kinin formation and kininogen depletion in rats after intravenous injection of ellagic acid. Brit. J. Pharmacol. **31**, 390 (1967).
Greeff, K.: Der Kininogengehalt des Plasmas beim experimentellen Schock. In: Neue Aspekte der Trasylol-Therapie, S. 135, hrsg. von R. Gross u. G. Kroneberg. Stuttgart: Schattauer 1966.
— Scharnagel, K.: Plasmakinine als Vermittler der Vasodilatation bei Wärmeeinwirkung. Med. Pharmacol. exp. **15**, 68 (1966).
— — Lühr, R., Strobach, H.: Die Abnahme des Kininogengehaltes des Plasmas beim toxischen, anaphylaktischen und anaphylaktoiden Schock. Naunyn-Schmiedebergs Arch. exp. Path. Pharmak. **253**, 235 (1966).
Greenbaum, L. M., Hosoda, T.: The liberation of a dialysable precursor of bradykinin by pepsin. Pharmacologist **5**, 263 (1963a).
— — Studies on the isolation of bradykininogen. Biochem. Pharmacol. **12**, 325 (1963b).
— Yamafuji, K., Hosoda, T.: Studies on the peptic degradation of bovine bradykininogen. Biochem. Pharmacol. **14**, 411 (1965).
Gross, E., Witkop, B.: Selective cleavage of the methionyl peptide bonds in the ribonuclease with cyanogen bromide. J. Amer. chem. Soc. **83**, 1510 (1961).
Habermann, E.: Über Zusammenhänge zwischen esterolytischen und pharmakologischen Wirkungen von Jararacagift, Kallikrein und Thrombin. Naunyn-Schmiedebergs Arch. exp. Path. Pharmak. **236**, 492 (1959).
— Über pH-bedingte Modifikationen des kininliefernden α-Globulins (Kininogen) aus Rinderserum und das Molekulargewicht von Kininogen I. Biochem. Z. **337**, 440 (1963).
— Isolierung, pharmakologische Eigenschaften, Strukturaufklärung und Spaltung peptischer kininliefernder Fragmente (PKF) aus Rinderserum-Kininogen. Naunyn-Schmiedebergs Arch. exp. Path. Pharmak. **251**, 187 (1965).
— Enzymatic kinin release from kininogen and from low-molecular compounds. In: Hypotensive peptides, p. 116, ed. by E. G. Erdös, N. Back and F. Sicuteri. Berlin-Heidelberg-New York: Springer 1966a.

Habermann, E.: Strukturaufklärung kininliefernder Peptide aus Rinderserum-Kininogen. Naunyn-Schmiedebergs Arch. exp. Path. Pharmak. **253**, 474 (1966b).
— Zur Frage der Beziehung zwischen Kininsystem und allergischen Prozessen. Dtsch. Med. Wschr. **93**, 40 (1968a).
— Inhibitors of kallikrein and other proteinases from animal blood. Ann. N.Y. Acad. Sci. **146**, 479 (1968b).
— Blennemann, G.: Zum Mechanismus der Kininfreilegung aus der gereinigten Vorstufe und kininliefernden Teilsequenzen. Naunyn-Schmiedebergs Arch. exp. Path. Pharmak. **247**, 324 (1964a).
— — Über Substrate und Reaktionsprodukte der kininbildenden Enzyme Trypsin, Serum- und Pankreaskallikrein sowie von Crotalusgift. Naunyn-Schmiedebergs Arch. exp. Path. Pharmak. **249**, 357 (1964b).
— — Müller, B.: Charakterisierung und Reinigung peptischer kininliefernder Fragmente (PKF) sowie von „Pepsitocin" aus Rinderserumkininogen. Naunyn-Schmiedebergs Arch. exp. Path. Pharmak. **253**, 444 (1966).
— Helbig, J.: Cleavage of kininogen by cyanogen bromide and enzymes. A procedure for determining position and structure of the kinin-yielding sequence. Naunyn-Schmiedebergs Arch. exp. Path. Pharmak. **255**, 20 (1966).
— — Untersuchungen zur Struktur des Rinderserum-Kininogens unter Verwendung von Bromcyan und Carboxypeptidase B. Naunyn-Schmiedebergs Arch. exp. Path. Pharmak. **258**, 160 (1967).
— Klett, W.: Reinigung und einige Eigenschaften eines Kallikreins aus Schweineserum. Biochem. Z. **346**, 133 (1966).
— — Rosenbusch, G.: Partielle Reinigung und einige Eigenschaften eines Kininogens aus Rinderblut. Hoppe-Seylers Z. physiol. Chem. **332**, 121 (1963).
— Müller, B.: Zur enzymatischen Spaltung peptischer kininliefernder Fragmente (PKF) sowie von Rinderserum-Kininogen. Naunyn-Schmiedebergs Arch. exp. Path. Pharmak. **253**, 464 (1966).
— Rosenbusch, G.: Reinigung und Spaltung von Kininogen aus Rinderblut. Naunyn-Schmiedebergs Arch. exp. Path. Pharmak. **243**, 357 (1962).
— Sailer, F., Müller, J.: Nachweis und Bedeutung der Kinine im Schock. Schocksymposium, Freiburg 1969 (im Druck).
— Schuck, S.: Einige Beziehungen zwischen „Pepsitocin" und Plasmakininen. Naturwissenschaften **51**, 61 (1964).
Helbig, J.: Über die kininliefernde Sequenz von Rinderserum-Kininogen; präparative und analytische Untersuchungen mit Hilfe von Enzymen und Bromcyan. Thesis Würzburg 1968.
Henriques, O. B., Gapanhuk, E., Kauritcheva, N., Budnitskaya, B.: Methionyl-lysyl-bradykinin release from plasma kininogen by plasmin. Biochem. Pharmacol. **18**, 1788 (1969).
— Kauritcheva, N., Kuznetsova, V., Astrakan, M.: Substrates of kinin-releasing enzymes isolated from horse plasma. Nature (Lond.) **215**, 1200 (1967).
— Picarelli, Z. P., Ferraz de Oliveira, M. C.: Partial purification of the plasma substrate for the bradykinin-releasing enzyme from the venom of *Bothrops jararaca*. Biochem. Pharmacol. **11**, 707 (1962).
Hochstrasser, K., Werle, E.: Über kininliefernde Peptide aus pepsinverdauten Rinderplasmaproteinen. Hoppe-Seylers Z. physiol. Chem. **348**, 177 (1967).
Holman, G., Lowe, J. S., Morley, J. S., Smithers, M. J.: The substrate specificity of guinea-pig plasma kallikrein. Biochem. biophys. Res. Commun. **33**, 140 (1968).
Horton, E. W.: The assay of kallikrein in urine. J. Physiol. (Lond.) **142**, 36P (1958).
Jacobsen, S.: Substrates for plasma kinin-forming enzymes in human, dog and rabbit plasmas. Brit. J. Pharmacol. **26**, 403 (1966a).
— Substrates for plasma kinin-forming enzymes in rat and guinea pig plasma. Brit. J. Pharmacol. 28, 64 (1966b).
— Observations on the content of kininogen, kallikrein and kininase in lymph from hind limbs of dogs and rabbits. Brit. J. Pharmacol. **27**, 213 (1966c).
— Kriz, M.: Some data on two purified kininogens from human plasma. Brit. J. Pharmacol. **29**, 25 (1967).
— Waaler, B. A.: The effect of scalding on the content of kininogen and kininase in limb lymph. Brit. J. Pharmacol. **27**, 222 (1966).
Jahrreiss, R., Habermann, E.: Isolierung und Struktur peptischer kininliefernder Peptide aus Rinderserum. Naunyn-Schmiedebergs Arch. Pharmak. **264**, 172 (1969a).
— — In vitro investigations on some components of the kinin system (kininogen, serum kallikrein, Hageman factor), and their interaction. Symposium on cardiovascular actions of kinins. Fiesole 1969b (in press).

KATO, H., NAGASAWA, S., SUZUKI, T.: Relationship between tertiary structure and kinin-yielding ability of bovine kininogen. Biochem. biophys. Res. Commun. **27**, 163 (1967a).
— SUZUKI, T.: The location and nature of the linkage of kinin moiety in bovine kininogen II. Biochem. biophys. Res. Commun. **32**, 800 (1968).
— — IKEDA, K., HAMAGUCHI, K.: Physicochemical properties of bovine kininogen II. J. Biochem. (Tokyo) **62**, 591 (1967b).
KATORI, M., SHIGEI, T.: Failure of kinin formation by glass powder in rat plasma after injection of bromelain. Jap. J. Pharmacol. **18**, 277 (1968).
LECOMTE, J.: Consommation des kininogènes plasmatiques au cours du choc anaphylactique du lapin. C. R. Soc. Biol. (Paris) **155**, 1411 (1961).
— Sur les propriétés des kininogènes de plasma du rat "in vivo". Bull. Soc. roy. Sci. Liège **37**, 358 (1968a).
— Absence d'action antianaphylactique de l'acide ellagique chez le lapin. C. R. Soc. Biol. (Paris) **162**, 807 (1968b).
— Rôle accessoire des kininogènes dans le déterminisme du choc anaphylactique du rat. C. R. Soc. Biol. (Paris) **162**, 1014 (1968c).
— Action de quelques enzymes kinin-formateurs sur le choc anaphylactique du lapin. Bull. Soc. Roy. Sci. Liège **36**, 480 (1968d).
— DAMAS, J.: Sur le rôle des kininogènes dans le syndrome déclenché par les dextrans chez le rat. Arch. int. Pharmacodyn. **176**, 403 (1968).
LEME, J., SCHAPOVAL, E. E. S., ROCHA E SILVA, M.: Factors influencing the development of local swelling induced in the rat paw by macromolecular compounds and heating. In: Bradykinin and related kinins, p. 213, ed. by M. ROCHA E SILVA and H. ROTHSCHILD. São Paulo 1967.
LEWIS, G. P.: Active polypeptides derived from plasma proteins. Physiol. Rev. **40**, 647 (1960).
MARGOLIS, J.: Quantitative studies of kinin-releasing enzymes in plasma. In: Hypotensive peptides, p. 198, ed. by E. G. ERDÖS, N. BACK and F. SICUTERI. Berlin-Heidelberg-New York: Springer 1966.
— BISHOP, E.: Studies on plasma kinins. I. The composition of the kininogen complex. Aust. J. exp. Biol. med. Sci. **41**, 293 (1963).
— BRUCE, S., STARZECKI, B., HORNER, G. J., HALMAGYI, D. F. J.: Release of bradykinin-like substance (BKLS) in sheep by venom of *Crotalus atrox*. Aust. J. exp. Biol. med. Sci. **43**, 237 (1965).
MEYER, A.: Die Wirkung von Trasylol bei Schockzuständen. In: Neue Aspekte der Trasylol-Therapie, S. 142, hrsg. von R. GROSS u. G. KRONEBERG. Stuttgart: Schattauer 1966.
MONGAR, J. L., PERERA, B. A. V.: The role of a chymotrypsin-like enzyme in histamine release from rat mast cells. J. Physiol. (Lond.) **162**, 70P (1962).
MORLEY, J. S.: The nature of the linkage of kinin in kininogens. Biochem. biophys. Res. Commun. **33**, 841 (1968).
MOURI, T.: A method for the estimation of human plasma kininogens I and II. Tohoku J. exp. Med. **98**, 147 (1969).
NAGASAWA, S., HORIUCHI, K., YANO, M., SUZUKI, T.: Partial purification of bovine plasma kallikrein activated by contact with glass. J. Biochem. (Tokyo) **62**, 398 (1967).
— MIZUSHIMA, Y., SATO, T., IWANAGA, S., SUZUKI, T.: Studies on the chemical nature of bovine bradykininogen. Determinations of amino acid, carbohydrate, amino and carboxyl terminals. J. Biochem. (Tokyo) **60**, 643 (1966).
NAGEL, M., KARL-SCHUCH, W., RAHMANZADAH, R.: Untersuchungen zur zusätzlichen Proteaseninhibitortherapie bei der septischen Peritonitis. In: Neue Aspekte der Trasylol-Therapie, Bd. 2, S. 129, hrsg. von R. MARX, H. IMDAHL u. G. L. HABERLAND. Stuttgart u. New York: Schattauer 1968.
NIES, A. S., FORSYTH, R. P., WILLIAMS, H. E., MELMON, K. L.: Contribution of kinins to endotoxin shock in unanesthetized rhesus monkeys. Circulat. Res. **22**, 155 (1968).
NORTHROP, J. H., KUNITZ, E.: In: ABDERHALDEN, Handbuch der biologischen Arbeitsmethoden, Bd. IV/2, S. 2213. Berlin: Urban & Schwarzenberg 1936.
NUGENT, F. W., ZUBERI, S., BULAN, M. B.: Kinin precursor in experimental pancreatitis. Proc. Soc. exp. Biol. (N.Y.) **130**, 566 (1969).
PERITI, P., GASPARRI, F.: Bradykininogen in the blood of women during pregnancy, labor, and puerperium. In: Hypotensive peptides, p. 536, ed. by E. G. ERDÖS, N. BACK and F. SICUTERI. Berlin-Heidelberg-New York: Springer 1966.
— — Cancer chemotherapy and blood kininogen content. Symposium on cardiovascular actions of kinins. Fiesole 1969 (in press).
PIERCE, J. V.: Structural features of plasma kinins and kininogens. Fed. Proc. **27**, 52 (1968).
— WEBSTER, M. E.: The purification and some properties of two different kallidinogens from human plasma. In: Hypotensive peptides, p. 130, ed. by E. G. ERDÖS, N. BACK and F. SICUTERI. Berlin-Heidelberg-New York: Springer 1966.

Rocha e Silva, M., Beraldo, W. T., Rosenfeld, G.: Bradykinin, a hypotensive and smooth muscle stimulating factor released from plasma globulin by snake venoms and by trypsin. Amer. J. Physiol. **156**, 261 (1949).

Rothschild, A. M.: Pharmacodynamic properties of cellulose sulfate and related polysaccharides—a group of bradykinin-releasing compounds. In: Bradykinin and related kinins, p. 197, ed. by M. Rocha e Silva and H. Rothschild. São Paulo 1967.

— Some pharmacodynamic properties of cellulose sulfate, a kininogen-depleting agent in the rat. Brit. J. Pharmacol. **33**, 501 (1968a).

— Role of anaphylatoxin and of bradykinin in passive cutaneous anaphylaxis against heterologous precipitating antibody in the rat. Proceedings 3rd Int. Pharmacol. Meeting, São Paulo 1966, **11**, 83 (1968b).

— Castania, A.: Endotoxin shock in dogs pretreated with cellulose sulfate, an agent causing partial plasma kininogen depletion. J. Pharm. Pharmacol. **20**, 77 (1968).

— Gascon, L. A.: Effect of agar on bradykininogen levels and esterolytic activity in rat plasma. Experientia (Basel) **21**, 208 (1965).

Rothschild, Z., Rosa, A. T., Rothschild, A. M.: On a plasminogen activator induced in rat plasma by cellulose sulphate, an activator of the kinin-generating system. Acta physiol. Lat.-amer. (in press) (1969).

Ryan, J. W., Moffat, J. G., Thompson, A. G.: Role of bradykinin system in acute hemorrhagic pancreatitis. Arch. Surg. **91**, 14 (1965).

— Thompson, A. G., Moffat, J. G.: Role of bradykinin in the development of acute pancreatitis. Nature (Lond.) **204**, 1212 (1964).

Sardesai, V. M., Walt, A. J.: Proteolytic reaction in endotoxin shock. Symposium on cardiovascular actions of kinins. Fiesole 1969 (in press).

Schachter, M.: Some properties of kallidin, bradykinin and wasp venom kinin. In: Polypeptides which affect smooth muscles and blood vessels, p. 241, ed. by M. Schachter. London: Pergamon press 1960a.

— (ed.): Polypeptides which affect smooth muscles and blood vessels, p. 325. London: Pergamon press 1960b.

Scharnagel, K., Greeff, K.: Änderung des Kininogengehaltes des Plasmas bei Hypoxie und lokaler Ischämie. Naunyn-Schmiedebergs Arch. exp. Path. Pharmak. **253**, 81 (1966).

Schwick, H. G., Heimburger, N., Haupt, H.: Antiproteinasen des Humanserums. Z. ges. inn. Med. **21**, 1 (1966).

Seidel, G., Vogt, W.: Kininogenspezifität von acetonaktiviertem menschlichem Plasmakallikrein. Naunyn-Schmiedebergs Arch. Pharmak. exp. Path. **262**, 135 (1969).

Sicuteri, F., Franchi, G., Bianco, P. L. del, Fanciullacci, M.: Some physiological and pathological roles of kininogen and kinins. In: Hypotensive peptides p. 522, ed. by E.G. Erdös, N. Back and F. Sicuteri. Berlin-Heidelberg-New York: Springer 1966.

Starr, M. S., West, G. B.: Further evidence for the involvement of kinin in anaphylactic shock in the rat. Brit. J. Pharmacol. **37**, 178 (1969).

Suzuki, T., Iwanaga, S., Nagasawa, S., Sato, T.: Purification and properties of bradykininogen and of the bradykinin-releasing and destroying enzymes in snake venom. In: Hypotensive peptides, p. 149, ed. by E. G. Erdös, N. Back and F. Sicuteri. Berlin-Heidelberg-New York: Springer 1966.

— — Sato, T., Nagasawa, S., Kato, H., Yano, M., Horiuchi, K.: Biochemical properties of kininogens and kinin releasing enzymes. In: Bradykinin and related kinins, p. 27, ed. by M. Rocha e Silva and H. Rothschild. São Paulo 1967.

Urbanitz, D., Sailer, F., Habermann, E.: In vivo investigations on the role of the kinin system in tissue injury and shock syndromes. Symposium on cardiovascular actions of kinins. Fiesole 1969b (in press).

— Wiegand, H., Habermann, E.: Zur Frage der Bedeutung des Kininsystems beim thermischen Ödem der Rattenpfote. Naunyn-Schmiedebergs Arch. Pharmak. **264**, 476 (1969a).

Vogt, W.: Demonstration of the presence of two separate kinin-forming systems in human and other plasma. In: Hypotensive peptides, p. 185, ed. by E. G. Erdös, N. Back and F. Sicuteri. Berlin-Heidelberg-New York: Springer 1966.

— Wawretschek, W.: Weitere Untersuchungen zur Existenz zweier kininbildender Systeme in menschlichem Plasma. Naunyn-Schmiedebergs Arch. exp. Path. Pharmak. **260**, 223 (1968).

Webster, M. E., Clark, W. R.: Significance of the kallikrein-kallidinogen-kallidin system in shock. Amer. J. Physiol. **197**, 406 (1959).

— Pierce, J. V.: The nature of the kallidins released from human plasma by kallikreins and other enzymes. Ann. N.Y. Acad. Sci. **104**, 91 (1963).

Werle, E.: The chemistry and pharmacology of kallikrein and kallidin. In: Polypeptides which stimulate plain muscle, p. 20, ed. by J. H. Gaddum. Edinburgh 1955.

Werle, E.: Kininogenspiegel im menschlichen Serum nach Verkehrsunfällen. In: Neue Aspekte der Trasylol-Therapie, S. 176, hrsg. von R. Gross u. G. Kroneberg. Stuttgart: Schattauer 1966a.
— Kininogenspiegel und Blutdruck beim Schock. In: Neue Aspekte der Trasylol-Therapie, S. 177, hrsg. von R. Gross u. G. Kroneberg. Stuttgart: Schattauer 1966b.
— Götze, W., Keppler, A.: Über die Wirkung des Kallikreins auf den isolierten Darm und eine neue darmkontrahierende Substanz. Biochem. Z. **289**, 217 (1937).
— Hochstrasser, K.: Versuche zur Isolierung eines niedermolekularen Kininogens. Hoppe-Seylers Z. physiol. Chem. **332**, 322 (1963).
— — Trautschold, I.: Studies on bovine plasma kininogen, ornitho-kallikrein, and ornithokinin. In: Hypotensive peptides, p. 105, ed. by E. G. Erdös, N. Back and F. Sicuteri. Berlin-Heidelberg-New York: Springer 1966.
— Leysath, G., Schmal, A.: Über das Verhalten des Kininogenspiegels nach Nieren- und nach Nebennierenexstirpation bei der Ratte. Hoppe-Seylers Z. physiol. Chem. **349**, 107 (1968).
— Trautschold, I.: Colostrokinin und seine Bildung durch Kallikreine. Z. Biol. **111**, 169 (1960).
Wiegershausen, B., Henninghausen, G., Klausch, B.: The level of kininogen in man and animal during gestation. Symposium on cardiovascular actions of kinins. Fiesole 1969a (in press).
— — — Körber, H. G., Hauzeur, F.: Kininogen level in myocardial infarction. Symposium on cardiovascular actions of kinins. Fiesole 1969b (in press).
— — — Paegelow, I.: Kininogen content of plasma in man and animals during pregnancy, p. 4. Abstracts, 5th FEBS Meeting, Prague 1968a.
— Klausch, B., Henninghausen, G., Sosat, R.: Der Kininogenspiegel von Ratten und Kaninchen während der Gestation. Experientia (Basel) **24**, 1128 (1968b).
— Paegelow, I., Walter, H.: Kininogen in Fruchtwasser und Serum. Naunyn-Schmiedebergs Arch. exp. Path. Pharmak. **257**, 76 (1967).
Yano, M., Kato, H., Nagasawa, S., Suzuki, T.: An improved method for the purification of kininogen II from bovine plasma. J. Biochem. (Tokyo) **62**, 386 (1967a).
— Nagasawa, S., Horiuchi, K., Suzuki, T.: Separation of a new substrate, kininogen I, for plasma kallikrein in bovine plasma. J. Biochem. (Tokyo) **62**, 504 (1967b).

Kininases*

E. G. Erdös and H. Y. T. Yang

With 6 Figures

Kininases are enzymes that inactivate kinins. This chapter will survey them together with other enzymes that can convert some of the longer analogs of bradykinin to the nonapeptide.

The rapid disappearance of kinins was observed simultaneously with the discovery of kallidin and bradykinin. Werle et al. (1937) saw that substance DK (later known as kallidin) once released by kallikrein was inactivated quickly on standing. Bradykinin was assumed to be destroyed by trypsin that liberated the peptide from dog plasma globulin in the first place (Rocha e Silva et al., 1949). Subsequently it was established that liberation and inactivation of kinins are independent processes occurring in the same crude system *in vitro*. Kallidin was inactivated by an agent in serum (Werle et al., 1937). Bradykinin activity was destroyed by the chymotrypsin contamination in the trypsin used (Werle and Berek, 1950; Werle et al., 1950; Werle, 1953), by snake venom (Rocha e Silva et al., 1949) or by serum (Rocha e Silva, 1951).

Kininases are widely distributed in nature, as shown in Table 1. The sources of kininases range from human blood to microorganisms. Some of these enzymes were purified and the peptide bond cleaved by them was identified, but other kininases have been used as crude extracts in biological experiments. Only those enzymes that are of possible physiological or practical importance will be discussed here in detail.

Table 1. *Sources of enzymes that inactivate bradykinin and kallidin*

Contaminating enzymes in kininogenases (e.g. in trypsin, kallikrein, snake venom)
Biological fluids (e.g. blood, urine, lymph, lung edema fluid)
Tissue extracts (e.g. pancreas, kidney)
Purified proteases (e.g. carboxypeptidase B, chymotrypsin)
Plants, bacteria, molds (e.g. bromelain, *E. coli*, *Ps. Aerug.*, *Cl. histol.*, "Dymal")

A. Blood

In the circulating blood, red blood cells, leukocytes, thrombocytes, and plasma contain active kininases. One of the characteristics of bradykinin and kallidin is the rapid inactivation of the peptides in normal plasma, contrary to the relative stability of other peptides, such as vasopressin. This homeostatic mechanism is a major factor in determining the duration of their action. Plasma and sera of various

* Some of the experiments described here were supported by Grant HE 08764 from the National Institutes of Health, United States Public Health Service.

animals hydrolyze kinins at different rates. Guinea pig serum is especially active in this respect (Werle et al., 1937; Werle and Hambuechen, 1943; Klett, 1962). Cohn fractions IV-1 and IV-4 of plasma which contain bradykininogen also inactivate kinins (Van Arman, 1955; Erdös and Sloane, 1962).

I. Carboxypeptidase N

The mechanism of inactivation of kinins in blood was characterized after the peptides became available in synthetic form. The first enzyme to be described in 1961 was a carboxypeptidase found in fraction IV-1 of human plasma and was named carboxypeptidase N (Erdös, 1961, 1962). The enzyme cleaves the carboxyl terminal arginine of the peptides. The removal of Arg^9 from bradykinin was shown by the sequential use of paper chromatography and electrophoresis. The inactivation of bradykinin was inhibited by various chelating agents, thus the enzyme is a metallopeptidase. Of the metal ions tested, Co^{2+} enhanced and Cd^{2+} inhibited the *in vitro* hydrolysis of bradykinin. In the presence of cobalt chloride the rate of hydrolysis of bradykinin by carboxypeptidase N of human plasma fraction IV-1 about doubled (Erdös and Sloane, 1962), and in rabbit serum (Erdös et al., 1963b) it was also enhanced.

The hydrolysis of bradykinin by human plasma fraction IV-1 and by unfractionated rabbit serum proceeds quite similarly (Erdös et al., 1963b). (This may be attributed to the lack of kininase II in both preparations.) From bradykinin substrate 1 ml human blood serum released 0.13 μmole arginine/min, and rabbit serum 0.15 μmole (Paskhina and Trapeznikova, 1967). The first-order reaction rate constant of the hydrolysis of bradykinin by human fraction IV-1 was $k = 0.024\ min^{-1}$ (Erdös and Sloane, 1962).

Table 2. *Carboxypeptidase N in activity in blood sera or plasma* (E. G. Erdös et al., 1964b, 1967a)

	Activity (μmole/min per ml)		
	HLL		HLAa
Human	0.79	0.80 [b]	3.01
Swine	1.01		5.2
Ox	0.26		
Newborn calf	0.43		
Rabbit	0.28	0.26 [b]	
Guinea pig	0.70		
Rat	1.02		
Cat	1.04		
Chicken	0.45		
Alligator	trace [a]		
Frog	0.28		
Turtle	0.87		
Carp	0.56		
Earthworm	trace [a]		

[a] Activity shown with peptide mapping only.
[b] Paskhina and Trapeznikova (1967).
HLL = hydrolysis of hippuryl-L-lysine by sera or plasma in presence of 1×10^{-4} M $CoCl_2$.
HLAa = hydrolysis of hippuryl-L-argininic acid by serum.

In addition to kinins, carboxypeptidase N cleaves shorter peptide substrates, including substrates of pancreatic carboxypeptidase B. The rate of hydrolysis of hippuric acid derivatives in human plasma decreased in the order: hippuryl-L-lysine (HLL), hippuryl-L-arginine (HLA), and hippuryl-L-ornithine. In a routine assay the enzyme activity was determined by measuring the hydrolysis of HLL after the enzyme was pre-equiliberated with $CoCl_2$. This metal ion increases the hydrolysis of HLL about 6-fold in man and 1.5-fold in rabbit (SHIMONAEVA, 1967). Table 2 shows the rate of hydrolysis of HLL in human and animal plasma. Human serum cleaves HLL only about 9% faster than heparinized plasma (ERDÖS et al., 1964b). Differences in the rate of cleavage of lysine from HLL by sera of various animals (Table 2) are smaller than the differences encountered when the inactivation of bradykinin is measured in bioassay. For example, guinea pig serum inactivates bradykinin much faster than human plasma. In a series of experiments, the relative kininase activities of the various untreated serum samples decreased in this order: guinea pig, dog, alligator, rabbit (ERDÖS et al., 1963b). Rat serum also breaks down bradykinin rapidly (FASCIOLO, 1964), whereas the kininase level in bovine serum is low (WERLE et al., 1937; FREY et al., 1968). Some of the discrepancies between the rate of hydrolysis of HLL and the rapidity of inactivation of bradykinin may have been caused by the presence of a second kininase in plasma.

In addition, some peptides representing C-terminal fragments of bradykinin not only served as substrates of carboxypeptidase N but also of other kininases originating from blood or kidney. The N-terminal end of the peptides was acetylated to avoid an unspecific attack by aminopeptidases. Arginine was cleaved from Ac-L-Phe-L-Arg and from Ac-L-Ser-Pro-L-Phe-L-Arg (ERDÖS et al., 1964b; ERDÖS and YANG, 1966) by plasma and kidney carboxypeptidases.

Like other peptidases, carboxypeptidase N has an esterase action in that it cleaves the ester substrate hippuryl-L-argininic acid (HLAa, *o*-benzoyl-glycyl-α-L-hydroxyl-δ-guanidino-*n*-valeric acid). For the determination of carboxypeptidase N activity, assaying the esterase instead of the peptidase action offers some advantages. The enzyme with HLAa substrate does not require preincubation with cobalt chloride, and the activity can be determined in 5 μl plasma in 5 minutes in the ultraviolet spectrophotometer with 0.25 μmole substrate (ERDÖS et al., 1967a). Human serum cleaved HLAa at a rate of 3 μmoles/min per ml serum; swine serum enzyme was more active, splitting 5.2 μmoles. TRAPEZNIKOVA and PASKHINA (1968) used Cbo-L-Phe-L-argininic acid as substrate, and this ester was also hydrolyzed faster than the peptide substrates.

Table 3. *Purification of the carboxypeptidase N of human plasma*

Steps	Relative specific activity			
	peptidase[a]	esterase[b]	kininase[c]	HLL[a] (% yield)
1. Plasma	1.0	1.0		100
2. Ammonium sulf. ppt (30–55%)	2.9	2.8	1.0	88
3. DEAE-Sephadex 1	110			35
4. DEAE-Sephadex 2	252	212	67	14

Substrates:
[a] Hippuryl-L-lysine.
[b] Hippuryl-L-argininic acid.
[c] Bradykinin.
The hydrolysis of hippuryl-L-lysine and hippuryl-L-argininic acid was calculated as μmole substrate hydrolyzed in 1 min by 1 mg enzyme protein (ERDÖS et al., 1967a).

Carboxypeptidase N was prepared (ERDÖS et al., 1964b, 1967a) by precipitating it from the plasma with ammonium sulfate, followed by dialysis against cobalt chloride solution. The enzyme was further purified by repeated DEAE-Sephadex column chromatographies. The peptidase activity increased 252-fold over the native plasma, while the esterase activity was enhanced 212-fold (Table 3). When the ammonium sulfate precipitate was taken as a starting material there was a proportional increase in the kininase activity. The kininase, peptidase, and esterase activities could not be separated because they migrated as a single peak in Pevikon zone electrophoresis at two different pH values. The starting material for electrophoresis was a human globulin fraction precipitated with ammonium sulfate. Similar results were obtained by Trapeznikova and Paskhina (1968), using zone electrophoresis.

Paskhina and Trapeznikova (1967) purified carboxypeptidase N from human and from rabbit sera. The activity of the purified human enzyme increased 80-fold and the rabbit enzyme about 60-fold as assayed with HLL substrate. In a later publication 273- and 130-fold purifications were reported (Trapeznikova and Paskhina, 1968). In other purification attempts the kininase activity of rabbit serum was concentrated 15 to 20-fold (Shimonaeva, 1967) and of guinea pig serum about 30-fold (Klett, 1962).

The K_m for carboxypeptidase N of human serum with HLL was 1.4 to 1.6×10^{-3} M (Erdös et al., 1964b; Trapeznikova and Paskhina, 1968) and with HLAa it was 1×10^{-4} (Erdös et al., 1967a). The K_m values for the enzyme with L-Pro-L-Phe-L-Arg and HLA were 1.3×10^{-3} M and 1.2×10^{-2} M (Trapeznikova and Paskhina, 1968).

The pH optimum of the carboxypeptidase N with HLL substrate is about 7.5 (Erdös et al., 1964b; Trapeznikova and Paskhina, 1968) and it decreases above 8. The optimal pH is slightly higher with the ester substrate and gives a broader peak in the alkaline range. The activity below pH 7 depends on the selection of the buffer. For example, the enzyme activity drops much more steeply in the acid milieu in a phosphate buffer than in an acetate buffer (Erdös et al., 1964b; the problem is discussed in detail on p. 313 of this chapter). When sodium chloride was added to the phosphate buffer, bradykinin was irreversibly inactivated much faster in guinea pig serum at various pH values (Aarsen and Kemp, 1963).

Metal ions influence the peptidase and esterase activities of carboxypeptidase N differently. For example, added $CoCl_2$ has no effect on the hydrolysis of HLAa, while $NiSO_4$ inhibits it. On the other hand, both metal ions enhance the cleavage of HLL by carboxypeptidase N (Erdös et al., 1964b, 1967a).

Plasma kininases are irreversibly inactivated by acid or heat treatment because they lose activity when incubated at pH 2–3 or at a temperature above 56° (Horton, 1959a; Frey et al., 1968). The enzymatic activity increases with the temperature up to 37° and then drops sharply. Five minutes of heating at 56° lowered the activity of a purified carboxypeptidase N preparation by 80% and 10 minutes in a boiling water bath inactivated it completely (Trapeznikova and Paskhina, 1968). Because of these properties crude kininogens were frequently prepared by a combination of heating and acidifying this plasma protein substrate to eliminate the contaminating kininases.

Carboxypeptidase N of human or animal plasma, although it hydrolyzes the peptide bond of basic carboxyl terminal amino acids just as carboxypeptidase B does, can be definitely distinguished from the pancreatic enzyme. For example, for peptidase activity the swine pancreatic carboxypeptidase B requires zinc as cofactor and added cadmium enhances the esterase activity. Both metals, however, inhibit plasma carboxypeptidase N from various sources including swine serum (Erdös et al., 1963b, 1964b, 1967a; Erdös, 1966a; Yang and Erdös, 1967). In addition EDTA inhibits carboxypeptidase N but not carboxypeptidase B. HLA is hydrolyzed faster than HLL by the pancreatic enzyme, while the opposite is true for the plasma enzyme. Cobalt ions have quantitatively different effects on the two carboxypeptidases.

Kallidin is also a substrate of carboxypeptidase N (ERDÖS et al., 1963b). Although it was claimed first that kallidin was more stable in plasma than bradykinin, later it was found that the inactivation of the two peptides proceeds at a similar rate. The kinin that was more stable in plasma and was mistakenly thought to be kallidin turned out to be Met-Lys-bradykinin (LEWIS, 1963; ELLIOTT and LEWIS, 1965).

Among the various bradykinin homologs, Lys^9-bradykinin is hydrolyzed by guinea pig serum kininase at the same rate as bradykinin (ERDÖS et al., 1967c).

In order to delay the very rapid breakdown of bradykinin in blood plasma, more resistant depsipeptide analogs were synthesized. In these compounds one or more of the amide bonds are replaced by an ester bond; they contain glycolic acid residues instead of the corresponding amino acid (RAVDEL et al., 1967). A related peptide, Gly^6-$PhLac^8$-bradykinin (glycyl^6-phenyllactic acid^8-bradykinin), had a vasodepressor effect two to three times longer than bradykinin itself. The peptide is hydrolyzed by carboxypeptidase N somewhat more slowly than is the parent compound. In contrast, other depsipeptides are cleaved faster by carboxypeptidase N (Table 4; PASKHINA and TRAPEZNIKOVA, 1967). Perhaps the longer-acting depsipeptide is either more resistant to kininase II than bradykinin or it is inactivated less in the pulmonary circulation.

Table 4. *Rate of hydrolysis of bradykinin and its depsipeptide analogs by partially purified preparations of kininase from human and rabbit blood serum*[a]

Enzyme	Bradykinin	$Glyc^4$-bk	$Glyc^6$-bk	$Diglyc^{4,6}$-bk	$Phenlac^8$-$glycyl^6$-bk
Human kininase	0.056	0.075	0.097	—	0.045
Rabbit kininase	0.10	0.14	0.25	0.084[b]	0.065

[a] According to PASKHINA and TRAPEZNIKOVA (1967) (μmole Arg/min per mg).
[b] Single determination.

No carboxypeptidase A activity was found in plasma when either the peptide substrate (ERDÖS et al., 1964b) or the ester substrate of this enzyme was used (ERDÖS et al., 1967a; TRAPEZNIKOVA and PASKHINA, 1968).

In addition to kinins, other peptides may serve as naturally occurring substrates of carboxypeptidase N. For example, blood of animals that do not have plasma kallikrein or kininogen (e.g. frog or carp) still contains kininase activity (ERDÖS et al., 1964b, 1967b, 1968a, and unpublished).

NG and VANE (1968) suggested that carboxypeptidase N may be important in converting angiotensin I to angiotensin II in the lung. Our unpublished exploratory studies, however, do not seem to support this hypothesis.

Bovine kininogen I of YANO et al. (1967) holds bradykinin at the C-terminal end of protein. Possibly in the native plasma kininogen, Arg^9 of bradykinin is sterically not accessible to carboxypeptidase N. During purification, however, *o*-phenanthroline had to be added, presumably to protect the kininogen against kininases, otherwise the purified kininogen I released very little active kinin.

Fibrin formation in blood is preceded by the release of fibrinopeptides from fibrinogen. Both peptides A and B contain arginine at the C-terminal end, which was cleaved by added pancreatic carboxypeptidase B. In contrast, human serum liberated arginine quickly from the B peptide and slowly and incompletely from the A peptide. Fibrinopeptide B without the C-terminal arginine was isolated from clotted fibrinogen supernatant (TEGER-NILSSON and BLOMBÄCK, 1967; TEGER-NILSSON, 1968). These experiments raise the possibility that some native plasma proteins might be substrates also of carboxypeptidase N.

II. Kininase II

As mentioned above, carboxypeptidase N was first found in Cohn fraction IV-1 of human plasma. During purification of the enzyme from native human plasma,

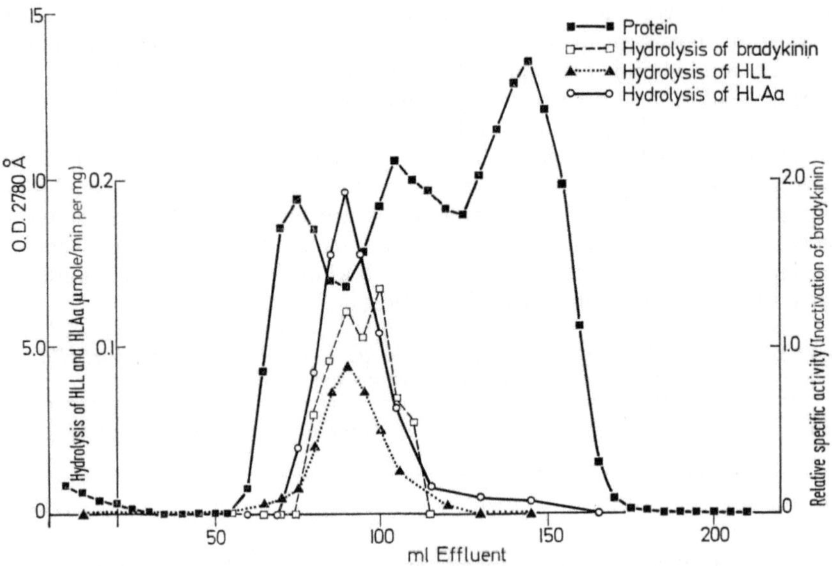

Fig. 1. Sephadex G-200 filtration of human plasma kininases. Fifteen ml fresh heparinized human plasma was filtered through a 3.5×46 cm column. A 0.05 M phosphate buffer, pH 7, containing 0.5 mole/liter of sodium chloride was the eluent; 5-ml fractions were collected every 30 min. HLL, Hippuryl-L-lysine. HLAa, hippuryl-L-argininic acid (YANG and ERDÖS, 1967)

it was precipitated with ammonium sulfate and dialyzed against a dilute solution of cobalt chloride, then chromatographed on columns (ERDÖS et al., 1963b). The kininase activity of the purified preparation and of the Cohn fraction was due to the presence of carboxypeptidase N. The method of purification of plasma kininase was changed later, and the starting material was obtained by means of gel filtration of fresh human plasma through a Sephadex G-200 column. The active fraction hydrolyzed both the ester and peptide substrates of carboxypeptidase; however, the kininase peak was broader than could be expected of the carboxypeptidase N activity alone (Fig. 1). When the kininase was further purified on a DEAE-Sephadex column, two enzymes were separated (YANG and ERDÖS, 1967) (Fig. 2). One was identical with carboxypeptidase N, but the other was different. For the sake of brevity carboxypeptidase N was called kininase I in the report, the second enzyme kininase II. Apparently, kininase II was inactivated in the previous experiments when the plasma proteins were fractionated by Cohn's procedure or by the method mentioned above. Chromatographic experiments with bradykinin and shorter peptide substrates such as Ac-L-Ser-L-Pro-L-Phe-L-Arg proved that kininase II breaks a different bond than does kininase I (Table 5) because kininase II inactivates bradykinin by cleaving the link between Pro[7] and Phe[8], thus removing the dipeptide, phenylalanylarginine, from the carboxyl terminal end of bradykinin. Although the enzyme acted as an endopeptidase, it was inhibited by chelating agents just as exopeptidases are. Some inhibitors of kininase I such as arginine, $CdSO_4$, and EACA are inactive against kininase II (Table 6). Trasylol had no effect on the enzyme. The bond specificity and inhibition

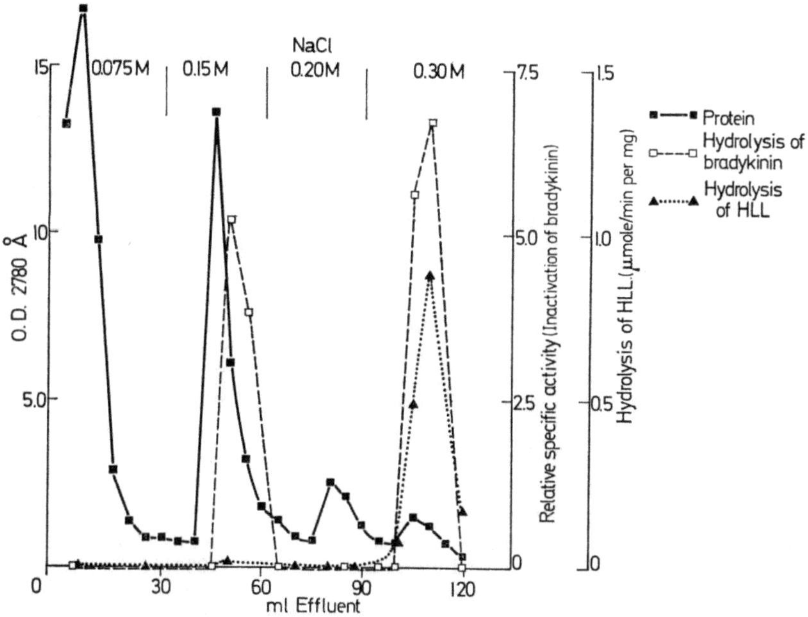

Fig. 2. Separation of the two kininases on a DEAE-Sephadex A-50 column. Three hundred mg protein obtained after gel filtration was purified on a 1×30 cm column. Fractions were eluted step by step by increasing the concentration of sodium chloride in a 0.02 M phosphate buffer, pH 6.8; 5 ml was collected every 30 min. The activity eluted with 0.3 M sodium chloride contained kininase I (carboxypeptide N). Kininase II moved with the fraction that was eluted with 0.15 M sodium chloride. HLL, Hippuryl-L-lysine (Yang and Erdös, 1967)

pattern of kininase II are very similar to those of a swine kidney microsomal enzyme named peptidase P (Erdös and Yang, 1967a, b, c), thus possibly kininase II originates from the kidney (p. 301). Kininase I and II can be found in the blood plasma of various laboratory animals. Man and most animals seem to have both kininases; only rabbit and pigeon plasma lack kininase II among those tested (Erdös et al., 1968a).

Table 5. *Site of action of some kininases*

	1 H-Arg-	2 Pro-	3 Pro-	4 Gly-	5 Phe-	6 Ser-	7 Pro-	8 Phe-	9 Arg-OH
Chymotrypsin						↑			↑
Carboxypeptidases (B, N, kidney, catheptic)									↑
Peptidase P, kininase II (kidney, plasma)								↑	
Prolidase (imidopeptidase; kidney, erythrocytes)		↑							
Snake venoms					↑	↑			
Bromelain					↑	↑			

Table 6. *Inhibitors of kininases in vitro (inhibition, +; no inhibition, −)*

Inhibitor	Enzyme (source and type)	Inhi-bition	Reference
Metal ion-binding agents			
EDTA	Plasma or sera, man, animals; carboxyp. N (kininase I)	+	Armstrong et al. (1955); Erdös (1962); Aarsen and Kemp (1962); Erdös and Sloane (1962); Margolis and Bishop (1962); Ferreira and Rocha e Silva (1962); Bishop and Margolis (1963); Erdös et al. (1963b); Jacobsen (1966b); Garbe (1967); Paskhina and Trapeznikova (1967)
	Kininase II, man	+	Yang and Erdös (1967)
	Erythrocytes, man	−	Erdös et al. (1963b); Amundsen and Nustad (1964)
	Leukocytes, man	−	Schwab (1962); Zachariae et al. (1966)
	Carboxyp., kidney	+	Erdös and Yang (1966,
	Peptidase P, kidney	+	1967a, c)
	Lymph, dog	+	Jacobsen (1966a)
	Brain, rat	+	Iwata et al. (1969)
	Some microbial kininases	+	Amundsen and Rugstad (1965)
1,10-Phenanthroline	Kininases of peptidyl amino acid hydrolase type (carboxyp.)	+	Erdös (1962); Erdös et al. (1963b); Erdös and Yang (1966); Erdös (1966a); Garbe (1967)
	Kininase II, plasma	+	Yang and Erdös (1967)
	Peptidase P, kidney	+	Erdös and Yang (1967a)
	Kininase from *Pseud. aer.*	+	Rugstad (1967b)
2,2-Dipyridyl	Erythrocytes, man	+	Erdös et al. (1963b); Amundsen and Nustad (1964)
	Plasma, man	+	Amundsen and Nustad (1964)
	Leukocytes, rabbit	+	Greenbaum and Kim (1967)
	Carboxypeptidase, kidney	+	Erdös and Yang (1966)
8-Hydroxyquinoline	Plasma, man, animals	+	Ferreira and Rocha e Silva (1962); Garbe (1967); Rocha e Silva et al. (1967)
	Kidney	+	Carvalho and Diniz (1964)
8-Hydroxyquinoline-5-sulfonic acid	Serum, man	+	Erdös and Wohler (1963a, b)
Cysteine	Plasma or sera, various	+	Werle and Grunz (1939); Van Arman (1955); Erdös (1962); Erdös and Sloane (1962); Erdös et al. (1963b)

Table 6 (continued)

Inhibitor	Enzyme (source and type)	Inhibition	Reference
Cysteine	Tissues, various	+	PICARELLI et al. (1962)
	Leukocytes, rabbit	—	GREENBAUM and KIM (1967)
	Snake venom	+	HAMBERG and DEUTSCH (1958)
BAL	Plasma, man	+	ERDÖS and WOHLER (1963b); GARBE (1967)
	Plasma, rat	+	FERREIRA and ROCHA E SILVA (1962); ROCHA E SILVA (1963)
	Kidney, swine	+	ERDÖS and YANG (1966)
	Kininase from *Pseud. aer.*	+	RUGSTAD (1967b)
2-Mercaptoethanol	Plasma, man	+	ERDÖS and WOHLER (1963b); ERDÖS et al. (1967a)
Thioglycolic acid	Plasma, rat, man	+	FERREIRA and ROCHA E SILVA (1962); WERLE et al. (1964); FREY et al. (1968)
Citrate	Plasma, bovine	+	KLETT (1962)
Metal ions			
Heavy metals, various	Plasma, various	+	ERDÖS (1962); ERDÖS and SLOANE (1962); ERDÖS et al. (1963b, 1964b)
	Erythrocytes, man	+	ERDÖS et al. (1963b); AMUNDSEN and NUSTAD (1964)
	Leukocytes, rabbit, man	+	ZCHARIAE et al. (1966); GREENBAUM and KIM (1967)
	Brain, rabbit	+	CAMARGO and GRAEFF (1969)
	Kininase from *Pseud. aer.*	+	RUGSTAD (1967b)
$CdSO_4$	Carboxyp. N (kininase I)	+	ERDÖS and SLOANE (1962); ERDÖS et al. (1964b, 1967a), TRAPEZNIKOVA and PASKHINA (1968)
	Kininase II	—	YANG and ERDÖS (1967)
$HgCl_2$	Carboxyp. N (kininase I)	+	ERDÖS et al. (1964); YANG and ERDÖS (1967)
	Kininase II	+	YANG and ERDÖS (1967)
	Erythrocytes, man	+	ERDÖS et al. (1963b)
Products of hydrolysis of substrate and related compounds			
Arginine, benzoylarginine	Carboxyp. N (kininase I)	+	ERDÖS 1962; ERDÖS and SLOANE (1962)
Arginine	Kininase II	—	YANG and ERDÖS (1967)
EACA	Carboxyp. N (kininase I)	+	ERDÖS (1962); ERDÖS and SLOANE (1962)
	Carboxyp. N, rabbit	+	PASKHINA and TRAPEZNIKOVA (1967)

Table 6 (continued)

Inhibitor	Enzyme (source and type)	Inhibition	Reference
	Kininase II	—	YANG and ERDÖS (1967)
	Serum, guinea pig	—	ERDÖS et al. (1963b)
	Erythrocytes, man	—	ERDÖS et al. (1963b)
	Plasma, man	+	MARGOLIS and BISHOP (1962)
	Intestine, guinea pig	+	DOLESCHEL and AUERSWALD (1966)
H-Phe-Arg-OH	Carboxyp. N (kininase I)	+	YANG and ERDÖS (1967)
	Kininase II	+	
H-Phe-Ser-Pro-Phe-Arg-OH	Plasma, man	+	GARBE (1967)
Argininic acid	Carboxyp. N (esterase)	+	ERDÖS et al. (1967a)
δ-Amino-*n*-valeric acid	Carboxyp. N (kininase I)	+	ERDÖS (1962); ERDÖS and SLOANE (1962)
Lysine Heptoic acid Pimelic acid	Plasma, man	+	BISHOP and MARGOLIS (1963)
Inhibitors of proteinases (peptidyl peptide hydrolases). E. g.: Trasylol, SBTI, OMTI, DFP	Most kininases, various origin	—	ERDÖS (1962); ERDÖS et al. (1963b)
DFP	Leukocytes, man	—	SCHWAB (1962)
	Leukocytes, rabbit	+	GREENBAUM and KIM (1967)
	Brain, rabbit	+	CAMARGO and GRAEFF (1969)
Trasylol	Brain, rabbit	+	CAMARGO and GRAEFF (1969)
	Leukocytes, rabbit	+	CHANG et al. (1969)
Miscellaneous compounds			
p-Chloromercuriphenylsulfonic acid (PCMS)	Carboxyp. N (kininase I)	—	ERDÖS et al. (1963b)
	Erythrocytes, man	+	ERDÖS et al. (1963b)
Tosyl-phe-chloromethylketone (TPCK)	Leukocytes, rabbit	+	CHANG et al. (1969)
p-Chloromercuribenzoic acid (PCMB)	Kininase from *Pseud. aer.*	+	RUGSTAD (1967b)
	Liver	+	FREY et al. (1968)
Bradykinin-potentiating factor (BPF)	Plasma, guinea pig	+	FERREIRA (1966)
	Whole blood, dog	+	FERREIRA and VANE (1967b)
β-Mercaptoethylamine	Carboxyp. P, kidney	+	ERDÖS and YANG (1966)
Sodium bisulfite	Catheptic, spleen	+	GREENBAUM and YAMAFUJI (1966)
Iodosobenzoic acid	Erythrocytes, man	+	ERDÖS et al. (1963b)
Iodoacetic acid	Catheptic, spleen	+	GREENBAUM and YAMAFUJI (1966)
Disulfiram	Erythrocytes, man, rat	+	DYRUD et al. (1965)
	Plasma, man	—	JENSEN et al. (1965a)
Cortisol and some other related drugs	Erythrocytes, man, rat	+	DYRUD et al. (1965)
	Plasma, man	+	

Table 6 (continued)

Inhibitor	Enzyme (source and type)	Inhibition	Reference
Chlorpromazine	Brain extracts	+	KRIVOY and KROGER (1964)
	Catheptic enzyme, spleen	—	GREENBAUM and YAMAFUJI (1966)
Urgocyton	Erythrocytes, liver	+	AMUNDSEN et al. (1964)
	Kidney	+	ERDÖS and YANG (1966)

These experiments provided additional evidence to show that in various animals the complete plasma kallikrein–kinin–kininase system exists in two different forms.

Another enzyme that cleaves off a dipeptide from the C-terminal end is the angiotensin I-converting enzyme. Purified kininase II preparations contain converting enzyme activity indicating that the two enzymes are very closely related (YANG, JENSSEN and ERDÖS, unpublished observation).

III. Blood Cells

In addition to plasma, the cellular elements of blood contain kininases. Hemolyzed red blood cells inactivate kinins rapidly at a neutral pH. The enzyme in erythrocytes was inhibited by agents (e.g. $CoCl_2$, PCMS) which do not block plasma carboxypeptidase (ERDÖS et al., 1963b; AMUNDSEN and NUSTAD, 1964; p. 310), and, conversely, some inhibitors of plasma kininases (e.g. EDTA, EACA) were inactive against the erythrocyte kininase. The enzyme had no carboxypeptidase activity since it did not hydrolyze HLA (ERDÖS et al., 1963b). It is, however, a metalloenzyme because 1,10-phenanthroline inhibits it. After it was established that plasma and erythrocyte kininases are not identical, combined biological and chemical studies were carried out to characterize the erythrocyte enzyme. The results indicated that the enzyme in question was an imidopeptidase (prolidase). During the hydrolysis of bradykinin, the arginine released (Arg^1) was converted to ornithine by an arginase (EC 3.5.3.1) present in red blood cells. Kallidin, which was also inactivated rapidly by the hemolyzed red cells, presumably had to be converted to bradykinin by an aminopeptidase present, and hydrolyzed by the same enzyme as bradykinin (ERDÖS et al., 1963b). It can be safely assumed that erythrocytes contain other kininases besides an imidopeptidase.

Thrombocytes contain traces of carboxypeptidase activity (ERDÖS et al., 1964b), as shown by the slow hydrolysis of HLL.

Many investigators have studied kininases originating from granulocytes. The enzyme from human or rabbit polymorphonuclear leukocytes is not identical with the plasma enzyme because the leukocyte kininase is inhibited by different agents (SCHWAB, 1962; ZACHARIAE et al., 1966; GREENBAUM and KIM, 1967; Table 7). Its activity per cell is of the same order of magnitude as that of red blood cell kininase (ZACHARIAE et al., 1966). The optimal pH for rabbit or human leukocyte kininases is around or above the neutral pH (ZACHARIAE et al., 1966; GREENBAUM and KIM, 1967; MELMON and CLINE, 1967a, b). The "neutral" kininase activity of human cells disrupted by sonication stayed mainly in the final supernatant instead of in a particulate fraction after centrifugations (GREENBAUM and KIM, 1967; MELMON and CLINE, 1967b), but a granular fraction has a kininase active at pH 5.5 (MELMON and CLINE, 1968). Lysosomes from bovine leukocytes also contain an enzyme that cleaves bradykinin at a neutral pH (Hegner, 1968). The kininase of granulocytes does not hydrolyze carboxypeptidase substrates (Greenbaum, 1967; Yamafuji and Carrara, 1968) and it is assumed to cleave bradykinin somewhere in the middle of the peptide chain.

Table 7. *Effect of inhibitors of kininases on the hypotensive activity of bradykinin in the guinea pig* (Erdös and Wohler, 1963b)

Inhibitor		No. of experiments	Dose of inhibitor (mg/kg)	Dose of bradykinin (μg/kg)	Drop in mean blood pressur	
					before[a] (%)	after[a] (%)
I	2-Mercaptoethanol	15	67 (45–83)[b]	1.0 (0.03–2.0)	10 (0–24)	42 (20–55)
II	β-Mercaptoethylamine	11	90 (50–165)	0.8 (0.4–1.2)	10 (0–20)	16 (7–37)
III	3-Mercaptopropionic acid	13	41 (25–74)	1.1 (0.5–1.8)	13 (0–25)	44 (33–57)
IV	α-Thioglycerol	13	242 (108–429)	0.6 (0.3–1.7)	11 (0–26)	32 (20–52)
V	2,3-Dimercaptopropanol (BAL)	15	16 (5–31)	0.9 (0.3–1.8)	13 (0–28)	48 (31–58)
VI	Diethyldithiocarbamic acid	13	71 (25–100)	1.2 (0.3–2.0)	13 (0–20)	38 (22–58)
VII	L-Penicillamine	13	130 (37–200)	1.2 (0.4–2.2)	11 (6–23)	23 (12–41)
VIII	8-Hydroxy-5-quinoline sulfonic acid	9	126 (50–165)	0.5 (0.3–0.6)	5 (0–13)	31 (23–42)
IX	Ca-EDTA	8	175 (162–198)	0.9 (0.5–1.2)	8 (7–17)	27 (18–33)
X	Glutathione	4	88 (66–111)	1.2 (1.1–1.2)	10 (0–19)	24 (20–30)

[a] Injection of inhibitor.
[b] Range.

Because the kininase activity per white blood cells does not exceed that of erythrocytes (Zachariae et al., 1966), the contribution of leukocyte kininase to the total activity of these enzymes in the blood must be negligible. It may be of greater importance after the extravasation of the cells (p. 314).

In contrast to granulocytes, human lymphocytes had no kininases (Melmon and Cline 1967b).

B. Other Biological Fluids

The presence of kininases was also observed in biological fluids other than blood, such as urine (Frey et al., 1950; Werle and Erdös, 1954; Horton, 1959b; Gaddum and Guth, 1960; Innerfield et al., 1963; Erdös et al., 1964b); lymph (Schachter, 1960; Edery and Lewis, 1963; Erdös et al., 1964b; Jacobsen, 1966a); bile, colostrum (Amundsen and Nustad, 1965); strangulation fluid from ileum (Amundsen, 1966); ascites (Werle and Grunz, 1939; Erdös and Melmon, 1966, unpublished); and synovial fluid (Eisen, 1966; Katori, 1967; Lewis, 1968). Very little was found in the cerebrospinal fluid (Sicuteri et al., 1965).

An enzyme that inactivates kinins occurs in saliva, where it may originate from the squamous epithelial cells of oral mucous membrane (Amundsen and

NUSTAD, 1964). The inhibition pattern of the epithelial enzyme suggests similarities to the enzyme in human erythrocytes. Salivary glands of rats and mice are rich in kallikrein and also in a kininase (ERDÖS et al., 1968b; CHIANG et al., 1968). The kininase was also present in the kallikrein-containing granules.

Only a few of the kininases of the various fluids were characterized. An ammonium sulfate precipitate of human urine, rat lymph (ERDÖS et al., 1964b), and ascites (ERDÖS and MELMON, unpublished observation) contained a carboxypeptidase, possibly carboxypeptidase N. In addition to carboxypeptidase N (kininase I), human urine has some peptidase P (kininase II) activity (YANG and ERDÖS, unpublished observations).

C. Tissues

Homogenized tissues from various sources inactivate kinins (WERLE et al., 1937; ERDÖS, 1966a). Several homogenized organ extracts are rich in kininases with higher activity per milligram protein than in plasma. Pancreas, kidney, and lung are especially active. Various types of cells, just like various subcellular fractions, inactivate bradykinin at a different rate. For example, cells from the gastric mucosa are much less active than cells from the mucosa of the small intestine (AMUNDSEN and NUSTAD, 1965).

In the homogenized pancreas the kininase action was attributed to three enzymes—chymotrypsin, an aminopeptidase, and a carboxypeptidase (WERLE et al., 1950). Subsequent studies showed pancreatic carboxypeptidase B to be the most potent kininase (ERDÖS, 1962; p. 304).

Kidney also contains several kininases. Many investigators (WERLE et al., 1937; FREY et al., 1950; HAMBERG and ROCHA E SILVA, 1954; FASCIOLO, 1964; CARVALHO and DINIZ, 1964) noticed that homogenized kidney inactivated bradykinin and kallidin. In order to distinguish histamine from crude bradykinin, HAMBERG and ROCHA E SILVA (1954), studied the differences between kidney kininase and histaminase. They found that in contrast to histaminase, the kininase in the crude kidney withstood 62° for 10 minutes and its pH optimum was above 7.

Our first approach to the problem consisted of investigating the role of various subcellular fractions of the homogenized rat kidney. The inactivation of bradykinin by these extracts was assayed on the isolated rat uterus. Most of the activity of the homogenized rat kidney was concentrated in a fraction that sedimented with the microsomal fraction (ERDÖS and YANG, 1966; ERDÖS, 1966b) (Fig. 3). The low activity of the lysosomal fraction was attributed to microsomal contamination, and hardly any kininase was found in the soluble fraction. This is in contrast to the high rate of destruction of bradykinin activity by the soluble, final supernatant fraction of the homogenized rat liver as found by AMUNDSEN and NUSTAD (1965) and confirmed by ERDÖS and YANG (1966).

The enzymatic activity in the kidney was much higher than in blood plasma or in the liver. The enzyme in the microsomal fractions of rat kidney is active at a neutral but not at an acid pH. Practically all the enzymatic activity ceases at pH 5. Subsequently, three kininases originating from the swine kidney were characterized; one is a prolidase (imidopeptidase) that cleaves the Arg^1-Pro^2 bond of the peptide (ERDÖS and YANG, 1966; ZUBER, 1966). The enzyme preparations used (ERDÖS and YANG, 1966) were less active than the two other kininases, which were partially purified from homogenized swine kidney cortex.

Acetone-dried kidney powder still contained at least two kininases capable of hydrolyzing bradykinin, as shown by chemical and biological techniques

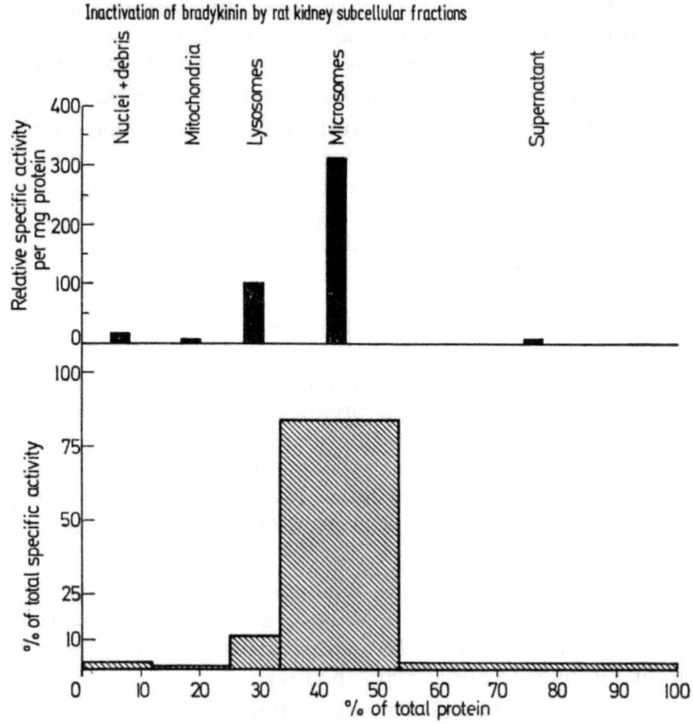

Fig. 3. Rat kidney was homogenized in 0.25 M sucrose. The inactivation of bradykinin was measured on the isolated rat uterus. Fraction 1: nuclei plus cell debris. Fraction 2: heavy mitochondria. Fraction 3: light mitochondria plus lysosomes. Fraction 4: microsomes. Fraction 5: final supernatant. Most of the activity was located in the microsomal fraction (Erdös and Yang, 1966)

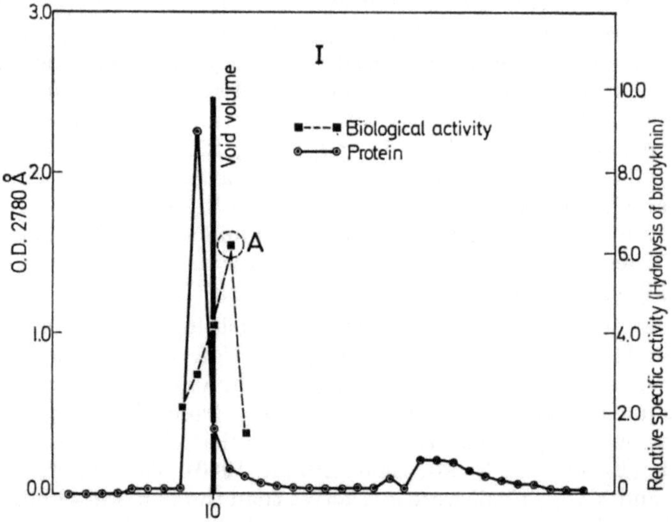

Fig. 4. Second gel filtration of the swine kidney microsomal kininase (peptidase P) on Sephadex G-150 column in presence of 0.15% deoxycholate in 0.1 N NaCl and 0.05 M Tris, pH 7.4. Abscissa: number of fractions collected (Erdös and Yang, 1967a)

(ERDÖS and YANG, 1966). Heating an extract from this powder at 62° for 10 minutes destroyed about 75% of the total kininase action but left a carboxypeptidase intact that cleaved bradykinin. The kidney carboxypeptidase split the Ac-L-Phe-L-Arg substrate much faster than HLA or HLL. Thus it behaved differently from the carboxypeptidases of human and swine plasma or of swine pancreas, because these enzymes release a basic C-terminal amino acid from peptides in which the amino acid preceding arginine is either a protected phenylalanine or glycine. Swine kidney carboxypeptidase liberates C-terminal arginine faster at the concentration of the substrates used (10^{-2} M) when it is linked to phenylalanine, that is, to an aromatic amino acid. The inhibition pattern of this kidney carboxypeptidase indicated that the enzyme was different from pancreatic carboxypeptidase B (FOLK et al., 1960) or from plasma carboxypeptidase N (Table 6).

It was also found that heating the kidney extract destroyed a kininase that was not identical with carboxypeptidase. This enzyme was extracted from a kidney microsomal fraction with deoxycholate and was solubilized by repeated gel filtration on a Sephadex G-150 column (ERDÖS and YANG, 1967a) (Fig. 4). This kininase was named peptidase P. Similar to plasma kininase II, it inactivated bradykinin by cleaving the Pro^7-Phe^8 bond, thus by removing a phenylalanyl-arginine dipeptide from the C-terminal end (Table 5). The enzyme is, however, different from other mammalian endopeptidases (peptidyl peptide hydrolases) but may be identical with kininase II (p. 294). The kininases found in the kidney were active at a neutral pH. They were inhibited by chelating agents such as EDTA, 1,10-phenanthroline, and BAL, but were not effected by *p*-chloromercuriphenyl sulfonic acid. Inhibitors of endopeptidases (Trasylol and DFP) were equally inactive. 2-Mercaptoethylamine, an activator of cathepsins, inhibited peptidase P (Table 6; ERDÖS and YANG, 1966).

As for other tissues, hydrolysis of bradykinin by the lung has been recently scrutinized. Homogenized lung inactivates bradykinin somewhat more slowly than kidney (TRAUTSCHOLD, 1965; FREY et al., 1968). A sediment of the homogenized dog lung obtained at 105,000 *g* in 60 minutes in the centrifuge destroyed bradykinin activity; this activity was blocked by EDTA (BAKHLE, 1968).

In comparison to other tissues, nervous tissues had less kininase action (FASCIOLO, 1964; GROSU and GRECICA, 1965). This activity was studied in extracts from different parts of the central nervous system. In dog brain all regions investigated contained appreciable and equal quantities of kininase, except for white matter, which contained less. Large amounts of kininases were found in the dorsal spinal roots and ganglia (HOOPER, 1963). Kininase activity in an extract from acetone-dried brain was attributed to a carboxypeptidase-type enzyme (KRIVOY and KROGER, 1964). When homogenized rabbit brain was fractionated in the centrifuge, two thirds of the activity was in the final supernatant, the rest was fairly evenly distributed among the particulate fractions (HORI, 1968; CAMARGO and GRAEFF, 1969). Homogenized rat brain yielded similar results (IWATA et al., 1969).

Catheptic enzymes also can inactivate kinins, but at an acid pH. For example, beef spleen contains catheptic carboxypeptidases that are activated by cysteine. The enzyme preparation used cleaved arginine from bradykinin; however, phenylalanine also was found at the same time in the incubation mixture. The release of phenylalanine was attributed to the subsequent action of a second catheptic carboxypeptidase present in the source of enzyme (GREENBAUM and YAMAFUJI, 1966). Another catheptic kininase was discovered in crude extracts of liver (FREY et al., 1968).

D. Purified Proteolytic Enzymes

(peptidyl peptide, peptidyl-amino acid, and α-amino-acyl-peptide hydrolases)

Kinins are inactivated by some proteinases. Among them two pancreatic enzymes—namely carboxypeptidase B and chymotrypsin—are the most important. Other enzymes (some commercially available) that may act as kininases are reviewed by Prado elsewhere in this volume (p. 156). These include subtilisin BPN (Nargarse) (EC 3.4.4.16), ficin (EC 3.4.4.12), papain (EC 3.4.4.10), and *St. griseus* protease (Pronase), but their site of action in the kinin molecule has not been determined.

In the initial studies when bradykinin was released by trypsin (EC 3.4.4.4), the enzyme also inactivated the peptide owing to a contamination by chymotrypsin (EC 3.4.4.5; Werle et al., 1950; Rocha e Silva, 1951; Werle, 1953; p. 157). Another kininogenase, commercial kallikrein (Padutin; Werle et al., 1950; Werle and Berek, 1950) destroyed kinin activity because it contained carboxypeptidase B (EC 3.4.2.2) as a contamination (Erdös et al., 1962).

Commercially available chymotrypsin was used by many investigators during the 1950s to inactivate the kinin content of crude extracts and thereby to differentiate the peptides from other biologically active substances. Proteolytic enzymes were also applied in degradation studies with purified or synthetic peptides to establish their amino acid sequence. Chymotrypsin (Elliott et al., 1960; Boissonnas et al., 1960a, b) hydrolyzes the Phe^{8}-Arg^{9} bond of bradykinin quickly and the Phe^{5}-Ser^{6} bond slowly. A carboxypeptidase preparation released Arg^{9} first and then Phe^{8} from bradykinin (Zuber and Jaques, 1960). The first activity was due to carboxypeptidase B and the second to carboxypeptidase A (EC 3.4.2.1), which must have been also present. Leucine aminopeptidase (EC 3.4.1.1) did not attack the N-terminal Arg^{1}-Pro^{2} bond of bradykinin (Boissonnas et al., 1960b). In biological studies bradykinin was also resistant to leucine aminopeptidase (Erdös, 1962), but it was inactivated by a partially purified prolidase (imidopeptidase, p. 301). The latter enzyme destroyed the activity of bradykinin by cleaving the N-terminal arginine (Erdös and Yang, 1966). Stem bromelain (EC 3.4.4.24) destroyed the activity as assayed on the guinea pig ileum and hydrolyzed the peptide at the Phe^{5}-Ser^{6} and Gly^{4}-Phe^{5} bonds (Enomoto et al., 1967). Table 5 shows the bonds broken by some of the enzymes mentioned.

In biological studies Erdös (1962) and Erdös et al. (1963b) noted the very rapid inactivation of bradykinin and kallidin by purified swine pancreatic carboxypeptidase B *in vitro*. Even the partially purified enzyme was 50 to 100 times faster in this respect than crystallized chymotrypsin. This estimate is probably quite conservative and should be corrected upward when the two enzymes are compared on the basis of the same degree of purity. Because of the very fast hydrolysis of the C-terminal arginine of bradykinin by carboxypeptidase B and the relatively higher specificity of the enzyme than chymotrypsin has, carboxypeptidase B has been frequently employed to identify kinin type peptides in crude extracts.

Since purified carboxypeptidase B is labile and must be kept frozen, attempts have been made to stabilize the preparations. The stability of purified carboxypeptidase B was increased by lyophilizing it in glycine. The activity of the resulting dry powder did not change even when it was kept on a laboratory shelf (Erdös and Yang, 1966). A more promising approach consisted of binding carboxypeptidase B to water-insoluble polymers. The enzyme was coupled to the copolymer of maleic anhydride and ethylene according to the method of Levin et al. (1964). The resulting preparation was kept without loss of activity in the refrigerator under buffer (Chiang et al., 1968). Carboxypeptidase B polymer when suspended in solution rapidly inactivated bradykinin (CHIANG et al., 1968; MIWA et al., 1969; ERDÖS et al., 1969). The enzyme can be collected from suspension by short centrifugation and used again. Other methods of stabilizing carboxypeptidase B included binding the enzyme to Sepharose or to water-soluble polymer or adsorbing it on colloidal silica and subsequently cross-linking it with glutaraldehyde (YANG, LEVIN, and ERDÖS, unpublished, and SEKI et al., 1970).

I. Use of Carboxypeptidase B *in vivo*

In contrast to such agents as histamine, 5-HT, and acetylcholine, no specific antagonists of kinins have yet been found which can block their effects in a wide

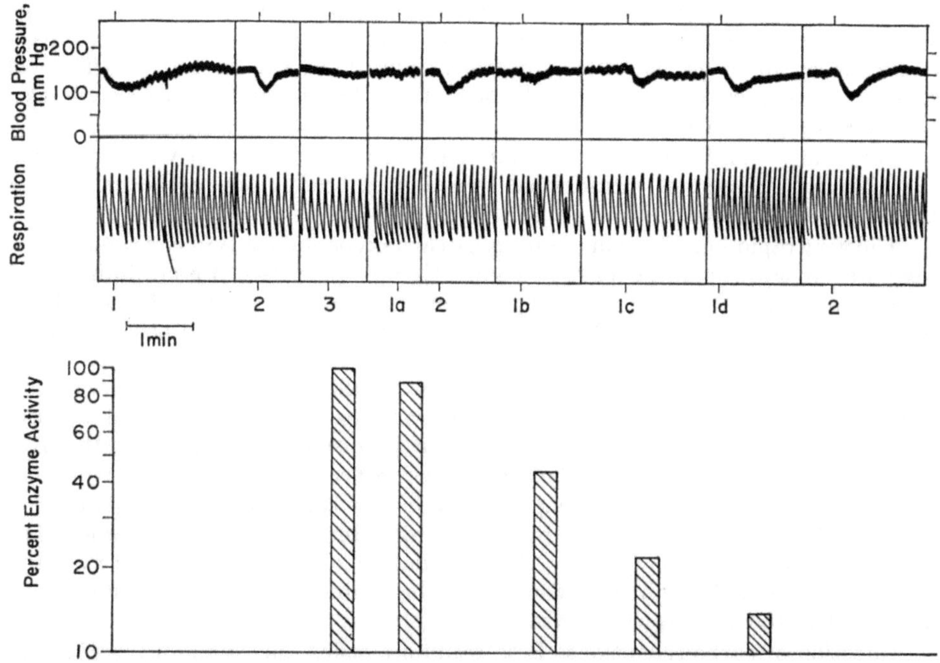

Fig. 5. Return of the effect of bradykinin and decrease in circulating carboxypeptidase B level in blood in a 2.5-kg female cat. Doses of i.v. injections per kg body weight: (1) 18 µg bradykinin; (2) 0.56 µg histamine; (3) 3.8 mg (269 U) carboxypeptidase B. Injections 1a, 1b, 1c, and 1d were given 5, 50, 80, and 110 minutes after the administration of the enzyme. Vertical bars show enzyme activity in plasma (ERDÖS et al., 1963a)

range of tests in various experimental animals. The observation of the very rapid hydrolysis of bradykinin by purified hog pancreatic carboxypeptidase B *in vitro* (ERDÖS, 1962), however, led to the application of this enzyme *in vivo* (ERDÖS et al., 1963a, b). Intravenous injection of carboxypeptidase B blocked the cardiovascular effects of bradykinin or kallidin in guinea pigs, cats, dogs, rabbits, rats, and even in an alligator (ERDÖS et al., 1963a, b; ERDÖS and YANG, 1966). Larger doses were needed, however, to block the activity of Met-Lys-bradykinin (ERDÖS and YANG, 1966) or Lys^9-bradykinin (ERDÖS et al., 1967c). When, instead of carboxypeptidase B, carboxypeptidase A or chymotrypsin was injected, these enzymes had no effect on kinin action. The hypotension caused by acetylcholine, substance P, or eledoisin was not influenced by pretreatment with carboxypeptidase B (ERDÖS et al., 1963b).

In the cat, after a single i.v. injection of carboxypeptidase B, the level of the enzyme decreases in the blood exponentially. The half-life of the enzyme is about 30 minutes; it is about 20 minutes in the rabbit. The decrease in the level of the circulating enzyme and the return of the hypotensive effect of injected bradykinin are closely related (ERDÖS et al., 1963a; Fig. 5). From the rate of disappearance of carboxypeptidase B after a single 2 mg/kg i.v. injection, a maintenance dose was calculated (ERDÖS and YANG, 1966). Starting 20 minutes after the first injection, 15% of the original dose of the enzyme was given in the femoral vein of cats at 10-min intervals, and the high level of carboxypeptidase B was maintained in blood with the resulting complete block of the hypotensive effect of bradykinin. (The peptide was injected every 15 minutes into the contralateral femoral vein.) When the administration of carboxypeptidase B was stopped, the effect of the peptide began to return. Thus repeated i.v. injection of carboxypeptidase B can block the effects of bradykinin in the cat for hours. Effects of kininogenases such as kallikrein (ERDÖS et al., 1963b) and trypsin were also abolished by pretreating animals with carboxypeptidase B.

Subcutaneous infiltration of the skin with carboxypeptidase B also diminished the effect of subsequent intradermal injection of bradykinin in the guinea pig (ERDÖS et al., 1963a).

The very rapid inactivation of kinins by carboxypeptidase B *in vitro* and *in vivo* suggested an additional use for the enzyme. Carboxypeptidase B was administered to men and animals under a variety of conditions where the importance of the release of bradykinin or kallidin in a physiological or pathological process was to be established. WEBSTER et al. (1967) infused carboxypeptidase B to dogs. Although it blocked the hemodynamic effects of kallidin, the decrease in vascular resistance that is seen during muscle contractions or after release of arterial occlusion was not altered by the simultaneous perfusion of the muscle with blood containing 6–40 μg of added carboxypeptidase B per ml.

Similar infusion of carboxypeptidase B in the cat submaxillary gland prevented the vasodilatation caused by bradykinin administered intra-arterially but not the vasodilatation caused by the stimulation of the chorda (SKINNER and WEBSTER, 1968). The authors concluded that kinin release is unlikely to be important in the two processes mentioned.

Injection of carboxypeptidase B to rabbits blocked the hypotensive effect of bradykinin but not that of i.v. injection of endotoxin (ERDÖS and MIWA, 1968). From these experiments it was concluded that the endotoxin effect in the rabbit is not connected with kinin release in the initial phase of shock.

Intra-articular injection of bradykinin raises the pressure in knee joints of dogs. This could be prevented by pretreatment with carboxypeptidase B, but some other signs of inflammation could not. Based on these studies PHELPS et al. (1966), denied the importance of bradykinin in arthritic inflammation. In contrast MELMON et al. (1967) indicated that bradykinin may play a role in gouty arthritis. By using carboxypeptidase B they relieved the increase in the temperature of the knee joint that follows intra-articular injection of bradykinin to dogs. Pretreatment of rat paw with carboxypeptidase B reduced the swelling caused by carrageenin in this mode of inflammation experiment (VAN ARMAN et al., 1968).

II. Fate of Injected Carboxypeptidase B

When exogenous carboxypeptidase B disappears from the circulation of various animals, it is taken up by the tissues. Injected carboxypeptidase B was recovered in active form from the kidney of dog, cat, guinea pig, and rat (ERDÖS and YANG,

1966; ERDÖS et al., 1967c). Highest concentrations were found in the guinea pig and rat kidney. Homogenized kidneys of nine guinea pigs that were injected with carboxypeptidase B hydrolyzed HLA at the rate of 3.3×10^{-2} μmole/min per mg kidney (range 0.7 to 9×10^{-2}). The concentration of the enzyme in the kidney of treated rats was about the same as in the guinea pig. Rat liver showed a significant activity, but the amount of enzyme recovered from the liver of other animals was negligible. Cat and dog kidney also concentrated from the blood a sizable fraction of the injected carboxypeptidase B. Large amounts of the enzyme were excreted in the urine of guinea pig, rat, and cat. Spleen, brain, and lung showed negligible activity, indicating that carboxypeptidase B was not removed from the circulation by these organs. When the renal arteries of a dog were ligated, injected carboxypeptidase B appeared in the lymph, and the half-life of the enzyme in the circulation was longer (WEBSTER et al., 1967). In nephrectomized rats 300 U of carboxypeptidase B blocked bradykinin effect for 1–2 hours (CROXATTO and CRUZATT, 1969). PHELPS et al. (1966) after their experiments recovered 30% of the dose of carboxypeptidase B injected into the knee joint of the dog. The blocking of bradykinin effect persisted for 5 hours.

E. Snake Venoms

Snake venoms contain both kininases and kininogenases, but the two activities do not follow parallel courses in the various venoms. The factor that inactivates bradykinin and the one that liberates it can be distinguished by heating snake venom (HAMBERG and ROCHA E SILVA, 1957). DEUTSCH and DINIZ (1955) studied a large number of venoms. *Crotalus atrox* venom was the most active in destroying bradykinin activity; *Agkistrodon piscivorus* and *A. contortix* venoms had no kininase. *A. halys blomhoffii* venom contains three proteinases. Of these, proteinase B was known to be a kininase because it broke a glycyl-phenylalanine bond in the peptide (SUZUKI et al., 1966). In addition some snake venoms cleave the phenylalanyl-serine linkage in bradykinin. *C. atrox*, *C. adamanteus*, and *Trimerusurus flavoridis* split two peptide bonds of the bradykinin molecule whereas the venoms of *A. contortrix*, *Bothrops jararaca*, and *Vipera russellii* hydrolyze only one peptide bond (Table 5). The kininases present in snake venoms are discussed in another part of this volume by SUZUKI and IWANAGA (p. 193).

F. Microorganisms

A commercial, partially purified collagenase preparation from *Clostridium histolyticum* inactivated bradykinin. Interestingly the enzyme splits the same Pro[7]-Phe[8] bond as kininase II of plasma or peptidase P of kidney (ERDÖS and SLOANE cf. ERDÖS, 1966a; ERDÖS and YANG, 1966). Clostridiopeptidase B (EC 3.4.4.20) from *A. histolyticum* hydrolyzes the lysyl-arginine and the arginyl-proline bonds in Met-Lys-bradykinin (MITCHELL, 1968).

The supernatant fluid of *Pseudomonas aeruginosa* (*Ps. aer.*) cultures contains strong kininase activity, while *Escherichia coli* and β-hemolytic streptococci give negative results. All three microbial suspensions were active after ultrasonic treatment (AMUNDSEN and RUGSTAD, 1965).

The kininase from *Ps. aer.* was studied in detail by RUGSTAD (1966, 1967a, b, c), who purified it about 170-fold by gel filtration (RUGSTAD, 1967a). The molecular weight of this kininase is about 50,000 (RUGSTAD, 1967b). It is inhibited by *o*-phenanthroline, BAL, $ZnCl_2$, and PCMS (Table 6). The enzyme has a pH optimum of about 7.5 and its activity diminishes above or below this value. The kininase inactivated bradykinin, kallidin, and phyllokinin (bradykinyl-isoleucyl-tyrosine) as well. Thin-layer chromatography and electrophoresis indicated that either the Phe^5-Ser^6 or the Phe^8-Arg^9 bond of bradykinin may be cleaved first. *Ps. aer.* kininase had no carboxypeptidase activity (RUGSTAD, 1967c).

Intravenous injection of this kininase significantly reduced the effect of bradykinin on the systemic blood pressure of the rat. The enzyme was stable in blood *in vitro* (RUGSTAD, 1967a) or when added to the blood perfusate of isolated rat lung (NILSEN and RUGSTAD, 1968). The enzyme had a half-life of about 20 minutes in the circulation of the rat after i.v. injection (RUGSTAD, 1967b); such administration significantly reduced the effect of bradykinin injected i.v.

A commercial proteolytic enzyme prepared from a mold (Dymal) also destroyed kinin activity *in vitro* (WERLE and ERDÖS, 1954). Disintegrated *Trypanosoma brucei* had a weak kininase action (BOREHAM, 1968).

G. Fate of Kinins in Circulation

Bradykinin has a very short half-life in blood. MCCARTHY et al. (1965) found a $t_{1/2}$ of 0.27 minute during the passage of dog blood through an extracorporeal system, and the value for kallidin was only slightly higher, 0.32 minute. The half-life of bradykinin in cat blood was about the same as in dog blood (FERREIRA and VANE, 1967a). Based on the circulatory effects of the peptide (SAAMELI and ESKES, 1962) calculated half-life in women to be shorter than 0.5 minute.

BUMPUS et al. (1964) indicated that infused labeled bradykinin which escaped inactivation in the circulation of the rat was taken up mainly by the kidney, where it was rapidly inactivated. Liver had about one fourth of the radioactivity of the kidney, and other organs contained even less labeled peptide or its metabolites. After half an hour most of the radioactive peptide and its fragments were excreted in the urine. In infused, nephrectomized rats, tritiated bradykinin was taken up mostly by the liver, then by the lung, salivary gland, spleen, heart, and uterus respectively (KHAIRALLAH, personal communication).

Many organs inactivate kinins if the peptides are injected into the vessel leading into the organ. For example, bradykinin or kallidin had to be given in doses 2 to 5 times higher into the mesenteric vein than into the femoral vein for an equally hypotensive response in the systemic arterial blood pressure (ERDÖS and YANG, 1966). This discrepancy in required doses could probably be explained by the increased inactivation of the peptide during passage through the splanchnic circulation or the liver. Infusion of bradykinin into the artery of human forearm did not increase the peptide level in venous blood for any considerable period. This also suggests a very rapid disappearance of the peptide from the circulation. The capillaries may be important both in the removal and in the inactivation of bradykinin (SICUTERI et al., 1963; ALLWOOD and LEWIS, 1964).

Recent studies showed that, in addition to hydrolysis in blood, the area of the pulmonary circulation plays a prominent role in inactivating kinins after i.v. injection or infusion. The importance of this process was first emphasized in a short communication by KRONEBERG and STOEPEL (1963). An interesting approach was developed by VANE and his associates (VANE, 1969). Using the blood-bathed organ technique, which allows the continuous bioassay of substances in circulating blood, they estimated the half-lives of peptides and amines in the circulation. In their experiments with kinins, a strip of cat jejunum was superfused with the arterial blood of a cat (FERREIRA and VANE, 1967a, b, c). When bradykinin was infused into various vascular beds of the cat, several areas destroyed the activity of infused bradykinin including the head, the liver, and the kidney. Most impressive was the lung, which rendered 80% of the peptide inactive during a single passage. This was confirmed by BIRON in rats and dogs (1968).

The fate of labeled bradykinin in the pulmonary circulation of the rat was studied also by RYAN et al. (1968). They perfused the lung with LOCKE's solution instead of blood. The metabolites of bradykinin leaving the pulmonary circulation were collected and analyzed. The authors concluded that bradykinin was hydrolyzed by enzymes in or near the endothelium of the pulmonary blood vessels. The first bond broken in the peptide has not yet been definitely established. Imidopeptidase, carboxypeptidase, and chymotrypsin-like enzymes were considered to be involved (STEWART and ROBLERO, 1967; RYAN et al., 1968). Polistes kinin, the longer analog of bradykinin, was more stable in the pulmonary circulation than the parent compound (p. 590; STEWART, 1968).

The rapid inactivation of the peptides in plasma and the effect of passage through the pulmonary circulation may explain in part why after i.v. administration of kinins only a fraction reaches the peripheral vascular bed and why injection of the peptides into the artery of the autoperfused hind limb of the dog requires much smaller amounts to cause vasodilatation than do i.v. injections (ERDÖS, 1966a).

H. Inhibitors of Kininases

The use of inhibitors *in vitro* played an essential part in characterizing kinins and kininases. Until bradykinin and kallidin became available in synthetic form, only isolated observations were made on the inhibition of kininases. For example, cysteine preserved the activity of both kallidin (WERLE and GRUNZ, 1939) and bradykinin (VAN ARMAN, 1955), and EDTA prolonged the existence of a pain-producing substance in plasma (ARMSTRONG et al., 1955) that later was shown to be identical with bradykinin (p. 445). Systematic studies of the inhibition pattern of various kininases started in 1961 (ERDÖS, 1961, 1962). The inhibitors found since can be grouped as chelating agents, metal ions, compounds structurally related to the products of hydrolysis of the substrates, and miscellaneous compounds. Evidently this classification is somewhat arbitrary because some agents would qualify under various headings (Table 6).

Among the sequestering compounds EDTA is used frequently as an inhibitor (ERDÖS et al., 1963b). Depending on the source of blood, there are some differences in the inhibition pattern of the plasma enzymes. Human plasma kininases are inhibited by EDTA (ERDÖS, 1962; YANG and ERDÖS, 1967), while some animal serum or plasma enzymes are more resistant (ERDÖS et al., 1963b; ROCHA E SILVA et al., 1967).

Higher concentrations of EDTA, for example, inhibited rat plasma kininase in JACOBSEN's experiments (1966b), although the agent failed to do that at a lower concentration (FERREIRA and ROCHA E SILVA, 1962; ROCHA E SILVA et al., 1967). Red blood cell kininase was not affected by 7.10^{-3} EDTA. Since both plasma and red blood cell enzymes require a metal ion cofactor, as shown by the effect of 1,10-phenanthroline on the kininases, the differences in inhibition by these sequestering agents are probably caused by structural, steric dissimilarities (ERDÖS et al., 1963b). 1,10-Phenanthroline is a very potent inhibitor of various kininases that are metal dependent. These include the exopeptidase-type enzymes (mostly peptidyl amino acid hydrolases) of blood and tissues. Kininase II (peptidase P), that does not belong to exopeptidases in the strict sense, since it breaks a bond one amino acid residue removed from the peptide bond at the C-terminal end, is also inhibited by 1,10-phenanthroline. This compound has been frequently used to preserve the activity of a kinin after its release *in vitro*, otherwise the kininases present in most crude systems would prevent a quantitative assay of the peptide (ERDÖS et al., 1967b; GARBE, 1967; ERDÖS and MIWA, 1968). For the same purpose MOVAT and DI LORENZO (1968; MOVAT et al., 1968) employed diethyldithiocarbamate (ERDÖS and WOHLER, 1963a, b).

Other sequestering agents, such as 8-hydroxyquinoline or 2,2-dipyridyl, were also used as inhibitors (Table 6). The application of cysteine and related SH compounds as kininase blockers can interfere with bioassay *in vitro*, since they potentiate bradykinin effect on isolated smooth muscle preparations.

The sensitivity of kininases to heavy metal ions varies. This property helps to differentiate, for example, kininase I from II in human plasma. Kininase I (carboxypeptidase N) is strongly inhibited by $CdSO_4$, while kininase II is resistant (YANG and ERDÖS, 1967). $CoCl_2$ accelerates the hydrolysis of bradykinin in plasma but blocks it in the hemolyzed red blood cells (ERDÖS et al., 1963b). $HgCl_2$ seems to be a generally good inhibitor; for example, the I_{50} for carboxypeptidase N is 4×10^{-5} M. $CdSO_4$ has the lowest I_{50}; it inhibited 50% of the hydrolysis of HLAa by carboxypeptidase N, at a 2×10^{-7} M concentration (YANG and ERDÖS, 1967). The metal was, however, less effective when used with a purified kininase preparation (TRAPEZNIKOVA and PASKHINA, 1968). Other metal ions such as Mn^{2+} or Zn^{2+} also inhibited some kininases (ERDÖS et al., 1963b). The kininases from leukocytes are very sensitive to copper or zinc ions (ZACHARIAE et al., 1966; GREENBAUM and KIM, 1967).

Among compounds that are structurally similar to or identical with the products of hydrolysis of substrates of kininases, arginine was the first to be tested. Arginine (ERDÖS, 1962) and benzoylarginine ($I_{50} = 10^{-4}$ M) inhibit carboxypeptidase N (ERDÖS et al., 1964b), but arginine is inactive against kininase II of human plasma (YANG and ERDÖS, 1967). The latter enzyme is inhibited by phenylalanylarginine, the dipeptide cleaved from bradykinin. Argininic acid, the product of the hydrolysis of the ester substrate (HLAa) by carboxypeptidase N, has an I_{50} of 4×10^{-5} M (ERDÖS et al., 1967a). Because of the application of EACA to clinical subjects, the inhibition of carboxypeptidase N by this agent is of interest (ERDÖS, 1962; MARGOLIS and BISHOP, 1962; ERDÖS and SLOANE, 1962). This type of compound was first used as an inhibitor of pancreatic carboxypeptidase B by FOLK in 1956. The blocking of kinin metabolism in plasma by EACA is not related to the known effect of the compound on plasminogen because AMCHA, a more potent plasminogen inhibitor, is inactive against plasma kininases (ERDÖS and YANG, unpublished). EACA inhibited carboxypeptidase because it is structurally related to lysine. EACA was also reported to potentiate kinin formation (ARMSTRONG and STEWART, 1960a, b), but this was not confirmed by MARGOLIS and BISHOP (1962). Some other compounds of similar structure were also inhibitors (Table 6).

Agents that react with SH group of enzymes, such as PCMS, inhibit erythrocyte kininase but not plasma enzymes (ERDÖS et al., 1963b). These compounds are useful for distinguishing kininases from various sources. Kininase from liver (FREY et al., 1968) and a catheptic carboxypeptidase of the spleen (GREENBAUM and YAMAFUJI, 1966) are inhibited by a mercaptide-forming reagent, while lung kininase (FREY et al., 1968) or kidney carboxypeptidase (YANG and ERDÖS, 1966) are not. Chlorpromazine was reported to inhibit kininase from brain and other sources (KRIVOY and KROGER, 1964), but this was attributed later to the presence of sodium bisulfate in the drug preparation (GREENBAUM and YAMAFUJI, 1966).

Inhibitors of proteinases (peptidyl peptide hydrolases) are generally inactive against most kininases tested. An exception to this are the effects of DFP and

Trasylol on rabbit granulocyte (Greenbaum and Kim, 1967; Chang et al., 1969) and rabbit brain (Camargo and Graeff, 1969) kininases. Urgocyton, a not yet clearly identified fluorescent material from liver, preserves the activity of bradykinin against some of the kininases (Amundsen et al., 1964) including the kidney (Yang and Erdös, 1966). The possibility exists that urgocyton acts as a chelating agent because when $CoCl_2$ is added to a kidney enzyme–urgocyton complex, the inhibitor effect disappears and the activity of the enzyme is restored by the metal ion (Yang and Erdös, 1966). Venom of *Bothrops jararaca* contains a small molecular weight material (BPF) that potentiates bradykinin *in vivo*, presumably by inhibition of kininases. This was also shown in various plasmas *in vitro* (Ferreira, 1966; Ferreira and Vane, 1967b; see also p. 312) (Table 7).

Inhibition *in vivo*

The very rapid inactivation of kinins in the circulation made the search for *in vivo* inhibitors of the kininases obvious. In 1939 Werle and Grunz had already injected cysteine to enhance the circulatory effects of substance DK (kallidin) in laboratory animals. When carboxypeptidase N was characterized in human plasma fraction IV-1 (Erdös, 1961, 1962; Erdös and Sloane, 1962), *in vitro* inhibitors of the enzyme were used extensively. The inhibition studies *in vitro* led to the application of some of these agents to guinea pigs (Erdös and Wohler, 1963a, b) and to other animals. They are mostly metal-binding agents; thiols were especially effective. Rocha e Silva and his associates were the first to suggest the use of BAL *in vivo* to enhance the effects of kinin (Ferreira et al., 1962; Ferreira and Rocha e Silva, 1962; Rocha e Silva, 1963; Corrado, 1963). This inhibitor, however, has too many toxic side effects. In the guinea pig other agents such as 2-mercaptoethanol and mercaptopropionic acid were very well tolerated after i.v. administration. Not all of the *in vitro* inhibitors acted *in vivo*, but nine prolonged the hypotension caused by bradykinin in the guinea pig (Erdös and Wohler, 1963a, b; Table 7). Among thio compounds, those with a free alcohol or carboxyl group were the most potent. Some inhibitors were tested and found equally active with kallidin. Because guinea pigs have the highest plasma kininase level among laboratory animals, and these compounds effectively prevent the *in vitro* enzymatic hydrolysis of kinins, it was assumed that their *in vivo* action is also based on enzyme inhibition. (It should be mentioned, however, that thio compounds also potentiate the *in vitro* effect of kinins on the smooth muscles. This potentiation cannot be attributed to the inhibition of kininases alone) (Erdös, 1966a). After the administration of the inhibitors, the drop in systemic arterial blood pressure caused by bradykinin or kallidin was bigger and longer lasting. The effect of other hypotensive agents such as histamine and eledoisin was not influenced. The increased sensitivity to kinins in guinea pig pretreated with an inhibitor was abolished by an i.v. injection of purified carboxypeptidase B (Erdös and Wohler, 1963b). Because the cardiovascular effects of bradykinin in the guinea pig increase for some time after the injection of an inhibitor such as 2-mercaptoethanol (Erdös and Wohler, unpublished), it can be assumed that in addition to inhibition of the inactivation of kinins in blood, some kininases in tissues are also blocked. Here the area of pulmonary (Vane, 1969) or splanchnic circulation may be involved. Of the other agents that contained no thiol groups, Ca-EDTA and 8-hydroxy-5-quinoline sulfonic acid potentiated bradykinin effects in the guinea pig (Erdös and Wohler, 1963a, b).

The hemodynamic effects of various kinin analogs such as Gly^6-bradykinin (Erdös and Wohler, 1963b) and Lys^9-bradykinin or Lys^{10}-kallidin (Erdös et al., 1967c), were also increased after pretreatment of guinea pig with an inhibitor.

In the dog 2- to 5-fold greater doses of bradykinin are required for the same hypotensive effect if given in a tributary of the superior mesenteric vein instead of the femoral vein. After pretreatment with BAL (Erdös, 1966b; Erdös and Yang, 1966) the activity of bradykinin injected into either vein was greatly enhanced. This was particularly noticeable after bradykinin was administered in the mesenteric vein, thus the difference between the effects of kinin injection via the two routes became smaller.

The action of inhibitors is different in the various experimental animals. 2-Mercaptoethanol, for example, is very efficient in the rat, although within a narrower dose range than in the guinea pig (Erdös and Yang, 1966). Stewart and his colleagues (Stewart and Roblero, 1967; Ryan et al., 1968) blocked in part the pulmonary inactivation of bradykinin in the rat with 2-mercaptoethanol. Since in some of their experiments the rat lung was perfused with a salt solution instead of blood, the site of action of the inhibitor must have been in the tissues, perhaps in the vascular endothelium. BAL also potentiated bradykinin in the rat (Jensen et al., 1965b).

Mercaptoacetic acid (Werle et al., 1964), diethyldithiocarbamic acid, and 8-hydroxy-5-quinoline sulfonic acid (Erdös, unpublished results 1964; Erdös, 1966a) prolonged the hypotensive effect of kinins in the dog. Intraperitoneal injections of BAL potentiated bradykinin effect in the rabbit (Erdös, unpublished results 1963). Mercaptoacetic acid increased the effect of kallikrein, but somewhat surprisingly that of angiotensin in the dog as well (Werle et al., 1964).

Venom of the Brazilian snake *Bothrops jararaca* and of some other snakes contains a factor (BPF) that potentiates various actions of bradykinin on the isolated smooth muscles or on the systemic arterial blood pressure (Ferreira, 1965, 1966). The factor was partially purified and it is probably a peptide. The activity of the factor was demonstrated in various animals. For example, it is known that eledoisin is 8 times more potent than bradykinin in the cat and 20–50 times more in the dog in lowering the blood pressure. After injection of BPF the difference in dosage was abolished in the cat and reduced to about 1:2 ratio in the dog (Ferreira, 1966; Amorim et al., 1967). When synthetic bradykinin was injected in combination with BPF the hypotensive phase was much prolonged, just as is seen in guinea pigs after the administration of various other kininase inhibitors (Erdös and Wohler, 1963a, b). BPF also increased the cerebral vasodilatation caused by bradykinin or kallidin in the dog (Graeff et al., 1965) or coronary vasodilatation in the guinea pig (Antonio, 1967). Intraventricular injection of bradykinin to cats produced tranquilization, according to the report of Graeff et al. (1967); these results were more consistent after the injection of BPF.

It was suggested that the action of BPF was related to the inhibition of enzymatic inactivation of bradykinin (Ferreira, 1966; Ferreira and Vane, 1967b). Using the blood-bathed organ technique Ferreira and Vane showed that more of the i.v. injected bradykinin reached the arterial side of the circulation in the cat treated with BPF than in the controls. Although BPF inhibited 34% of the inactivation of bradykinin by homogenized dog lung in Bakhle's experiment (1968), this inhibition was not specific. BPF was an even more potent inhibitor of the angiotensin-converting enzyme.

Recently several peptides were separated from *Bothrops jararaca* venom. One of them, the tetrapeptide PCA-Lys-Trp-Ala-Pro was synthesized. The peptide potentiated the effect of bradykinin *in vitro*, its activity *in vivo*, however, was slight (Greene, Stewart and Ferreira, to be published).

J. Activities of Kininases in Various Conditions

The destruction of bradykinin and kallidin by human blood was studied in a variety of states. Owing to the differences in methods of determination used, and to the existence of several kininases, the literature on the subject can be exasperatingly confusing.

Experiments in which kininase activity was measured in plasma of pregnant women yielded controversial results. EFFKEMANN and WERLE (1941) and ARMSTRONG and STEWART (1960b) did not observe any increase in blood enzyme level, while CENTARO et al. (1963) and WERLE in a later paper (1960) noticed that pregnant blood serum or plasma destroys kinins faster than does normal blood. The level of the enzyme in the newborn was lower than in the mother. In the experiments of MELMON et al. (1968), however, the difference between neonatal and adult plasma was not statistically significant.

ERDÖS et al. (1964a, 1965) studied the hydrolysis of HLL by carboxypeptidase N in the blood serum of thirty pregnant women. Carboxypeptidase N level was significantly higher (1.07 μmoles per min/ml) in pregnant than in non pregnant subjects (0.77) and lower than normal in the newborn (0.45). When the esterase activity of the enzyme was measured with HLAa, it increased gradually during pregnancy (ERDÖS et al., 1967a) from 3.71 μmoles per min/ml in the first trimester to 4.74 in the third trimester.

The hydrolysis of HLL in the blood sera of several hundred clinical subjects was also assayed. Patients with cirrhosis of the liver had lower values, while neoplastic clinical subjects had higher values than healthy individuals. The enzyme level in men suffering from gastrointestinal diseases, allergic conditions, or renal diseases fell within the normal range (ERDÖS et al., 1965).

Many attempts were made to link changes in kininase levels to specific pathological conditions. It has been known (WERLE et al., 1937) that the activity of the plasma enzymes ceases at a low pH, for example at 2 (HORTON, 1959a). EDERY and LEWIS (1962) and LEWIS (1963) pointed out (p. 000) the importance of the lower activity of the enzyme below pH 7. According to these authors, kininogenases would still liberate kinins rapidly at a pH where the destruction of bradykinin might be slowed down by even a slightly acid milieu. In inflammation, the lowered pH of the tissues may lead to the accumulation of the peptide and aggravation of the existing symptoms. Although this hypothesis is an attractive one, it has to be confirmed in a more comprehensive system. The enzymatic hydrolysis of bradykinin was measured here in a phosphate buffer. The effect of pH on kinin hydrolysis in this medium depends very much on the chloride ion concentration (AARSEN and KEMP, 1963). In general, the pH curve of a metallopeptidase such as carboxypeptidase is determined to a large extent by the choice of buffer used (WOLFF et al., 1962; ERDÖS et al., 1964b). ERDÖS et al. (1964b, 1967a) found significant carboxypeptidase N activity with both peptide and ester substrates below pH 7, and in the experiments of others (KLETT, 1962; ABE et al., 1965; WATANABE, 1967), the destruction of bradykinin activity dropped less precipitously below neutral pH than in the studies of EDERY and LEWIS. (It was also stated that salivary kallikrein would have a broad pH optimum between 7.8 and 6 (LEWIS, 1963), but the activity of a kallikrein and a kininase preparation decreased below neutrality in a parallel manner (TRAUTSCHOLD and RÜDEL, 1963).

ZACHARIAE et al. (1967) injected autologous plasma into the subcutaneous space of man and animals. This led to kinin formation that was enhanced by a lowering of the pH to 6.3. The kinin accumulation might have been caused by a decreased inactivation of the kinin but also by a diminished inhibition of the plasma kininogenases by plasma inhibitors at the acid pH.

The role of kininases originating from granulocytes in inflammation has recently been discussed. These kininases were assumed to be of importance in removing accumulated kinin from the site of inflammation (Greenbaum and Kim, 1967; Melmon and Cline, 1967a). The release of kininases from leukocytes in synovial fluid in arthritic inflammation was thought to be one of these conditions. Jasani et al. (1967), Katori (1967), and Lewis (1968) found, however, that the kininase activity in synovial fluid does not originate from cellular elements but from plasma. Thus their experiments negate the proposed role for leukocyte kininases.

Shock is another condition where the release and removal of kinins may be of importance. During anaphylactic shock neither the quantity of kininase that appeared in guinea pig lung perfusate increased (Brocklehurst and Lahiri, 1963) nor the carboxypeptidase N activity changed significantly in guinea pig blood (Erdös et al., 1964b). Kininase level was normal in dogs in endotoxin shock (Massion and Erdös, 1966; Erdös et al., 1967a), but kininase action increased in dog plasma during anaphylactic shock (Back et al., 1966, 1968) and in monkey plasma in lethal endotoxin shock (Nies et al., 1968). Dextran shock or anaphylactic shock did not affect the kininases significantly in the rat (Dawson et al., 1966; Ankier and Starr, 1967).

Scalding the hind leg of dog raises the concentration of the various components of the kallikrein–kininogen system in lymph, including the kininase (Edery and Lewis, 1963; Jacobsen and Waaler, 1966).

Infusion of epinephrine to man lowered the kinin level in blood with a concomitant rise in kininase activity (Mashford and Zacest, 1967). Epinephrine was also described as increasing the inactivation of bradykinin in blood *in vitro*. This effect was blocked by added phenoxybenzamine. Serum kininase level in rat did not change after the removal of kidneys or adrenals (Werle et al., 1968). In the dog, ischemia of the kidney brought about an increased excretion of a urinary kininase (Vichi, 1968).

Kininase activity in venous blood of various patients was studied by a group of investigators at Tohoku University using bio-assay to determine the destruction of bradykinin effect (Abe et al., 1965; Watanabe et al., 1966; Watanabe, 1967). Patients with hyperthyroidism and liver diseases had higher than normal values. In pancreatitis, normal enzyme level was found by Erdös et al. (1965) and by Watanabe (1967), but Nugent et al. (1966) reported higher values in blood of dogs. The reported decreased kininase action in some asthmatic persons (Sicuteri et al., 1963b) was not confirmed by others (Tewksbury and Marschke, 1966; Briseid et al., 1968). The level of the aminopeptidase that can convert kallidin to bradykinin and its inhibition pattern were also normal in these patients (Berrens, 1968a, b).

K. Conversion of Kinins

The metabolism of the longer analogs of bradykinin such as kallidin or Met-Lys-bradykinin is somewhat different from that of the nonapeptide, since cleaving off the N-terminal lysine or methionyl-lysine may lead to the release of bradykinin. However, the situation is not analogous to the angiotensin system, where the decapeptide angiotensin I has to be converted to the vasoactive octapeptide angiotensin II before becoming active. Kallidin is active in its own right both *in vitro* and *in vivo*. In some animals it is even more hypotensive than bradykinin (ERDÖS, 1966b). Nevertheless, blood plasma contains an aminopeptidase that can convert kallidin to bradykinin. This was shown simultaneously by WEBSTER and PIERCE (1963) and by ERDÖS et al. (1963b). WEBSTER and PIERCE (1963) incubated 12.5 μg of kallidin with human plasma. After paper chromatography the reaction mixture was eluted from the paper and yielded two active peaks at Rf values similar to those of kallidin and bradykinin. This was taken as an indication that kallidin was converted to bradykinin. ERDÖS et al. (1963b) incubated 0.5 mg kallidin with diluted human plasma. The plasma was pretreated with $MnSO_4$ to partially inhibit carboxypeptidase N and to enhance the activity of an aminopeptidase attacking the bond of the N-terminal lysine of kallidin. The incubation mixture was separated in peptide mapping. Human plasma released lysine and yielded a spot that migrated just as bradykinin did and was biologically active (ERDÖS et al., 1963b; ERDÖS, unpublished). Simultaneously, plasma also partially inactivated the peptides by releasing an arginine, presumably from the C-terminal end. Less arginine was liberated when EACA was added to inhibit a kininase present in plasma. Although the experimental conditions used by WEBSTER and PIERCE and ERDÖS et al. were different, ERDÖS concluded that only a fraction of the available kallidin is converted to bradykinin prior to its inactivation by kininases. Since both kallidin and bradykinin are inactivated equally fast, kallidin may serve simultaneously as a substrate of the converting aminopeptidase and inactivating kininases (ERDÖS, 1966a). This statement is indirectly corroborated by the findings of OATES and MELMON (1966). Metastatic carcinoid tumor contains kallikrein that releases kallidin (MELMON et al., 1965) which is in turn converted to bradykinin (OATES et al., 1966). Blood of carcinoid patients had elevated bradykinin levels, but in the experiments done in *in vitro* only a fraction of the kallidin added to the plasma was recovered as bradykinin (OATES et al., 1966; OATES and MELMON, 1966; OATES and BUTLER, 1967).

HOPSU et al. (1966a, b, c, d, e) found in the liver of various laboratory animals an enzyme, called aminopeptidase B, that splits naphthylamides of lysine and arginine. It also occurs in various other tissues and is activated by chloride ions. The enzyme liberated lysine from kallidin but did not hydrolyze bradykinin (HOPSU et al., 1966e). BERRENS (1968a, b) studied the hydrolysis of L-lysyl-2-naphthylamide in human sera. He assumed that the naphthylamidase activity is identical with that of the kallidin-converting enzyme. This naphthylamidase was inhibited by atopic allergens, chelating agents, a sugar complex of EACA, and by SBTI, but not by Trasylol. The level of the enzyme was about the same in blood of normal and allergic subjects.

Some analogs of bradykinin having additional amino acids at the C-terminal end can also be converted to active kinin. The cleaving of the Arg^9-Ser^{10} bond of the "minimum substrate" and in the longer derivatives by kininogenases are discussed elsewhere by HABERMANN (p. 250). Carboxypeptidase A can degrade a kininogen fragment containing six more additional amino acids at the C-terminal end of bradykinin to an active kinin by sequential removal of the carboxyl terminal amino acids (HABERMANN, p. 263).

Phyllokinin (p. 592) is bradykinyl-isoleucyl-tyrosine-*o*-sulfate. The terminal dipeptide of this kinin is rapidly cleaved off by trypsin (ANASTASI et al., 1966). Rabbit plasma removes the same dipeptide *in vitro*, and that action must be attributed to a trypsin-like enzyme. Plasma does not contain a carboxypeptidase A-type enzyme (ERDÖS et al., 1964b, 1967a), thus a sequential removal of the two amino acids *in vivo* by a carboxypeptidase and the conversion of phyllokinin or another derivative with a nonbasic amino acid in the 10th position (e.g. bradykinyl-glycine) to bradykinin by a carboxypeptidase in the blood stream is unlikely (Erdös and Yang, 1967b).

A bradykinin derivative, which has an additional basic amino acid, arginine in the 10th position, was synthesized by Stewart and Woolley (1966). The peptide has only 4% of the activity of bradykinin. In our experiments human plasma carboxypeptidase N, which attacks basic C-terminal amino acids, converted this decapeptide to an active agent by liberating bradykinin. (The possibility of such enzymatic conversion was already assumed by Anastasi et al., 1966.) The released kinin is subsequently inactivated by the same enzyme. 1,10-Phenanthroline or EDTA inhibited the reaction (Fig. 6; Erdös and Yang, 1967b).

Some purified proteolytic enzymes can liberate bradykinin not only from the protein substrate kininogen but also from some longer kinin analog peptides.

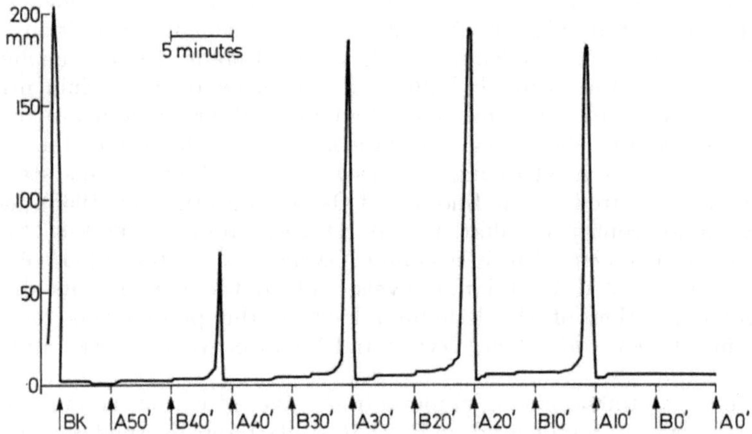

Fig. 6. Release of bradykinin from bradykinyl-arginine by plasma carboxypeptidase N and subsequent inactivation of bradykinin. Source of enzyme was human plasma globulin precipitated with ammonium sulfate. A: 0.1 μg/ml bradykinyl-arginine incubated with carboxypeptidase at pH 7.4. B: same as A, but contained 1.10^{-3} M 1,10-phenanthroline. Bk = bradykinin control, 0.04 ng/ml bath. The figure shows the direction of the chart paper of the recorder. Samples were withdrawn at regular intervals and the inactivation of the peptide was followed on the isolated rat uterus (Erdös and Yang, 1967b)

Trypsin can convert kallidin to bradykinin (Webster and Pierce, 1963; Nicolaides et al., 1963; Erdös et al., 1963b). Kallidin, however, is a rather poor substrate for trypsin, and not more than 5 to 14% of a given amount was converted to bradykinin (Webster and Pierce, 1963; Habermann and Blennemann, 1964). Commercial trypsin preparations can also destroy some of the available kallidin during incubation, owing to contamination or endogenous chymotryptic activity (Werle, 1953; Erdös et al., 1963b; Webster and Gilmore, 1965). Met-Lys-Bradykinin can be easily converted to bradykinin by trypsin, serum kallikrein, or snake venom (Habermann and Blennemann, 1964; Schröder, 1964; Elliott et al., 1965), but the release of bradykinin from kininogen is much faster than that from the undecapeptide (Habermann and Blennemann, 1964). Met-Lys-Bradykinin, however, is hydrolyzed by leucine aminopeptidase; the first two N-terminal bonds of the peptide are broken by the purified enzyme (Schröder, 1964).

References

AARSEN, P., KEMP, A.: Influence of metals on the activity of a bradykinin-destroying enzyme kininase. Brit. J. Pharmacol. **19**, 442 (1962).

— — Effect of pH and chloride ions on plasma kininase activity. Nature (Lond.) **198**, 687 (1963).

ABE, K., WATANABE, N., KUMAGAI, N., MIWA, I., MOURI, K., SEKI, T., OIKAWA, A., YOSHINAGA, K.: Assay of kininase activity in human blood. Tohoku J. exp. Med. **86**, 77 (1965).

ALLWOOD, M. J., LEWIS, G. P.: Bradykinin and forearm blood flow. J. Physiol. (Lond.) **170**, 571 (1964).

AMORIM, D. S., MANCO, J. C., FERREIRA, S. H., TANAKA, A., CARDOSO, S. S.: Hemodynamic effects of bradykinin potentiated by a factor contained in the *Bothrops jararaca* venom. Comparative results with eledoisin. Acta physiol. lat.-amer. **17**, 258 (1967).

AMUNDSEN, E.: Kinin formation and destruction in fluid produced by a strangulated segment of ileum in the rat. In: Hypotensive peptides, p. 474, ed. by E. G. ERDÖS, N. BACK and F. SICUTERI. Berlin-Heidelberg-New York: Springer 1966.

— NUSTAD, K.: Kinin-forming and destroying activities of saliva. Brit. J. Pharmacol. **23**, 440 (1964).

— — Kinin-forming and destroying activities of cell homogenates. J. Physiol. (Lond.) **179**, 479 (1965).

— RUGSTAD, H. E.: Influence of some pathogenic bacteria on kinin formation and destruction. Brit. J. Pharmacol. **25**, 67 (1965).

— WAALER, B. A., DEDICHEN, J., LALAND, P., LALAND, S., THORSDALEN, N.: Kininase inhibition by a fluorescent substance prepared from liver. Nature (Lond.) **203**, 1245 (1964).

ANASTASI, A., ERSPAMER, V., BERTACCINI, G., CEI, J. M.: A bradykinin-like endecapeptide of the skin of *Phyllomedusa rohdei*. In: Hypotensive peptides, p. 76, ed. by E. G. ERDÖS, N. BACK and F. SICUTERI. Berlin-Heidelberg-New York: Springer 1966.

ANKIER, S. I., STARR, M. S.: The importance of plasma kinins in the anaphylactoid reaction in rats. Brit. J. Pharmacol. **31**, 331 (1967).

ANTONIO, A.: The coronary vasodilator effect of bradykinin. In: Symposium on Vasoactive Polypeptides: Bradykinin and Related Kinins, p. 87, ed. by M. ROCHA E SILVA and H. A. ROTHSCHILD. São Paulo 1967.

ARMAN, C. G. VAN: Interrelationships among some peptide precursors. In: Polypeptides which stimulate plain muscle, p. 103, ed. by J. H. GADDUM. London 1955.

— NUSS, G. W., WINTER, C. A., FLATAKER, L.: Proteolytic enzymes as mediators of pain. In: Pharmacology of pain, p. 25, ed. by R. K. S. LIM, D. ARMSTRONG and E. G. PARDO. Oxford: Pergamon Press 1968.

ARMSTRONG, D., JEPSON, J. B., KEELE, C. A., STEWART, J. W.: Activation by glass of pharmacologically active agents in blood of various species. J. Physiol. (Lond.) **129**, 80 (1955).

— STEWART, J. W.: Formation of plasma kinin in human plasma by ε-amino caproic acid and certain related compounds. J. Physiol. (Lond.) **154**, 19P (1960a).

— — Spontaneous plasma kinin formation in human plasma collected during labour. Nature (Lond.) **188**, 1193 (1960b).

BACK, N., WILKENS, H., STEGER, R.: Fibrinolysis and vasoactive peptides in anaphylaxis. In: Hypotensive peptides, p. 485, ed. by E. G. ERDÖS, N. BACK and F. SICUTERI. Berlin-Heidelberg-New York: Springer 1966.

— — — Proteinases and proteinase inhibitors in experimental shock states. Ann. N.Y. Acad. Sci. **146**, 491 (1968).

BAKHLE, Y. S.: Conversion of angiotensin I to angiotensin II by cell-free extracts of dog lung. Nature (Lond.) **220**, 919 (1968).

BERRENS, L.: Levels of lysyl- and arginyl-naphthylamidase in sera of normal and allergic subjects. Clin. chim. Acta **20**, 170 (1968a).

— Inhibition of serum naphthylamidases by atopic allergens. Clin. chim. Acta **22**, 239 (1968b).

BIRON, P.: Pulmonary extraction of bradykinin and eledoisin. Rev. canad. Biol. **27**, 75 (1968).

BISHOP, E., MARGOLIS, J.: Studies on plasma kinins. II. Some properties of the kinin-destroying enzyme. Aust. J. exp. Biol. med. Sci. **41**, 307 (1963).

BOISSONNAS, R. A., GUTTMANN, ST., JAQUENOUD, P.-A.: Synthèse de la L-arginyl-L-prolyl-L-prolyl-glycyl-L-phenylalanyl-L-séryl-L-prolyl-L-phénylalanyl-L-arginine, un nonapeptide présentant les proprietés de la bradykinine. Helv. chim. Acta **43**, 1349 (1960a).

— — — Synthèse de la L-arginyl-L-prolyl-L-prolyl-glycyl-L-phenylalanyl-L-seryl-L-phenylalanyl-L-arginine. Distinction entre cet octapeptide et la bradykinine. Helv. chim. Acta **43**, 1481 (1960b).

BOREHAM, P. F. L.: *In vitro* studies on the mechanism of kinin formation by trypanosomes. Brit. J. Pharmacol. **34**, 598 (1968).

Briseid, K., Dyrud, O. K., Lange-Nielsen, F.: Determination of factors of the plasma kinin system in plasma substrate specimens from patients with specific, exogenous allergies. Acta allerg. (Kbh.) **23**, 413 (1968).

Brocklehurst, W. E., Lahiri, S. C.: Formation and destruction of bradykinin during anaphylaxis. J. Physiol. (Lond.) **165**, 39 P (1963).

Bumpus, F. M., Smeby, R. R., Page, I. H., Khairallah, P. A.: Distribution and metabolic fate of angiotensin II and various derivatives. Canad. med. Ass. J. **90**, 190 (1964).

Camargo, A. C. M., Graeff, F. G.: Subcellular distribution and properties of the bradykinin inactivation system in rabbit brain homogenates. Biochem. Pharmacol. **18**, 548 (1969).

Carvalho, I. F., Diniz, C. R.: Kinin-forming enzyme (kininogenin) in rat kidney. Ann. N.Y. Acad. Sci. **116**, 912 (1964).

Centaro, A., Periti, P., Sicuteri, F.: Bradykininogen and bradykininase in blood of women during labour. Sett. med. **51**, Suppl. 1, 70 (1963).

Chang, J., Stella, R., Greenbaum, L. M.: Trasylol inhibition of leucocyte kininases. Fed. Proc. **28**, 799 (1969).

Chiang, T. S., Erdös, E. G., Miwa, I., Tague, L. L., Coalson, J. J.: Isolation from a salivary gland of granules containing renin and kallikrein. Circulat. Res. **23**, 507 (1968).

Corrado, A. P.: Recent investigations of the pharmacology of bradykinin and their physiopathological implications. Sett. med. **51**, Suppl. 1, 30 (1963).

Croxatto, H., Cruzatt, H.: Ineffectiveness of carboxypeptidase B in inhibiting the pressor effect of incubated human plasma. Experientia (Basel) **25**, 59 (1969).

Dawson, W., Starr, M. S., West, G. B.: Inhibition of anaphylactic shock in the rat by antihistamines and ascorbic acid. Brit. J. Pharmacol. **27**, 249 (1966).

Deutsch, H. F., Diniz, C. R.: Some proteolytic activities of snake venoms. J. biol. Chem. **216**, 17 (1955).

Doleschel, W., Auerswald, W.: On the mechanism of potentiation of kinins by inhibitors of the fibrinolytic system. Experientia (Basel) **22**, 540 (1966).

Dyrud, O. K., Rinvik, S. F., Jensen, K. B.: Effects of inhibitors on the *in vitro* inactivation of bradykinin by various kininases. Acta pharmacol. (Kbh.) **23**, 235 (1965).

Edery, H., Lewis, G. P.: Inhibition of plasma kininase activity at slightly acid pH. Brit. J. Pharmacol. **19**, 299 (1962).

— — Kinin-forming activity and histamine in lymph after tissue injury. J. Physiol. (Lond.) **169**, 568 (1963).

Effkemann, G., Werle, E.: Die körpereigenen uteruswirksamen und kreislaufaktiven Wirkstoffe im Schwangerenorganismus. Arch. Gynäk. **171**, 1 (1941).

Eisen, V.: Urates and kinin formation in synovial fluid. Proc. roy. Soc. Med. **59**, 302 (1966).

Elliott, D. F., Lewis, G. P.: Methionyl-lysyl-bradykinin, a new kinin from ox blood. Biochem. J. **95**, 437 (1965).

— — Horton, E. W.: The structure of bradykinin—a plasma kinin from ox blood. Biochem. Biophys. Res. Commun. **3**, 87 (1960).

Enomoto, T., Mineshita, S., Oh-Ishi, S., Shigei, T.: Kininase activity of stem bromelain. Jap. J. Pharmacol. **17**, 331 (1967).

Erdös, E. G.: Enzymes that inactivate active polypeptides. Biochem. Pharmacol. **8**, 112 (1961).

— Enzymes that inactive polypeptides. In: Metabolic factors controlling duration of drug actions, p. 159, ed. by B. B. Brodie and E. G. Erdös. Oxford: Pergamon Press 1962.

— Hypotensive peptides, bradykinin, kallidin and eledoisin. Advanc. Pharmacol. **4**, 1 (1966a).

— Release and inactivation of kinins. Gastroenterology **51**, 893 (1966b).

— Cano, G., Yang, H. Y. T.: Hypotensive effect of Lys^9-bradykinin in the guinea pig. Biochem. Pharmacol. **16**, 1035 (1967c).

— McMennamin, M. A., Wohler, J. R.: Presence of carboxypeptidase B in crude kallikrein (Padutin) preparations. Life Sci. **1**, 765 (1962).

— Miwa, I.: Effect of endotoxin shock on the plasma kallikrein-kinin system of the rabbit. Fed. Proc. **27**, 92 (1968).

— — Graham, W. J.: Studies on the evolution of plasma kinins. Kinins of reptilian and avian blood. Life Sci. **6**, 2433 (1967b).

— Renfrew, A. G., Sloane, E. M., Wohler, J. R.: Enzymatic studies on bradykinin and similar peptides. Ann. N.Y. Acad. Sci. **104**, 222 (1963b).

— Seki, T., Yang, H. Y. T., Tague, L. L.: Use of insoluble polymers of enzymes in kinin metabolism. Pharmacol. Res. Commun. **1**, 152 (1969).

— Sloane, E. M.: An enzyme in human blood plasma that inactivates bradykinin and kallidins. Biochem. Pharmacol. **11**, 585 (1962).

— — Wohler, I. M.: Carboxypeptidase in blood and other fluids. I. Properties, distribution and partial purification of the enzyme. Biochem. Pharmacol. **13**, 893 (1964b).

Erdös, E. G., Tague, L. L., Miwa, I.: Kallikrein in granules of the submaxillary gland. Biochem. Pharmacol. **17**, 667 (1968b).
— Westerman, M. P., Moritz, I. E.: Presence of a carboxypeptidase in blood sera. In: XI. Colloquium on Protides of Biological Fluids, 1963, p. 524, ed. by H. Peeters. Amsterdam: Elsevier 1964a.
— Wohler, I. M., Levine, M. I., Westerman, M. P.: Carboxypeptidase in blood and other fluids. Values in human blood in normal and pathological conditions. Clin. chim. Acta **11**, 39 (1965).
— Wohler, J. R.: Inhibitors of the *in vivo* enzymatic inactivation of bradykinin and kallidin. Life Sci. **2**, 270 (1963a).
— — Inhibition *in vivo* of the enzymatic inactivation of bradykinin and kallidin. Biochem. Pharmacol. **12**, 1193 (1963b).
— — Levine, M. I.: Blocking of the *in vivo* effects of bradykinin and kallidin with carboxypeptidase B. J. Pharmacol. exp. Ther. **142**, 327 (1963a).
— Yang, H. Y. T.: Inactivation and potentiation of the effects of bradykinin. In: Hypotensive peptides, p. 235, ed. by E. G. Erdös, N. Back and F. Sicuteri. Berlin-Heidelberg-New York: Springer 1966.
— — An enzyme in microsomal fraction of kidney that inactivates bradykinin. Life Sci. **6**, 569 (1967a).
— — Metabolism of bradykinin and related peptides. In: Symposium on Vasoactive Polypeptides: Bradykinin and Related Kinins, p. 239, ed. by M. Rocha e Silva and H. A. Rothschild. São Paulo 1967b.
— — Enzymes in blood and tissues that inactivate plasma kinins. Symposium of Tanabe Amino Acid Foundation, Osaka. J. clin. Sci. **3**, 605 (1967c).
— — Miwa, I.: Kininases. Hoppe-Seylers Z. physiol. Chem. **349**, 928 (1968a).
— — Tague, L. L., Manning, N.: Carboxypeptidase in blood and other fluids: III. The esterase activity of the enzyme. Biochem. Pharmacol. **16**, 1287 (1967a).
Fasciolo, J. C.: Formation and destruction of plasma kinins. Acta physiol. lat.-amer. **14**, 170 (1964).
Ferreira, S. H.: A bradykinin-potentiating factor (BPF) present in the venom of *Bothrops jararaca*. Brit. J. Pharmacol. **24**, 163 (1965).
— Bradykinin-potentiating factor. In: Hypotensive peptides, p. 356, ed. by E. G. Erdös, N. Back and F. Sicuteri. Berlin-Heidelberg-New York: Springer 1966.
— Corrado, A. P., Rocha e Silva, M.: Potenciacao do efeito hipotensor da bradicinina por inibicao do enzima bradicininolitico plasmatico. Ciencia e Cult. **14**, 238 (1962).
— Rocha e Silva, M.: Potentiation of bradykinin by dimercaptopropanol (BAL) and other inhibitors of its destroying enzyme in plasma. Biochem. Pharmacol. **11**, 1123 (1962).
— Vane, J. R.: The disappearance of bradykinin and eledoisin in the circulation and vascular beds of the cat. Brit. J. Pharmacol. **30**, 417 (1967a).
— — The detection and estimation of bradykinin in the circulating blood. Brit. J. Pharmacol. **29**, 367 (1967b).
— — Half-lives of peptides and amines in the circulation. Nature (Lond.) **215**, 1237 (1967c).
Folk, J. E.: New pancreatic carboxypeptidase. J. Amer. chem. Soc. **78**, 3541 (1956).
— Piez, K. A., Carroll, W. R., Gladner, J. A.: Carboxypeptidase B. IV. Purification and characterization of the porcine enzyme. J. biol. Chem. **235**, 2272 (1960).
Frey, E. K., Kraut, H., Werle, E.: Kallikrein Padutin. Stuttgart: Ferdinand Enke 1950.
— — — Vogel, R., Zickgraf-Rüdel, G., Trautschold, I.: Das Kallikrein-Kinin-System und seine Inhibitoren. Stuttgart: Ferdinand Enke 1968.
Gaddum, J. H., Guth, P. S.: A comparison of the kallikrein-kinin system in sheep and dogs. Brit. J. Pharmacol. **15**, 181 (1960).
Garbe, G.: Quantitative Kininogenbestimmung in menschlichem Plasma. Naunyn-Schmiedebergs Arch. exp. Path. Pharmak. **256**, 112 (1967).
Graeff, F. G., Corrado, A. P., Pela, I. R., Capek, R.: Actions of bradykinin upon the central nervous system. In: Symposium on Vasoactive Polypeptides: Bradykinin and Related Kinins, p. 97, ed. by M. Rocha e Silva and H. A. Rothschild. São Paulo 1967.
— Ferreira, S. H., Corrado, A. P., Rocha e Silva, M.: Potentiation of the cerebral vascular action of bradykinin by the "Bradykinin potentiating factor" (BPF) in the dog. Experientia (Basel) **21**, 607 (1965).
Greenbaum, L. M.: Studies on the metabolism of bradykinin in inflammation. In: Symposium on Vasoactive Polypeptides and Inhibitors of Proteolytic Enzymes, p. 56. Tokyo 1967.
— Kim, K. S.: The kinin-forming and kininase activities of rabbit polymorphonuclear leucocytes. Brit. J. Pharmacol. **29**, 238 (1967).
— Yamafuji, K.: The *in vitro* inactivation and formation of plasma kinins by spleen cathepsins. Brit. J. Pharmacol. **27**, 230 (1966).

Grosu, L., Grecica, E.: Activitatea esterazica, kininoformatoare si kininolitica a sistemului nervous central inainte si dupa excitarea unor nervi aferenti. Fiziol. norm. si pat. **11**, 279 (1965).
Habermann, E., Blennemann, G.: Über Substrate und Reaktionsprodukte der kininbildenden Enzyme Trypsin, Serum- und Pankreaskallikrein sowie von Crotalusgift. Arch. Exp. Pathol. Pharmakol. **249**, 357 (1964).
Hamberg, U., Deutsch, H. F.: A large scale preparation of bradykinin. Arch. Biochem. **76**, 262 (1958).
— Rocha e Silva, M.: Studies on the enzymatic inactivation of bradykinin. Acta physiol. scand. **30**, 215 (1954).
— — On the release of bradykinin by trypsin and snake venoms. Arch. int. Pharmacodyn. **110**, 222 (1957).
Hegner, D.: Isolierung und Enzymbestand von Granula aus polymorphkernigen Leukozyten des peripheren Rinderblutes. Hoppe-Seylers Z. physiol. Chem. **349**, 544 (1968).
Hooper, K. C.: The enzymic inactivation of some physiologically active polypeptides by different parts of the nervous system. Biochem. J. **88**, 398 (1963).
Hopsu, V. K., Makinen, K. K., Glenner, G. G.: A peptidase (aminopeptidase B) from cat and guinea pig liver selective for N-terminal arginine and lysine residues. I. Purification and substrate specificity. Acta chem. scand. **20**, 1225 (1966a).
— — — A peptidase (aminopeptidase B) from cat and guinea pig liver selective for N-terminal arginine and lysine residues. II. Modifier characteristics and kinetic studies. Acta chem. scand. **20**, 1231 (1966b).
— — — Purification of a mammalian peptidase selective for N-terminal arginine and lysine residues: aminopeptidases B. Arch. Biochem. **114**, 557 (1966c).
— — — Characterization of aminopeptidase B: substrate specificity and affector studies. Arch. Biochem. **114**, 567 (1966d).
— — — Formation of bradykinin from kallidin-10 by aminopeptidase B. Nature (Lond.) **212**, 1271 (1966e).
Hori, S.: The presence of bradykinin-like polypeptides, kinin-releasing and -destroying activity in brain. Jap. J. Physiol. 18, 772 (1968).
Horton, E. W.: The estimation of urinary kallikrein. J. Physiol. (Lond.) **148**, 267 (1959a).
— Human urinary kinin excretion. Brit. J. Pharmacol. **14**, 125 (1959b).
Innerfield, I., Gimble, F. S., Blincoe III, E.: Peptidase activity in rat urine following orally given proteases. Life Sci. **2**, 671 (1963).
Iwata, H., Shikimi, T., Oka, T.: Pharmacological significances of peptidase and proteinase in the brain (report I)—Enzymatic inactivation of bradykinin in rat brain. Biochem. Pharmacol. 18, 119 (1969).
Jacobsen, S.: Observations on the content of kininogen, kallikrein and kininase in lymph from hind limbs of dogs and rabbits. Brit. J. Pharmacol. **27**, 213 (1966a).
— Substrates for plasma kinin-forming enzymes in rat and guinea-pig plasmas. Brit. J. Pharmacol. **28**, 64 (1966b).
— Waaler, B. A.: The effect of scalding on the content of kininogen and kininase in limb lymph. Brit. J. Pharmacol. **27**, 222 (1966).
Jasani, M. K., Katori, M., Lewis, G. P.: Origin of kinin enzymes and intracellular enzymes in the synovial fluid of rheumatoid patients. J. Physiol. (Lond.) **190**, 26P (1967).
Jensen, K. B., Dyrud, O. K., Rinvik, S. F.: Depressor effect of Padutin (hog pancreas kallikrein) in rats treated with disulfiram. Acta pharmacol. (Kbh.) **22**, 196 (1965b).
— Rinvik, S. F., Venneröd, A. M.: Experiments on the *in vitro* inactivation of plasma kinins by carboxypeptidase B, plasma kininase or erythrocyte kininase in the presence of disulfiram. Acta pharmacol. (Kbh.) **22**, 187 (1965a).
Katori, M.: Origin of kinin enzymes and intracellular enzymes in the synovial fluid of rheumatoid patients. In: Symposium on Vasoactive Polypeptides and Inhibitors of Proteolytic Enzymes, p. 84. Tokyo 1967.
Klett, W.: Über Reinigung und Reaktionsbedingungen von Kininase und Kininogen. Inaug.-Diss. Würzburg 1962.
Krivoy, W., Kroger, D.: The preservation of bradykinin by phenothiazines *in vitro*. Brit. J. Pharmacol. **22**, 329 (1964).
Kroneberg, G., Stoepel, K.: Vergleichende Untersuchungen über die Kreislaufwirkung von Kallikrein (Padutin), Kallidin und Bradykinin. Naunyn-Schmiedebergs Arch. exp. Path. Pharmak. **245**, 284 (1963).
Levin, Y., Pecht, M., Goldstein, L., Katchalski, E.: A water-insoluble polyanionic derivative of trypsin. I. Preparation and properties. Biochemistry **3**, 1905 (1964).
Lewis, G. P.: Pharmacological actions of bradykinin and its role in physiological and pathological reactions. Ann. N.Y. Acad. Sci. **104**, 236 (1963).
— Kinins in chronic inflammation. Advanc. exp. Med. Biol. **2**, 595 (1968).

MARGOLIS, J., BISHOP, E. A.: Interrelations between different mechanisms of release of biologically active peptides from blood plasma. Nature (Lond.) **194**, 749 (1962).
MASHFORD, M. L., ZACEST, R.: Effect of adrenaline on blood kinin levels and blood kininase activity in man. Circulat. Res., Suppl. III., **20** and **21**, 111–183 (1967).
MASSION, W. H., ERDÖS, E. G.: The effects of ATP and a proteolytic enzyme inhibitor in irreversible shock. Shock Tour and Symposium at F.A.A. Aeronautical Center 1964. J. Okla. med. Ass. **59**, 467 (1966).
MCCARTHY, D. A., POTTER, D. E., NICOLAIDES, E. D.: An *in vivo* estimation of the potencies and half-lives of synthetic bradykinin and kallidin. J. Pharmacol. exp. Ther. **148**, 117 (1965).
MELMON, K. L., CLINE, M. J.: Kallikrein activator and kininase in human granulocytes. A model of inflammation. In: Symposium on Vaso-Active Polypeptides: Bradykinin and related kinins, p. 223, ed. by M. ROCHA E SILVA and H. A. ROTHSCHILD. São Paulo 1967a.
— — Interaction of plasma kinins and granulocytes. Nature (Lond.) **217**, 90 (1967b).
— — The interaction of leukocytes and the kinin system. Biochem. Pharmacol. **17**, Suppl., p. 271 (1968).
— — HUGHES, T., NIES, A. S.: Kinins: possible mediators of neonatal circulatory changes in man. J. clin. Invest. **47**, 1295 (1968).
— LOVENBERG, W., SJOERDSMA, A.: Characteristics of carcinoid tumor kallikrein. Identification of lysyl-bradykinin as a peptide it produces *in vitro*. Clin. chim. Acta **12**, 292 (1965).
— WEBSTER, M. E., GOLDFINGER, S. E., SEEGMILLER, J. E.: The presence of a kinin in inflammatory synovial effusion from arthritides of varying etiologies. Arthr. and Rheum. **10**, 13 (1967).
MITCHELL, W. M.: Hydrolysis at arginylproline in polypeptides by clostridiopeptidase B. Science **162**, 374 (1968).
MIWA, I., ERDÖS, E. G., SEKI, T.: Separation of peptide components of urinary kinin (Substance Z). Proc. Soc. exp. Med. (N.Y.) **131**, 768 (1969).
MOVAT, H. Z., DI LORENZO, N. L.: Activation of the plasma kinin system by antigen-antibody aggregates. I. Generation of permeability factor in guinea pig serum. Lab. Invest. **19**, 187 (1968).
— — TRELOAR, M. P.: Activation of the plasma kinin system by antigen-antibody aggregates. II. Isolation of permeability-enhancing and kinin-releasing fractions from activated guinea pig serum. Lab. Invest. **19**, 201 (1968).
NG, K. K. F., VANE, J. R.: Fate of angiotensin I in the circulation. Nature (Lond.) **218**, 144 (1968).
NICOLAIDES, E. D., DEWALD, H. A., CRAFT, M. K.: The synthesis of kinin analogues. Ann. N.Y. Acad. Sci. **104**, 15 (1963).
NIES, A. L., FORSYTH, R. P., WILLIAMS, H. E., MELMON, K. L.: Contribution of kinins to endotoxin shock in unanesthetized rhesus monkeys. Circulat. Res. **23**, 155 (1968).
NILSEN, K. H., RUGSTAD, H. E.: Stability of a kininase of microbial origin in the blood perfusates of an isolated rat lung preparation. Life Sci. **7**, 921 (1968).
NUGENT, F. W., ATENDIDO, W. A., BULAN, M. B., MACDONALD, A. J.: Kininase activity in experimental pancreatitis. Nature (Lond.) **211**, 207 (1966).
OATES, J. A., BUTLER, T. C.: Pharmacologic and endocrine aspects of carcinoid syndrome. Advanc. Pharmacol. **5**, 109 (1967).
— MELMON, K. L.: Biochemical and physiologic studies of the kinins in carcinoid syndrome. In: Hypotensive peptides, p. 565, ed. by E. G. ERDÖS, N. BACK and F. SICUTERI. Berlin-Heidelberg-New York: Springer 1966.
— PETTINGER, W. A., DOCTOR, R. B.: Evidence for the release of bradykinin in carcinoid syndrome. J. clin. Invest. **45**, 173 (1966).
PASKHINA, T. S., TRAPEZNIKOVA, S. S.: Cleavage of depsipeptide analogs of bradykinin by kininase (carboxypeptidase N) from human and rabbit serum. Biokhimiya **32**, 527 (1967).
PHELPS, P., PROCKOP, D. J., MCCARTY, D. J.: Crystal induced inflammation in canine joints. III. Evidence against bradykinin as a mediator of inflammation. J. Lab. clin. Med. **68**, 433 (1966).
PICARELLI, Z. P., HENRIQUES, O. B., OLIVEIRA, M. C. F.: Potentiation of bradykinin action on smooth-muscle by cysteine. Experientia (Basel) **18**, 77 (1962).
RAVDEL, G. A., FILATOVA, M. P., SHCHUKINA, L. A., PASKHINA, T. S., SUROVIKINA, M. S., TRAPEZNIKOVA, S. S., EGOROVA, T. P.: 6-Glycine-8-phenyllactic acid bradykinin. Its synthesis, biological activity, and splitting by kininase (carboxypeptidase N). J. Med. Chem. **10**, 242 (1967).
ROCHA E SILVA, M.: Bradykinin—mechanism of its release by trypsin and kallikrein. Arch. int. Pharmacodyn. 88, 271 (1951).
— The physiological significance of bradykinin. Ann. N.Y. Acad. Sci. **104**, 190 (1963).

Rocha e Silva, M., Beraldo, W. T., Rosenfeld, G.: Bradykinin, a hypotensive and smooth muscle stimulating factor released from plasma globulin by snake venoms and by trypsin. Amer. J. Physiol. **156**, 261 (1949).
— Reis, M. L., Ferreira, S. H.: Release of kinins from fresh plasma under varying experimental conditions. Biochem. Pharmacol. **16**, 1665 (1967).
Rugstad, H. E.: Kininase production by some microbes. Brit. J. Pharmacol. **28**, 315 (1966).
— Purification of a kinin-inactivating enzyme from cultures of *Pseudomonas aeruginosa*. Brit. J. Pharmacol. **30**, 134 (1967a).
— Characterization of a plasma kinin-inactivating enzyme produced by *Pseudomonas aeruginosa*. Brit. J. Pharmacol. **30**, 425 (1967b).
— Degradation of plasma kinins by an enzyme from *Pseudomonas aeruginosa*. Brit. J. Pharmacol. **31**, 401 (1967c).
Ryan, J. W., Roblero, J., Stewart, J. M.: Inactivation of bradykinin in the pulmonary circulation. Biochem. J. **110**, 795 (1968).
Saameli, K., Eskes, T. K. A. B.: Bradykinin and cardiovascular system: estimation of half-life. Amer. J. Physiol. **203**, 261 (1962).
Schachter, M.: Some properties of kallidin, bradykinin and wasp venom kinin. In: Polypeptides which affect smooth muscles and blood vessels, p. 232, ed. by M. Schachter. Oxford 1960.
Schröder, E.: Über Peptidsynthesen. Synthese von Methionyl-Lysyl-Bradykinin, einem Kinin aus Rinderblut. Experientia (Basel) **20**, 39 (1964).
Schwab, J.: Kininases in leucocytes and other tissues. Nature (Lond.) **195**, 345 (1962).
Seki, T., Yang, H. Y. T., Levin, Y., Jenssen, T. A., Erdös, E. G.: Application of water-insoluble complexes of kininogenases, inhibitors and kininases to kinin research. Advanc. exp. Med. Biol. (in press).
Shimonaeva, E. E.: Some properties of carboxypeptidase N from rabbit blood serum. Vop. med. Khim **13**, 105 (1967).
Sicuteri, F., Fanciullacci, M., Anselmi, B.: Bradykinin release and inactivation in man. Int. Arch. Allergy **22**, 77 (1963b).
— — del Bianco, P. L., Anselmi, B.: Bradichininasi nel liquido cefalo-rachidiano dell'uomo. Boll. Soc. ital. Biol. sper. **41**, 464 (1965).
— Periti, P., Anselmi, B., Fanciullacci, M.: Livelli plasmachininici nell'unomo dopo somministrazione endovenosa ed endoarteria di bradichinina sintetica e naturale. Boll. Soc. Ital. Biol. Sper. **39**, 314 (1963a).
Skinner, N. S., Jr., Webster, M. E.: Kinins, beta-adrenergic receptors and functional vasodilatation in the submaxillary gland of the cat. J. Physiol. (Lond.) **195**, 505 (1968).
Stewart, J. M.: Synthesis and pharmacology of polistes kinin, a bradykinin homolog. Fed. Proc. **27**, 534 (1968).
— Roblero, J.: Studies on the pulmonary inactivation of bradykinin. In: Symposium on Vasoactive Polypeptides and Inhibitors of Proteolytic Enzymes, p. 52. Tokyo 1967.
— Woolley, D. W.: Bradykinin analogs. In: Symposium on Vasoactive Polypeptides: Bradykinin and Related Kinins, p. 7, ed. by M. Rocha e Silva and H. A. Rothschild. São Paulo 1966.
Suzuki, T., Iwanaga, S., Nagasawa, S., Sato, T.: Purification and properties of bradykininogen and of the bradykinin-releasing and -destroying enzymes in snake venom. In: Hypotensive peptides, p. 149, ed. by E. G. Erdös, N. Back and F. Sicuteri. Berlin-Heidelberg-New York: Springer 1966.
Teger-Nilsson, A.-C.: Degradation of human fibrinopeptides A and B in blood serum *in vitro*. Acta chem. Scand. **22**, 3171 (1968).
— Blömback, B.: Degradation of human fibrinopeptides in serum. Acta chem. scand. **21**, 307 (1967).
Tewksbury, D. A., Marschke, G. R.: Kininase activity in asthmatic serum. Int. Arch. Allergy **30**, 538 (1966).
Trapeznikova, S. S., Paskhina, T. S.: The isolation, purification, and properties of carboxypeptidases (kininases) from human and rabbit blood serum. Biokhimiya **33**, 1012 (1968).
Trautschold, I.: Enzyme und Inhibitoren der Bildung und des Abbaues gefäßaktiver Polypeptide (Kinine). Habil.-Schr. Munich 1965.
— Rüdel, G.: Neuere Ergebnisse auf dem Gebiet der Plasmakinine. Klin. Wschr. **41**, 297 (1963).
Vane, J. R.: The release and fate of vaso-active hormones in the circulation. Brit. J. Pharmacol. **35**, 209 (1969).
Vichi, F. L.: Enzymuria following acute renal ischemia in dogs. Experientia (Basel) **24**, 1219 (1968).

WATANABE, N.: Kininase activity in human blood in normal and pathological conditions. Tohoku J. exp. Med. **92**, 63 (1967).
— ABE, K., KUMAGAI, N., MOURI, T., SEKI, T., YOSHINAGA, K.: Kininase activity in human blood. Tohoku J. exp. Med. **89**, 383 (1966).
WEBSTER, M. E., GILMORE, J. P.: The estimation of the kallidins in blood and urine. Biochem. Pharmacol. **14**, 1161 (1965).
— PIERCE, J. V.: The nature of the kallidins released from human plasma by kallikreins and other enzymes. Ann. N.Y. Acad. Sci. **104**, 91 (1963).
— SKINNER, N. S., Jr., POWELL, W. J., Jr.: Role of the kinins in vasodilatation of skeletal muscle of the dog. Amer. J. Physiol. **212**, 553 (1967).
WERLE, E.: Über Kallidin und Bradykinin. Arch. int. Pharmacodyn. **92**, 427 (1953).
— Kallikrein, kallidin and related substances. In: Polypeptides which affect smooth muscles and blood vessels, p. 199, ed. by M. SCHACHTER. Oxford 1960.
— BEREK, U.: Über Kallidin. Biochem. Z. **320**, 136 (1950).
— ERDÖS, E. G.: Über eine neue blutdrucksenkende, darm- und uteruserregende Substanz im menschlichen Urin. Naunyn-Schmiedebergs Arch. exp. Path. Pharmak. **223**, 234 (1954).
— GÖTZE, W., KEPPLER, A.: Über die Wirkung des Kallikreins auf den isolierten Darm und über eine neue darmkontrahierende Substanz. Biochem. Z. **289**, 217 (1937).
— GRUNZ, M.: Zur Kenntnis der darmkontrahierenden, uteruserregenden und blutdrucksenkenden Substanz Dk. Biochem. Z. **301**, 429 (1939).
— HAMBUECHEN, R.: Zur Kenntnis der blutdrucksenkenden und spasmolytischen Wirkung des Kallikreins und der Substanz Dk. Naunyn-Schmiedebergs Arch. exp. Path. Pharmak. **201**, 311 (1943).
— HOCHSTRASSER, K., TRAUTSCHOLD, I., LEYSATH, G.: Wirkung von Thioglykolsäure auf Kininogen und Kininase. Hoppe-Seylers Z. physiol. Chem. **337**, 286 (1964).
— KEHL, R., KOEBKE, K.: Über Trypsin, Chymotrypsin, Kallidin und Bradykinin. Biochem. Z. **321**, 213 (1950).
— LEYSATH, G., SCHMAL, A.: Über das Verhalten des Kininogenspiegels nach Nieren- und nach Nebennierenexstirpation bei der Ratte. Hoppe-Seylers Z. physiol. Chem. **349**, 107 (1968).
WOLFF, E. C., SCHIRMER, E. W., FOLK, J. E.: The kinetics of carboxypeptidase B activity. 1. Kinetic parameters. J. biol. Chem. **237**, 3094 (1962).
YAMAFUJI, K., CARRARA, M. C.: Studies on the kininase activity of rabbit polymorphonuclear leucocytes. Fed. Proc. **27**, 533 (1968).
YANG, H. Y. T., ERDÖS, E. G.: Second kininase in human blood plasma. Nature (Lond.) **215**, 1402 (1967).
YANO, M., NAGASAWA, S., HORIUCHI, K., SUZUKI, T.: Separation of a new substrate, kininogen-I, for plasma kallikrein in bovine plasma. J. Biochem. **62**, 504 (1967).
ZACHARIAE, H., MALMQUIST, J., OATES, J. A.: Kininase in human polymorphonuclear leukocytes. Life Sci. **5**, 2347 (1966).
— — — PETTINGER, W.: Studies on the mechanism of kinin formation in inflammation. J. Physiol. (Lond.) **190**, 81 (1967).
ZUBER, H.: Observations on the use of enzymes in the analysis of peptides. In: Peptides, p. 189, ed. by L. ZERVAS. Oxford: Pergamon Press 1966.
— JAQUES, R.: Isolierung von Bradykinin aus Rinderplasma nach Einwirkung von Schlangengift (*Bothrops jararaca*). Helv. chim. Acta **43**, 1128 (1960).

Chapter 6: Kinins

Section A: hysiological and Pharmacological Actions

Structure-Activity Relationships of Kinins

E. SCHRÖDER

The elucidation of the structure of bradykinin by ELLIOTT et al. (1960) and of kallidin by WERLE et al. (1961) and independently by PIERCE and WEBSTER (1961), as well as the synthesis of these two naturally occurring polypeptides by BOISSONNAS et al. (1960; cf. GUTTMANN et al., 1962), PLESS et al. (1962), and NICOLAIDES and colleagues (1961) stimulated subsequent intensive research work. The use of larger amounts of synthetic material made an exact quantitative determination of the various pharmacological effects possible, such as action on smooth muscles *in vitro* and on extravasal smooth muscles *in vivo*, bronchoconstriction, action on the heart and the vascular system, and influence on renal blood flow, stomach secretion, pain sensation, and leukocyte emigration. The large number of biological effects that can be demonstrated in extremely low doses raised many questions about the importance of the kinins in the physiological and pathological processes (STÜRMER, 1966; WIEGERSHAUSEN and PAEGELOW, 1966; ERDÖS, 1966; WERLE, 1967; HABERMANN, 1968). Peptide chemists already engaged with modifications of natural molecules became interested in clarifying the following problems: Which chemically functional or nonfunctional groups are essential for biological activity, or what special structural requirements are responsible for an attachment to a hypothetical receptor? Related to this is the search for specific inhibitors of bradykinin, which could be decisive for investigations of the participation of kinins as mediator substances in physiological–pathological processes. A further goal for the chemist is to differentiate the various activities, i.e. to reduce unpleasant side effects to a minimum by chemical modifications or to prolong the most interesting activities, which are only of short duration when the original molecule is applied. An improvement of this kind is possible if the structure of the natural peptide is modified in such a way that the *in vivo* enzymatic degradation of the peptide chain is blocked without destruction of the active centers of the molecule.

The research work on systematic alteration primarily of bradykinin but also of kallidin was started in 1961–62 and is still in progress. To date more than 170 kinin analogs have been described, which may be classified into the following groups:

Bradykinin Analogs

1. With modified functional groups.
2. Obtained by replacement of one or more amino acids.
3. Obtained by shortening of the peptide chain.
4. Obtained by C-terminal lengthening of the peptide chain and by inserting amino acids.

5. Obtained by N-terminal shortening and C-terminal lengthening of the peptide chain.
6. Obtained by N-terminal lengthening of the peptide chain (kallidin analogs).
7. Obtained by N-terminal lengthening of the peptide chain with more than one amino acid (Met-Lys-bradykinin analogs).

Various research groups characterized the synthetic analogs by testing them on the isolated rat uterus, isolated guinea pig ileum, the blood pressure of rabbit, guinea pig, and mouse. In special cases a measurement of the effect on the blood flow in dog hind limb was carried out. Another favored assessment was the bronchoconstrictor test in guinea pigs. To demonstrate an antibradykinin effect, the inhibition of contraction of the isolated rat uterus or isolated guinea pig ileum induced by bradykinin was used. Depending on the individual test methods, only a general statement can be made whether an analog is highly active, slightly active, or inactive in a given test. Comprehensive comparisons often are difficult because similar compounds were investigated in only one or in different test systems. In spite of these disadvantages, a number of conclusions can be drawn from the structure–activity relationship on the basis of the presently known analogs.

According to the classification made above, all the analogs, with the corresponding literature references, are compiled in Table 1 at the end of this paper. As reference compound, bradykinin is used with a fixed activity of 1.

A. Modified Functional Groups

The functional groups of bradykinin exert different influences on biological activity. While a blocking of the C-terminal carboxyl function reduces the biological activity on the isolated rat uterus to $^1/_{100}$ (*3*)[1], the selective N-terminal acetylated product (*1*)[1] still has an activity half that of bradykinin. The elimination of the basic guanido function of the Arg^1 and Arg^9 residues[2] by introduction of nitro groups (*4*) results in a decrease of activity to $^1/_{100}$ (compare replacement of the arginine residues by other amino acids). The substitution of the aliphatic hydroxyl function of the serine residue in position 6 (*2*) shows different effects in the two test systems used. The bronchoconstrictor activity is much more reduced than the activity on the guinea pig blood pressure.

B. Replacement of One or More Amino Acids

The exchange of the Arg^1 residue by the neutral amino acids glycine (*8*) and alanine (*5*) results in a very strong decrease in activity on rabbit blood pressure and on rat uterus (to $<^1/_{1000}$ and $<^1/_{1500}$ of the original value). By substitution of the basic amino acids lysine (*9*) or ornithine (*10*), the activity on guinea pig blood pressure is only slightly reduced ($^1/_{10}$ and $^1/_{50}$ respectively). Less active is Cit^1-bradykinin (*6*). Substitution of the Arg^9 residue by glycine (*101*) or alanine (*98*), as in the case of the corresponding changes in position 1, causes a decrease of activity to $<^1/_{1000}$ that of bradykinin. In contrast Cit^9- (*100*), His^9- (*102*), Orn^9- (*104*) and Lys^9-bradykinin (*103*) are moderately effective analogs of bradykinin. These compounds are slightly more active than the corresponding deriva-

1. The number of the compound in the table.
2. For the abbreviations of the amino acids essentially those suggested by the IUPAC-IUB-Commission on Biochemical Nomenclature, in Hoppe-Seylers Z. physiol. Chem. **348**, 256, 262 (1967), have been adopted. For D-amino acids the uncapitalized abbreviation is used in the table.

Table 1. *Synthetic analogs*

No.	Variation in position	Name	Amino acid sequences
		Bradykinin	H-Arg-Pro-Pro-Gly-Phe-Ser-Pro-Phe-Arg-OH 1 2 3 4 5 6 7 8 9
(1) ***Bradykinin analogs with modified functional groups***			
1	1	(Ac-Arg)[1]-bradykinin	Ac-*Arg*-Pro-Pro-Gly-Phe-Ser-Pro-Phe-Arg-OH
2	6	(O-Carbamyl-L-Ser)[6]-bradykinin	H-Arg-Pro-Pro-Gly-Phe-*Ser*(CONH$_2$)-Pro-Phe-Arg-OH
(2) ***Bradykinin analogs obtained by replacement of one or more amino acids***			
3	9	(Arg-NH$_2$)[9]-bradykinin	H-Arg-Pro-Pro-Gly-Phe-Ser-Pro-Phe-*Arg*-NH$_2$
4	1 + 9	Arg(NO$_2$)[1]-Arg(NO$_2$)[9]-bradykinin	H-Arg(NO$_2$)-Pro-Pro-Gly-Phe-Ser-Pro-Phe-Arg(NO$_2$)-OH
5	1	Ala[1]-bradykinin	H-*Ala*-Pro-Pro-Gly-Phe-Ser-Pro-Phe-Arg-OH
6	1	Cit[1]-bradykinin	H-*Cit*-Pro-Pro-Gly-Phe-Ser-Pro-Phe-Arg-OH
7	1	Glu[1]-bradykinin	H-*Glu*-Pro-Pro-Gly-Phe-Ser-Pro-Phe-Arg-OH
8	1	Gly[1]-bradykinin	H-*Gly*-Pro-Pro-Gly-Phe-Ser-Pro-Phe-Arg-OH
9	1	Lys[1]-bradykinin	H-*Lys*-Pro-Pro-Gly-Phe-Ser-Pro-Phe-Arg-OH
10	1	Orn[1]-bradykinin	H-*Orn*-Pro-Pro-Gly-Phe-Ser-Pro-Phe-Arg-OH
11	2	Ala[2]-bradykinin	H-Arg-*Ala*-Pro-Gly-Phe-Ser-Pro-Phe-Arg-OH
12	2	pro[2]-bradykinin	H-Arg-*pro*-Pro-Gly-Phe-Ser-Pro-Phe-Arg-OH
13	2	Sar[2]-bradykinin	H-Arg-*Sar*-Pro-Gly-Phe-Ser-Pro-Phe-Arg-OH
14	2	Val[2]-bradykinin	H-Arg-*Val*-Pro-Gly-Phe-Ser-Pro-Phe-Arg-OH
15	1 + 2	Pro[1]-Arg[2]-bradykinin	H-*Pro-Arg*-Pro-Gly-Phe-Ser-Pro-Phe-Arg-OH
16	3	Ala[3]-bradykinin	H-Arg-Pro-*Ala*-Gly-Phe-Ser-Pro-Phe-Arg-OH
17	3	Gly[3]-bradykinin	H-Arg-Pro-*Gly*-Gly-Phe-Ser-Pro-Phe-Arg-OH
18	3	Lys[3]-bradykinin	H-Arg-Pro-*Lys*-Gly-Phe-Ser-Pro-Phe-Arg-OH
19	3	Pip[3]-bradykinin	H-Arg-Pro-*Pip*-Gly-Phe-Ser-Pro-Phe-Arg-OH
20	3	pro[3]-bradykinin	H-Arg-Pro-*pro*-Gly-Phe-Ser-Pro-Phe-Arg-OH
21	3	Sar[3]-bradykinin	H-Arg-Pro-*Sar*-Gly-Phe-Ser-Pro-Phe-Arg-OH

of bradykinin and kallidin

Biological activities						
Rat uterus (isolated)	Guinea pig ileum (isolated)	Rabbit blood pressure	Guinea pig blood pressure	Guinea pig broncho-constriction	Antibradykinin activity	References
$1 \cdot 10^{-10}$ g/ml =1	$1 \cdot 10^{-9}$ g/ml =1	$5 \cdot 10^{-8}$ g/kg =1	$2 \cdot 10^{-7}$ g/kg =1	$2 \cdot 10^{-7}$ g/ml =1	—	CERLETTI et al. (1961) DEWALD and NICOLAIDES (1964), BODANSZKY et al. (1962)
1/2	—	—	—	—	—	STEWART and WOOLLEY (1966, 1967)
—	—	—	—	<1/2,000	—	NICOLAIDES et al. (1963a)
—	—	—	1/75	<1/500		DEWALD et al. (1963)
1/100	—	—	—	—	—	ERDÖS (cited by STEWART and WOOLLEY (1967)
1/100	—	—	—	—	—	BODANSZKY et al. (1962, 1963a)
<1/1,500	<1/1,500	~1/1,000	—	—	—	SCHRÖDER (1965a, b)
1/600	—	—	—	—	—	BODANSZKY et al. (1962, 1963a)
1/400	—	—	<1/100 (rat)	—	—	ONDETTI (1963)
—	—	—	1/250	<1/2,000		NICOLAIDES et al. (1963a, b)
—	—	—	1/300	<1/2,000	—	NICOLAIDES et al. (1963c)
1/1,500	—	1/1,000	—	—	—	SCHRÖDER (1965b)
—	—	—	1/10	1/62	—	NICOLAIDES et al. (1963a, c)
1/500	1/150 to 1/300	1/250	—	—	—	SCHRÖDER (1964b, 1965b)
—	—	—	1/50	1/1,000	—	NICOLAIDES et al. (1963a, c)
1/300	1/150	1/200	—	—	—	SCHRÖDER (1964c, 1965b)
1/500	—	—	—	—	—	STEWART and WOOLLEY (1966, 1967)
—	1/2.5	1/3—1/4 (blood flow dog hind limb)	1/2	—	—	YANAIHARA et al. (1967)
1/100	1/500	1/200	—	—	—	SCHRÖDER and HEMPEL (1964)
~1/500	~1/1,500	~1/1,500	—	—	—	SCHRÖDER et al. (1964), SCHRÖDER (1965b)
1	1	1	—	—	—	SCHRÖDER (1964c, 1965b)
—	1/7	—	—	—	none	SUZUKI and ABIKO (1967b)
—	1/1,000	—	—	—	none	SUZUKI and ABIKO (1967a)
—	—	—	1/2,000	<1/2,000	—	NICOLAIDES et al. (1963a)
1/10,000	—	—	—	—	—	STEWART and WOOLLEY (1966, 1967)
—	1/1.5	1/10—1/20 (blood flow dog hind limb)	1	—	—	YANAIHARA et al. (1967)

Table 1

No.	Variation in position	Name	Amino acid sequences
22	3	Val^{3}-bradykinin	H-Arg-Pro-*Val*-Gly-Phe-Ser-Pro-Phe-Arg-OH
23	2 + 3	Sar^{2}-Sar^{3}-bradykinin	H-Arg-*Sar*-*Sar*-Gly-Phe-Ser-Pro-Phe-Arg-OH
24	2 + 3	pro^{2}-pro^{3}-bradykinin	H-Arg-*pro*-*pro*-Gly-Phe-Ser-Pro-Phe-Arg-OH
25	4	Ala^{4}-bradykinin	H-Arg-Pro-Pro-*Ala*-Phe-Ser-Pro-Phe-Arg-OH
26	4	β-Ala^{4}-bradykinin	H-Arg-Pro-Pro-*β-Ala*-Phe-Ser-Pro-Phe-Arg-OH
27	4	Glyco^{4}-bradykinin	H-Arg-Pro-Pro-*Glyco*-Phe-Ser-Pro-Phe-Arg-OH
28	4	Ileu^{4}-bradykinin	H-Arg-Pro-Pro-*Ileu*-Phe-Ser-Pro-Phe-Arg-OH
29	4	Pro^{4}-bradykinin	H-Arg-Pro-Pro-*Pro*-Phe-Ser-Pro-Phe-Arg-OH
30	4	Sar^{4}-bradykinin	H-Arg-Pro-Pro-*Sar*-Phe-Ser-Pro-Phe-Arg-OH
31	4	Ser^{4}-bradykinin	H-Arg-Pro-Pro-*Ser*-Phe-Ser-Pro-Phe-Arg-OH
32	4	Val^{4}-bradykinin	H-Arg-Pro-Pro-*Val*-Phe-Ser-Pro-Phe-Arg-OH
33	5	Ala^{5}-bradykinin	H-Arg-Pro-Pro-Gly-*Ala*-Ser-Pro-Phe-Arg-OH
34	5	phe^{5}-bradykinin	H-Arg-Pro-Pro-Gly-*phe*-Ser-Pro-Phe-Arg-OH
35	5	Tyr^{5}-bradykinin	H-Arg-Pro-Pro-Gly-*Tyr*-Ser-Pro-Phe-Arg-OH
36	5	(H_2N-Val)^{5}-bradykinin	H-Arg-Pro-Pro-Gly-*H_2N-Val*-Ser-Pro-Phe-Arg-OH
37	6	Ala^{6}-bradykinin	H-Arg-Pro-Pro-Gly-Phe-*Ala*-Pro-Phe-Arg-OH
38	6	β-Ala^{6}-bradykinin	H-Arg-Pro-Pro-Gly-Phe-*β-Ala*-Pro-Phe-Arg-OH
39	6	Cys^{6}-bradykinin	H-Arg-Pro-Pro-Gly-Phe-*Cys*-Pro-Phe-Arg-OH
40	6	Gly^{6}-bradykinin	H-Arg-Pro-Pro-Gly-Phe-*Gly*-Pro-Phe-Arg-OH
41	6	Glyco^{6}-bradykinin	H-Arg-Pro-Pro-Gly-Phe-*Glyco*-Pro-Phe-Arg-OH
42	6	Lys(Tos)^{6}-bradykinin	Tos | H-Arg-Pro-Pro-Gly-Phe-*Lys*-Pro-Phe-Arg-OH
43	6	Phe^{6}-bradykinin	H-Arg-Pro-Pro-Gly-Phe-*Phe*-Pro-Phe-Arg-OH
44	6	Sar^{6}-bradykinin	H-Arg-Pro-Pro-Gly-Phe-*Sar*-Pro-Phe-Arg-OH
45	6	ser^{6}-bradykinin	H-Arg-Pro-Pro-Gly-Phe-*ser*-Pro-Phe-Arg-OH

(continued)

Biological activities						
Rat uterus (isolated)	**Guinea pig ileum (isolated)**	**Rabbit blood pressure**	**Guinea pig blood pressure**	**Guinea pig broncho-constriction**	**Antibradykinin activity**	**References**
—	~1/1,500	1/125	—	—	—	SCHRÖDER and HEMPEL (1964)
—	1/20	1/50 (blood flow dog hind limb)	1/3—1/5	—	—	YANAIHARA et al. (1967)
1/10,000	—	—	—	—	—	STEWART and WOOLLEY (1967)
<1/1,500	<1/1,500	1/300	—	—	—	SCHRÖDER et al. (1964), SCHRÖDER (1965b)
—	1/5 (mouse)	—	—	—	none	SUZUKI and ABIKO (1966)
1/100 to 1/200	—	—	—	—	—	SHCHUKINA et al. (1965)
—	1/1,000	—	—	—	none	SUZUKI and ABIKO (1967c)
—	<1/800	~1/200	—	—	—	SCHRÖDER and HEMPEL (1964)
~1/800	1/500	1/125	—	—	—	SCHRÖDER and HEMPEL (1964)
—	<1/800	~1/200	—	—	—	SCHRÖDER and HEMPEL (1964)
—	1/500	—	—	—	none	SUZUKI and ABIKO (1967c)
1/1,000	<1/1,500	~1/1,000	—	—	—	SCHRÖDER (1964a, 1965b)
—	1/16	—	—	—	—	SCHNABEL and MEIENHOFER (1964)
—	—	—	1/40	1/30	—	NICOLAIDES and LIPNIK (1966)
1/500	1/150	1/300	—	—	—	SCHRÖDER (1965b), SCHRÖDER et al. (1964)
1/300	—	—	—	—	—	NOWAK (1966)
—	—	—	1/60	1/1,000	—	NICOLAIDES and LIPNIK (1966)
1/10	1/5	1/10	—	—	—	SCHRÖDER (1964c, 1965b)
—	1/20 (mouse)	—	—	—	antagonized ~20% by $1 \cdot 10^{-6}$ g/ml of ileum contraction	SUZUKI and ABIKO (1966)
—	1/5	—	—	—	—	SCHNABEL and MEIENHOFER (1964)
1	—	—	—	—	—	BODANSZKY et al. (1963a, b)
1/10	1/3—1	1/2—1	—	—	—	SCHRÖDER (1964a, 1965b)
1/100 to 1/200	—	—	—	—	—	SHCHUKINA et al. (1965)
1/2,000	—	—	—	—	—	STEWART and WOOLLEY (1966)
1/1,000	—	—	—	—	—	STEWART and WOOLLEY (1966)
<1/1,500	1/1,500	1/1,000	—	—	—	SCHRÖDER (1965b)
—	—	—	1/2.5	1/40	—	NICOLAIDES et al. (1963a), DEWALD et al. (1963)

Table 1

No.	Variation in position	Name	Amino acid sequences
46	6	Thr^{6}-bradykinin	H-Arg-Pro-Pro-Gly-Phe-*Thr*-Pro-Phe-Arg-OH
47	3 + 6	Ala^{3}-Gly^{6}-bradykinin	H-Arg-Pro-*Ala*-Gly-Phe-*Gly*-Pro-Phe-Arg-OH
48	3 + 6	Gly^{3}-Gly^{6}-bradykinin	H-Arg-Pro-*Gly*-Gly-Phe-*Gly*-Pro-Phe-Arg-OH
49	3 + 6	Gly^{3}-Ser(Ac)^{6}-bradykinin	Ac H-Arg-Pro-*Gly*-Gly-Phe-*Ser*-Pro-Phe-Arg-OH
50	3 + 6	Lys^{3}-Ser(Ac)^{6}-bradykinin	Ac H-Arg-Pro-*Lys*-Gly-Phe-*Ser*-Pro-Phe-Arg-OH
51	3 + 6	Sar^{3}-Gly^{6}-bradykinin	H-Arg-Pro-*Sar*-Gly-Phe-*Gly*-Pro-Phe-Arg-OH
52	4 + 6	β-Ala^{4}-β-Ala^{6}-bradykinin	H-Arg-Pro-Pro-*β-Ala*-Phe-*β-Ala*-Pro-Phe-Arg-OH
53	4 + 6	β-Ala^{4}-Ser(Ac)^{6}-bradykinin	Ac H-Arg-Pro-Pro-*β-Ala*-Phe-*Ser*-Pro-Phe-Arg-OH
54	4 + 6	Ileu^{4}-Ser(Ac)^{6}-bradykinin	Ac H-Arg-Pro-Pro-*Ileu*-Phe-*Ser*-Pro-Phe-Arg-OH
55	4 + 6	Ileu^{4}-Thr^{6}-bradykinin	H-Arg-Pro-Pro-*Ileu*-Phe-*Thr*-Pro-Phe-Arg-OH
56	4 + 6	Ileu^{4}-Thr(Ac)^{6}-bradykinin	Ac H-Arg-Pro-Pro-*Ileu*-Phe-*Thr*-Pro-Phe-Arg-OH
57	4 + 6	Leu^{4}-Thr^{6}-bradykinin	H-Arg-Pro-Pro-*Leu*-Phe-*Thr*-Pro-Phe-Arg-OH
58	4 + 6	Leu^{4}-Thr(Ac)^{6}-bradykinin	Ac H-Arg-Pro-Pro-*Leu*-Phe-*Thr*-Pro-Phe-Arg-OH
59	4 + 6	Ser^{4}-Gly^{6}-bradykinin	H-Arg-Pro-Pro-*Ser*-Phe-*Gly*-Pro-Phe-Arg-OH
60	4 + 6	Val^{4}-Ser(Ac)^{6}-bradykinin	Ac H-Arg-Pro-Pro-*Val*-Phe-*Ser*-Pro-Phe-Arg-OH
61	4 + 6	Val^{4}-Thr^{6}-bradykinin	H-Arg-Pro-Pro-*Val*-Phe-*Thr*-Pro-Phe-Arg-OH
62	4 + 6	Val^{4}-Thr(Ac)^{6}-bradykinin	Ac H-Arg-Pro-Pro-*Val*-Phe-*Thr*-Pro-Phe-Arg-OH
63	5 + 6	Ala^{5}-Gly^{6}-bradykinin	H-Arg-Pro-Pro-Gly-*Ala*-*Gly*-Pro-Phe-Arg-OH
64	5 + 6	Pro^{5}-Gly^{6}-bradykinin	H-Arg-Pro-Pro-Gly-*Pro*-*Gly*-Pro-Phe-Arg-OH
65	7	Ala^{7}-bradykinin	H-Arg-Pro-Pro-Gly-Phe-Ser-*Ala*-Phe-Arg-OH
66	7	Asn^{7}-bradykinin	H-Arg-Pro-Pro-Gly-Phe-Ser-*Asn*-Phe-Arg-OH
67	7	Gly^{7}-bradykinin	H-Arg-Pro-Pro-Gly-Phe-Ser-*Gly*-Phe-Arg-OH
68	7	His^{7}-bradykinin	H-Arg-Pro-Pro-Gly-Phe-Ser-*His*-Phe-Arg-OH

(continued)

Biological activities						
Rat uterus (isolated)	Guinea pig ileum (isolated)	Rabbit blood pressure	Guinea pig blood pressure	Guinea pig broncho-constriction	Antibradykinin activity	References
—	—	—	1/2	<1/500	—	DEWALD et al. (1963)
1	1/3	1/10	—	—	—	SCHRÖDER and HEMPEL (1964)
1/3	—	—	—	—	—	STEWART and WOOLLEY (1964)
1/50	1/5	1/6	—	—	—	SCHRÖDER and HEMPEL (1964)
—	1/4	—	—	—	none	SUZUKI and ABIKO (1967b)
—	1/100	—	—	—	none	SUZUKI and ABIKO (1967b)
—	1/5	—	—	—	none	SUZUKI and ABIKO (1967b)
—	3/1,000	—	—	—	none	SUZUKI and ABIKO (1967a)
—	1/5	—	—	—	none	SUZUKI and ABIKO (1967b)
—	inactive by $9 \cdot 10^{-6}$ g/ml (mouse)	—	—	—	none	SUZUKI and ABIKO (1966)
—	1/100 (mouse)	—	—	—	none	SUZUKI and ABIKO (1966)
—	3/1,000	—	—	—	none	SUZUKI and ABIKO (1967c)
—	1/1,000	—	—	—	none	SUZUKI and ABIKO (1967c)
—	1/1,000	—	—	—	none	SUZUKI and ABIKO (1967c)
—	1/250	—	—	—	none	SUZUKI and ABIKO (1967c)
—	inactive	—	—	—	none	SUZUKI and ABIKO (1967c)
—	1/100	1/100	—	—	—	SCHRÖDER et al. (1964), SCHRÖDER (1965b)
—	inactive	—	—	—	none	SUZUKI and ABIKO (1967c)
—	1/500	—	—	—	none	SUZUKI and ABIKO (1967c)
—	1/500	—	—	—	none	SUZUKI and ABIKO (1967c)
—	<1/1,500	1/200	—	—	—	SCHRÖDER and HEMPEL (1964)
—	—	<1/1,000	—	—	—	SCHRÖDER and HEMPEL (1964)
1/80	1/100	<1/1,000	—	—	—	SCHRÖDER (1964c 1965b)
—	—	—	1/1,000	0	—	NICOLAIDES et al. (1963a)
1/100	—	—	—	—	—	BODANSZKY et al. (1963a, b)
—	<1/1,500	~1/1,000	—	—	—	SCHRÖDER and HEMPEL (1964)

Table 1

No.	Variation in position	Name	Amino acid sequences
69	7	pro^{7}-bradykinin	H-Arg-Pro-Pro-Gly-Phe-Ser-*pro*-Phe-Arg-OH
70	7	Sar^{7}-bradykinin	H-Arg-Pro-Pro-Gly-Phe-Ser-*Sar*-Phe-Arg-OH
71	1 + 7	(Ac-Arg)^{1}-pro^{7}-bradykinin	*Ac-Arg*-Pro-Pro-Gly-Phe-Ser-*pro*-Phe-Arg-OH
72	2 + 7	pro^{2}-pro^{7}-bradykinin	H-Arg-*pro*-Pro-Gly-Phe-Ser-*pro*-Phe-Arg-OH
73	3 + 7	pro^{3}-pro^{7}-bradykinin	H-Arg-Pro-*pro*-Gly-Phe-Ser-*pro*-Phe-Arg-OH
74	2 + 3 + 7	pro^{2}-pro^{3}-pro^{7}-bradykinin	H-Arg-*pro-pro*-Gly-Phe-Ser-*pro*-Phe-Arg-OH
75	2 + 3 + 7	Sar^{2}-Sar^{3}-Sar^{7}-bradykinin	H-Arg-*Sar-Sar*-Gly-Phe-Ser-*Sar*-Phe-Arg-OH
76	8	Ala^{8}-bradykinin	H-Arg-Pro-Pro-Gly-Phe-Ser-Pro-*Ala*-Arg-OH
77	8	phe^{8}-bradykinin	H-Arg-Pro-Pro-Gly-Phe-Ser-Pro-*phe*-Arg-OH
78	8	Phe(F)^{8}-bradykinin	F H-Arg-Pro-Pro-Gly-Phe-Ser-Pro-*Phe*-Arg-OH
79	8	phe(F)^{8}-bradykinin	F H-Arg-Pro-Pro-Gly-Phe-Ser-Pro-*phe*-Arg-OH
80	8	*m*-CF_3Phe^{8}-bradykinin	H-Arg-Pro-Pro-Gly-Phe-Ser-Pro-*m-CF₃Phe*-Arg-OH
81	8	Tyr^{8}-bradykinin	H-Arg-Pro-Pro-Gly-Phe-Ser-Pro-*Tyr*-Arg-OH
82	1 + 8	(Ac-Arg)^{1}-Tyr(Me)^{8}-bradykinin	Me *Ac-Arg*-Pro-Pro-Gly-Phe-Ser-Pro-*Tyr*-Arg-OH
83	5 + 8	phe^{5}-phe^{8}-bradykinin	H-Arg-Pro-Pro-Gly-*phe*-Ser-Pro-*phe*-Arg-OH
84	5 + 8	phe^{5}-Tyr^{8}-bradykinin	H-Arg-Pro-Pro-Gly-*phe*-Ser-Pro-*Tyr*-Arg-OH
85	5 + 8	Tyr(Me)^{5}-Tyr(Me)^{8}-bradykinin	Me Me H-Arg-Pro-Pro-Gly-*Tyr*-Ser-Pro-*Tyr*-Arg-OH
86	1 + 5 + 8	(Ac-Arg)^{1}-Tyr(Me)^{5}-Tyr(Me)^{8}-bradykinin	Me Me *Ac-Arg*-Pro-Pro-Gly-*Tyr*-Ser-Pro-*Tyr*-Arg-OH
87	6 + 8	Gly^{6}-PhLac^{8}-bradykinin	H-Arg-Pro-Pro-Gly-Phe-*Gly*-Pro-*PhLac*-Arg-OH

(continued)

Biological activities						
Rat uterus (isolated)	Guinea pig ileum (isolated)	Rabbit blood pressure	Guinea pig blood pressure	Guinea pig broncho-constriction	Antibradykinin activity	References
1/75	—	—	—	—	—	STEWART and WOOLLEY (1966)
15/1,000	—	—	—	—	—	STEWART and WOOLLEY (1967)
—	1/8	1/10—1/15 (blood flow dog hind limb)	1/3	—	—	YANAIHARA et al. (1967)
1/1,000	—	—	—	—	—	STEWART and WOOLLEY (1966)
1/10,000	—	—	—	—	—	STEWART and WOOLLEY (1967)
$1 \cdot 10^{-5}$	—	—	—	—	—	STEWART and WOOLLEY (1967)
1/200,000	—	—	—	—	85% at 20 μg/ml	STEWART and WOOLLEY (1966, 1967)
—	1/100	1/200 (blood flow dog hind limb)	1/25	—	—	YANAIHARA et al. (1967)
~1/1,500	~1/1,000	~1/1,000	—	—	—	SCHRÖDER (1964c, 1965b)
—	—	—	1/4	1/60	—	NICOLAIDES et al. (1963a)
—	—	—	1/4	1/20	—	NICOLAIDES et al. (1963b)
—	1/1,000	—	—	—	—	SCHNABEL and MEIENHOFER (1964)
—	—	—	1.5	1.4	—	NICOLAIDES et al. (1963a)
—	—	—	1.5	1.4	—	NICOLAIDES et al. (1963b)
—	—	—	1/3	1/100	—	NICOLAIDES et al. (1963b)
—	—	—	2/3	1/3	—	NICOLAIDES and LIPNIK (1966)
—	1/5	—	—	—	—	SCHNABEL and MEIENHOFER (1964)
1/3	—	—	—	—	—	STEWART and WOOLLEY (1966)
—	<1/1,000	—	—	—	—	SCHNABEL and MEIENHOFER (1964)
—	5/1,000	—	—	—	—	SCHNABEL and MEIENHOFER (1964)
1/3	—	—	—	—	90% at $1 \cdot 10^{-6}$ rat uterus	STEWART and WOOLLEY (1966)
1/4	—	—	—	—	50% at $1 \cdot 10^{-6}$ rat uterus	STEWART and WOOLLEY (1966)
1/2	—	~2	4.5 (rat)	—	—	RAVDEL et al. (1967)

Table 1

No.	Variation in position	Name	Amino acid sequences
88	6 + 8	Gly^{6}-Tyr(Me)^{8}-bradykinin	Me | H-Arg-Pro-Pro-Gly-Phe-*Gly*-Pro-*Tyr*-Arg-OH
89	6 + 8	Thr^{6}-Leu^{8}-bradykinin	H-Arg-Pro-Pro-Gly-Phe-*Thr*-Pro-*Leu*-Arg-OH
90	1 + 6 + 8	(Ac-Arg)^{1}-Gly^{6}-Tyr(Me)^{8}-bradykinin	Me | *Ac-Arg*-Pro-Pro-Gly-Phe-*Gly*-Pro-*Tyr*-Arg-OH
91	5 + 6 + 8	Leu^{5}-Gly^{6}-Leu^{8}-bradykinin	H-Arg-Pro-Pro-Gly-*Leu*-*Gly*-Pro-*Leu*-Arg-OH
92	5 + 6 + 8	Leu^{5}-Thr^{6}-Leu^{8}-bradykinin	H-Arg-Pro-Pro-Gly-*Leu*-*Thr*-Pro-*Leu*-Arg-OH
93	5 + 6 + 8	Tyr(Me)^{5}-Asn^{6}-Tyr(Me)^{8}-bradykinin	Me Me | | H-Arg-Pro-Pro-Gly-*Tyr*-*Asn*-Pro-*Tyr*-Arg-OH
94	5 + 6 + 8	Tyr(Me)^{5}-Gly^{6}-Tyr(Me)^{8}-bradykinin	Me Me | | H-Arg-Pro-Pro-Gly-*Tyr*-*Gly*-Pro-*Tyr*-Arg-OH
95	2 + 4 + 6 + 8	Phe^{2}-Ser^{4}-Gly^{6}-Pro^{8}-bradykinin "Retrobradykinin"	H-Arg-*Phe*-Pro-*Ser*-Phe-*Gly*-Pro-*Pro*-Arg-OH
96	2 + 4 + 6 + 8	phe^{2}-ser^{4}-Gly^{6}-pro^{8}-bradykinin all-D-retro-bradykinin	H-arg-*phe*-pro-*ser*-phe-*Gly*-pro-*pro*-arg-OH
97	2—8	Arg-heptagly-Arg	H-Arg-*Gly*-*Gly*-*Gly*-*Gly*-*Gly*-*Gly*-*Gly*-Arg-OH
98	9	Ala^{9}-bradykinin	H-Arg-Pro-Pro-Gly-Phe-Ser-Pro-Phe-*Ala*-OH
99	9	arg^{9}-bradykinin	H-Arg-Pro-Pro-Gly-Phe-Ser-Pro-Phe-*arg*-OH
100	9	Cit^{9}-bradykinin	H-Arg-Pro-Pro-Gly-Phe-Ser-Pro-Phe-*Cit*-OH
101	9	Gly^{9}-bradykinin	H-Arg-Pro-Pro-Gly-Phe-Ser-Pro-Phe-*Gly*-OH
102	9	His^{9}-bradykinin	H-Arg-Pro-Pro-Gly-Phe-Ser-Pro-Phe-*His*-OH

(continued)

Biological activities						
Rat uterus (isolated)	Guinea pig ileum (isolated)	Rabbit blood pressure	Guinea pig blood pressure	Guinea pig broncho-constriction	Antibradykinin activity	References
1/4	—	—	—	—	—	Stewart and Woolley (1966)
bradykinin-like activity	—	—	—	—	—	Stewart (1963)
1/100	—	—	—	—	—	Stewart and Woolley (1964)
1/3	—	—	—	—	30% at 0.001 μ/ml rat uterus	Stewart and Woolley (1966)
1/50,000	—	—	—	—	—	Stewart and Woolley (1966)
slight activity	—	—	—	—	in small doses rat uterus	Stewart (1963)
1/30,000	—	—	—	—	—	Stewart and Woolley (1964)
1/200	—	—	—	—	30% at $1 \cdot 10^{-5}$ rat uterus	Stewart and Woolley (1966)
1/15	—	—	—	—	50% at $1 \cdot 10^{-6}$ rat uterus	Stewart and Woolley (1966)
inactive up to 10^{-5}	—	—	—	—	—	Vogler et al. (1962)
inactive up to $8 \cdot 10^{-5}$	—	—	—	—	—	Lande (1962)
1/5,000	—	—	—	—	—	Bodanszky et al. (1963a)
1/30,000	—	—	—	—	—	Stewart and Woolley (1966)
inactive up to 10^{-5} g/ml	—	—	—	—	none	Vogler and Lanz (1966)
0	—	—	—	—	—	Bodanszky et al. (1963a, b)
1/500	<1/800	<1/1,000	—	—	—	Schröder (1964c, 1965b)
1/1,000	—	—	—	—	—	Stewart and Woolley (1966)
1/400	—	—	—	—	—	Bodanszky et al. (1962, 1963a)
1/400	—	—	<1/100 (rat)	—	—	Ondetti (1963)
—	—	—	1/20	1/1,000	—	Nicolaides et al. (1963a) DeWald and Nicolaides (1964)
<1/1,500	<1/1,500	~1/1,000	—	—	—	Schröder (1965b)
—	—	—	1/20	1/2,000	—	Nicolaides et al. (1963a)
—	—	—	1/20	<1/2,000	—	DeWald and Nicolaides (1964)
—	~1/500	~1/1,000	—	—	—	Schröder and Hempel (1964)

Table 1

No.	Variation in position	Name	Amino acid sequences
103	9	Lys^{9}-bradykinin	H-Arg-Pro-Pro-Gly-Phe-Ser-Pro-Phe-*Lys*-OH
104	9	Orn^{9}-bradykinin	H-Arg-Pro-Pro-Gly-Phe-Ser-Pro-Phe-*Orn*-OH
105	1 + 9	Cit^{1}-Cit^{9}-bradykinin	H-*Cit*-Pro-Pro-Gly-Phe-Ser-Pro-Phe-*Cit*-OH
106	1 + 9	Dab^{1}-Dab^{9}-bradykinin	H-*Dab*-Pro-Pro-Gly-Phe-Ser-Pro-Phe-*Dab*-OH
107	1 + 9	Lys^{1}-Lys^{9}-bradykinin	H-*Lys*-Pro-Pro-Gly-Phe-Ser-Pro-Phe-*Lys*-OH
108	1 + 9	Lys^{1}-Lys(BOC)^{9}-bradykinin	BOC | H-Lys-Pro-Pro-Gly-Phe-Ser-Pro-Phe-*Lys*-OH
109	6 + 9	Cys^{6}-Orn^{9}-bradykinin	H-Arg-Pro-Pro-Gly-Phe-*Cys*-Pro-Phe-*Orn*-OH
110	7 + 9	Phe^{7}-Lys^{9}-bradykinin	H-Arg-Pro-Pro-Gly-Phe-Ser-*Phe*-Phe-*Lys*-OH
111	7 + 8 + 9	Phe^{7}-Arg^{8}-Pro^{9}-bradykinin	H-Arg-Pro-Pro-Gly-Phe-Ser-*Phe-Arg-Pro*-OH
112	1 + 5 + 6 + 8 + 9	arg^{1}-phe^{5}-ser^{6}-phe^{8}-arg^{9}-bradykinin	H-*arg*-Pro-Pro-Gly-*phe-ser*-Pro-*phe-arg*-OH
113	3 + 4 + 5 + 6 + 7 + 8	Lys^{3}-Val^{4}-Gly^{5}-Leu^{6}-Gly^{7}-Ala^{8}-bradykinin	H-Arg-Pro-*Lys-Val-Gly-Leu-Gly-Ala*-Arg-OH
114	1—9	all-D-bradykinin	H-*arg-pro-pro*-Gly-*phe-ser-pro-phe-arg*-OH

(3) *Bradykinin analogs obtained by shortening the peptide chain*

No.	Variation in position	Name	Amino acid sequences
115	1	Des-(Arg^{1})-bradykinin	H-□-Pro-Pro-Gly-Phe-Ser-Pro-Phe-Arg-OH
116	1 + 2	Des-(Arg^{1})-pro^{2}-bradykinin	H-□-*pro*-Pro-Gly-Phe-Ser-Pro-Phe-Arg-OH
117	3	Des-(Pro^{3})-bradykinin	H-Arg-Pro-□-Gly-Phe-Ser-Pro-Phe-Arg-OH
118	1 + 3	Des-(Arg^{1})-pro^{3}-bradykinin	H-□-Pro-*pro*-Gly-Phe-Ser-Pro-Phe-Arg-OH
119	1 + 6	Des-(Arg^{1})-Thr^{6}-bradykinin	H-□-Pro-Pro-Gly-Phe-*Thr*-Pro-Phe-Arg-OH
120	1 + 6	Des-(Arg^{1})-Lys(Tos)^{6}-bradykinin	Tos | H-□-Pro-Pro-Gly-Phe-*Lys*-Pro-Phe-Arg-OH
121	1 + 6	Des-(Arg^{1})-Phe^{6}-bradykinin	H-□-Pro-Pro-Gly-Phe-*Phe*-Pro-Phe-Arg-OH
122	7	Des-(Pro^{7})-bradykinin	H-Arg-Pro-Pro-Gly-Phe-Ser-□-Phe-Arg-OH
123	1 + 7	Des-(Arg^{1})-pro^{7}-bradykinin	H-□-Pro-Pro-Gly-Phe-Ser-*pro*-Phe-Arg-OH
124	1 + 2 + 3 + 7	Des-(Arg^{1})-pro^{2}-pro^{3}-pro^{7}-bradykinin	H-□-*pro-pro*-Gly-Phe-Ser-*pro*-Phe-Arg-OH

(continued)

Biological activities

Rat uterus (isolated)	Guinea pig ileum (isolated)	Rabbit blood pressure	Guinea pig blood pressure	Guinea pig broncho-constriction	Antibradykinin activity	References
1/500	1/5	1/10—1/30	2.9	—	—	SCHRÖDER (1964b, 1965b), ERDÖS et al. 1967
—	1/100	1/400	—	—	—	SCHRÖDER et al. (1964)
<1/5,000	—	—	—	—	—	BODANSZKY et al. (1962, 1963a)
<1/5,000	—	—	<1/100 (rat)	—	—	ONDETTI (1963)
inactive up to 10^{-4}	—	—	—	—	—	VOGLER et al. (1962)
<1/1,500	<1/1,500	1/500	—	—	—	SCHRÖDER (1964b, 1965b)
<1/1,500	<1/1,500	<1/1,000	–	–	–	SCHRÖDER (1964b, 1965b)
—	1/1,000	—	—	—	—	SCHNABEL and MEIENHOFER (1964)
—	<1/10,000	—	—	—	—	SCHNABEL and MEIENHOFER (1964)
<1/300	1/150	<1/1,000	—	—	—	SCHRÖDER (1965b)
1/10,000	—	—	—	—	—	STEWART and WOOLLEY (1966)
—	1/1,000 (mouse)	—	—	—	—	SUZUKI (1966)
1/200,000	—	—	—	—	—	STEWART and WOOLLEY (1966)
—	inactive up to 10^{-5} g/ml	—	—	—	—	VOGLER and LANZ (1966)
—	—	—	1/80	<1/2,000	—	NICOLAIDES et al. (1963a, c)
1/1,000	—	—	—	—	—	STEWART and WOOLLEY (1966)
1/20	1/100	—	—	—		GUTTMANN and BOISSONNAS (1961)
1/100,000	—	—	—	—	—	STEWART and WOOLLEY (1966)
1/3,000	—	—	—	—	—	STEWART and WOOLLEY (1966)
1/20,000	—	—	—	—	—	STEWART and WOOLLEY (1966)
1/3,000	—	—	—	—	—	STEWART and WOOLLEY (1966)
inactive up to 10^{-5}	inactive up to 10^{-5}	—	—	—	—	BOISSONNAS et al. (1960), SCHWYZER et al. (1960), NICOLAIDES and DEWALD (1960)
1/3,000	—	—	—	—	—	STEWART and WOOLLEY (1966)
1/500,000	—	—	—	—	50% at $1 \cdot 10^{-5}$ rat uterus	STEWART and WOOLLEY (1966)

Table 1

No.	Variation in position	Name	Amino acid sequences
125	3 + 7	Des-(Pro^{3}-Pro^{7})-bradykinin	H-Arg-Pro-□-Gly-Phe-Ser-□-Phe-Arg-OH
126	3 + 4 + 7	Des-(Pro^{7})-Gly^{3}-Pro^{4}-bradykinin	H-Arg-Pro-*Gly*-*Pro*-Phe-Ser-□-Phe-Arg-OH
127	4 + 5 + 7	Des-(Pro^{7})-Phe^{4}-Gly^{5}-bradykinin	H-Arg-Pro-Pro-*Phe*-*Gly*-Ser-□-Phe-Arg-OH
128	1 + 6 + 8	Des-(Arg^{1})-Gly^{6}-Tyr(Me)^{8}-bradykinin	H-□-Pro-Pro-Gly-Phe-*Gly*-Pro-*Tyr*(Me)-Arg-OH
129	1 + 6 + 8	Des-(Arg^{1})-Thr^{6}-Leu^{8}-bradykinin	H-□-Pro-Pro-Gly-Phe-*Thr*-Pro-*Leu*-Arg-OH
130	1 + 6 + 8	Des-(Arg^{1})-Tyr(Me)^{6}-Tyr(Me)^{8}-bradykinin	H-□-Pro-Pro-Gly-Phe-*Tyr*(Me)-Pro-*Tyr*(Me)-Arg-OH
131	1 + 5 + 6 + 8	Des(Arg^{1})-Leu^{5}-Thr^{6}-Leu^{8}-bradykinin	H-□-Pro-Pro-Gly-*Leu*-*Thr*-Pro-*Leu*-Arg-OH
132	1 + 5 + 6 + 8	Des-(Arg^{1})-Tyr(Me)^{5}-Asn^{6}-Tyr(Me)^{8}-bradykinin	H-□-Pro-Pro-Gly-*Tyr*(Me)-*Asn*-Pro-*Tyr*(Me)-Arg-OH
133	1 + 5 + 6 + 8	Des-(Arg^{1})-Tyr(Me)^{5}-Gly^{6}-Tyr(Me)^{8}-bradykinin	H-□-Pro-Pro-Gly-*Tyr*(Me)-*Gly*-Pro-*Tyr*(Me)-Arg-OH
134	9	Des-(Arg^{9})-Bradykinin	H-Arg-Pro-Pro-Gly-Phe-Ser-Pro-Phe-□-OH
135	1 + 9	Des-(Arg^{1}-Arg^{9})-bradykinin	H-□-Pro-Pro-Gly-Phe-Ser-Pro-Phe-□-OH
136	1 + 9	Des-(Arg^{1})-arg^{9}-bradykinin	H-□-Pro-Pro-Gly-Phe-Ser-Pro-Phe-*arg*-OH
(4) *Bradykinin analogs obtained by C-terminal lengthening of the peptide chain and by inserting amino acids*			
137	4	(Gly-Gly)^{4}-bradykinin	H-Arg-Pro-Pro-Gly-*Gly*-Phe-Ser-Pro-Phe-Arg-OH
138	9	(Arg-Arg)^{9}-bradykinin	H-Arg-Pro-Pro-Gly-Phe-Ser-Pro-Phe-Arg-*Arg*-OH
139	9	(Arg-Gly)^{9}-bradykinin	H-Arg-Pro-Pro-Gly-Phe-Ser-Pro-Phe-Arg-*Gly*-OH
140	6 + 9	Gly^{6}-(Phe-Arg)^{9}-bradykinin	H-Arg-Pro-Pro-Gly-Phe-*Gly*-Pro-Phe-*Phe*-Arg-OH
141	5 + 8 + 9	Tyr(Me)^{5}-Tyr(Me)^{8}-(Arg-Phe)^{9}-bradykinin	H-Arg-Pro-Pro-Gly-*Tyr*(Me)-Ser-Pro-*Tyr*(Me)-Arg-*Phe*-OH
142	5 + 8 + 9	Tyr(Me)^{5}-Tyr(Me)^{8}-(Arg-Gly)^{9}-bradykinin	H-Arg-Pro-Pro-Gly-*Tyr*(Me)-Ser-Pro-*Tyr*(Me)-Arg-*Gly*-OH
143	9	(Arg-Ser-Val-Gln)^{9}-bradykinin	H-Arg-Pro-Pro-Gly-Phe-Ser-Pro-Phe-Arg-*Ser*-*Val*-*Gln*-OH
144	9	[Arg-Ile-Tyr(SO_4)]^{9}-bradykinin = phyllokinin	H-Arg-Pro-Pro-Gly-Phe-Ser-Pro-Phe-Arg-*Ile*-*Tyr*(SO_3H)-OH

(continued)

Biological activities						
Rat uterus (isolated)	Guinea pig ileum (isolated)	Rabbit blood pressure	Guinea pig blood pressure	Guinea pig broncho-constriction	Antibradykinin activity	References
—	inactive up to $2{,}6 \cdot 10^{-6}$	—	—	—	—	GUTTMANN and BOISSONNAS (1961)
inactive up to 10^{-5}	inactive up to 10^{-5}	—	—	—	—	GUTTMANN and BOISSONNAS (1961)
inactive up to 10^{-5}	inactive up to 10^{-5}	—	—	—	—	GUTTMANN and BOISSONNAS (1961)
1/1,000	—	—	—	—	—	STEWART and WOOLLEY (1966)
1/150,000	—	—	—	—	100% at 50 µg/ml rat uterus	STEWART and WOOLLEY (1966)
1/1,000	—	—	—	—	—	STEWART and WOOLLEY (1966)
inactive	—	—	—	—	—	STEWART and WOOLLEY (1964)
1/1,000	—	—	—	—	—	STEWART and WOOLLEY (1966)
1/4,000	—	—	—	—	—	STEWART and WOOLLEY (1966)
—	—	—	1/2,000	1/2,000	—	NICOLAIDES et al. (1963a), DEWALD and NICOLAIDES (1964)
—	—	—	1/2,000	1/2,000	—	NICOLAIDES et al. (1963a)
1/500,000	—	—	—	—	50% at $1 \cdot 10^{-5}$ rat uterus	STEWART and WOOLLEY (1966)
—	—	—	1/10	1/10	—	NICOLAIDES and LIPNIK (1966)
1/25	—	—	—	—	—	STEWART and WOOLLEY (1966)
1/150	—	—	—	—	—	STEWART and WOOLLEY (1966)
1/5,000	—	—	—	—	—	STEWART and WOOLLEY (1966)
1/1,500	—	—	—	—	—	STEWART and WOOLLEY (1966)
1/5,000	—	—	—	—	—	STEWART and WOOLLEY (1966)
2/1,000	—	3/100	—	—	—	cited in STEWART and WOOLLEY (1967)
1-2	—	1	—	—	—	cited in STEWART and WOOLLEY (1967)

Table 1

No.	Variation in position	Name	Amino acid sequences
(5) *Bradykinin analogs obtained by N-terminal shortening and C-terminal lengthening of the peptide chain*			
145	1 + 9	Des-(Arg^1)-(Arg-Arg)^9-bradykinin	H-□-Pro-Pro-Gly-Phe-Ser-Pro-Phe-Arg-*Arg*-OH
146	1 + 9	Des-(Arg^1)-(Arg-Gly)^9-bradykinin	H-□-Pro-Pro-Gly-Phe-Ser-Pro-Phe-Arg-*Gly*-OH
147	1 + 6 + 9	Des(Arg^1)-Gly^6-(Phe-Arg)^9-bradykinin	H-□-Pro-Pro-Gly-Phe-*Gly*-Pro-Phe-*Phe*-Arg-OH
			Me Me
148	1 + 5 + 8 + 9	Des-(Arg^1)-Tyr(Me)^5-Tyr(Me)^8-(Arg-Gly)^9-bradykinin	H-□-Pro-Pro-Gly-*Tyr*-Ser-Pro-*Tyr*-Arg-*Gly*-OH
(6) *Bradykinin analogs obtained by N-terminal lengthening of the peptide chain* (kallidin and kallidin analogs)			
149		Kallidin	H-Lys-Arg-Pro-Pro-Gly-Phe-Ser-Pro-Phe-Arg-OH
			1 2 3 4 5 6 7 8 9 10
150	1	Arg^1-kallidin	H-*Arg*-Arg-Pro-Pro-Gly-Phe-Ser-Pro-Phe-Arg-OH
151	1	Glu^1-kallidin	H-*Glu*-Arg-Pro-Pro-Gly-Phe-Ser-Pro-Phe-Arg-OH
152	1	Gly^1-kallidin	H-*Gly*-Arg-Pro-Pro-Gly-Phe-Ser-Pro-Phe-Arg-OH
153	1	Orn^1-kallidin	H-*Orn*-Arg-Pro-Pro-Gly-Phe-Ser-Pro-Phe-Arg-OH
154	1	Phe^1-kallidin	H-*Phe*-Arg-Pro-Pro-Gly-Phe-Ser-Pro-Phe-Arg-OH
155	2	Lys^2-kallidin	H-Lys-*Lys*-Pro-Pro-Gly-Phe-Ser-Pro-Phe-Arg-OH
156	7	Gly^7-kallidin	H-Lys-Arg-Pro-Pro-Gly-Phe-*Gly*-Pro-Phe-Arg-OH
			F
157	9	Phe(F)^9-kallidin	H-Lys-Arg-Pro-Pro-Gly-Phe-Ser-Pro-*Phe*-Arg-OH
158	10	Lys^{10}-kallidin	H-Lys-Arg-Pro-Pro-Gly-Phe-Ser-Pro-Phe-*Lys*-OH
159	2 + 10	Lys^2-Lys^{10}-kallidin	H-Lys-*Lys*-Pro-Pro-Gly-Phe-Ser-Pro-Phe-*Lys*-OH
			Me
160	1 + 7 + 9	Gly^1-Gly^7-Tyr(Me)^9-Kallidin	H-*Gly*-Arg-Pro-Pro-Gly-Phe-*Gly*-Pro-*Tyr*-Arg-OH
161	2—4 + 6—10	(L-Lys)^1-all-D-kallidin	H-Lys-*arg-pro-pro*-Gly-*phe-ser-pro-phe-arg*-OH
162	1—10		H-Phe-Gly-Pro-Phe-Arg-Lys-Arg-Pro-Pro-Gly-OH
163	1—10	Gly^7-cyclo-kallidin	→Lys-Arg-Pro-Gly- Arg-Phe-Pro-Gly-Phe←
(7) *Bradykinin analogs obtained by N-terminal lengthening of the peptide chain with more than one amino acid* (methionyl-lysyl-bradykinin and methionyl-lysyl-bradykinin analogs)			
164		Met-Lys-bradykinin	H-Met-Lys-Arg-Pro-Pro-Gly-Phe-Ser-Pro-Phe-Arg-OH
			1 2 3 4 5 6 7 8 9 10 11

(continued)

Biological activities						
Rat uterus (isolated)	Guinea pig ileum (isolated)	Rabbit blood pressure	Guinea pig blood pressure	Guinea pig broncho-constriction	Antibradykinin activity	References
1/200	—	—	—	—	—	STEWART and WOOLLEY (1966)
1/10,000	—	—	—	—	—	STEWART and WOOLLEY (1966)
1/10,000	—	—	—	—	—	STEWART and WOOLLEY (1966)
1/100,000	—	—	—	—	—	STEWART and WOOLLEY (1966)
~1/2—2/3	1/3 ± 1/10	1.9 ± 0.4	1/2—2/3 (cat)	—	—	PLESS et al. (1962)
~1/2—2/3	1/3 ± 1/10	1.9 ± 0.4	3.3 ± 0.8 (rat)	—	—	STÜRMER and BERDE (1963)
—	—	—	2/3	1/3	—	NICOLAIDES et al. (1961)
1/10	1	2	—	—	—	SCHRÖDER and GIBIAN (1964)
1	1/10	1/3—1/4	—	—	—	SCHRÖDER and HEMPEL (1964)
—	1/3	—	1—1/2	—	—	YANAIHARA and SEKIYA (1967)
1—2	1	1/2—1/3	—	—	—	SCHRÖDER and HEMPEL (1964)
—	—	—	2—4	4	—	NICOLAIDES and LIPNIK (1966)
1/10	1/3	1/5—1/10	—	—	—	SCHRÖDER and GIBIAN (1964), SCHRÖDER (1965b)
1	1/2	1/5	—	—	—	SCHRÖDER (1965b)
—	—	—	1/20	1/500	—	NICOLAIDES et al. (1963a)
1.4—1	—	—	—	—	—	BODANSZKY et al. (1963b)
~1/10	~1/10	2—3	—	—	—	SCHRÖDER and HEMPEL (1964)
—	—	—	2/3	1/3	—	NICOLAIDES et al. (1963a)
1/500	1/100	1.5	2/3	—	—	SCHRÖDER (1965b), ERDÖS et al. (1967)
inactive	—	—	—	—	—	WÜNSCH et al. (1964)
1/5	—	—	—	—	—	STEWART and WOOLLEY (1966)
$1 \cdot 10^{-5}$	—	—	—	—	—	STEWART and WOOLLEY (1967)
inactive	—	—	—	—	—	SCHNABEL and MEIENHOFER (1964)
—	—	—	inactive	—	—	MEIENHOFER (1966)
1/4	1/4	—	—	1/4	—	ELLIOTT et al. (1963)
1/3	1/3	2—3	—	—	—	SCHRÖDER (1964d, 1965b)

Table 1

No.	Variation in position	Name	Amino acid sequences
165	1 + 2	[BOC-Met-Lys(BOC)-Arg]¹-bradykinin	BOC-Met-*Lys*(BOC)-Arg-Pro-Pro-Gly-Phe-Ser-Pro-Phe-Arg-OH
166	1	(Eti-Lys-Arg)¹-bradykinin	H-*Eti*-Lys-Arg-Pro-Pro-Gly-Phe-Ser-Pro-Phe-Arg-OH
167	1	(Lys-Lys-Arg)¹-bradykinin	H-*Lys*-Lys-Arg-Pro-Pro-Gly-Phe-Ser-Pro-Phe-Arg-OH
168	1	(met-Lys-Arg)¹-bradykinin	H-*met*-Lys-Arg-Pro-Pro-Gly-Phe-Ser-Pro-Phe-Arg-OH
169	1	(Phe-Lys-Arg)¹-bradykinin	H-*Phe*-Lys-Arg-Pro-Pro-Gly-Phe-Ser-Pro-Phe-Arg-OH
170	1	(Ser-Lys-Arg)¹-bradykinin	H-*Ser*-Lys-Arg-Pro-Pro-Gly-Phe-Ser-Pro-Phe-Arg-OH
171	1	(Lys-Lys-Lys-Arg)¹ bradykinin	H-*Lys*-*Lys*-Lys-Arg-Pro-Pro-Gly-Phe-Ser-Pro-Phe-Arg-OH
172	1	(Ser-Lys-Met-Lys-Arg)¹-bradykinin	H-*Ser*-*Lys*-Met-Lys-Arg-Pro-Pro-Gly-Phe-Ser-Pro-Phe-Arg-OH
173	8	(Met-Lys-Arg)¹-Gly⁸-bradykinin	H-Met-Lys-Arg-Pro-Pro-Gly-Phe-*Gly*-Pro-Phe-Arg-OH

tives with changes in position 1. Therefore the arginine residue in position 1 seems to be somewhat more important than that in position 9.

The simultaneous exchange of the arginine residue in positions 1 and 9 as in Cit^1-Cit^9-bradykinin (*105*), Dab^1-Dab^9-bradykinin (*106*), and Lys^1-Lys^9-bradykinin (*107*) leads to very low activity. Among these analogs, Lys^1-Lys^9-bradykinin shows the highest activity but less than the $Arg(NO_2)^1$-$Arg(NO_2)^9$ compound (*4*). Summarizing the data from all analogs modified in position 1 or 9 or 1 and 9, one can conclude that neither the basicity nor structural features alone are responsible for the full biological activity, but that both characteristics are necessary. The necessity of a basic residue seems to be more pronounced in position 1 than in position 9.

The amino acid in position 2, proline, was exchanged for alanine, D-proline, sarcosine or valine (compounds *11–14*). The proline residue in position 3 was exchanged for alanine, glycine, lysine, pipecolic acid, D-proline, sarcosine, or valine (compounds *16–22*). In case of D-Pro^2-, D-Pro^3-, and Lys^3-bradykinin, inactive products were found. Ala^2- and Val^2-bradykinin (*11, 14*) show medium activity ($^1/_{200}$ that of bradykinin) on rabbit blood pressure. The activity on smooth muscle organs is in the range $^1/_{100}$–$^1/_{500}$.

With Ala^3-bradykinin (*16*) on isolated rat uterus, guinea pig ileum, and rabbit blood pressure, a fully active analog was synthesized. Additional highly active compounds are Sar^2- and Sar^3-bradykinin (*13, 21*) which show on guinea pig ileum, guinea pig blood pressure, and the blood flow of the dog hind limb from $^1/_{10}$ up to full activity. Both analogs differ only slightly in the individual tests.

The replacement of the proline residues in positions 2 and 3 must be compared with the exchange of the proline residue in position 7. Of high activity is Sar^7-bradykinin (*70*) on guinea pig blood pressure ($^1/_3$), on guinea pig ileum ($^1/_8$) and on the blood flow of dog hind limb ($^1/_{10}$–$^1/_{15}$), though the values are somewhat lower than with the corresponding Sar^2 and Sar^3 derivatives (*13, 21*). Much lower

(continued)

Biological activities						
Rat uterus (isolated)	Guinea pig ileum (isolated)	Rabbit blood pressure	Guinea pig blood pressure	Guinea pig broncho-constriction	Antibradykinin activity	References
< 1/150	<1/150	1/300	—	—	—	SCHRÖDER (1964d, 1965b)
1/5	1/2	1.5—2	—	—	—	SCHRÖDER (1965a)
1/2	1/5	8—10	—	—	—	SCHRÖDER (1965a)
—	—	2—3	—	—	—	SCHRÖDER (1965a)
1	1/15	1.5—2	—	—	—	SCHRÖDER (1965a)
1	1/10	2—3	—	—	—	SCHRÖDER (1965a)
1/5	1/5	8—10	—	—	—	SCHRÖDER (1965a)
1/8	1/80	1	—	—	—	SCHRÖDER (1965a)
—	—	2.5	—	—	—	SCHRÖDER (1965a)

is the activity of Ala^7-bradykinin (*65*) compared with Ala^2- and Ala^3-bradykinin (*11*, *16*). Gly^3-bradykinin (*17*) shows an activity $^1/_7$ that of bradykinin on guinea pig ileum, Gly^7-bradykinin (*67*) a value of $^1/_{100}$ an isolated rat uterus. Gly^2-bradykinin has not been described in the literature. As a result of the specific exchange of the proline residue in positions 2, 3, and 7 by sarcosine, alanine, or glycine residues, one can deduce that the order of importance of the proline residues for biological activity is as follows: Pro^7 > Pro^2 > Pro^3. The activity of the analogs has the following order: Ala^3 > Sar^3 > Sar^2 > Gly^3 > Sar^7 > Gly^7 > Ala^2 > Ala^7, which demonstrates very clearly the different influence of individual amino acid residues in different positions. The somewhat higher activity exhibited by one or the other sarcosine-containing analogs would suggest that imide linkages between positions 1 and 2 and 6 and 7 contribute to the structural requirements which are necessary for the full bradykinin activity.

Other changes in position 7, i.e. Asn^7-bradykinin (*66*), His^7-bradykinin (*68*), and D-Pro^7-bradykinin (*69*), cause a decrease in activity to $<^1/_{1000}$ that of bradykinin. As is expected, the introduction of two and three D-proline residues leads to the inactive products (*72*, *73*, *74*).

Changes in position 4 result in a medium reduction of bradykinin activity on rabbit blood pressure to $^1/_{125}$ to $^1/_{300}$, as was demonstrated in the case of Ala^4- (*25*), Pro^4- (*29*), Sar^4- (*30*), and Ser^4-bradykinin (*31*). With these derivatives the decrease in activity is more pronounced in smooth muscle organs ($^1/_{500}$–$^1/_{1500}$). A contrast is β-Ala^4-bradykinin (*26*) with an activity $^1/_5$ that of bradykinin on isolated mouse ileum. The Sar^4 derivative (*30*) shows different effects on the blood pressure of rabbit and guinea pig.

The phenylalanine residue in position 5 seems to be essential for full bradykinin activity. The Ala^5-bradykinin (*33*) has very low values of $^1/_{1000}$ and less. The higher activity of Tyr^5-bradykinin (*35*) should be taken perhaps as an indication of the importance of the aromatic ring system in this position. Remarkable is the relatively high activity of D-Phe^{5}-bradykinin (*34*) on isolated guinea pig ileum ($>^{1}/_{16}$), guinea pig blood pressure ($^{1}/_{40}$), and guinea pig bronchoconstriction ($^{1}/_{30}$). By comparison the D-Phe^{8}-bradykinin (*77*) has an activity of $^{1}/_{1000}$ on guinea pig ileum.

An exchange of the residue in position 6 by several other amino acids results in highly active analogs. The most active compound is Gly^{6}-bradykinin (*40*) which possesses practically the full bradykinin activity on the isolated rat uterus and guinea pig ileum. Only slightly less active in these tests are Ala^{6}- (*37*), β-Ala^{6}- (*38*), Cys^{6}- (*39*), and Thr^{6}-bradykinin (*46*). Even an inversion of the configuration, as was carried out with the synthesis of D-Ser^{6}-bradykinin (*45*), has a potency of $^{1}/_{2.5}$ that of bradykinin on guinea pig blood pressure.

In position 8 primarily the influence of a substitution of the phenylalanine residue on biological activity was investigated. Substitution in the *p*-position by a fluorine atom, Phe(F)^{8}-bradykinin (*78*), increases the activity on guinea pig blood pressure and bronchoconstriction to 1.5 times the value that of bradykinin, as has been demonstrated by Nicolaides et al. (1963a, b). Change of configuration, D-Phe^{8}-bradykinin (*77*), the concurrent change of configuration and *p*-substitution, D-Phe(F)^{8}-bradykinin (*79*), and substitution in the *m*-position by the trifluoromethyl group, Phe(m-CF_3)^{8}-bradykinin (*80*), cause only a very small decrease ($^{1}/_{4}$ to $^{2}/_{3}$ of the original value) in the activity on guinea pig blood pressure or bronchoconstriction (*78, 80*). Tyr^{8}-bradykinin (*81*) was tested only on isolated guinea pig ileum, where it possesses $^{1}/_{5}$ of the bradykinin activity. Exchange of the Phe^{8} residue by a nonaromatic amino acid produces a very considerable decrease in activity (Ala^{8}-bradykinin, *76*). The replacement of the amide bond by an ester bond as it was carried out with the synthesis of Gly^{6}-PheLac^{8}-bradykinin (*87*) leads to an effect three times longer and two to four times greater on blood pressure than bradykinin has.

Modification of the bradykinin molecule by exchange of two amino acids leads, in the case of the following compounds, to active derivatives: Sar^{2}-Sar^{3}-bradykinin (*23*), Ala^{3}-Gly^{6}-bradykinin (*47*), Sar^{3}-Gly^{6}-bradykinin (*51*), Gly^{6}-Tyr(Me)^{8}-bradykinin (*88*), and Tyr(Me)^{5}-Tyr(Me)^{8}-bradykinin (*85*), which have $^{1}/_{3}$ to $^{1}/_{20}$ the activity of bradykinin in different tests. In all these cases single exchanges in position 3 or 6 had already led to compounds with full or nearly full potency. A second group of analogs, Ser^{4}-Gly^{6}-bradykinin (*59*), Gly^{3}-Gly^{6}-bradykinin (*48*), and β-Ala^{4}-Ser(Ac)^{6}-bradykinin (*53*), has activities about $^{1}/_{100}$ that of bradykinin. Other compounds with concurrent exchange of two amino acids, e.g. the derivatives (*24, 50, 52, 63, 64, 71, 72, 83, 106, 109, 110*), are practically inactive (values of $^{1}/_{1000}$ or less).

Among analogs with concurrent exchange of three amino acids or two amino acids and a simultaneous acetylation of the N-terminal amino group, Tyr(Me)^{5}-Gly^{6}-Tyr(Me)^{8}-bradykinin (*94*), (Ac-Arg)^{1}-Tyr(Me)^{5}-Tyr(Me)^{8}-bradykinin (*86*), and (Ac-Arg)^{1}-Gly^{6}-Tyr(Me)^{8}-bradykinin (*90*) still exhibit activities of $^{1}/_{4}$ to $^{1}/_{15}$ of the parent compound on isolated rat uterus.

Changing bradykinin in more than three positions leads to the formation of virtually inactive products (*95, 113*).

C. Shortening of the Peptide Chain

The shortening of the peptide chain or shortening of the peptide chain with simultaneous exchange of amino acids resulted in slightly active (*177*) or inactive products (compounds *115–136*).

D. C-Terminal Lengthening of the Peptide Chain or Inserting Amino Acids

In this group of bradykinin analogs (Arg-Arg)^9-bradykinin (*138*) has an activity of $^1/_{25}$ on isolated rat uterus. With (Gly-Gly)^4-bradykinin (*137*) a compound with $^1/_{10}$ bradykinin activity on guinea pig blood pressure and bronchoconstriction was obtained. Of moderate potency is (Arg-Gly)^9-bradykinin (*139*). As a naturally occurring bradykinin analog, the undecapeptide phyllokinin (*144*), H-Arg-Pro-Pro-Gly-Phe-Ser-Pro-Phe-Arg-Ile-Tyr(SO_3H)-OH, isolated from the skin of *Phyllomedusa rohdei*, has the same effect as bradykinin on rabbit blood pressure.

E. N-Terminal Shortening and C-Terminal Lengthening of the Peptide Chain

Very few analogs of this type were synthesized; among these Des-(Arg^1)-(Arg-Arg)^9-bradykinin (*145*) demonstrates some activity on the isolated rat uterus.

F. N-Terminal Lengthening of the Peptide Chain (Kallidin Analogs)

Elongation of the bradykinin molecule at the N-terminal residue by a lysine leads to the formation of kallidin (*149*). Compared with bradykinin, the activity on smooth muscle organs is reduced, while the action on blood pressure, varying with the species, is potentiated. Only a few analogs of kallidin have been synthesized so far.

Replacement of the N-terminal lysine residue of kallidin by various other amino acids results only in a small decrease of activity—1 to $^1/_{10}$ of the original values, depending on the tests used—(compounds *150–154*). Modification in those positions which were known to cause only minor alterations in potency in the case of bradykinin have practically the same effect on kallidin (*149*)—e.g. Gly^7-kallidin (*156*) and Phe(F)^9-kallidin (*157*). The exchange of the Arg^2 residue with lysine, Lys^2-kallidin (*155*), decreases the activity on guinea pig blood pressure to $^1/_{20}$. This is reminiscent of Lys^1-bradykinin (*9*), where the same activity is reduced to $^1/_{10}$. The bronchoconstrictor activity, however, is affected more severely. Lys^{10}-kallidin (*158*) is somewhat more active on rabbit blood pressure than is bradykinin. A decrease in activity, however, was observed for smooth muscle organs. This behavior corresponds roughly to Lys^9-bradykinin (*103*).

G. N-Terminal Lengthening of the Peptide Chain with More than One Amino Acid

After incubation at pH 7.5 of the acid-treated pseudoglobulin fraction of bovine plasma, Elliott et al. (1963) were able to isolate a kinin which was different from bradykinin and kallidin. The structure of this new kinin which does not naturally occur was postulated as methionyl-lysyl-bradykinin (*164*) and soon thereafter confirmed by synthesis (Schröder, 1964d). The activity of this undecapeptide is about $^1/_3$ on isolated smooth muscle organs and 2- to 3-fold on rabbit blood pressure in comparison with bradykinin. Other not naturally occurring kinins were isolated by Habermann (1965) during his study of kinin release from a precursor kininogen. By incubation of a highly purified kininogen with pepsin and successive chromatography it was possible to isolate a tetradecapeptide and a pentadecapeptide of the following structures:

H-Met-Lys-Arg-Pro-Pro-Gly-Phe-Ser-Pro-Phe-Arg-Ser-Val-Gln-OH

H-Met-Lys-Arg-Pro-Pro-Gly-Phe-Ser-Pro-Phe-Arg-Ser-Val-Gln-Val-OH

Both peptides were synthesized (Schröder cited by Habermann, 1966); the natural and synthetic compounds are substrates for all kinin-forming enzymes (trypsin, snake venom, and kallikrein).

Two other low molecular-weight peptides were isolated by Hochstrasser and Werle (1967) after the digestion of bovine plasma proteins with pepsin. Their sequences are:

H-Ser-Arg-Met-Lys-Arg-Pro-Pro-Gly-Phe-Ser-Pro-Phe-Arg-OH

H-Gly-Arg-Met-Lys-Arg-Pro-Pro-Gly-Phe-Ser-Pro-Phe-Arg-OH

Some analogs of Met-Lys-bradykinin were prepared by exchange of the N-terminal Met residue, e.g. for ethionine (*166*), D-methionine (*168*), phenylalanine (*169*), and serine (*170*). These compounds, compared with bradykinin, show a 2- to 3-fold increase in activity on rabbit blood pressure. The activity on smooth muscle organs is slightly decreased. Compared with Met-Lys-bradykinin (*164*) itself these analogs are equipotent. Very potent analogs could be found with $(\text{Lys-Lys-Arg})^1$-bradykinin (*167*) and $(\text{Lys-Lys-Lys-Arg})^1$-bradykinin (*171*), where an 8- to 10-fold increase in the potency on rabbit blood pressure was observed. As in the case of bradykinin and kallidin, the exchange of the serine residue in position 8 by glycine has no influence on the blood pressure activity.

To summarize the structure–activity data, the following general statements can be made:

(1) The terminal arginine residues may be exchanged with other basic amino acids or amino acids closely resembling the structural features of arginine. Only limited decrease in activity will result. The Arg^1 residue seems to be more important than the Arg^9 residue. A simultaneous replacement of both arginine residues considerably reduces the activity. An exchange of the arginine residues by neutral amino acids leads to inactive products.

(2) The proline residues in positions 2, 3, and 7 can be replaced by sarcosine, alanine, or glycine, retaining the complete or nearly complete activity. Other amino acids cause a greater decrease in activity. The most potent derivatives are those that are modified in position 3. The importance of the proline residues may be arranged in the order $\text{Pro}^7 > \text{Pro}^2 > \text{Pro}^3$.

(3) In position 4 only the introduction of β-alanine or sarcosine results in active compounds.

(4) Alteration in position 5 brings about a strong reduction of the biological potency.

(5) A replacement of the Ser^6 residue by glycine retains the biological activity; only a slight reduction was observed with threonine, alanine, β-alanine, and cysteine in this position.

(6) The *p*-substitution of the Phe^8 residue by fluorine, or the *p*-substitution by an OH-group (tyrosine residue), or the *m*-substitution by a trifluoromethyl group has very little effect on the activity. Nonaromatic residues in this position gave inactive products.

(7) A replacement of the natural L-amino acids by the corresponding D forms leads to inactive products, with the exception of D-Ser^6 and D-Phe^8 analogs.

(8) An exchange of two amino acids in the bradykinin molecule can be made in positions 2 and 3 or 3 and 6 with almost no loss in activity. A somewhat greater reduction in potency can be observed by simultaneous exchange in positions 4 and 6.

(9) N-Terminal shortening of the bradykinin peptide chain, omission of amino acids, and N-terminal shortening together with C-terminal elongation lead to inactive products.

(10) Among several C-terminal elongated bradykinin molecules only the $(Arg\text{-}Arg)^9$ analog possesses a rather high activity. The naturally occurring phyllokinin is a derivative with full bradykinin activity.

(11) Kallidin can be modified in position 1 without considerable loss of activity. Replacement of the Ser^7 position by glycine and the Phe^9 residue by *p*-fluorophenylalanine causes practically no change in activity by analogy with the same modifications with the bradykinin molecule.

(12) Met-Lys-bradykinin can be modified in position 1 or 8 without a loss of activity. $(Lys\text{-}Lys\text{-}Arg)^1$- and $(Lys\text{-}Lys\text{-}Lys\text{-}Arg)^1$-bradykinin are the most potent analogs as far as is known.

(13) As an attempt to classify the effect of the individual residues of the bradykinin molecule in terms of influence on biological activity, the following series can be postulated:

$$7,8>1>9>5>4>2>3>6$$

Although there exists as yet no conception of the secondary structure of the bradykinin molecule, one can assume that a randomly coiled structure is most probable. From the available biological data of the analogs, it can be concluded that basic N-terminal residues are responsible for the attachment to a hypothetic receptor but that the basicity is not the only prerequisite. In this connection, homoarginine analogs would be of interest. Moreover, the aromatic residues in positions 5 and 8 are of additional importance, the Pro^7 residue perhaps contributing to a special folding of the molecule. Among a number of analogs, alteration of the bradykinin molecule by residues which had an obligatory effect on conformation, such as changes in glycine or proline, also exhibited for instance a very pronounced effect in the binding of these analogs to antibodies of a branch-chain copolymer of bradykinin and poly-L-lysine (evaluated by a radioimmuno assay technique (SPRAGG et al., 1967).

H. Bradykinin Analogs with Prolonged and Differentiated Activities

Among the various activities of the kinins, the action on blood presssure is the most interesting. Some workers have investigated the possibility of a clinical application (GERSMEYER and SPITZBARTH, 1961; KONTOS et al., 1964). A disadvantage is the very short duration of action as well as side reactions (e.g. action on smooth muscle organs or pain sensation). The chemists engaged in the synthesis of kinin analogs sought to modify the naturally occurring molecule in such a way that the very rapid enzymatic degradation *in vivo* could be prevented. An intensive degradation occurs physiologically through the action of a blood plasma kininase (carboxypeptidase N) at the C-terminal end, by splitting the Phe^8-Arg^9 bond (ERDÖS, 1966). Investigations by SHCHUKINA et al. (1965) had shown that, for example, glycolic $acid^6$-bradykinin (*41*) as well as glycolic $acid^4$-bradykinin (*27*) has an activity of $^1/_{100}$–$^1/_{200}$ that of bradykinin. That means that the replacement of an amide bond by the spatially and electronically similar ester group does not completely abolish biological activity. As a consequence of this observation, Ravdel et al. (1967) synthesized Gly^6-PheLac^8-bradykinin (*87*) and found that the vasodepressor effect of this compound in rats and rabbits lasts two to three times longer and is four and two times greater, respectively, than that of bradykinin. Degradation studies with kininases prepared from human and rabbit serums demonstrated that the rate of hydrolysis by this enzyme preparation is about 20 to 35% lower than that of bradykinin. These experiments show that it is possible, in principle, to retain and prolong the biological activity of the bradykinin molecule, although unfortunately not sufficiently up to the present time, to be of clinical interest.

In some analogs a differentiation of activity on smooth muscles and blood pressure activity was attained (e.g. compounds *103, 158*), i.e. primarily derivatives modified at the C-terminal, as far as can be seen from the limited number of analogs that were checked in several tests.

None of the efforts to synthesize analogs yielded an orally active kinin — a desirable feature that is expected from most modern drugs.

I. Bradykinin Analogs with Inhibitory Activity

One of the main efforts in the present research is to elucidate the role of kinins in inflammatory processes—rheumatic diseases, allergic reactions, asthma, etc. This might be accomplished if a specific inhibitor of bradykinin could be found. Among a great number of compounds of different structures, bradykinin analogs were also tested for their inhibitory potency. The most promising inhibitory effects are expected from analogs containing D-amino acid residues, especially compounds such as all-D-bradykinin (*114*), retrobradykinin (*95*), and all-D-retrobradykinin (*96*); but no indication of bradykinin antagonism could be observed. With a number of other analogs such as *38, 74, 85, 86, 90, 92, 93, 94, 124, 129*, and *136* in relatively high doses, inhibitory effects on the bradykinin action on smooth muscle could be detected; none of these compounds is of really practical interest, however.

K. Summary

After surveying some 170 synthetic analogs of bradykinin and kallidin, ideas about the parts of the structure that may be responsible for biological activity have been formulated, but so far it has not been possible to prepare analogs of unequivocal practical interest, i.e. analogs with prolonged activity on blood pressure or specific bradykinin inhibitors. Only a few of the experiments point toward this development.

References

Bodanszky, M., Ondetti, M. A., Rubin, B., Piala, J. J., Fried, J., Sheehan, J. T., Birkhimer, C. A.: Biologically active citrulline peptides. Nature (Lond.) **194**, 485 (1962).

— — Sheehan, J. T., Lande, S.: Synthetic peptides related to bradykinin. Ann. N.Y. Acad. Sci. **104**, 24 (1963a).

— Sheehan, J. T., Ondetti, M. A., Lande, S.: Glycine analogs of bradykinin. J. Amer. chem. Soc. **85**, 991 (1963b).

Boissonnas, R. A., Guttmann, S., Jaquenoud, P. A.: Synthèse de la L-arginyl-L-prolyl-L-prolyl-glycyl-L-phénylalanyl-L-séryl-L-prolyl-L-phénylalanyl-L-arginine, un nonapeptide présentant les propriétés de la bradykinine. Helv. chim. Acta **43**, 1349 (1960).

Cerletti, A., Stürmer, E., Konzett, H.: Bradykinin; Strukturaufklärung, Synthese, physiologisch-pharmakologische Grundlagen. Dtsch. med. Wschr. **86**, 678 (1961).

DeWald, H. A., Craft, M. K., Nicolaides, E. D.: The synthesis of 6-O-carbamyl-L-serine, 6-D-serine and 6-L-threonine bradykinin. J. med. Chem. **6**, 741 (1963).
— Nicolaides, E. D.: The synthesis of 9-citrulline, 9-histidine, and 9-desarginine bradykinin. J. med. Chem. **7**, 50 (1964).
Elliott, D. F., Lewis, G. P., Horton, E. W.: The structure of bradykinin—a plasma kinin from ox blood. Biochem. biophys. Res. Commun. **3**, 87 (1960).
— — Smyth, D. G.: A new kinin from ox blood. Biochem. J. **87**, 21 p (1963).
Erdös, E. G.: Hypotensive peptides: bradykinin, kallidin, and eledoisin. Advan. Pharmacol. **4**, 1 (1966).
— Cano, G., Yang, H. Y. T.: Hypotensive effect of Lys[9]-bradykinin in the guinea pig. Biochem. Pharmacol. **16**, 1035 (1967).
Gersmeyer, E. F., Spitzbarth, H.: Über Kreislaufwirkungen von synthetischem Bradykinin beim Menschen und beim wachen Hund. Klin. Wschr. **39**, 1227 (1961).
Guttmann, S., Boissonnas, R. A.: Synthèse d'analogues structuraux de la bradykinine. Helv. chim. Acta **44**, 1713 (1961).
— Pless, J., Boissonnas, R. A.: Nouvelle synthèse de la bradykinine. Helv. chim. Acta **45**, 170 (1962).
Habermann, E.: Isolierung, pharmakologische Eigenschaften, Strukturaufklärung und Spaltung peptischer kininliefernder Fragmente (PKF) aus Rinderserum-Kininogen. Naunyn-Schmiedebergs Arch. exp. Path. Pharmak. **251**, 187 (1965).
— Enzymatic kinin release from kininogen and from low-molecular compounds. In: Hypotensive peptides, p. 116, ed. by E. G. Erdös, N. Back, and F. Sicuteri. Berlin-Heidelberg-New York: Springer 1966.
— Zur Frage der Beziehungen zwischen Kininsystemen und allergischen Prozessen. Dtsch. med. Wschr. **93**, 40 (1968).
Hochstrasser, K., Werle, E.: Über kininliefernde Peptide aus pepsinverdauten Rinderplasmaproteinen. Hoppe-Seylers Z. physiol. Chem. **348**, 177 (1967).
Kontos, H. A., Magee, J. H., Shapiro, W., Patterson, J. L., Jr.: General and regional circulatory effects of synthetic bradykinin in man. Circulat. Res. **14**, 351 (1964).
Lande, S.: Retrobradykinin: A peptide with the reverse sequence of bradykinin. J. org. Chem. **27**, 4558 (1962).
Meienhofer, J.: Synthese von Gly[7]-cyclo-kallidin. Justus Liebigs Ann. Chem. **691**, 218 (1966).
Nicolaides, E. D., Craft, M. K., DeWald, H. A.: The synthesis of 8-D-phenylalanine-, 8-*p*-fluoro-L-phenylalanine, and 8-*p*-fluoro-D-phenylalanine-bradykinin. J. med. Chem. **6**, 524 (1963b).
— DeWald, H. A.: Synthesis and biological properties of L-arginyl-L-prolyl-L-prolyl-glycyl-L-phenylalanyl-L-seryl-L-phenylalanyl-L-arginine, an octapeptide related to bradykinin. Nature (Lond.) **187**, 773 (1960).
— — Studies on the synthesis of polypeptides: Bradykinin. J. org. Chem. **26**, 3872 (1961).
— — Craft, M. K.: The synthesis of kinin analogues. Ann. N.Y. Acad. Sci. **104**, 15 (1963a).
— — — The synthesis of 1-lysine, 1-ornithine, 1-citrulline, 1-glutamic acid, and 1-desarginine bradykinin. J. med. Chem. **6**, 739 (1963c).
— — McCarthy, D. A.: The synthesis of a biologically active decapeptide having the structure proposed for kallidin. II. Biochem. biophys. Res. Commun. **6**, 210 (1961).
— Lipnik, M.: Synthetic bradykinin analogs. J. med. Chem. **9**, 958 (1966).
Nowak, K.: Synteza tyrozynowego analogu bradykininy (tyrozylo[5]–bradykininy) [Synthesis of the tyrosine analog of bradykinin (Tyr[5]-bradykinin)]. Roczn. Chem. **40**, 1051 (1966).
Ondetti, M. A.: Citrulline-containing analogs of bradykinin. J. med. Chem. **6**, 10 (1963).
Pierce, J. V., Webster, M. E.: Human plasma kallidins: Isolation and chemical studies. Biochem. biophys. Res. Commun. **5**, 353 (1961).
Pless, J., Stürmer, E., Guttmann, S., Boissonnas, R. A.: Kallidin, Synthese und Eigenschaften. Helv. chim. Acta **45**, 394 (1962).
Ravdel, G. A., Filatova, M. P., Shchukina, L. A., Paskhina, T. S., Surovikina, M. S., Trapeznikova, S. S., Egorova, T. P.: 6-Glycine–8-phenyllactic acid bradykinin. Its synthesis, biological activity, and splitting by kininase (carboxypeptidase N). J. med. Chem. **10**, 242 (1967).
Schnabel, E., Meienhofer, J.: Discussion. In: Proceedings, 7th European Symposium on Peptides, Budapest, 1964.
Schröder, E.: Über Peptidsynthesen. XVII. Synthese von Gly[6]-Bradykinin und Ala[5]-Bradykinin. Justus Liebigs Ann. Chem. **673**, 186 (1964a).
— Über Peptidsynthesen. XX. Synthese weiterer Bradykinin-Analoga. Justus Liebigs Ann. Chem. **673**, 220 (1964b).
— Über Peptidsynthesen. XXIV. Alanyl-Analoga des Bradykinins. Justus Liebigs Ann. Chem. **679**, 207 (1964c).

Schröder, E.: Über Peptidsynthesen. Synthese von Methionyl–Lysyl–Bradykinin, einem Kinin aus Rinderblut. Experientia (Basel) **20**, 39 (1964d).
— Synthese und biologische Aktivität bradykininwirksamer Undeca-, Dodeca- und Trideca-peptide. Experientia (Basel) **21**, 271 (1965a).
— Struktur-Aktivitäts-Beziehungen bei bradykinin-analogen Polypeptiden. In: Peptides. Proceedings of the 6th European Symposium, p. 253, ed. by L. Zervas. London: Pergamon Press 1965b).
— Gibian, H.: Über Peptidsynthesen. XVI. Synthese von Orn^1–Kallidin und Kallidin. Justus Liebigs Ann. Chem. **673**, 176 (1964).
— Hempel, R.: Bradykinin, kallidin, and their synthetic analogues. Experientia (Basel) 20, 529 (1964).
— Petras, H.-S., Klieger, E.: Über Peptidsynthesen. XXV. Synthese von Pro^1-Arg^2–, Ala^4-, Ser^4-Gly^6-, Tyr^5- und Orn^9-Bradykinin. Justus Liebigs Ann. Chem. **679**, 221 (1964).
Schwyzer, R., Rittel, W., Sieber, P., Kappeler, H., Zuber, H.: Synthese von L-arginyl-L-prolyl-L-prolyl-glycyl-L-phenylalanyl-L-seryl-L-phenylalanyl-L-arginin (Bradykinin?). Helv. chim. Acta **43**, 1130 (1960).
Shchukina, L. A., Ravdel, G. A., Filatova, M. P., Zhuze, A. L.: Depsipeptide analogues of biologically active peptides. II. Acta chim. Acad. Sci. hung. **44**, 205 (1965).
Spragg, J., Schröder, E., Stewart, J. M., Austen, K. F., Haber, E.: Structural requirements for binding to antibody of sequence variants of bradykinin. Biochemistry **6**, 3933 (1967).
Stewart, J. M.: Structural analogs of bradykinin. Biochem. Pharmacol. **12**, 180 (1963).
— Woolley, D. W.: Threonine analogs of bradykinin designed as antimetabolites. Biochemistry **3**, 700 (1964).
— — The search for peptides with specific antibradykinin activity. In: Hypotensive peptides, p. 23, ed. by E. G. Erdös, N. Back, and F. Sicuteri. Berlin-Heidelberg-New York: Springer 1966.
— — Bradykinin analogs. In: Internat. Symposium on Vasoactive Polypeptides: Bradykinin and Related Kinins, p. 7, ed. by M. Rocha e Silva and H. A. Rothschild. São Paulo 1967.
Stürmer, E.: Plasmakinine. Schweiz. med. Wschr. **96**, 1667 (1966).
— Berde, B.: A pharmacological comparison between synthetic bradykinin and synthetic kallidin. J. Pharmacol. exp. Ther. **139**, 38 (1963).
Suzuki, K.: Synthesis of peptides related to the C-terminus of B-peptide of ox co-fibrin (positions 16–21, 15–21, and 13–21). Chem. Pharm. Bull. **14**, 909 (1966).
— Abiko, T.: Synthesis of β-alanine-containing analogs of bradykinin. Chem. Pharm. Bull. **14**, 1017 (1966).
— — Synthesis of 3-L-lysine-bradykinin and its O-acetyl compound. Chem. Pharm. Bull. **15**, 536 (1967a).
— — Synthesis of 3-sarcosine-, 3-glycine-, and 3-L-alanine-6-glycine-bradykinin and 3-glycine-bradykinin. Chem.. Pharm. Bull. **15**, 1212 (1967b).
— — Synthesis of 4-L-valine-6-L-threonine-, 4-L-isoleucine-6-L-threonine-, 4-L-leucin-6-L-threonine-, 4-L-valine-, and 4-L-isoleucine-bradykinin and their O-acetyl compounds. Chem. Pharm. Bull. **15**, 1508 (1967c).
Vogler, K., Lanz, P.: Synthesis of all-D-isomers in the bradykinin series. In: Hypotensive peptides, p. 14, ed. by E. G. Erdös, N. Back, and F. Sicuteri. Berlin-Heidelberg-New York: Springer 1966.
— — Lergier, W.: Synthese des Bradykininanalogen mit umgekehrter Aminosäuresequenz. Helv. chim. Acta **45**, 561 (1962).
Werle, E.: Plasmakinine. Dtsch. med. Wschr. **92**, 1573 (1967).
— Trautschold, I., Leysath, G.: Isolierung und Struktur des Kallidins. Hoppe-Seylers Z. physiol. Chem. **326**, 174 (1961).
Wiegershausen, B., Paegelow, I.: Die Rolle der Kinine im pathologischen Geschehen. Dtsch. Gesundh.-Wes. **21**, 2092 (1966).
Wünsch, E., Heidrich, H.-G., Grassmann, W.: Synthese von $Lys^{1,9}$-Bradykinin und $Lys^{2,10}$-Kallidin. Chem. Ber. **97**, 1818 (1964).
Yanaihara, N., Sekiya, M.: Synthesis of l-glutamic acid kallidin. Chem. Pharm. Bull. **15**, 82 (1967).
— — Takagi, K., Kato, H., Ishimura, M., Nagao, T.: Syntheses of bradykinin analogs containing sarcosine residues and their biological activities. Chem. Pharm. Bull. **15**, 110 (1967).

Effect of Kallikrein on the Cardiovascular System*

GERHARD A. BRECHER and GÜNTHER F. BROBMANN

With 4 Figures

In principle there are no fundamental differences between the effects of kallikrein and of the kinins on the cardiovascular system. Kallikrein does not act directly on the responsive tissues which initiate changes in the circulation but affects them through the liberation of kinins. The release of kinins from kallikrein is brought about by enzymatic processes which take varying periods of time, lasting but a few seconds. For this reason the onset of all reactions to kallikrein is somewhat delayed in comparison to that elicited by kinins. In addition, the reactions to kallikrein fade away more slowly than those resulting from kinins, because the latter are rapidly inactivated by enzymes.

Contrary to the kinins, which are demonstrated with difficulty in their active form in blood, it has been shown conclusively that kallikrein is present in its active form in variuos tissues. The human pancreas contains 10% of active kallikrein and the salivary glands even 100% of the active form (WERLE and VON RODEN, 1936). In blood, however, kallikrein is present only as an inactive precursor which is activated by trypsin and other proteinases (see p. 82). The chemical interrelations between kallikrein and the liberated kinins in blood may help to explain the essential similarity of the cardiovascular reactions, which differ mainly in their time course and quantity. Since the definition of the kallikrein unit is based on neither the quantity nor the origin of the substance but on a functional test, the different action of various types of kallikrein on the circulation cannot be distinguished. This is due to the pecularity of the definition, i.e. one kallikrein unit (KU) is that amount which lowers carotid blood pressure to the same extent as 5 ml of pooled human urine (FREY et al., 1950).

It is also important to realize that there are different types of kallikreins in various species and that the reactions of one species depend upon the source of the substance from other species. This area has not been explored extensively as yet. Although the primary interest lies in the study of the kallikrein–kinin mechanism in man, it is nevertheless of theoretical interest to understand the mechanisms in animals. Mammals appear to have the largest number of organs containing kallikrein. Some of these are enumerated in Table 1.

A kallikrein–kinin system has been described in birds as well as in mammals. However, bird kallikrein is inactive in mammals, as was established in 1936 by WERLE and HÜRTER. Furthermore, it has been found that the avian kinin system is not affected by mammalian kallikrein (WERLE et al., 1966). Even in the venom glands of snakes a kininogenase has been described which may be identical with kallikrein. Parenthetically, it should be mentioned that the venom glands of the snakes correspond to salivary glands in other vertebrae (WERLE et al., 1950; see p. 193). In the subsequent discourse attention will be focused on the action

* This work was supported in part by USPHS Research Grant HE 03796 from the National Heart Institute.

Table 1. *Content of kallikrein in glands and blood in adult organisms.* (Modified from WERLE et al., 1960)

Organ	Species	Content
Submandibular gland	man	1—2
(KU/g fresh material)	cat	15—100
	pig	25—60
	dog	6—40
	rat	3,000
	mouse	200
Pancreas	man	25
(KU/g fresh material)	cat	20
	pig	20—40
	dog	20—100
	rat	70
	mouse	4
Blood	cat	0.6
(KU/ml serum)	pig	2—10
	dog	1.2

of kallikrein, although in many instances reference to kinin activity cannot be avoided. Hence, for details of cardiovascular reactions to kinins the chapter of HADDY et al. should be consulted (p. 362). The action of kallikrein will be presented according to regions of the circulatory system.

A. In vitro Responses of Isolated Vasculature

Because of the unavoidable artificiality of the conditions, it is in general difficult to arrive at meaningful conclusions from experiments on isolated vessels or strips of vasculature (FREY et al., 1950). Discrepancies of findings of various investigators may very well be the result of differences in techniques, kallikrein concentration, depth of preceding anesthesia, or other factors. The majority of authors (WERLE and STUECKER, 1956; KOVALCIK, 1962; KONZETT and BAUER, 1966; KEATINGE, 1966) report a dilatation of capillaries and the smaller arterioles ranging from 0.04 to 0.1 mm in diameter, but a contraction of all larger arteries, e.g. aorta and pulmonary and coronary arteries. On the other hand, FELIX (1939) observed a relaxation of strips from the subclavian artery, pulmonary vein, and coronary sinus.

B. Vascular Reactions in the Skin

Whereas in isolated vessel preparations the results were somewhat nonuniform despite simple methodology, the findings in skin reactions all point, remarkably, in the same direction, independent of various investigative techniques. All observers agree that skin blood flow increases upon administration of kallikrein and kinins. The findings follow: (1) Through direct observation of the rabbit ear it was demonstrated that upon intravenous injection of kallikrein the skin became first somewhat pale and thereafter flushed (FREY et al., 1935; SACKERS, 1936). Microscopic examination of the vessels in the rabbit ear revelaed dilatation of arterioles and capillaries. When epinephrine was injected prior to kallikrein administration the stasis of blood in the contracted vessels initiated by epinephrine was overcome by kallikrein (FREY et al., 1935; SACKERS, 1936). In order to exclude any effects of radiant energy on the blood flow, suitable filters were used (Leitz skin microscope; FRIEDLÄNDER, 1931; FREY, 1931).

(2) Blood flow to the skin was determined in a skin vein of a dog with Rein's thermostromuhr and found to increase from 8 to 17 ml per minute after an injection of 16 KU (SCHNEIDER and SPRINGORUM, 1939). The quantitative values may not be accurate because it has now been recognized that the thermostromuhr indicates directional rather than quantitative changes (GREGG, 1948; ASCHOFF, 1955). (3) The skin temperature was used to estimate blood flow changes. The earliest experiments were performed with mercury thermometers, the sensitivity of which was enhanced by a spiral winding of the column touching the skin (WERLE and MULTHAUPT, 1937; MULTHAUPT, 1937). An increase of human skin temperature after intravenous and intramuscular administration of kallikrein

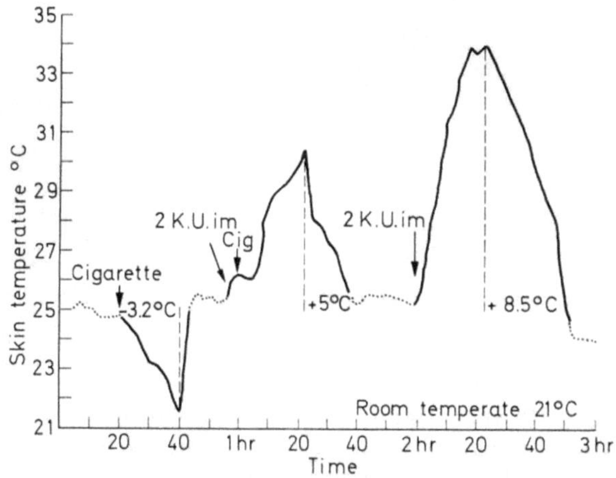

Fig. 1. Changes in skin temperature after use of nicotine and after injections of kallikrein

was found by these workers. The results were particularly striking after administration of nicotine, which led to a lowering of the temperature (WRIGHT and MOFFAT, 1934) (Fig. 1). (4) Changes in skin blood flow were also estimated with the aid of photo cells. For this purpose filters were inserted which permitted only the passage of infrared light so as to eliminate differences in the spectral absorption bands of arterial and venous blood. Intravenous and intramuscular injection of kallikrein consistently reduced the photo current, which was interpreted as an increase in blood flow.

All more recent experiments on skin blood flow were undertaken with kinins. The results are qualitatively identical with those with kallikrein (FOX et al., 1960, 1961; EHRINGER et al., 1961; BERGAMASCHI and GLÄSSER, 1964; TAKACS and ALBERT, 1965). In this connection it is also of interest to note that skin transplants, which were poorly supplied with blood and appeared cyanotic, definitely became redder after injection of kallikrein into the basal area of the transplant (LORENZ, 1946; LINDEMANN, 1947).

C. Vascular Reactions in Skeletal Muscle

Some testing for changes in skeletal muscle blood supply was undertaken with methods involving both the skin and the underlying tissues, e.g. plethysmographic methods. The extremity of a pig was enclosed in a suitable pletysmograph. The pressure in the plethysmograph rose when kallikrein was injected

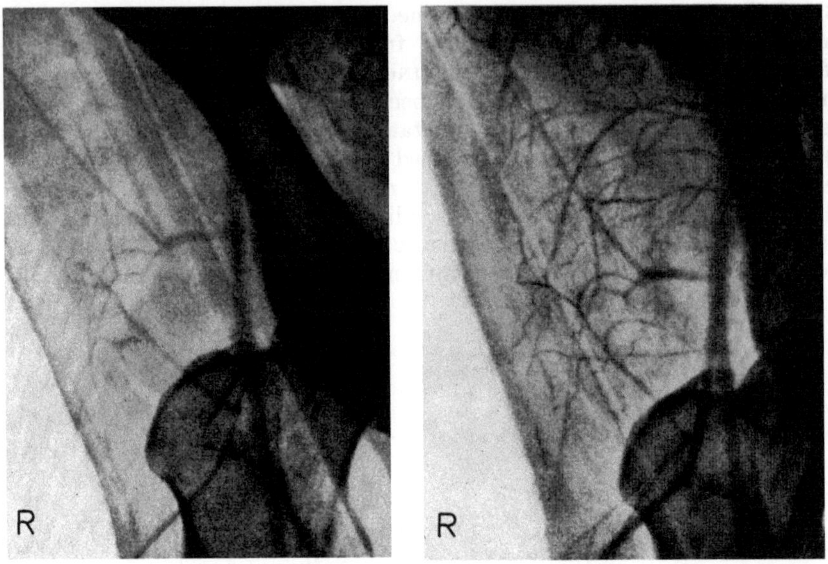

Fig. 2. Angiography of vessels in the leg of a dog before (left) and after (right) i.m. injection of kallikrein

into the limb, indicating a volume increase probably resulting from vasodilatation (Frey and Kraut, 1928). Striking vasodilatation in extremities could also be demonstrated with arteriography subsequent to intra-arterial kallikrein injection (see Fig. 2). It appeared from an increase of tissue temperature that kallikrein can double the blood supply to muscle in man (Golenhofen et al., 1958). From the evidence presented in the above experiments it is, however, not possible to decide whether the changes were caused by local increases in blood *volume* or by greater blood *flow*.

D. Behavior of Coronary Vessels

Kallikrein as well as kinins appear to dilate the coronary vessels. Kallikrein action was studied in a Starling heart–lung preparation to eliminate potential central autonomic effects. Upon injection of 3 to 5 units the coronary sinus outflow increased by 80% over the control value (Fig. 3). Repetition resulted in similar effects which diminished gradually until tachyphylaxis intervened (Krayer and Rühl, 1931). These results were confirmed by others who also compared the reactions to kallikrein with those to histamine. Although the arterial blood pressure declined in both cases, the coronary sinus flow became enhanced only after kallikrein injection, whereas it remained unchanged after histamine was given. The heart rate stayed constant in both the heart–lung preparation and damaged hearts. This may indicate the absence of an inotropic effect by kallikrein (Frey and Kraut, 1928; Hochrein and Keller, 1931; Schneider and Springorum, 1939). Similar conclusions were reached from the injection of 0.05 to 0.2 KU into a Langendorf rabbit heart preparation. Coronary flow increased by 75%, but the heart rate and the amplitude of contractions remained constant. These studies with the isolated heart differ from experiments in the intact organism which may respond to extracardiac influence after kallikrein (Wiethaup, 1932; Greene, 1936; Felix, 1939). More recent studies using kinins instead of kallikrein are in good agreement with reports referred to above (ROCHA E SILVA, 1962; ANTONIO and ROCHA E SILVA, 1962; PARRATT and GRAYSON, 1963; COLLIER, 1963; PARRATT, 1964; SCHRÖDER and HEMPEL, 1964; MOOG and FISCHER, 1964a, b; HEEG and MENG, 1965; SCHOLTHOLT et al., 1965; NAKANO, 1965; LOCHNER and PARRATT, 1966).

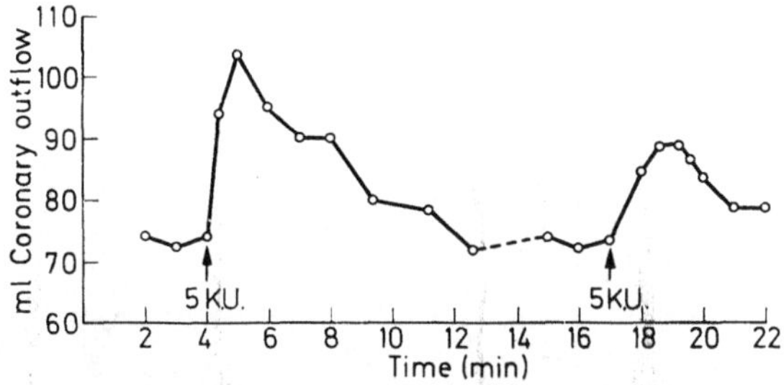

Fig. 3. Coronary outflow in a dog heart–lung preparation after injection of kallikrein

E. Kallikrein Activity in the Cerebral and Ocular Circulation

The bulk of the material relating to the circulation of the brain is treated in the chapter by SICUTERI (p. 482), who concentrated his attention primarily on bradykinin action. At this place, however, it may be valuable to add a few brief comments to some aspects of the action of kallikrein alone, particularly as they are of historical interest.

As early as 1928 it had been demonstrated by means of a plethysmograph that injection of 2 KU increased the volume of the exposed dog brain markedly, subsequent to a fleeting volume reduction. Concomitantly, mean carotid blood pressure declined. From this observation it was concluded that the cerebral vessels are directly influenced by kallikrein (FREY and KRAUT, 1928). Furthermore, intravenously administered kallikrein or bradykinin raised cerebrospinal fluid pressure in man. This could be interpreted to have resulted from intracranial arteriolar vasodilatation (REEKE and WERLE, 1935; SICUTERI, 1963). In this case carotid pressure declined likewise. In dogs, kallikrein enhanced blood volume flow in the internal carotid artery as estimated with Rein's thermostromuhr (KELLER, 1930; SCHNEIDER and SPRINGORUM, 1939).

Of great interest is the therapeutic potential of kallikrein in cases of visual impairment related to disturbances in retinal blood supply. Within 1 to 3 minutes, intravenous injection of 4 KU produces dilatation and greater filling with increased pulsation of the human retinal arteries and veins (FELIX, 1939). Systematic measurements in eighty normal persons revealed that the diameter of the retinal arteries increased 15 to 30 minutes after injection of 20 to 40 KU, reaching a maximum (7 to 12%) after 60 to 90 minutes and lasting from 6 to 8 hours (HOLLOWICH and WETHMAR, 1958); 100 units of inactivated kallikrein (Komplex-Padutin) even caused the diameter to increase by 21%, which may explain the favorable therapeutic effects on the retina and optic nerve in the circulatory disorders as well as in cases of degenerations of the macula (HOLLOWICH and WETHMAR, 1958; HOLLOWICH et al., 1967).

F. Pulmonary Vessels

When compared to the rather pronounced effects on the vessels of the greater circulation, the action of kallikrein on the smooth musculature of the lung vessels seems to be neither striking nor consistent. This is also in agreement with most of the results of recent work with kinins (LECOMTE and TROQUET, 1960; BISHOP et al., 1963, 1965; COLLIER, 1963; KLUPP and KONZETT, 1963; MOOG and GREEFF, 1963; MOOG and FISCHER, 1964a, b; GREEFF and MOOG, 1964, 1965; KLUPP and KONZETT, 1965; NAKANO, 1965; HAUGE et al., 1966; KONZETT and BAUER, 1966). In open-chest dogs with positive pressure respiration the neutral and bronchial blood and air supply were eliminated in two lobes of the lung. A lung plethysmograph showed a small volume increase after administration of 2 KU.

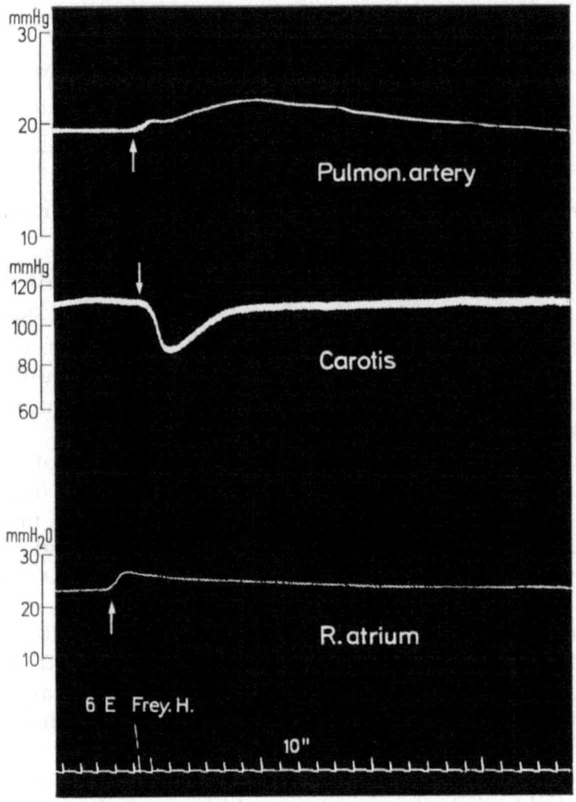

Fig. 4. Effect of 6 units of kallikrein on pressures in the pulmonary and carotid arteries and the right atrium of the cat

Larger dosages did not enhance but merely prolonged the reaction. Pulmonary arterial pressure rose slightly, whereas there was a simultaneous and remarkable drop in carotid arterial pressure (FREY and KRAUT, 1938).

When kallikrein was applied to cats under urethan anesthesia the pulmonary arterial pressure rose slightly, concomitant with right atrial pressure (KRAYER and RÜHL, 1931) (Fig. 4). KRAYER and RÜHL concluded from these observations that an increased venous return and greater right ventricular stroke volume probably accounted for the pulmonary arterial pressure rise, rather than a pulmonary resistance increase as had been surmised by previous authors (FREY and KRAUT, 1938). Although he demonstrated only the action of bradykinin, NAKANO's work (1965) lent weight to the interpretation of KRAYER and RÜHL; he kept venous return constant and found that pulmonary arterial pressure remained unchanged.

G. Changes of the Heart and in the Greater Circulation

I. Heart Rate

One to several units of kallikrein injected in man and animals increased the heart rate consistently. The threshold dosage for cardiac acceleration is slightly less than that for lowering the arterial blood pressure (FREY et al., 1935; FREY and KRAUT, 1938). When kallikrein is injected into a vein, the heart rate accelerates with increasing dosages, but not in proportion to them (FREY et al., 1935). Histamine elicited the same reactions, except that it produced extrasystoles at higher dosages (FREY et al., 1935). Slow intravenous infusion (40 to 80 KU per 5–6 hours) barely increased the heart rate (LOEWENECK and MADLENER, 1937), whereas intramuscular application did not alter the cardiac frequency at all (FREY et al., 1935). In the dog, 5 KU accelerated the heart rate from 90 to 260/min. On the other hand, 80 "parts" of histamine, which lowered blood pressure to the same value as 5 units of kallikrein, did not produce such high rates (SCHNEIDER and SPRINGORUM, 1939). An attempt to elucidate the reasons for the increase in heart rate was made by KRAYER and RÜHL (1931). In a denervated Starling heart–lung preparation they found only insignificant changes in heart beat frequency, contrary to the striking heart rate acceleration observed in the intact dog. They were cautious in their conclusion by stating merely that the acceleration cannot be explained by a direct effect upon the heart.

II. Mean Blood Pressure

Kallikrein lowers mean blood pressure in man and animals. The extent of the drop depends upon the dosage; e.g. in the anesthetized dog intravenous injection of 0.01 to 0.1 KU/kg lowers the pressure by 20 to 40% and 0.5 to 1.0 unit by 60%. The onset occurs after 5 to 10 seconds and reaches its maximum 10 to 30 seconds thereafter. The relationship of the extent of the blood pressure decrease and the amount of kallikrein infused per minute represents an exponential function—i.e. 8 units have the same effect as 40 units. The larger the dosage the longer lasting will be the effect (FREY and KRAUT, 1938). The blood pressure reduction is apparently not mediated through autonomic nervous impulses from centers in the brain. In rabbits and cats it occurs also after severing the brain stem above or below the medulla oblongata. Atropinization has no influence (FELIX, 1939). In normal man the arterial pressure drops immediately after kallikrein injection, although the individual responses vary greatly. If 5 to 30 KU are applied intramuscularly the pressure declines after some 15 to 30 minutes for a duration of 2 to 3 hours (FREY et al., 1935). If kallikrein is continuously infused into anesthetized dogs the blood pressure drops at first rather quickly, but then it increases again slightly and remains above the lowest level in some cases. If such an infusion lasts for a long time the response of the tissues to kallikrein diminishes. As an explanation, it is suggested that the kininogen level in the blood decreases progressively (WERLE, 1964). After discontinuing the infusion the pressure rises gradually. The circulation in dogs remains unaffected when smaller amounts than the threshold dose (0.25 KU/min) are continuously infused (FREY and KRAUT, 1928). This could be interpreted to mean that, on account of the rapid kallikrein and kinin inactivation, an insufficient concentration of kinins is reached to evoke hypotension. Prolonged administration of large amounts of kallikrein gradually abrogates the response to kallikrein, because the kinin precursor is apparently waning (WERLE, 1964).

III. Pulse Pressure

Whereas there can be no doubt about the validity of the changes in mean arterial blood pressure reported above, the changes in pulse pressure (difference between systolic and diastolic pressures) recorded thus far suffer from methodological inadequacies. Most the work was undertaken with the Frank-Petter spring manometer or other devices with poor fidelity (mainly from overshoot). This was clearly recognized at the time by the authors (Frey and Kraut, 1928), who pointed out the qualitative nature of the finding and the impossibility of arriving at quantitations. It is suggested by the writers of this chapter that some of this very interesting work be repeated or expanded with modern technology which assures high-fidelity recordings.

Nevertheless, despite the limited recording techniques, some information can be gained from the tracings. In most cases the pulse pressure increases while the heart rates remain constant or are accelerated. Generally, the diastolic pressure declines more than the systolic rises, which obviously results in a drop of the mean pressure. The lowest threshold value is 0.005 to 0.01 KU/kg (i.v.) in the dog. Increasing dosages lead to progressively greater pulse pressures up to a maximum reached at about 1 KU/kg. Young dogs respond better in this respect than old ones. At injection dosages ranging from 0.04 to 0.1 KU/kg the effect lasts about 2 minutes and at larger dosages 10 minutes or longer. Injection of 1 KU/kg every 15 minutes kept the increase almost level for 5 hours, with a slight decrease in pulse pressures in the subsequent 2 hours. However, when several amounts (3–5 KU) are injected in rather short intervals, the effect diminishes progressively. Slow infusion of kallikrein in low concentrations has little effect even if the accumulated total amount is large (Frey and Kraut, 1928; Krayer and Rühl, 1931).

In normal man intravenous injection quickly provokes a greater drop of systolic than of diastolic pressures, hence narrowing the pulse pressure. About 20 minutes later the systolic pressure increases substantially while the diastolic still declines, with a net effect of an occasional pulse pressure widening beyond the pre-experimental values. Many of these peculiarities may be explainable through the counter-regulatory processes (Frey et al., 1935; Sackers, 1936).

H. Overall Effects

The effects of kallikrein on the entire greater circulation must obviously be those of an integration of changes in the individual organs. Although in the lesser circulation, through which the same amount of blood flows as through the greater circulation, the tissue uniformity leads to a rather consistent overall response, this cannot be expected in the greater circulation. The complexity of the organs perfused and the discrepancies in the responses determine the resultant overall picture. This picture is best gained from mean blood pressure changes in the aorta. In this instance, and in future work on pulse pressure, many valuable studies are now possible because of the advent of physically accurate modern registration techniques which include direct measuring devices such as electromagnetic flowmeters at the root of the aorta, catheter tip manometers, cardiac X-ray cinematography, etc.

We still can arrive at several valid conclusions from the older work, if we take into consideration its technical limitations. Extrapolations from carotid arterial flow measurements with Ludwig's stromuhr indicate that subsequent to a fleeting decrease there is a consistent increase in cardiac output when kallikrein is injected. The effects wane slowly (Frey and Kraut, 1928).

Recently a much longer-lasting blood flow enhancement through peripheral vessels with a concomitant cardiac output increase has been achieved by KRONEBERG et al. (1965) through the use of the kallikrein inhibitor complex. The kallikrein which is freed by splitting of the complex liberates kinins over an appreciable period. The influence on the circulation is rather protracted. A note of caution may not be amiss, however, because rapid injection of large amounts of kallikrein can lead to states similar to circulatory collapse when pulse frequency and cardiac output decrease and tissue perfusion is diminished.

Recent interest has focused more on kinins rather than on kallikrein. Nevertheless, the latter may still offer scientific and therapeutic possibilities that would warrant additional investigations.

J. Brief Remarks Concerning Therapeutic Applications

In man, kallikrein produces a vasodilatation of the vessels in the coronary, skin, and muscle circulation and hence a better perfusion of the respective organs. Kallikrein may therefore be indicated in the treatment of inadequate perfusion of these peripheral vascular beds. Of particular significance is the vasodilatation of the ophthalmic and retinal vessels, which can improve retinal ischemia or hyposchemia. Whereas the above-mentioned therapeutic measures are well established, the useful action of kallikrein on the myocardium is debatable. Some investigators deny a direct effect upon the myocardium (NAKANO, 1965), but others suspect that there might be such an effect (BISHOP et al., 1965).

References

ANTONIO, A.: On the nature of the inotropic effect of bradykinin. Abstract no 472 III. Internat. Pharmacol. Congr. Sao Paulo 1966.

— ROCHA E SILVA, M.: Coronary vasodilatation produced by bradykinin on isolated mammalian heart. Circulat. Res. **11**, 910 (1962).

ASCHOFF, J.: Wärmeübergang an strömendes Blut. Pflügers Arch. ges. Physiol. **201**, 264 (1955).

BERGAMASCHI, M., GLÄSSER, A. H.: Peripheral vasodilator action of eledoisin, bradykinin, and nitroglycerin in anesthetized dogs. Circulat. Res. **15**, 371 (1964).

BISHOP, J. M., HARRIS, P., SEGEL, N.: The effect of synthetic bradykinin on the pulmonary and systematic circulation in man. J. Physiol. (Lond.) **163**, 372 (1963).

— — — The circulatory effects of bradykinin in normal subjects and patients with chronic bronchitis. Brit. J. Pharmacol. **25**, 456 (1965).

COLLIER, H. O. J.: The action and antagonism of kinins on bronchioles. Ann. N.Y. Acad. Sci. **104**, 290 (1963).

EHRINGER, H., HERZOG, P., KONZETT, H.: Über die Wirkung von synthetischem Bradykinin auf die Durchblutung der Extremitäten des Menschen. Helv. physiol. pharmacol. Acta **19**, 866 (1961).

FELIX, J.: An experimental study of the action of padutin (kallikrein). Acta med. scand. **83**, 1 (1939).

FOX, R. H., GOLDSMITH, R., KIDD, D. J., LEWIS, G. P.: Bradykinin as a vasodilator in man. J. Physiol. (Lond.) **154**, 16P (1960).

— — — — Bradykinin as a vasodilator in man. J. Physiol. (Lond.) **157**, 589 (1961).

FREY, E. K.: Über ein neues inneres Sekret des Pankreas, das Kreislaufhormon Kallikrein und seine therapeutische Verwendung. Dtsch. Z. Chir. **233**, 481 (1931).

— KRAUT, H.: Ein neues Kreislaufhormon und seine Wirkung. Naunyn-Schmiedebergs Arch. exp. Path. Pharmak. **133**, 1 (1928).

— — WERLE, E.: Kallikrein, Padutin, p. 6. Stuttgart: Ferdinand Enke 1950.

— WERLE, E., SACKERS, E.: Über die Wirkung intravenöser und intramuskulärer Kallikreininjektionen beim Menschen. Z. ges. exp. Med. **96**, 404 (1935).

FRIEDLÄNDER, R.: Über die Wirkung des Kallikreins auf die Gefäße. Inaug.-Diss. Düsseldorf 1931.

Golenhofen, K., Hensel, H., Papenberg, J.: Über die Wirkung von aktivem und inaktiviertem Kallikrein auf die Muskel- und Hautdurchblutung des Menschen. In: Leistungen und Ergebnisse der Neuzeitlichen Chirurgie, p. 49, 1958.
Greeff, K., Moog, E.: Vergleichende Untersuchungen über die bronchokonstriktorische und gefäßkonstriktorische Wirkung des Bradykinins, Histamins und Serotonins an isolierten Lungenpräparaten. Naunyn-Schmiedebergs Arch. exp. Path. Pharmak. **248**, 204 (1964).
— — Zur bronchokonstriktorischen Wirkung des Bradykinins. Klin. Wschr. **43**, 51 (1965).
Greene, C. W.: Dilatation of coronary vessels by certain extracts and drugs. J. Pharmacol. exp. Ther. **57**, 98 (1936).
Gregg, D. E.: Thermostromuhr. In: Methods in medical research, vol. 1, p. 89. Chicago: Year Book Publ. 1948.
Hauge, A., Lunde, P. K. M., Waaler, B. A.: The effect of bradykinin, kallidin and eledoisin upon the pulmonary vascular bed of an isolated blood-perfused rabbit lung preparation. Acta physiol. scand. **66**, 269 (1966).
Heeg, E., Meng, K.: Die Wirkung des Bradykinins, Angiotensins und Vasopressins auf Vorhof, Papillarmuskel und isoliert durchströmte Herzpräparate des Meerschweinchens. Naunyn-Schmiedebergs Arch. exp. Path. Pharmak. **250**, 35 (1965).
Hochrein, M., Keller, J. C.: Die Beeinflussung des Kreislaufes durch Organextrakte (sog. Kreislaufhormone). Naunyn-Schmiedebergs Arch. exp. Path. Pharmak. **159**, 438 (1931).
Hollowich, F., Jünemann, G., Damaske, E.: In: H. Schievelbein, Nikotin. Stuttgart: Georg Thieme 1967.
— Wethmar, A.: In: Leistungen und Ergebnisse der neuzeitlichen Chirurgie, p. 68. Stuttgart: Georg Thieme 1958.
Keatinge, W. R.: Electrical and mechanical responses of vascular smooth muscle to vasodilator agents and vasoactive polypeptides. Circulat. Res. 18, 641 (1966).
Keller, C. J.: Untersuchungen über die Gehirndurchblutung. I. Mitt. Gibt es eine Autonomie der Gehirngefäße? Naunyn-Schmiedebergs Arch. exp. Path. Pharmak. **154**, 357 (1930).
Klupp, H., Konzett, H.: Zur Wirkung von Bradykinin und Kallidin auf den Druck in der Arteria pulmonalis. Naunyn-Schmiedebergs Arch. exp. Path. Pharmak. **246**, 19 (1963).
— — Der Einfluß von Bradykinin und Kallidin auf den Druck in der Arteria pulmonalis. Naunyn-Schmiedebergs Arch. exp. Path. Pharmak. **249**, 471 (1965).
Konzett, H., Bauer, G.: The action of hypotensive polypeptides on the pulmonary arterial pressure. In: Hypotensive peptides, p. 375, ed. by E. G. Erdös, N. Back, and F. Sicuteri. Berlin-Heidelberg-New York: Springer 1966.
Kovalcik, V.: Effect of bradykinin on isolated coronary arteries. Nature (Lond.) **196**, 174 (1962).
Krayer, O., Rühl, A.: Über die Wirkung einer reinen Gefäßerweiterung auf den Gesamtkreislauf. Naunyn-Schmiedebergs Arch. exp. Path. Pharmak. **162**, 70 (1931).
Kroneberg, G., Stoepel, K., Pütter, J.: Kreislaufuntersuchungen über die Pharmakodynamik des Kallikrein-Kinin-Systems am Hund. Naunyn-Schmiedebergs Arch. exp. Path. Pharmak. **251**, 183 (1965).
Lecomte, J., Troquet, L.: Antagonisme entre bradykinine et phenylbutazone chez le lapin. C. R. Soc. Biol. (Paris) **154**, 1115 (1960).
Lindemann, A.: Leitfaden der Chirurgie und Orthopädie der Kiefer und des Mundes. Liefg. 5. Leipzig: J. A. Barth 1947.
Lochner, W., Parratt, J. R.: A comparison of the effects of locally and systemically administered kinins on coronary blood flow and myocardial metabolism. Brit. J. Pharmacol. **26**, 17 (1966).
Loeweneck, M., Madlener, M.: Intravenöse Dauerinfusion von Padutin. Dtsch. Z. Chir. **248**, 700 (1937).
Lorenz, O.: Die Wiederherstellung der Ober- und Unterlippe durch den Nasolabiallappen. Med. Klin. **17**, 379 (1946).
Moog, E., Fischer, J.: Vergleich der Wirkung verschiedener biogener Amine und Polypeptide auf den arteriellen und venösen Lungenkreislauf. Naunyn-Schmiedebergs Arch. exp. Path. Pharmak. **247**, 325 (1964a).
— — Die Wirkung des Histamins, Serotonins, Bradykinins, Eledoisins und Hypertensins auf isoliert durchströmte Arterien-, Venen- und Bronchienpräparate der Meerschweinchenlunge. Naunyn-Schmiedebergs Arch. exp. Path. Pharmak. **249**, 384 (1964b).
— Greeff, K.: Der Einfluß verschiedener biogener Amine und Polypeptide auf die Gefäß- und Bronchialmuskulatur isoliert durchströmter Meerschweinchenlungen. Naunyn-Schmiedebergs Arch. exp. Path. Pharmak. **246**, 16 (1963).
Multhaupt, G.: Padutin und Hauttemperatur. Inaug.-Diss. Düsseldorf 1937.

NAKANO, J.: Effects of synthetic bradykinin on the cardiovascular system. Arch. int. Pharmacodyn. **157**, 1 (1965).
PARRATT, J. R.: A comparison of the effects of the plasma kinins, bradykinin and kallidin, on myocardial blood flow and metabolism. Brit. J. Pharmacol. **22**, 34 (1964).
— GRAYSON, J.: The effect of bradykinin on blood flow and heat production in the myocardium. Experientia (Basel) **19**, 161 (1963).
REEKE, T., WERLE, E.: Die Wirkung intravenöser Kallikreingaben auf den Liquordruck. Z. ges. exp. Med. **36**, 398 (1935).
ROCHA E SILVA, M.: Definition of bradykinin and other kinins. Biochem. Pharmacol. **10**, 3 (1962).
SACKERS, E.: Über die Wirkung intravenöser und intramuskulärer Kallikreininjektionen. Inaug.-Diss. Düsseldorf 1936.
SCHNEIDER, D., SPRINGORUM, P. W.: Über die Kreislaufwirkung des Padutins. Langenbecks Arch. klin. Chir. **194**, 373 (1939).
SCHOLTHOLT, J., BUSSMANN, W. D., HIRCHE, H. J., LOCHNER, W., PARRATT, J.: Die Wirkung von Adeninnucleotiden und Plasmakininen auf die Coronardurchblutung und ihre Bedeutung bei der physiologischen Regulation. Pflügers Arch. ges. Physiol. **283**, Referat 54, Frühjahrstagung 1965.
SCHRÖDER, E., HEMPEL, R.: Bradykinin, kallidin and their synthetic analogues. Experientia (Basel) **20**, 529 (1964).
SICUTERI, F.: Prophylactic treatment of migraine by means of lysergic acid derivatives. Triangel **6**, 116 (1963).
TAKACS, L., ALBERT, K.: Action of bradykinin on cardiac output and blood distribution of rats. Arch. int. Pharmacodyn. **155**, 117 (1965).
WERLE, E.: Biochemische Betrachtungen zur Regulierung der Gewebsdurchblutung. Ärztl. Forsch. **18**, 281 (1964).
— HOCHSTRASSER, K., TRAUTSCHOLD, J.: Studies of bovine plasma kininogen, ornithokallikrein, and ornitho-kinin. In: Hypotensive peptides, p. 105, ed. by E. G. ERDÖS, N. BACK, and F. SICUTERI. Berlin-Heidelberg-New York: Springer 1966.
— HÜRTER, J.: Über Ornithokallikrein. I. Mitt. Über kreislaufaktive Substanzen der Vögel. Biochem. Z. **285**, 176 (1936).
— KEHL, R., KOEBKE, K.: Über Trypsin, Chymotrypsin, Kallidin und Bradykinin. Biochem. Z. **321**, 213 (1950).
— MULTHAUPT, G.: Über einen einfachen Nachweis der peripheren Gefäßwirkung des Padutins. Münch. med. Wschr. **79**, 407 (1937).
— RODEN, P. v.: Über das Vorkommen von Kallikrein in den Speicheldrüsen und im Mundspeichel. Biochem. Z. **286**, 213 (1936).
— STUECKER, F.: In: F. STUECKER, Inaug.-Diss. Med. Fakultät Univ. München, 1956.
— VOGEL, R., LENRODT, J.: Über den Kallikreingehalt der Glandula submandibularis während der Entwicklung einiger Säugerarten und nach der Abbindung des Ductus Whartoni. Arch. int. Pharmacodyn. **126**, 182 (1960).
WIETHAUP, H.: Die Beeinflussung der Digitaliswirkung durch coronarerweiternde Mittel. Naunyn-Schmiedebergs Arch. exp. Path. Pharmak. **168**, 554 (1932).
WRIGHT, J., MOFFAT, D.: Die Wirkung des Tabaks auf die peripheren Gefäße. Weitere Untersuchungen. J. Amer. med. Ass. **103**, 318 (1934).

The Effect of the Kinins on the Cardiovascular System

F. J. Haddy, T. E. Emerson Jr., J. B. Scott* and R. M. Daugherty Jr.

With 2 Figures

The kinins produce dramatic effects on the cardiovascular system, the two most pronounced being hypotension on systemic administration and water efflux from small blood vessels on local administration. In this review, these two effects are presented in two separate sections. In the first, the determinants of blood pressure are briefly reviewed. This is followed by an attempt to systematically analyze the action of the kinins on each of these determinants. The same format is used in the second section on water efflux. It is hoped that this method of presentation will accomplish more for the reader than would a simple listing of the effects of the kinins on the cardiovascular system.

A. General Effects on the Cardiovascular System

The kinins have been shown to lower systemic arterial pressure in all species tested (Holdstock et al., 1957; Elliott et al., 1960; Konzett and Stürmer, 1960; Holtz et al., 1962; Erspamer and Glässer, 1963; Stürmer and Berde, 1963a, b, c; Parratt, 1964; Elliott and Lewis, 1965).

Mean systemic arterial pressure is immediately determined by cardiac output and total peripheral vascular resistance. The determinants of these two variables have been considered in detail in a previous communication (Haddy and Scott, 1966) and therefore will be only briefly reviewed here. The immediate mechanical determinants of cardiac output are stroke volume and stroke frequency. Stroke volume is in turn determined by resistance to ejection, end diastolic ventricular volume, and ventricular strength (defined as the ratio stroke work/diastolic ventricular volume; the "stronger" ventricle performs more work at a given diastolic ventricular volume and hence initial fiber length). Diastolic ventricular volume is influenced by (1) filling pressure (atrial pressure), (2) diastolic filling time (a function of cardiac frequency), (3) ventricular compliance, and (4) the resistance to blood flow through the atrioventricular valves.

Total peripheral vascular resistance, the other immediate determinant of systemic arterial blood pressure, is influenced by blood viscosity, blood vessel radius, and blood vessel length. Blood vessel radius can change through active and passive mechanisms (an active change in radius is here defined as any change in caliber resulting from alteration in the contractile state of the smooth muscle in the vessel wall).

Table 1 presents studies in which at least cardiac output and arterial blood pressure were measured during intravenous infusion of bradykinin. It is evident that the fall in systemic arterial pressure is associated with a rise in cardiac output. Thus the fall in pressure results from a decrease in total peripheral resistance. Of the three components of resistance (viscosity, length, radius), it appears that only changes in radius are applicable to the fall in resistance seen

* Established Investigator of the American Heart Association.

Table 1. *General effects of intravenous bradykinin infusion on the cardiovascular system*

Infusion rate (µg/kg/min)	No.	Q	f	vs	PAS	PVS	RTS	PAP	PVP	RTP	Reference
Unanesthetized man											
0.4	19	↑	↑↔	↑	↓↔		↓				Kontos et al. (1964)
0.4—1.6	10	↑	↑	↑	↓		↓	↔		↓	De Freitas et al. (1964)
0.3—0.8	6	↑	↑	↑	↓	↔	↓	↔	↔[a]	↔	Bishop et al. (1965)
0.5—1.0	11	↔	↑	↓	↓		↓				Feruglio et al. (1964)
Anesthetized dog											
2.5	8	↑	↑		↓↔	↓	↓	↔		↓	Rowe et al. (1963)
10.0	33	↑	↔	↑	↓	↑	↓	↔	↔	↓↔	Emerson (1967)
1.0	14	↑	↑	↔	↓	↔	↓	↓↔		↓	Amorim et al. (1967)
0.5—1.0	12	↔	↔		↓		↔	↔		↔	Anguissola et al. (1966)
2.5	8	↑	↑	↓	↓		↓	↓		↓	Maxwell et al. (1962)
Anesthetized rat											
12.5 and 25.0	10	↑	↔	↑	↓		↓				Rosas et al. (1965)
28.0 and 63.0	13	↑			↓		↓				Takacs and Albert (1965)
25.0	10	↑			↓		↓				Arcidiacono et al. (1966)

[a] Pulmonary artery wedge pressure.

Q = cardiac output, f = stroke frequency, vs = stroke volume, PAS = systemic arterial pressure, PVS = systemic venous pressure, RTS = total systemic resistance, PAP = pulmonary arterial pressure, PVP = pulmonary venous pressure, RTP = total pulmonary resistance, ↑ = increase, ↓ = decrease, ↔ = no change, ↑↔ = increase with return to control, ↓↔ = decrease with return to control.

Table 2. *Effects of intravenous infusion of*

	Hand		Calf		Fore-arm or fore-limb		Skele-tal mus-cle		Skin		Kid-ney		Splanch-nic bed		Liver		Gut		Spleen		Coro-nary bed	
	R[a]	F[a]	R	F	R	F	R	F	R	F	R	F	R	F	R	F	R	F	R	F	R	F
Man																						
	↓	↑			↔	↔[b]					↔	↔										
		↑				↑																
													↓	↔								
											↔	↔										
				↔																		
Dog																						
																					↓	↑
																					↓	↑
					↓	↔	↓	↔	↓	↔												
											↔	↔									↓	↑
																					↓[c]	↑[d]
											↔	↔										
																					↓	↑
Rat																						
									↔	↓	↔	↔			↓	↑	↓	↑	↓	↑	↓	↑
									↔[e]	↔	↓	↑			↓	↑	↓	↑			↓	↑

[a] R = resistance; F = flow.
[b] Increased at a higher infusion rate.
[c] Same response in monkey, chimpanzee, cat, and rabbit.

with bradykinin. Hematocrit does not change (AMORIM et al., 1967) or increases slightly (ROWE et al., 1963), and there is no reason to suspect significant changes in vessel length. Thus total peripheral resistance falls because of an increase in blood vessel radius. This likely occurs mainly at the arteriolar level. While microscopic observations apparently have not been made during intravenous infusion, arteriolar dilatation has been directly observed on local administration (BAEZ and ORKIN, 1963; ZWEIFACH, 1964a, 1966; HYMAN and PALDINO, 1966; ALTURA, 1967). The increase in radius undoubtedly results from relaxation of vascular smooth muscle (active vasodilatation) since it occurs in the face of a fall in arterial transmural pressure.

The increase in cardiac output results from elevation of stroke frequency and, in most studies, stroke volume (Table 1). As indicated above, stroke volume is determined by resistance to ejection, myocardial strength, and diastolic ventricular volume. The fall in total peripheral resistance (and hence arterial pressure) would by itself increase stroke volume. While neither strength nor diastolic ventricular volume has been definitively examined in the intact animal, there are indications that at least one of the variables might work in concert with the fall in resistance to elevate stroke volume. Small increases in left ventricular contractile force (strain gauge arch) have been observed after intravenous injection in the open-chest dog (NAKANO, 1965; HARRISON et al., 1968). Such a response could result from an increase in strength, increase in diastolic ventricular volume, or both. With regard to diastolic ventricular volume, intravenous infusion causes a decrease in filling time (inferred from the increase in cardiac frequency) and very little change in filling pressure. While there are no studies of ventricular compliance and valvular resistance, there is little reason to believe that these *bradykinin on systemic organ resistance and flow*

Brain		Carcass		Adrenals		Pancreas		Salivary gland		Reference
R	F	R	F	R	F	R	F	R	F	
										KONTOS et al. (1964)
										FOX et al. (1961)
										FERUGLIO et al. (1964)
										GILL et al. (1965)
										COFFMAN and JAVETT (1963)
										MAXWELL et al. (1962)
										ROWE et al. (1963)
										DAUGHERTY et al. (1968)
↔	↔									ANGUISSOLA et al. (1966)
										PARRATT (1964)
										MURPHY et al. (1965)
										LOCHNER and PARRATT (1966)
↓	↑	↓	↑	↓	↑	↓	↔	↑	↓	ARCIDIACONO et al. (1966)
										TAKACS and ALBERT (1965)

[d] Same response in monkey, chimpanzee, and cat but did not change in rabbit.
[e] Decreased at a higher infusion rate.

change. Thus indirect evidence does not suggest an increase in diastolic ventricular volume. On the other hand, there is indirect evidence suggesting an increase in myocardial strength. Right and left ventricular work sometimes increase despite no change or a fall in right and left ventricular filling time and pressure (ROWE et al., 1963; DE FREITAS et al., 1964; BISHOP et al., 1965), at least at low infusion rates. Furthermore, left ventricular filling pressure often does not rise despite an increase in venous return (EMERSON, 1967). It should be noted that in some studies (Table 1) stroke volume did not change or actually fell. Examination of these studies shows that this was associated with a large increase in cardiac frequency. This suggests that in these studies an abbreviated filling time reduced diastolic ventricular volume, thereby reducing stroke volume (despite the decrease in ejection resistance and presumed increase in strength).

Bradykinin, in physiological concentrations, has little effect on frequency and strength of the isolated heart (ANTONIO and ROCHA E SILVA, 1962; RUBIN et al., 1963; NAKANO, 1965). Neither does it alter the rate of change of intraventricular pressure on intracoronary infusion in the intact dog (LOCHNER and PARRATT, 1966). Thus the increase in cardiac frequency and strength seen in the intact animal on intravenous infusion apparently results indirectly (see below).

Most of the systemic organs contribute to the fall in total peripheral vascular resistance and hence to the fall in systemic arterial pressure. Table 2 shows that intravenous infusion of bradykinin reduces the resistance to blood flow through the hand, skeletal muscle, carcass, splanchnic, liver, gut, spleen, adrenal, pancreas, and coronary vascular beds. Resistance sometimes also falls in the forelimb, skin, cerebral and renal vascular beds. One group of investigators, utilizing rubidium clearance, report an increase in salivary gland resistance. Coronary resistance is also decreased by intravenous kallidin infusion in a variety of species (Parratt, 1964), as is renal resistance in the dog (Murphy et al., 1965). Intravenous injection of hog kallikrein apparently decreases coronary resistance in the rabbit (Parratt, 1964).

Blood flow is increased during intravenous infusion of bradykinin (Table 2) in the carcass, hand, liver, gut, spleen, adrenal, and coronary vascular beds (coronary flow responds variably in the rabbit). Flow is sometimes increased in the forelimb, brain, and kidney beds but does not change greatly in calf skeletal muscle, pancreas, and splanchnic beds. It is sometimes decreased in the skin bed. Salivary gland flow has been reported to decrease. Nutritive or capillary blood flow, as measured by the disappearance rate of Na^{131}, apparently does not change in calf skeletal muscle of man (Coffman and Javett, 1963). Intravenous infusion of kallidin also increases coronary blood flow in all species (Parratt, 1964), but it does not change renal blood flow in the dog (Murphy et al., 1965). Intravenous injection of hog kallikrein fails to increase coronary flow in the rabbit (Parratt, 1964).

Associated with the increase in coronary blood flow induced by intravenous infusion of bradykinin in the dog is an increase in myocardial oxygen consumption (Maxwell et al., 1962; Rowe et al., 1963; Anguissola et al., 1966; Lochner and Parratt, 1966) and sometimes a slight rise in arterial oxygen content (Maxwell et al., 1962; Rowe et al., 1963), the latter possibly due to a splenic discharge. Coronary sinus oxygen content does not change (Maxwell et al., 1962; Rowe et al., 1963; Anguissola et al., 1966) and neither is there an appreciable effect on coronary sinus oxygen tension (Lochner and Parratt, 1966). This suggests that the increased myocardial oxygen utilization is precisely met by an increased oxygen supply. Cardiac efficiency, the ratio of work to oxygen consumption, has been reported not to change (Rowe et al., 1963) or fall (Maxwell et al., 1962; Anguissola et al., 1966). The oxygen content of deep forearm venous blood of man was found to decrease in three subjects and increase in one subject (Kontos et al., 1964). Intravenous infusion of bradykinin or kallikrein apparently does not affect renal venous oxygen tension (Murphy et al., 1965). Intravenous infusion of kallidin, like bradykinin, increases myocardial oxygen consumption without affecting coronary sinus oxygen tension, at least when the infusion rate is slow; at more rapid infusion rates, sinus tension may actually rise (Lochner and Parratt, 1966).

There have been no studies on pre- and postcapillary resistances during intravenous infusion. However, to judge from the magnitude of the fall in total systemic resistance, precapillary resistance undoubtedly falls. The resistances to blood flow through large veins in skin and muscle of the dog forelimb do not change greatly during intravenous infusion of bradykinin despite a large fall in total forelimb resistance (Daugherty et al., 1968). Compliance of veins in the human hand, however, has been reported to increase (Kontos et al., 1964). Capillary hydrostatic pressure and absolute blood volume have not been measured. It seems likely that the distribution of the blood volume between the arterial and venous sides of the systemic circulation is altered. Dilatation of resistance vessels would translocate blood from arteries to veins, thereby contributing to the increase in venous return to the heart (Emerson, 1967).

The reduction in the regional resistances results from a direct relaxing action of the kinins on vascular smooth muscle. A direct action is supported by a wealth of evidence. Intra-arterial administration produces a fall in the resistances to blood flow through the coronary (Antonio and Rocha e Silva, 1962; Rocha e Silva, 1963; Rubin et al., 1963; Nakano, 1965; Lochner and Parratt, 1966), renal (GOLDBERG et al., 1965; NAKANO, 1965; BARRACLOUGH and MILLS, 1965; MURPHY et al., 1965; FURUYAMA et al., 1966), whole forelimb (RAHE et al., 1963; NAKANO, 1965; DAUGHERTY et al., 1968), whole hindlimb (GERSMEYER and SPITZBARTH, 1961; VAN ARMAN and MILLER, 1961; BERGAMASCHI and GLÄSSER, 1964; ROSAS et al., 1965; NAKANO, 1965; NAKANO and KUSAKARI, 1966; DIANA et al., 1967), whole hindquarters (MCCARTHY et al., 1965), forearm (ALLWOOD and LEWIS, 1964), calf (COFFMAN and JAVETT, 1963), hand (KONTOS et al., 1964; COFFMAN, 1966), skeletal muscle (GERSMEYER and SPITZBARTH, 1961; PALDINO et al., 1962; HIRVONIN et al., 1964; BERGAMASCHI and GLÄSSER, 1964; KJELLMER and ODELRAM, 1965; HYMAN and PALDINO, 1966; HYMAN and BALLARD, 1966; WEBSTER et al., 1967; EMERSON et al., 1967; DAUGHERTY et al., 1968), skin (GERSMEYER and SPITZBARTH, 1961; BERGAMASCHI and GLÄSSER, 1964; HYMAN and PALDINO, 1966; DAUGHERTY et al., 1968), superior mesenteric (CHOU et al., 1965; BOIJSEN and REDMAN, 1966), ileal (CHOU and DABNEY, 1967; HADDY et al., 1967), stomach (JACOBSON, 1964, 1965), bronchial (WAALER, 1961), internal carotid (GERSMEYER and SPITZBARTH, 1961), and salivary gland (BHOOLA et al., 1965) vascular beds (for additional information on glands see chapter 6A, p. 389). Topical application produces, by microscopic observation, dilatation of arterioles in skeletal muscle (HYMAN and PALDINO, 1966; MAJNO et al., 1967), mesentery (BAEZ and ORKIN, 1963; HYMAN and PALDINO, 1966; ZWEIFACH, 1966; ALTURA, 1967), and skin (HYMAN and PALDINO, 1966). In contrast to the findings during intravenous infusion, intra-arterial infusion of bradykinin increases skeletal muscle nutritional flow as measured by the disappearance rate of diffusible substances injected into the tissue (PALDINO et al., 1962; COFFMAN and JAVETT, 1963). On the other hand, digital blood flow in man has been reported to decrease during intrabrachial infusion of bradykinin or kallidin (BURCH and DE PASQUALE, 1962; DE PASQUALE and BURCH, 1966). It is of interest that isolated blood vessels and some vascular beds perfused with artificial fluids also respond to bradykinin with constriction (GUTH et al., 1963; MOOG and FISCHER, 1964; SHIMAMOTO et al., 1966; WIEGERSHAUSEN, 1966; NORTHOVER, 1967).

In addition to vasodilatation, intracoronary administration of bradykinin produces an increase in myocardial oxygen consumption and coronary sinus oxygen tension (LOCHNER and PARRATT, 1966). Since bradykinin does not seem to have a direct stimulating effect on cardiac muscle (see above), the mechanism of the increase in myocardial oxygen consumption is not readily apparent. It may be indirect, perhaps related to coronary flow. Possibly the increase in flow washes out depressing metabolites, thereby increasing contractile force and oxygen consumption. Increase in force and oxygen consumption are known to occur when flow is artificially elevated (GREGG, 1963; BACANER et al., 1965; SCOTT et al., 1965; DAUGHERTY et al., 1967) and a large bradykinin-induced increase in coronary flow is associated with an increase in force in the hypodynamic isolated heart (ANTONIO and ROCHA E SILVA, 1962). Intrarenal administration of bradykinin also raises renal venous oxygen tension (MURPHY et al., 1965).

Kallidin, on local administration, produces similar effects. Intracoronary infusion decreases coronary resistance and increases coronary flow, myocardial oxygen consumption, and coronary sinus oxygen tension (LOCHNER and PARRATT, 1966). Intrarenal administration decreases renal resistance and increases renal blood flow and renal venous oxygen tension (WEBSTER and GILMORE, 1964; MURPHY et al., 1965).

It is apparent that the changes in resistance and flow seen during local administration are not always seen during intravenous infusion. While intravenous infusion lowers total peripheral resistance, the drop in resistance is not uniformly distributed. In fact, a resistance decrease may not be seen in some beds (Table 2). However, since total peripheral resistance falls there is almost always a fall in blood pressure. The effect on flow in a particular bed then depends upon the relationship between the change in arterial pressure and the change in resistance of the bed. For example, intravenous infusion of bradykinin does not affect flow through the forelimb even though forelimb resistance falls because of a proportionate fall in blood pressure (Daugherty et al., 1968). On the other hand, coronary flow almost always increases (Table 2) because the fall in resistance is out of proportion to the fall in pressure. The net change in resistance in a given vascular bed during intravenous infusion is the result of several forces. These probably include the direct effect of the agent on vascular smooth muscle, indirect effects on vascular smooth muscle mediated through nerves and other vasoactive agents, and effects due to change in transmural pressure. For example, catecholamine release would tend to further dilate the coronary vascular bed but would antagonize the dilatation in the renal vascular bed.

Several investigators have noted that the blood pressure depression during intravenous infusion of bradykinin may not be maintained (Montague et al., 1963; Rowe et al., 1963; Feruglio et al., 1964; Kontos et al., 1964; Parratt, 1964; Rosas et al., 1965; Emerson, 1967). This apparently results at least in part from a waning of the effect on total peripheral resistance (Montague et al., 1963; Bishop et al., 1965; Rosas et al., 1965; Emerson, 1967). Furthermore, intravenous injection may be followed by an overshoot in blood pressure (Konzett and Stürmer, 1960; Croxatto and Belmar, 1961; Olmsted and Page, 1962; Feldberg and Lewis, 1964; Lecomte et al., 1964; Mason and Melmon, 1965; Pearson and Lang, 1967; Miele and De Natale, 1967; Lang and Pearson, 1968). These findings suggest that this depressor agent, like others, evokes compensatory responses. At least four compensatory mechanisms must be entertained: (1) enhanced sympathicoadrenal activity, (2) cardioparasympathetic inhibition, (3) enhanced kininase activity, and (4) autoregulation.

With respect to the first, the fall in blood pressure is enhanced in magnitude and duration and the overshoot is abolished by treatment with reserpine (Rocha e Silva et al., 1960; Rowe et al., 1963; Nakano, 1965), phenoxybenzamine (Rocha e Silva et al., 1960), chlorpromazine[1] (Rocha e Silva et al., 1960), or hexamethonium (Lang and Pearson, 1968)[2]. The increase in heart rate is less pronounced after pronethalol (Bishop et al., 1965), reserpine (Rowe et al., 1963; Nakano, 1965), and after combined blockade with atropine, phenoxybenzamine, and MJ-1999 (Harrison et al., 1968). The increase in contractile force is converted to a decrease by reserpine (Nakano, 1965), and the initial decrease in forearm venous compliance is abolished by guanethidine (Mason and Melmon, 1965). The overshoot in blood pressure is also reduced or abolished after adrenalectomy and is enhanced after denervation of the carotid sinuses (Lang and Pearson, 1968). Furthermore, in spinal and decerebrate cats, only a depressor response is seen (Lang and Pearson, 1968). Studies in guanethidine-

1. In addition to effects on the nervous system, studies *in vitro* suggest that these agents may also inhibit the destruction of bradykinin (Krivoy and Kroeger, 1964).

2. Pentolinium (Croxatto and Belmar, 1961; Montague et al., 1963; Rosas et al., 1965) and guanethidine (Miele and De Natale, 1967) convert a depressor response to a pressor response in the rat. The pressor response is associated with a greater increase in cardiac output and a lesser decrease in total peripheral resistance. Under this condition, the increase in cardiac output is out of proportion to the decrease in total peripheral resistance, resulting in a rise rather than a fall in blood pressure.

pretreated rats also suggest an adrenal medullary discharge (MIELE and DE NATALE, 1967).

While catecholamine blood levels and action potentials in sympathetic nerves have not been measured, these studies suggest that the kinins activate the sympathicoadrenal system. The question then arises as to how the agents initiate this activity. Does activation occur reflexly via the baroreceptors or does it result from direct effects on the central nervous system, sympathetic ganglia, or adrenal medulla?

Hypotension per se is known to produce activation of the sympathicoadrenal system via the baroreceptors (HEYMANS and NEIL, 1958). While this seems to be a likely mechanism for activation of the sympathicoadrenal system during kinin infusion, this question has not been critically examined. It is known, however, that the overshoot in pressure following intravenous injection of bradykinin is enhanced after partial baroreceptor denervation (LANG and PEARSON, 1968). Other investigators have suggested that pain receptors are activated on intra-arterial injection of the kinins (GUZMAN et al., 1962). Whether this occurs on intravenous administration is unknown.

As already mentioned, intravenous injection of bradykinin in spinal and decerebrate cats produces only a depressor response (LANG and PEARSON, 1968). Furthermore, injection of bradykinin into the lateral ventricle produces a more persistent fall in blood pressure than when the same amount is given intravenously. Finally, intracarotid injection in an amount without effect on intravenous administration causes a depressor response (ROCHA E SILVA et al., 1960). From these observations the authors suggest that bradykinin can act centrally, and it is possible that such an action is mediated via the sympathicoadrenal system.

The question of a direct stimulating effect on the adrenal medulla has been studied more thoroughly. Close arterial injection of the kinins has been reported to produce an adrenal medullary discharge (LECOMTE et al., 1961; FELDBERG and LEWIS, 1964, 1965; POISNER and DOUGLAS, 1965; STASZEWSKA-BARCZAK and VANE, 1967; ROBINSON, 1967), though this is not always seen (VOGT, 1965; COMLINE et al., 1968). A direct stimulating effect of bradykinin on sympathetic ganglia has also been observed (LEWIS and REIT, 1965; TRENDELENBURG, 1966).

Finally, it is possible that the kinins release catecholamines at the tissue level (MONTGOMERY and KROEGER, 1967). However this does not seem to be the case in the heart (LOCHNER and PARRATT, 1966).

With respect to the other possible compensatory mechanisms, a baroreceptor-induced cardioparasympathetic inhibition deserves attention. Interestingly enough, central stimulation of parasympathetic centers acting on heart rate is claimed for bradykinin (BUCKLEY et al., 1963). It has been observed that the concentration of bradykinin in forearm venous blood during constant infusion into the brachial artery is not maintained, suggesting activation of kininase mechanisms (ALLWOOD and LEWIS, 1964). That these mechanisms are normally quite active is suggested by the fact that the half-life *in vivo* of bradykinin is estimated to be approximately 30 seconds (SAAMELI and ESKES, 1962; McCARTHY et al., 1965). It is also possible that in some vascular beds the fall in resistance is antagonized via the autoregulatory phenomenon, the increase in flow removing tissue vasodilator metabolites. Autoregulation should occur whenever the flow to metabolism ratio is increased (HADDY and SCOTT, 1968). That the ratio does increase in some organs during intravenous infusion is suggested by the observations that (1) right atrial oxygen content and saturation rise (see below); (2) cardiac output increases (Table 1) in the face of little change in total body oxygen consumption (see below).

The kinins do not appear to produce striking effects on the pulmonary circulation. Bradykinin, infused intravenously into the intact animal, produces no change (Rowe et al., 1963; Bishop et al., 1965; Anguissola et al., 1966; Emerson, 1967; Amorim et al., 1967) or a small fall (Maxwell et al., 1962) in pulmonary artery pressure. Pulmonary artery wedge pressure also does not seem to change greatly (Table 1); neither does left atrial pressure in the venous return preparation (Emerson, 1967). Pulmonary vascular resistance has been reported to fall (Maxwell et al., 1962; Rowe et al., 1963; De Freitas et al., 1964; Amorim et al., 1967; Emerson, 1967) or not to change (Bishop et al., 1965; Anguissola et al., 1966). In the dog venous return preparation, the fall in resistance does not occur when flow is held constant (Emerson, 1967). Bradykinin reduces the resistance to flow through the isolated blood-perfused dog (fetal, puppy, and adult) lung (Waaler, 1961; Grega et al., 1969) but elevates resistance in the isolated blood-perfused rabbit lung (Hauge et al., 1966b). Thus in the intact animal the net resistance response during intravenous infusion could be the result of (1) a direct effect on the pulmonary blood vessels, (2) an indirect effect on pulmonary blood vessels via evoked changes in nerve activity and concentrations of circulating hormones (see above), and (3) passive effects due to changes in transmural pressure subsequent to the rise in cardiac output.

There appear to be no studies of pulmonary blood volume during intravenous infusion in the intact animal.

Total body oxygen consumption does not change (Kontos et al., 1964; De Freitas et al., 1964; Bishop et al., 1965; Anguissola et al., 1966) or rises slightly (Rowe et al., 1963) during intravenous infusion. Right atrial oxygen content (Rowe et al., 1963) and saturation (Amorim et al., 1967) apparently increase.

Summary

The kinins act directly upon peripheral arterioles to produce vasodilatation and hypotension and act indirectly on the heart to produce an increase in cardiac output. The peripheral vasodilatation decreases the resistance to left ventricular ejection and probably translocates blood from the arterial to the venous side of the circulation. These two effects, in association with evoked sympathico-adrenal excitation and perhaps parasympathetic inhibition, increase the cardiac output.

Flow does not increase in all organs, indicating that the effect on the peripheral blood vessels is not uniform. The vasodilatation clearly involves the precapillary vessels, but definitive information on the postcapillary vessels, capillary hydrostatic pressure, and blood volume is lacking. The rise in output results from an increase in stroke frequency and, most often, stroke volume. The increase in stroke volume apparently results from the decrease in ejection resistance and from an evoked increase in myocardial strength. The literature does not indicate whether changes in initial fiber length are also involved in the increase in stroke volume. Both branches of the autonomic nervous system may participate in the increase in frequency and strength.

Relative to the systemic circulation, effects on the pulmonary circulation are minimal.

B. Effects on Transvascular Movement of Water

Local administration of bradykinin, kallidin, or kallikrein, like local administration of histamine, clearly causes rapid efflux of fluid from systemic vascular beds. Water efflux has been demonstrated by a number of techniques including

(1) inspection and palpation of the limb after intra-arterial infusion (KONTOS et al., 1964) or intradermal injection (WITTE et al., 1961; GREAVES and SHUSTER, 1967); (2) measurement of limb weight (RAHE et al., 1963; DIANA et al., 1967; DAUGHERTY et al., 1968), volume (KONTOS et al., 1964; KJELLMER and ODELRAM, 1965) or girth (ALLWOOD and LEWIS, 1964) during intra-arterial infusion; (3) measurement of hindpaw volume after injection under the plantar skin (STÜRMER and CERLETTI, 1961; GILFOIL and KLAVINS, 1965); and (4) measurement of hind limb lymph flow on intra-arterial infusion (STÜRMER, 1966). An increased rate of appearance of protein extravascularly in skin on intra-arterial infusion or intradermal injection and in hindlimb lymph on intra-arterial infusion also suggests enhanced water efflux (see below).

In accordance with the Starling-Landis hypothesis (STARLING, 1896; LANDIS and PAPPENHEIMER, 1963), an increase in the net rate of fluid movement out of the microvasculature can result from (1) increase in the transmural hydrostatic

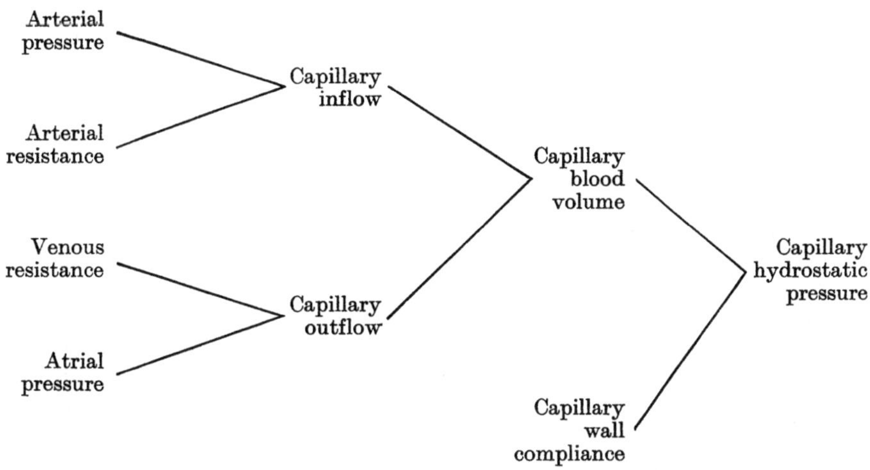

Fig. 1. Immediate and remote determinants of capillary hydrostatic pressure

pressure gradient, (2) decrease in the transmural colloid osmotic pressure gradient, and (3) a combination of (1) and (2). Under these conditions, the outward rate of movement also increases as a function of the microvasculature surface area.

Fig. 1 shows that capillary hydrostatic pressure, one determinant of the transmural hydrostatic pressure gradient, can increase subsequent to (1) rise in aortic pressure, (2) fall in the resistance to flow through precapillary (arterial) vessels, (3) rise in the resistance to flow through postcapillary (venous) vessels, and (4) rise in right atrial pressure (HADDY and SCOTT, 1966). The first two changes increase capillary inflow whereas the latter two changes decrease capillary outflow. These changes in inflow and outflow in turn increase capillary blood volume, one of the two immediate determinants of capillary hydrostatic pressure. All four variables are relevant to systemic administration of vasoactive agents while only precapillary and postcapillary resistances are relevant when administration is local in amounts without general effects. As indicated above, the resistances are determined by the calibers of arteries and veins (which can change actively or passively) and by blood viscosity. The determinants of hydrostatic pressure shown in Fig. 1 can equally well be applied to the venule.

A rise in the transmural hydrostatic pressure gradient can also result from a fall in tissue hydrostatic pressure subsequent, for example, to enhanced absorption of tissue fluid into lymphatic vessels. Whether this is ever a cause of increased water efflux from capillaries is unknown.

A rise in the transmural hydrostatic pressure gradient can occur in the face of a rise in tissue hydrostatic pressure provided the capillary hydrostatic pressure rises more or in the face of a fall in capillary hydrostatic pressure provided tissue hydrostatic pressure falls more.

A decrease in the transmural colloid osmotic pressure gradient and hence an increase in the net fluid movement out of the capillary can occur either because of a fall in the colloid osmotic pressure of plasma, a rise in the colloid osmotic pressure of tissue fluids, or changes in both which are in the same direction but disproportionate.

Since plasma colloid osmotic pressure is a function of the plasma protein concentration, this pressure may fall because of protein loss or water gain by the plasma. Similarly, tissue fluid colloid osmotic pressure may rise either because of protein gain or water loss by tissue fluid. A discussion of the determinants of plasma and tissue fluid protein and water contents is for the most part beyond the scope of this presentation. Within its scope, however, is the change in tissue fluid protein concentration that occurs on alteration of the permeability of the capillary and venule to plasma proteins. An increase in the protein permeability of these structures will raise the concentration of the protein in tissue fluid and hence increase net fluid movement out of the microvascular system.

As has been pointed out previously (LANDIS, 1945–47; VISSCHER et al., 1956) the permeability of the capillary wall is not easy to measure. The rate of movement of small molecules across the wall is theoretically a function of transmural concentration gradient, transmural hydrostatic pressure gradient, and the permeability of the wall. Particularly troublesome is the possibility that the wall permeability to protein may change as a function of the transmural hydrostatic pressure gradient. Thus in order to determine whether an intervention that increases permeability does so by a direct effect on the membrane or indirectly via a change in pressure, it is important to know the protein efflux rate as a function of capillary transmural pressure before and during the intervention. This is crucial if the intervention happens to be one that raises capillary hydrostatic pressure. Under this condition it is possible that an increased rate of protein efflux might be mistakenly attributed to a direct effect of the intervention on the permeation characteristics of the membrane when in fact it wholly or in part resulted indirectly from the rise in pressure.

The classical studies of LANDIS leave little room for doubt that normal capillary membranes under low pressures are only slightly permeable to plasma proteins. This slight permeability may vary from region to region. Studies in the isolated perfused hindlimb of the dog suggest that skeletal muscle capillaries have pores of fairly uniform radius in the range 35 to 45 Å (PAPPENHEIMER, 1953). These may not be anatomic entities since, by electron microscopy, pores are not visible in the capillaries of muscle, lung, and central nervous system. Pores have however been identified in kidney, intestinal villi, endocrine glands, liver, and spleen, being quite sizable in the last two (BENNETT et al., 1959). The appearance of intravenously injected dextrans in leg, cervical, and hepatic lymph suggests that there are leaks permitting passage of particles up to 350 Å (GROTTE, 1956).

With respect to the question of the effect of distension on protein permeability, high pressures have not been studied by the direct methods of LANDIS. While studies using indirect methods are not conclusive (VISSCHER et al., 1956; LANDIS and PAPPENHEIMER, 1963), they suggest that some microvascular surface becomes more permeable to macromolecules as microvascular pressure is elevated (LANDIS et al., 1932; WASSERMAN et al., 1955; SHIRLEY et al., 1957; ROWLEY, 1964; ARESKOG et al., 1968). Any increase in permeability apparently occurs mainly at the level of the venous capillary and venule. These vessels seem to be more distensible than capillaries (BAEZ et al., 1960; ZWEIFACH, 1964a) and more permeable to protein at a given pressure (HAUCK and SCHRÖER, 1968; INTAGLIETTA, 1968). These features may be related to ultrastructural peculiarities. RHODIN (1968) reports that in the rabbit subdermal vascular bed, venous capillaries have an endothelial lining in which there are frequent fenestrations and many small vesicles relative to the arterial capillary.

The surface area available for water transfer can increase either through distension of microvascular vessels already open, through an opening of those that are closed, or both. Thus a rise in microvascular transmural pressure might increase surface area through the first mechanism, particularly at the level of the venule. Opening a closed precapillary sphincter would increase area at all microvascular levels downstream to the sphincter. Obviously the addition of vessels in which the forces do not favor net water efflux will not contribute to edema formation.

The available evidence, while by no means conclusive, suggests that the increase in net fluid movement out of the capillary on local administration of the kinins results both from an increase in the transmural hydrostatic pressure gradient and from a decrease in the transmural colloid osmotic pressure gradient. A contributing factor might be an increase in the microexchange surface area. The evidence for these changes is for the most part indirect. The conclusion that the kinins raise the transmural hydrostatic pressure gradient is deduced from the following observations: (1) the water gain seems to be flow-linked; (2) the water gain is associated with a rise in small vein pressure; (3) water gain does not occur when the capillary hydrostatic pressure is maintained below plasma colloid osmotic pressure.

With respect to the first type of indirect evidence, intravenous infusion of bradykinin does not cause the forelimb to gain weight nor does it increase total blood flow (DAUGHERTY et al., 1968). On the other hand, the filtration seen on intra-arterial infusion is associated with a large increase in blood flow (Fig. 2) and this filtration is attenuated if flow is not allowed to increase (RAHE et al., 1963; DAUGHERTY et al., 1968). Bradykinin, in doses that reduce vascular resistance, also fails to cause edema in the isolated hindlimb preparation perfused at constant flow (DIANA et al., 1967). However, edema does occur in preparations perfused at constant flow when the infusion rate is raised to high levels (RAHE et al., 1963; KJELLMER and ODELRAM, 1965; DIANA et al., 1967). When the infusion is stopped in all these preparations, enhanced rates of filtration vanish as rapidly as the vasodilator response. Of particular relevance to the question of an increase in the transmural hydrostatic pressure gradient is the observation that at least part of the increase in total flow produced by kinins traverses microcirculatory exchange surfaces (PALDINO et al., 1962; HYMAN and PALDINO, 1966; ZWEIFACH, 1966). This observation is also relevant to the question of surface area and is therefore described in detail below.

The second type of indirect evidence suggesting an increase in the transmural hydrostatic pressure gradient is more definitive. The edema seen in the dog forelimb on intra-arterial administration of bradykinin is associated with small vein pressures as high as 28 mm Hg in skin (RAHE et al., 1963; DAUGHERTY et al., 1968) and 43 mm Hg in muscle (Daugherty et al., 1968). Average values for skin and muscle small-vein pressures at two infusion rates are presented in Fig. 2. Since small-vein pressures represent minimal values for capillary hydrostatic pressure, the finding of a raised small-vein pressure further substantiates the conclusion that the kinins raise capillary hydrostatic pressure. When flow is held constant, small-vein pressures do not rise and the edema is

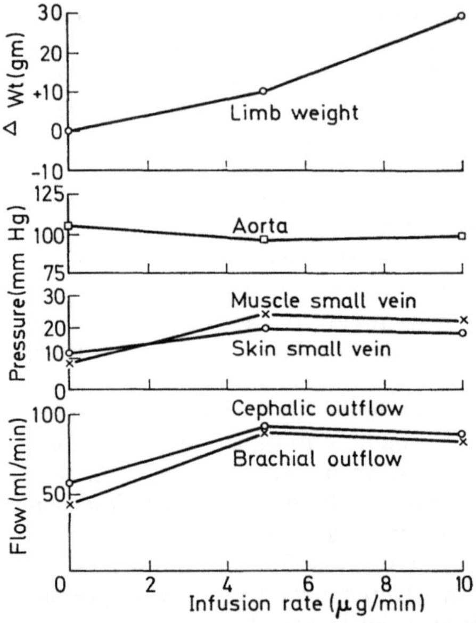

Fig. 2. Average effects of intra-arterially infused bradykinin on weight, small-vein pressures in skin and muscle, and venous outflows from muscle (brachial) and skin (cephalic) of the forelimb of the anesthetized dog ($n = 10$). Limbs were naturally perfused with nerves intact. Measurements were made in the steady state after each infusion rate had been maintained for 1.5 min. (For details, see Daugherty et al., 1968)

greatly attenuated. Intravenous infusion, which fails to produce edema, also fails to raise small-vein pressures.

Finally, particularly compelling indirect evidence that an increase in the net hydrostatic pressure gradient is a factor of importance in the kinin-induced gain in tissue water is provided by studies in isolated fetal and puppy lungs. These preparations do not develop edema despite rapid infusion of bradykinin when perfusion pressure is held constant at 12 mm Hg (Grega et al., 1969). Thus edema does not occur in this tissue when capillary hydrostatic pressure is not permitted to exceed plasma colloid osmotic pressure (see below for another similar study).

These three lines of indirect evidence strongly suggest that the kinins cause tissue water gain in part through their effect on microvascular hydrostatic pressure. It therefore seems appropriate to consider the possible mechanisms of such a pressure rise (Fig. 1). As already pointed out, aortic and right atrial pressures need not be considered when agents are administered locally in amounts without general action. Thus the effect of the kinins on microvascular pressure must be mediated via change in precapillary and/or postcapillary resistances. Numerous studies show that local administration of the kinins produces a large fall in total resistance in most systemic vascular beds (see section on general effects) without doubt resulting mainly from a fall in arterial resistance. For microvascular pressure not to rise in the face of this fall in arterial resistance, there would have to be a proportionate fall in venous resistance. Studies, for the most part, do not support a proportionate fall in venous resistance.

In the dog forelimb, hindlimb, and mesenteric circulations intra-arterial infusion of bradykinin or kallidin produces very little changes or only a slight fall in the resistance to flow through the larger veins (RAHE et al., 1963; CHOU et al., 1965; DIANA et al., 1967; DAUGHERTY et al., 1968). In the study presented in Fig. 2, intra-arterial infusion of bradykinin at 5 and 10 μg/min reduced total resistance without greatly affecting the resistances to flow through the larger veins in both skin and muscle despite an increase in venous intraluminal pressures (DAUGHERTY et al., 1968). Furthermore, in the isolated calf muscle preparation of cats perfused at constant flow, intra-arterial infusion of bradykinin (7 μg/min) has little effect on total vascular volume despite a large fall in total resistance (KJELLMER and ODELRAM, 1965). In the same preparation, other vasodilators (acetylcholine and ATP) increase vascular volume. Constriction of larger veins has even been observed in rat subcutaneous tissue and in rabbit ear after local application of bradykinin (ROWLEY, 1964; GUTH et al., 1966; BOBBIN and GUTH, 1968). On the other hand, small muscular venules (roughly 50 μ) in rat mesentery respond to topical application with dilatation (ZWEIFACH, 1966; ALTURA, 1967), sometimes to an extent proportionately greater than the feeding arteriole (ZWEIFACH, 1966). Whether this venular dilatation is active or passive is unknown. It has been suggested (BOBBIN and GUTH, 1968) that venous constriction is not seen on intra-arterial infusion because of the short half-life of the kinins in blood. In any event, while total postcapillary resistance has not yet been directly measured during local administration of the kinins, the available evidence indicates that it does not fall in proportion to precapillary resistance. A large fall in arterial resistance in the face of very little change in venous resistance or an actual rise in venous resistance would raise microvascular blood volume and pressure (Fig. 1)[3].

Analogous changes are seen on local administration of histamine. This agent causes rapid water efflux on local administration (T. LEWIS, 1927) but not on systemic administration (DEYRUP, 1944; REMINGTON and BAKER, 1958). The water efflux seen on local administration is flow-linked (LEWIS, 1927; RAHE et al., 1963; DAUGHERTY et al., 1968) and is associated with elevated small-vein pressures (HADDY, 1960; RAHE et al., 1963; DAUGHERTY et al., 1968; DIANA et al., 1968). Histamine does not produce edema in the isolated fetal and puppy lung perfused at a pressure of 12 mm Hg (GREGA et al., 1969). It therefore seems relevant to the mechanisms of kinin edema to review the changes in microvascular pressure that follow local administration of histamine. In the case of histamine, capillary hydrostatic pressure in human skin has been measured directly by micropuncture (LANDIS, 1929–31). Intradermal administration raises arteriolar capillary hydrostatic pressure to between 32 and 50 mm Hg and venous capillary pressure to between 27 and 39. Evidence from other local studies suggests that this rise in capillary hydrostatic pressure results from a fall in arterial resistance which is out of proportion to the fall in venous resistance. While topical application produces dilatation of muscular venules in rat mesentery (ALTURA, 1967) and intra-arterial infusion lowers resistance to flow through large veins in the isolated

3. At constant inflow, a fall in arterial resistance without a change in venous resistance could affect microvascular pressure only through a redistribution of flow. It is of interest that small-vein pressure does not rise, and edema is attenuated under this condition (RAHE et al., 1963; DIANA et al., 1967; DAUGHERTY et al., 1968).

dog hindlimb (Diana et al., 1968), intra-arterial infusion at rates without general effects has very little effect on the resistance to flow through large veins in the dog forelimb (Haddy, 1960; Rahe et al., 1963; Daugherty et al., 1968). Measurements of vascular volume suggest very little effect on postcapillary resistance in skeletal muscle (Kjellmer and Odelram, 1965), even in preparations that appear to respond with venous dilatation to other vasodilator substances (acetylcholine and ATP). Furthermore, venous constriction has been observed in other preparations (Inchley, 1926; Lee, 1957; Rowley, 1964).

The evidence that the colloid osmotic pressure gradient decreases after local administration of the kinins is also entirely indirect. As indicated above, the increase in net fluid movement out of the capillary is associated with an increase in the rate of appearance of extravascular protein. This has been demonstrated by measuring the size of skin stain at the site of intracutaneous injection of kinins in animals with plasma proteins labeled with pontamine sky blue (Bhoola et al., 1960), Evans blue (Konzett and Stürmer, 1960; Erdös et al., 1963; Carr and Wilhelm, 1964; Zweifach, 1966) or trypan blue (Rocha e Silva, 1940; Rubin et al., 1963), by observing the appearance of blueing of limb skin on intra-arterial injection in animals with circulating Evans blue (Berkinshaw-Smith et al., 1962), and by observing the spread of fluorescence in mesenteric interstitial fluid on topical application in animals with circulating fluorochromated plasma proteins (Witte et al., 1961). In addition, it has been shown that intra-arterial infusion of bradykinin increases lymph flow and protein concentration in the hindleg of the dog (Stürmer, 1966). These findings may be interpreted to mean that the filtrate and the interstitial fluid have higher than usual protein concentrations.

In order to determine whether the concentration of protein in the filtrate does in fact increase, simultaneous measurements of the efflux rates of protein and water from the microvessels would be needed. The effect on concentration of protein in interstitial fluid could be determined by sampling interstitial fluid and measuring the variable directly or by calculating the variable from measurements of tissue fluid water and protein content (the problems encountered in estimating capillary permeability to protein from lymph protein concentration have been presented previously (Visscher et al., 1956). Such studies are not available for the kinins, but it has been demonstrated that they increase the efflux rate of macromolecules such as colloid gold, 25–100 Å (Frimmer, 1961) and carbon particles, 200 Å (Rowley, 1964; Majno et al., 1967) from the microvessels. Furthermore, the edema produced by intra-arterially infused bradykinin in isolated constantly perfused cat skeletal muscle disappears more slowly than the edema produced by acetylcholine and ATP (Kjellmer and Odelram, 1965). In the latter study it was also observed that bradykinin increases the capillary filtration coefficient (ml/min/mm Hg/100 g), and this was concluded to result from both an increase in capillary surface area and an increase in capillary permeability. The latter was considered to be the case because (1) the capillary filtration coefficient during bradykinin infusion was higher than that due to increased surface area alone, i.e. the coefficient exceeded the coefficient obtained during exercise which produced comparable vasodilatation; (2) the volume remained elevated after discontinuance of the infusion. It should be pointed out, however, that large-vein pressure rather than capillary hydrostatic pressure was utilized in the calculation of the capillary filtration coefficient.

Such calculations must be interpreted with caution, particularly when drugs capable of producing venomotion are infused. In such studies it is always necessary to estimate the fraction of the applied venous pressure which is transmitted to the capillary, and there is always the added danger that the very agent under study might change the true fraction by altering venous compliance. Furthermore, while filtration may be a linear function of capillary pressure over the lower range of pressures (LANDIS and PAPPENHEIMER, 1963), this has not yet been proven to be the case for higher pressures (see above). Thus, even if the agent does not alter the fraction of applied venous pressure transmitted to the capillary, interpretation of the calculated coefficient is still difficult if the agent is one potentially capable of raising capillary hydrostatic pressure. With respect to the second criterion for enhanced permeability, slow disappearance of the edema at best indicates only that the tissue fluid has a high protein concentration but sheds no light on the mechanism of its occurrence.

While the observations on the penetration of carbon particles and the disappearance rate of edema strongly suggest that the interstitial fluid protein concentration actually increases, more direct measurements, such as those carried out with histamine, are needed before this can be stated with complete assurance. Histamine, in greater than threshold doses, apparently produces an increase in the extravascular concentration of protein in rat skin. The relative net efflux of water and protein was studied by comparing the water increment calculated on the basis of radioactive protein accumulation with the actual increment in the water content of the tissue determined by measurements of wet and dry tissue weights (ASCHEIM and ZWEIFACH, 1962). At the threshold dose, the skin appeared to gain more water than protein. At higher doses the increment of tissue water and protein approached that of plasma, and at the highest doses the ratio of protein to tissue water actually exceeded that of plasma, indicating either an accelerated removal of water from the site or a differential protein retention by the skin. With the intermediate and higher doses, the protein concentration of interstitial fluid was clearly elevated. Direct measurements suggest this is also the case for interstitial fluid in the histamine wheal of human skin (T. LEWIS, 1927). Hence, at least in high concentrations, histamine appears to decrease the transmural colloid osmotic pressure gradient.

With respect to the possible mechanisms whereby bradykinin could induce an increase in tissue fluid protein concentration, recent studies in the lung are of interest. Isolated rabbit lungs perfused with blood at constant inflow and infused with 6 to 200 μg bradykinin/min fail to show weight changes indicative of net outward transvascular fluid movement; nor does bradykinin change the rate of filtration seen when capillary pressure is elevated by raising left atrial pressure (HAUGE et al., 1966a). Similarly, when isolated fetal and puppy lungs are perfused at a constant pressure which is less than plasma colloid osmotic pressure, bradykinin does not produce lung edema (GREGA et al., 1969). This is also true for histamine. In addition, when the lung is perfused at a constant pressure sufficient to cause steady filtration, histamine does not increase the rate of filtration (GREGA et al., 1969). Thus these studies fail to provide evidence for a direct effect of bradykinin or histamine on microvascular membranes and indirectly support the hypothesis that the apparent increase in interstitial fluid protein concentration in systemic organs is secondary to effects of increased pressure on the membrane.

In this regard several other studies are of interest. ROWLEY (1964) observed that local administration of bradykinin, histamine, or serotonin causes venous constriction in rat subcutaneous tissue. This was associated with venular dilatation and penetration of 200-Å carbon particles between the junctions of the endothelial cells lining the venules at the site of injection. The duration of the increased penetration was short and corresponded with the duration of the venous constriction. Drug antagonists which inhibited venous constriction also inhibited increased penetration. In perfusion experiments, an elevated venous pressure produced venular dilatation and increased venular penetration equal to that produced by the three agents. Furthermore, during retrograde perfusion of hindquarters, the agents did not increase the penetration of the particles. These observations suggested to the investigator that the increased penetration during normal perfusion results from an elevated pressure in the venules which drain the constricted veins.

It has, however, been reported that venous constriction is only rarely seen in the small veins of striated muscle (Majno et al., 1967). Vessels of the exposed rat and rabbit cremaster were photographed during topical application of histamine, serotonin, and bradykinin; the occurrence of vascular leakage was tested by intravenous injection of carbon black. The first observed event was arteriolar dilatation. This was followed by labeling of the venules with carbon and inconstant venular dilatation. Constriction of a small vein was observed in only 1 of 76 experiments (these investigators did observe transient constriction of larger veins on topical application of bradykinin in an everted skin flap preparation similar to the one used by Rowley). It was concluded that venous spasm cannot account for the leakage, though such leakage may be enhanced by venous spasm whenever it may occur. As an alternative mechanism, the authors proposed a direct effect on the venular endothelium which induces it to contract, and the sequence was described as follows: "There is an immediate dilatation of the arterioles, which will raise the pressure in both capillaries and venules. At the same time, the endothelial cells of the venules respond by contraction; since they contract in a vessel under high pressure, their pulling does not result in a decrease in diameter of the lumen, but in a partial detachment of the intercellular connections. If the larger veins contract this may help to raise the intravenular pressure, as does the arteriolar dilatation; but it is not a necessary event." This proposal is similar to one made by Zweifach (1964a) except he interprets the endothelial change as swelling.

With regard to the question of venous constriction, it has been observed in the rat mesenteric circulation (Zweifach, 1964b, 1966; Weiner and Altura 1967) that bradykinin and serotonin have a synergistic action characterized by intense venular spasm followed by capillary stasis and extravasation of red cells through defects in the walls of the postcapillary venules. The synergism appears to be peculiar to this combination of agents. It was proposed that the rhexis of the postcapillary collecting venules is brought about by a local increase of intravascular pressure as a consequence of severe venular constriction (Weiner and Altura, 1967).

Finally, both direct and indirect studies indicate that local administration of the kinins increases the microvascular surface available for exchange. Topical application or intra-arterial administration of bradykinin to the mesentery of the rat produces, by direct observation, a widening of and an increase in flow through the arterioles and opens precapillary sphincters to increase flow through a large number of capillaries (Hyman and Paldino, 1966; Zweifach, 1966). The changes following topical and intra-arterial administration to the mouse skeletal muscle are not greatly different (Hyman and Paldino, 1966). Close intra-arterial injection increases the clearance of diffusible substances as well as total blood flow in the skinned hindleg of the cat (Paldino et al., 1962), in the spinotrapezius muscle of the rat (Paldino et al., 1962), and in the calf muscle of man (Coffman and Javett, 1963). Hence local application of bradykinin increases nutritional blood flow, at least in skeletal muscle and mesentery.

This will enhance the effects of a rise in transmural hydrostatic pressure gradient and a fall in transmural colloid osmotic pressure gradient on water efflux from the microvascular system.

Summary

The available evidence, while far from conclusive, suggests that the kinins increase net fluid movement out of the microvascular system both by increasing the transmural hydrostatic pressure gradient and by decreasing the transmural colloid osmotic pressure gradient and that the effects of these two changes are enhanced by an increase in the surface area for filtration. A major question still unanswered concerns the mechanism of the decrease in the colloid osmotic pressure gradient. Is the apparent increase in tissue fluid protein concentration the result of a direct effect on the microvascular membrane or does it arise indirectly via elevated microvascular pressures? Is there a primary effect on the membrane, resulting in passage of protein into tissue fluid thereby raising tissue fluid colloid osmotic pressure and hence enhancing water efflux? Or is the membrane effect secondary to arteriolar dilatation and possibly venous constriction, causing increased microvascular blood volume, pressure, and hence protein permeability? In short, does increased protein permeability result from a primary effect on the membrane, on the vascular smooth muscle, or on both? Studies of the lung fail to provide evidence for a direct effect on the membrane and thus suggest that more attention should be given the possible role of pressure in systemic organs.

References

ALLWOOD, M. J., LEWIS, G. P.: Bradykinin and forearm blood flow. J. Physiol. (Lond.) **170**, 571 (1964).

ALTURA, B. M.: Evaluation of neurohumoral substances in local regulation of blood flow. Amer. J. Physiol. **212**, 1447 (1967).

AMORIM, D. S., MANCO, J. C., FERREIRA, S. H., TANAKA, A., CARDOSO, S. S.: Hemodynamic effects of bradykinin potentiated by a factor contained in the "Bothrops jararaca" venom. Comparative results with eledoisin. Acta physiol. lat-.amer. **17**, 258 (1967).

ANGUISSOLA, A. B., FERUGLIO, F. S., CAMPUS, S., CHIANDUSSI, L., PANDOLFO, G., BERT, G.: The effects of eledoisin and bradykinin on the general and visceral circulation. In: Hypotensive peptides, p. 430, ed. by E. G. ERDÖS, N. BACK and F. SICUTERI. Berlin-Heidelberg-New York: Springer 1966.

ANTONIO, A., ROCHA E SILVA, M.: Coronary vasodilation produced by bradykinin on isolated mammalian heart. Circulat. Res. **11**, 910 (1962).

ARCIDIACONO, F. G., REININGER, E. J., SAPIRSTEIN, L. A.: Effect of bradykinin on total peripheral resistance and regional vascular resistance in the rat. In: 4th European Conf. on Microcirculation, p. 29, ed. by H. HARDERS. Basel and New York: S. Karger 1966.

ARESKOG, N. H., ARFORS, K. E., ARTURSON, G., GROTTE, G., MALMBERG, P.: The transport of macromolecules across the blood lymph barrier. In: Abstracts, p. 6, Internat. Conf. on Microcirculation, Gothenberg, Sweden, 1968.

ARMAN, C. G. VAN, MILLER, L. M.: Close similarity and minor differences between bradykinin and kallidin. J. Pharmacol. exp. Ther. **131**, 366 (1961).

ASCHEIM, E., ZWEIFACH, B. W.: Quantitative studies of protein and water shifts during inflammation. Amer. J. Physiol. **202**, 554 (1962).

BACANER, M. B., LIOY, F., VISSCHER, M. B.: Induced changes in heart metabolism as a primary determinant of heart performance. Amer. J. Physiol. **209**, 519 (1965).

BAEZ, S., LAMPORT, H., BAEZ, A.: Pressure effects in living microscopic vessels. In: Flow properties of blood, ed. by A. COPLEY and G. STAINSBY. New York, N.Y.: Pergamon Press 1960.

— ORKIN, L. R.: Effects of anesthetic on the response of the microcirculation to circulating humors. Anesthesiology **24**, 568 (1963).

BARRACLOUGH, M. A., MILLS, I. H.: Effect of bradykinin on renal function. Clin. Sci. **28**, 69 (1965).

Bennett, H. S., Luft, J. H., Hampton, J. C.: Morphological classification of vertebrate blood capillaries. Amer. J. Physiol. **196**, 381 (1959).
Bergamaschi, M., Glässer, A. H.: Peripheral vasodilator action of eledoisin, bradykinin and nitroglycerin in anesthetized dogs. Circulat. Res. **15**, 371 (1964).
Berkinshaw-Smith, E. M. I., Morgan, R. S., Payling Wright, G.: Permeability response of cerebral and cutaneous blood vessels to vasoactive agents. Nature (Lond.) **196**, 173 (1962).
Bhoola, K. D., Calle, J. D., Schachter, M.: The effect of bradykinin, serum kallikrein and other endogenous substances on capillary permeability in the guinea-pig. J. Physiol. (Lond.) **152**, 75 (1960).
— Morley, J., Schachter, M., Smaje, L. H.: Vasodilatation in the submaxillary gland of the cat. J. Physiol. (Lond.) **179**, 172 (1965).
Bishop, J. M., Harris, P., Segel, N.: The circulatory effects of bradykinin in normal subjects and patients with chronic bronchitis. Brit. J. Pharmacol. **25**, 456 (1965).
Bobbin, R. P., Guth, P. S.: Venoconstriction action of bradykinin. J. Pharmacol. exp. Ther. **160**, 11 (1968).
Boijsen, E., Redman, H. C.: Effect of bradykinin on celiac and superior mesenteric angiography. Invest. Radiol. **1**, 422 (1966).
Buckley, J. P., Bickerton, R. K., Halliday, R. P., Kato, H.: Central effects of peptides on the cardiovascular system. Ann. N.Y. Acad. Sci. **104**, 299 (1963).
Burch, G. E., De Pasquale, N. P.: Bradykinin, digital blood flow, and the arteriovenous anastomoses. Circulat. Res. **10**, 105 (1962).
Carr, J., Wilhelm, D. L.: The evaluation of increased vascular permeability in the skin of guinea-pigs. Aust. J. exp. Biol. med. Sci. **42**, 511 (1964).
Chou, C. C., Dabney, J. M.: Interrelation of ileal wall compliance and vascular resistance. Amer. J. dig. Dis. **12**, 1198 (1967).
— Frohlich, E. D., Texter, E. C., Jr.: A comparative study of the effects of bradykinin, kallidin II and eledoisin on segmental superior mesenteric resistance. J. Physiol. (Lond.) **176**, 1 (1965).
Coffman, J. D.: The effect of aspirin on pain and hand blood flow responses to intra-arterial injection of bradykinin in man. Clin. Pharmacol. Ther. **7**, 26 (1966).
— Javett, S. L.: Calf blood flow and oxygen usage during bradykinin infusions. J. appl. Physiol. **18**, 1003 (1963).
Comline, R. S., Silver, M., Sinclair, D. G.: The effects of bradykinin, angiotensin and acetylcholine on the bovine adrenal medulla. J. Physiol. (Lond.) **196**, 339 (1968).
Croxatto, H., Belmar, J.: Hypertensive effects of bradykinin in rats. Nature (Lond.) **192**, 879 (1961).
Daugherty, R. M., Jr., Scott, J. B., Dabney, J. M., Haddy, F. J.: Local effects of O_2 and CO_2 on limb, renal and coronary vascular resistances. Amer. J. Physiol. **213**, 1102 (1967).
— — Emerson, T. E., Jr., Haddy, F. J.: Comparison of iv and ia infusion of vasoactive agents on dog forelimb blood flow. Amer. J. Physiol. **214**, 611 (1968).
De Freitas, F. M., Faraco, E. Z., De Azevedo, D. F.: General circulatory alterations induced by intravenous infusion of synthetic bradykinin in man. Circulation **29**, 66 (1964).
De Pasquale, N. P., Burch, G. E.: Digital vascular responses to intra-arterial injections of bradykinin, kallidin and eledoisin in man. Circulation **34**, 211 (1966).
Deyrup, I. J.: Circulatory changes following subcutaneous injection of histamine in dogs. Amer. J. Physiol. **142**, 158 (1944).
Diana, J. N., Colantino, R., Haddy, F. J.: Transcapillary fluid movement during vasopressin and bradykinin infusion. Amer. J. Physiol. **212**, 456 (1967).
— Schwinghamer, J., Young, S.: Direct effect of histamine on arterial and venous resistance in isolated dog hindlimb. Amer. J. Physiol. **214**, 494 (1968).
Elliott, D. F., Horton, E. W., Lewis, G. P.: Actions of pure bradykinin. J. Physiol. (Lond.) **153**, 473 (1960).
— Lewis, G. P.: Methionyl-lysyl-bradykinin, a new kinin from ox blood. Biochem. J. **95**, 437 (1965).
Emerson, T. E., Jr.: Changes of venous return and other hemodynamic parameters during bradykinin infusion. Amer. J. Physiol. **212**, 1455 (1967).
— Daugherty, R. M., Jr., Scott, J. B., Haddy, F. J.: Local effect of bradykinin on resistance to blood flow through isolated gracilis muscle. Unpublished observations (1967).
Erdös, E. G., Wohler, J. R., Levine, M. I.: Blocking of the in vivo effects of bradykinin and kallidin with carboxypeptidase B. J. Pharmacol. exp. Ther. **142**, 327 (1963).
Erspamer, V., Glässer, A.: The action of eledoisin on the systemic arterial blood pressure of some experimental animals. Brit. J. Pharmacol. **20**, 516 (1963).

FELDBERG, W., LEWIS, G. P.: The action of peptides on the adrenal medulla release of adrenaline by bradykinin and angiotensin. J. Physiol. (Lond.) **171**, 98 (1964).
— — Further studies on the effects of peptides on the suprarenal medulla of cats. J. Physiol. (Lond.) **178**, 239 (1965).
FERUGLIO, F. S., GRECO, F., CESANO, L., INDOVINA, D., SARDI, G., CHIANDUSSI, L.: Effect of drug infusion on the systemic and splanchnic circulation. I. Bradykinin infusion in normal subjects. Clin. Sci. **26**, 487 (1964).
FOX, R. N., GOLDSMITH, R., KIDD, J. D., LEWIS, G. P.: Bradykinin as a vasodilator in man. J. Physiol. (Lond.) **157**, 589 (1961).
FRIMMER, M.: Beeinflussung der Durchlässigkeit von Blutcapillaren der Kaninchenhaut für Makromoleküle durch einige biogene, gefäßaktive Substanzen. Naunyn-Schmiedebergs Arch. exp. Path. Pharmak. **242**, 390 (1961).
FURUYAMA, T., SUZUKI, C., SAITO, H., ONOZAWA, Y., SHIOJI, R., RIKIMARU, S., ABE, K., YOSHINAGA, K.: Effect of bradykinin and eledoisin on renal function in the dog. Tohoku J. exp. Med. **89**, 69 (1966).
GERSMEYER, E. F., SPITZBARTH, H.: Über Kreislaufwirkungen von synthetischem Bradykinin beim Menschen und beim wachen Hund. Klin. Wschr. **39**, 1227 (1961).
GILFOIL, T. M., KLAVINS, I.: 5-Hydroxytryptamine, bradykinin and histamine as mediators of inflammatory hyperesthesia. Amer. J. Physiol. **208**, 867 (1965).
GILL, J. R., JR., MELMON, K. L., GILLESPIE, L., JR., BARTTER, F. C.: Bradykinin and renal function in normal man: Effects of adrenergic blockade. Amer. J. Physiol. **209**, 844 (1965).
GOLDBERG, L. I., DOLLERY, C. T., PENTECOST, B. L.: Effects of intrarenal infusions of bradykinin and acetylcholine on renal blood flow. J. clin. Invest. **44**, 1052 (1965).
GREAVES, M., SHUSTER, S.: Responses of skin blood vessels to bradykinin, histamine and 5-hydroxytryptamine. J. Physiol. (Lond.) **193**, 255 (1967).
GREGA, G., SCOTT, J. B., DAUGHERTY, R. M., JR., HADDY, F. J.: Mechanism of edema formation by bradykinin and histamine. Fed. Proc. **28**, 646 (1969).
GREGG, D. E.: Effect of coronary perfusion pressure or coronary flow on oxygen usage of the myocardium. Circulat. Res. **13**, 497 (1963).
GROTTE, G.: Passage of dextran molecules across the blood lymph barrier. Acta chir. scand., Suppl. **211** (1956).
GUTH, P. S., BOBBIN, R., CANO, G., AMARO, J.: Venoconstriction induced by bradykinin in the rabbit ear. In: Hypotensive peptides, p. 396, ed. by E. G. ERDÖS, N. BACK, and F. SICUTERI. Berlin-Heidelberg-New York: Springer 1966.
— CANO, G., JARAMILLO, J.: The effect of bradykinin on vascular smooth muscle. Ann. N.Y. Acad. Sci. **104**, 69 (1963).
GUZMAN, F., BRAUN, C., LIM, R. K. S.: Visceral pain and the pseudoaffective response to intra-arterial injection of bradykinin and other algesic agents. Arch. int. Pharmacodyn. **136**, 353 (1962).
HADDY, F. J.: Effect of histamine on small and large vessel pressures in the dog foreleg. Amer. J. Physiol. **198**, 161 (1960).
— CHOU, C. C., SCOTT, J. B., DABNEY, J. M.: Intestinal vascular responses to naturally occurring vasoactive substances. Gastroenterology **52**, 444 (1967).
— SCOTT, J. B.: Cardiovascular pharmacology. Ann. Rev. Pharmacol. **6**, 49 (1966).
— — Current evaluation of the roles of metabolically linked vasoactive chemicals in local regulation of blood flow. Physiol. Rev. **48**, 688 (1968).
HARRISON, D. C., HENRY, W. L., PASSO, B., MILLER, H. A.: Circulatory response to bradykinin before and after autonomic nervous system blockade. Amer. J. Physiol. **214**, 1035 (1968).
HAUCK, G., SCHRÖER, H.: The transmural passage of proteins in the terminal stream bed in relation to the "gradient of vascular permeability." In: Abstracts, p. 75, Internat. Conf. on Microcirculation, Gothenburg, Sweden, 1968.
HAUGE, A., LUNDE, P. K. M., WAALER, B. A.: Bradykinin and pulmonary vascular permeability in isolated blood-perfused rabbit lungs. In: Hypotensive peptides, p. 385, ed. by E. ERDÖS, N. BACK, and F. SICUTERI. Berlin-Heidelberg-New York: Springer 1966a.
— — — The effect of bradykinin, kallidin and eledoisin upon pulmonary vascular bed of an isolated blood perfused rabbit lung preparation. Acta physiol. scand. **66**, 269 (1966b).
HEYMANS, C., NEIL, E.: Reflexogenic areas of the cardiovascular system. London: J. and A. Churchill Ltd. 1958.
HIRVONIN, L., KOROBKIN, M., SONNENSCHEIN, R. R., WRIGHT, D. L.: Depression of contractile force of skeletal muscle by intra-arterial vasodilator drugs. Circulat. Res. **14**, 525 (1964).
HOLDSTOCK, D. J., MATHIAS, A. P., SCHACHTER, M.: A comparative study of kinin, kallidin, and bradykinin. Brit. J. Pharmacol. **12**, 149 (1957).
HOLTZ, B., HEICHE, B., BARCK, S.: Bradykinin and kallidin. Experientia (Basel) **18**, 184 (1962).

Hyman, C., Ballard, K. W.: Effect of bradykinin on blood flow in skeletal muscle of pentolinium-blocked cats. Proc. Soc. exp. Biol. Med. (N.Y.) **121**, 932 (1966).
— Paldino, R. T.: Influence of intravascular and topically administered bradykinin on microcirculation of several tissues. In: 4th European Conf. on Microcirculation, ed. by H. Harders. Basel and New York: S. Karger 1966.
Inchley, O.: Histamine shock. J. Physiol. (Lond.) **61**, 282 (1926).
Intaglietta, M.: Pressure permeability relation in the rabbit omentum capillaries. In: Abstracts, p. 86, Internat. Conf. on Microcirculation, Gothenburg, Sweden, 1968.
Jacobson, E. D.: Hemodynamic effects of bradykinin and gastrin in the stomach. Amer. Heart J. **68**, 214 (1964).
— The circulation of the stomach. Gastroenterology **48**, 85 (1965).
Kjellmer, I., Odelram, H.: The effect of some physiological vasodilators on the vascular bed of skeletal muscle. Acta physiol. scand. **63**, 94 (1965).
Kontos, H. A., Magee, J. H., Shapiro, W., Patterson, J. L.: General and regional circulatory effects of synthetic bradykinin in man. Circulat. Res. **14**, 351 (1964).
Konzett, H., Stürmer, E.: Biological activity of synthetic polypeptides with bradykinin-like properties. Brit. J. Pharmacol. **15**, 544 (1960).
Krivoy, W., Kroeger, D.: The preservation of bradykinin by phenothiazines in vitro. Brit. J. Pharmacol. **22**, 329 (1964).
Landis, E. M.: Micro-injection studies of capillary blood pressure in human skin. Heart **15**, 209 (1929–31).
— Capillary permeability and the factors affecting the composition of capillary filtrate. Ann. N.Y. Acad. Sci. **46**, 713 (1945–47).
— Jonas, L., Angevine, M., Erb, W.: The passage of fluid and protein through the human capillary wall during venous congestion. J. clin. Invest. **11**, 717 (1932).
— Pappenheimer, J. R.: Exchange of substances through the capillary wall. In: Handbook of physiology, sect. II: Circulation, vol. II. Washington: Amer. Physiol. Soc. 1963.
Lang, W. J., Pearson, L.: Studies on the pressor responses produced by bradykinin and kallidin. Brit. J. Pharmacol. **32**, 330 (1968).
Lecomte, J., Troquet, J., Cession-Fossion, A.: Sur la nature de l'hypertension arterielle provoquée par la bradykinine et la kallidin. Arch. int. Pharmacodyn. **147**, 518 (1964).
— — Dresse, A.: Stimulation medullo-surrenalienne par la bradykinine. Arch. int. Physiol. Biochim. **69**, 89 (1961).
Lee, J. S.: Microscopic observations on the action of histamine on small blood vessels. Amer. J. Physiol. **190**, 503 (1957).
Lewis, G. P., Reit, E.: The action of angiotensin and bradykinin on the superior cervical ganglion of the cat. J. Physiol. (Lond.) **179**, 538 (1965).
Lewis, T.: The blood vessels of the human skin and their responses. London: Shaw 1927.
Lochner, W., Parratt, J. R.: A comparison of the effects of locally and systemically administered kinins on coronary blood flow and myocardial metabolism. Brit. J. Pharmacol. **26**, 17 (1966).
Majno, G., Gilmore, V., Leventhal, M.: On the mechanism of vascular leakage caused by histamine-type mediators. Circulat. Res. **21**, 833 (1967).
Mason, D. T., Melmon, K. L.: Effects of bradykinin on forearm venous tone and vascular resistance in man. Circulat. Res. **17**, 106 (1965).
Maxwell, G. M., Elliott, R. B., Kneebone, G. M.: Effects of bradykinin on the systemic and coronary vascular bed of the intact dog. Circulat. Res. **10**, 359 (1962).
McCarthy, D. A., Potter, D. E., Nicolaides, E. D.: An *in vivo* estimation of the potencies and half-lives of synthetic bradykinin and kallidin. J. Pharmacol. exp. Ther. **148**, 117 (1965).
Miele, E., De Natale, G.: Modification of pressor effects of some vasoactive polypeptides in the rat by guanethidine, propanolol and related agents. Brit. J. Pharmacol. **29**, 8 (1967).
Montague, D., Rosas, R., Bohr, D. F.: Bradykinin: Vascular relaxant, cardiac stimulant. Science **141**, 907 (1963).
Montgomery, E. H., Kroeger, D. C.: Bradykinin relaxation of duodenum. Fed. Proc. **26**, 465 (1967).
Moog, E., Fischer, J.: Die Wirkung des Histamins, Serotonins, Bradykinins, Eledoisins und Hypertensins auf isoliert durchströmte Arterien-, Venen- und Bronchienpräparate der Meerschweinchenlunge. Naunyn-Schmiedebergs Arch. exp. Path. Pharmak. **249**, 384 (1964).
Murphy, G. P., Homsy, E. G., Scott, W. W.: Evaluation of pharmacologically induced renal vasodilation. J. surg. Res. **5**, 525 (1965).
Nakano, J.: Effects of synthetic bradykinin on the cardiovascular system. Arch. int. Pharmacodyn. **157**, 1 (1965).
— Kusakari, T.: Effect of bradykinin and eledoisin on the regional circulation. Angiology **17**, 333 (1966).

Northover, B. J.: The effect of anti-inflammatory drugs on vascular smooth muscle. Brit. J. Pharmacol. **31**, 483 (1967).
Olmsted, F., Page, I. H.: Hemodynamic effects of eledoisin, kallidin II, and bradykinin in unanesthetized dogs. Amer. J. Physiol. **203**, 951 (1962).
Paldino, R. L., Hyman, C., Lenthall, J.: Bradykinin-induced increase in total and effective blood flow in skeletal muscle. Circulat. Res. **11**, 847 (1962).
Pappenheimer, J. R.: Passage of molecules through capillary walls. Physiol. Rev. **33**, 387 (1953).
Parratt, J. R.: A comparison of the effects of the plasma kinins, bradykinin and kallidin, on myocardial blood flow and metabolism. Brit. J. Pharmacol. **22**, 34 (1964).
Pearson, L., Lang, W. J.: A comparison in conscious and anesthetized dogs of the effect on blood pressure of bradykinin, eledoisin and kallikrein. Europ. J. Pharmacol. **2**, 83 (1967).
Poisner, A. M., Douglas, W. W.: The requirement for calcium in adrenomedullary secretion evoked by histamine, serotonin, angiotensin and bradykinin. Fed. Proc. **24**, 488 (1965).
Rahe, G., Russell, T., Scott, J., Haddy, F.: Comparison of vasodilator and edemogenic actions of bradykinin and histamine in dog forelimb. Clin. Res. **11**, 54 (1963).
Remington, J. W., Baker, C. H.: Blood and plasma specific gravity changes during acute alterations in hemodynamics in splenectomized dogs. Circulat. Res. **6**, 146 (1958).
Rhodin, J. A. G.: Ultrastructural differences between arterial and venous capillaries. In: Abstracts, p. 130, Internat. Conf. on Microcirculation, Gothenburg, Sweden, 1968.
Robinson, R. L.: Stimulation of the catecholamine output of the isolated perfused adrenal gland of the dog by angiotensin and bradykinin. J. Pharmacol. exp. Ther. **156**, 252 (1967).
Rocha e Silva, M.: Kallikrein and histamine. Nature (Lond.) **145**, 591 (1940).
— The physiological significance of bradykinin. Ann. N.Y. Acad. Sci. **104**, 190 (1963).
— Couado, A. P., Ramos, A. O.: Potentiation of duration of the vasodilator effect of bradykinin by sympatholytic drugs and by reserpine. J. Pharmacol. exp. Ther. **128**, 217 (1960).
Rosas, R., Montague, D., Gross, M., Bohr, D. F.: Cardiac action of vasoactive polypeptides in the rat. Circulat. Res. **16**, 150 (1965).
Rowe, G. G., Afonso, S., Castillo, C. A., Lioy, F., Lugo, J. E., Crumpton, C. W.: The systemic and coronary hemodynamic effects of synthetic bradykinin. Amer. Heart J. **65**, 656 (1963).
Rowley, D. A.: Venous constriction as the cause of increased vascular permeability produced by 5-hydroxytryptamine, histamine, bradykinin and 48/80 in the rat. Brit. J. Path. **45**, 56 (1964).
Rubin, B., Waugh, M. H., Loffan, R. J., O'Keefe, E., Craver, B. N.: Effects on smooth muscle and blood vessels of polypeptides related to bradykinin and to kallidin. Proc. Soc. exp. Biol. Med. (N.Y.) **113**, 328 (1963).
Saameli, K., Eskes, T. K. A. B.: Bradykinin and the cardiovascular system. Amer. J. Physiol. **203**, 261 (1962).
Scott, J. B., Daugherty, R. M., Jr., Dabney, J. M., Haddy, F. J.: Role of chemical factors in regulation of flow through kidney, hindlimb and heart. Amer. J. Physiol. **208**, 813 (1965).
Shimamoto, T., Numano, F., Fiyita, T., Ishioka, T., Atsumi, T.: Treatment of experimental and human atherosclerosis with bradykinin-antagonist, pyridinolcarbamate: A preliminary report. In: Hypotensive peptides, p. 506, ed. by E. G. Erdös, N. Back, and F. Sicuteri. Berlin-Heidelberg-New York: Springer 1966.
Shirley, H. H., Wolfram, C. G., Wasserman, K., Mayerson, H. S.: Capillary permeability to macromolecules: Stretched pore phenomenon. Amer. J. Physiol. **190**, 189 (1957).
Starling, E. H.: On the absorption of fluids from the connective tissue spaces. J. Physiol. (Lond.) **19**, 312 (1896).
Staszewska-Barczak, J., Vane, J. R.: The release of catecholamines from the adrenal medulla by peptides. Brit. J. Pharmacol. **30**, 655 (1967).
Stürmer, E.: The influence of intra-arterial infusions of synthetic bradykinin on flow and composition of lymph in dogs. In: Hypotensive peptides, p. 368, ed. by E. G. Erdös, N. Back, and F. Sicuteri. Berlin-Heidelberg-New York: Springer 1966.
— Berde, B.: A pharmacological comparison between synthetic bradykinin and synthetic kallidin. J. Pharmacol. exp. Ther. **139**, 38 (1963a).
— — A comparative pharmacological study of synthetic eledoisin and synthetic bradykinin. J. Pharmacol. exp. Ther. **140**, 349 (1963b).
— — Bradykinin und Eledoisin, vergleichende pharmakologische Untersuchungen. Naunyn-Schmiedebergs Arch. exp. Path. Pharmak. **246**, 21 (1963c).
— Cerletti, A.: Das Bradykininödem der Rattenpfote. Helv. physiol. pharmacol. Acta **19**, C 32 (1961).
Takacs, L., Albert, K.: Action of bradykinin on cardiac output and blood distribution in rats. Arch. int. Pharmacodyn. **155**, 117 (1965).

Trendelenburg, U.: Observations on the ganglion-stimulating action of angiotensin and bradykinin. J. Pharmacol. exp. Ther. 154, 418 (1966).
Visscher, M. B., Haddy, F. J., Stephens, G.: The physiology and pharmacology of lung edema. Pharmacol. Rev. 8, 389 (1956).
Vogt, M.: Release of medullary amines from the isolated perfused adrenal gland of the dog. Brit. J. Pharmacol. 24, 561 (1965).
Waaler, B. A.: Effect of bradykinin in the isolated perfused dog lung preparation. J. Physiol. (Lond.) 157, 475 (1961).
Wasserman, K., Lobb, L., Mayerson, H. S.: Capillary permeability to macromolecules. Circulat. Res. 3, 594 (1955).
Webster, M. E., Gilmore, J. P.: Influence of kallidin-10 on renal function. Amer. J. Physiol. 206, 714 (1964).
— Skinner, N. S., Jr., Powell, W. J., Jr.: Role of the kinins in vasodilatation of skeletal muscle of the dog. Amer. J. Physiol. 212, 553 (1967).
Weiner, R., Altura, B. M.: Serotonin-bradykinin synergism in the mammalian capillary bed. Proc. Soc. exp. Biol. Med. (N.Y.) 124, 494 (1967).
Wiegershausen, B.: Pharmacodynamics of bradykinin-vasoconstriction in the hindlimb of cat. In: Abstracts, p. 186, Third Internat. Congr. of Pharmacol., 1966.
Witte, S., Schricker, K. T., Schmid, E.: Zur Wirkung von synthetischem Bradykinin auf die Gefäßpermeabilität. Arzneimittel-Forsch. (Drug Res.) 11, 619 (1961).
Zweifach, B. W.: Microcirculatory aspects of tissue injury. Ann. N.Y. Acad. Sci. 116, 831 (1964a).
— The behavior of the vascular barrier during tissue injury. Bibl. anat. (Basel) 4, 21 (1964b).
— Microcirculatory effects of polypeptides. In: Hypotensive peptides, p. 451, ed. by E. G. Erdös, N. Back, and F. Sicuteri. Berlin-Heidelberg-New York: Springer 1966.

Effects of Bradykinin on the Kidney and Gastrointestinal Organs

EUGENE D. JACOBSON

A. Kidney

The action of kinins on renal water diuresis is variable and is influenced by the route of administration and the animal species employed. Excretion of sodium appears to depend upon the dosage of polypeptide used. Excretion of other electrolytes is increased by bradykinin. Renal blood flow and blood volume are augmented by injection of the kinin through both local and distant cardiovascular events. There are interesting, albeit speculative, neuroendocrine relationships in the regulation of renal functions by steroid and polypeptide hormones, which may involve kinins or kallikrein.

Urinary kinin and bradykinin caused antidiuresis in dogs and rats (WERLE and ERDÖS, 1954; BARAC, 1957; STÜRMER and BERDE, 1963). The antidiuretic response appeared to be mediated through the release of vasopressin from the posterior pituitary (ROCHA E SILVA, JR., and MALNIC, 1964). In addition, bradykinin diminished glomerular filtration rate (GILL et al., 1965). Intravenous or intraperitoneal routes of injection were used in the preceding reports. When kinins or kallikrein were administered intra-arterially in dogs, a diuretic response was observed (SZAKÁLL, 1932; HEIDENREICH et al., 1964; KÖVER et al., 1968). In man, intravenous infusion of bradykinin was also diuretic (MERTZ, 1963a, b, 1967a, b; GILL et al., 1965) and augmented clearance of PAH and inulin and osmolal clearance (MERTZ, 1967a, b).

Sodium excretion was increased in human subjects by intravenous doses of 100 ng/min per kilogram body weight (GILL et al., 1965). At four times this dose there was no further loss of cation. This was not, however, confirmed in dogs (KÖVER et al., 1968). Excretion of potassium and total solute was increased by kallidin and bradykinin (WEBSTER and GILMORE, 1964; HEIDENREICH et al., 1964; BARRACLOUGH and MILLS, 1965).

Bradykinin is a potent arteriolar dilator in the kidney, as in other organs (GOLDBERG et al., 1965; NAKANO, 1965; BARRACLOUGH and MILLS, 1965; MURPHY et al., 1965; FURUYANA et al., 1966; FREED et al., 1968; KÖVER et al., 1968). Systemic infusion of bradykinin increases renal blood flow (MERTZ, 1963a, b; BARER, 1963; GILL et al., 1965), and both bradykinin and kallidin increase renal volume (STÜRMER and BERDE, 1963). These actions of the polypeptides are probably accountable on the basis of an increased cardiac output, direct dilator action on arteriolar smooth muscle, and an increase in capillary filtration (see p. 370).

Vasoactive polypeptides interact with corticosteroid hormones (ROSAS, 1963), induce release of vasopressin (ROCHA E SILVA, JR., and MALNIC, 1964) and catecholamines (LECOMTE et al., 1961; FELDBERG and LEWIS, 1964, 1965; POISNER and DOUGLAS, 1965; STASZEWSKA-BARCZAK and VANE, 1967; ROBINSON, 1967), and may involve the angiotensin system (GILL et al., 1965). Actions of some polypeptides on renal function may be secondary to release of these agents. There is suggestive evidence implicating release of polypeptides in renal hypertensive disease (ROSAS, 1963; DOLLERY et al., 1965a, b). However, the role of kinins in renal function during health and disease remains a matter for future experimentation.

B. Gastrointestinal Organs

Among the substances present in gastrointestinal tissue are gastrin and kallikrein. It has been amply demonstrated that gastrin meets certain necessary physiological criteria, permitting the conclusion that gastrin is a normal direct chemical regulator of gastrointestinal function, especially secretion. These criteria include: (1) the polypeptide is normally present in a specific anatomical locus, the antral mucosa (EDKINS, 1905; KOMAROV, 1938); (2) ablation of this tissue depresses gastric secretory function (LANGLOIS and GROSSMAN, 1950); (3) physiological stimuli, such as vagal stimulation or food in the stomach, induce the release of gastrin and subsequent increase in secretory rate (PE THIEN and SCHOFIELD, 1959); (4) prevention of gastrin release after activating the vagi reduces the secretory response (ANDERSON and OLBE, 1964); (5) infusion of exogenous synthetic or extracted gastrin mimics all known effects of endogenous gastrin release (GROSSMAN, 1968); and (6) the effects of gastrin are observable in the denervated or innervated stomach (GROSSMAN, 1968).

Aside from its physical presence in the stomach (JOHANSON and MARTINSON, 1963; FREY et al., 1968), kallikrein does not meet the criteria outlined above for gastrin. Like histamine, serotonin, heparin, prostaglandins, and many other agents, kallikrein is present in the wall of the gut, but its function in the normal life of the enteric organs awaits delineation.

Bradykinin is a powerful vasodilator in both the stomach (JACOBSON, 1964) and the circulation of the gut (see p. 367 and SHEHADEH et al., 1969). It is a more potent arteriolar dilator than gastrin, histamine, or acetylcholine in these vascular beds. In the mesenteric vasculature, dilator responses were observed with intra-arterial doses as low as 100 ng/min. Cessation of drug infusion was followed by restoration of normal blood flow within a few minutes.

In the stomach, intra-arterial bradykinin caused an increased volume of secretion, but the pH rose, indicating a transudation of extracellular fluid from the mucosa rather than true secretion of acid (JACOBSON, 1964). Systemic infusion of bradykinin had no effect on either gastric secretion or mucosal blood flow (personal observation).

There is evidence that kallikrein is present in the normal pancreas (HILTON and JONES, 1968; FREY et al., 1968), and possibly that it may be released from that organ in pancreatitis (THAL et al., 1963). A role has also been claimed for bradykinin in several diseases involving the gut, i.e., carcinoid, dumping syndrome, and septic shock (p. 550).

For many years it was believed that the chemical mediator causing gastrointestinal symptoms and flushing of the skin in carcinoid syndrome was 5-hydroxytryptamine. Recent evidence (ZEITLIN and SMITH, 1966a, b; MELMON, 1968) implicates bradykinin in the characteristic skin flushing with carcinoid tumors. Serum bradykinin concentrations were elevated during flushing and intravenous infusion of exogenous bradykinin induced skin flushes. Metastatic carcinoid tumor in the liver contained kallikrein. Of interest was the conclusion that serotonin (and not bradykinin) was responsible for the gastrointestinal symptoms of carcinoid (see p. 563).

Similarly, in dumping syndrome the hypotension and flushing of the skin after eating were accompanied by a marked increase in venous free kinin concentration and a concomitant fall in kininogen levels (ZEITLIN and SMITH, 1966a, b BROCKLEHURST and ZEITLIN, 1967). Free kinin activity in plasma during symptomatic dumping was similar to that of synthetic bradykinin.

In shock produced by prolonged occlusion of the superior mesenteric artery, or by bacterial endotoxin, venous blood draining from the gut contained kinin-like material (KOBOLD and THAL, 1963). The investigators speculated that ischemic cell damage in the gut may release proteolytic enzymes from lysosomes which then elaborate dilator kinins and further aggravate the shock state. Fluid from a strangulated segment of ileum in the rat contained kinin-like material (AMUNDSEN, 1966).

These studies by no means prove that kinins are the responsible agents in gastrointestinal disease. They do, however, suggest that disturbances in kinin metabolism may be part of some gastrointestinal diseases, either early or late in the pathogenesis. In any event, these leads should invite further clinical investigations into possible pathogenetic mechanisms involving biologically active polypeptides.

References

AMUNDSEN, E.: Kinin formation and destruction in fluid produced by a strangulated segment of ileum in the rat. In: Hypotensive peptides, p. 474, ed. by E. G. ERDÖS, N. BACK and F. SICUTERI. Berlin-Heidelberg-New York: Springer 1966.

ANDERSON, S., OLBE, L.: Inhibition of gastric acid response to sham feeding in Pavlov pouch dogs by acidification of antrum. Acta physiol. scand. 61, 55 (1964).

BARAC, G.: Effet rénal de la bradykinine chez le chien. C. R. Soc. Biol. (Paris) 151, 1771 (1957).

BARER, G. R.: The action of vasopressin, a vasopressin analogue (PLV_2), oxytocin, angiotensin, bradykinin and theophylline ethylene diamine on renal blood flow in the anaesthetized cat. J. Physiol. (Lond.) 169, 62 (1963).

BARRACLOUGH, M. A., MILLS, I. H.: Effect of bradykinin on renal function. Clin. Sci. 28, 69 (1965).

BROCKLEHURST, W. E., ZEITLIN, I. J.: Determination of plasma kinin and kininogen levels in man. J. Physiol. (Lond.) 191, 417 (1967).

DOLLERY, C. T., GOLDBERG, L. I., PENTECOST, B. L.: Effects of intrarenal infusions of bradykinin and acetylcholine on renal blood flow in man. Clin. Sci. 29, 433 (1965a).

— PENTECOST, B. L., GOLDBERG, L. I., BRECKENRIDGE, A. M.: The action of renal vasodilators on the hypertensive kidney. In: Internat. Club on Arterial Hypertension, p. 411, ed. by P. MILLIER and P. TCHERDOKOFF. Paris: Premiere Reunion 1965b.

EDKINS, J. S.: On the chemical mechanism of gastric secretion. Proc. roy. Soc. B 76, 376 (1905).

FELDBERG, W., LEWIS, G. P.: The action of peptides on the adrenal medulla; release of adrenaline by bradykinin and angiotensin. J. Physiol. (Lond.) 171, 98 (1964).

— — Further studies on the effects of peptides on the suprarenal medulla of cats. J. Physiol. (Lond.) 178, 239 (1965).

FREED, T. A., NEAL, M. P., JR., VINIK, M.: The effect of bradykinin on renal arteriography. Amer. J. Roentgenol. 102, 776 (1968).

FREY, E. K., KRAUT, H., WERLE, E., VOGEL, R., ZICKGRAF-RÜDEL, G., TRAUTSCHOLD, I.: Das Kallikrein-Kinin-System und seine Inhibitoren, p. 23. Stuttgart: Enke 1968.

FURUYANA, T., SUZUKI, C., SAITO, H., ONOZAWA, Y., SHIOJI, R., RIKIMARU, S., ABE, K., YOSHINAGA, K.: Effect of bradykinin and eledoisin on renal function in the dog. Tohoku J. exp. Med. 89, 69 (1966).

GILL, J. R., JR., MELMON, K. L., GILLESPIE, L., JR., BARTTER, F. C.: Bradykinin and renal function in normal man: effects of adrenergic blockade. Amer. J. Physiol. 209, 844 (1965).

GOLDBERG, L. I., DOLLERY, C. T., PENTECOST, B. L.: Effects of intrarenal infusions of bradykinin and acetylcholine in renal blood flow. J. clin. Invest. 44, 1052 (1965).

GROSSMAN, M. I.: Gastrointestinal hormones. Med. Clin. N. Amer. 52, 1297 (1968).

HEIDENREICH, O., KELLER, P., KOOK, Y.: Die Wirkungen von Bradykinin und Kallidin auf die Nierenfunktion des Hundes. Naunyn-Schmiedebergs Arch. exp. Path. Pharmak. 247, 243 (1964).

Hilton, S. M., Jones, M.: The role of plasma kinin in functional vasodilation in the pancreas. J. Physiol. (Lond.) **195**, 521 (1968).
Jacobson, E. D.: Hemodynamic effects of bradykinin and gastrin in the stomach. Amer. Heart J. **68**, 214 (1964).
Johanson, G., Martinson, J.: Release of a plasma kinin-forming enzyme from the stomach of the cat. Acta physiol. scand., Suppl. **213**, 59, 71 (1963).
Kobold, E. E., Thal, A. P.: Quantitation and identification of vasoactive substances liberated during various types of experimental and clinical intestinal ischemia. Surg. Gynec. Obstet. **117**, 315 (1963).
Köver, G., Szöcs, E., Temlev, E.: Effect of bradykinin on renal function. Acta physiol. Acad. Sci. hung. **33**, 11 (1968).
Komarov, S. A.: Gastrin. Proc. Soc. exp. Biol. (N.Y.) **38**, 514 (1938).
Langlois, K., Grossman, M. I.: Effect of surgical extirpation of the pyloric portion of the stomach on the response of the fundic glands to histamine and urecholine in dogs. Amer. J. Physiol. **163**, 38 (1950).
Lecomte, J., Iroquet, J., Dresse, A.: Stimulation medullo-surrénalienne par la bradykinine. Arch. int. Physiol. Biochim. **69**, 89 (1961).
Melmon, K. L.: Kinins—one of many mediators of the carcinoid spectrum. Gastroenterology **55**, 545 (1968).
Mertz, D. P.: Bradykinin und Nierenfunktion. Verh. dtsch. Ges. Kreisl.-Forsch. **29**, 177 (1963a).
— Renotrope Wirkungen von synthetischem Bradykinin. Naunyn-Schmiedebergs Arch. exp. Path. Pharmak. **244**, 405 (1963b).
— Der Einfluß von Kinin-Hormonen auf den Vorgang der Harnverdünnung und Harnkonzentrierung. Arzneimittel-Forsch. **17**, 376 (1967a).
— Über den Einfluß von Kinin-Hormonen auf den Vorgang der Harnverdünnung und Harnkonzentrierung. Arzneimittel-Forsch. **17**, 440 (1967b).
Murphy, G. P., Homsey, E. G., Scott, W. W.: Evaluation of pharmacologically induced renal vasodilatation. J. Surg. Res. **5**, 525 (1965).
Nakano, J.: Effects of synthetic bradykinin on the cardiovascular system. Arch. int. Pharmacodyn. **157**, 1 (1965).
Pe Thien, M., Schofield, B.: Release of gastrin from the pyloric antrum following vagal stimulation by sham feeding in dogs. J. Physiol. (Lond.) **148**, 291 (1959).
Poisner, A. M., Douglas, W. W.: The requirement for calcium on adrenomedullary secretion evoked by histamine, serotonin, angiotensin and bradykinin. Fed. Proc. **24**, 488 (1965).
Robinson, R. L.: Stimulation of the catecholamine output of the isolated perfused adrenal gland of the dog by angiotensin and bradykinin. J. Pharmacol. exp. Ther. **156**, 252 (1967).
Rocha e Silva, M., Jr., Malnic, G.: Release of antidiuretic hormone by bradykinin. J. Pharmacol. exp. Ther. **146**, 24 (1964).
Rosas, R. B.: Vasoactive peptides and substrates and their relation to protein handling by the kidney. Circul. Res. **12**, 573 (1963).
Shehadeh, Z., Price, W. E., Jacobson, E. D.: Effects of vasoactive agents on intestinal blood flow and motility in the dog. Amer. J. Physiol. **216**, 386 (1969).
Staszewska-Barczak, J., Vane, J. R.: The release of catecholamines from the adrenal medulla by peptides. Brit. J. Pharmacol. **30**, 655 (1967).
Stürmer, E., Berde, B.: A pharmacological comparison between synthetic bradykinin and synthetic kallidin. J. Pharmacol. exp. Ther. **139**, 38 (1963).
Szakáll, A.: Über die Wirkung intravenöser Kallikreinzufuhr auf den tierischen Organismus. Naunyn-Schmiedebergs Arch. exp. Path. Pharmak. **166**, 301 (1932).
Thal, A. P., Kobold, E. E., Hollenberg, M. J.: The release of vasoactive substances in acute pancreatitis. Amer. J. Surg. **105**, 708 (1963).
Webster, M. E., Gilmore, J. P.: Influence of kallidin-10 on renal function. Amer. J. Physiol. **206**, 714 (1964).
Werle, E., Erdös, E. G.: Über eine neue blutdrucksenkende, darm- und uteruserregende Substanz im menschlichen Urin. Naunyn-Schmiedebergs Arch. exp. Path. Pharmak. **223**, 234 (1954).
Zeitlin, I. J., Smith, A. N.: A relation between kinins and the dumping syndrome. Lancet **1966**a **II**, 896.
— — 5-Hydroxyindoles and kinins in the carcinoid and dumping syndromes. Lancet **1966**b **II**, 986.

The Physiological Role of Glandular Kallikreins

S. M. HILTON

With 3 Figures

A. Early Ideas

Evidence has been accumulating for some time that different glands of several mammalian species contain substances of protein nature which can have powerful vasodepressor effects. These substances can be readily extracted from the glandular tissues and appear in an active form in their secretions. It was only natural

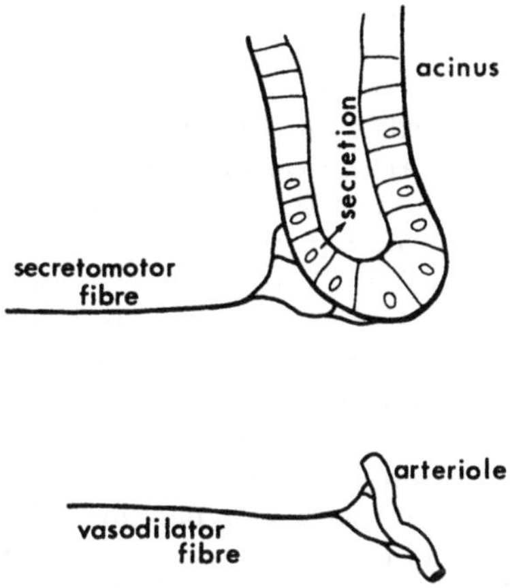

Fig. 1. Diagrammatic representation of the classical idea of separate secretomotor and vasodilator innervations of the submandibular salivary gland

that these findings should lead to speculation, some of it quite early, about their possible physiological role. Thus, the first ideas about what are now known as the kinin systems were propounded under a different name. In their earliest definitive work, KRAUT et al. (1930) had shown that extracts of pancreas and pancreatic juice owed their vasodepressor activity to a material of protein nature which they called kallikrein (see p. 2). Having found a similar substance in extracts of blood and urine, they put forward the idea that they were dealing with a new vasodilator hormone which was secreted by the pancreas, circulated in the blood stream in an inactive form, and then excreted. Physiological and clinical interest in this notion waned, but WERLE and his colleagues carried on to show that, in part at least, the action of kallikrein was due to the release of a hypotensive substance from plasma (WERLE et al., 1937; WERLE and BEREK, 1948).

The next suggestion for a physiological role for kallikrein was made in a brief note by UNGAR and PARROT (1936). Cat saliva had been found to contain a vasodepressor substance (SECKER, 1934) which was not acetylcholine (FELDBERG and GUIMARAIS, 1935). UNGAR and PARROT (1936) showed that there were similarities between this substance and pancreatic kallikrein, and they proposed that the substance found in saliva was the mediator of the vasodilator nerve fibers to the salivary gland. They thus seemed to accept what may be regarded as the classical view (Fig. 1) that there were vasodilator, as well as secretomotor, fibers in the nerve supply to the submandibular salivary gland; but they raised the question whether the vasodilator fibers might in fact be kallikreinergic. The work of HEIDENHAIN (1872) had established that the secretory, but not the vasodilator, effect of nerve stimulation was blocked by atropine. UNGAR and PARROT had therefore proposed an original solution of the problem of the atropine-resistant vasodilatation. With the acceptance of the humoral theory of transmission at efferent nerve endings, however, and the universal finding that acetylcholine is the transmitter at the endings of the postganglionic nerve fibers of the parasympathetic nerve system, this early idea was forgotten.

B. Kinins as Mediators of Functional Vasodilatation in Glands

I. Cat Submandibular Salivary Gland

More recently the kinin system has again been associated with local vasodilatation in glands, but in a rather different way. In the course of a re-investigation of the cause of the vasodilatation occurring in the submandibular salivary gland on stimulation of the chorda tympani (HILTON and LEWIS, 1955a), evidence was advanced to show, first, that the vasodilator agent was certainly more stable than acetylcholine and, second, that this agent appeared in the tissue fluid after glandular activity and was eliminated in the lymphatic drainage from the gland. The evidence, quite simply, was that if the chorda was stimulated for the first 15 seconds of a 1-minute period of circulatory arrest, by occlusion of the artery and vein, the hyperemia seen on re-establishing the circulation was at least as great as that seen after chorda stimulation alone. A similar result was obtained if the gland was activated by a close arterial injection of acetylcholine, the humoral transmitter of the secretomotor nerve endings. It could be demonstrated, in control experiments, that the reactive hyperemia following a 1-minute period of vascular occlusion alone was trivial by comparison, and that the direct vasodilator action of acetylcholine would not outlast such a period of circulatory arrest.

If the chorda was stimulated during a period of venous occlusion, which would, if anything, increase the flow of lymph from the gland, subsequent removal of the venous clamp was not followed by any hyperemia. Only after lymphatic drainage from the gland had been abolished by carefully separating it from the surrounding tissues could the stable vasodilator material be retained within the gland by occlusion of the venous outflow alone. Therefore, even if acetylcholine, released from secretomotor nerve endings, is making a contribution to the vasodilatation within the active gland, some other vasodilator substance is formed in the tissue fluid which is much more stable and which is eliminated via the lymphatic drainage.

These findings seemed to provide an exciting prospect for anyone engaged in the search for the chemical cause of functional vasodilatation. This phenomenon, so well known in the case of skeletal muscle, had been investigated for more than eighty years without any concrete evidence coming to hand. Now, for the first time, there was solid evidence in the case of a glandular organ for the formation of a relatively stable vasodilator substance consequent upon activity. This idea goes right back to the investigations of BARCROFT (1914) which had revealed that stimulation of the chorda increases the metabolic activity of the gland, even when secretion has been abolished by atropine; for these findings had led him to the conclusion that the vasodilatation which occurs in this gland under these conditions, as well as during or after sympathetic stimulation, is secondary to the secretory activity and is, in other words, a true functional vasodilatation.

The next step in the investigation of HILTON and LEWIS (1955b) was to look for the vasodilator agent in venous effluent from the activated gland. No such material was found in the venous blood coming from the gland, but when the gland was perfused with LOCKE's solution and the effluent collected during and immediately after a period of chorda stimulation, it was found to possess strong vasodilator activity. It was shown that this was not due to an actual vasodilator substance in the effluent but to some material that produced the vasodilator substance from some fraction of the plasma. This substance, which

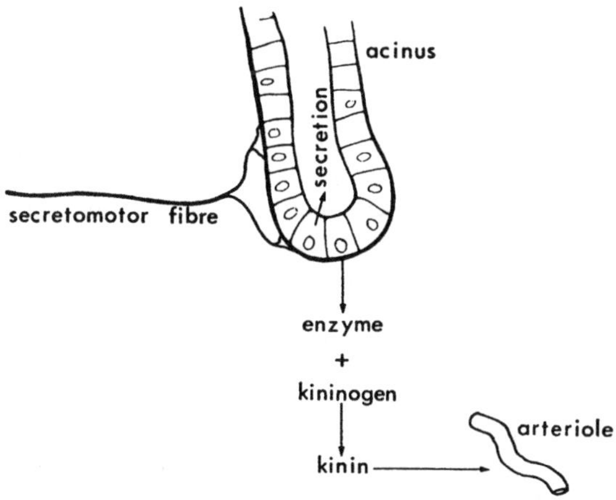

Fig. 2. Diagrammatic representation of the indirect mediation of functional vasodilatation in the activated submandibular salivary gland by kinin formation

was also produced by the action of saliva on plasma, proved to be indistinguishable from bradykinin. Thus the hypothesis was established, as illustrated in Fig. 2, that when the gland was activated by secretomotor nerve stimulation, not only was enzyme released into the secretion, but it also passed into the interstitial fluid where it reacted with the plasma proteins present to form kinin, which then produced local dilatation of the resistance vessels in the gland. In later experiments, the effluent of glands perfused with LOCKE's solution was assayed for kinin-forming activity (HILTON and LEWIS, 1956) and the output of kinin-forming enzyme was found to be increased as readily by a close arterial injection of acetylcholine as it was by stimulation of the chordolingual nerve. The increase in activity was, if anything, even greater when the gland was activated by norepinephrine. Thus, in every situation in which glandular activity was accompanied by local vasodilatation the evidence showed kininogenase to be released into the interstitial fluid of the gland where, under conditions of normal circulation, plasma kinin would be formed.

Even in the atropinized glands, where the output of kininogenase was no longer increased by close arterial injections of acetylcholine, it was still increased by chorda stimulation, though this increase was naturally smaller than that seen without atropine. This supplements other evidence that atropine does not prevent the acetylcholine released from the secretomotor nerve endings from having some metabolic effects in the salivary gland, as already shown by Barcroft (1914) in the case of oxygen consumption and Anrep and Cannan (1922) in the case of glucose consumption. The gland does not produce overt secretion, but some of the biochemical processes normally associated with the secretory activity are stimulated, among which is release of kinin-forming enzyme. When summing up the results of these experiments, Hilton and Lewis (1957) concluded that functional vasodilatation in the submandibular salivary gland is mediated by kinin formation, and the question was posed whether there really are separate parasympathetic vasodilator nerve fibers to the resistance vessels of the gland. More than that, it seemed reasonable to ask whether it might not be found that functional vasodilatation in all glandular organs and tissues might not be similarly mediated. In the outcome this has proved to be so.

II. Cat Pancreas

An important glandular organ to be considered from this point of view was the pancreas, for this, after all, was the original source of kallikrein, the classical kinin-forming enzyme. Further, it would be no surprise to find that kininogenase would be released by the exocrine elements of this organ into the tissue fluid of the gland, as it is so well known that pancreatic enzymes can appear in the blood stream when this organ has received a powerful stimulus to secretion. When the vascular responses of the pancreas were examined to various secretory stimuli (Hilton and Jones, 1968), it was found that the blood flow increased about 60% on vagal stimulation, in confirmation of the previous report of Gayet and Guillaumie (1930). Highly purified secretin did not cause any increase in flow, nor did it even give rise to a significant capillary dilatation. Pancreozymin was found to be the most potent vasodilator stimulus, increasing the flow up to 5-fold. Although pancreozymin has not yet been purified as highly as secretin, the vasodilator effect found in these experiments was almost certainly localized to the pancreas, since the response was so great within the organ itself, but was obtained without any fall of arterial blood pressure.

This then was a situation which could provide a critical test of the theory relating kinin formation to functional vasodilatation, for dilatation had been obtained with two types of stimulation but not with the third. In the event, when the effluent from the perfused pancreas was examined for kinin-forming activity before and after these three different stimuli, it was found that acetylcholine led to considerable release of kininogenase, that pancreozymin was equally effective, but that secretin had no such action. These results seem to provide a good test of the theory relating kinin formation to functional vasodilatation in glands; since, first, it has never been suggested that there are vasodilator nerve fibers running to the pancreas, second, pancreozymin could hardly be producing dilatation through such nerve fibers, and, finally, it could hardly be a coincidence that evidence for kinin formation in the gland is found only when the gland is activated by those forms of stimulation that cause vasodilatation. It needs only to be added that, in the cat submandibular salivary gland also, where functional vasodilatation occurs on sympathetic as well as chorda stimulation (and in the latter case even after atropine), these are the stimuli which cause release of the kininogenase.

III. Sweat Glands in Human Skin

There seems little room for doubt that in both these glandular organs, under the conditions where functional vasodilatation occurs, plasma kinin will be formed in the interstitial fluid and will make a major contribution to the vascular response. This is exactly what was found by Fox and Hilton (1958) in an investigation of yet another glandular tissue, the human forearm skin, using a slightly different experimental technique. The mechanism being studied was that underlying the active vasodilatation occurring in the skin of the human forearm during body heating. This is, of course, accompanied by sweating, and human forearm sweat has high kinin-forming activity (Fox and Hilton, 1956). In order to see whether kinin is formed in the subcutaneous tissue space when the sweat gland is activated, it was not possible to use the perfusion technique which had been employed in acute experiments on anaesthetized cats. Fox and Hilton (1958) therefore devised a method which may be called subcutaneous tissue space perfusion, whereby buffered saline solution was introduced into this space through a needle with multiple perforations along its length, and a fairly constant proportion of this fluid was withdrawn via a second, similar needle parallel to the first. Under these conditions, the skin and subcutaneous tissue still had a blood supply and hence a supply of substrate for the kininogenase. The fluid withdrawn under resting conditions contained some kinin which could be accounted for on the basis of dilution of the plasma proteins present. When the trunk and legs of the subject where heated sufficiently to cause sweating on the exposed forearm, the kinin content of the fluid was greatly increased, up to five times the resting value, without any detectable increase on total protein. As in the salivary gland and pancreas, the kinin so formed could fully account for the active dilatation of the vessels of the skin which occurs under these conditions.

C. Criteria for the Theory

For any substance to be considered to have a particular transmitter function, certain criteria have to be met. Those which are frequently emphasized are (1) the presence of the substance at the proposed site of release, (2) evidence for release of the substance under the conditions in which the responses are observed, and (3) the reproduction of the responses, qualitatively at least, by the hypothetical transmitter substance. These indeed, are the criteria traditionally employed when gauging the validity of the case for any substance as a humoral transmitter across synapses in the peripheral or central nervous system. But the same criteria should be employed in the cases of functional vasodilatation that have been considered in this paper. As an example the cat submandibular salivary gland may be taken, for this has been the most thoroughly investigated. The evidence for the presence of kininogenases in the acinar cells of the gland does not need to be repeated. Also, as shown above, there is strong evidence for the release of these enzymes into the tissue fluid of the active gland. Finally, the kinins themselves are powerful vasodilator substances, they are more stable than acetylcholine, and they possess one further and significant property bearing on the local vascular response, i.e. the increased capillary permeability to large molecules which they are known to cause. This has been shown by the development of blueing in areas of skin and mesentery of animals in which an intravenous injection of Evan's blue has been followed by a local injection of bradykinin (Schachter, 1960; Zweifach, 1966) and by the fact that intra-arterial infusion of bradykinin will cause an increased flow of lymph, with an increased protein content (Stürmer, 1966). After intravenous injection of Evans' blue, stimulation of the chorda leads rapidly to blueing of the submandibular salivary gland (Hilton, 1960). Thus the kinin-forming system fulfills all the criteria required for a mediator of functional vasodilatation in this gland. No other single substance would fulfill all these criteria, and it may also be important to add that vasodilator nerve fibers acting through the release of acetylcholine would not have the required effect on capillary permeability.

D. Arguments Against the Theory

I. Arguments Based on Presence or Absence of Kallikreins

All these positive findings have to be taken into account by any critic of the theory relating kinins to functional vasodilatation in glandular organs and tissues. Nevertheless, a review of the publications of the most active of these critics (cf. Schachter, 1966; Schachter and Beilenson, 1968) shows no mention of them. The arguments in these publications rest on different grounds. The first put forward was that the secretions and extracts of some glands do not contain kininogenases (Schachter, 1960; Bhoola et al., 1962). This argument, although raised seriously by the authors concerned, is hardly relevant to the immediate question, for as was pointed out previously by Hilton (1960, 1962), functional vasodilatation does not occur in all glands, and even in the glands in which it does occur is not seen in response to all secretory stimuli. As stated by Hilton and Jones (1968), if there is no vasodilatation, there is no need to look for a vasodilator agent. In 1960 Schachter argued that kinins were unlikely to play a role in functional vasodilatation in the pancreas, since Werle and Urhahn (1940) had found little or no active kallikrein in pancreatic secretion. As it turned out, when the situation in the pancreas was examined critically, not only was good evidence found for kinin formation under conditions in which functional vasodilatation occurred (which is the main question in hand), but it was also confirmed, as a by-product of the investigation, that pancreatic juice does contain active kallikrein, though this can be obscured by the presence in the juice of a kininase, which is almost certainly carboxypeptidase B (Hilton and Jones, 1968).

II. Arguments Based on "Perfectionist" View of Humoral Transmitter Theory

The next objections are all in the same category, insofar as they belong to the general type of finding that has long been adduced against the theory of humoral transmission anywhere in the nervous system. They run as follows: (1) the vasodilator effect of a close arterial injection of saliva into the gland does not duplicate exactly the vasodilatation produced by stimulation of the chordolingual nerve (Bhoola et al., 1965); (2) close arterial infusion of a large dose of bradykinin into the gland desensitizes the gland more to a subsequent injection of a smaller dose of bradykinin than it does to stimulation of the chordolingual nerve (Bhoola et al., 1965); (3) in cats which have received an intravenous injection of the kininase, carboxypeptidase B, the vasodilator effect of intra-arterial bradykinin in small doses can be abolished, while the dilatation following stimulation of the chorda tympani remains unchanged (Skinner and Webster, 1968).

In fact, if this type of evidence were accepted at its face value, it would not be possible to believe that acetylcholine was a transmitter even at the neuromuscular junction. Regarding the first objection, there is hardly any experimental situation in which local administration of a transmitter substance can mimic exactly the natural effect of nerve stimulation. Regarding the second, it is a familiar experience to anyone carrying out class demonstrations of the role of acetylcholine in neuromuscular transmission that, after a close arterial injection of acetylcholine to a muscle, there is commonly a period of 5 to 10 minutes during which the response to a similar dose of acetylcholine is much depressed while that to motor nerve stimulation appears quite normal. Finally, whereas the administration of cholinesterase might block the reaction of skeletal muscle even to a large dose of acetylcholine injected close arterially, it could hardly be expected to have any effect on the action of the transmitter released by the nerve endings at the neuromuscular junction, where the concentration of cholinesterase is already exceedingly high. To refer more specifically to the situation in the salivary gland, the kininase activity of lymph is also high, yet kinin can be formed within it. In short, none of these findings should be in any way surprising.

It was once hoped that more rigorous criteria even than those already listed could be applied to substances considered likely candidates as humoral transmitters, but this is now known to be a rather futile pursuit. It was proposed that any agent which depressed or facilitated the response of the hypothetical transmitter substance would also act in the same sense on the effect of nerve stimulation; and it is from such a lack of parallelism that BHOOLA et al. (1965) and SKINNER and WEBSTER (1968) have tried to argue. But there is a peculiar lack of logic, particularly in the former instance, since BHOOLA et al. maintain that the vasodilatation in the cat submandibular salivary gland is produced by vasodilator fibers that are cholinergic but are not blocked by atropine, in doses which fully block the vasodilator response to close arterial injections of acetylcholine.

III. Arguments Based on Attempts to Deplete the Substrate or Enzyme

SCHACHTER and his colleagues have brought forward two further arguments against the participation of kinins in functional vasodilatation in the cat submandibular salivary gland. One is based upon an attempt to deplete the substrate available in the gland for glandular kallikrein, and the other is an attempt to deplete the gland of the enzyme itself, after which procedures the response to chorda stimulation is tested. The former argument was elaborated by BHOOLA et al. (1965) on the basis of experiments in which the gland had been perfused for several hours with horse serum, which does not contain a suitable substrate for cat salivary kallikrein. It was presumably hoped that the substrate for this enzyme which is normally present in the interstitial fluid of the gland would be removed from the tissue spaces as the foreign plasma proteins diffused in; but this was not tested. The authors state that in six out of eight such experiments they were able to demonstrate vasodilator responses to chorda stimulation. However, even to obtain these responses they usually had to add physostigmine, in addition to norepinephrine, to the horse serum used to perfuse the gland. It seems curious that in the interpretation of the results no account was taken of the fact that, in the presence of physostigmine, acetylcholine released by the secretomotor nerve fibers will be protected and therefore able to diffuse freely through the interstitial fluid of the gland to act directly upon the resistance vessels. This experiment therefore does not provide evidence in favor of specific vasodilator nerve fibers, as the authors claimed.

In the study reported by BEILENSON et al. (1965) advantage was taken of the finding of WERLE and TRAUTSCHOLD (1963) that, if the duct of the submandibular salivary gland is tied, the concentration of several intracellular enzymes falls sharply within a few days, one of the enzymes so affected being kallikrein itself. BEILENSON et al. (1965) repeated this maneuver, and then examined the effect of chordolingual stimulation on the blood flow through the gland with a much reduced kallikrein content. They reported that the vasodilatation was normal, and concluded that it could not have been caused by bradykinin. When Hilton and Torres (1967) repeated these experiments, they obtained a similar result; the only difference they found between the effect of chorda stimulation in glands with tied ducts and normal glands was that the responses were more variable in the former, there being some in which the vasodilator response was very small and some in which it was very large, compared with normal control glands. Further investigation, however, revealed another and most interesting difference between the two sets of glands. This was a selective increase in sensitivity to bradykinin which was invariably found in glands whose duct had been tied for several days. The dose–response curve was displaced to the left and was much steeper. This change was of such extent that the dose of bradykinin injected close arterially which was needed to reproduce the response to 10-second chorda stimulation was ten times smaller in the glands with tied ducts than in normal glands. The vasodilator responses to close arterial injections of acetylcholine were unchanged. Therefore, we have a situation in these glands in which the atrophic processes taking place lead to a reduction in glandular kallikrein and simultaneously to a selective increase in vascular sensitivity to bradykinin. The latter speaks very strongly in favor of the postulated role of kinin as the mediator of the vasodilator response during glandular activity. The fact that the two changes (reduction of enzyme and increased sensitivity to kinin) are occurring simultaneously will also account for the greater variability of the vasodilator response in the glands with tied ducts.

In these experiments of Hilton and Torres (1967), kallikrein was always found in the saliva from the glands whose duct had been tied, the mean value being 3% of the activity in saliva from normal glands. Thus this procedure alone by no means completely depletes the gland of kallikrein. An attempt was made to reduce this kinin content still further by taking advantage of the fact that sympathetic stimulation causes a particularly large output of kininogenase into the salivary secretion, as this might provide a more effective depletion of the enzyme in the glands with ligated ducts. In these glands, therefore, the chorda was stimulated before and after prolonged sympathetic stimulation. It was then seen that the vasodilator response was always reduced. So this effect of chorda stimulation can indeed be impaired if the glandular content of kallikrein is lowered sufficiently.

E. New Evidence for the Theory, in a Gland with a Blood Supply

A critical review of the arguments and evidence brought forward against the postulated role of kinins as the mediators of functional vasodilatation in glands has thus shown that only one appeared to have a firm foundation; and when this particular experimental situation was looked at carefully, evidence was revealed which exactly fitted the original theory. Moreover, none of the direct evidence has been challenged. Some skepticism might still remain, however, on the grounds that the glands have had to be artificially perfused in order to detect the increase in kininogenase enzyme, which would ordinarily be released into the interstitial fluid and probably never reach the blood stream. In recent experiments, advantage has been taken of the fact that there are two substrates for kininogenase in both plasma and lymph (Jacobsen, 1966a, b), which can be assayed independently. In the cat, one of these (substrate 2) is acted upon exclusively by glandular kallikreins (Gautvik, unpublished observations). By examining the concentration of this substrate in venous blood from the submandibular salivary gland, it is therefore possible to tell whether glandular kallikrein has been released into the tissue fluid of the gland; for if it is so released, it will act on the substrate therein and consequently the level of the substrate in the plasma will fall in turn. When such assays were carried out and the chorda stimulated, it was found that substrate 2 was reduced up to 60% during and immediately after glandular activity. As a control, the concentration of substrate 1, which is acted upon exclusively by plasma kallikrein, was also assayed and this was found to be unaffected by chorda stimulation (GAUTVIK et al., 1968).

This has shown that in the salivary gland with an arterial blood supply, kallikrein does pass into the interstitial fluid on chorda stimulation. Indeed all the positive results quoted in this paper show that kinin is formed in the interstitial fluid of several glands during secretory activity, and it must therefore be playing a role in causing the vascular concomitants of this activity. Indeed, the only question left is whether a contribution to this vasodilatation could be

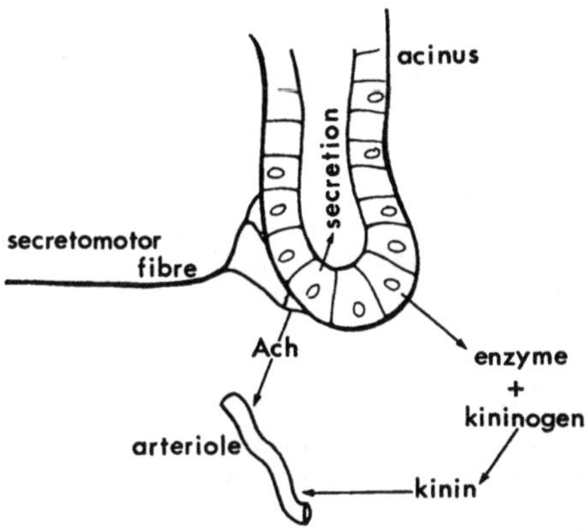

Fig. 3. Diagrammatic representation of a possible way whereby acetylcholine may contribute to the vasodilatation caused by kinin formation in the active gland

made by acetylcholine released from secretomotor nerve endings. This possibility, which is indicated in the diagram of Fig. 3, cannot be ignored, particularly in view of the recent histological findings suggestive of parasympathetic nerve endings in close relation to muscular blood vessels (GARRETT, 1966a, b). Indeed it might even be thought likely, because of the lack of an organized structure as at the neuromuscular junction, which seems designed to prevent the acetylcholine from leaking away.

Nevertheless, an argument against this possibility still remains: this rests on the fact that acetylcholine causes a dilatation of veins whereas venodilatation is not a feature of the vascular response to chorda stimulation. On the other hand, the effect of bradykinin on veins is, if anything, constrictor.

F. Other Possible Physiological Roles for Kinins

In conclusion, it is still fascinating to pursue the question whether kininogenases have any other function in glandular organs and tissues. The general suggestion has been made that these enzymes may have some exocrine function (SCHACHTER, 1960; BHOOLA, 1968), though the particular function has not been specified. This is conceivable in the case of the salivary gland and the pancreas. Indeed, HILTON and LEWIS (1955b) speculated whether the salivary enzyme might act on proteins in food to produce gastrin-releasing material and so promote gastric digestion. But this idea would not hold good for the enzyme in sweat, nor for that which is known to appear in the urine and seems to be elaborated in the kidney (Beraldo et al., 1956). If we are to seek some significant function for this enzyme which is to apply in every case where it is found, then it must surely be to some aspect of the secretory process itself that we should look. It was with this in mind that the suggestion was previously made (Hilton, 1962) that these enzymes may play a role in the secretory process itself by altering the permeability of the secretory cell membrane so as to facilitate the transfer of secreted materials. There is, at present, no evidence either to support or to refute such an idea, though the ubiquity of the enzyme in secretory structures makes it an attractive possibility.

References

Anrep, G. V., Cannan, R. K.: The metabolism of the salivary glands. III. The blood sugar metabolism of the submaxillary gland. J. Physiol. (Lond.) **57**, 1 (1922).

Barcroft, J.: The respiratory function of the blood, p. 138. Cambridge: University Press 1914.

Beilenson, S., Schachter, M., Smaje, L. H.: Kallikrein in the submaxillary gland of the cat. J. Physiol. (Lond.) **177**, 61 (1965).

Beraldo, W. T., Feldberg, W., Hilton, S. M.: Experiments on the factor in urine forming substance U. J. Physiol. (Lond.) **133**, 558 (1956).

Bhoola, K. D.: Intracellular distribution of submaxillary kallikrein. J. Physiol. (Lond.) **196**, 431 (1968).

— May May Yi, R., Morley, J., Schachter, M.: Release of kinin by an enzyme in the accessory sex glands of the guinea-pig. J. Physiol. (Lond.) **163**, 269 (1962).

— Morley, J., Schachter, M., Smaje, L. H.: Vasodilatation in the submaxillary gland of the cat. J. Physiol. (Lond.) **179**, 172 (1965).

Feldberg, W., Guimarais, J. A.: Some observations on salivary secretion. J. Physiol. (Lond.) **85**, 15 (1935).

Fox, R. H., Hilton, S. M.: Sweat gland activity as a contributory factor to heat vasodilatation in the human skin. J. Physiol. (Lond.) **133**, 68 (1956).

— — Bradykinin formation in human skin as a factor in heat vasodilatation. J. Physiol. (Lond.) **142**, 219 (1958).

Garrett, J. R.: The innervation of salivary glands. III. The effect of certain experimental procedures on cholinesterase-positive nerves in glands of the cat. J. roy. micr. Soc. **86**, 1 (1966a).

— The innervation of salivary glands. IV. The effect of certain experimental procedures on the ultrastructure of nerves in glands of the cat. J. roy. micr. Soc. **86**, 15 (1966b).

Gautvik, K. M., Hilton, S. M., Torres, S. H.: Consumption of the plasma substrate for glandular kallikrein on activation of the submandibular salivary gland. J. Physiol. (Lond.) **197**, 22—23P (1968).

Gayet, R., Guillaumie, M.: Les réactions vasomotrices du pancréas étudiées par la mesure des débits sanguins. C. R. Soc. Biol. (Paris) **103**, 1106 (1930).

Heidenhain, R.: Über die Wirkung einiger Gifte auf die Nerven der Glandula submaxillaris. Pflügers Arch. ges. Physiol. **5**, 309 (1872).

Hilton, S. M.: Plasma kinin and blood flow. In: Polypeptides which affect smooth muscles and blood vessels, p. 258, ed. by M. Schachter. London: Pergamon Press 1960.

— Local mechanisms regulating peripheral blood flow. Physiol. Rev. **42**, 265 (1962).

— Jones, M.: The role of plasma kinin in functional vasodilatation in the pancreas. J. Physiol. (Lond.) **195**, 521 (1968).

— Lewis, G. P.: The cause of the vasodilatation accompanying activity in the submandibular salivary gland. J. Physiol. (Lond.) **128**, 235 (1955a).

— — The mechanism of the functional hyperaemia in the submandibular salivary gland. J. Physiol. (Lond.) **129**, 253 (1955b).

— — The relationship between glandular activity, bradykinin formation and functional vasodilatation in the submandibular salivary gland. J. Physiol. (Lond.) **134**, 471 (1956).

— — Functional vasodilatation in salivary gland. Brit. med. Bull. **13**, 189 (1957).

— Torres, S. H.: Bradykinin and functional vasodilatation in the submandibular salivary gland in the cat. J. Physiol. (Lond.) **189**, 69P (1967).

JACOBSEN, S.: Observations on the content of kininogen, kallikrein and kininase in lymph from hind limbs of dogs and rabbits. Brit. J. Pharmacol. **27**, 213 (1966a).
— Substrates for plasma kinin-forming enzymes in rat and guinea-pig plasmas. Brit. J. Pharmacol. **28**, 64 (1966b).
KRAUT, H., FREY, E. K., WERLE, E.: Der Nachweis eines Kreislaufhormons in der Pankreasdrüse. Hoppe-Seylers Z. physiol. Chem. **189**, 97 (1930).
SCHACHTER, M.: Some properties of kallidin, bradykinin and wasp venom kinin. In: Polypeptides which affect smooth muscles and blood vessels, p. 232, ed. by M. SCHACHTER. London: Pergamon Press 1960.
— Kallikrein and vasodilatation in the salivary gland. In: Hypotensive peptides, p. 275, ed. by E. G. ERDÖS, N. BACK, and F. SICUTERI: Berlin-Heidelberg-New York: Springer 1966.
— BEILENSON, S.: Mediator of vasodilatation in the submaxillary gland. Fed. Proc. **27**, 73 (1968).
SECKER, J.: The humoral control of the secretion by the submaxillary gland of the cat following chorda stimulation. J. Physiol. (Lond.) 81, 81 (1934).
SKINNER, N. S., WEBSTER, M. E.: Submaxillary gland blood flow: The role of kinins and β-adrenergic receptors. Fed. Proc. **27**, 76 (1968).
STÜRMER, E.: The influence of intra-arterial infusions on synthetic bradykinin on flow and composition of lymph in dogs. In: Hypotensive peptides, p. 368, ed. by E. G. ERDÖS, N. BACK, and F. SICUTERI. Berlin-Heidelberg-New York: Springer 1966.
UNGAR, G., PARROT, J.-L.: Sur la présence de la callicréine dans la salive, et la possibilité de son intervention dans la transmission chimique de l'influx nerveux. C. R. Soc. Biol. (Paris) **122**, 1052 (1936).
WERLE, E., BEREK, U.: Zur Kenntnis des Kallikreins. Angew. Chem. **60** A, 53 (1948). [Cit. by G. P. LEWIS, in: Active polypeptides derived from plasma proteins. Physiol. Rev. **40**, 647 (1960).]
— GÖTZE, W., KEPPLER, A.: Über die Wirkung des Kallikreins auf den isolierten Darm und über eine darmkontrahierende Substanz. Biochem. Z. **289**, 217 (1937). [Cit. by G. P. LEWIS, in: Active polypeptides derived from plasma proteins. Physiol. Rev. **40**, 647 (1960).]
— TRAUTSCHOLD, I.: Kallikrein, kallidin, kallikrein inhibitors. Ann. N.Y. Acad. Sci. **104**, 117 (1963).
— URHAHN, K.: Über den Aktivitätszustand des Kallikreins in der Bauchspeicheldrüse. Biochem. Z. **304**, 387 (1940).
ZWEIFACH, B. W.: Microcirculatory effects of polypeptides. In: Hypotensive peptides, p. 451, ed. by E. G. ERDÖS, N. BACK, and F. SICUTERI. Berlin-Heidelberg-New York: Springer 1966.

Vasodilatation in the Submaxillary Gland of the Cat, Rabbit, and Sheep

M. SCHACHTER

With 9 Figures

A. Introduction

This chapter will discuss the possible role of kallikrein as mediator of functional hyperemia in the salivary glands.

Salivary kallikrein was first described by WERLE and RODEN (1936) and shortly afterward was shown to exert its vasodilator and other effects by releasing an active fragment from a protein substrate in plasma, apparently by a proteolytic action (WERLE et al., 1937). UNGAR and PARROT (1936) were quick to recognize that such a substance in the submaxillary gland might explain the puzzling resistance to atropine of the vasodilatation accompanying parasympathetic nerve stimulation in this organ, and since they found that the hypotensive action of salivary kallikrein in the cat was atropine resistant, they suggested that kallikrein was the mediator of this vasodilatation produced by chorda tympani nerve stimulation. This suggestion extended BARCROFT'S (1914) view that functional vasodilatation was caused by the secretory metabolic activity of the gland cells; furthermore, it implicated kallikrein as the hitertho unidentified metabolic mediator of the vasodilatation. The view that kallikrein released into the interstitial fluid during secretion is the physiological mediator of functional dilatation, not only in the salivary glands but also in sweat, pancreatic, and other glands, has since been maintained by some workers (HILTON and LEWIS, 1955a, b, 1956, 1958; FOX and HILTON, 1958; HILTON, 1960; HILTON and JONES, 1968), but was opposed by others (SCHACHTER, 1960; BHOOLA et al., 1962, 1965; MORLEY et al., 1966; SCHACHTER and BEILENSON, 1968; BEILENSON et al., 1968; SKINNER and WEBSTER, 1968).

SCHACHTER and his colleagues first questioned the *generalization* that kinin-releasing enzymes provide the mechanism regulating functional hyperemia. Thus, of the large number of glands examined in the guinea pig, only the submaxillary and prostate glands contained a kininogenase in an active form (BHOOLA et al., 1962). Also, whereas this enzyme in the guinea pig's salivary gland released kinin from human and other mammalian plasmas, it failed to do so from guinea pig plasma. Further, the prostate gland of man, dog, cat, rabbit, and rat, unlike that of the guinea pig, does not contain a kininogenase. These observations made untenable the conclusion that kinin-releasing enzymes afford a general mechanism for functional hyperemia in glands.

Since the conditions required for the intervention of kallikrein (an abundance of enzyme in the gland and its substrate in plasma and interstitial fluid) in functional hyperemia do exist in the submaxillary gland, SCHACHTER and his colleagues studied the possible relationship between kallikrein in the submaxillary gland and vasodilatation in the cat, rabbit, and sheep. The results of their studies are presented below:

B. Experiments on the Cat

The following pertinent observations have been made by SCHACHTER and colleagues which have a bearing on the possible role of kallikrein in the submaxillary gland of the cat. None of the observations is consistent with the view that kallikrein mediates the profound increase in blood flow that accompanies the secretion produced by stimulation of the chorda tympani nerve.

(1) The close arterial injection of saliva into a submaxillary gland with natural circulation does not duplicate the vasodilatation produced by stimulation of the

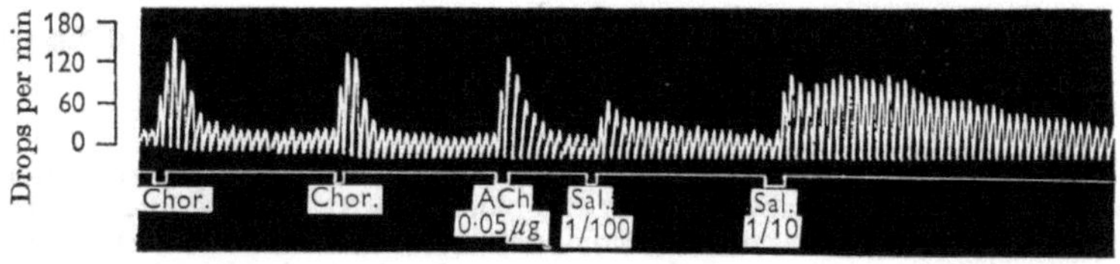

Fig. 1. Record of blood flow in cat submaxillary gland (natural circulation). Comparison of vasodilator effects of close-arterial injections of saliva (*Sal.*), acetylcholine (*ACh.*), and chorda lingual nerve stimulation (*Chor.*). The numbers indicate the amount of ACh. or the dilution of the injected saliva. (From BHOOLA et al., 1965)

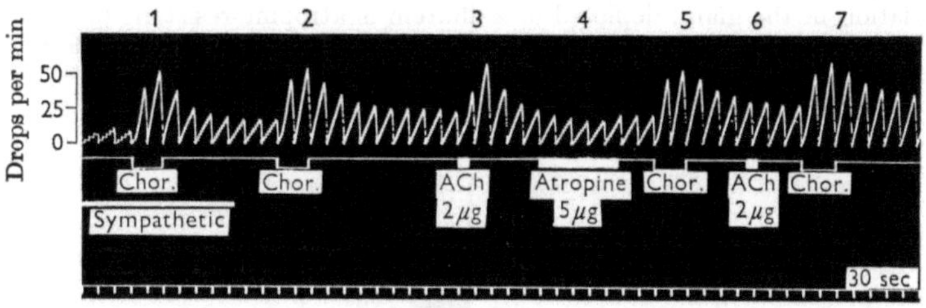

Fig. 2. Atropine-resistant vasodilatation (*5* and *7*) in a cat submaxillary gland perfused with horse serum (from which cat saliva fails to release kallidin); eserine 1:250,000 (w/v) present throughout. Vasodilatation was produced both on chorda lingual stimulation, either alone (*2*, *5*, and *7*), or when combined with cervical sympathetic stimulation (*1*) to increase "basal" vasoconstriction, and after atropine given at *4*. Note that atropine blocks the effect of close-arterial injection of ACh. (From BHOOLA et al., 1965)

chorda lingual nerve. The increased blood flow produced by injection of saliva is always slower in onset; it is never as great as that obtained by nerve stimulation (or by injected acetylcholine or bradykinin), and it is more protracted. Further, whereas marked duplication of the vasodilator response to nerve stimulation or to injections of acetylcholine is readily obtained, a progressive reduction of the vasodilatation occurs quickly with repeated injections of saliva. Some of these observations are seen in the experiment shown in Fig. 1.

(2) After desensitization of the gland's blood vessels to a standard dose of bradykinin by close-arterial infusion of high concentrations of this substance, the equivalent vasodilator response to chorda lingual nerve stimulation or to injection of acetylcholine is reduced to a much lesser degree (BHOOLA et al., 1965).

(3) It is possible to produce a maximal, atropine-resistant vasodilatation by stimulation of the chorda lingual nerve when the gland has been perfused for as long as 3 hours with horse serum, from which cat saliva fails to release kinin. Under these conditions, close-arterial injection of saliva fails to cause vasodilatation, indicating the unavailability of kininogen in the preparation. Nonetheless, a maximal vasodilatation can be produced by chorda lingual nerve stimulation at this time (Fig. 2).

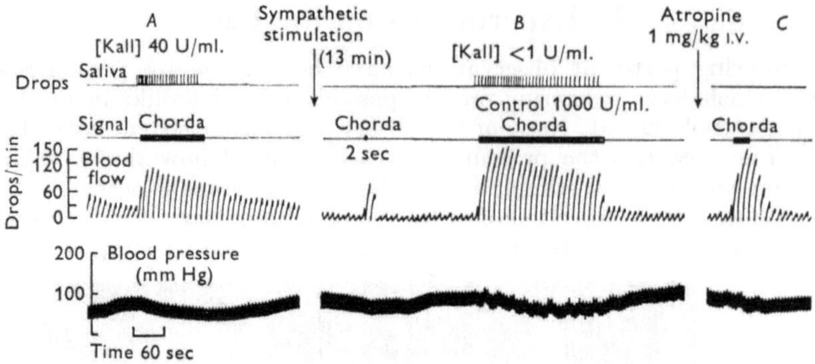

Fig. 3A–C. Blood flow and salivary secretion in a cat's submaxillary gland after depletion of kallikrein. A Record of salivary secretion and blood flow 3 days after duct ligation. Chorda saliva contains only 40 KU/ml, but the accompanying vasodilatation is normal. B Between A and B the sympathetic nerve was stimulated for 13 min to further deplete the gland of kallikrein. A marked vasodilatation is obtained in response to only 2 sec of chorda stimulation. A more prolonged chorda stimulation produces a maximal vasodilatation, although kallikrein is undetectable (<1 KU/ml) in the accompanying secretion. Saliva obtained from the contralateral gland at the same time contains 1,000 KU/ml. C The vasodilatation in response to chorda stimulation in the gland depleted of kallikrein is atropine-resistant (as in the normal gland) but salivary secretion is blocked. (From BEILENSON et al., 1968)

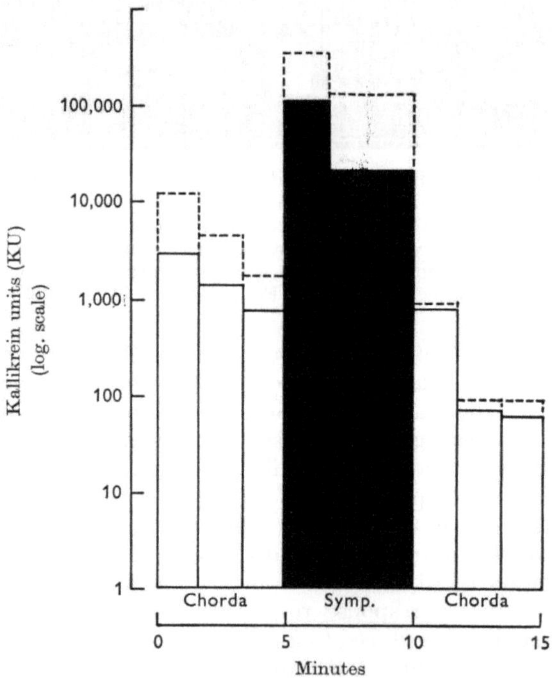

Fig. 4. Comparison of the effects of chorda lingual and sympathetic nerve stimulation on concentration and output of kallikrein in saliva from a cat's submaxillary gland (5 drops of saliva were rejected between samples 3 and 4, and between 5 and 6). Chorda lingual and sympathetic nerve stimulation were stopped for 20 sec after each 10-sec period of stimulation. Abscissae indicate durations of actual nerve stimulation, excluding intervals of interruption. ⬚ Kallikrein concentration, KU/ml. □ or ■ Kallikrein output, KU/min. (From BEILENSON et al., 1968)

(4) BEILENSON et al. (1968) were able to deplete the cat's submaxillary gland of kallikrein either by ligation of the duct for several days or by duct ligation plus subsequent sympathetic nerve stimulation. Such glands still responded to chorda lingual nerve stimulation with a normal atropine-resistant vasodilatation, although kallikrein was undetectable in the saliva obtained during this stimulation or in the gland itself after the vasodilatation (Fig. 3).

(5) Whereas stimulation of the chorda lingual nerve to the submaxillary gland causes marked vasodilatation, stimulation of the sympathetic nerve, which causes vasoconstriction, produces saliva with a far greater concentration of kallikrein (Fig. 4).

(6) Whereas there is a close parallelism between curves showing the rate of secretion of saliva and vasodilatation at different frequencies of nerve stimulation,

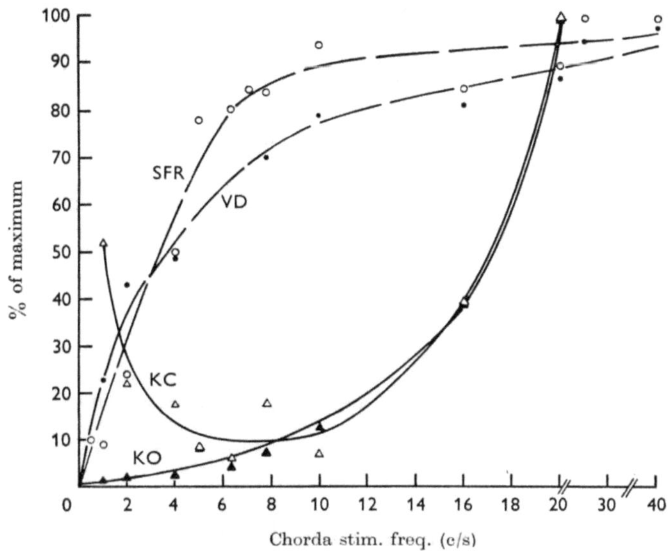

Fig. 5. Cat's submaxillary gland. Relationship between frequency of chorda nerve stimulation and (0) saliva flow rate (*SFR*); ● vasodilatation (*VD*); ▲ kallikrein output in saliva (*KO*); and △ kallikrein concentration in saliva (*KC*). The sequence of the different frequencies of stimulation was randomized in each experiment. SFR (ml/min), each measurement is the mean of nine experiments. VD (ml/min), each measurement is the mean of five experiments. KO and KC (KU/min and KU/ml) respectively, each measurement is the mean of five experiments. (From BEILENSON et al., 1968)

the curves of the output and concentration of kallikrein in the saliva for the same frequencies of nerve stimulation are distinctly different from the others. Thus, when the chorda lingual nerve is stimulated at a frequency of 8 cps, whereas the salivary flow rate and vasodilatation are near their highest, the concentration and output of kallikrein in saliva are near their lowest values (Fig. 5).

(7) After injection of carboxypeptidase B, a potent inactivator of kinins, hyperemia normally produced by the infusion of bradykinin close-arterially was blocked, whereas the vasodilator response to nerve stimulation, even at minimal levels of stimulation, was unaffected (Fig. 6) (SKINNER and WEBSTER, 1968). Similar results have been obtained by BEILENSON, MORIWAKI, and SCHACHTER (unpublished).

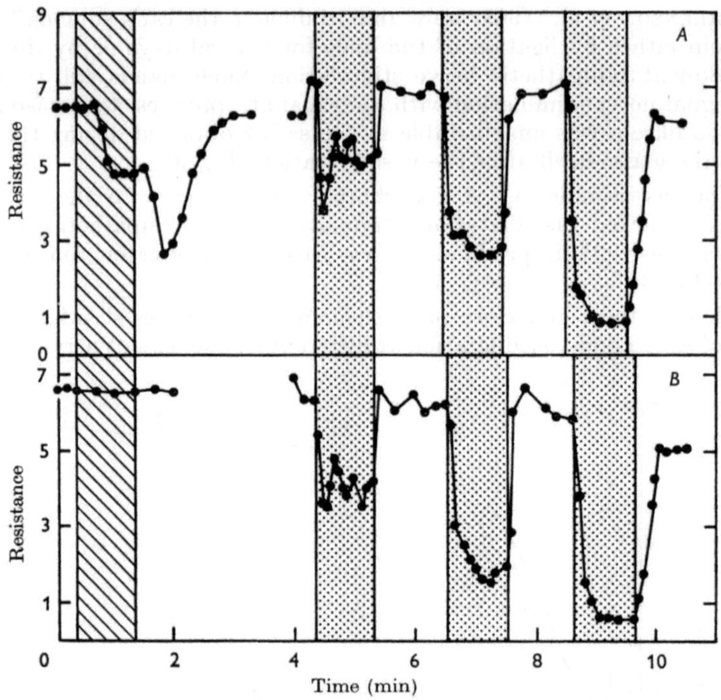

Fig. 6. Effect of carboxypeptidase B on vasodilatation induced by infusion of bradykinin and chorda tympani nerve stimulation. Resistance (mm Hg·ml flow)$^{-1}$ 100 g^{-1}·min^{-1}) plotted against time. The 60-sec periods of bradykinin infusion at 2.7 μg/min (left: hatched areas) and nerve stimulation (right: stippled areas) are shown. Stimulation voltage, 2.0 V; impulse duration, 0.5 msec; and stimulation frequencies, 2/sec, 3/sec, 5/sec, respectively. Panel A = without carboxypeptidase B; Panel B = with carboxypeptidase B (130 μg/ml blood). (From SKINNER and WEBSTER, 1968)

C. Experiments on the Rabbit

In contrast to the cat and dog, experiments on the submaxillary gland of the rabbit (MORLEY et al., 1966) have demonstrated a parallel sensitivity of parasympathetic-induced secretion and vasodilatation to atropine. Fig. 7 illustrates the sensitivity of the chorda-induced vasodilatation to atropine whereas both the sympathetic vasoconstriction and after-dilatation are unaffected. Fig. 8 shows the parallel inhibition of secretion and vasodilatation in the same rabbit by atropine. The effective dose of atropine varied considerably in different rabbits, probably due to the marked differences in the concentration of atropinase in the plasma of different rabbits (SAWIN and GLICK, 1943). Bradykinin itself was relatively ineffective in causing vasodilatation in the gland when injected close-arterially.

D. Experiments on the Sheep

In unpublished experiments on lambs and sheep, BEILENSON, SMAJE, and SCHACHTER found that the secretion and vasodilatation induced by parasympathetic nerve stimulation in the parotid gland were equally sensitive to inhibition by atropine. In the submaxillary gland, however, although the secretion was readily blocked by atropine (as in the parotid), the vasodilatation was resistant.

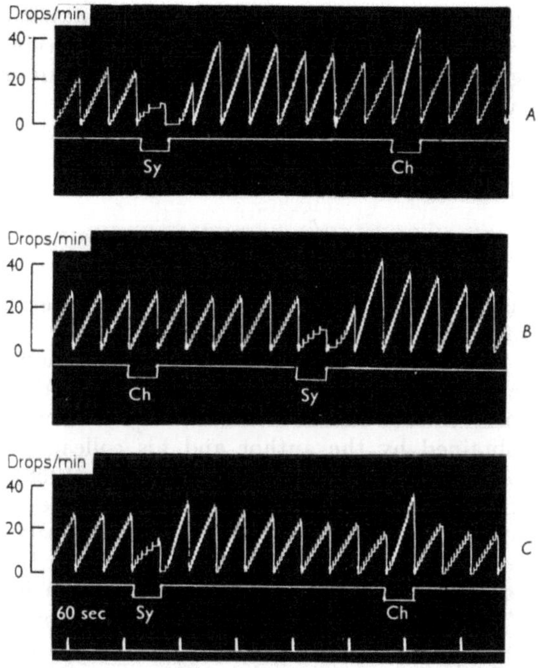

Fig. 7 A–C. Record of blood flow in submaxillary gland of rabbit (4.3 kg) showing vascular responses to chorda lingual (*Ch*), and sympathetic (*Sy*), nerve stimulation. A Control. B 35 min after atropine (250 µg/kg i.v.). C 6 min after eserine (250 µg/kg i.v.). (From MORLEY et al., 1966)

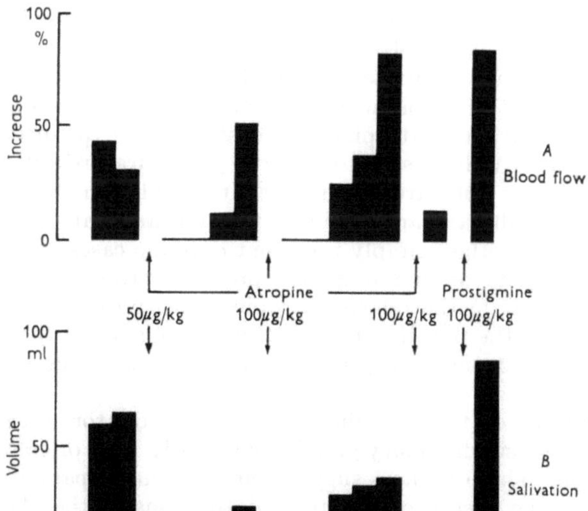

Fig. 8 A and B. The parallel effects of intravenous injections of atropine and prostigmine on the vasodilatation (A), and salivation (B) in the submaxillary gland of a rabbit (4.7 kg) caused by stimulation of the chorda lingual nerve for 30 sec. Time scale as in Fig. 2. (From MORLEY et al., 1966)

Thus, in three animals, both the secretion and vasodilatation were completely blocked in the parotid gland after the intravenous injection of atropine in a dose of 100–200 μg/kg. In the submaxillary gland of four animals, however, whereas the parasympathetic secretion was blocked by atropine in doses of 100–200 μg/kg i.v., the accompanying vasodilatation was not blocked by doses ranging from 1,000–6,850 μg/kg. Similar results were obtained when both glands were compared in the same animals.

E. Discussion

The observations in the cat, particularly the occurrence of a maximal vasodilatation on chorda lingual nerve stimulation when (a) the gland had been perfused for hours with a medium which contained no substrate for salivary kallikrein, or (b) the gland with normal circulation had been depleted of kallikrein, must be taken to indicate that kallikrein is not required for this vasodilatation. The other results obtained by the author and his colleagues also lead to this conclusion. The observation of SKINNER and WEBSTER (1968), confirmed in our laboratory, that whereas the marked vasodilatation in the gland produced by close-arterial infusion of bradykinin is "blocked" completely by carboxypeptidase B, that produced by chorda lingual nerve stimulation is unaffected, is also convincing evidence against a significant role of kallikrein in the mediation of this vasodilatation. Evidence that the arterioles of the parotid and submaxillary glands of the cat are innervated by parasympathetic as well as sympathetic nerve fibers has recently been presented by GARRETT (1966a, b) on the basis of electronmicroscopic and histochemical studies. GARRETT states, "The present investigation shows quite conclusively that the vessels in the parotid receive a dual innervation. The evidence is a little less complete for the submandibular gland because of the inability to perform postganglionic parasympathectomy, but it is nevertheless fairly conclusive, for nerves were always detected in the vessels at all stages after extremely radical postganglionic sympathetic denervations, and these results are supported by cholinesterase studies".

The experiments on the rabbit which demonstrate the parallel sensitivity of secretion and vasodilatation of atropine are most readily explained by assuming that true vasodilator as well as secretory nerve fibers are present in the chorda tympani nerve, and that both are cholinergic. It would seem probable that this vasodilatation in the submaxillary gland of the dog and cat on the one hand, and of the rabbit on the other, simply represent extreme cases of the well-known variation in the sensitivity of cholinergic receptors to atropine (AMBACHE, 1955). The extreme discrepancy in the relative atropine sensitivities of the parasympathetic vasodilatation in the parotid and submaxillary glands of the sheep suggest that a thorough microscopic study of the blood vessels in these glands might prove enlightening.

A new explanation of the atropine-resistant vasodilator effects of chorda stimulation in the cat's submaxillary gland has recently been offered by SKINNER and WEBSTER (1968). These authors suggest that the major part of chorda vasodilatation is due to the presence of adrenergic neurons in the chorda tympani nerve which cause vasodilatation via β-adrenergic receptors that are present in the blood vessels. According to SKINNER and WEBSTER, the vasodilatation produced by chorda lingual nerve stimulation is suppressed by propranolol (a β-receptor blocking drug) in parallel with the block by propranolol of the vasodilatation produced by isoproterenol injected into the gland close-arterially. This view is questioned by BEILENSON and SCHACHTER (1968), who in part confirm the observations of SKINNER and WEBSTER with propranolol but maintain that although large doses of propranolol can reduce chorda vasodilatation, they also reduce the action of acetylcholine in parallel. Furthermore, BEILENSON and SCHACHTER (1968) have shown that in a cat pretreated with reserpine, the secretory and vasomotor actions of sympathetic stimulation on the submaxillary

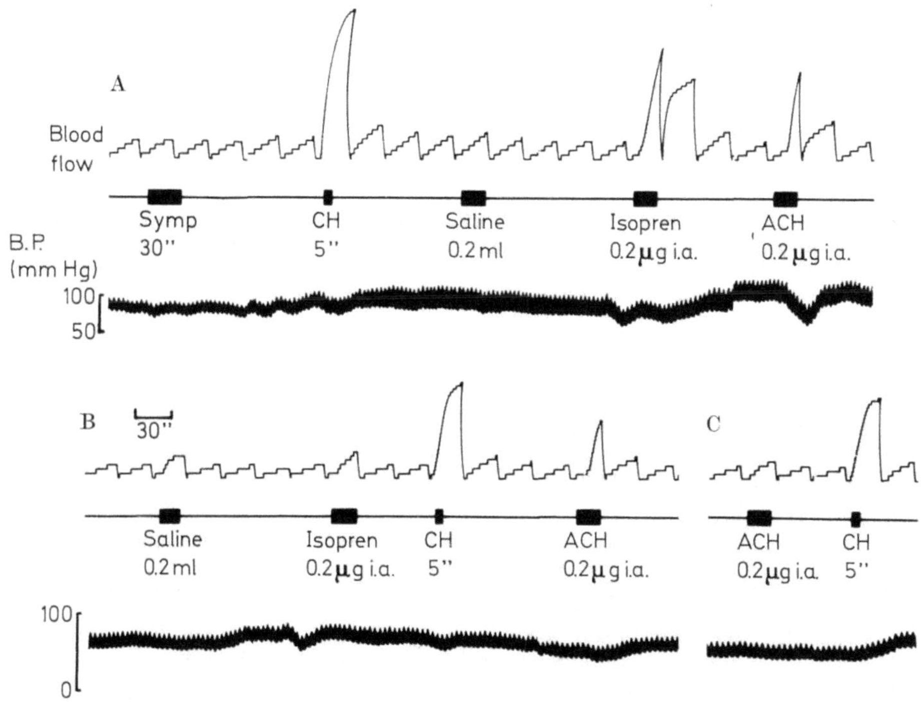

Fig. 9 A–C. Cat (2.1 kg) treated 24 hr previously with reserpine (1 mg/kg s.c.). A Sympathetic nerve stimulation for 30 sec is without effect after reserpine whereas chorda lingual nerve stimulation produces typical vasodilatation. Injections of isoproterenol (isoprenaline, 0.2 μg) and acetylcholine (0.2 μg) close-arterially produce marked dilatation. Control injection of saline (0.2 ml) is without effect. Between A and B, propranolol (20 μg) was injected close-arterially. B Propanolol blocks the effect of isoproterenol. In this experiment the effects of chorda lingual nerve stimulation and acetylcholine injection are proportionally reduced by propranolol. Between B and C, atropine (20 μg) was injected close-arterially. The effect of injected acetylcholine is now completely blocked and there is a slight reduction in the effect of chorda lingual nerve stimulation. (From SCHACHTER and BEILENSON, 1968)

gland are absent, whereas chorda vasodilatation is normal. These results are shown in Fig. 9.

It is the author's opinion that further electronmicroscopic anatomical studies, extending those of GARRETT (1966a, b), and attempting to relate structural detail to the many new physiological observations, are desirable. It would be of interest to study the parasympathetic innervation of blood vessels (as described by GARRETT for the cat) in the rabbit, where parasympathetic vasodilatation, unlike that in the cat, is sensitive to atropine. For similar reasons, it would be desirable to carry out studies comparing the vascular innervation of the parotid and submaxillary glands in the sheep.

In the author's opinion the significance of kallikrein in the salivary glands remains an intriguing but as yet unsolved problem.

References

AMBACHE, N.: The uses and limitations of atropine for pharmacological studies on autonomic effectors. Pharmacol. Rev. **7**, 467 (1955).

BARCROFT, J.: The respiratory function of the blood. London: University Press 1914.

BEILENSON, S., SCHACHTER, M., SMAJE, L. H.: Secretion of kallikrein and its role in vasodilatation in the submaxillary gland. J. Physiol. (Lond.) **199**, 303 (1968).

BHOOLA, K. D., MAY MAY YI, R., MORLEY, J., SCHACHTER, M.: Release of kinin by an enzyme in the accessory sex glands of the guinea-pig. J. Physiol. (Lond.) **163**, 269 (1962).

— MORLEY, J., SCHACHTER, M., SMAJE, L. H.: Vasodilatation in the submaxillary gland of the cat. J. Physiol. (Lond.) **179**, 172 (1965).

FOX, R. H., HILTON, S. M.: Bradykinin formation in human skin as a factor in heat vasodilatation. J. Physiol. (Lond.) **142**, 219 (1958).

GARRETT, J. R.: The innervation of salivary glands. III. The effects of certain experimental procedures on cholinesterase-positive nerves in glands of the cat. J. roy. micr. Soc. **86**, 1 (1966a).

— The innervation of salivary glands. IV. The effects of certain experimental procedures on the ultrastructure of nerves in glands of the cat. J. roy. micr. Soc. **86**, 15 (1966b).

HILTON, S. M.: Plasma kinin and blood flow. In: Polypeptides which affect smooth muscles and blood vessels, ed. by M. SCHACHTER. London: Pergamon Press 1960.

— JONES, M.: The role of plasma kinin in functional vasodilatation in the pancreas. J. Physiol. (Lond.) **195**, 521 (1968).

— LEWIS, G. P.: The cause of the vasodilatation accompanying activity in the submandibular gland. J. Physiol. (Lond.) **128**, 235 (1955a).

— — The mechanism of the functional hyperaemia in the submandibular salivary gland. J. Physiol. (Lond.) **129**, 253 (1955b).

— — The relationship between glandular activity, bradykinin formation and functional vasodilatation in the submandibular salivary gland. J. Physiol. (Lond.) **134**, 471 (1956).

— — Vasodilatation in the tongue, and its relationship to plasma kinin formation. J. Physiol. (Lond.) **144**, 532 (1958).

MORLEY, J., SCHACHTER, M., SMAJE, L. H.: Vasodilatation in the submaxillary gland of the rabbit. J. Physiol. (Lond.) **187**, 595 (1966).

SAWIN, P. B., GLICK, D.: Atropinesterase, a genetically determined enzyme in the rabbit. Proc. nat. Acad. Sci. (Wash.) **29**, 55 (1943).

SCHACHTER, M.: Some properties of kallidin, bradykinin and wasp venom kinin. In: Polypeptides which affect smooth muscles and blood vessels, ed. by M. SCHACHTER. London: Pergamon Press 1960.

— BEILENSON, S.: Mediator of vasodilatation in the submaxillary gland. Fed. Proc. **27**, No 1, 73 (1968).

SKINNER, N. S., WEBSTER, M. E.: Submaxillary gland blood flow: The role of kinins and β-adrenergic receptors. J. Physiol. (Lond.) **195**, 505 (1968).

UNGAR, G., PARROT, J. L.: Sur la presence de la callicreine dans la salive, et la possibilité de son intervention dans la transmission chimique de l'influx nerveux. C. R. Soc. Biol. (Paris) **122**, 1052 (1936).

WERLE, E., GÖTZE, W., KEPPLER, E.: Über die Wirkung des Kallikreins auf den isolierten Darm und über eine neue darmkontrahierende Substanz. Biochem. Z. **289**, 217 (1937).

— RODEN, P. v.: Über das Vorkommen von Kallikrein in den Speicheldrüsen und im Mundspeichel. Biochem. Z. **286**, 213 (1936).

Kinins and Ventilation of the Lungs

H. O. J. Collier

A. Introduction

Kinins influence mammalian lungs both directly and indirectly. In several species, kinins lessen the volume of air entering the lungs during spontaneous or artificial ventilation *in vivo* and, in the guinea pig, they are also effective in isolated preparations of lungs or tracheobronchial muscle. In some species also, kinins raise the pressure in the pulmonary artery and constrict isolated pulmonary blood vessels. Kinins affect, too, the rate and depth of the ventilatory movements of ribs and diaphragm.

Several of the effects of kinins on lungs are puzzling and some are paradoxical. For example, although bradykinin constricts the airways of the isolated lungs of the guinea pig, it is ineffective in several other species. Likewise, inhaled bradykinin in aerosol causes bronchoconstriction in some asthmatic patients, but not in others or in normal individuals. Again, bradykinin is at least as effective as histamine in the isolated lung of the guinea pig, but it is much less effective than histamine on the isolated trachea of this species. Likewise, in the artificially ventilated guinea pig, bradykinin lessens the volume of air entering the lungs, but dilates the trachea. Also in the artificially ventilated guinea pig, bradykinin is detectably effective at a lower dose than is histamine or 5-hydroxytryptamine; yet, with increasing doses, the response to bradykinin increases less than does the response to the other bronchoconstrictor agents and it never reaches so high a maximum. Yet again, bradykinin embarrasses respiration in the guinea pig when injected intravenously or intracardially but is ineffective when given intraperitoneally or by inhalation.

The paradoxes extend to the antagonism of kinin effects on the lungs. Thus aspirin very readily blocks the effect of kinins on lung volume in the artificially ventilated guinea pig, even after destruction of the central nervous system and blockade of β-receptors for adrenaline; yet aspirin shows a feebler effect in preparations of isolated trachea and is ineffective against bradykinin in rabbit lung and in some other responses of the guinea pig to kinins *in vivo*.

Not only do kinins affect lungs, but lungs affect kinins. For example, bradykinin is rapidly destroyed while passing through lungs (p. 417), and again, when the lungs isolated from a sensitized guinea pig are challenged, kallikrein is liberated (p. 416). The potent effects of the lungs on kinins, as well as those of kinins on the lungs, suggest that these peptides play a part in the natural reactions of this organ, at least in some species.

We do not fully understand these complex and sometimes paradoxical effects. This review attempts to outline what is known, to appraise and to interpret the experiments upon which this knowledge is based and to set down the evidence that kinins are involved in some natural reactions of the lungs of the guinea pig and perhaps man.

B. Responses of Lungs to Kinins

Because the responses of the lungs to kinins depend upon the species of animal and the type of preparation in which they are tested and even upon the route by which the kinin is administered, the effects of kinins on particular lung preparations will be considered separately. Likewise, because drugs may modify these responses only in some situations, the effects of drugs are best considered while the responses of particular preparations are discussed.

I. Tracheobronchial Muscle in vitro

Bradykinin contracts the isolated trachea of the guinea pig, but not that of the rabbit or the isolated bronchial muscle of dog or man (Hawkins, 1952; Bhoola et al., 1962). As might be expected, the trachea of the guinea pig contracted more slowly in response to bradykinin than to histamine. Bradykinin was less potent than histamine and its dose-response line was flatter and reached a lower maximal response than did histamine. Bradykinin also tended to induce tachyphylaxis in the trachea. Nonsteroidal anti-inflammatory drugs, such as amidopyrine and phenylbutazone, relaxed the trachea, and antagonized the response to bradykinin more effectively than that to histamine; but the sharp selectivity towards bradykinin shown by such drugs *in vivo* was not seen in the isolated trachea (Bhoola et al., 1962).

II. Isolated Lungs

Bradykinin strongly constricts the airways of the isolated whole lungs of the guinea pig, whether these are perfused via the pulmonary artery (Collier et al., 1960; Moog and Greeff, 1963; Greeff and Moog, 1964; Aarsen, 1966) or via the trachea (Bhoola et al., 1962; Aarsen, 1966) or whether the lungs are part of a heart–lung preparation (Carpi et al., 1962). In some experiments, bradykinin had, weight for weight, roughly the same bronchoconstrictor potency as histamine (Collier et al., 1960; Bhoola et al., 1962; Aarsen, 1966). In other experiments bradykinin was more potent than histamine (Moog and Greeff, 1963; Greeff and Moog, 1964; Aarsen, 1966).

Carpi et al. (1962) found that phenylbutazone blocked the bronchoconstrictor response of the heart–lung preparation of the guinea pig to bradykinin. Moog and Greeff (1963) and Greeff and Moog (1964) found that aspirin and phenylbutazone blocked the response to bradykinin, but not that to histamine or to 5-hydroxytryptamine. Aarsen (1966) failed to obtain this blocking effect with either drug.

Bradykinin does not constrict the airways of the isolated lungs of several species other than the guinea pig. Greeff and Moog (1964) observed no bronchoconstriction in rat or cat lungs *in vitro*. In rabbit isolated lungs, perfused with blood via the pulmonary artery, neither bradykinin nor kallikrein, administered in the blood, induced bronchoconstriction (Hauge et al., 1966). Likewise, in an isolated preparation of dog lungs perfused with blood, bradykinin (injected into the pulmonary or bronchial circulation) either did not affect the airways or slightly dilated them (Waaler, 1961).

In some of the above-mentioned experiments on isolated lungs, the effects of kinins on the blood vessels were also tested. In the isolated lungs of both guinea pig and rabbit, bradykinin and kallikrein constricted the pulmonary blood vessels (Carpi et al., 1962; Greeff and Moog, 1964; Hauge et al., 1966). In the isolated lungs of the dog, on the contrary, bradykinin dilated both the pulmonary and bronchial blood vessels (Waaler, 1961).

III. Artifically Ventilated Preparations in vivo

Kinins in the Konzett-Rössler Preparation. The effects of kinins on the airways have been studied in artifically ventilated preparations of the guinea pig, rabbit, cat, and rat *in vivo*. Most investigators have used the preparation of Konzett and Rössler (1940), in which the lungs are intermittently inflated with a pump of fixed stroke volume. When a predetermined pressure (usually about 10 cm water) is exceeded during inflation, the air overflows into a volume recorder. The overflow volume is thus inversely related to the volume of air entering the lungs. An increase in overflow volume will hence reflect a decrease in lung volume at a fixed maximal inflation pressure. Such a decrease will mainly depend on a fall in lung compliance, which can result from a constriction followed by a collapse of the smaller airways, or from changes in surface tension at the alveolar–air interface or, again, from lung edema or vascular congestion (Widdicombe, 1963). Changes that are rapid in onset and reversible seem unlikely to depend on edema. With substances shown to contract the isolated tracheobronchial muscle of the species under test, an increase in lung compliance after their intravenous injection is likely, at least in part, to reflect a constriction of the finer branches of the bronchial tree.

In the Konzett-Rössler preparation of the guinea pig, small intravenous doses of bradykinin (0.1–1 μg/kg), after a latency of about 6 seconds cause a relatively slow and very prolonged increase in air overflow volume (Collier et al., 1959, 1960; Elliott et al., 1960; Konzett and Stürmer, 1960; Bisset and Lewis, 1962; Berry and Collier, 1964). Kallidin had an effect similar to bradykinin but was slightly less potent (Bhoola et al., 1962).

Bradykinin remained effective after the administration of atropine, after transection of the vagi, or after destruction of the central nervous system (Collier and Shorley, 1960; Berry and Collier, 1964; Collier et al., 1966). These findings show that, in this preparation, the increase of air overflow induced by bradykinin is not mediated reflexly or by stimulation of cholinergic bronchoconstrictor fibers.

By the intravenous route, bradykinin was roughly as potent as was histamine in the Konzett-Rössler preparation of the guinea pig, but the slope of the dose response curve was flatter and the maximum response was lower than that for histamine (Collier et al., 1960, 1965; Bisset and Lewis, 1962). When dropped onto the pleural surface of the exposed lungs, bradykinin also increased air overflow volume in the Konzett-Rössler preparation, but by this route it was effective at a lower dose than was histamine, suggesting that bradykinin has a particularly potent action on smooth musculature in the neighborhood of the alveoli (Bhoola et al., 1962).

The effect of intravenous bradykinin on the Konzett-Rössler preparation of the guinea pig readily shows tachyphylaxis, particularly in some animals (Collier et al., 1960; Elliott et al., 1960). Kallidin was cross-tachyphylactic with bradykinin (Collier and James, 1967). The two kinins also showed cross-tachyphylaxis in their effect on the pulmonary circulation of the rabbit (Hauge et al., 1966).

Bradykinin also increases air overflow volume when injected intravenously in the Konzett-Rössler preparation of the cat (Konzett and Stürmer, 1960) and of the rabbit and rat (Bhoola et al., 1962). The potency of bradykinin in the rabbit was roughly comparable with its potency in the guinea pig; but it was low in the cat and still lower in the rat.

Modification by Drugs of the Konzett-Rössler Response. Relatively few types of drugs have so far been found to modify the effect of bradykinin in the Konzett-Rössler preparation of the guinea pig *in vivo*. Most drugs that antagonize bradykinin in this preparation are either nonsteroidal anti-inflammatory agents of the aspirin group or nonspecific bronchodilators. The main potentiators of bradykinin are drugs that antagonize adrenaline.

All anti-inflammatory drugs of the group exemplified by aspirin and phenylbutazone so far tested have antagonized bradykinin in the Konzett-Rössler preparation; but benzydamine, the corticosteroids, and the quinoline antimalarials are inactive (Collier et al., 1959, 1960, 1968; Collier and Shorley, 1960, 1963; Berry and Collier, 1964; Simke et al., 1967; Jahn and Wagner-Jauregg, 1968). Like drugs of the aspirin group, 2,4-dinitrophenol uncouples oxidative phosphorylation, but it was inactive in the antibradykinin test (Collier et al., 1968). Morphine, hexamethonium, atropine, and the antihistamines did not antagonize bradykinin in this test (Collier and Shorley, 1960; Berry and Collier, 1964; Simke et al., 1967). Simke and co-workers (1967) have reported that chlorpromazine and phenoxybenzamine also antagonized the effect of bradykinin, but Collier and co-workers (1968) could not confirm this, although they found that phenelzine and mebanazine were weak antagonists.

In the Konzett-Rössler preparation of the guinea pig, aspirin and like-acting drugs did not lessen responses to acetylcholine, angiotensin, eledoisin, histamine, 5-hydroxytryptamine, or substance P (Collier and Shorley, 1960; Bhoola et al., 1962; Stürmer and Berde, 1963); but they did also antagonize a slow-reacting substance in anaphylaxis (SRS-A), adenosine triphosphate (Berry and Collier, 1964; Collier et al., 1966), and arachidonic acid (Berry, 1966). The antagonism is therefore selective, but not specific.

The antagonism of bradykinin and SRS-A by these anti-inflammatory drugs is potent — by the intravenous route, aspirin was effective at 1–2 mg/kg and meclofenamate was effective at 62.5–125 μg/kg. Over a certain range, the dose of bradykinin required to produce a given response was directly related to the dose of aspirin or fenamate (Collier and Shorley, 1960, 1963; Collier et al., 1968). When this relationship was tested at very high doses of aspirin, however, it broke down and no practical dose of aspirin would suppress the effect of a very high dose of bradykinin (Collier and Shorley, 1963).

The antagonism of bradykinin by aspirin or fenamates occurred in the Konzett-Rössler preparation after vagotomy or destruction of the central nervous system and after adrenalectomy or blockade of β-receptors for adrenaline (Collier and Shorley, 1960; Berry and Collier, 1964; Collier et al., 1966, 1968). The antagonism therefore appears to be a local one, but Aarsen (1966) failed to obtain it in isolated preparations of guinea pig lung and it was difficult to show in the guinea-pig isolated trachea (Bhoola et al., 1962). The antagonism was also not seen in some other responses of the guinea-pig (Collier and Shorley, 1960; Lewis, 1963) or in the response to bradykinin of the Konzett-Rössler preparation of the rabbit or rat (Bhoola et al., 1962). This antagonism therefore remains a rather curious and isolated phenomenon. Its mechanism is not explained, but the conclusion has been reached that "aspirin and like-acting drugs block a route leading to or from the specific receptors for the agonists [kinins, SRS-A, ATP and arachidonic acid], rather than blocking these receptors themselves" (Collier et al., 1966). Collier (1969) has suggested that the common point in the route that aspirin blocks might be a carrier mechanism whereby agonists of this group reach their receptors on bronchial muscle, or, alternatively, it might be the release of an unidentified broncho-active substance through which all of these agonists act upon bronchial muscle.

A less selective antagonism of bradykinin-induced airway constriction is that exerted by general bronchodilators of the type of adrenaline (COLLIER et al., 1960) and prostaglandin E_2 (ROSENTHALE et al., 1968).

Drugs that block β-receptors for adrenaline shift the dose–response line of bradykinin to the left and raise the maximal response obtainable (COLLIER et al., 1965; COLLIER, 1966; SIMKE et al., 1967). Other drugs that inhibit adrenergic mechanisms, such as guanethidine and reserpine, also enhanced the response to bradykinin (SIMKE et al., 1967). SIMKE and co-workers also record the enhancement of bradykinin-induced constriction of the airways with ε-amino-n-caproic acid (EACA), which inhibits the enzymatic destruction of bradykinin (ERDÖS, 1966), and with amethopterin. The activity of amethopterin suggests that it too may inhibit kininases.

IV. Action and Antagonism of Kinins in Other Preparations

GJURIS and WESTERMANN (1965) have studied the action and antagonism of kinins in the anesthetized guinea pig placed in a whole-body plethysmograph. In artificially ventilated animals, paralyzed with succinylcholine, both bradykinin and kallidin reduced the inflation volume. The dose–response curve of bradykinin was very flat compared with the curve of eledoisin or 5-hydroxytryptamine. With bradykinin, the maximal reduction of inflation volume was not more than 50%, whereas, with eledoisin and 5-hydroxytryptamine, 100% reduction of inflation volume was obtainable. Low doses of bradykinin were readily antagonized by isoproterenol, adrenaline, aspirin, or phenylbutazone; but higher doses of bradykinin were not antagonized by any of these drugs.

JAMES (1969) has studied the action and antagonism of bradykinin in a guinea pig preparation in which a part of the trachea is separated from the rest of the bronchial tree. The animal is artificially ventilated through a cannula in the pulmonary part of the bronchial tree. Pressures in the separate segment of trachea and in the laryngeal end of the pulmonary part of the bronchial tree are independently recorded. In this preparation, intravenous bradykinin lowered pressure inside the separated tracheal segment, whereas it raised pressure inside the pulmonary part of the bronchial tree. A similar dose of bradykinin, given into the arch of the aorta so as to reach the bronchial artery, lowered pressure in the tracheal segment but did not change pressure in the rest of the bronchial tree.

The effect of bradykinin on the trachea was abolished by propranolol, but not changed by meclofenamate. The effect of bradykinin on the pulmonary part of the bronchial tree was enhanced by propranolol and abolished by meclofenamate. These experiments suggest that bradykinin has a dual action on the airways of the guinea pig, dilating the trachea through an adrenergic mechanism and constricting pulmonary airways served by the pulmonary artery.

V. Spontaneously Breathing Preparations

Laboratory Animals. In the conscious, intact guinea pig, an intracardial injection of bradykinin induced severe and long-lasting dyspnea; but administration of up to 20 mg/kg by the intraperitoneal route or of up to 2% solution of bradykinin by inhalation as an aerosol did not cause any respiratory distress (HERXHEIMER and STRESEMANN, 1961).

The responses to bradykinin of the spontaneously breathing guinea pig are complex. For example, in a lightly anesthetized animal, prepared for recording tracheal flow and tidal volume, intravenous bradykinin increased, whereas histamine lessened, tracheal flow and tidal volume; but, after β-receptors for adrenaline were blocked with propanolol, the same dose of bradykinin had an effect like that of histamine, except that it was less intense and more prolonged (Collier and James, 1969).

The bronchograms of Jänkälä and Virtama (1963), obtained in spontaneously breathing, lightly anesthetized guinea pigs and rabbits, explain how bradykinin may reduce tracheal flow and tidal volume after treatment with propranolol, because these bronchograms showed that bradykinin (1–600 μg/kg i.v.) constricted the respiratory bronchioles without narrowing larger airways. From mathematical considerations, such a localized constriction would lessen chiefly the volume of air inhaled (Weibel, 1963; Green, 1966) and hence would reduce tracheal flow and tidal volume.

In the guinea pig and rabbit, lightly anesthetized and breathing spontaneously, kinins induce changes in the rate and amplitude of ventilation, as recorded with a whole-body plethysmograph. Small intravenous doses of bradykinin (0.5–4 μg/kg i.v.) and slightly larger doses of kallidin induced a tachypnea that was prevented by cutting or cooling the vagi or by drugs of the aspirin group (Gjuris et al., 1964a; Gjuris and Westermann, 1965; Marquardt, 1966).

Although Gjuris and co-workers (1964a) claimed that bradykinin-induced tachypnea was not prevented by isoproterenol, Marquardt (1966) showed that isoproterenol prevented both the tachypnea and the accompanying burst of impulses in the vagus nerve that followed injection of bradykinin. From this and other experiments, Marquardt concluded that the tachypnea is probably a reflex response to the constriction of the airways elicited by kinins. This conclusion is consistent with the fact previously noted (Collier, 1965) that seven drugs of the group of aspirin and phenylbutazone had very similar potencies in blocking the tachypnea induced by bradykinin in the spontaneously breathing guinea pig (Gjuris et al., 1964a) as they had in antagonizing bradykinin-induced airway constriction in the artificially ventilated animal (Berry and Collier, 1964).

In the spontaneously breathing guinea pig and rabbit, higher doses of kinins arrest respiration in the expiratory position (Gjuris et al., 1964b; Gjuris and Westermann, 1965; Marquardt, 1966). In inducing this effect, kallidin was more effective than bradykinin, and both were more effective by the intracarotid than by the intrajugular route of injection (Gjuris et al., 1964b). Cutting both vagi enhanced, rather than blocked, the effect; but aspirin or phenylbutazone prevented it (Gjuris et al., 1964b; Marquardt, 1966). The mechanism of this apnea is unknown, but it presumably arises from an effect of kinins on sensory or nervous structures served by the carotid arteries.

Man. The demonstration that bradykinin induces airway constriction in the guinea pig (Collier et al., 1959) led Herxheimer and Stresemann (1961) to test bradykinin aerosol in man. They found that it reduced the vital capacity of chronic asthmatics, but at the same concentration (0.5%) it was ineffective in normal individuals.

This finding has been confirmed and extended in several studies. Stresemann (1963) reported that an aerosol of 0.5% bradykinin, inhaled for 20–100 seconds, lowered the vital capacity in 48 of 53 chronic asthmatics by 8–47% (mean 17%). The effect reached a peak in about 5 minutes and disappeared within about 25 minutes. In seven normal individuals, inhalation of bradykinin for up to 300 seconds was ineffective, and in two individuals an intravenous dose of 3 or 5 μg/kg failed to lower vital capacity. The effect was lessened by antipyretic drugs, by mepyramine, and by atropine, but these drugs also increased to about the same extent the vital capacity in asthmatics not treated with bradykinin (STRESEMANN, 1963). In 5 of 15 asthmatics, ethanol, taken by mouth between exposures to bradykinin aerosol, more than doubled the fall in vital capacity induced by bradykinin (HERXHEIMER and STRESEMANN, 1963).

LECOMTE et al. (1962) reported that in five normal subjects inhalation of an aerosol of 0.8% bradykinin did not increase airway resistance, although it provoked a prickling sensation in the upper airways and a facial flush. In four of six asthmatics, an 0.8% aerosol of bradykinin increased airway resistance by more than 50%. GIRARD and MORET (1963) essentially confirmed the above findings. VARONIER and PANZANI (1968) observed that an aerosol of 0.1% bradykinin significantly diminished peak flow in 14 of 16 asthmatic children, but in none of 15 normal controls.

VI. The Release of Catecholamines

Release from the Adrenals. Kinins indirectly affect airway function through their ability to release catecholamines, either from the adrenals or by stimulation of sympathetic ganglia. This explains both the potentiation of kinins by some antagonists of adrenaline and some of the paradoxical self-antagonistic effect exerted by kinins (COLLIER, 1966). This effect was probably first observed by LECOMTE and co-workers (1961, 1964) in the rat and rabbit; but it has been more fully explored in other species.

In the cat, 50 ng of bradykinin or 1 ng of angiotensin, injected into the abdominal aorta, released catecholamines from the adrenal glands (FELDBERG and LEWIS, 1964). Using the blood-bathed organ technique, in which blood flowing in an extracorporeal loop of the circulation, is superfused over test tissues with different sensitivities to adrenaline and noradrenaline, STASZEWSKA-BARCZAK and VANE (1967) have studied this effect further. Their experiments showed that the catecholamine released was adrenaline. In the cat, by the intra-arterial route, angiotensin was more effective than histamine and histamine more effective than bradykinin, weight for weight, in releasing adrenaline. In the dog, bradykinin was more effective than angiotensin or histamine. Eledoisin released adrenaline in the dog, but not in the cat. In the hands of FELDBERG and LEWIS (1964), bradykinin was slightly more effective than kallidin, but this order of potency was reversed in the hands of STASZEWSKA-BARCZAK and VANE (1967).

The blood-bathed organ technique has also been used to study the release of catecholamines by bradykinin and other substances in the guinea pig (PIPER et al., 1967; PIPER and VANE, 1967). In this species, adrenaline is the main catecholamine released into the circulation. Bradykinin was effective by the intravenous or the intra-arterial route and by the latter it released adrenaline without inducing bronchoconstriction (PIPER et al., 1967). To liberate 0.1 μg of adrenaline, the following intravenous doses were required: angiotensin, 0.37 μg; bradykinin, 0.75 μg; histamine 4.4 μg (PIPER and VANE, 1967). Whereas kinins liberate adrenaline from the adrenal gland of the rat, rabbit, cat, dog and guinea pig, bradykinin released little or no catecholamine from the adrenal gland of the calf (COMLINE et al., 1968).

Stimulation of a Ganglion. Bradykinin, kallidin, and angiotensin stimulate the superior cervical ganglion of the cat (LEWIS and REIT, 1965, 1966; TRENDELENBURG, 1966) as also do acetylcholine, histamine, 5-hydroxytryptamine, and adrenaline. Weight for weight, angiotensin was rather more active than bradykinin, histamine, or 5-hydroxytryptamine (Lewis and Reit, 1966). Morphine blocked stimulation due to bradykinin, angiotensin, or 5-hydroxytryptamine but not that due to adrenaline or nicotine (Lewis and Reit, 1966; Trendelenburg, 1966). Whereas morphine was effective against angiotensin and bradykinin at the superior cervical ganglion, it was but slightly effective at the adrenal medulla and ineffective against the changes that these peptides induce in blood pressure (Lewis and Reit, 1966). Although both bradykinin and angiotensin were blocked by morphine, their receptors on the ganglion cells are different, because the two peptides were not cross-tachyphylactic (Lewis and Reit, 1965). Relatively large intra-arterial doses of bradykinin stimulated the superior cervical ganglion of the dog and rabbit (Lewis and Reit, 1966).

Self-Antagonism of Kinins. The release of adrenaline and the stimulation of sympathetic ganglia tend to oppose the direct effect of kinins on the bronchioles. Bradykinin-induced airway constriction is therefore self-antagonizing and is much potentiated by blockade of β-receptors for adrenaline (Collier et al., 1965; Collier, 1966; James, 1969). The self-antagonism may be great enough for the adrenergic effect to outweigh the direct effect of kinin, as in the trachea of the guinea pig *in vivo*, which relaxes to bradykinin, except after β-receptor blockade (James, 1969). The readiness with which kinins release catecholamines when they reach the superior cervical ganglion and the adrenal medulla has led to the suggestion (Collier, 1966) that this release is a mechanism to protect the body against the systemic spread of kinins liberated locally at a site of injury.

C. The Role of Kinins in Airway Function

That kinins are highly effective in constricting the airways of the guinea pig and of the human asthmatic raises the question whether these peptides help to mediate airway constriction in response to irritants or to antigens in the guinea pig or man. Several groups of workers have reported results bearing on this question. In anaphylaxis of the guinea pig, the kinin concentration of the blood rose (Brocklehurst and Lahiri, 1962; Lahiri, 1962) (p. 541). Subsequently, the kininogen concentration fell (Lahiri, 1962; Brocklehurst and Lahiri, 1963; Greeff et al., 1966). When the isolated lungs of sensitized guinea pigs were challenged with antigen, kallikrein was liberated (Brocklehurst and Lahiri, 1962; Jonasson and Becker, 1966). In severe bronchial asthma in man, Abe and co-workers (1967) have found a raised kinin concentration in the blood. Dolovich et al. (1968) have reported that secretions of the respiratory tract of some sufferers from asthma, hay fever, and bronchitis contained a kinin-like substance. Di Mattei (1967) has detected kininogen and kinin in extracts of human lung adenocarcinoma.

Experiments with drugs in sensitized guinea pigs provide further evidence of the participation of kinins in anaphylactic bronchoconstriction. Aspirin or meclofenamate significantly lessened the bronchoconstriction that immediately follows intravenous challenge and each synergized with mepyramine in so doing (Collier et al., 1963, 1968; Collier and James, 1967). Since both these anti-inflammatory drugs antagonize not only kinins but also a slow-reacting bronchoconstrictor substance liberated in anaphylaxis (Berry and Collier, 1964; Collier et al., 1968), their effectiveness does not prove that kinins participate in anaphylactic bronchoconstriction. That specific desensitization to bradykinin also lessened the bronchoconstrictor response shows that kinins are involved in it (Collier and James, 1967).

FERREIRA and VANE (1967) found that bradykinin was quickly destroyed while passing in the pulmonary circulation through the lungs of the cat. This finding supports the view that kinins play a part in lung function, because a powerful mechanism of destruction tends to exist alongside the site of action of a local hormone.

D. Summary and Conclusion

Kinins affect tracheobronchial smooth muscle in different ways and to different extents, according to the site of the muscle, the type of test preparation used, and the species and pathological condition of the subject. Among laboratory animals, the guinea pig has been most fully studied in the responses of its ventilatory mechanism to kinins. Bradykinin contracts feebly the isolated trachea of the guinea pig and it relaxes the trachea *in vivo*, because it releases catecholamines. In this species, kinins strongly constrict the finer twigs of the bronchial tree, both *in vitro* and *in vivo*, and they also contract the interstitial smooth muscle of the pleural surface of the lung. The net effect of kinins on the guinea pig airways is thus to lessen lung compliance and to reduce the inflation volume. Kallidin is slightly less effective than bradykinin, and the two kinins are cross-tachyphylactic.

Kinins also reduce the inflation volume of the lungs of the anesthetized rabbit, cat, and rat *in vivo*, the last two species being rather insensitive in this respect. Kinins tend to relax tracheobronchial muscle in the dog. In all species in which they have been tested, except the calf, kinins liberate adrenaline form the adrenal medulla and stimulate a sympathetic ganglion. Differences between the extents of catecholamine release and of contractant action on the tracheobronchial smooth muscle may help to account for the different response of the airways of each species to kinins. Inhaled bradykinin induces an attack of asthma in the human chronic asthmatic, but it does not affect ventilation in normal persons.

Probably as a result of the bronchiolar constriction, kinins induce in the guinea pig a reflex tachypnea, which depends upon the integrity of the vagi. Large intravenous or smaller intracarotid doses of kinins induce an apnea, which does not depend on the vagi and is presumably mediated through the central nervous system.

Aspirin and like-acting drugs in low doses inhibit bronchoconstriction and some other effects of kinins on pulmonary ventilation in the guinea pig *in vivo*. The antagonism of bronchoconstriction is not specific towards kinins but selective towards these and a few other active endogens. The antagonism by antipyretic drugs of kinin-induced bronchoconstriction is dose-related over a limited range of doses and it does not depend on central nervous or on adrenergic mechanisms; but it has paradoxical features that distinguish it from the type of specific antagonism at receptors thought to obtain, for example, with histamine and antihistamine drugs. The proposal has been made that the antagonism by antipyretic drugs of kinins and some other agonists in guinea pig lungs *in vivo* occurs at a common point on a route leading to or from the specific receptors for the agonists affected, rather than at the receptors themselves. The suggestion has been made that such a common point could be a carrier mechanism or the release of an unidentified intermediate transmitter substance.

There is good evidence that the release of kinins plays a part in anaphylactic bronchoconstriction in the guinea pig and some evidence that kinins may be involved in human bronchial asthma.

References

Aarsen, P. N.: The influence of analgesic antipyretic drugs on the responses of guinea-pig lungs to bradykinin. Brit. J. Pharmacol. **27**, 196—204 (1966).

Abe, K., Watanabe, N., Kumagai, N., Mouri, T., Seki, T., Yoshinaga, K.: Cicurlating plasma kinin in patients with bronchial asthma. Experientia (Basel) **23**, 626 (1967).

Berry, P. A.: Slow-reacting substance in anaphylaxis (SRS-A), its release, actions and antagonism. Ph.D. Thesis. Council of National Academic Awards, London, p. 91–93 (1966).

— Collier, H. O. J.: Bronchoconstrictor action and antagonism of a slow-reacting substance from anaphylaxis of guinea-pig lung. Brit. J. Pharmacol. **23**, 201–216 (1964).

Bhoola, K. D., Collier, H. O. J., Schachter, M., Shorley, P. G.: Action of some peptides on bronchial muscle. Brit. J. Pharmacol. **19**, 190–197 (1962).

Bisset, G. W., Lewis, G. P.: A spectrum of pharmacological activity in some biologically active peptides. Brit. J. Pharmacol. **19**, 168–182 (1962).

Brocklehurst, W. E., Lahiri, S. C.: The production of bradykinin in anaphylaxis. J. Physiol. (Lond.) **160**, 15–16P (1962).

— — Formation and destruction of bradykinin during anaphylaxis. J. Physiol. (Lond.) **165**, 39–40P (1963).

Carpi, A., Klupp, H., Konzett, H.: Über die Bradykinin-Wirkung am Herz-Lungen-Präparat des Meerschweinchens. Naunyn-Schmiedebergs Arch. exp. Path. Pharmak. **243**, 356 (1962).

Collier, H. O. J.: Some pharmacological correlates of anti-inflammatory activity. A study of nonsteroidal anti-inflammatory drugs as antagonists of local hormones. In: Nonsteroidal anti-inflammatory drugs, p. 139–150, ed. by S. Garattini, and N. M. G. Dukes. Amsterdam: Excerpta Medica 1965.

— Self-antagonism of bronchoconstriction induced by bradykinin and angiotensin. In: Hypotensive peptides, p. 305–313, ed. by E. G. Erdös, N. Back, and F. Sicuteri. Berlin-Heidelberg-New York: Springer 1966.

— A pharmacological analysis of aspirin. Advanc. Pharmacol., **7**, 333—405 (1969).

— Hammond, A. R., Whiteley, B.: Anti-anaphylactic action of acetylsalicylate in guinea-pig lung. Nature (Lond.) **200**, 176–178 (1963).

— Holgate, J. A., Schachter, M., Shorley, P. G.: An apparent bronchoconstrictor action of bradykinin and its suppression by some anti-inflammatory agents. J. Physiol. (Lond.) **149**, 54–55P (1959).

— — — — The bronchoconstrictor action of bradykinin in the guinea-pig. Brit. J. Pharmacol. **15**, 290–297 (1960).

— James, G. W. L.: Humoral factors affecting pulmonary inflation during acute anaphylaxis in the guinea-pig. Brit. J. Pharmacol. **30**, 283–301 (1967).

— — Humoral factors in airway function, with particular reference to anaphylaxis in the guinea-pig. In: The physiology and pharmacology of the airways, ed. by A. Bouhuys. Springfield, Ill.: Thomas 1969.

— — Piper, P. J.: Intensification by adrenalectomy or by β-adrenergic blockade of the bronchoconstrictor action of bradykinin in the guinea-pig. J. Physiol. (Lond.) **180**, 13–14P (1965).

— — — Antagonism by fenamates and like-acting drugs of bronchoconstriction induced by bradykinin or antigen in the guinea-pig. Brit. J. Pharmacol. **34**, 76–87 (1968).

— — Schneider, C.: Antagonism by aspirin and fenamates of bronchoconstriction and nociception induced by adenosine-5′-triphosphate. Nature (Lond.) **212**, 411–412 (1966).

— Shorley, P. G.: Analgesic antipyretic drugs as antagonists of bradykinin. Brit. J. Pharmacol. **15**, 601–610 (1960).

— — Antagonism by mefenamic and flufenamic acids of the bronchoconstrictor action of kinins in the guinea-pig. Brit. J. Pharmacol. **20**, 345–351 (1963).

Comline, R. S., Silver, M., Sinclair, D. G.: The effects of bradykinin, angiotensin and acetylcholine on the bovine adrenal medulla. J. Physiol. (Lond.) **196**, 339–350 (1968).

Di Mattei, P.: Occurrence of bradykinin in human pulmonary carcinoma. Biochem. Pharmacol. **16**, 909–911 (1967).

Dolovich, J., Back, N., Arbesman, C. E.: The presence of bradykinin-like activity in nasal secretions from allergic subjects. J. Allergy (Abstr.) **41**, 103 (1968).

Elliott, D. F., Horton, E. W., Lewis, G. P.: Actions of pure bradykinin. J. Physiol. (Lond.) **153**, 473–480 (1960).

Erdös, E. G.: Hypotensive peptides. Bradykinin, kallidin and eledoisin. Advanc. Pharmacol. **4**, 1–90 (1966).

Feldberg, W., Lewis, G. P.: The action of peptides on the adrenal medulla. Release of adrenaline by bradykinin and angiotensin. J. Physiol. (Lond.) **171**, 98–108 (1964).

FERREIRA, S. H., VANE, J. R.: The disappearance of bradykinin and eledoisin in the circulation and vascular beds of the cat. Brit. J. Pharmacol. **30**, 417–424 (1967).
GIRARD, J. P., MORET, P.: Action de la sérotonine et de la bradykinine en aérosols chez les asthmatiques. Helv. med. Acta **30**, 520–526 (1963).
GJURIS, V., HEICKE, B., WESTERMANN, E.: Über die Stimulierung der Atmung durch Bradykinin und Kallidin. Naunyn-Schmiedebergs Arch. exp. Path. Pharmak. **247**, 429–444 (1964a).
— — — Apnoe nach Bradykinin und Kallidin. Naunyn-Schmiedebergs Arch. exp. Path. Pharmak. **248**, 540–551 (1964b).
— WESTERMANN, E.: Bronchoconstrictor action of bradykinin, kallidin and eledoisin. Nature (Lond.) **205**, 402–404 (1965).
GREEFF, K., MOOG, E.: Vergleichende Untersuchungen über die bronchoconstrictorische und gefäßconstrictorische Wirkung des Bradykinins, Histamins und Serotonins an isolierten Lungenpräparaten. Naunyn-Schmiedebergs Arch. exp. Path. Pharmak. **248**, 204–215 (1964).
— SCHARNAGEL, K., LÜHR, R., STROBACH, H.: Die Abnahme des Kininogengehaltes des Plasmas beim toxischen, anaphylaktischen und anaphylaktoiden Schock. Naunyn-Schmiedebergs Arch. exp. Path. Pharmak. **253**, 235–245 (1966).
GREEN, M.: How big are the bronchioles? St Thom. Hosp. Gaz. **63**, 136–139 (1966).
HAUGE, A., LUNDE, P. K. M., WAALER, B. A.: The effect of bradykinin, kallidin and eledoisin upon the pulmonary vascular bed of an isolated blood-perfused rabbit lung preparation. Acta physiol. scand. **66**, 269–277 (1966).
HAWKINS, D. F.: Pharmacological studies of bronchial and intestinal muscle in relation to anaphylaxis and asthma. Ph.D. Thesis, University of London, p. 250–251, 367; 1952.
HERXHEIMER, H., STRESEMANN, E.: The effect of bradykinin aerosol in guinea-pigs and in man. J. Physiol. (Lond.) **158**, 38–39P (1961).
— — Bradykinin and ethanol in bronchial asthma. Arch. int. Pharmacodyn. **144**, 315–318 (1963).
JÄNKÄLÄ, E. O., VIRTAMA, P.: Bronchographic demonstration of the bronchoconstrictor effect of bradykinin in the guinea-pig. Ann. Med. exp. Fenn. **41**, 436–440 (1963).
JAHN, U., WAGNER-JAUREGG, T.: Vergleich von zwei neuen Klassen antiphlogistischer Substanzen im Collier-Test. Arzneimittel-Forsch. 18, 120–121 (1968).
JAMES, G. W. L.: The use of the *in vivo* trachea preparation of the guinea-pig to assess drug action on lung. J. Pharm. Pharmacol. **21**, 379–386 (1969).
JONASSON, O., BECKER, E. L.: Release of kallikrein from guinea pig lung during anaphylaxis. J. exp. Med. **123**, 509–522 (1966).
KONZETT, H., RÖSSLER, R.: Versuchsanordnung zu Untersuchungen an der Bronchialmuskulatur. Naunyn-Schmiedebergs Arch. exp. Path. Pharmak. **195**, 71–74 (1940).
— STÜRMER, E.: Biological activity of synthetic polypeptides with bradykinin-like properties. Brit. J. Pharmacol. **15**, 544–551 (1960).
LAHIRI, S. C.: The activation of kinins by antigen-antibody reactions. Ph.D. Thesis. Edinburgh University, p. 66–87, 1962.
LECOMTE, J., PETIT, J. M., MÉLON, J., TROQUET, J., MARCELLE, R.: Propriétés bronchoconstrictrices de la bradykinine chez l'homme asthmatique. Arch. int. Pharmacodyn. **137**, 232–235 (1962).
— TROQUET, J., CESSION-FOSSION, A.: Sur la nature de l'hypertension artérielle provoquée par la bradykinine et la kallidine. Arch. int. Pharmacodyn. **147**, 518–524 (1964).
— — DRESSE, A.: Stimulation médullo-surrénalienne par la bradykinine. Arch. int. Physiol. **69**, 89–91 (1961).
LEWIS, G. P.: Kinin antagonism and kinin formation. In: Salicylates: An International Symposium, p. 134–137, ed. by A. ST. J. DIXON, B. K. MARTIN, M. J. H. SMITH, and P. N. H. WOOD. London: Churchill 1963.
— REIT, E.: The action of angiotensin and bradykinin on the superior cervical ganglion of the cat. J. Physiol. (Lond.) **179**, 538–553 (1965).
— — Further studies on the actions of peptides on the superior cervical ganglion and suprarenal medulla. Brit. J. Pharmacol. **26**, 444–460 (1966).
MARQUARDT, H.: Zur Frage der Entstehung der vagal-reflektorischen Bradykinin-Tachypnoe. Naunyn-Schmiedebergs Arch. exp. Path. Pharmak. **253**, 207–220 (1966).
MOOG, E., GREEFF, K.: Der Einfluß verschiedener biogener Amine und Polypeptide auf die Gefäß- und Bronchialmuskulatur isoliert durchströmter Meerschweinchenlungen. Naunyn-Schmiedebergs Arch. exp. Path. Pharmak. **246**, 16–17 (1963).
PIPER, P. J., COLLIER, H. O. J., VANE, J. R.: Release of catecholamines in the guinea-pig by substances involved in anaphylaxis. Nature (Lond.) **213**, 838–840 (1967).
— VANE, J. R.: The assay of catecholamines released into the circulation of the guinea-pig by angiotensin. J. Physiol. (Lond.) 188, 20–21P (1967).

Rosenthale, M. E., Dervinis, A., Begany, A. J., Lapidus, M., Gluckman, M. I.: Bronchodilator activity of the prostaglandin PGE_2. Pharmacologist **10**, 175 (1968).
Simke, J., Graeme, M. L., Sigg, E. B.: Bradykinin induced bronchoconstriction in guinea-pigs and its modification by various agents. Arch. int. Pharmacodyn. **165**, 291–301 (1967).
Staszewska-Barczak, J., Vane, J. R.: The release of catecholamines from the adrenal medulla by peptides. Brit. J. Pharmacol. **30**, 655–667 (1967).
Stresemann, E.: Die Wirkung von Bradykinin-Aerosol auf die Atmung des Menschen und des Meerschweinchens und der Einfluß verschiedener Substanzen auf den experimentellen Bradykinin-Bronchospasmus. Acta allerg. (Kbh.) 18, 235–255 (1963).
Stürmer, E., Berde, B.: A comparative pharmacological study of synthetic eledoisin and synthetic bradykinin. J. Pharmacol. exp. Ther. **140**, 349–355 (1963).
Trendelenburg, U.: Observations on the ganglion-stimulating action of angiotensin and bradykinin. J. Pharmacol. exp. Ther. **154**, 418–425 (1966).
Varonier, H. S., Panzani, R.: The effect of inhalation of bradykinin on healthy and atopic (asthmatic) children. Int. Arch. Allergy **34**, 293–296 (1968).
Waaler, B. A.: The effect of bradykinin in an isolated perfused dog lung preparation. J. Physiol. (Lond.) **157**, 475–483 (1961).
Weibel, E. R.: Morphometry of the human lung, p. 110–143. Berlin-Göttingen-Heidelberg: Springer 1963.
Widdicombe, J. G.: Regulation of tracheobronchial smooth muscle. Physiol. Rev. **43**, 1–37 (1963).

The Effect of Bradykinin and Kallidin on Smooth Muscle

EDWARD J. WALASZEK

The actions of bradykinin, kallidin, and related substances are, of necessity, assayed primarily on smooth muscle since at present this is the only way to quantitatively assess potency. Thus most of the published literature on these polypeptides refers, in part, to their actions on smooth muscle. This section deals primarily in modes of action on smooth muscle and includes the antagonists and potentiators of the kinins on smooth muscle. Bioassay techniques and activity comparisons with other kinins are covered elsewhere.

A. Actions of Kinins on Smooth Muscle in vitro

Although most of the reported effects of bradykinin and kallidin were published in the last twenty years, we must remember that some of the pioneer work with kallikrein goes back forty years. Reports on the response of smooth muscle to kallikrein are difficult to interpret in that in some cases it may be due to the production of the kinin; however, it may also be due to a direct action of the enzyme kallikrein.

WERLE (1936) reported that isolated dog intestine contracts with 0.03 unit of kallikrein in a 50-ml bath. A small stimulation was noted on rat and pig intestine. Further work (WERLE et al., 1937) reported contraction of the human appendix and isolated cat intestine. In one of the excellent figures published one can see that the effect took place after 1 minute and the peak effect occurred 7 minutes after administration. It seems more than likely that the enzyme was producing a kinin from some available substrate even though this was an isolated preparation. Furthermore, evidence was shown (WERLE, 1936) that the boiled enzyme did not produce a contraction. LABORIT (1964) reported no stimulation on rabbit intestine with kallikrein.

Bradykinin and kallidin possess powerful and stimulating effects *in vitro* on smooth muscle of rat uterus and guinea pig ileum (ROCHA E SILVA et al., 1949; WERLE, 1955; KONZETT and STÜRMER, 1960; STÜRMER and BERDE, 1963a, b). This contraction is considerably slower than that of histamine or acetylcholine and usually requires at least 1 minute contact time. The threshold dose for bradykinin is 1 ng/ml on the guinea pig ileum and 0.03 ng/ml on the rat uterus (CERLETTI et al., 1961). The rat uterus is by far the most sensitive preparation and is widely used for testing bradykinin and bradykinin-like substances (ELLIOTT et al., 1960). The real usefulness of smooth muscle preparations is for differentiating the various peptides, and for this the rat uterus is the least discriminating of the available preparations (BISSET and LEWIS, 1962). Weight for weight, bradykinin is as active as histamine on guinea pig ileum and slightly less active than oxytocin on rat uterus (KONZETT and STÜRMER, 1960; ELLIOTT et al., 1960). On the basis of molecular weight, bradykinin is more potent than either histamine or acetylcholine.

The rabbit uterus is inhibited by bradykinin (ERSPAMER and ERSPAMER, 1962); however, others report contraction of the rabbit uterus but not on a regularly elicited basis (STÜRMER and BERDE, 1963b). Large concentrations are necessary in order to contract the isolated human myometrium (BERDE and SAAMELI, 1961). The cat uterus is also stimulated.

The rabbit duodenum and rabbit large intestine are stimulated by bradykinin (ERSPAMER and ERSPAMER, 1962), but the duodenum is much more sensitive. Kallidin was also more active than bradykinin on the rabbit duodenum, which is the only isolated tissue that contracts and demonstrates this difference. ROCHA E SILVA (1962) reported a relaxation of the rabbit intestine. ELLIOTT et al. (1960) and KONZETT and STÜRMER (1960) reported relaxations followed by contractions. Using the rabbit jejunum WALASZEK and HUGGINS (1959) observed a slight relaxation followed by contraction. Some consideration must be given to the possibility that these results may be related to a mechanical effect. If the muscle is weighted down sufficiently one will see a slight relaxation followed by contraction. If the muscle is not weighted and the lever is set to record relaxations, the predominant effect would be one of relaxation. On the isolated human ileum longitudinal strips contracted with bradykinin while the circular strips relaxed. On the isolated human colon a relaxation followed by a contraction was obtained (FISHLOCK, 1966).

The smooth muscle of the rat duodenum and rat colon is relaxed by bradykinin (HORTON, 1959; GADDUM and HORTON, 1959). This important fact makes the rat duodenum the smooth muscle of choice in discriminating between different polypeptides. The threshold concentration of bradykinin on this preparation is 0.1 ng/ml.

The hen rectal caecum also responds with relaxation to bradykinin and kallidin, but here kallidin is more potent (BISSET and LEWIS, 1962; STÜRMER and BERDE, 1963a). It is claimed that this effect is due to chloretone present in the solvent for pure bradykinin (HAMBERG, 1964). This is not substantiated by the other investigators.

Isolated rabbit aorta is not affected by bradykinin (ROCHA E SILVA, 1962), nor is the spirally-cut isolated cat carotid arterial strip (HUGGINS and WALASZEK, 1960). Contraction of the circular muscles of ox pulmonary arteries was obtained with bradykinin by KLUPP and KONZETT (1965). Isolated coronary artery from sheep was also contracted by bradykinin (KOVALCIK, 1962). Isolated veins were contracted by bradykinin (GULATI et al., 1968) at a concentration of 10 μg/ml (SUTTER, 1965). GOKHALE et al. (1966) demonstrated that the isolated human umbilical artery was contracted by bradykinin. They also reported that aspirin blocked the effect of bradykinin.

Recently FERREIRA and VANE (1967) studied a number of isolated organs of cat, rat, rabbit, and guinea pig. They concluded that rat duodenum and cat jejunum were the most sensitive to bradykinin. The cat jejunum, in their hands, responded to as little as 0.1 ng/ml. The cat jejunum was used previously by ERSPAMER and ERSPAMER (1962) and SCHACHTER (1956).

Guinea pig vas deferens contracts with a concentration of 30 ng/ml of bradykinin (GRAHAM and AL KATIB, 1966).

B. Action of Kinins on Smooth Muscle in vivo

FREY and KRAUT (1928) reported a strong contraction of dog intestine *in situ* upon injecting intravenously 5–10 units of kallikrein. In decapitated cats 2 units of kallikrein cause relaxation of cat intestine *in situ* (FELIX, 1934). No change in peristaltic activity was reported by WERLE (1934) when kallikrein was injected intravenously in anesthetized guinea pigs.

In vivo bradykinin inhibits intestinal motility in dog (Levy, 1963) and in cat (Türker et al., 1964). This inhibition was blocked by antihistaminics and atropine in dogs and by pretreatment with reserpine in cats.

Winkler et al. (1965) reported an inhibition followed by an increase in intestinal motility after injecting bradykinin into the abdominal aorta. Similar results were obtained on cats and rabbits after injections of bradykinin and kallidin; however, only inhibition was seen after i.v. infusion (1–3 μg/kg/min) (Bauer et al., 1966a).

In vitro the rat uterus is the most sensitive preparation to bradykinin, but *in vivo* the uterus of rat, rabbit, and cat are less sensitive. Bradykinin appears to be almost inactive on the rabbit uterus (Fregnan and Glässer, 1964). No oxytocic effect was reported when women in labor received bradykinin (Berde and Saameli, 1961). In addition, it has no milk-ejecting activity (Bisset and Lewis, 1962; Bisset et al., 1967). Bradykinin affects the ureter of dogs and rats but does not affect urine flow (Catacutan-Labay and Boyarsky, 1966).

Bradykinin administered intravenously causes bronchoconstriction in the guinea pig (Collier et al., 1960). It would seem that there is a specific receptor site for bradykinin, as its activity is much greater than that found for histamine or acetylcholine. This effect may be indirect since it is not as pronounced in the isolated organ (Collier et al., 1960; Konzett and Stürmer, 1960; Shorley and Collier, 1960).

This bronchoconstriction was not observed in perfused lungs of dogs, and bradykinin exerts no effect on the isolated rabbit and human bronchial muscles (Bhoola et al., 1962).

C. Mode of Action of Kinins on Smooth Muscle

A definitive mode of action for bradykinin on smooth muscles has not been established (Khairallah and Page, 1961). In using the isolated guinea pig ileum (Day and Vane, 1963), and differentiating bradykinin from the action of other drugs, the conclusion was reached that the effect of bradykinin is a direct one on the muscle. This opinion is shared by Khairallah and Page (1961). Zar (1966), using denervated and innervated guinea pig ileum, concluded that bradykinin had direct action on smooth muscle. These results were confirmed by Gershon (1967) when he demonstrated that tetrodotoxin, eserine, and hyoscine do not affect the maximal response of bradykinin. Besides the direct effect there may exist an indirect cholinergic mechanism. The evidence rests on an inhibition of bradykinin responses by atropine and morphine and a potentiation by eserine (Wiegershausen et al., 1964).

Huidobro (1963) demonstrated that $CaCl_2$ was necessary for the contractile response by bradykinin. We do know that release of catecholamine by peptide from adrenals of cats depends on the presence of calcium ions (Poisner and Douglas, 1966).

Bradykinin was found to depress or abolish the peristaltic reflex and its action here was postulated to be on the cholinoceptive synapses (Beleslin et al., 1964).

A cross-tachyphylaxis is seen between bradykinin and kallidin and between eledoisin, substance P, and physalaemin but not between these two groups on the guinea pig ileum. This is evidence for chemical and physical similarity between the peptides in each group (Lembeck and Fischer, 1967).

The effect of pH on responses to bradykinin was studied on the guinea pig ileum (Walaszek and Dyer, 1966). They compared the action of a number of peptides and correlated their actions with their isoelectric point. Thus bradykinin with an isoelectric point of 10–10.5 had its greatest biological activity at pH 6–7 while angiotensin with an isoelectric point of 6.3 had its greatest biological activity at pH 9–10.

The conformation of bradykinin is not dependent on internal hydrogen bonding since incubation of the peptide with urea and arginine had no effect on the subsequent contractile response of the uterus to bradykinin (Khairallah and Page, 1963). This was confirmed (Walaszek et al., 1968) by using D_2O and urea.

The bradykinin receptor on the rat fundal strip was found to be heat stable (Ehrenpreiss and Fleisch, 1968). Treatment of the muscle with urea produced a significant decrease in the activity of the bradykinin receptor. Antonio (1968) studied the mechanisms of the relaxing effect of bradykinin on isolated rat duodenum. Bradykinin is 200 times as potent as epinephrine and β and α adrenergic blocking agents did not antagonize the relaxation due to bradykinin. Thus the relaxant effect of bradykinin on the rat duodenum cannot be mediated by a local release of catecholamines. Contrary results were obtained by Montgomery (1968) in a preliminary paper; however, more definitive results need to be reported before this view can be accepted. Fishlock (1966) reported that pronethalol did block the relaxation seen with bradykinin on the isolated human ileum. Low-calcium Tyrode's solution antagonized the relaxing effect of bradykinin on the rat duodenum and dose-dependent contractions to bradykinin were then observed (Antonio, 1968).

D. Antagonists of Kinins on Smooth Muscle

At the present time we possess no specific antagonist to bradykinin and kallidin. Specific antagonists would resolve many problems in this area and could provide clues which, in turn, could lead to conclusions as to the mechanism of action and possible physiological roles of these kinins. In addition, a specific antagonist could perhaps be a useful therapeutic agent in diseases and conditions in which bradykinin and kallidin may play a role.

The stimulating action of bradykinin and kallidin upon the smooth muscle of the guinea pig is resistant to atropine, to antihistamines and to paralyzing concentrations of nicotine (Ambache and Rocha e Silva, 1951; Werle, 1955; Walaszek et al., 1963). The bradykinin effect was also not affected by morphine or BOL-148 (Walaszek et al., 1963). The inhibitory phase of bradykinin and kallidin on rabbit intestine is blocked by morphine but not by atropine, local anesthetics, adrenergic agents, ganglionic blockers, guanethidine, and phenylbutazone. In rat intestine the inhibitory effect is not blocked by the above compounds or morphine (Bauer et al., 1966b).

The number of compounds which have been tried and found to be unsuccessful must be legion. It certainly would be worthwhile to solicit a list of such compounds which could be published as a guide to future workers.

The most comprehensive work on antagonists is that of Rocha e Silva and Leme (1963, 1964, 1965). Essentially, they found that some phenothiazines and imipramine can act as antagonists. Leme and Rocha e Silva (1965) in a detailed paper indicated that cyproheptadine was a noncompetitive antagonist of bradykinin. Some dibenzocycloheptene derivatives and thiaxanthene derivatives were competitive antagonists. The benzodiazepine, cycloalkindole and dibenzazepine derivatives acted as noncompetitive antagonists. Methixene was also reported as a competitive antagonist, but van Riezen (1966) reports that by his procedure methixene was a noncompetitive antagonist. All of these antagonism studies were on the guinea pig ileum. Other compounds reported include dicyclomine (McGRATH et al., 1964), chlorpromazine (MARIANI, 1961), conopharyngine (CARROLL and STARMER, 1967), and 48/80 (PATON, 1951).

In general, the search for antagonists among closely related peptides has been disappointing. A few have been found that antagonize the action of bradykinin on the uterus. These are summarized well by STEWART and WOOLLEY (1964, 1965) and STEWART (1968).

One of the more successful antagonists to bradykinin and kallidin *in vivo* has been carboxypeptidase B (ERDÖS et al., 1963). This enzyme can metabolize the peptides very rapidly and hence prevents their action.

Brief mention should be made of the antagonism of the bronchoconstriction of bradykinin in guinea pig by anti-inflammatory agent (COLLIER and SHORLEY, 1960; COLLIER, 1962). This important area is reviewed separately in this volume.

Urine of various species has been reported to contain a lipid-soluble substance that antagonizes bradykinin on the guinea pig ileum and elsewhere (KOVACS and MELVILLE, 1963). Lysolecithin can effectively antagonize the action of bradykinin on smooth muscle; however, it also antagonizes most of the known agonists (MIDDLETON and PHILLIPS, 1963). Khellin, apiin, and hesperitin can antagonize bradykinin on the guinea pig ileum and on the development of paw edema by bradykinin in rats (LEME and WALASZEK, 1967). The antagonism between khellin and bradykinin seems to be competitive while hesperitin and apiin blocked bradykinin in a competitive manner.

It is reported by ROCHA E SILVA and LEME (1963) that phenoxybenzamine first potentiates and subsequently antagonizes the stimulant action of bradykinin on the guinea pig ileum. Using isolated guinea pig vas deferens GRAHAM and AL KATIB (1966) demonstrated elegantly that the ethanolamine compounds derived from 2-halogenoalkylamine compounds (phenoxybenzamine type) potentiate bradykinin while their imine or carbonium ion antagonizes bradykinin. This explains well the initial potentiation followed by antagonism that is seen with phenoxybenzamine. The antagonism was nonspecific since histamine, acetylcholine, and norepinephrine responses were also reduced or abolished at concentrations that antagonized bradykinin.

E. Potentiators of Kinins on Smooth Muscle

Many compounds have been described that potentiate the effects of kinins *in vivo* and *in vitro*. One group consists primarily of thiol compounds. These include cysteine, BAL, thioglycolic acid, and mercaptoethanol (FERREIRA and ROCHA E SILVA, 1962; PICARELLI et al., 1962; ERDÖS and WOHLER, 1963a, b). All of these compounds are inhibitors of the enzymatic metabolism of bradykinin and their *in vivo* effects are probably related to this fact (ERDÖS and WOHLER, 1963a, b). They also potentiate the contraction of bradykinin on the guinea pig ileum, and here the mechanism of potentiation is not clear. It may be related to destruction of bradykinin, but the enzymatic metabolism of bradykinin is very slow in the guinea pig ileum (PICARELLI et al., 1962). This relation of potentiation to enzymatic inhibition is also not supported by the experiments of TEWKSBURY (1968), who obtained potentiation after a maximal response. In quite high concentrations (AUERSWALD and DOLESCHEL, 1967) the thiol compounds can inhibit the kinins on the guinea pig ileum while in low concentrations the potentiation is confirmed. CÎRSTEA (1965) has another explanation for the potentiation which, in essence, involves rupture of disulfide bridges with a subsequent unfolding of protein macromolecules which increase the number of bradykinin receptors available. Another alternative explanation was proposed in which the potentiation is seen as a cholinergic mechanism (Potter and Walaszek, 1968). Antihistaminics and ganglionic blocking agents do not antagonize the potentiation, but morphine, tetrodotoxin, and high concentrations of atropine can antagonize the potentiation of bradykinin on the guinea pig ileum by cysteine.

A series of cysteine analogs were synthesized which demonstrated that the group essential for activity is the amino while the sulfhydryl group probably tends to govern potency. Esterification of the carboxyl group resulted in compounds 4–8 times more potent than cysteine. S-benzhydryl cysteine inhibited the potentiation and was in its own right an inhibitor of bradykinin responses (Walaszek and Potter, 1969).

Tetraethylammonium potentiates the effect of bradykinin on the guinea pig ileum (Khairallah and Page, 1961) and on the rat uterus (Capek and Knesslova, 1959). LSD can also potentiate bradykinin, angiotensin, and substance P on the guinea pig ileum (Smith and Walaszek, 1962).

Another group of potentiators is protein in nature. Trypsin, chymotrypsin, papain, and chymotrypsinogen increase the sensitivity of the guinea pig ileum and rat uterus to kinins (Edery, 1964, 1965). This seems to be quite specific for kinins, as other polypeptides are not affected. This mechanism is obscure; however, it has been shown that chymotrypsin releases histamine from the guinea pig ileum (Gilfoil and Kelly, 1966), but it is rather doubtful that this mechanism operates on the rat uterus.

An interesting discovery was the bradykinin-potentiating factor which is an alcohol-soluble fraction of the venom of *Bothrops jararaca* (Ferreira and Rocha e Silva, 1965; Ferreira, 1965). This factor is probably a polypeptide as its activity is destroyed by proteolytic enzymes. It can potentiate bradykinin *in vivo* and *in vitro* and can also potentiate eledoisin and angiotensin on the guinea pig ileum and oxytocin on the rat uterus.

Sensitization of guinea pig ileum to the action of bradykinin can also be accomplished by trypsin hydrolysates of ox and rabbit plasma (Aarsen, 1968). Peptide B, which is released by the action of thrombin on fibrinogen, potentiates the effect of bradykinin on the rat uterus (Gladner et al., 1963; Gladner, 1966). All of these peptide potentiators may be physiologically important in sensitizing tissue receptors to bradykinin and kallidin.

It has been suggested that the mechanism of bradykinin potentiation by peptide and protein hydrolysates is due to competitive inhibition of carboxypeptidase B or carboxypeptidase-like enzymes (enzymes responsible) for the metabolism of bradykinin and that this inhibition may depend on the presence of arginine and/or lysine on the carboxyl end of the peptide fragments (Hamberg et al., 1968).

References

Aarsen, P. N.: Sensitization of guinea-pig ileum to the action of bradykinin by trypsin hydrolysate of ox and rabbit plasma. Brit. J. Pharmacol. **32**, 453 (1968).

Ambache, N., Rocha e Silva, M.: Analysis of certain interactions of nicotine with bradykinin and histamine. Brit. J. Pharmacol. **6**, 68 (1951).

Antonio, A.: The relaxing effect of bradykinin on intestinal smooth muscle. Brit. J. Pharmacol. **32**, 78 (1968).

Auerswald, W., Doleschel, W.: On the potentiation of kinins by sulfhydrylic compounds. Arch. int. Pharmacodyn. **168**, 188 (1967).

Bauer, G., Gmeiner, R., Winkler, H.: Über die Wirkung synthetischer Polypeptide auf den Darm in situ. Arch. int. Pharmacodyn. **159**, 373 (1966a).

— Ziegler, E., Konzett, H.: Zur Hemmwirkung von Kininen and isolierten Darmpräparaten. Naunyn-Schmiedebergs Arch. exp. Path. Pharmak. **254**, 235 (1966b).

BELESLIN, D. B., BOGADNOVIC, S. BI., RADMANOVIC, B. Z.: The possible site of action of bradykinin on the peristaltic reflex of the isolated guinea pig ileum. Arch. int. Pharmacodyn. **147**, 43 (1964).

BERDE, B., SAAMELI, K.: Effect of bradykinin on uterine activity. Nature (Lond.) **191**, 83 (1961).

BHOOLA, K. D., COLLIER, H. O. J., SCHACHTER, M., SHORLEY, P. G.: Actions of some peptides on bronchial muscle. Brit. J. Pharmacol. **19**, 190 (1962).

BISSET, G. W., CLARK, B. J., HALDAR, J., HARRIS, M. C., LEWIS, G. P., ROCHA E SILVA, M.: The assay of milk-ejecting activity in the lactating rat. Brit. J. Pharmacol. **31**, 537 (1967).

— LEWIS, G. P.: A spectrum of pharmacological activity in some biological active peptides. Brit. J. Pharmacol. **19**, 168 (1962).

CAPEK, R., KNESSLOVA, V.: Die Wirkung von TEAE auf die Bradykininkontraktion des isolierten Rattenuterus. Naunyn-Schmiedebergs Arch. exp. Path. Pharmak. **236**, 161 (1959).

CARROLL, P. R., STARMER, G. A.: Studi s on the pharmacology of conopharyngine, an indole alkaloid of the voacanga series. Brit. J. Pharmacol. **30**, 173 (1967).

CATACUTAN-LABAY, P., BOYARSKY, S.: Effect on ureteral peristalsis. Science **151**, 78 (1966).

CERLETTI, A., STÜRMER, E., KONZETT, H.: Bradykinin: Information on its structure, synthesis, and physiologic-pharmacological basis. Dtsch. med. Wschr. **86**, 678 (1961).

CÎRSTEA, M.: Potentiation of some bradykinin effects by thiol compounds. Brit. J. Pharmacol. **25**, 405 (1965).

COLLIER, H. O. J.: Antagonists of bradykinin. Biochem. Pharmacol. **10**, 47 (1962).

— HOLGATE, J. A., SCHACHTER, M., SHORLEY, P. G.: The bronchoconstrictor action of bradykinin in the guinea-pig. Brit. J. Pharmacol. **15**, 290 (1960).

— SHORLEY, P. G.: Analgesic antipyretic drugs as antagonists of bradykinin. Brit. J. Pharmacol. **15**, 601 (1960).

DAY, M., VANE, J. R.: An analysis of the direct and indirect actions of drugs on the isolated guinea pig ileum. Brit. J. Pharmacol. **20**, 150 (1963).

EDERY, H.: Potentiation of the action of bradykinin on smooth muscle by chymotrypsin and trypsin. Brit. J. Pharmacol. **22**, 371 (1964).

— Further studies of the sensitization of smooth muscle to the action of plasma kinins by proteolytic enzymes. Brit. J. Pharmacol. **24**, 485 (1965).

EHRENPREISS, S., FLEISCH, J. H.: Alteration in vasoactive polypeptide receptor activity of rat fundal strip by heat and urea. Fed. Proc. **27**, 70 (1968).

ELLIOTT, D. F., HORTON, E. W., LEWIS, G. P.: Actions of pure bradykinin. J. Physiol. (Lond.) **153**, 473 (1960).

ERDÖS, E. G., WOHLER, J. R.: Inhibitors of the "in vivo" effects of bradykinin and kallidin. Life Sci. **2**, 270 (1963a).

— — Inhibition "in vivo" of the enzymatic inactivation of bradykinin and kallidin. Biochem. Pharmacol. **12**, 1193 (1963b).

— — LEVINE, M. I.: Blocking of the "in vivo" effects of bradykinin and kallidin with carboxypeptidase B. J. Pharmacol. exp. Ther. **142**, 327 (1963).

ERSPAMER, V., ERSPAMER, G. F.: Pharmacological actions of eledoisin on extravascular smooth muscle. Brit. J. Pharmacol. **19**, 337 (1962).

FELIX, J.: A clinical and experimental study of the action of tissue extracts on the circulatory system: An experimental study of the action of Padutin (kallikrein). Acta med. scand. **83**, 328 (1934).

FERREIRA, S. H.: A bradykinin-potentiating factor (BPF) present in the venom of *Bothrops jararaca*. Brit. J. Pharmacol. **24**, 163 (1965).

— ROCHA E SILVA, M.: Potentiation of bradykinin by dimercaptopropanol (BAL) and other inhibitors of its destroying enzyme in plasma. Biochem. Pharmacol. **11**, 1123 (1962).

— — Potentiation of bradykinin and eledoisin by BPF (bradykinin potentiating factor) from *Bothrops jararaca* venom. Experientia (Basel) **21**, 347 (1965).

— VANE, J. R.: The detection and estimation of bradykinin in the circulating blood. Brit. J. Pharmacol. **29**, 367 (1967).

FISHLOCK, D. J.: Effect of bradykinin on the human isolated small and large intestine. Nature (Lond.) **212**, 1533 (1966).

FREGNAN, G. B., GLÄSSER, A. H.: Activity of eledoisin, other polypeptides and ergometrine on the uterus *in situ* of rabbit and other animal species. J. Pharm. Pharmacol. **16**, 744 (1964).

FREY, E. K., KRAUT, H.: Ein neues Kreislaufhormon und seine Wirkung. Naunyn-Schmiedebergs Arch. exp. Path. Pharmak. **133**, 1 (1928).

GADDUM, J. H., HORTON, E. W.: The extraction of human urinary kinin (Substance Z) and its relation to the plasma kinins. Brit. J. Pharmacol. **14**, 117 (1959).

GERSHON, M. D.: Effects of tetrodotoxin on innervated smooth muscle preparations. Brit. J. Pharmacol. **29**, 259 (1967).

Gilfoil, T. M., Kelly, C. A.: Mechanism of action of chymotrypsin on plain muscle. Brit. J. Pharmacol. 27, 120 (1966).
Gladner, J. A.: Potentiation of the effect of bradykinin. In: Hypotensive peptides, p. 344, ed. by E. G. Erdös, N. Back, and F. Sicuteri. Berlin-Heidelberg-New York: Springer 1966.
— Murtaugh, P. A., Folk, J. E., Laki, K.: Nature of peptides released by thrombin. Ann. N.Y. Acad. Sci. 104, 47 (1963).
Gokhale, S. D., Gulati, O. D., Kelkar, L. V., Kelkar, V. V.: Effect of some drugs on human umbilical artery *in vitro*. Brit. J. Pharmacol. 27, 332 (1966).
Graham, J. D. P., Al Katib, H.: The effect of 2-halogenoalkylamines on the biological activity of some peptides. Brit. J. Pharmacol. 27, 377 (1966).
Gulati, O. D., Parikh, H. M., Umar, M. S.: Receptors for noradrenaline and histamine in the rabbit's posterior vena cava. Brit. J. Pharmacol. 32, 87 (1968).
Hamberg, U.: Structure and biological activity of bradykinin. Ann. Acad. Sci. fenn. 106, 12 (1964).
— Elg, P., Stelwagen, P.: On the mechanism of bradykinin potentiation. In: Advances in experimental medicine and biology, pharmacology of hormonal polypeptides and proteins, vol. 2, p. 626, ed. by N. Back, L. Martini, and R. Paoletti. New York: Plenum Press 1968.
Horton, E. W.: Human urinary kinin excretion. Brit. J. Pharmacol. 14, 125 (1959).
Huggins, C. G., Walaszek, E. J.: Depressor polypeptides. Amer. Heart J. 60, 976 (1960).
Huidobro, H. V.: The role of calcium in the effect of bradykinin on smooth muscle. Biochem. Pharmacol. 12 (Suppl.), 180 (1963).
Khairallah, P. A., Page, I. H.: Mechanism of action of angiotensin and bradykinin on smooth muscle *in situ*. Amer. J. Physiol. 200, 51 (1961).
— — Effects of bradykinin and angiotensin on smooth muscle. Ann. N.Y. Acad. Sci. 104, 212 (1963).
Klupp, H., Konzett, H.: Der Einfluß von Bradykinin und Kallidin auf den Druck in der Arteria pulmonalis. Naunyn-Schmiedebergs Arch. exp. Path. Pharmak. 249, 479 (1965).
Konzett, H., Stürmer, E.: Biological activity of synthetic polypeptides with bradykinin-like properties. Brit. J. Pharmacol. 15, 544 (1960).
Kovacs, B. A., Melville, K. I.: Antihistamine and antibradykinin effects of normal urine extracts. Nature (Lond.) 198, 1060 (1963).
Kovalcik, V.: Effect of bradykinin on isolated coronary arteries. Nature (Lond.) 196, 174 (1962).
Laborit, H., Leterrier, F., Massart, A., Baron, C.: Contribution à l'étude pharmacologique de la Padutine (Kallikreine pancreatique). Agressologie 5, 623 (1964).
Lembeck, F., Fischer, G.: Gekreuzte Tachyphylaxie von Peptiden. Naunyn-Schmiedebergs Arch. exp. Path. Pharmak. 258, 452 (1967).
Leme, J. G., Rocha e Silva, M.: Competitive and non-competitive inhibition of bradykinin on the guinea pig ileum. Brit. J. Pharmacol. 25, 50 (1965).
— Walaszek, E. J.: Antagonists of pharmacologically active polypeptides: Effects on guinea pig ileum and inflammation. Pharmacologist 7, No 2, 242 (1967).
Levy, B.: The intestinal inhibitory response to oxytocin, vasopressin and bradykinin. J. Pharmacol. exp. Ther. 140, 356 (1963).
Mariani, L.: Drugs antagonistic to bradykinin. Boll. Soc. ital. Biol. sper. 37, 1481 (1961).
McGrath, W. R., Lewis, R. E., Kuhn, W. L.: The dual mode of the antispasmodic effect of dicyclomine hydrochloride. J. Pharmacol. exp. Ther. 146, 354 (1964).
Middleton, E., Jr., Phillips, G. B.: Effects of lysolecithin on the smooth muscle stimulating activity of histamine, acetylcholine, 5-HT, anaphylactic, slow-reacting substance and bradykinin. Nature (Lond.) 198, 758 (1963).
Montgomery, E. H.: The response of the rat duodenum to bradykinin. Proc. Western Pharmacol. Soc. 11, 51 (1968).
Paton, W. D. M.: Compound 48/80: A potent histamine liberator. Brit. J. Pharmacol. 6, 499 (1951).
Picarelli, Z. P., Henriques, O. B., Oliveira, M. C.: Potentiation of bradykinin action on smooth-muscle by cysteine. Experientia (Basel) 18, 77 (1962).
Poisner, A. M., Douglas, W. W.: The need for calcium in adrenomedullary secretion evoked by biogenic amines, polypeptides, and muscarinic agents. Proc. Soc. exp. Biol. (N.Y.) 123, 62 (1966).
Potter, D. E., Walaszek, E. J.: Potentiation of the bradykinin response by cysteine: Mechanism of action. Fed. Proc. 27, 662 (1968).
Riezen, H. van: Methixene: A non-competitive antagonist of bradykinin. J. Pharm. Pharmacol. 18, 688 (1966).

ROCHA E SILVA, M.: Definition of bradykinin and other kinins. Biochem. Pharmacol. **10**, 3 (1962).
— BERALDO, W. T., ROSENFELD, G.: Bradykinin, a hypotensive and smooth muscle stimulating factor released from plasma globulin by snake venom and trypsin. Amer. J. Physiol. **156**, 261 (1949).
— LEME, J. G.: Antagonists of bradykinin. Med. exp. (Basel) 8, 287 (1963).
— — On some antagonists of bradykinin. Naunyn-Schmiedebergs Arch. exp. Path. Pharmak. **250**, 167 (1964).
— — Antagonists of bradykinin. In: Recent advances in the pharmacology of toxins. Proc. II. Internat. Pharmacol. Congr., vol. 9, p. 33, ed. by HELENA RASKOVA. Oxford: Pergamon Press 1965.
SCHACHTER, M.: A delayed contracting effect of serum and plasma due to the release of a substance resembling kallidin and bradykinin. Brit. J. Pharmacol. **11**, 111 (1956).
SHORLEY, P. G., COLLIER, H. O. J.: Direct comparisons of the synthetic nonapeptide with trypsin bradykinin. Nature (Lond.) **188**, 999 (1960).
SMITH, C. M., WALASZEK, E. J.: Interaction of substance P and other smooth muscle stimulants with LSD-25 on the guinea pig ileum. Arch. int. Pharmacodyn. **138**, 429 (1962).
STEWART, J. M.: Structure-activity relationships in bradykinin-analogues. Fed. Proc. **27**, 63 (1968).
— WOOLLEY, D. W.: Threonine analogs of bradykinin designed as antimetabolites. Biochemistry **3**, 700 (1964).
— — The search for peptides with specific anti-bradykinin activity. Biochem. Pharmacol. **14**, 1399 (1965).
STÜRMER, E., BERDE, B.: A pharmacological comparison between synthetic bradykinin and synthetic kallidin. J. Pharmacol. exp. Ther. **139**, 38 (1963a).
— — A comparative pharmacological study of synthetic eledoisin and synthetic bradykinin. J. Pharmacol. exp. Ther. **140**, 349 (1963b).
SUTTER, M. C.: The pharmacology of isolated veins. Brit. J. Pharmacol. **24**, 742 (1965).
TEWKSBURY, D. A.: Studies on the mechanism of bradykinin potentiation. Arch. int. Pharmacodyn. **173**, 426 (1968).
TÜRKER, K., KIRAN, B. K., KAYMAKCALAN, S.: The effects of synthetic bradykinin on intestinal motility in different laboratory animals and its relation to catecholamines. Arch. int. Pharmacodyn. **151**, 260 (1964).
WALASZEK, E. J., DYER, D.: Polypeptide receptor mechanism: Influence of pH. In: Hypotensive spolypeptide, p. 329, ed. by E. G. ERDÖS, N. BACK, and F. SICUTERI. Berlin-Heidelberg-New York: Springer 1966.
— — GASCON, A. L.: Polypeptide receptor mechanisms. Fed. Proc. **27**, 67 (1968).
— HUGGINS, C. G.: Substance A: A hypertensive polypeptide from Fraction IV-4 of plasma protein. J. Pharmacol. exp. Ther. **126**, 258 (1959).
— — SMITH, C. M.: Drugs that modify actions of pharmacologically active polypeptides. Ann. N.Y. Acad. Sci. **104**, 281 (1963).
— POTTER, D. E.: Amino acid derivatives: An approach to the study of potentiation and antagonism of pharmacologically active polypeptides. Pharm. Res. Comm. **1**, 204 (1969).
WERLE, E.: Zur Kenntnis des Haushalts des Kallikreins. Biochem. Z. **269**, 415 (1934).
— Die Wirkung des Kallikrein (=Padutin) auf den isolierten Darm. Klin. Wschr. **15**, 848 (1936).
— The chemistry and pharmacology of kallikrein and kallidin. In: Polypeptides which stimulate plain muscle, p. 20, ed. by J. H. GADDUM. Edinburgh: E. & S. Livingstone 1955.
— GÖTZE, W., KEPPLER, A.: Über die Wirkung des Kallikreins auf den isolierten Darm und über eine neue darmkontrahierende Substanz. Biochem. Z. **289**, 217 (1937).
WIEGERHAUSEN, B., STOPP, G., EICHSTÄDT, M.: Zum Mechanismus der Bradykininwirkung am Meerschweinchendarm. Acta biol. med. germ. **12**, 443 (1964).
WINKLER, H., BAUER, G., GMEINER, R.: Zur Wirkung von Bradykinin, Kallidin und Eledoisin auf den Katzen- und Kaninchen-Darm *in situ*. Naunyn-Schmiedebergs Arch. exp. Path. Pharmak. **250**, 459 (1965).
ZAR, M. A.: Factors influencing the output of acetylcholine. D. Phil. Thesis. University of Oxford (1966).

Effect of Bradykinin on the Central Nervous System

Edward J. Walaszek

At the present time the effects of bradykinin on the central nervous system (CNS) have not been definitely established. In general, it would seem difficult to ascribe an effect of a peptide on the CNS since its penetration of the blood–brain barrier would be limited. The most definitive work on penetration into the CNS was done by Bumpus et al. (1964). These workers administered tritiated bradykinin to rats and studied its distribution. The bulk of the bradykinin was found in the kidney, liver, and urine; however, the amount in the brain was equal to that found in heart tissue. Thirty minutes after the intravenous infusion of bradykinin the brain had the least amount of radioactivity, being 20% of that found in heart tissue, and at no time was it higher in brain than in blood. Electrophoretic mobility was also studied to ascertain if it was bradykinin or its metabolites, and at 30 minutes no unchanged bradykinin was detected. On this basis one can assume that only a very small amount can penetrate the brain even when infused in large doses.

Using cross-circulation experiments in dogs, Buckley et al. (1963) were able to demonstrate that bradykinin elicits central cardiovascular effects. The responses were variable and unpredictable, and the authors concluded that bradykinin appears to stimulate central parasympathetic centers.

Severs et al. (1967) reported that the pressor effects of angiotensin injected into the lateral ventricle of the cat were abolished by lesions at the high midbrain levels. This observation should be extended to bradykinin.

Of some interest are the experiments (Corrado et al., 1959; Rocha e Silva, 1960) demonstrating that bradykinin injected intraventricularly to cats causes tranquilization. This state in cats is also characterized by relative immobility. The tranquilization and catatonic state were confirmed by Capek (1962). He also injected bradykinin intraventricularly to mice and reported a state of excitation that caused some mice to jump to remarkable heights and induced convulsions in some. It was also reported that bradykinin decreased the seizure threshold to metrazol, strychnine, and electroshock-induced convulsions. Zetler (1956), with subcutaneous administration of large amounts of bradykinin to mice, was not able to demonstrate an effect in experimentally-induce catatonia or tremor. All these results were with crude bradykinin. Investigators who used pure or synthetic bradykinin (Heath, 1963; Horton, 1963; Lewis, 1963) were unable to demonstrate any central effect. Rocha e Silva (1963) pointed out that variable results were also obtained with pure bradykinin; he attributed this to the rapid destruction of the peptide. More consistent results were obtained if animals were pretreated with cysteine.

Other possible central effects of bradykinin measured by electroencephalography were also reported (Corrado et al., 1963). Bradykinin has been reported to increase the acetylcholine content in the brain of mice (Beaulnes and Ling, 1968).

KRIVOY et al. (1963) concluded that bradykinin may modulate nervous excitability and this could be one of the physiological roles of bradykinin. In general, bradykinin depressed excitability. Correlation of neurologic and oxytocic actions of bradykinin and related nonapeptides were studied with no definitive result (KRIVOY et al., 1961). Bradykinin belongs to the group of non-nicotinic ganglion-stimulating agents (TRENDELENBURG, 1966) (p. 369).

Intracarotid injection of bradykinin affects the respiration (ROCHA E SILVA, 1963). Whether this is a central effect or is due to cerebral vasodilator activity is not known. Evidence for a central effect has been established (PIERI and MARRAZZI, 1964) in that bradykinin inhibits synaptic transmission in the transcallosal pathway without affecting the circulation appreciably. This possible central effect of bradykinin and kallidin on respiration (GJURIS et al., 1964a, b) was reported by other workers (p. 414). The evidence for the central action lies in differences between intracarotid and intravenous injections of bradykinin. It was demonstrated previously that vagotomy and denervation of carotid bodies do not abolish this effect of bradykinin (ROCHA E SILVA, 1960). Of possible interest in penetration of peptides into brain tissue is the observation that Gly^6 derivative of bradykinin stimulates respiration of cats and guinea pigs more than the parent compound (ERDÖS et al., 1963).

Bradykinin may be involved in transmitting pain, but this area is reviewed elsewhere (p. 434). Very little has been done in relating pathways in the CNS to this phenomenon (KEELE and ARMSTRONG, 1964).

CHAPMAN et al. (1959) have reported studies on the neurohumoral features of the axon reflex. They perfused the subcutaneous space of the forearm with normal saline before and after the induction of the axon reflex by noxious stimulation. Aliquots of the perfusate were assayed for the ability to stimulate the isolated rat uterus or relax the rat duodenum. A 2- to 3-fold increase, both in total volume of perfusate and in its activity, was observed during the axon reflex flare as assayed on the rat uterus. CHAPMAN et al. suggest their data support the view that a protease is liberated locally after noxious stimulation, and this enzyme reacts with the globulin of the interstitial fluid to form a polypeptide which increases capillary permability, lowers pain threshold, induces vasodilatation and edema, and produces other reactions relevant to the inflammatory response. These authors indicated that the polypeptide may be bradykinin; however, their implications would be more strongly supported if they had presented data showing parallel assays of the active material which standard bradykinin on two or more sensitive test systems.

CHAPMAN and WOLFF (1959) have carried out studies to ascertain whether and under what conditions an enzymatic vasodilator system is present in the central nervous system. Cerebrospinal fluid was collected from subjects with (1) active disease of the central nervous system; (2) inactive, nonprogressive, or no disease of the central nervous system; (3) vascular headache of the migraine type; (4) sustained nervous stimulation and pain arising from disorders of the legs or pelvic organs; and (5) disease syndromes classified as chronic schizophrenia. The fluid was bioassayed on the isolated rat uterus before (type I response) and after (type II response) incubation with bovine globulin. Subjects in categories 1, 3, 4, and 5 showed a positive type II response in a significant number of instances, which would suggest the appearance in the cerebrospinal fluid of any enzyme capable of reaction with a globulin to produce a pharmacologically active substance as measured on the rat uterus and a vasodepressor reaction in the anesthetized cat. These authors suggest that the polypeptide bradykinin is formed in type II response. However, until further proof of the character of this material one must be cautious in its evaluation as bradykinin. They suggest that the protease-polypeptide system may be inplicated in local vasomotor control within the central nervous system and, when in excess, the components of the system may be relevant to disease.

CHAPMAN et al. (1963) summarized much of the evidence for kinin formation as governed by neural activity. They have named it neurokinin, and RAMOS et al. (1963a, b, c) indicate that it is different from bradykinin. Other investigators disagree with these findings (KEELE and ARMSTRONG, 1964). A protease forming a vasodilator polypeptide was found in cerebrospinal fluid by COPPEN and LEWIS (1961), while others were unable to find a protease (HAMBERG, 1960).

SICUTERI (1967) believes that bradykinin is one of many factors in migraine headache. He was able to demonstrate the presence of a bradykinin-like substance in the cerebrospinal fluid and, further, could produce a headache by introducing a small quantity of bradykinin into the spinal fluid of patients (p. 482).

Many workers demonstrated the circulatory antidiuretic effect of bradykinin. The results of ROCHA E SILVA, JR., and MALNIC (1964) suggest that bradykinin releases antidiuretic hormone (vasopressin) from hypothalamic areas or the posterior pituitary. Convincing evidence was the antidiuretic effect with intracarotid injections of bradykinin doses that were inactive intravenously and the abolishment of the bradykinin response in dogs with diabetes insipidus. Thus the antidiuretic effect is due to release of the antidiuretic hormone by a central effect of bradykinin.

References

BEAULNES, A., LING, G. M.: Effect of angiotensin and bradykinin on brain acetylcholine. Fed. Proc. **27**, (2), 471 (1968).

BUCKLEY, J. P., BICKERTON, R. K., HALLIDAY, R. P., KATO, H.: Central effects of peptides on the cardiovascular system. Ann. N.Y. Acad. Sci. **104**, 299 (1963).

BUMPUS, F. M., SMEBY, R. R., PAGE, I. H., KHAIRALLAH, P. A.: Distribution and metabolic fate of angiotensin II and various derivatives. Canad. med. Ass. J. **90**, 190 (1964).

CAPEK, R.: Some effects of bradykinin on the central nervous system. Biochem. Pharmacol. **10**, 61 (1962).

CHAPMAN, L. F., GOODELL, H., WOLFF, H. G.: Increased inflammatory reaction induced by central nervous system activity. Trans. Ass. Amer. Phycns **72**, 84 (1959).

— RAMOS, A. O., GOODELL, H., WOLFF, H. G.: Evidence for kinin formation resulting from neural activity evoked by noxious stimulation. Ann. N.Y. Acad. Sci. **104**, 248 (1963).

— WOLFF, H. G.: Studies of proteolytic enzymes in cerebrospinal fluid. Arch. intern. Med. **103**, 86 (1959).

COPPEN, A. J., LEWIS, G. P.: An enzyme forming vasodilator polypeptides in human cerebrospinal fluid. J. Neurochem. **7**, 155 (1961).

CORRADO, A. P., CAPEK, R., FERREIRA, S. H., ROCHA E SILVA, M.: EEG analysis of the central effects of bradykinin. Ciencia e Cult. (S. Paulo) **15**, 271 (1963).

— RAMOS, A. O., ROCHA E SILVA, M.: The central action of bradykinin. Ciencia e Cult. (S. Paulo) **11**, 165 (1959).

ERDÖS, E. G., WOHLER, J. R., LEVINE, M. I.: Blocking of the *in vivo* effects of bradykinin and kallidin with carboxypeptidase B. J. Pharmacol. exp. Ther. **142**, 327 (1963).

GJURIS, V., HEICKE, B., WESTERMANN, E.: Über die Stimulierung durch Bradykinin und Kallidin. Naunyn-Schmiedebergs Arch. exp. Path. Pharmak. **247**, 429 (1964a).

— — — Apnoe nach Bradykinin und Kallidin. Naunyn-Schmiedebergs Arch. exp. Path. Pharmak. **248**, 540 (1964b).

HAMBERG, U.: Cerebrospinal fluid and bradykinin release. Biochem. Pharmacol. **3**, 169 (1960).

HEATH, R. G.: Discussion. Ann. N.Y. Acad. Sci. **104**, 311 (1963).

HORTON, E. W.: The role of bradykinin in the peripheral nervous system. Ann. N.Y. Acad. Sci. **104**, 250 (1963).

KEELE, C. A., ARMSTRONG, D.: Substances producing pain and itch. London: Edward Arnold, Ltd. 1964.

Krivoy, W. A., Bodansky, M., Lande, S.: Neurological and oxytocic action of some nonapeptides related to bradykinin. Biochem. Pharmacol. **12**, Suppl. 179 (1961).
— Lane, M., Kroeger, D. C.: The action of certain polypeptides on synaptic transmission. Ann. N.Y. Acad. Sci. **104**, 312 (1963).
Lewis, G.: Discussion. In: Proc. 1st Int. Pharmacol. Meeting, vol. 9, p. 65, ed. by B. Uvnäs. New York: Pergamon Press 1963.
Pieri, L., Marrazzi, A. S.: Cerebral synaptic effect of bradykinin and analogs. Fed. Proc. **23**, 124 (1964).
Ramos, A. O., Chapman, L. F., Ramos, L.: Neurokinin from cerebrospinal fluid. I. Some pharmacological properties. Arch. int. Pharmacodyn. **146**, 501 (1963a).
— — — Zileli, T.: Neurokinin from cerebrospinal fluid. III. Reciprocal actions with some drugs. Arch. int. Pharmacodyn. **146**, 511 (1963c).
— Giesbrecht, A. M., Ramos, L.: Neurokinin from cerebrospinal fluid. II. Chromatographic studies. Arch. int. Pharmacodyn. **146**, 507 (1963b).
Rocha e Silva, M.: Biochemistry and pharmacology of bradykinin. In: Polypeptides which affect smooth muscles and blood vessels, p. 210, ed. by M. Schachter. Oxford: Pergamon Press 1960.
— The physiological significance of bradykinin. Ann. N.Y. Acad. Sci. **104**, 190 (1963).
— Corrado, A. P., Ramos, A. O.: Potentiation of duration of the vaso-dilator effects of bradykinin by sympatholytic drugs and by reserpine. J. Pharmacol. exp. Ther. **128**, 217 (1960).
Rocha e Silva, M., Jr., Malnic, G.: Release of antidiuretic hormone by bradykinin. J. Pharmacol. exp. Ther. **146**, 24 (1964).
Severs, W. B., Daniels, A. E., Buckley, J.P.: On the central hypertensive effect of angiotensin II. Int. J. Neuropharmacol. **6**, 199 (1967).
Sicuteri, F.: Vasoneuroactive substances and their implication in vascular pain. Res. clin. Stud. Headache **1**, 6 (1967).
Trendelenburg, U.: Observations on the ganglionic-stimulating action of angiotensin and bradykinin. J. Pharmacol. exp. Ther. **154**, 418 (1966).
Zetler, G.: Wirkungsunterschied zwischen den Polypeptiden Bradykinin und Substanz P am Zentralnervensystem. Naunyn-Schmiedebergs Arch. exp. Path. Pharmak. **229**, 148 (1956).

Section B: Pathological Role

Pain

DÉSIRÉE ARMSTRONG

With 21 Figures

A. Introduction

Almost without exception man is familiar with the experience we call "pain". It is a matter of concern because of its frequent, though not infallible, warning of personal damage or danger, arousing protective reflexes and courses of action. From PLATO and ARISTOTLE until about the time of AVICENNA, in the 11th century (see DALLENBACH, 1939; K. D. KEELE, 1962; PROCACCI, 1969) it was regarded as a "passion of the soul" believed to result from "overstimulation" of any of the senses. Avicenna's suggestion of its being a separate sense was borne out experimentally by the work of SCHIFF (1858), who by appropriate cord section was able to distinguish touch and pain as separate events following separate tracts and not mutually extinguishable. Even later, GOLDSCHEIDER (1916) still adhered to the physical overstimulation theory but limited his ideas to those of "pressure overstimulation". He was opposed, chiefly by von FREY (1922), who not only believed pain to be a separate sense but also that it was mediated by receptor organs of its own—free nerve endings. This does not imply that pain is the only sensation initiated by stimulation of free nerve endings (NAFE and WAGONER, 1937; SJÖQUIST, 1938). WEDDELL (1947) showed that some presumed pain-nerve endings are connected to myelinated nerve fibers (rapidly conducting) and some to unmyelinated (slowly conducting) nerve fibers. HEAD (1920), WOOLLARD et al. (1940), IGGO (1962), and others suggest that the complete pain picture will be modified by the relative distribution of stimulation between the peripheral nerve elements affected, and that the general distribution of stimulation in space, peripherally, will also affect the mental picture as a whole.

The usual concomitant of noxious stimulation is the arousal of withdrawal reflexes and these have often been used to detect and assess the presence or absence of pain. It should be noted however that the noxious element may be removed from "pain" stimulation and that the absence of withdrawal reflexes is not necessarily the *sine qua non* of analgesia.

Several aspects of chemically induced pain in relation to tissue damage are particularly interesting. HARDY et al. (1952) observed that in the case of pain induced by heat on the skin, the pain threshold and tissue injury threshold temperatures coincide (about 45°). This suggests that the pain-stimulating factor might well be damaged tissue proteins.

The fact that above-threshold pain is proportional to temperature (rather than to the duration of exposure and tissue injury) suggested to these workers that destruction and "repair" of protein (or formation and destruction of the pain-producing agent) may be taking place simultaneously. On brief exposure to high temperatures where marked pain is felt, though injury is negligible, production of the pain-producing agent far outweighs, for the moment, its destruction. Thus pain stimulation is related to the rate of protein alteration. The observations of HARDY et al. are in keeping with the studies of HENRIQUES on thermal changes of proteins and enzymes in relation to tissue injury (HENRIQUES, 1947; MORITZ and HENRIQUES, 1947). They are also in keeping with the known potentiality of plasma proteins to form and destroy polypeptide pain-producing material rapidly under suitable conditions (ARMSTRONG, 1957; HARDY, 1962; ARMSTRONG et al., 1967).

LIM and GUZMAN (1968) indicate that pain occurs in tissue damage at times of inflammation, and natural chemical repair in that tissue indicates that repair forces are called into action. They say that the function of the pain receptor is not so much to signal the impact of injury at the time it is inflicted but to signal the occurrence of ischemia and hypoxia or the development of inflammation. Studying the work of LAVRENKO (1938), WOOLLARD et al. (1940), and WHITE and SWEET (1955), LIM wrote in 1960 that probably both fast and slow pain receptors are present in visceral or deep areas as well as in cutaneous areas, and that the difference between visceral and cutaneous pain is the preponderance of slow pain in visceral and of fast pain in cutaneous injury. The difference will tend to disappear with the severity and duration of the injury and the corresponding degree of inflammation that develops.

Concerning visceral pain LIM (1966) notes that bradykinin can stimulate both fast and slow pain fibres. He presents evidence, moreover, that the *pain receptor is a specific, somesthetic chemoreceptor paravascularly situated.* Bradykinin injected into the splenic artery excites activity in splenic afferents with conduction velocities ranging from 0.3 to 9.0 meters per second (group IV or C fibers) and 13 to 55 meters per second (group III or A-gamma-delta fibers). It is probable that some or all of the smaller fibers are associated with the mediation of pain, and that fast and slow pain fibers are as much a part of the visceral pain system as they are of the cutaneous.

The identification of the receptors for pain as *chemoreceptors* reaffirms the MÜLLER doctrine (1843) of nerve specificity and lends support to the proposition that three modalities—mechanical, thermal, and chemical—are concerned in somestheses. The current trend to question the specificity of somesthetic afferents, based on the finding that some single-fiber (and multifiber, using DOUGLAS and RITCHIE'S antidromic occlusion technique) preparations may be activated by more than one mode of stimulation, disregards the existence of the organized specific receptors (MEISSNER, KRAUSE, VATER-PACINI corpuscles and end bulbs; MERKEL, RUFFINI, and hair-follicle nerve endings with terminal disks) as well as those of the unorganized receptors with free-branching terminals that respond to only one stimulus modality—mechanical, thermal, or chemical. In the case of some of the receptors with slow conduction rate (C-fiber stems), there is doubt whether bimodal response may not come from the receptor with one stimulus, and from the stem axons with the other. The denial of specificity has stimulated a search for a system of coding to convey information from the periphery to the brain.

The Paravascular Sensory Nerve Endings as the Chemoreceptors for Pain

The generalized distribution throughout the body of a *bradykinin-sensitive chemoreceptor that evokes pain on stimulation by the algensic peptides, and on stimulation of its stem axons and receptor terminals by nociceptive stimuli and also by non-nociceptive stimuli after ischemic and inflammatory sensitization, suggests it is the sole receptor for the mediation of pain.* Since bradykinin is readily destroyed by kininase in plasma and lymph, it may be inferred that its target organ cannot be far away; and since it evokes pain on intra-arterial injection throughout the body, the pain receptors may be assumed to be situated close to the capillaries. The "paravascular" afferent or sensory nerves that accompany blood vessels nearly everywhere to join the peripheral plexus and end in free-branching unmyelinated terminals in the connective tissue spaces surrounding capillaries and venules in skin and other organs are ubiquitous enough to fill the role of chemoreceptors for pain. Since contraction of plain muscle in the spleen by epinephrine does not cause pain, the receptors for pain are not mechano-sensitive.

According to LIM, the superficial or cutaneous paravascular chemoreceptors, which evoke immediate cutaneous pain, form the first line of warning in a defense

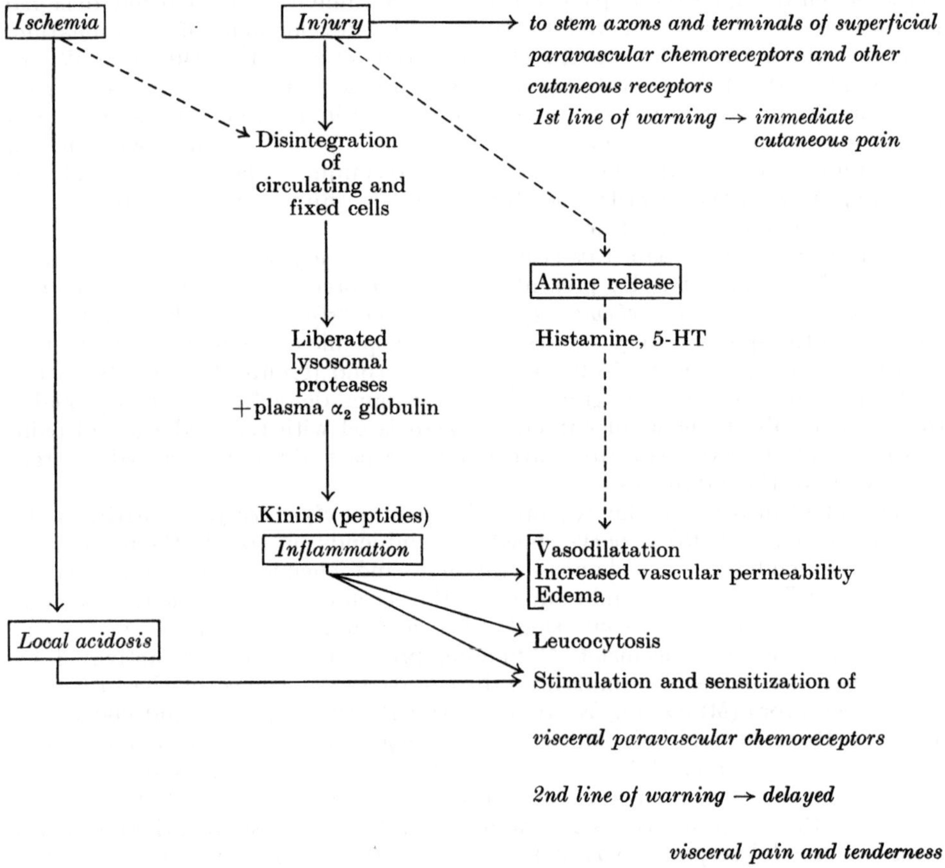

Fig. 1. The postulated role of ischemia, injury, and inflammation in the genesis of pain. (From LIM, 1966)

system to limit the effect of injury or disease to the organism (Fig. 1). Injury inevitably evokes immediate pain through accidental stimulation of axons, as well as receptors, of this system, along with some of the tactile-sensing and temperature-sensing systems. If, however, inflammation occurs after injury, the following events ensue: vasodilatation, primarily of venules, and increased vascular permeability and leakage; discharge of amines; aggregation of circulating cells with liberation of lysosomal enzymes, one of which may act on α_2 globulin in plasma to form inflammatory peptides like bradykinin, or the enzyme may be liberated from an inactive precursor in plasma by physical means such as contact with a suitable surface. Such peptides not only produce the characteristic signs of inflammation but also they may sensitize the chemoreceptors and their axons. The deep or visceral paravascular chemoreceptors, which induce delayed visceral pain and tenderness, form the second line of warning, alerting the organism to the sequelae of the injury and disease (Fig. 1). This concept is essentially Sir THOMAS LEWIS' "nocifensor" hypothesis (T. LEWIS, 1937a, b, 1942) applied to both cutaneous and visceral pain, but differs in that normal dorsal root neurons terminating in the paravascular receptors are involved. The work of LIM and colleagues seems to have provided us with an experimentally based theory of pain stimulation which unifies concepts of pain of both cutaneous and visceral origin. It is not incompatible with the views of SHERRINGTON (1906).

If chemoreceptors mediate pain, and the peripheral analgesics act by blocking these receptors, then pain caused by injury acting upon the axons of the pain receptors would not be blocked by the peripheral analgesics. The central analgesics, however, not being able to distinguish between impulses coming from receptors or axons, would block (or inhibit) all impulses regardless of their origin, and thus appear to be "stronger" than the "weaker" peripheral analgesics (LIM et al., 1964).

Thus PLATO, ARISTOTLE, AVICENNA, SCHIFF, GOLDSCHEIDER, VON FREY, SHERRINGTON, HEAD, and others have all contributed to our present-day concepts of pain mechanisms. All were right in part. It is likely that LIM also is right in part, but his concepts with their experimental basis provide an excellent ground and stimulus for further studies.

A moderate number of human chemalgogenic studies based on the nature of the stimulus rather the receptor have been reported. The modern experiments date from GRÜTZNER (1894) who, like many others (e.g. LINDAHL, 1961), concentrated on the direct effects of simple compounds and agents such as KCl, acids, and alkalis.

THUNBERG (1902) and VON FREY (1922) suggested that the (immediate) pain of injury was related to the mediation of intrinsic chemical agents. Participation of endogenous mediators in pain of gastric ulcer and intermittent claudication was discussed by T. LEWIS et al. (1931); and in hyperalgesia by LEWIS and HESS (1933), ROSENTHAL and MINARD (1939), ROSENTHAL (1950), ADDIS et al. (1950), C. A. KEELE and ARMSTRONG (1964), ROCHA E SILVA (1964a, b), GRAHAM et al. (1965). The hyperalgesic or "'susceptible' state is not the immediate result of injury but of ensuing inflammation. It is caused by the liberation of some tissue substance which acts on the pain nerve endings" (T. LEWIS and HESS, 1933; ADDIS et al., 1950). In 1950 the preliminary ideas for experimental studies of chemalgogens, to be put into operation the following year and reported in KEELE and ARMSTRONG (1964), were being organized, and assessment, measurement, and recording of pain were our first problems.

The verbal report of the subjective experience, obtained under carefully controlled conditions, is the fundamental basis of all studies of pain and, like many other investigators of pain (see GOETZ et al., 1943; HARDY et al., 1952; BEECHER, 1957), we have utilized such reports in all our work on the production of pain by chemical agents (see also C. A. KEELE, 1962; KEELE and ARMSTRONG, 1968; R. SMITH, 1962). Since we are dealing mainly with pain of mild or moderate severity, in circumstances that arouse little or no apprehension in our experimental subjects, objective accompaniments of pain, such as changes in blood pressure, heart rate, rate of breathing, and electrical resistance of the skin, are slight or absent, and it is very unusual to provoke movements of withdrawal from the site of stimulation. The electroencephalogram shows no specific changes during pain perception (BENJAMIN and IVY, 1949).

However, although we regard the evidence from human experience as the primary source of information about pain, we also accept, at one remove as it were, information obtained from animal experiments. For example, experiments in which an irritant such as mustard oil is applied to the eyes of rabbits to produce an acute inflammatory reaction characterized by conjunctival vasodilatation and chemosis (Bruce, 1913) may be presumed to be painful. When Jancsó (1960) applied 0.5% alcoholic capsaicin solution to rats' ears it caused intense hyperemia, vigorous scratching of the ear, and reflex muscle twitches. In this case Jancsó found the same solution caused intensive burning pain, accompanied by bright-red hyperemia with edema, when applied to human facial skin. The link between human and animal observations cannot be closer and, if ever one is justified in saying that animals feel pain comparable to the human experience, it is in such a case as this. Injection of algogenic agents such as bradykinin into unanesthetized guinea pigs' skin evokes biting, licking, or scratching directed to the site of injection, as well as more general reactions such as squeaking and various undirected movements (Collier and Lee, 1963). These nociceptive responses may also be assumed to indicate an experience of pain.

Responses in anesthetized, decerebrate, or spinal animals are more difficult to interpret. However, when reactions occur in lightly anesthetized animals to substances which evoke pain in man, it seems likely that they are relevant to our field of study. Intra-arterial injection to dogs of algogens such as lactic acid (Burget and Livingston, 1931), hypertonic saline (Moore and Singleton, 1933; Moore and Moore, 1933; Moore, 1934; and Moore et al., 1934), ACh, KCl, and bradykinin (Lim, 1960; Guzman et al., 1962) provoke a "pseudo-affective" response characterized by vocalization, struggling, hypernea, and a rise in arterial blood pressure. Calma and Wright (1947) noted that intrathecal injection or application of pain-producing concentrations of KCl or hypertonic saline to exposed posterior nerve roots in chloralosed cats caused a reflex rise in blood pressure, dilatation of the pupil, changes in breathing and alterations in spinal reflexes.

Electrophysiological observations on chemalgogenic agents have been disappointing. There is no decisive evidence for the existence of exclusively nociceptive nerve fibers, and the pattern of activity responsible for pain is not known (Bowsher and Albe-Fessard, 1962; Keele and Armstrong, 1964; Albe-Fessard, 1968).

The importance of the participation of man as a subject in pain studies (Sherrington, 1900), the essential differentiation between pain on the one hand and pain-induced behavior on the other (e.g. see Edwards, 1950), the employment at the time of the pain sensation of easy to make and relatively easy to interpret pain charts (K. D. Keele, 1948; Hewer and C. A. Keele, 1948; C. A. Keele and Armstrong, 1964), and the suggestion of C. A. Keele to use a skin blister base whereby chemalgogenic comparisons might safely be made on the same group of nerve endings, have all promoted pain studies (Lim and Guzman, 1968). Experiments in animals basic to the study of analgesics for use in man have been developed by Lim, Collier, Blane and their collaborators, and by others. During this period bradykinin was purified and then synthesized. Its ability to stimulate pain in concentrations of about 10 mμmoles upward (CBA test) or in doses of 1 or 2 μg per man (for example, i.a., Burch and de Pasquale, 1962, and Coffman, 1966; i.v., Sicuteri and his colleagues, 1964—1968; or i.p., Lim, 1960—1968), and the enormous kinin-generating power of the human plasma, make it a compound well worth serious study. In view of the rapid rate of destruction of kinin *in vivo*, examination of the chemical environment of the milieu interne will be essential.

Each man's pain experience may not be identical with that of the next. Great care must be taken in the selection of subjects, both animal and human, as ill health may affect sensitivity, metabolism, and other reactions. A severe pain which the recipient knows is going to be of short duration (or which he himself can terminate) is far more tolerable than a less severe pain of unknown duration. The investigator must know the objectives and limitations of his proposed pain researches; he can then select and instruct his subjects accordingly.

My colleagues and I, believing in the value of behavior as proposed in the Declaration of Helsinki and in the Recommendations of the Medical Research Council, London, concerning clinical research (M.R.C. 1953, 1962/63), adhere to them. Because the chief initial objective in many of the expermients has been the causation of pain, those authors whose works on man are described here have been asked if they would sign the following statement.

"To the best of my knowledge the experiments on man which have been recorded in my writings:

1. Have been on non-dependent adults who have been, in the best sense of the term, volunteers.

2. The nature and consequences of the desired experiments were clearly explained to the subjects by a responsible person who was not the subject's physician or surgeon, and were also understood by both subject and experimenter.

3. The experimenter, who was not the subject's physician or surgeon, was well qualified to deal adequately with all foreseeable untoward effects and also with some unexpected ones."

The objective of the letter was to establish that in cited articles an ethic not obviously contrary to my own was being employed.

Concerning work on animals, though some countries employ protective measures, there is no universality of procedure. In Britain a license is required to permit animal experimentation. The operator and also the department in which he works are inspected by the goverment, to which each is independently responsible. In addition, disapproved behavior on the part of an operator would terminate or at least seriously jeopardize the permit of a whole department to continue any animal experimentation.

B. Pain Induced by Kinins. Experimental Methods. Quality of Pain

I. The Cantharidin Blister Area in Man (CBA)

The pain-producing actions of the plasma kinins (PPS, pain-producing substance) and later bradykinin were first described by ARMSTRONG et al. (1952, 1953a, b, 1954, 1957).

The method is simple and the results are reproducible. Moreover, it is our preference to make the results comparative. In this technique a blister is raised on the volar surface of the forearm, the raised epidermis is cut off, and test solutions are poured onto the denuded base. The base of a blister raised by heat or friction is, in general, equally suitable and gives the same results (Fig. 2), but the procedure for making the blister is more complicated and its eventual production and depth are uncertain. Unless one has a specific reason for doing otherwise, using a blister base raised by cantharidin for testing chemical excitants of (cutaneous) pain appears to be a justified procedure (KEELE and ARMSTRONG, 1964; LIM and GUZMAN, 1968).

This cantharidin blister area technique was studied by ARMSTRONG and KEELE and their collaborators for over ten years, and was the basis of several publications, a University of London thesis, and a monograph (Keele and Armstrong, 1964) which describes the CBA technique in detail.

Up to 10 or 12 applications may be made in one experimental session without causing fatigue. The blister area is sensitive to pain-producing solutions throughout the day after application of the cantharidin plaster, and on occasions we have used a blister area for two days, during which as many as 40 to 50 applications have been made.

The pain and itch thus experienced are measured and recorded almost simultaneously with their occurrence. We used a numerical scale for subjective estimates

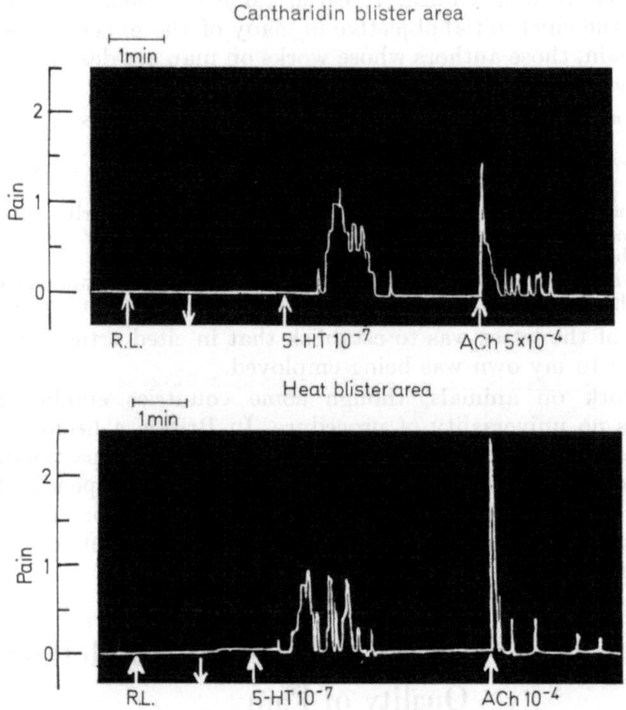

Fig. 2. Blister bases formed after cantharidin and after a heat burn. Pain responses to ACh, 5-HT, and Locke's solution (*R.L.*). (Concentrations in g/ml). (From Armstrong et al., 1953a)

as follows (Armstrong et al., 1953a, b). Pain: 0 = none; 1 = slight; 2 = moderate; 3 = severe; 4 = very severe.

"We regard this merely as an ordinal scale (Stevens, 1951) and leave our subjects to work out the values for themselves. There is considerable variation in sensitivity from one person to another, and the words here used are arbitrary. We do not feel that it is possible to attain great accuracy in pain recording but in our experiments on the blister base we have obtained graded responses to increasing concentrations of any given pain-producing solution. In such experiments most subjects can readily distinguish $^1/_2$ and even $^1/_4$ units of pain intensity. The scale is not regarded as an equal interval one, i.e. the difference between 0 and 1 cannot be equated with that between 2 and 3. We use a 2-unit scale for recording itch. During an experiment we make separate notes on sensations which cannot be classified as pain or itch" (Keele and Armstrong, 1964).

Graphic recording of the pain was used because descriptive methods take a little longer to produce (see below) and because accurate interpretation of them, especially in quantity, was extraordinarily difficult and tedious. K. D. Keele (1948) introduced the pain chart as a means of recording pain at intervals in patients, and Hewer and C. A. Keele (1948) adapted this for recording rapid changes in the intensity of experimental ischemic pain.

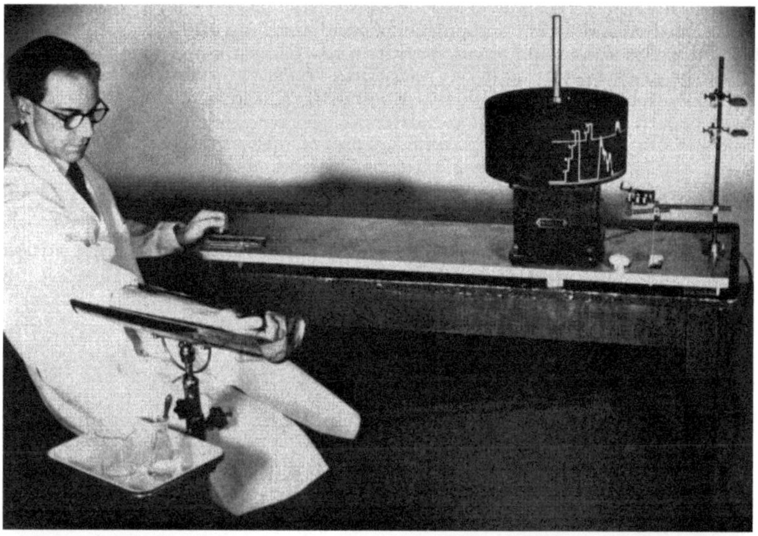

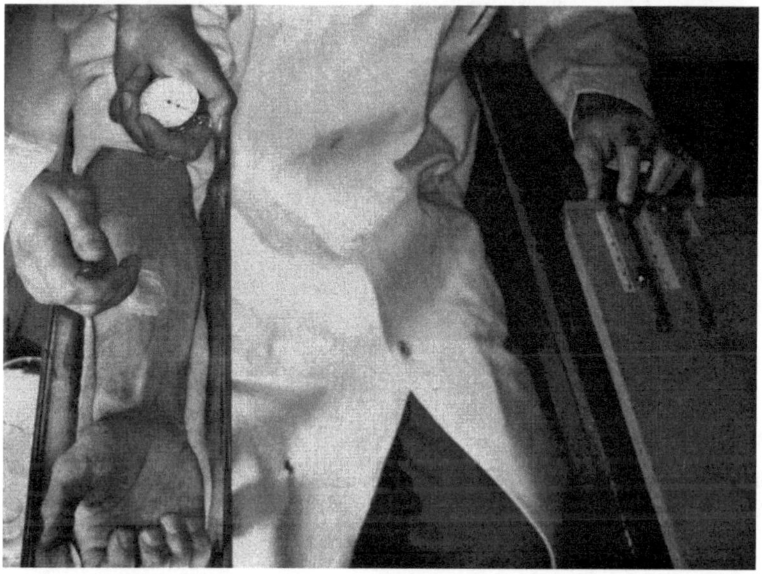

Fig. 3. *Above:* Graphic recording of subjective estimate of pain. Pain-producing solutions are applied to an exposed blister base on the right forearm. The subject moves a pointer, with his left hand, along a scale marked 0, 1, 2, 3, 4, to indicate the intensity of pain as described. The pointer is connected by a thread and pulley to a writing lever which makes a record on a moving smoked drum. *Below:* Blister area surrounded by wax, with application of test solution. Subject's left hand is ready to move pointer along scale

Fig. 3 shows the apparatus we used to record subjective estimates of pain. The arrangement is such that the subject cannot see the shape of the record he is making. These permanent records show the time of onset, rate of rise to peak, and the intensity and duration of pain and itch at a glance. The latent period between application of a solution and onset of pain is timed.

In addition to the graphic time-intensity curve, other information is noted, such as the feeling of warmth that may occur with applications of low concentrations of certain pain-producing substances, e.g. KCl and 5-HT, to the blister base. Objective manifestations such as pallor of the blister base after epinephrine, or weal and flare after histamine, are also noted.

Cantharidin is the anhydride of cantharidic acid. It occurs in a concentration of not less than 0–6% in the dried beetle *Cantharis vesicatoria* (*Lytta vesicatoria*) which is also known as cantharides, blistering beetle, Spanish fly, Russian flies, and meloides. Cantharidin is found too in Mylabris beetle, known as Chinese blistering beetle or Indian blistering beetle (MARTINDALE, 1958), and very likely in many other species of blistering beetle (SWARTS and WANAMAKER, 1946). Cantharides and other blistering agents have been used since the second century A.D. (BROCKBANK, 1954).

The cantharidin plasters denude the skin down to the basal layer of the epidermis. Onto such a preparation the test and control (also bathing) solutions were poured in manner very similar to that employed in the isolated organ techniques

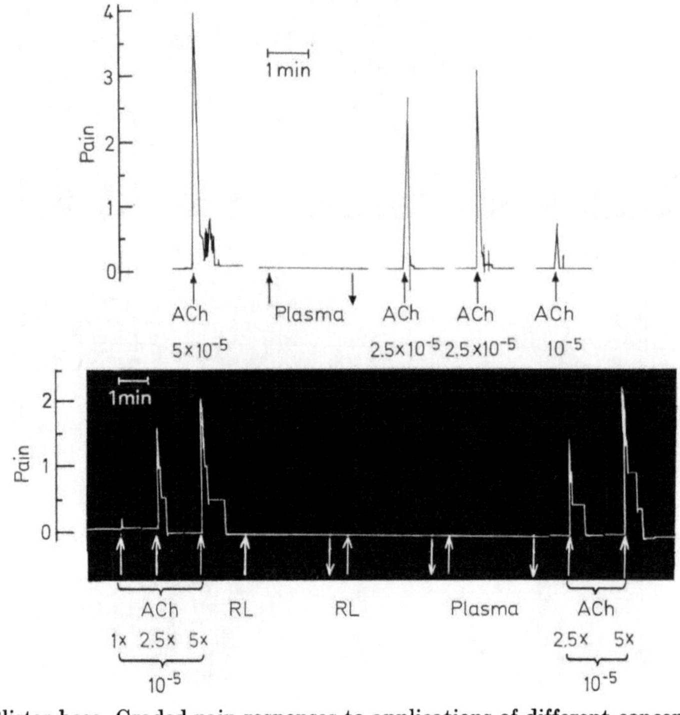

Fig. 4. Blister base. Graded pain responses to applications of different concentrations of ACh (expressed as g/ml) in two subjects. *R.L.* LOCKE's solution. Plasma from heparinized blood. Ordinate = pain scale as described in text. Test solutions applied at 10-min intervals and left on for 1 min. (From ARMSTRONG et al., 1953a)

of pharmacology. Since bathing and test solution do not mix, the area having been dried of almost all superficial excess moisture, the technique also resembles that of superfusion (MONGAR, 1955).

As with isolated organ work a rest interval is necessary for recovery of sensitivity, between administrations. A rest period of about 10 minutes has been found suitable in general. The area recovered from administrations of acetylcholine within this period. Due to the good recovery which the area makes to this substance, acetylcholine has been used concurrently and in addition to the specific chemical standards. Almost all volunteers provide useful experiments. Fig. 4 shows typical discrimination between concentrations of acetylcholine by two respective subjects. The main characteristics of the acetylcholine-induced pain are the same for each subject, e.g. immediate onset, usually flash-like increase to peak intensity and rapid decline, and needle-like pain without heat or burning sensation and without aftermath of sensation except for an occasional "flick" of itch. Upon the characteristics of the pain of a particular chemical type are superimposed the lesser characteristics of the individual (Fig. 4). In this way an observer is enabled to detect the chemical substance and the person who has been the subject, in a record. These greater and lesser characteristics of the record may be analogous respectively to language and handwriting.

Pain responses to 5-HT are shown in Fig. 5 (Armstrong, 1958). The characteristics of 5-HT-induced pain are quite different from those of acetylcholine-induced pain. They are, however, similar to those induced by adenosine compounds, bradykinin, or PPS. The pain is burning in character (see also below), is delayed in onset from about 10–40 seconds or more (average, 20–25 seconds), is slow

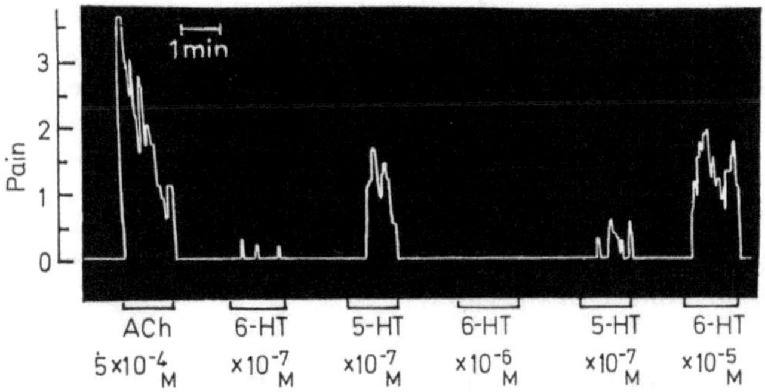

Fig. 5. Comparison of algogenic potencies of 5- and 6-hydroxytryptamines. (From Armstrong, 1958)

mounting, often in stages, to a peak during about one minute, and, if the solution be left on the blister base test area for longer than the usual 1–2 minutes, exposure time, its slow decline from the "peak" plateau can be traced.

The 5-HT-induced pain further resembles that caused by bradykinin in that complete recovery of the test area does not usually occur within a 10 minute rest period. Tachyphylaxis ensues, especially when concentrations of either agent, of approximately 0.5 μg-ml, i.e. μM and 0.5 μM respectively or higher are used (see also Keele and Armstrong, 1964 and below). Nevertheless, by employing a technique used in Fig. 5 the relative pain-producing potencies of analogs of the substances, especially those that induce tachyphylaxis within our experimental conditions, can be estimated.

Although 5-HT and bradykinin produce similar pain when they are applied to the blister base, bradykinin and related agents have a characteristic of inducing *after-pain*, which is often intense, during and especially after their removal, by gentle washing off, from the area. This characteristic would help a subject or an observer to guess at the nature of the agent that had been applied. The phenomenon can occur also after subthreshold applications for pain production.

Tissue injuries liberate 5-HT and bradykinin-like substances in addition to histamine (T. Lewis, 1927, 1942; Rosenthal and Minard, 1939). The pain-producing actions of histamine are qualitatively and quantitatively different from 5-HT and bradykinin. Its effective concentrations are very high (e.g. 5×10^{-3} to 5×10^{-4} M) (Armstrong, 1957; Keele and Armstrong, 1964). The direct pain-producing actions of histamine are probably not of great significance. The 5-HT and bradykinin-like agents, on the other hand, are several thousand-fold more effective in inducing pain on the human blister base than is histamine and thus may well be of physiopathological importance. Though effective concentrations of 5-HT for moderate pain production are low (about 10^{-6} M), bradykinin is at least ten times more active, and its threshold concentrations for pain production range from about 10^{-8} to 10^{-7} M.

ELLIOTT et al. (1960a); ELLIOTT and LEWIS (1965), and BISSET and LEWIS (1962) described the pain induced by bradykinin on the blister area as "burning" in character. BISSET and LEWIS stress the contrast in the sensations aroused by the bradykinin and those by histamine, itching being the predominant feature with the histamine (cf. T. LEWIS, 1927, 1942; ROSENTHAL and MINARD, 1939; EMMELIN and FELDBERG, 1947; ARMSTRONG, 1957; KEELE and ARMSTRONG, 1964).

The burning quality of kinin-induced pain has been emphasized by C. A. KEELE repeatedly. The immediate smarting pain of ACh is different in character from the delayed burning, pricking pain of 5-HT and plasma PPS. The former feels more "superficial" than the latter (KEELE, 1958). On the blister base the typical immediate smarting pain produced by ACh is different in character from the delayed duller pain of 5-HT and PPS (KEELE, 1957). The delayed pain of thermal burns is commonly described as "burning" because of the nature of the stimulus that causes it.

Concerning the pain of burning, i.e. application of thermal stimuli, HARDY (1962) points out that 44°–46° was the lowest temperature found capable of producing observable damage in the skin.

II. The Pain Experience with Bradykinin Applied to Man by Other Techniques

CORMIA and DOUGHERTY (1960) injected *crude bradykinin intradermally* more than fifty times in seven subjects. On most occasions a burning pain after slight delay occurred, also some itch. The latter may perhaps be due to the subjects' having a full complement of fairly normal or intact nerve endings at the site of injection (perhaps unlike the CBA subjects) and also perhaps to impurities present in the crude bradykinin. There was flare present, but no whealing. In close vicinity to injection, hypoalgesia was present; surrounding this, hyperalgesia existed (see below for their injections of kallikrein). HARPMAN and ALLEN (1959) also injected crude bradykinin to man (see also KEELE and ARMSTRONG, 1964). Others who have injected bradykinin intradermally to man are WITTE et al. (1961) and MITCHELL and KRELL (1964).

The pain description of BURCH and DE PASQUALE (1962) following *intra-arterial* injection of bradykinin also involved a "burning" element, thus the pain was localized to the arm and involved the entire extremity distal to the site of injection in the antecubital fossa. The pain was usually most intense at the site of injection but in several subjects was most intense in the fingertips. The pain was described as burning by all (10) subjects. The onset of pain occurred within 30 seconds of injection. It reached maximum intensity at about 45 seconds and disappeared completely in 60–120 seconds. A residual sensation of warmth, which lasted from 120 to 180 seconds, was present in the fingertips. COFFMAN (1966) produced similar effects in his subjects by intra-arterial injection. In addition they felt warmth before and after the pain, and throbbing in the fingers at time of peak pain. In the CBA experiments we frequently experience warmth preceding the rise of the pain; the time sequences are very similar, then on washing off of the kinin solution strong resurgence of burning pain occurs. LIM et al. (1967) found stinging or burning pain on intradermal injection of bradykinin, but subcutaneous or intramuscular injections did not cause pain. With *intraperitoneal injections* in man, however, descriptions referred to "cramp", "colic", or pressure. This may represent a different series of events peripherally, or merely a different central representation. Whereas BURCH and DE PASQUALE and COFFMAN produced marked pain by injecting a few micrograms of bradykinin intra-arterially, FOX et al. (1961) produced only feelings of swelling, warmth, and transient unpleasantness or pain (KEELE and ARMSTRONG, 1964), and SICUTERI produced no pain with bradykinin in the human hand-vein preparation which had not been pretreated with 5-HT.

III. Other Findings with CBA

HOLDSTOCK et al. (1957), describing the actions of their purified wasp kinin (SCHACHTER and THAIN, 1954), found it more potent than ACh, with a threshold about 20 μg/ml. The sensation of itchiness frequently occurred with lower concentrations of the kinin preparation or when pain decreased on prolonged contact with the solution. Itch sensation with pure kinins has been an infrequent observation in our experiments. The "after-pain" referred to above is quite distinct from this and is quite "painful". BHOOLA (1961), using highly purified bradykinin (100 μg/ml) on the blister area, also found it produced more intense pain than an equal concentration (w/v) of acetylcholine and with a longer latent period before the pain ensued. The bradykinin-induced pain then lasted at least twice as long as acetylcholine-induced pain (75–150 seconds).

Other workers who have used the cantharidin blister area for the study of pain production by plasma kinins include MARGOLIS (1958b), EISEN (1961, 1963), HORTON (1963), and KIYOHARA (1967). ARCANGELI produced cantharidin blisters in man in order to use the fluid for intradermal injection to humans to compare the activities of this agent with those of burn blister fluid, plasma, and synthetic bradykinin (ARCANGELI et al., 1966).

Since these two similarly algogenic agents, 5-HT and bradykinin, may sometimes arise together in pathological fluids, ARMSTRONG et al. (1953), in order to distinguish them, used the isolated rat uterus.

The PPS was the first of the algogenic bradykinin-like substances of the human body to be investigated. In 1951 the first of a series of experiments on various chemalgogens were made in our laboratories. It was nearly ten years before bradykinin was synthesized. The years between were spent differentiating our agent from 5-HT, classifying it chemically, and studying its timecourse of appearance and disappearance and conditions of arousal in human and animal plasma.

In 1955 we were privileged to have Professor ROCHA E SILVA working with us in our laboratories where he underwent both PPS pain and that due to highly purified bradykinin (ANDRADE and ROCHA E SILVA, 1956). Parallel quantitative assays were also performed (ROCHA E SILVA, 1960; KEELE and ARMSTRONG, 1964). The opinion was reached that the pain stimulant arising in human plasma on its exposure to glass, and which was extractable in ethyl alcohol was indeed bradykinin-like. HABERMANN (1966), studying the chemistry chromatographically, was of like opinion. Thus it is reasonable to assume that bradykinin has been produced. (For certain differences between pain-producing actions of glass-exposed human plasma and bradykinin see under "Tachyphylaxis".)

The polypeptide pain-producing substance was found in our aspirates of cantharidin blister fluid, heat burn blister fluid, insect bite blister fluid, rheumatoid arthritis fluid (Fig. 6), inflammatory pleural effusion (Fig. 6), hydrocele fluid, and blood plasma, but not in cardiac edema fluid or cerebrospinal fluid. The pain was similar to that of the delayed pain of thermal burns.

It was found that the presence of glass or certain other foreign surfaces was necessary for formation of the algogenic agent which did not appear if the collecting vessels and all utensils were siliconed or made of polyethylene. The active principle is destroyed within a few minutes in plasma at room temperature, (20° or higher, e.g. 37°). Cooling to 0° would preserve the active principle longer (e.g. 0.5 hour), and storage at −20° would preserve it indefinitely. The incomplete absence, in fact growing concentrations, of PPS, plasma kinin, in our samples of plasma at +20° was noted. This was believed to be due to a spontaneous, intrinsic kinin-forming process (Armstrong et al., 1957). It was also believed that this kinin-forming action would be slowed by cooling (p. 449). Hence fresh plasma

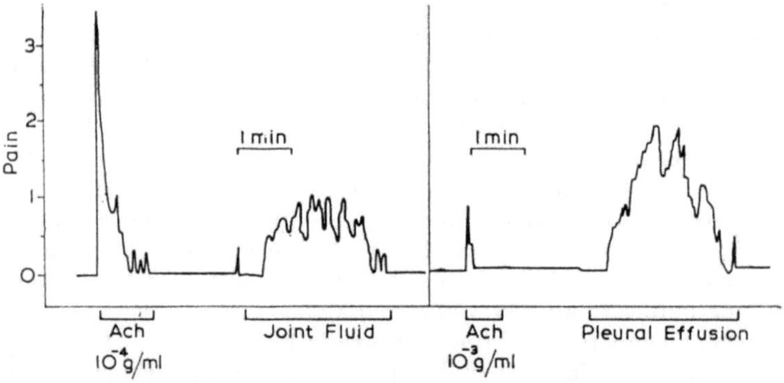

Fig. 6. Pain responses in blister area to applications of (a) joint fluid from a patient with rheumatoid arthritis, and (b) a pleural effusion of inflammatory type. (From Armstrong et al., 1957)

samples in our early work were stored during experiment at 0°. They were discarded when, by the appearance of fair amounts of kinin, it became unreasonable to continue to refer to them as "preactive" (Armstrong et al., 1957; cf. Armstrong and Mills, 1965).

The screening tests on the isolated rat uterus were of great assistance (cf. also "Structure in Relation to Action" section, below). Smooth muscle stimulating and pain-producing properties appear contemporaneously in plasma exposed to glass. The dual activities also arise when the plasma kinin is induced by other means, e.g. ε-amino-n-caproic acid (EACA) and related compounds (cf. Nakahara and Tokita, 1967). The arisal of kinins when plasma is exposed to other treatments, e.g. dilution (20-fold) or cold (37–0°), (Figs. 7 and 8), can likewise be measured against bradykinin by the smooth muscle technique.

Many other methods have been used to produce kinins. We have chosen to study kinin formation which involved, if possible, minimum interference with the plasma. We have therefore concentrated mainly on studies of the "spontaneous" effects of cooling or heating (37–0°, and 37–50°) the preactive plasma in closed polythene containers, and their modification by chemical interference. We have also compared these effects with those obtained with $(NH_4)_2\ SO_4$ precipitation; dilution; acidification and exposure to glass. Eisen has studied plasma kinin formation induced by sodium urate crystals, and the kinin levels and pain in rheumatoid arthritic and other joint fluids (Eisen, 1966; Eisen and Keele, 1966; Keele, 1966; Eisen, 1969; see also Faires and McCarthy, 1962; Goldfinger et al., 1964; Melmon et al., 1967).

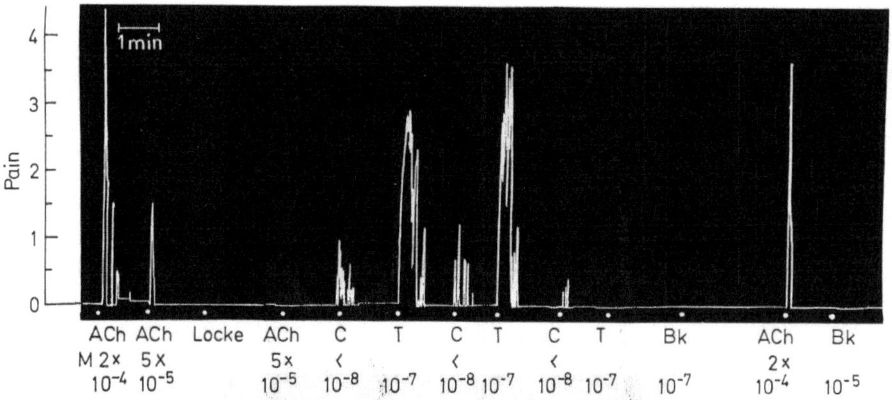

Fig. 7. Blister base. Pain responses to alcoholic extracts of the subject's own diluted plasma. C = control, made at $t = 5$ min; T = test made after 2 hr, 20°. The plasma had been diluted 20-fold in water. Prior to administration the EtOH and water were evaporated off and the extract brought back to plasma volume by added half-strength LOCKE's solution

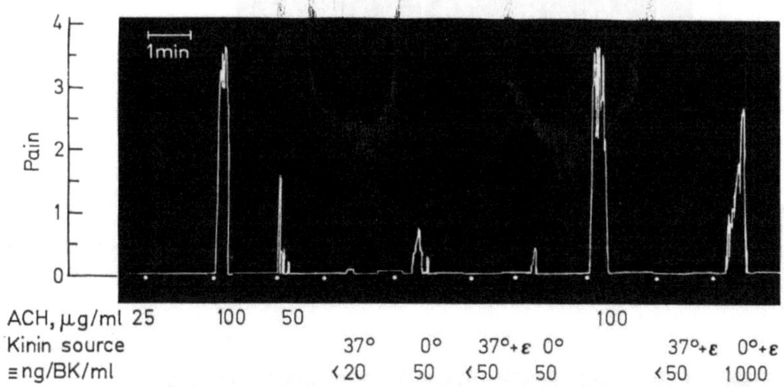

Fig. 8. Blister base. Pain responses to alcoholic extracts of the subject's own plasma (normal) which had been kept at the temperatures indicated in the absence or presence (= + ε) of kininase inhibitor ε-amino caproic acid. Prior to administration the EtOH was evaporated and the extract brought back to plasma volume by addition of half-strength LOCKE's solution

Fig. 9 shows pain production by (burn) blister fluid which had been aspirated to a glass syringe. The agent was labile, as shown in the lower record (ARMSTRONG et al., 1957; KEELE and ARMSTRONG, 1964).

When however the fresh, "preactive" (see above reference) blood plasma (heparinized or citrated) or serum is collected into siliconed or polythene apparatus (or stored in a blood vessel) it is not algogenic. Exposure to glass produces a peptide chemalgogen (PPS) (ARMSTRONG et al., 1953a, b, 1954) that subsequently disappears. The concurrent appearance and decline of other kinin-like properties were also shown.

The appearance of the PPS kinin of plasma can be inhibited by SBTI (soybean trypsin inhibitor), 1 mg/ml (ARMSTRONG et al., 1955, 1957). However, the algogenic or uterotonic actions of PPS, once it is formed, are not inhibited by SBTI (MARGOLIS, 1958b). It can also be inhibited by the presence of hexadimethrine bromide (or protamine sulfate) whose actions are independent of the presence of heparin (ARMSTRONG and STEWART, 1962; cf. ERDÖS, 1966). For this inhibition

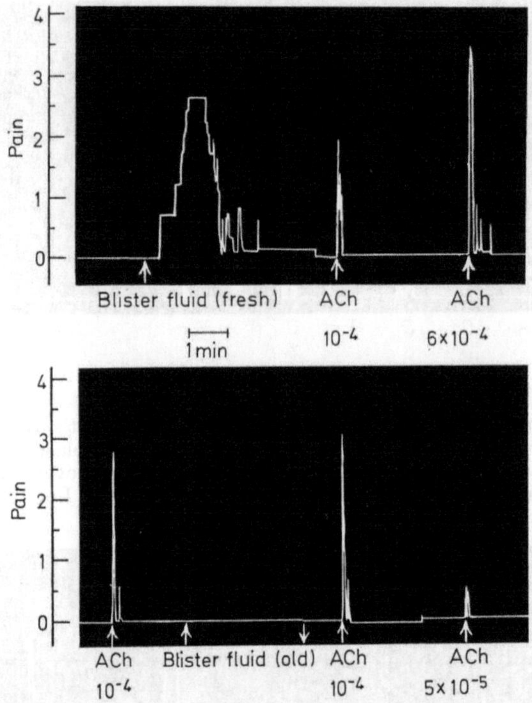

Fig. 9. Record of pain responses to fresh and old blister fluid. Cantharidin blister base. (a) Fresh blister fluid aspirated from the cantharidin blister 25 min before it was applied to the base. Latent period between application and onset of pain, 18 sec. (b) Sample of same blister fluid applied 4 hr after aspiration. (From ARMSTRONG et al., 1953a)

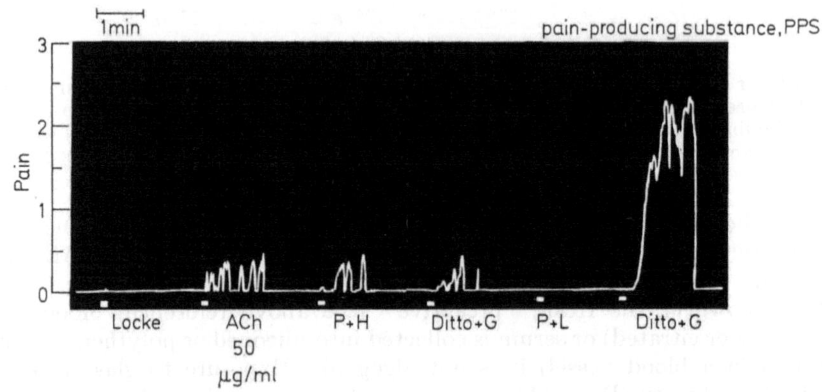

Fig. 10. Blister base. Pain responses to the subject's own plasma P, which has been exposed to glass G, in the presence or absence of hexadimethrine bromide (H, Polybrene; 5×10^{-4} g/ml)

(against the action of large glass surface) high concentrations of hexadimethrine bromide are required—e.g. about 1 mg/ml. EISEN (1964) has demonstrated that the hexadimethrine bromide inhibits kinin formation by inhibiting the activation of factor XII (Hageman factor) at the glass surface. Hexadimethrine bromide does not inhibit the response of either smooth muscle or the pain area to formed kinin. Fig. 10 shows the absence of pain response to fresh plasma which contained hexadimethrine bromide at the time of exposure to clean glass, and the presence of marked pain in the control experiment using Locke's solution.

Algogenic plasma kinin also appears within a few minutes when preactive human plasma, at room temperature (20°), is exposed to EACA (or related compounds) and the "formation" of this too is inhibited by the presence of hexadimethrine bromide. However, in this case extremely low concentrations of the agent (which is a polymer with a molar weight between 6,000 and 10,000) are required—e.g. 10^{-8} to 10^{-7} μg/ml (Armstrong and Stewart, 1960b, 1962). SBTI (1 mg/ml) inhibits this "formation" of kinin.

As Schachter (1956) showed, dilution of human plasma (say 10- or 20-fold) produces kinin. Fig. 7 shows that the kinin formed by dilution is, unlike some kinins (see Table 1), an algogenic one. The kinin was extracted in EtOH from the diluted plasma. Sicuteri and his colleagues (1964, 1965b) have infused the diluted plasma to their 5-HT-sensitized human hand-vein substrate and found it to be pain-producing (Fig. 11).

Table 1. *Synthetic kinins, man; pain-producing potency of analogs of bradykinin*
H-Arg^1-Pro^2-Pro^3-Gly^4-Phe^5-Ser^6-Pro^7-Phe^8-Arg^9-OH

Test	Potency		Reference
Cantharidin blister area	Absent[a]	(1) Des-Pro^7	Keele and Armstrong (1964)
		(2) Retro L	Armstrong (1967–1968)
		(3) Retro D	Armstrong and J. M. Stewart (1968)
		(4) $BkNH_2$	As for (2)
		(5) Des-Arg^9	As for (3)
		(6) D-Arg^9	As for (3)
	Reduced[b]	Bk-Arg	As for (3)
		Bk-Gly	As for (3)
		Acetyl- Bk	As for (3)
		8a.a.Gly-Bk[d]	As for (3)
	High[c]	Bk	Elliott et al. (1960a); Keele and Armstrong (1964)
		Kallidin	Armstrong and Mills (1963)
		Gly-Bk	As for (3)
		Met-Lys-Bk	Elliott and Lewis (1965)
Intradermal injection	Reduced	Kallidin (Lys-Bk)	Marra et al. (1966)
Hand-vein substrate	Reduced	Kallidin (Lys-Bk)	Sicuteri et al. (1964) Sicuteri et al. (1965b)

[a] Normally or always absent at 10^{-5} M concentration.
[b] Present at 10^{-5} M.
[c] Present at 10^{-6} M, or lower, concentration.
[d] Polistes kinin = eight amino acids Gly-Bk = Pyroglu-Thr-Asn-Lys-Lys-Lys-Leu-Arg-Gly-Bk.

Cooling the human plasma (37–0°) produces a reversible thermal activation of the plasma kinin-forming system (Armstrong and Mills, 1965). The activity present at 20 or 0° in normal human plasma (Armstrong et al., 1957) is augmented in parturition plasmas in which high concentrations (e.g. 1–5 μg/ml or more) of plasma kinin and rapid depletion of kininogen occur (Armstrong and Stewart, 1960a; Armstrong et al., 1966). In contrast, the system of plasma kinin-forming enzyme is relatively little insulted by the cooling (Armstrong et al., 1967),

CENTARO et al., 1959; WEBSTER and PIERCE, 1960; DINIZ and CARVALHO, 1963).

The kinin formed by the cooling process (37–0°) is a pain-producing one. Fig. 8 shows the pain produced by the kinin extracted from normal human plasma kept at body temperature (37°) and from that exposed to cold (0°). EACA (0.12 M) which, in addition to inhibiting the activation of plasminogen to plasmin and plasmin's actions, inhibits plasma kininase but does not cause pain (ALKJAERSIG et al., 1959; ERDÖS and SLOANE, 1962; ERDÖS et al., 1963a; ARMSTRONG and STEWART, 1960b), was added to prevent digestion of the formed kinin. In general, plasma kinin does not form, neither does the kininogen level deplete markedly in normal human serum or plasma which is kept at 37° until 24–48 hours or longer have elapsed (cf. PENSKY et al., 1961). Precautions to obtain bacteriological sterility have not been taken here, but sterility had no effect in other experiments. We believe that the kinin-generating, kininogen-depleting effects of cooling upon the plasma are due to a molecular unfolding or disaggregation

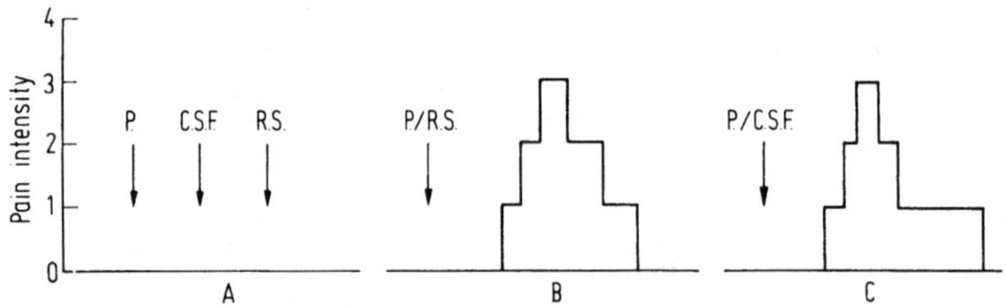

Fig. 11. "Hand-vein substrate". The pain-producing effects of released kinins when fresh plasma, diluted (1 in 10) with RINGER's solution (B) and with cerebrospinal fluid (C) on a 5-HT vein substrate are shown. Identical amounts of plasma, cerebrospinal fluid, and RINGER's solution, given individually, do not produce pain (A). (From SICUTERI, 1967)

within the kinin-forming enzyme system (KAUZMANN, 1959; NÉMETHY and SCHERAGA, 1962; ARMSTRONG and MILLS, 1965; DONALDSON and RATNOFF, 1965).

When EACA is present, the rate of kinin formation in fresh human serum is also usually very close to zero at 37° and it increases as the plasma or serum temperature falls toward 0°. At each temperature the rate of fall of the kininogen level in the EACA-containing samples does not differ from those without the EACA. When assayed on various tissues (ELLIOTT and LEWIS, 1965) against synthetic bradykinin, this EACA-formed kinin behaves very similarly. It is pain producing (see ARMSTRONG and STEWART, 1960b). In the presence of EACA at 0° the accumulation of kinin in normal human plasmas is about as rapid as in the parturition plasmas without EACA. Levels equivalent to several μg synthetic bradykinin/ml plasma or serum are usually obtained in 1 to 2 hours at 0°. It would appear that we are dealing with the kinin induced by cold.

Although kinin has been observed in heated plasma (37–50°) the first outstanding feature of these hot plasmas stored in closed polythene vessels is their relative reluctance to burst into kinin formation. Agent(s) promoting kinin formation are produced during the heating. The conditions for their production and the specificity of their actions are at present not known. The heated plasmas can burst into kinin formation on cooling. Their sensitivity is such that the kinin is then generated rapidly at higher temperatures (e.g. 20°, 37°) than occur in unheated plasmas (ARMSTRONG et al., 1967).

IV. Bradykinin-Induced Pain in Animals

In addition to other references in the text, those who have administered bradykinin to animals by various routes, e.g. intradermal, arterial, venous, peritoneal, intrathecal, mainly to develop tests for analgesic agents, include: BRAUN et al. (1961; dogs and man); EMELE and SHANAMAN (1963; mice); COLLIER et al. (1964; mice); WHITTLE (1964; mice); DICKERSON et al. (1965; dogs and mice); DEFFENU et al. (1966; rats); BLANE (1967, 1968) and BLANE and DUGDALL (1968; rats and mice); SICUTERI (1968a; rabbits and man); and LIM and GUZMAN (1968; guinea pigs, rats, dogs, cats, man). See also pp. 454 and 456.

C. Structure-Action Relationships

I. Bradykinin Analogs

1. Action in Man

Students of the comparative activities of synthetic bradykinin analogs on the cantharidin blister area (see Table 1 and 2) have included KEELE and ARMSTRONG (1964)[1], ELLIOTT and LEWIS (1965)[2], ARMSTRONG and J. M. STEWART (1967–1968)[3] (Figs. 12, 13, 14). The CBA has also been used to observe the algogenic potencies of kinin preparations in various relatively pure states (Figs. 7, 8). By comparing their actions with those of the known synthetic kinins, an enlightened guess as to their structure may be made (ARMSTRONG et al., 1957[4]; HOLDSTOCK et al., 1957[5]; ARMSTRONG and MILLS, 1963[6]; 1965[7]; KEELE and ARMSTRONG, 1964[1]; ARMSTRONG, 1967–1968[8]) (Table 2).

Table 2. *Pain production in man by kinins in states of relative purity applied to the cantharidin blister area*

Kinin[a]	Experimenters[b]	Potency
Bradykinin		
ANDRADE and ROCHA E SILVA, 1956)	ARMSTRONG, KEELE and ROCHA E SILVA (unpublished, 1955)	+++
ELLIOTT et al., 1960b, c, 1961; BOISSONNAS et al., 1960	ELLIOTT et al. (1960a) (1), (2)	
Kinin induced by glass PPS	(4), (1)	+++
Kinin induced by cold (37—0°)	(7)	+++
Kinin induced by dilution (e. g. 20-fold)	(8)	+++
Kinin released by KFS[c] (kinin E)	(6)	+++
Kinin F	(6)	++
Kinin S	(6)	++
Kinin released by *Crotalus atrox* venom	(8)	+++
Kinin of *Vespa vulgaris*	(5)	++ to +++

[a] Kinins used by ARMSTRONG and colleagues were applied to the blister base in concentrations equivalent to those arising in the respective parent plasmas. Assumed that the kinins may be bradykinin or closely related, their bradykinin equivalent concentrations were evaluated against it as a standard on the isolated rat uterus. On this basis their algogenic potencies with respect to bradykinin on the CBA preparation were then determined.
[b] See text.
[c] Kinin-forming substance (ARMSTRONG and MILLS, 1964). See Fig. 15.

Other routes of administration of bradykinin analogs to man have included intradermal injection (Marra et al., 1966; Arcangeli et al., 1966), and intravenous injection to a vein on the dorsum of the hand after its presensitization with 5-HT (Sicuteri et al., 1964, 1965; Table 3).

Marra and colleagues (1966) describe the pain of both bradykinin and kallidin as "burning". According to Sicuteri (1965), with bradykinin the latency between onset of pain and intensity of action bears an inverse and clear relationship.

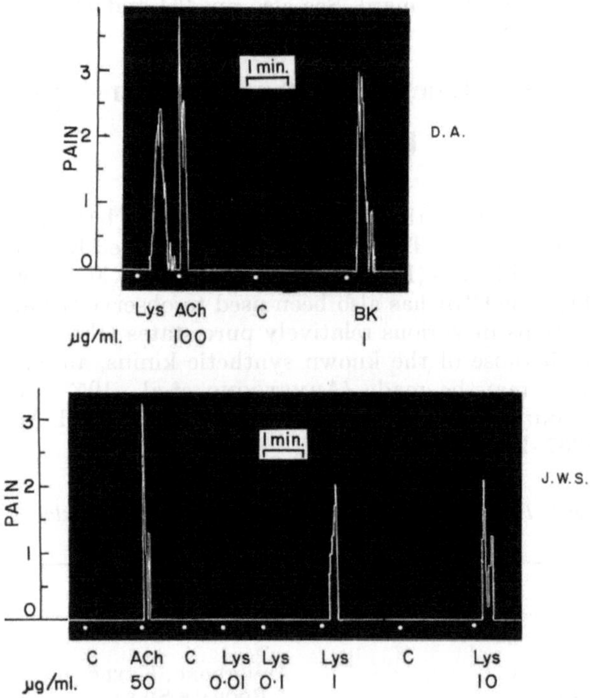

Fig. 12. CBA pain tests in man. Two subjects, one female, the author, upper record; one a male medical colleague, lower record. Ordinates: Subjective pain scale. Abscissae: time. Lys = kallidin; ACh = acetylcholine; C = control = Locke's solution; Bk = bradykinin. Note both subjects suffered pain of "moderate" intensity at a concentration of kallidin of 10^{-6} M, suggesting similarity of effective threshold concentration for pain induction

In Sicuteri's experiments, without pretreatment of the vein the kinins did not cause pain; 5-HT alone caused only a slight paresthesia and burning itch (Table 3).

Administration of Impure Kinins to Humans. The studies of Keele and Armstrong and colleagues, Galletti et al. (1960), and Marra et al. (1960) are concerned with the detection of the algogenic properties of the body fluids. Their later work on the unpurified fluids (Marra et al., 1966), has been an assay of the PPS, formed by exposure of the human plasma to glass, against bradykinin. Arcangeli, on the other hand, has compared the whole nature of the algogenic behaviour of bradykinin with those of the blister fluids and plasma (Arcangeli et al., 1966). The solutions were injected (intra?) dermally to the volar surface of the forearm. The responses were characterized by delayed (40–50 sec) "burning" pain and by hyperalgesia. Burn blister fluid was active even when kept in siliconed

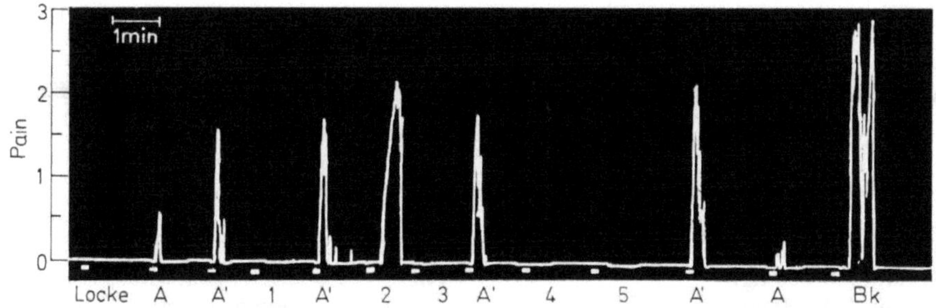

Fig. 13. CBA pain test in man. Ordinates as previously described. 1 = All DBk; 2 = BkArg; 3 = BkDes Arg[9]; 4 = BkDArg[9]; 5 = Retro L Bk; Bk = bradykinin: each was administered at 10^{-5} M concentration in LOCKE's solution. A and A' = acetylcholine 10^{-4} and 2×10^{-4} M, respectively. (From ARMSTRONG and J. M. STEWART, 1967/68)

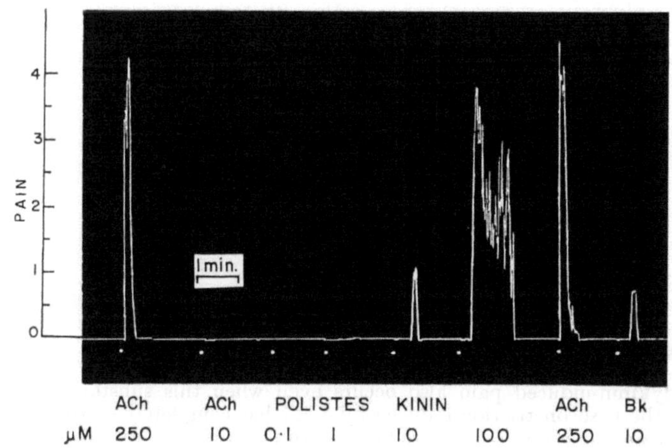

Fig. 14. CBA pain test on the author. Ordinates as previously described. ACh = acetylcholine; Polistes kinin = the pure synthetic 18-amino acid compound (see text) dissolved in LOCKE's solution; Bk = bradykinin. (From ARMSTRONG and J. M. STEWART, 1967/68)

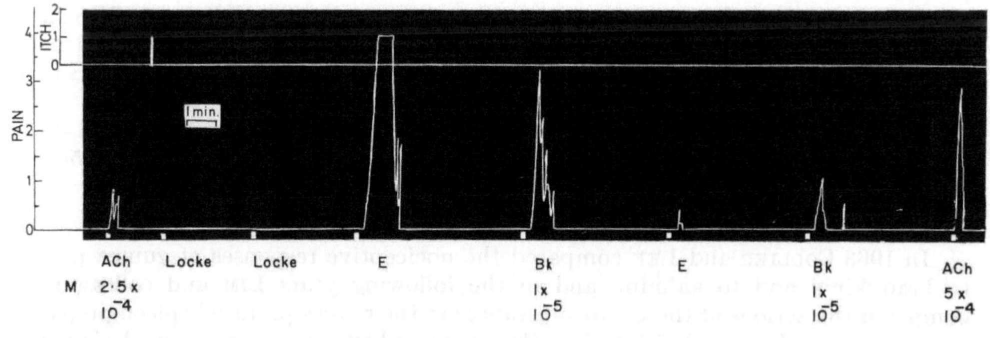

Fig. 15. CBA pain test in man (normal plasma); itch is also recorded. First ordinate = subjective pain scale; second ordinate = subjective scale of itch. Abscissa = time. ACh = acetylcholine; Locke = LOCKE's solution. E = extracted kinin from reaction of KFS (kinin-forming substance, ARMSTRONG and MILLS, 1964) with normal human plasma. Bk = bradykinin

Table 3. *Pain effect. Injections into veins presensitized with 5-HT*. (See SICUTERI and colleagues, 1964, 1965, 1967; SICUTERI, 1967, 1968a)

Agent	Pretreatment of vein				Effect
	no pre-treatment	saline	5-HT (50–100 ng)	other	
5-HT	yes				− to ±
Bradykinin (50–500 ng)		yes			−
Bradykinin (50–500 ng)			yes		+++
Bradykinin (50–500 ng)				norepinephrine 5-HT + methyl 1-lysergic acid butanol-amide (anti-vasoconstrictor)[a]	+++
Kallidin			yes		++
Kallikrein			yes		+++
Angiotensin	yes				−
Angiotensin			yes		−
Eledoisin	yes				−
Eledoisin			yes		−
Histamine	yes				− to ±
Histamine			yes		− to ±
KCl	yes				+
KCl			yes		+++
Oxytocin			yes		−
Plasma diluted × 10–25			yes		+++
PPS[b] (glass-exposed plasma)			yes		+++
Vasopressin			yes		−
Arginine-vasopressin			yes		−

[a] Severe bradykinin-induced pain also occurs even when this substance is introduced into a vein where the vasoconstriction induced by 5-HT has completely subsided.

[b] The normal response is quoted; occasionally a painless response (or nearly so) occurred.

apparatus, and the action was not changed by short (10 min) or long (8 hour) exposure to glass. The pain induced by the burn blister fluid lasted longer than that induced by the other agents, and the hyperalgesia lasted eight times as long (i.e. 16 hour).

As described in Table 3, SICUTERI and colleagues have injected the PPS in plasma to the hand-vein substrate and like bradykinin, but unlike eledoisin or angiotensin, it has induced strong pain on almost all occasions in the 5-HT-treated vein (SICUTERI, 1967).

The results in Tables 1, 2, and 3 should be compared with those obtained on other (smooth muscle) preparations (STEWART and WOOLLEY, 1966, and p. 458).

2. *Action in Animals*

In 1963 COLLIER and LEE compared the nociceptive responses of guinea pigs to bradykinin and to kallidin, and in the following years LIM and colleagues compared the actions of these two substances in their cross-perfused spleen preparations of dogs (LIM et al., 1964). The COLLIER and LIM experiments were designed to predict from animal experiments whether new substances would either cause pain or reduce pain in man. The solutions were injected to guinea pigs intradermally at several sites. Nine behavioral responses to strongly anisotonic solu-

Table 4. *Minimal doses of some endogenous substances eliciting pain or nociceptive responses in man, dog, and guinea-pig* (COLLIER and LEE, 1963)

Substance	Human skin		Dog[f], various sites of injection (μg)	Guinea pig, intradermal injection, μg/ml (actual dose in μg)
	on blister base (μg/ml)	injection (μg/ml)		
Bradykinin	0.1–1[a]	100[d]	0.1–6.3	10 (0.5)
Kallidin	1[b]			10 (0.5)
Acetylcholine	10–100[c]	1,000[e]	250–1,000	100–1,000 (5–50)
Histamine	1,000[c]	100[e]	25–300	100–1,000 (5–50)
5-Hydroxytryptamine	0.1–100[c]	100–1,000[e]	25–200	> 1,000 (> 50)

[a] ELLIOTT et al. (1960a). [b] ARMSTRONG, personal communication.
[c] ARMSTRONG et al. (1953a). [d] HERXHEIMER, personal communication.
[e] LINDAHL (1961).
[f] GUZMAN et al. (1962).

tions, normally painful to man, were observed with great frequency in the animals. Some were directed to the injection site and some not. All nine were used in a scoring system. The question arose: To what degree were the responses nociceptive and to what degree tangioceptive? A study of the parallelism of effectiveness of a range of tonicity changes in solutions injected and applied to man and to the guinea pig revealed sufficient similarity to justify the assumption that the guinea pigs' reactions were to stimulation of nociceptors. A study in the responses of the two species to solutions of various pH was also made for the same reason, and the two responses types were again found to correlate (LINDAHL, 1961; ARMSTRONG et al., 1953a). COLLIER and LEE found three facts to suggest that the responses to intradermal injection of bradykinin were also nociceptive. (1) The pattern of responses to bradykinin was indistinguishable from that to strongly anisotonic solutions; (2) bradykinin causes pain in man; (3) the responses of guinea pigs were suppressed by strong analgesics but not by weak analgesics or by anti-inflammatory agents or tranquilizers. With groups of guinea pigs, one for each concentration of bradykinin used (0.1, 1, 10, 100, 1,000 μg/ml), it was possible to draw fairly steep dose–response curves relating the drug concentration with the near nociceptive scores in each group. These curves were closely similar whether all nine nociceptive criteria or only the two directed to the site of injections were used. The minimally effective concentration (at 0.05-ml injection volume) was about 10 μg/ml of either agent, which is more than ten times the concentration normally required to elicit pain in man. This may well be related not only to activity of peripheral receptors for the kinin but also to central and integrative processes in the animal. Kallidin, effective at similar concentration, has a lower nociceptive score and thus seems to be significantly less active. Table 4 shows the effective concentrations of the two kinins in various species and also relative to other chemalgogens.

The main objective of LIM and his colleagues (GUZMAN et al., 1964) was the elucidation of the site of action of various narcotic and non-narcotic analgesic drugs by using bradykinin as a stimulant of visceral pain, the efficiency of which has been determined in previous work (BRAUN et al., 1961; GUZMAN et al., 1962). However, kallidin (1–2 μg) proved to be as active an algesic agent as bradykinin (1–2 μg) to induce the vocalization and somatic and autonomic responses characteristic of visceral pain (see WOODWORTH and SHERRINGTON, 1904).

II. Bradykinin Compared with Other Peptides

1. Action in Man

Cantharidin Blister Area. Numerous experiments on the human blister base have been reported by ARMSTRONG et al. (1954), ARMSTRONG (1957), and BISSET and LEWIS (1962). The results are summarized by KEELE and ARMSTRONG (1964); see Table 5.

Table 5. *Bradykinin and other peptides: man*

Algogenic effects of naturally occurring peptides applied to CBA. The compounds are placed in descending order of potency.

1. Substance P Bradykinin Kallidin	Active in concentrations of 10^{-7}–10^{-6} g/ml
2. Vasopressin Oxytocin	Active at about 10^{-5} g/ml
3. Angiotensin	Active at about 5×10^{-5} g/ml
4. Leucotaxine	Negligible activity at 10^{-3} g/ml (KEELE and ARMSTRONG, 1964)
5. Polistes kinin (PRADO et al., 1966; PISANO, 1966, 1967, 1968; NAKAJIMA and PISANO, 1968; J. M. STEWART, 1968b). Polistes kinin is active in concentrations of 10^{-5}–10^{-4} M.	

Table 6. *Bradykinin, substance P, and other chemalgogens: animals* (POTTER et al., 1962)

	Minimal vocalization dose in dogs
Substance P	0.57–4.3 μg
Bradykinin	1.25–3.5 μg
Histamine hydrochloride	100.0 μg
Acetylcholine bromide	200.0–750.0 μg
5-HT creatinine sulfate	300.0 μg
Potassium chloride	9.0–28 mg

Intradermal Injection. MARRA and colleagues compared the actions of bradykinin with kallidin, injected intradermally to the volar surface, with those of angiotensin and oxytocin administered in this way and with those of CO_2 snow applied to the skin surface (MARRA et al., 1966). Of the four peptides tested, the bradykinin (10^{-6} g/ml) and angiotensin (5×10^{-5} g/ml) manifested the greater algogenic activities, whereas kallidin and oxytocin, at concentrations of 10^{-6} g/ml and 10^{-5} g/ml, respectively, gave pain of relatively slight intensity. Bradykinin was the most active of the compounds, all of which provoked delayed, "burning" pain. Only the oxytocin solution produced also immediate pain of high intensity. The solution of angiotensin did not evoke immediate pain. All immediate pain was of brief duration and subsided before secondary pain and hyperalgesia ensued. The bradykinin produced a large hyperalgesic area. As for whealing and flare reactions, these seemed to be remarkable only with the oxytocin injections.

2. Action in Animals

LIM and GUZMAN (1968) refer to various kinins administered intra-arterially to dogs and also to other peptides—arginyl-8-vasopressin, lysyl-8-vasopressin angiotensin, and substance P. The peptides, kinin and others, were compared in their actions with those of acetylcholine, histamine, and 5-HT and were found to be far more potent. The comparison of the actions of substance P with those of bradykinin are discussed in detail (POTTER et al., 1962). It was injected to the femoral,

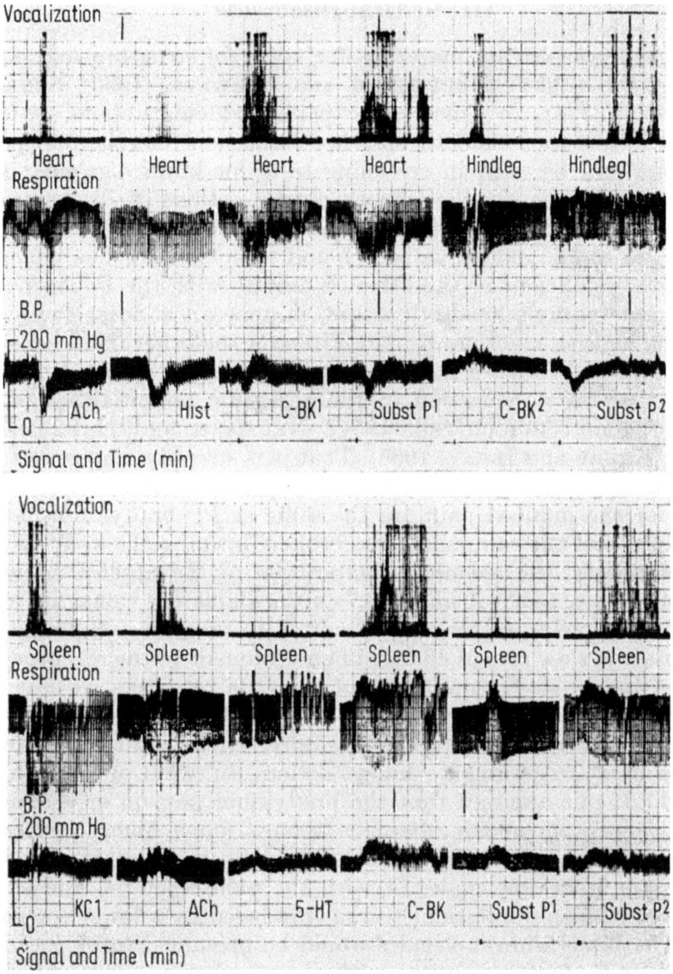

Fig. 16. *Above:* Pseudoaffective response (vocalization, respiratory, and blood pressure change) to intra-arterial injection of algesic agent in the heart (coronary artery) and hind leg (femoral artery) of the dog. Acetylcholine bromide or acetylcholine (250 μg in 0.25 ml), histamine hydrochloride or histamine (100 μg in 0.1 ml), natural bradykinin or C-Bk^1 (equiv. 3.5 μg synthetic bradykinin or S-Bk in 0.5 ml), substance P or substance P^1 (equiv. 0.57 μg P in 1.0 ml), C-Bk^2 (equiv. 2.5 μg S-Bk in 0.5 ml), substance P^2 (equiv. 1.43 μg P in 0.5 ml). Time on bottom line in minutes; background thin lines = 4 sec; thick lines = 20 sec. *Below:* Pseudoaffective response to intra-arterial injection of algesic agents into splenic artery of the dog. Potassium chloride (0.4 mg in 0.25 ml), acetylcholine (ACh) (500 μg in 0.5 ml), 5-hydroxytryptamine creatinine sulfate (5-HT) (300 μg in 0.3 ml), C-Bk (equiv. 1.25 μg S-Bk in 0.25 ml), substance P^1 (equiv. 2.86 μg P in 1.0 ml), substance P^2 (equiv. 4.29 μg P in 1.5 ml). Abbreviations and time as in upper figure. (From Potter et al., 1962)

splenic, or coronary artery of dogs which had previously been appropriately cannulated under anesthesia. The peptides were compared with the biologically active amines in doses necessary to evoke vocalization (Fig. 16). A comparison of activity on a weight basis, assumed that there are 35 units of substance P/μg material, shows that the range of just effective doses for substance P and bradykinin overlap, that substance P may be more active than bradykinin, and that the dose is much smaller than that for other algesic agents (Table 6; cf. Table 5).

III. General Discussion

Peptide syntheses provide materials for study of structure-activity relationships (Merrifield, 1964; Merrifield and Stewart, 1965; Schröder and Hempel, 1964) (p. 324). In general, the pain-producing actions of the analogs vary in parallel with their smooth muscle stimulation (or relaxing) properties—hence the latter can be used in screening tests for kinin algogens. This is not invariably the case. Whereas the smooth muscle actions of Bk-Arg and Bk-Gly are severely reduced, this does not appear to be equally true of the pain-producing action. So far, no compounds have been found to possess the one biological effect and be completely deficient of the other. Similarly with the Polistes wasp kinin, its smooth muscle stimulant activities are, in general, at least twice as high as for Bk, but the algogenic action of bradykinin on the other hand exceeds that of the Polistes kinin by *at least* a factor of 10 to 20. Once threshold concentrations are exceeded there is no question of the algogenic potentialities of this large peptide (Jaques and Schachter, 1954; Neumann and Habermann, 1956; Beard, 1963; Edery and Ishay, 1965). That it is strongly algogenic I can surely testify, but higher concentrations are necessary to be effective. Since the time relationships for the induced pain are the same as for bradykinin-induced pain, it seems unlikely that the compound was broken down by the body to Bk or even to Gly-Bk. Moreover, the chemical composition of the applied solution (about 0.2 ml is applied to a CBA of about 0.7 cm in diameter) would be expected to change relatively slowly as the ratio of active to inactive compound increased. This would result in slow rate of change of environment to the receptor-containing blister surface and in slow stimulation of the pain receptors. In our experience this results, for a given normally strong chemical stimulus when applied rapidly, in pain of low intensity (see Armstrong, 1957; Keele and Armstrong, 1964). Thus it is reasonable to assume a "direct" action. But what of the high concentrations required? If one assumes that the bradykinin portion of the molecule fits the "specific" receptors and is effective, then a much higher concentration of molecules of the unduly large substance would be required to ensure that the same number per unit time make fit with the pain receptors and so ensure an equal intensity of pain stimulations to that produced by a lower concentration of bradykinin. The bradykinin molecules would be presumed to fit the "bradykinin receptors" on their first encounter with them, whereas many of the Polistes kinin molecules would be likely to encounter these receptors opposed to them, thus reducing the effective algogenic potential. Differences in diffusion, transportation and metabolism may also occur and should be considered. (See also Edery and Lewis, 1962a; Walaszek and Dyer, 1966.) Though various other peptide types induce pain, Substance P is the only type, so far, that is equally or more active than bradykinin.

The significance of the intactness of the carboxyl end of the bradykinin molecule has been shown in our experiments; such "minor" changes as conversion to amide or the omission or even the use of the D-Arg^9 remove the algogenic property. The much lesser significance of the amino end is demonstrated in kallidin (Lys-Bk); Gly-Bk; and Met-Lys-Bk, all of which are highly active, and even acetyl Bk or Polistes kinin can certainly cause pain. This relative significance of the carboxyl end of the bradykinin molecule is in agreement with the observations of various authors in relation to its activity (p. 449) (Stewart and Woolley, 1965b; Stewart, 1968a). Stewart and Woolley drew attention to comparison of the significance of the intactness of the carboxyl end of the molecule in bradykinin with its similar significance for the activities of other peptides and even for activity of certain proteins, e.g. pancreatic ribonuclease. Comparative studies of pain production, and also of their enzymatic degradation to bradykinin, of Bk-Arg, Bk-Gly, on the one hand, and phyllokinin (bradykininyl-isoleucyl-tyrosine) on the other, would be valuable in elucidating the significance of the free C-terminal of bradykinin for pain production (ANASTASI et al., 1966, p. 591). The substances listed in Table 2 are all bradykinin-like. However, in view of the above discourse, it is not easy to give details of what this means in terms of structure. At least one of the substances, the PPS kinin, may be bradykinin (HABERMANN, 1966); at least one, the kinin E, appears not to be bradykinin. A third kinin, the one released in human plasma by *Crotalus atrox* (rattlesnake venom), is not produced in plasma which has been exhausted of its kininogen by the spontaneous production of the natural kinin induced by the cooling of human plasma (ARMSTRONG and STEWART, 1960a; ARMSTRONG and MILLS, 1965).

D. Characteristics of Pain Induced by Bradykinin

I. Tachyphylaxis

Bradykinin Dose-response Curves. Dose-response curves may be determined on tissues that have a constant background. Thus, for example, the responses of the CBA to pain stimulation by acetylcholine may readily be determined (the area recovers completely from the effects of moderate dosage within 10 minutes) and the dose-response curve obtained. In the case of ACh stimulation, it is very steep: doubling the dose greatly enhances the pain. When bradykinin or related agents are applied, progressive, type-specific insensitivity of the area develops (ELLIOTT, et al., 1960a; BISSET and LEWIS, 1962; KEELE and ARMSTRONG, 1964; ELLIOTT and LEWIS, 1965). Dose-response curves as such cannot be determined. To maintain equal intensity of response using the typical 10 minute interval, one must think in terms of tenfold increase of original concentration of kinin solution. This situation is similar to that occurring on repeated administration of 5-HT. Such depression as occurs with bradykinin on the CBA does not occur on isolated organ preparations or when the drug is administered to man causing him pain where blood flow is good (see below). LIM, administering the drug intraperitoneally to man, found the range of optimal doses for individual persons for pain production to be less than tenfold, with results clustered at the lower end of the scale, around 4 µg per subject. A few individuals neither responded at the upper limit of this scale nor did they respond to higher doses (LIM and GUZMAN, 1968). On the CBA, subjects generally respond well, recording pain of at least "medium intensity", to concentrations of bradykinin over the range 10^{-7} to 10^{-6} M.

Latent Period Preceding Bradykinin Response. Not only is a latent period observed when bradykinin stimulates isolated organs tissues but also when it is administered close to tissues in man which respond with pain. What is taking place during this latency is difficult to determine. Curiously, in pain studies, it occurs after different methods of administration and has been reported by numerous workers. The time sequences are also curiously similar. Is there some basic action governing this? Somehow it seems unlikely, as the methods of administration are so different.

Bradykinin Tachyphylaxis. Bradykinin tachyphylaxis, i.e. the rapid and specific self-"protection" of a tissue against rapidly repeated administration of the drug, has been a frequently remarked upon feature of bradykinin's actions. It has occurred principally in regard to pain stimulation, being less remarkable in relation, e.g., to smooth muscle stimulation. This tissue "protection" results in a smaller response to a given concentration of a drug upon its re-administration in that or even in a higher concentration within a short period (Fig. 15; cf. Figs. 7, 12).

Despite the fact that KEELE and ARMSTRONG and their collaborators did not emphasize the tachyphylaxis-inducing property of bradykinin, saying merely that development of refractoriness is "less marked", various authors reported tachyphylaxis (MARGOLIS, 1958; ELLIOTT et al., 1960a; BHOOLA, 1961; EISEN,

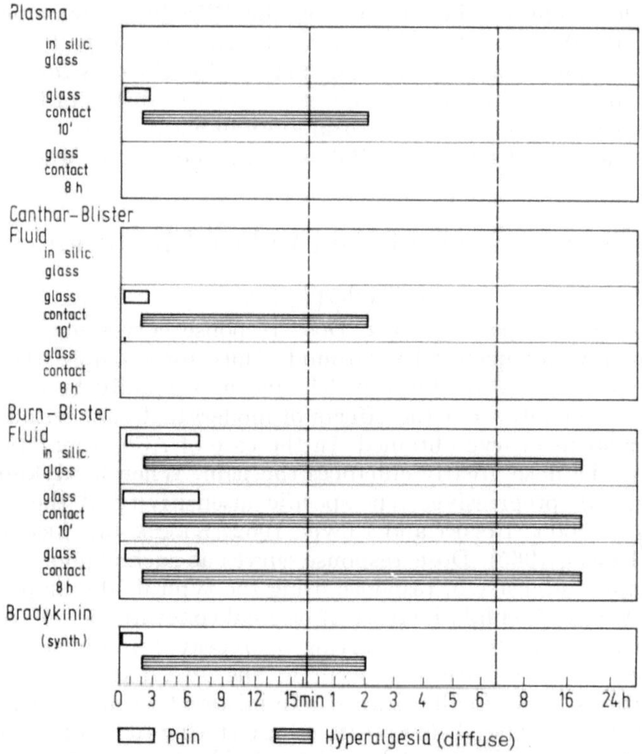

Fig. 17. Intradermal injections to man: recording of pain and hyperalgesia. Each of 5 subjects received each of the biological fluids and also bradykinin. Note that the burn blister fluid differs from the plasma, cantharidin blister fluid, and synthetic bradykinin. The prolonged hyperalgesia is attributed to stable algogens in the burn fluid, present in it *de novo*. (From ARCANGELI et al., 1966)

1961; BISSET and LEWIS, 1962; HORTON, 1963; ELLIOTT and LEWIS, 1965, who report strong tachyphylaxis). When we examined specifically for this property, on CBA tests, we have found it to be almost invariably present and well marked. On the other hand an almost equal number of authors have reported absence of tachyphylaxis to the repeated administrations (GUZMAN et al., 1964; SICUTERI and colleagues, 1964, 1965b; COFFMAN, 1966; SICUTERI, 1967, 1968a; LIM and GUZMAN, 1968).

The early reports on the tachyphylaxis concerned experiments on the CBA. Moreover, undue frequency of administration or variations in the frequency is probably not responsible for the modification of sensitivity on that tissue because, whether a 5-, 10-, or 30-minute interval is allowed between the administrations, the tissue infrequently recovers completely to concentrations of bradykinin of about 1 μmole even during the longer intervals. Even longer rest periods are experimentally impracticable because of the tendency of the area to heal and of the subject's central nervous system to forget the relative intensities of previous pain, by then distant in time. The tendency to tachyphylaxis is marked when the drug is administered to the CBA but not if it is injected intravascularly (COFFMAN, 1966; LIM and GUZMAN, 1968; SICUTERI, 1968a).

What of the PPS? When human plasma is exposed to glass a bradykinin-like agent (see also HABERMANN, 1966) is formed through the activation of Hageman factor and subsequent mediation of kinin-forming enzymes. The glass-exposed plasma, on the other hand, contains also kinin-forming enzymes. These, too, are algogenic when applied to the blister base. Thus repeated administrations of fresh aliquots of plasma freshly exposed to glass and then to the blister area may be expected to produce pain responses longer than when extracted PPS or bradykinin alone is applied. ARCANGELI et al. (1966, and Fig. 17) believe that the extended hyperalgesias obtained with burn blister fluid are due to stable substances of tissue origin. Perhaps "bradykinin-potentiating factors" take part (FERREIRA, 1965; AARSEN, 1968).

The interesting experiments and results of HORTON (1963), whose "pain-producing substance" failed to resemble synthetic bradykinin or trypsin-formed bradykinin when applied to the blister base (in that little tachyphylaxis occurred), also require explanation. Is HORTON (even with inactive control solutions) dealing with the same situation as KEELE and ARMSTRONG, who did not acidify their plasma or heat it to 96°? Until the nature of the kinins formed by these various means is determined, and the influences imposed on their responses by both the algogenic and other components of the medium are known, we cannot be certain of what is taking place. Perhaps more than one reason accounts for the findings. However, it seems clear that the acid + glass + heat treatment of human plasma results in a preparation of different algogenic properties from the plasma + trypsin + heat treatment in that the preparation in which glass was used, unlike synthetic bradykinin, produces little tachyphylaxis on the human blister base, according to HORTON's method.

II. Sensitization of Tissues

Various authors have reported sensitization of pain receptors to bradykinin. It should be noted that tachyphylaxis occurs. This involves specificity. A blister area depressed to bradykinin will thus respond to 5-HT, ACh, K^+, tonicity effects, etc. Likewise, one depressed to 5-HT will respond to Bk. The relation of various chemical agents, in particular 5-HT, to the inflammatory response is of interest since pain is one of the signs of inflammation. FELDBERG (1956) has pointed out the multiplicity of substances that might be liberated in cellular injury and thus be implicated in the response. On the one hand, while it is highly unlikely that any one mediator may be responsible for the inflammatory response, on the other it is perhaps possible to exclude some substances as possible mediators on grounds of inappropriate or insufficient distribution. Among them he has named acetylcholine, norepinephrine, epinephrine, and substance P. There is no mention of 5-HT but, on grounds of less specialized distribution than substance P, it might qualify for further inspection. G. P. LEWIS (1964b) refers to the activation of the plasma kinin-forming system by 5-HT, which is liberated in injury. In the same book MAJNO (1964) refers to the vascular leakage caused by the compound acting particularly in venules. This is most interesting in relation to the studies on 5-HT-bradykinin potentiation by SICUTERI et al. (1964, 1965b) in the human hand-vein substrate and by GILFOIL et al. (1963) and GILFOIL and KLAVINS (1965) in the

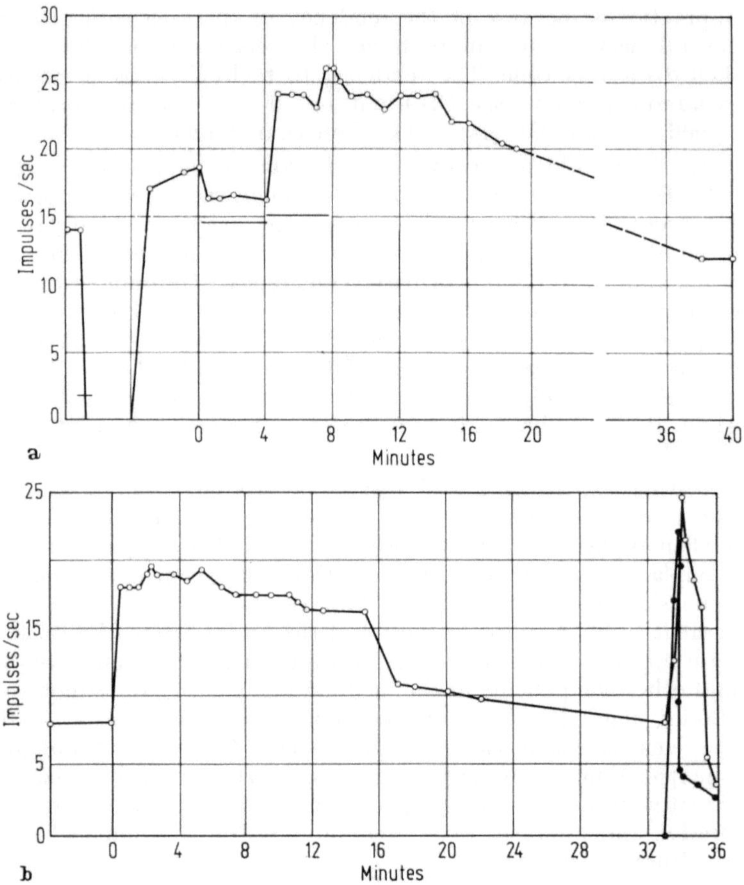

Fig. 18. The effect of (a) histamine pricked into the skin and (b) bradykinin and then a mixture of histamine and acetylcholine injected close-arterially, on the discharge of impulses in cutaneous afferent fibers from the saphenous nerve of the cat. The open circles in each graph show the rate of firing in a slowly adapting mechanoreceptor with a myelinated afferent fiber. In the upper graph there was a steady discharge which disappeared temporarily when superficial cuts were made in the skin. At zero time histamine (10^{-3} g/ml) was applied to the skin and caused an increase in the rate of steady firing in the fiber. The lower graph shows that the injection of 400 μg impure bradykinin also caused the acceleration of the steady discharge in a similar fiber. After 33 minutes a mixture of histamine (10 μg) and acetylcholine (24 μg) was injected. In addition to a strong excitatory action on the myelinated fiber there was also a discharge of impulses in several nonmyelinated fibers (filled circles) which had not been excited by the bradykinin. The injected histamine caused a depression of the steady discharge after the initial enhancement. (From Iggo, 1962)

rat paw, when considered in relation to the work of Lim on the perivascular location of the pain receptors. It may be that in man, increase in permeability in certain areas of the vascular bed may occur (Cotran and Majno, 1964). It is not likely that stasis is the chief cause of the 5-HT-bradykinin potentiation reported by Sicuteri and his colleagues, since low doses (e.g. 1–2 μg) were used and he produced some evidence, including also the use of methysergide (methyl 1-lysergic acid butanol amide) which, to the contrary, antagonized 5-HT constriction. Moreover, the vein sensitized by 5-HT remains so for days, whereas 5-HT vasoconstriction is short-lived (Sicuteri, 1968a). When some degree of stasis was present, ischemic effects would be added to the picture (see below), and these combined with an increase in permeability of the vessels might cause rapid access of relatively high concentrations of the Bk algogen to LIM's perivascular receptors and so cause high-intensity pain (cf. KEELE and ARMSTRONG, 1964). It is not very likely that a synergism of the type described by ZWEIFACH (1964) for 5-HT and catecholamines occurs. This does not rule out the possibility of some metabolic interactions or interference in the synergism. For example, the 5-HT could occupy nonspecific sites for Bk, thereby raising the effective concentration of the bradykinin (the sensitization is not specific; SICUTERI, 1968a). It should be noted that it is necessary to give the 5-HT *first*, followed by the bradykinin. Thus the 5-HT would appear to be the true sensitizer. The phenomenon of the potentiation is reported to be marked and powerful. The rapid rate of rise of concentration of chemalogen at its site of action is a probable mechanism participating in this interesting effect mediated by a common tissue constituent, 5-HT, liberated from blood platelets and other cells in injury and present with polypeptide in the sting of the common nettle and in wasp and hornet venoms (COLLIER and CHESHER, 1956; NEUMANN and HABERMANN, 1956; MATHIAS and SCHACHTER, 1958; JAQUES and SCHACHTER, 1954; BHOOLA et al., 1961; SCHACHTER, 1963, 1964). Hypersensitivities, chemically induced, have been reported in relation to ACh, 5-HT, and plasma kinins which have been shown to produce hyperalgesia to thermal stimuli in human skin (SKOUBY, 1951; OSTFELD et al., 1955; CHAPMAN et al., 1961; KEELE and ARMSTRONG, 1964; SICUTERI, 1968a). How they are determined is not known. However LIM (1960) makes interesting remarks on actions of certain analgesic agents (acetylsalicylic acid) and their modifications of congestion and blood flow (in zones where chemically stimulated pain is antagonized by them), suggesting that the *relief* of pain and resulting chemo-insensitivity of the receptors may be due to rendering the stimuli ineffective, perhaps by preventing stimulation, by some relatively simple means.

Just as it seems unlikely that inflammation is mediated by a single chemical agent, so with pain (KEELE and ARMSTRONG, 1964, p. 283). It is not certain that bradykinin is an exclusive pain stimulant for, according to IGGO (1962), when pricked into the skin or injected close-arterially into the saphenous artery of cats, while recording from cutaneous afferent fibers dissected from the saphenous nerve, almost without exception the nonmyelinated fibers tested were depressed by the chemicals (histamine, 5-HT, or bradykinin). Slowly adapting cutaneous mechanoreceptors with myelinated afferent fibers, however, showed only enhanced response (Fig. 18; see also FJALLBRANT and IGGO, 1961). IGGO states nonmyelinated fibers which had previously not been stimulated by bradykinin were nevertheless sensitive to other chemical agents (chemalgogens?). Thus the bradykinin depression of firing even on the individual type of fiber (nonmyelinated) was not general but selective. It may be that certain chemalgogens can alter the whole spectrum input to the CNS from a given location and so alter sensation (HEAD, 1920; LIM, 1966), thus one must follow the impulses centrally. This central search may turn out to be required for the complete analysis of pain (IGGO, 1962). The fact that bradykinin fails to stimulate certain fibers thought to be involved in pain transmission, or even depresses them, selectively or otherwise, does not *per se* necessarily indicate that it is not an agent promoting nociception even though it may not be acting, in these circumstances, peripherally, as a direct chemalgogen. LIM (1968) draws attention to the fact that in sensitization studies (physiological) control mechanisms should also be considered, as the inhibitory tracts play an important but not exclusive role in pain modulation. The alternative to a central mechanism of sensitization would be a peripheral change in the transducer mechanism of the receptor terminals, or in the state of the nerve membrane, allowing it to respond to any modality of stimulation at much lower thresholds than is effective in the normal axon. Whether the sensitization of the pain receptors in veins by 5-HT is local or central is not known. The fact that it is so curiously long-lasting suggests the possibility of a local damaging action to the tissues which outlasts the life span of the 5-HT in them. Whatever the action of the 5-HT, it is not possessed by bradykinin since reversing the order of administration of these drugs to a vein results in no sensitization.

Ischemia. This is another, and perhaps related, method of sensitizing tissues to the pain-producing actions of bradykinin. To what extent this is a concentration effect, due to reduced blood and tissue fluid flow, and how much due to accumulation and liberation of, e.g., 5-HT of various sensitizing metabolites — a chemalgogenic sensitization — is not known (ARCANGELI et al., 1963; PANERAI et al., 1964; GHETTI et al., 1965; SICUTERI, 1966; LIM and GUZMAN, 1968). The liberation of 5-HT and kinins under conditions of ischemia was also reported (BESSOU and LAPORTE, 1958; LIM, 1966).

Proteolytic Enzymes as Sensitizers to Kinin Action. Such sensitization to bradykinin and plasma kinin action in smooth muscle preparations has been reported by EDERY in relation to the action of trypsin, chymotrypsin, chymotrypsinogen, and papain (EDERY, 1964, 1965; EDERY and GRUNFELD, 1969). FERREIRA (1965, 1966) has shown that the kinin-producing *Bothrops jararaca* venom contains, in addition, a kinin-potentiating factor (BPF). The potentiating or sensitizing action of the enzymes in relation to pain production is a matter of conjecture. Some of them (e.g. trypsin and *B. jararaca* venom) are kinin producers. If they can also sensitize the kinin receptors to kinin or otherwise increase the effective concentration of kinin, a potent self-aggrandizing action would be in progress.

Bradykinin-potentiating Factors (e.g. BPF; FERREIRA, 1965, 1966). See p. 461 and p. 471 below.

E. Proteolytic Enzymes

That proteolytic enzymes applied to man are capable of inducing pain seems to be fairly well established. Production of moderate to severe pain by an application of trypsin to the human blister base was demonstrated by KEELE and ARMSTRONG (1964). Chymotrypsin in the same concentration (2×10^{-4} g/ml), failed to cause pain in the same test. As trypsin is a kinin-generating enzyme and chymotrypsin is not, it may be that pain is caused in the first instance with trypsin by the liberation of kinin from the blister base. It may be, however, that trypsin produces pain in its own right, i.e. independent of its production of kinin. This appears true for at least one other kinin-forming enzyme, the "Contact factor" of MARGOLIS (1958b). When the blister area is "depressed" by SBTI, the contact factor enzyme fails to cause pain, though the area is still responsive to already formed plasma kinin. MARGOLIS calls this a direct pain response due to this enzyme (see p. 86). EISEN, on the other hand, suggests the production of kinin-forming mechanisms not hitherto present, induced by the rubbing of an exposed blister base, and that these respond to added plasma by kinin formation and pain (EISEN, 1961). It is not easy to assess to what extent the pain-producing action is directly due to enzymatic factors and how much is due to the kinin formed. Slow liberation of kinin would be expected to produce pain of low intensity (KEELE and ARMSTRONG, 1964).

Several methods of plasma kinin formation involving the intrinsic mechanisms are promoted by the presence of heparin (ARMSTRONG and STEWART, 1962), though this agent in similar concentrations inhibited EISEN's responses. This is difficult to interpret. The inhibitory actions of the SBTI on EISEN's system may resemble those found by MARGOLIS, and MARGOLIS's experiments suggest that the action of the SBTI is not just directly analgesic one. EISEN used blister areas in which there was not a generalized hyperalgesic action, as the pain responses to acetylcholine were not enhanced by the rubbing (EISEN, 1961). Although EISEN's effects seem to suggest mainly enzymatic rather than mainly kinin actions, their potentiation by cell-rich plasma, perhaps by 5-HT, suggests kinin actions (SICUTERI et al., 1964, 1965b, 1967; SICUTERI, 1967, 1968a).

Plasmin, or streptolysin (Merck) preparations, applied to the blister area caused pain. The agent did not seem to be outstandingly potent in terms of threshold concentrations, or the pain intense. Whether the action is direct or not has not been determined (G. P. LEWIS, 1958, 1960; EISEN, 1961).

The pain-producing actions of saliva, a potent source of glandular kallikrein, are interesting for several reasons. First, it is common knowledge that animals, including man, lick sores gently and the saliva seems to act as a balm. Thus saliva *per se* cannot be claimed to be a pain-producing agent in the usual sense, and this despite its being a familiar and rich source of kininogenase. However, the pain induced by saliva on the blister area, when it occurs, is intense. KEELE and ARMSTRONG (1964) dialyzed the saliva against Locke's solution for some hours prior to experiment. The dialysate did not produce pain; the dialyzed saliva did. I suggest that the palliative actions of native saliva may be due not only to the presence of mucous secretions but perhaps also to some inhibitor(s) of the salivary kallikrein enzyme which is removed or inactivated by dialysis. In any case, under these circumstances the saliva certainly produces "good" pain.

Snake venoms may be classified, in general, as neurotoxic or proteolytic. To what extent the pain induced by the proteolytic venoms (e.g. *Bothrops jararaca*, *Crotalus atrox*, etc.) is a direct action is not known. Certainly the kinin formed by *C. atrox* (rattlesnake) venom introduced to human plasma is a pain-producing one as we have tested it on the CBA, and it does not arise if the venom is introduced to plasma previously depleted of its kininogen spontaneously by exposure to cold (ARMSTRONG and MILLS, 1965). However, we have not applied the venom itself to the CBA as we felt that the known high bacteriological contamination in venoms and their protein constituents rendered them unfit for this in humans. The *C. atrox* venom actively generates kinin when it is applied to human plasma (in μg/ml concentrations); the animal may inject 30–300 mg of venom per bite (WRIGHT and WRIGHT, 1957; DEUTSCH and DINIZ, 1956).

Some proteolytic and kinin-forming enzymes appear to be able to cause pain by the dual mechanisms of direct action, and indirect action through kinin formation. The direct action appears to be of short latency and to involve moderate to high intensity pain stimulation. Some inhibitions of this direct action of the enzyme by the SBTI have been reported.

Proteolytic enzymes are released in tissue damage (e.g. in burning; BELOFF and PETERS, 1945; UNGAR and DAMGAARD, 1954; GOODWIN et al., 1963; ROCHA E SILVA and ANTONIO, 1960; ROCHA E SILVA and ROSENTHAL, 1961; EDERY and LEWIS, 1962b, 1963; DE DUVE, 1964; JACOBSON and WAALER, 1966) and also may be presumed to be activated in acute pancreatitis. They are also liberated to the lumen of the gut in the course of digestion. To what extent they contribute to the pain of disease (e.g. in the gastrointestinal tract) either directly or indirectly (through kinin formation) remains to be assessed.

Eisen has found high concentrations of kinin-forming, kallikrein-like activity in concentrates of human antihemophilic factor which on infusion to humans produced various reactions including induction of pain at operation sites and pain in the back and sometimes in the chest. Further purification of the concentrates resulted in less pain and less kallikrein (Maycock et al., 1963; Eisen, 1965; Biggs et al., 1965). Sicuteri et al. (1967) report on the algogenic actions of intra-arterial and intra-venous administration of kallikrein and of trypsin and note the high sensitivity to intracarotid administration. Sicuteri (1968a) refers to the selectivity of response of the pain receptors of his hand-vein preparation toward certain peptides.

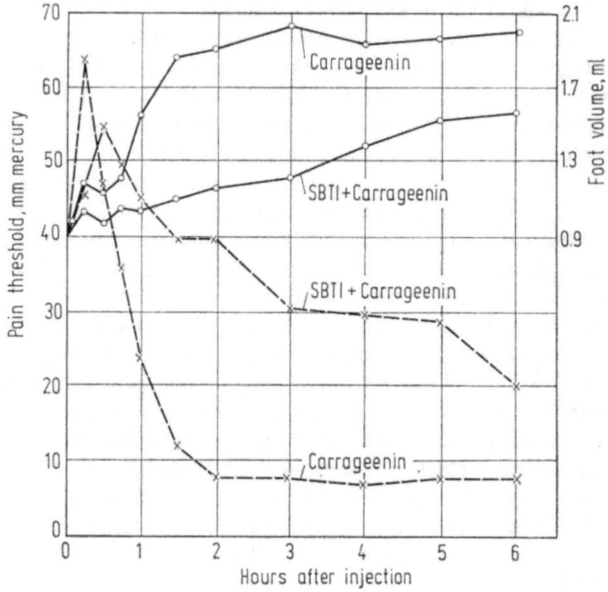

Fig. 19. Carrageenin inflammation influenced by soybean trypsin inhibitor (SBTI). Foot volume in solid lines (right-hand ordinates); pressures for pain threshold in dashed lines (left-hand ordinates). (From Van Arman et al., 1968)

He notes that kallikrein causes pain in this preparation and that there is an extended latency after administration till pain appears. Sicuteri (1968b) noted that Trasylol fails to modify the effects of bradykinin and synthetic kallidin given intravenously but is effective in blocking the vasomotor effects and headache caused by "threshold" doses of kallikrein.

Van Arman et al. (1968) pointed out that the swelling and pain of inflammation are not related in constant manner and suggest that different chemical mediators are involved in the two types of reaction. Carrageenin produces *both* swelling and pain. Evidence is presented by these authors against histamine or 5-HT as the main mediator in carrageenin inflammation and for the participation of bradykinin. The nature of the enzyme system involved is not clear but appears not to involve trypsin, and the mast cells do not seem to be mainly affected. Inhibition by SBTI of the lowering of the pain threshold induced by carrageenin is shown Fig. 19 (see also Van Arman et al., 1965).

Trypsin also caused depression of the pain threshold along with swelling in rat feet. Local administration of SBTI inhibited both phenomena. When indomethacin was used in place of SBTI, however, only the depression of the pain threshold was inhibited. This is interesting because it suggests that the sensitivity of the paravascular pain receptors of LIM and his colleagues is not modulated *per se* by the permeability changes of the blood vessels. Indomethacin did not inhibit the response of isolated smooth muscle to formed bradykinin, nor did it inhibit the formation of kinin in plasma by trypsin. It did not affect the permeability changes induced by trypsin. It would appear to act on the pain receptors reducing their sensitivity. In hand-vein substrate experiments the administration of indomethacin to the same vein did not modify the pain response to bradykinin (SICUTERI, 1964).

Kallikrein injected intradermally, like a number of other proteolytic enzymes injected in this way (e.g. trypsin, plasmin, mucunain), causes itch (ARTHUR and SHELLEY, 1955; CORMIA and DOUGHERTY, 1960; KEELE and ARMSTRONG, 1964).

For proteolytic enzymes as possible sensitizers to bradykinin action see p. 464.

F. Antagonisms

If bradykinin is responsible for mediation of pain or sensitization of pain receptors, the first type of antagonist for which one might seek would be a bradykinin-blocking agent. So far, out of the many peptides tried, those that have blocked bradykinin's action have also had excessively excitatory properties (STEWART and WOOLLEY, 1965a). It is necessary to fall back on inhibition of kinin formation (p. 213). Various natural inhibitors exist. Whereas the actions of plasma kallikrein are antagonized by the *SBTI* (p. 219), those of glandular sources and urine are not. The protein nature of the SBTI, and possibly also impurities, renders it unsuitable for systemic use in man. *Trasylol,* however, has been used in man (e.g. in acute pancreatitis) apparently with success and suitability in some cases only (p. 558).

Another SBTI-sensitive enzyme of the human plasma is the KFS of ARMSTRONG and MILLS (1964). It may act through the formation of plasma kallikrein.

Perhaps it would be possible to inhibit the formation of plasma kallikrein. Activation of Hageman factor at foreign surface can be inhibited by *hexadimethrine bromide* (Fig. 10; ARMSTRONG and STEWART, 1962; EISEN, 1964), as well as "activated" Hageman factor in solution (RATNOFF and MILES, 1962; EISEN, 1964). If certain types of inflammatory action are bradykinin mediated, then the reports of antagonism of them *in vivo* by means of hexadimethrine bromide are interesting (RATNOFF and MILES, 1962; EISEN, 1964; KELLETT, 1965; LEME et al., 1967). KELLETT found the hexadimethrine bromide active against a variety of inflammatory stimuli in the rat paw test and was about fifteen times more active than protamine (ARMSTRONG and STEWART, 1962). Against ultraviolet-induced erythema in the guinea pig it was effective at a dose level below that of phenylbutazone. It was about three times as active as cortisone acetate in suppressing the tuberculin reaction occurring in Mycobacterium B.C.G.-sensitized animals. LEME et al. (1967), using high concentrations of hexadimethrine bromide in the rat, were impressed by the degree of suppression of edema subsequently obtained to the locally applied stimuli of heat (45°) or injection of carrageenin or cellulose sulfate.

However, hexadimethrine bromide disrupts mast cells (KIMURA et al., 1959a, b). It liberates histamine in the skin of man and is a nephrotoxic agent (HALLER et al., 1962; BEALL, 1963; PATE and LEE, 1963). Ideally, therefore, in man it must be administered, if at all, in low concentrations, probably locally, to tissues of low histamine content or in the presence of an antihistamine drug such as mepyramine.

If the activation of the Hageman factor *in vivo* is inhibited by means of the dual operation of the warm (37°) state and the operation of the *C'1 esterase inhibitor* of Pensky et al. (1961), Levy and Lepow (1959), and Armstrong (1968, 1969), perhaps a specific agent of this type would be more active in suppressing inflammation with its hyperalgesia (see also Billingham et al., 1969).

It is possible to increase the destruction of bradykinin at sites where it may be acting. Reduction of carrageenin-induced inflammation, which is believed to be mediated or modulated through the kinin system, has been achieved by means of *carboxypeptidase B* (see Van Arman et al., 1965, 1968; Erdös et al., 1963b). Other possibilities include nonspecific antagonism of the pain induced by kinins peripherally or centrally, which may be mediated by recognized analgesic drugs like acetylsalicylic acid or morphine, or others (e.g. perhaps the amphetamines) whose potentialities for pain inhibition have not been appreciated till recent years.

Acetylsalicylic Acid, Morphine and Other Drugs

In addition to an inhibitory action on certain kinin-induced smooth muscle contraction (Collier and Lee, 1963), acetylsalicylic acid has been reported to antagonize bradykinin-induced pain. Collier and Lee (1963) used nociceptive responses of guinea pigs; Emele and Shanaman (1963) used tests in mice; Blane, (1967, 1968) used the technique of Deffenu et al. (1966) which involves injecting the stimulus (e.g. bradykinin) to the common carotid of unanesthetized rats by means of an implanted catheter. The stimulus causes dextro rotation of the rat's head (pain ?). Tachyphylaxis is not produced when the drug is administered at 15 minute intervals. If a suspected analgesic agent causes the rat to fail to turn its head on two successive administrations it is deemed to be effective. The antagonist may be administered by one of several routes. Compounds which antagonize writhing in mice also antagonize the intra-arterial administration of bradykinin (Blane, 1968). The writhing test used by Whittle (1964), Emele and Shanaman (1963), Pearl et al. (1968), and others is difficult to understand. In essence the procedure is as for the administration of bradykinin into man by Lim and his associates. Lim (1967) administers a low dose of bradykinin (e.g. 1, 2, or 4 μg) to man i.p. After a delay of less than one minute pain is experienced. Thus, in man, Lim's method does not differ significantly in results from those obtained on other human preparations (e.g. CBA tests or i.a. injections). However, in the Emele and Shanaman tests the mice receive more bradykinin than Lim gives to a man (though the dose may *appear* low enough—e.g. 2.5 μg). Nevertheless the peak of the writhing effect which ensues is greatly delayed (20 to 40 minutes). It is preceded by a latent period of about 10 minutes (Lim 5–20 seconds, not minutés, as in other tests after administration of the stimulus). Nevertheless the specificity of antagonism of this bradykinin-induced pain(?) by aspirin is higher than when the writhing stimulus is phenylquinone (21 mg aspirin/kg against 150 mg/ml when antagonism of the phenylquinone writhing is required). Carroll and Lim (1958) made an attempt to understand the writhing in rats and mice and to correlate "writhing" with "pain".

Lim and his colleagues have studied the effects of intraperitoneal bradykinin not only in animals but also in man, systematically noting against a time clock both objective and subjective manifestations of pain. Oral administration of aspirin (e.g. 650 mg) will antagonize this pain. This is a therapeutic dose level. Half the dose was ineffective, and doubling it increased depth and duration of analgesia, though it was clear that the major analgesic achievement had been reached by the 650 mg dose level. Of greater significance is the fact that local i.p. administration of the aspirin is effective in counteracting the bradykinin-induced pain when the algogen is likewise administered i.p., and does so at a dose level of about 5% of that required when the drug is administered orally. This would seem to point very strongly toward a peripheral site of action of aspirin in man related to its analgesic action (LIM et al., 1967).

It is possible that aspirin acts as a competitive antagonist to bradykinin (and certain other, apparently unrelated stimuli such as H^+ or K^+ ions), denying access of the chemalgogen to the pain receptor sites. Relative to bradykinin–aspirin antagonism it is interesting to note the effect of aspirin in endotoxin shock (HINSHAW et al., 1967) which may well be mediated via the blood vessels in this way. Evidence concerning the mode of action of the non-narcotic antipyretic analgesics has been summarized by LIM and GUZMAN (1968). Potentials evoked in the splanchnic nerve by intra-arterial injections of bradykinin into the spleen are blocked by aspirin but not by morphine. The vocalization response (to intrasplenic injection of bradykinin) of a recipient dog whose vasoisolated spleen with nerves intact is cross-perfused by the carotid and jugular of a donor dog, is blocked when aspirin is injected into the donor's circulation, but not when injected into the recipient's circulation; on the other hand, morphine blocks when given to the recipient but not when given to the donor. The vocalization response to intrasplenic injection of bradykinin is blocked by aspirin injected directly into the splenic artery at one tenth of the dose required to block when aspirin is given intravenously, or intraarterially into the brain via the brachiocephalic artery. Less morphine is required to block when given into the brachiocephalic artery than when given into the splenic artery.

It may be concluded from these experiments that the antipyretic analgesics or antalgics act peripherally by blocking impulse generation at the chemoceptors for pain, while the narcotic analgesics act centrally by blocking synaptic transmission.

Of great interest is the fact that when vocalization, induced in animals by means of intraperitoneal or intrasplenic administration of bradykinin, is stopped by analgesic drugs the blood pressure, heart rate, and respiratory changes also cease. Moreover, bradykinin-induced (pain) responses at other sites in the body are similarly reduced or abolished.

According to LIM (personal communication), aspirin blocks the pain response (vocalization, struggling, and biting) evoked in dogs by acetylcholine, by minimal mechanical and electrical stimulation after ischemic sensitization, and by minimal stimulation with hypertonic NaCl or KCl. The "pain" receptor may be excited by a variety of chemical agents (H^+ and K^+ ions, some amines, and the bradykinin peptides) and "blocked" by all the well-known antipyretic analgesics (salicylate, acetaminophen, aminopyrine, phenylbutazone). It is thus not obviously stereospecific, although the concept that the pain receptor is electrophilic is an oversimplification. The pain receptor, however, may be regarded as modality specific in being a *chemoreceptor*, and not a mechanoreceptor or a thermoreceptor.

Only the opiates are useful in relieving colic and physically induced pain; aspirin is not. Cutaneous pain caused by the intradermal injection of bradykinin is not blocked by aspirin; this confirms ARMSTRONG'S observation of bradykinin-evoked pain from the blister base. Postoperative wound pain (BEECHER et al., 1953; LASAGNA, 1961; KANTOR et al., 1964; SUNSHINE et al., 1964) and postpartum wound pain (ORKIN et al., 1957; DEKORNFELD et al., 1962) are antagonized by aspirin. With regard to T. LEWIS' ischemic pain (WEBSTER and MACWILLIAM, 1923; LEWIS et al., 1931; LEWIS, 1942), DENEAU et al. (1953) thought that ischemic muscle pain could be blocked by both narcotic and non-narcotic (antipyretic) analgesics, and more recently Beecher (Smith et al., 1966a, b) have used a submaximum effort tourniquet method for producing experimental pain in man which can be blocked by aspirin and morphine.

In observations *in vitro* of Lim on the contraction of guinea pig ileum or rat uterus by bradykinin, "antagonism" by aspirin occurred only in the toxic range, requiring nearly a milligram in a 5 ml-bath. *In vivo*, the ED_{50} for aspirin, administered intraperitoneally to dogs through the same tube that is used for bradykinin, is 0.8 (0.46–1.48) mg/kg i.p. In man, 20–40 mg (total dose) will block the bradykinin-evoked pain. It is probable that the pain is associated with gut contractions, as 50–60% of the subjects complained of cramping or colicky pain alone or associated with pressure, distention, or gas "pain" (Lim et al., 1967). The i.p. bradykinin-evoked pain is associated with gut contraction, but on the basis of experience with bradykinin applied on mesentery alone and intra-arterially in other parts of the body, bradykinin may also cause pain without evoking contraction, which is a separate effect (Lim, personal communication, 1967).

In the early days of our bradykinin studies we attempted to antagonize its actions on the CBA with aspirin, but a clear-cut antagonism was not demonstrated. It may be that with this CBA preparation where the nerve endings are truncated, we are stimulating more, and other, than the perivascular pain receptors of Lim. The same applies to physical pains and intestinal colic.

Thus pain "stimulation" may be of peripheral or central origin. Pain antagonism, likewise, may occur principally at peripheral sites (aspirin) or principally centrally (morphine). Finally, there is sensitization to encounter or injury and this too may take place owing to peripheral activities (stimulation of small nerve afferents—chemically or otherwise) and/or central activities (central disinhibition). The picture is not simple, but observations involving bradykinin have been helping to clarify it.

G. Discussion

Bradykinin does cause pain, as is shown in this article. Moreover the very low concentrations in which it is effective, from 10 nM upward, combined with the very high potentiality of the human plasma to generate kinins (concentrations up to 7 or 8 µM, and perhaps higher, can arise "spontaneously") make it an agent worthy of serious chemalgogenic studies. The work of Chapman et al. (1959–1961), Galletti et al. and Marra et al. (1960, 1966) and Ostfeld and Wolff and Ostfeld et al. (1955), Iggo (1962) raises the possibilities of its possessing an action which would result in hyperalgesia of tissues (Keele and Armstrong, 1964) The topic of bradykinin in disease as a whole is dealt with on p. 470.

Speaking against the participation of bradykinin-induced pain in disease is the tachyphylaxis which it, and also related substances, produces. However, several thoughts come to mind. (1) If the nicotine or succinylcholine-like actions of acetylcholine or excess muscarine-like actions had been the only ones demonstrated, acetylcholine would never have been recognized, even as a possible nerve transmitter. The agent, in this case, must be formed, removed, and be "formed" and act again to elicit its typical action. (2) When bradykinin tachyphylaxis or depression is present, the tissue is selectively depressed. This will affect the central somesthetic image. Moreover, it may still be stimulated by other agents or even be hyperalgesic. (3) When tissues have been presensitized (e.g. with 5-HT), low concentrations of bradykinin, previously inactive, then cause pain. It may be that bradykinin acts differently in low than in high concentrations. (4) Several observers (viz. SICUTERI, LIM, and COFFMAN) have reported that no tachyphylaxis occurs in experiments in which blood flow or tissue circulation is good. Thus the tachyphylaxis produced by bradykinin does not exclude the possibility that it is concerned in the mediation of pain.

If bradykinin participates in human disease, causing pain, one might expect to find *in vivo* concentrations, notwithstanding the high activity of plasma kininases (FERREIRA and VANE, 1967; YANG and ERDÖS, 1967). MELMON et al. (1967) noted that whereas normal plasma levels are less than 3 ng bradykinin equivalents per ml (ZACEST and MASHFORD, 1967; BROCKLEHURST and ZEITLIN, 1967), examination of 25 samples of joint fluid from 13 patients suffering from arthritides of varying etiology showed levels of 1.6–58 ng/ml. In two patients suffering from gouty arthritis an acute attack "resulted in" an increase in polypeptide

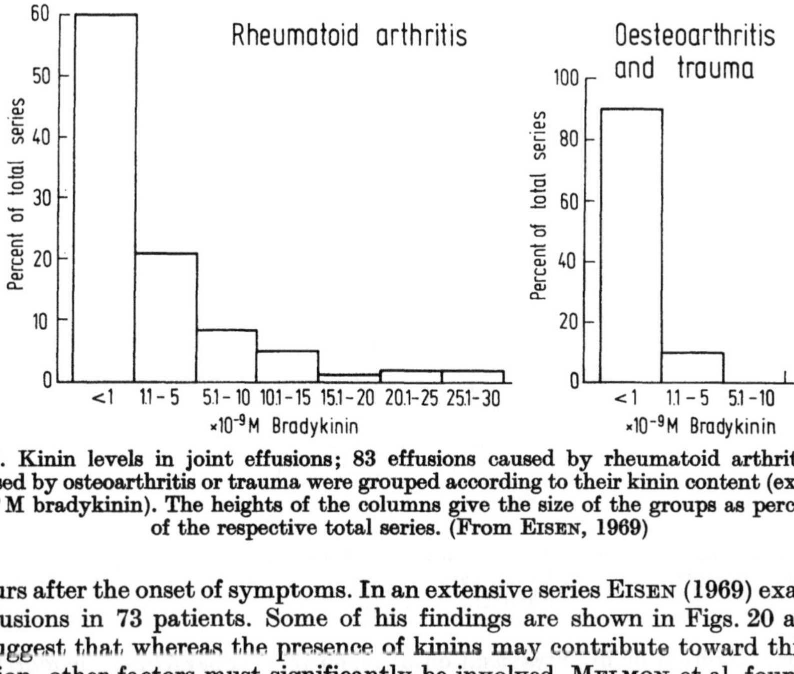

Fig. 20. Kinin levels in joint effusions; 83 effusions caused by rheumatoid arthritis, and 27 caused by osteoarthritis or trauma were grouped according to their kinin content (expressed as 10^{-9} M bradykinin). The heights of the columns give the size of the groups as percentages of the respective total series. (From EISEN, 1969)

24 hours after the onset of symptoms. In an extensive series EISEN (1969) examined 82 effusions in 73 patients. Some of his findings are shown in Figs. 20 and 21, and suggest that whereas the presence of kinins may contribute toward this pain situation, other factors must significantly be involved. MELMON et al. found that changes in kinin content of synovial fluid seemed to correlate well with symptoms in "selected individual patients" but that the clinical severity of an arthritis could not be predicted from knowledge of the kinin concentration in synovial fluid.

Effects of naturally occurring or injected kinins *in vivo* will be modified by the concurrence of various naturally occurring "bradykinin potentiating factors" (GLADNER et al., 1963; GLADNER, 1966; FERREIRA, 1965, 1966; AARSEN, 1968). If these substances are present when kinin is liberated, increased biological effects including pain production are to be expected. GLADNER'S factors arise in blood clotting and may therefore be presumed to be liberated in injury to tissues when kinin liberation is also suspected (MARGOLIS, 1958, 1963; DONALDSON and RATNOFF, 1965; NOSSEL and NIEMETZ, 1965; RATNOFF and ROSENBLUM, 1958; FAIRES and MCCARTHY, 1962). Fairly high concentrations seem to be necessary to potentiate kinin (pain not tested). Ferreira's BPF, bradykinin-potentiating factor, is interesting in that this peptide is effective *in vivo* (pain not tested) (concentration of a few μg/ml upward) and occurs in the pain-producing, kinin-producing *Bothrops jararaca* venom in concentrations as high as 10% of the dry weight of the venom (p. 465). The BPF, or like substances, may have use *in vivo* as analytical tools in examination of painful situations where bradykinin participation is suspected.

The work of SICUTERI and colleagues draws attention to the possible modification of pain of patients, e.g. through the participation of 5-HT in myocardial

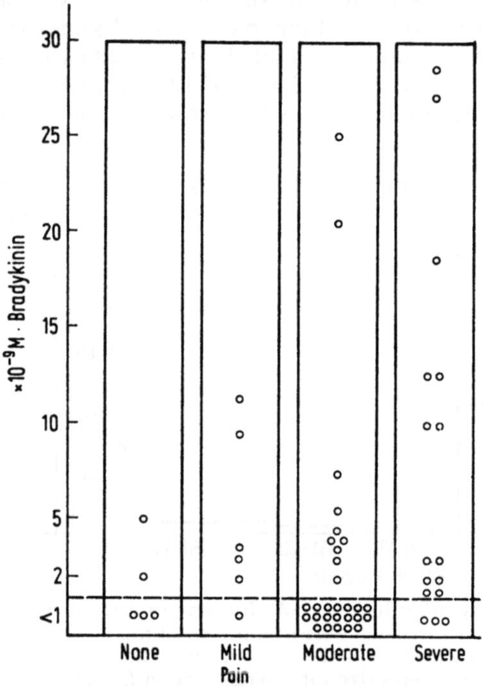

Fig. 21. The kinin concentrations in exudates from rheumatoid joints (given as 10^{-9} M bradykinin) were grouped according to the pain the patients felt in the joint before the fluid was removed. (From EISEN, 1969)

or other infarction or in extravasation of blood (e.g. subarachnoid hemorrhage). Using bradykinin as an experimental chemalgogen, the reader can from a useful basis from which he may organize his own experimental approaches.

Acknowledgments

I wish to express to the Middlesex Hospital Medical School, and also to Professor C. A. KEELE, my appreciation for their continued help toward our research projects. It was Dr. KEELE's stimulus and his idea of the use of the base of a cantharides blister which, along with the works of others, has led to the present outburst of chemalgogenic studies on various tissues.

I wish to acknowledge the help of Dr. R. K. S. LIM, Prof. E. GREPPI † and the University of Florence, Prof. M. ROCHA E SILVA, Dr. J. MARGOLIS, Dr. O. D. RATNOFF, Dr. DAVIE, and Drs. G. F. BLANE, C. R. DINIZ, V. EISEN, J. J. PISANO, L. PRADO, E. SCHRÖDER, J. M. STEWART, and K. VOGLER.

Permission to reproduce published figures is acknowledged with thanks to the authors and the editors and publishers of the following journals: *Acta Neurovegetativa, British Journal of Pharmacology, Journal of Physiology, Nature (London)*; and to the Athlone Press, London; Edward Arnold Ltd., London; S. Karger, Basle and New York; Little Brown and Co. Inc., Boston; E. & S. Livingstone Ltd., Edinburgh and London; Pergamon Press Inc., New York and London; Universities Federation for Animal Welfare, London.

References

AARSEN, P. N.: Sensitization of guinea-pig ileum to the action of bradykinin by trypsin hydrolysate of ox and rabbit plasma. Brit. J. Pharmacol. 32, 453 (1968).

ADDIS, H. ST. C. C., JEPSON, R. P., KELLGREN, J. H.: On the effect of arterial occlusion and venous congestion upon limb pain. Clin. Sci. 9, 271 (1950).

ALBE-FESSARD, D.: Central nervous mechanisms involved in pain and analgesia. In: Pharmacology of pain, p. 131, ed. by R. K. S. LIM, D. ARMSTRONG and E. G. PARDO. Proceedings of III. Int. Congr. of Pharmacology, vol. 9. Oxford: Pergamon Press 1968.

ALKJAERSIG, N., FLETCHER, A. P., SHERRY, S.: E-amino caproic acid; an inhibitor of plasminogen activation. J. biol. Chem. 234, 832 (1959).

ANASTASI, A., ERSPAMER, V., BERTACCINI, G., CEI, J. M.: A bradykinin-like endecapeptide of the skin of *Phyllomedusa rohdei*. In: Hypotensive peptides, p. 76, ed. by E. G. ERDÖS, N. BACK and F. SICUTERI. Berlin-Heidelberg-New York: Springer 1966.

ANDRADE, S. O., ROCHA E SILVA, M.: Purification of bradykinin by ion exchange chromatography. Biochem. J. 64, 701 (1956).

ARCANGELI, P., PANERAI, A., GHETTI, A.: Mediatori chimici ed arresto della circolazione arteriosa e venosa degli arti nell'uomo. Nota I. Liberazione di mediatori chimici ad attività utero-contraente durante la stasi venosa e sua inhibizione mediante l'ischemia preventiva. Rass. Neurol. veg. 17, 154 (1963).

— — — Differences between the pain-producing activities of plasma, burn blister fluid, cantharidin blister fluid and synthetic bradykinin. Acta neuroveg. (Wien) 28, 454 (1966).

ARMAN, C. G. VAN, BEGANY, A. J., MILLER, L. M., PLESS, H. H.: Some details of the inflammation caused by yeast and carrageenin. J. Pharmacol. exp. Ther. 150, 328 (1965).

— NUSS, G. W., WINTER, C. A., FLATAKER, L.: Proteolytic enzymes as mediators of pain. In: Pharmacology of pain, p. 25, ed. by R. K. S. LIM, D. ARMSTRONG and E. G. PARDO. Proceedings of III. Int. Congr. of Pharmacology, vol. 9. Oxford: Pergamon Press 1968.

ARMSTRONG, D.: The relation of pain production by tryptamines to their chemical structure. In: 5-Hydroxytryptamine, p. 140, ed. by G. P. LEWIS. London: Pergamon Press 1958.

— Unpublished observations 1967/68.

— The effects of temperature on the response of human plasma kinin-forming system to promoting and inhibiting agents. Brit. J. Pharmacol. 34, 670P (1968).

— Hageman factor and the spontaneous human plasma-kinin generation occurring in homogenous media. Activation and inactivation. In: Inflammation, biochemistry and drug interaction, p. 153 ed. by A. BERTELLI and J. C. HOUCK. Amsterdam: Excerpta Medica Foundation (1969).

— DRY, R. M. L., KEELE, C. A., MARKHAM, J. W.: Pain-producing substances in blister fluid and in serum. J. Physiol. (Lond.) 117, 4P (1952).

— — — — Observations on chemical excitants of cutaneous pain in man. J. Physiol. (Lond.) 120, 326 (1953a).

— HOBBIGER, F., JEPSON, J. B., KEELE, C. A.: Pain-producing substance in blister fluid. Abstracts of Communications, XIX. Int. Physiological Congr., Montreal 1953b.

— JEPSON, J. B., KEELE, C. A., STEWART, J. W.: Development of pain-producing substance in human plasma. Nature (Lond.) 174, 791 (1954).

— — — — Activation by glass of pharmacologically active agents in blood of various species. J. Physiol. (Lond.) 129, 80P (1955).

— — — — Pain-producing substance in human inflammatory exudates and plasma. J. Physiol. (Lond.) 135, 350 (1957).

ARMSTRONG, D. A. J.: Chemical excitants of cutaneous pain. University of London Thesis, 1957.

— MILLS, G. L.: Chemical characterization of kinins of human plasma. Nature (Lond.) 197, 490 (1963).

— — A highly purified kinin-forming enzyme from human plasma. Biochem. Pharmacol. 13, 1393 (1964).

— — The reversible cold-induced activation of the human plasma kinin-forming system between 37° and 0° C. J. Physiol. (Lond.) 179, 89 (1965).

— — SICUTERI, F.: Physiological influence on the liberation of human plasma kinin at low temperatures. In: Hypotensive peptides, p. 139, ed. by E. G. ERDÖS, N. BACK and F. SICUTERI. Berlin-Heidelberg-New York: Springer 1966.

— — STEWART, J. W.: Thermally induced effects on the kinin-forming system of native human plasma, 37°—0° C and 37°—50° C. In: Vaso-active polypeptides, bradykinin and related kinins, p. 167, ed. by M. ROCHA E SILVA and H. A. ROTHSCHILD. São Paulo 1967.

— STEWART, J. M.: Unpublished observations 1967/68.

— STEWART, J. W. Spontaneous plasma kinin formation in human plasma collected during labour. Nature (Lond.) 188, 1193 (1960a).

Armstrong, D. A. J., Stewart, J. W.: Formation of plasma kinin in human plasma by ε-amino caproic acid and certain related compounds. J. Physiol. (Lond.) **154**, 19P (1960b).
— — Anti-heparin agents as inhibitors of plasma kinin formation. Nature (Lond.) **194**, 689 (1962).
Arthur, R. P., Shelley, W. B.: The role of proteolytic enzymes in the production of pruritus in man. J. invest. Derm. **25**, 341 (1955).
Beall, A. C., Jr.: A comparison of the renal hemodynamic effects of protamine sulfate and hexadimethrine bromide as used for heparin neutralization. Cardiovasc. Res. Centre Bull. **1**, 76 (1963).
Beard, R. L.: Insect toxins and venoms. Ann. Rev. Entomol. **8**, 1 (1963).
Beecher, H. K.: The measurement of pain. Prototype for the quantitative study of subjective responses. Pharmacol. Rev. **9**, 59 (1957).
— Keats, A. S., Mosteller, E., Lasagna, L.: The effectiveness of oral analgesics (morphine, codeine, acetylsalisylic acid) and the problem of placebo "reactors" and "non-reactors". J. Pharmacol. exp. Ther. **109**, 393 (1953).
Beloff, A., Peters, R. A.: Observations upon thermal burns; the influence of moderate temperature burns upon a proteinase of skin. J. Physiol. (Lond.) **103**, 461 (1945).
Benjamin, F. B., Ivy, A. C.: Electroencephalographic changes associated with painful and non-painful peripheral stimulation. Proc. Soc. exp. Biol. (N.Y.) **72**, 420 (1949).
Bessou, P., Laporte, Y.: Activation des fibres afférentes amyéliniques d'origine musculaire. C. R. Soc. Biol. (Paris) **152**, 1587 (1958).
Bhoola, K. D.: Properties of kallikrein, kallidin and related substances. Thesis, University of London, 1961.
— Calle, J. D., Schachter, M.: Identification of acetylcholine, 5-hydroxytryptamine, histamine and a new kinin in hornet venom (*V. crabro*). J. Physiol. (Lond.) **159**, 167 (1961).
Biggs, R., Matthews, J. M., Rush, B. M., Johnstone, F. C., MacFarlane, R. G., Hayton Williams, D. S.: Further experience in the use of human antihaemophilic globulin (H.A. H.G.) for the control of bleeding after dental extractions in haemophilic patients. Lancet **1965 I**, 969.
Billingham, M. E. J., Robinson, B. V., Robson, J. M.: Partial purification of the anti-inflammatory factor(s) in inflammatory exudate. Brit. J. Pharmacol. **35**, 543 (1969).
Bisset, G. W., Lewis, G. P.: A spectrum of pharmacological activity in some biologically active peptides. Brit. J. Pharmacol. **19**, 168 (1962).
Blane, G. F.: Blockade of bradykinin-induced nociception in the rat as a test for analgesic drugs with particular reference to morphine antagonists. J. Pharm. Pharmacol. **19**, 367 (1967).
— A new laboratory model for evaluating analgesic and analgesic-antagonist drugs. In: Pain, p. 218, ed. by A. Soulairac, J. Cahn and J. Charpentier. London and New York: Academic Press 1968.
— Dugdall, D.: Interactions of narcotic antagonists and antagonist-analgesics. J. Pharm. Pharmacol. **20**, 447 (1968).
Boissonnas, R. A., Guttmann, St., Jaquenoud, P. A., Konzett, H., Stürmer, E.: Synthesis and biological activity of peptides related to bradykinin. Experientia (Basel) **16**, 326 (1960).
Bowsher, D. R., Albe-Fessard, D.: Patterns of somatosensory organization within the central nervous system. In: Assessment of pain in man and animals, p. 107, ed. by C. A. Keele and R. Smith. London: Livingstone 1962.
Braun, C., Guzman, F., Horton, E. W., Lim, R. K., Potter, G. D.: Visceral receptors, pain, bradykinin and analgesic agents. J. Physiol. (Lond.) **155**, 13P (1961).
Brockbank, W.: Ancient therapeutic arts. London: Heinemann 1954.
Brocklehurst, W. E., Zeitlin, I. J.: Determination of plasma kinin and kininogen levels in man. J. Physiol. (Lond.) **191**, 417 (1967).
Bruce, A. N.: Vasodilator axon reflexes. Quart. J. exp. Physiol. **6**, 339 (1913).
Burch, G. E., Pasquale, N. P. de: Bradykinin, digital blood flow, and the arteriovenous anastomoses. Circulat. Res. **10**, 105 (1962).
Burget, G. E., Livingston, W. K.: Pathway for visceral afferent impulses from the forelimb of the dog. Amer. J. Physiol. **97**, 249 (1931).
Calma, I., Wright, S.: Effects of intra-thecal injection of KCl and other solutions in cats. Excitatory action of K ions on posterior nerve root fibres. J. Physiol. (Lond.) **106**, 211 (1947).
Carroll, M. N., Jr., Lim, R. K. S.: Mechanism of phenylquinone writhing. Fed. Proc. **17**, 357 (1958).
Centaro, A., Laurentis, G. de, Periti, P.: Oxitocina nel sangue di donna in travaglio di parto. Boll. Soc. ital. Biol. sper. **35**, 1454 (1959).

Chapman, L. F., Goodell, H., Wolff, H. G.: Augmentation of the inflammatory reaction by activity of the central nervous system. Arch. Neurol. **1**, 557 (1959).
— Ramos, A. O., Goodell, H., Silverman, G., Wolff, H. G.: A humoral agent implicated in vascular headache of the migraine type. Arch. Neurol. **3**, 223 (1960).
— — — Wolff, H. G.: Neurohumoral features of afferent fibres in man. Their role in vasodilatation, inflammation and pain. Arch. Neurol. Psychiat. (Chic.) **4**, 617 (1961).
Coffman, J. D.: The effect of aspirin on pain and hand blood flow responses to intra-arterial injection of bradykinin in man. Clin. Pharmacol. Ther. **7**, 26 (1966).
Collier, H. O. J., Chesher, G. B.: Identification of 5-hydroxytryptamine in the sting of the nettle (*Urtica dioica*). Brit. J. Pharmacol. **11**, 186 (1956).
— Hammond, A. R., Horwood-Barrett, S., Schneider, C.: Rapid induction by acetylcholine, bradykinin and potassium of a nociceptive response in mice and its selective antagonism by aspirin. Nature (Lond.) **204**, 1316 (1964).
— Lee, I. R.: Nociceptive responses of guinea-pigs to intradermal injections of bradykinin and kallidin-10. Brit. J. Pharmacol. **21**, 155 (1963).
Cormia, F. E., Dougherty, J. W.: Proteolytic activity in development of pain and itching. Cutaneous reactions to bradykinin and kallikrein. J. invest. Derm. **35**, 21 (1960).
Cotran, R. S., Majno, G.: A light and electron microscopic analysis of vascular injury. Ann. N.Y. Acad. Sci. **116**, 750 (1964).
Dallenbach, K. M.: Pain; history and present status. Amer. J. Psychol. **52**, 331 (1939).
De Duve, C.: Lysosomes and cell injury. In: Injury, inflammation and immunity, p. 283, ed. by L. Thomas, J. W. Uhr and L. H. Grant. Baltimore: Williams & Wilkins Co. 1964.
Deffenu, G., Pegrassi, L., Lumachi, B.: The use of bradykinin-induced effects in rats as an assay for analgesic drugs. J. Pharm. Pharmacol. **18**, 135 (1966).
Dekornfeld, T. J., Lasagna, L., Frazier, T. M.: A comparative study of fine proprietary analgesic compounds. J. Amer. med. Ass. **182**, 1315 (1962).
Deneau, G. A., Waud, R. A., Gowdey, C. W.: A method for the determination of the effects of drugs on the pain threshold of human subjects. Canad. J. med. Sci. **31**, 387 (1953).
Deutsch, H. F., Diniz, C. R.: Some proteolytic activities of snake venoms. In: Venoms, p. 199, ed. by E. E. Buckley and N. Porges. Washington: Amer. Ass. for the Advancement of Science 1956.
Dickerson, G. D., Engle, R. T., Guzman, F., Rodgers, D. W., Lim, R. K. S.: The intraperitoneal bradykinin-evoked pain test for analgesia. Life Sci. **4**, 2063 (1965).
Diniz, C. R., Carvalho, I. F.: A micromethod for determination of bradykinin under several conditions. Ann. N.Y. Acad. Sci. **104**, 77 (1963).
Donaldson, V. H., Ratnoff, O. D.: Hageman factor. Alterations in physical properties during activation. Science **150**, 754 (1965).
Edery, H.: Potentiation of the action of bradykinin on smooth muscle by chymotrypsin, chymotrypsinogen and trypsin. Brit. J. Pharmacol. **22**, 371 (1964).
— Further studies of the sensitization of smooth muscle to the action of plasma kinins by proteolytic enzymes. Brit. J. Pharmacol. **24**, 485 (1965).
— Grunfeld, Y.: Sensitization of smooth muscle to plasma kinins. Effects of enzymes and peptides on various preparations. Brit. J. Pharmacol. **35**, 51 (1969).
— Ishay, I.: Pharmacologically active substances of the *Vespa orientalis* wasp venom. Proc. Israel Physiol. Pharmacol. Soc. **1**, 17 (1965).
— Lewis, G. P.: Inhibition of plasma kininase activity at slightly acid pH. Brit. J. Pharmacol. **19**, 299 (1962a).
— — Plasma kinin forming enzyme activity in lymph after injury. J. Physiol. (Lond.) **163**, 48P (1962b).
— — Kinin-forming activity and histamine in lymph after tissue injury. J. Physiol. (Lond.) **169**, 568 (1963).
Edwards, W.: Recent research on pain perception. Psychol. Bull. **47**, 449 (1950).
Eisen, V.: Modes of formation of human plasma kinins. Thesis University of London, 1961.
— Observations on intrinsic kinin-forming factors in human plasma. The effect of acid, acetone, chloroform, heat and euglobulin separation on kinin formation. J. Physiol. (Lond.) **166**, 496 (1963).
— Effect of hexadimethrine bromide on plasma kinin formation, hydrolysis of *p*-tosyl-L-arginine methyl ester and fibrinolysis. Brit. J. Pharmacol. **22**, 87 (1964).
— Studies on fibrinogen fractions isolated from human plasma by precipitation with cold ether. Brit. J. Haemat. **11**, 576 (1965).
— Urates and kinin formation in synovial fluid. Proc. roy. Soc. Med. **59**, 302 (1966).
— Kinin formation in human diseases. In: Lectures on the scientific basis of medicine, Ann. Reviews 1969, p. 146. London: The Athlone Press, University of London 1969.

Eisen, V., Keele, C. A.: Possible modes of kinin formation in some pathological states in man. In: Hypotensive peptides, p. 551, ed. by E. G. Erdös, N. Back and F. Sicuteri. Berlin-Heidelberg-New York: Springer 1966.
Elliott, D. F., Horton, E. W., Lewis, G. P.: Actions of pure bradykinin. J. Physiol. (Lond.) 153, 473 (1960a).
— — — The isolation of bradykinin, a plasma kinin from ox blood. Biochem. J. 78, 60 (1961).
— Lewis, G. P.: Methionyl-lysyl-bradykinin, a new kinin from ox blood. Biochem. J. 95, 437 (1965).
— — Horton, E. W.: The isolation of bradykinin, a plasma kinin from ox blood. Biochem. J. 74, 15P (1960b).
— — — The structure of bradykinin. Biochem. J. 76, 16P (1960c).
Emele, J. F., Shanaman, J.: Bradykinin writhing. A method for measuring analgesia. Proc. Soc. exp. Biol. (N.Y.) 114, 680 (1963).
Emmelin, N., Feldberg, W.: The mechanism of the sting of the common nettle (*Urtica urens*). J. Physiol. (Lond.) 106, 440 (1947).
Erdös, E. G.: Hypotensive peptides; bradykinin, kallidin and eledoisin. Advanc. Pharmacol. 4, 1 (1966).
— Renfrew, A. G., Sloane, E. M., Wohler, J. R.: Enzymatic studies on bradykinin and similar peptides. Ann. N.Y. Acad. Sci. 104, 222 (1963a).
— Sloane, E. M.: An enzyme in human blood plasma that inactivates bradykinin and kallidins. Biochem. Pharmacol. 11, 585 (1962).
— Wohler, J. R., Levine, M. L.: Blocking of the *in vivo* effects of bradykinin and kallidin with carboxypeptidase. B. J. Pharmacol. exp. Ther. 142, 327 (1963b).
Faires, J., McCarthy, D. J.: Acute arthritis in man and dog after intrasynovial injection of sodium urate crystals. Lancet 1962 II, 682.
Feldberg, W.: The role of mediators in the inflammatory tissue response. Int. Arch. Allergy 8, 15 (1956).
Ferreira, S. H.: A bradykinin-potentiating factor (BPF) present in the venom of *Bothrops jararaca*. Brit. J. Pharmacol. 24, 163 (1965).
— Bradykinin-potentiating factor. In: Hypotensive peptides, p. 356, ed. by E. G. Erdös, N. Back and F. Sicuteri. Berlin-Heidelberg-New York: Springer 1966.
— Vane, J. R.: The disappearance of bradykinin and eledoisin in the circulation and vascular beds of the cat. Brit. J. Pharmacol. 30, 417 (1967).
Fjallbrant, N., Iggo, A.: The effect of histamine, 5-hydroxytryptamine and acetylcholine on cutaneous afferent fibres. J. Physiol. (Lond.) 156, 578 (1961).
Fox, R. H., Goldsmith, R., Kidd, D. J., Lewis, G. P.: Bradykinin as a vasodilator in man. J. Physiol. (Lond.) 157, 589 (1961).
Frey, M. von: Versuche über schmerzerregende Reize. Z. Biol. 76, 1 (1922).
Galletti, R., Marra, N., Vecchiet, L.: Indagine analitica sulle manifestazioni algogene conseguenti all'introduzione per via intradermica di liquido di bolla e di essudato pleurico. Rass. Neurol. veg. 15, 200 (1960).
Ghetti, A., Arcangeli, P., Panerai, A.: Mediatori chimici ed arresto della circolazione arteriosa e venosa degli arti nell'uomo. Nota III. Variazioni del tasso di serotonina durante la stasi venosa, l'iperemia reattiva e la stasi venosa postischemica. Rass. Neurol. veg. 19, 143 (1965).
— Marra, N., Matassi, L., Vecchiet, L., Fini, F.: Confronto tra i fenomeni reattivi della cute prodotti dal plasma umano normale alla massima attivazione algogena e i fenomeni reattivi prodotti dalla bradichinina sintetica in concentrazioni scalari. Settim. med. 54, 387 (1966).
Gilfoil, T. M., Klavins, I.: 5-Hydroxytryptamine, bradykinin and histamine as mediators of inflammatory hyperesthesia. Amer. J. Physiol. 208, 867 (1965).
— — Grumbach, L.: Effects of acetylsalicylic acid on the edema and hyperesthesia of the experimentally inflammed rat's paw. J. Pharmacol. exp. Ther. 142, 1 (1963).
Gladner, J. A.: Potentiation of the effect of bradykinin. In: Hypotensive peptides, p. 344, ed. by E. G. Erdös, N. Back and F. Sicuteri. Berlin-Heidelberg-New York: Springer 1966.
— Murtaugh, P. A., Folk, J. E., Laki, K.: Nature of peptides released by thrombin. Ann. N.Y. Acad. Sci. 104, 45 (1963).
Goetz, F. R., Burrill, D. Y., Ivy, A. C.: A critical analysis of algesimetric methods with suggestions for a useful procedure. Quart. Bull. Northwestern Univ. Med. School 17, 280 (1943).
Goldfinger, S., Melmon, K. L., Webster, M. E., Sjoerdsma, A., Seegmiller, J. E.: The presence of a kinin-peptide in inflammatory synovial effusions. Arthr. and Rheum. 7, 311 (1964).
Goldscheider, A.: Das Schmerzproblem. Berlin: Springer 1916.

GOODWIN, L. G., JONES, C. R., RICHARDS, W. H. G., KOHN, J.: Pharmacologically active substances in the urine of burned patients. Brit. J. exp. Path. **44**, 551 (1963).
GRAHAM, R. C., EBERT, R. H., RATNOFF, O. D., MORES, J. M.: Pathogenesis of inflammation. II. *In vivo* observations of the inflammatory effects of activated Hageman factor and bradykinin. J. exp. Med. **121**, 807 (1965).
GRÜTZNER, P.: Über die chemische Reizung sensibler Nerven. Pflügers Arch. ges. Physiol. **58**, 69 (1894).
GUZMAN, F., BRAUN, C., LIM, R. K. S.: Visceral pain and the pseudoaffective response to intra-arterial injection of bradykinin and other algesic agents. Arch. int. Pharmacodyn. **136**, 353 (1962).
— — — POTTER, G. D., RODGERS, D. W.: Narcotic and non-narcotic analgesics which block visceral pain evoked by intra-arterial injection of bradykinin and other algesic agents. Arch. int. Pharmacodyn. **149**, 571 (1964).
HABERMANN, E.: Enzymatic kinin release from kininogen and from low-molecular compounds. In: Hypotensive peptides, p. 116, ed. by E. G. ERDÖS, N. BACK and F. SICUTERI. Berlin-Heidelberg-New York: Springer 1966.
HALLER, J. A., JR., RANSDELL, H. T., JR., STOWENS, D., RUBEL, W. F.: Renal toxicity of polybrene in open-heart surgery. J. thorac. cardiovasc. Surg. **44**, 486 (1962).
HARDY, J. D.: The pain threshold and the nature of pain sensation. In: Assessment of pain in man and animals, p. 170, ed. by C. A. KEELE and R. SMITH. London: Livingstone 1962.
— WOLFF, H. G., GOODELL, H.: Pain sensations and reactions. London: Ballière, Tindall & Cox 1952.
HARPMAN, J. A., ALLEN, R. T.: Neural activity and polypeptides. Brit. Med. J. **1959 I**, 1043.
HEAD, H., in conjunction with W. H. R. RIVERS, G. HOLMES, J. SHERREN, T. O. THOMPSON and G. RIDDOCH: Studies in neurology, vol. 1, p. 257. London: Oxford University Press 1920.
HENRIQUES, F. C.: Studies of thermal injury. V. The predictability and the significance of thermally induced rate processes leading to irreversible epidermal injury. Arch. Path. **43**, 489 (1947).
HEWER, A. J. H., KEELE, C. A.: A method of testing analgesics in man. Lancet **1948 II**, 683.
HINSHAW, L. B., SOLOMON, L. A., ERDÖS, E. G., REINS, D. A., GUNTER, B. J.: Effects of acetylsalicylic acid on the canine response to endotoxin. J. Pharmacol. exp. Ther. **157**, 665 (1967).
HOLDSTOCK, D. J., MATHIAS, A. P., SCHACHTER, M.: A comparative study of kinin, kallidin and bradykinin. Brit. J. Pharmacol. **12**, 149 (1957).
HORTON, E. W.: The role of bradykinin in the peripheral nervous system. Ann. N.Y. Acad. Sci. **104**, 250 (1963).
IGGO, A.: Non-myelinated visceral, muscular and cutaneous afferent fibres and pain. In: Assessment of pain in man and animals, p. 74, ed. by C. A. KEELE and R. SMITH. London: Livingstone 1962.
JACOBSEN, S., WAALER, B. A.: The effect of scalding on the content of kininogen and kininase in limb lymph. Brit. J. Pharmacol. **27**, 222 (1966).
JANCSÓ, N.: Role of the nerve terminals in the mechanism of inflammatory reactions. Bull. Millard Fillmore Hosp., Buffalo, N.Y. **7**, 53 (1960).
JAQUES, R., SCHACHTER, M.: The presence of histamine, 5-hydroxytryptamine and a potent, slow contracting substance in wasp venom. Brit. J. Pharmacol. **9**, 53 (1954).
KANTOR, T. G., MEISSNER, M., LASKA, G., SUNSHINE, A.: A computer program for the clinical study of analgesic compounds. Fed. Proc. **23**, 176 (1964).
KAUZMANN, W.: Some factors in the interpretation of protein denaturation. Advanc. Protein Chem. **14**, 1 (1959).
KEELE, C. A.: Chemical causes of pain and itch. Proc. roy. Soc. Med. **50**, 477 (1957).
— Causes of pain. In: Lectures on the scientific basis of medicine, Ann. Reviews 1958, p. 143. London: The Athlone Press, University of London 1958.
— Sensations aroused by chemical stimulation of the skin. In: Assessment of pain in man and animals, p. 28, ed. by C. A. KEELE and R. SMITH. London: Livingstone 1962.
— Measurement of response to chemically induced pain. In: Touch, heat and pain, p. 57, ed. by A. V. S. DE REUCK and J. KNIGHT. London: Churchill Ltd 1966a.
— Excitants of pain receptors. Acta neuroveg. (Wien) **28**, 392 (1966b).
— ARMSTRONG, D.: Substances producing pain and itch. London: Edward Arnold Ltd 1964.
— — Mediators of pain. In: Pharmacology of pain, p. 3, ed. by R. K. S. LIM, D. ARMSTRONG and E. G. PARDO. Proceedings of the III. Int. Congr. of Pharmacology, vol. 9. Oxford: Pergamon Press 1968.
KEELE, K. D.: The pain chart. Lancet **1948 II**, 6.
— Some historical concepts of pain. In: Assessment of pain in man and animals, p. 12, ed. by C. A. KEELE and R. SMITH. London: Livingstone 1962.

Kellett, D. N.: On the anti-inflammatory activity of protamine sulphate and of hexadimethrine bromide, inhibitors of plasma kinin formation. Brit. J. Pharmacol. **24**, 705 (1965).
Kimura, E. T., Young, P. R., Ebert, D. M.: Further studies on hexadimethrine bromide (Polybrene), an antiheparin agent. Toxicol. appl. Pharmacol. **1**, 560 (1959b).
— — Stein, R. J., Richards, R. K.: Some pharmacologic characteristics of hexadimethrine bromide (Polybrene), a new antiheparin agent. Toxicol. appl. Pharmacol. **1**, 185 (1959a).
Kiyohara, M.: Pain: its mechanism and clinical practice. Tokyo: Igaku Shoin Ltd. 1967.
Lasagna, L.: Analgesic drugs. Amer. J. med. Sci. **242**, 620 (1961).
Lavrenko, V. V.: Participation of sympathetic nerve fibres in the structure of sensory nerve endings. Byull. eksp. Biol. Med. **5**, 37 (1938).
Leme, J. G., Schapoval, E. S., Rocha e Silva, M.: Factors influencing the development of local swelling induced in the rat's paw by macromolecular compounds and heating. In: Vasoactive polypeptides: Bradykinin and related kinins, p. 213, ed. by M. Rocha e Silva and H. A. Rothschild. São Paulo 1967.
Levy, L. R., Lepow, I. H.: Assay and properties of serum inhibitor of C'1-esterase. Proc. Soc. exp. Biol. (N.Y.) **101**, 608 (1959).
Lewis, G. P.: Formation of plasma kinins by plasmin. J. Physiol. (Lond.) **140**, 285 (1958).
— Active polypeptides derived from plasma proteins. Physiol. Rev. **40**, 647 (1960).
— Plasma kinins and other vaso-active compounds in acute inflammation. Ann. N.Y. Acad. Sci. **116**, 847 (1964a).
— Role of peptide in the first stages of inflammation. In: Injury, inflammation and immunity, p. 242, ed. by L. Thomas, J. W. Uhr and L. H. Grant. Baltimore: Williams & Wilkins Co. 1964b.
Lewis, T.: The blood vessels of the human skin and their responses. London: Shaw 1927.
— Nocifensor system of nerves and its reactions. Brit. med. J. **1937a I**, 431.
— The effect of asphyxia and cocaine on nerves belonging to the nocifensor system. Clin. Sci. **3**, 59 (1937b).
— Pain. New York: Macmillan 1942.
— Hess, W.: Pain derived from the skin and the mechanism of its production. Clin. Sci. **1**, 39 (1933).
— Pickering, G. W., Rothschild, P.: Observations upon muscular pain in intermittent claudication. Heart **15**, 359 (1931).
Lim, R. K. S.: Visceral receptors and visceral pain. Ann. N.Y. Acad. Sci. **86**, 73 (1960).
— A revised concept of the mechanism of analgesia and pain. In: Pain, p. 117, ed. by R. S. Knighton and P. R. Dumke. Boston: Little Brown 1966.
— Pain mechanisms. Anaesthesiology **28**, 106 (1967),
— Neuropharmacology of pain and analgesia. In: Pharmacology of pain, p. 169, ed. by R. K. S. Lim, D. Armstrong and E. G. Pardo. Oxford: Pergamon Press 1968.
— Guzman, F.: Manifestations of pain in analgesic evaluation in animals and man. In: Pain, p. 119, ed. by A. Soulairac, J. Cahn and J. Charpentier. London and New York: Academic Press 1968.
— — Rodgers, D. W., Goto, K., Braun, C., Dickerson, C. D., Engle, R. J.: Site of action of narcotic and non-narcotic analgesics determined by blocking bradykinin-evoked visceral pain. Arch. int. Pharmacodyn. **152**, 25 (1964).
— Miller, D. G., Guzman, F., Rodgers, D. W., Rogers, R. W., Wang, S. K., Chao, P. Y., Shih, T. Y.: Pain and analgesia evaluated by the intraperitoneal bradykinin-evoked pain method in man. Clin. Pharmacol. Ther. **8**, 521 (1967).
Lindahl, O.: Experimental skin pain induced by injection of water-soluble substances in humans. Acta physiol. scand. **51**, Suppl. 179 (1961).
Majno, G.: Mechanisms of abnormal vascular permeability in acute inflammation. In: Injury, inflammation and immunity, p. 59, ed. by L. Thomas, J. W. Uhr and L. H. Grant. Baltimore: Williams & Wilkins Co. 1964.
Margolis, J.: Hageman factor in plasma foreign surface reactions. Nature (Lond.) **182**, 1102 (1958a).
— Activation of plasma by contact with glass. Evidence for a common reaction which releases plasma kinin and initiates coagulation. J. Physiol. (Lond.) **144**, 1 (1958b).
— The inter-relationship of coagulation of plasma and release of peptides. Ann. N.Y. Acad. Sci. **104**, 133 (1963).
Marra, N., Matassi, L., Vecchiet, L., Fini, F., Galletti, R.: I'l comportamento della reazione cutanea all'iniezione intradermica di alcuni peptidi biologicamente attivi. Bradichinina, callidina, ipertensina e ossitocina. Settim. med. **54**, 335 (1966).
— Vecchiet, L., Galletti, R.: Studio dei fenomeni dolorosi e reattivi della cute umana dopo iniezione intradermica di sangue, siero e plasma. Rass. Neurol. veg. **15**, 227 (1960).

MARTINDALE, W.: The extra pharmacopoeia, 24th ed., vol. I, p. 167. London: Pharmaceutical Press 1958.
MATHIAS, A. P., SCHACHTER, M.: The chromatographic behaviour of wasp venom kinin, kallidin, and bradykinin. Brit. J. Pharmacol. **13**, 326 (1958).
MAYCOCK, D. D'A., EVANS, S., VALLETT, L., COMBRIDGE, B., WOLF, P., MCGIBBON, N., FRENCH, E. E., WALLETT, L. H., DACIE, J. V., BIGGS, R., HANDLEY, D., MACFARLANE, R. C.: Further experience with a concentrate containing human anti-haemophilic factor. Brit. J. Haemat. **9**, 215 (1963).
MELMON, K. L., WEBSTER, M. E., GOLDFINGER, S. E., SEEGMILLER, J. E.: The presence of a kinin in inflammatory synovial effusion from arthritides of varying etiologies. Arthr. and Rheum. **10**, 13 (1967).
MERRIFIELD, R. B.: Solid-phase peptide synthesis III. An improved synthesis of bradykinin. Biochemistry **3**, 1385 (1964).
— STEWART, J. M.: Automated peptide synthesis. Nature (Lond.) **207**, 522 (1965).
MITCHELL, J. C., KRELL, R.: A study of the cutaneous effects of bradykinin. J. invest. Derm. **43**, 177 (1964).
MONGAR, J. L.: A study of two methods for testing local anaesthetics in man. Brit. J. Pharmacol. **10**, 240 (1955).
MOORE, R. M.: The stimulation of peripheral nerve-elements subserving pain-sensibility by intra-arterial injections of neutral solutions. Amer. J. Physiol. **110**, 191 (1934).
— MOORE, R. E.: Studies on the pain-sensibility of arteries. I. Some observations on the pain sensibility of arteries. Amer. J. Physiol. **104**, 259 (1933).
— — SINGLETON, A. O.: Experiments on the chemical stimulation of pain-endings associated with small blood vessels. Amer. J. Physiol. **107**, 594 (1934).
— SINGLETON, A. O.: Studies on the pain-sensibility of arteries. Amer. J. Physiol. **104**, 267 (1933).
MORITZ, A. R., HENRIQUES, F. C.: Studies of thermal injury. II. The relative importance of time and surface temperature in the causation of cutaneous burns. Amer. J. Path. **23**, 695 (1947).
M.R.C.: Medical Research Council duplicated paper No MRC. 53/649; Clinical investigations 1953. Also in Medical Ethics p. 151. London: Lloyd-Luke 1957.
M.R.C.: Responsibility in investigations on human subjects. In: The Report of the Medical Research Council for 1962/63 (Cmnd. 2382), p. 21.
MÜLLER, J.: Elements of Physiology, vol. 2, p. 1059 (trans. by W. BALY). London: Taylor & Walton 1843.
NAFE, J. P., WAGONER, K. S.: The insensitivity of the cornea to heat and pain derived from high temperatures. Amer. J. Psychol. **49**, 631 (1937).
NAKAHARA, M., TOKITA, T.: Capillary permeability effects of synovial fluid, AMCHA, E-ACA and prednisolone acetate. Nature (Lond.) **216**, 497 (1967).
NAKAJIMA, T., PISANO, J. J.: Structure of polistes kinin. In press (1968).
NÉMETHY, G., SCHERAGA, H. A.: The structure of water and hydrophobic bonding in proteins. III. The thermodynamic properties of hydrophobic bonds in proteins. J. phys. Chem. **66**, 1773 (1962).
NEUMANN, W., HABERMANN, E.: Paper electrophoresis separation of pharmacologically and biochemically active compounds of bee and snake venoms. In: Venoms, p. 171, ed. by E. E. BUCKLEY and N. PORGES. Washington: Amer. Ass. for the Advanc. of Science 1956.
NOSSEL, H. L., NIEMETZ, J.: A normal inhibitor of the blood coagulation contact reaction product. Blood **25**, 712 (1965).
ORKIN, L. R., JOSEPH, S. I., HELRICH, M.: Effects of mild analgesics on post-partum pain. A method for evaluating analgesics. N.Y. St. med. J. **57**, 71 (1957).
OSTFELD, A. M., REIS, D. J., GOODELL, H., WOLFF, H. G.: Headache and hydration. The significance of two varieties of fluid accumulation in patients with vascular headache of the migraine type. Arch. int. Med. **96**, 142 (1955).
— WOLFF, H. G.: Arterenol (norepinephrine) and vascular headache of the migraine type. Arch. Neurol. Psychiat. Chic. **74**, 131 (1955).
PANERAI, A., GHETTI, A., ARCANGELI, P.: Mediatori chimici ed arresto della circolazione arteriosa e venosa degli arti nell'uomo. Nota II. Liberazione di bradichinina durante la stasi venosa e sua inibizione mediante l'ischemia preventiva. Rass. Neurol. veg. **18**, 131 (1964).
PATE, J. W., LEE, W. H. Jr.: Polybrene and renal toxicity. J. thorac. cardiovasc. Surg. **46**, 390 (1963).
PEARL, J., ACETO, M. D., HARRIS, L. S.: Prevention of writhing and other effects of narcotics and narcotic antagonists in mice. J. Pharmacol. exp. Ther. **160**, 217 (1968).
PENSKY, J., LEVY, L. R., LEPOW, I. H.: Partial purification of a serum inhibitor of C'1-esterase. J. biol. Chem. **236**, 1674 (1961).

PISANO, J. J.: Wasp kinins. Mem. Inst. Butantan Symp. Int. **33** (2), 441 (1966).
— Studies on the structure of the major kinin in wasp venom. In: Vaso-active polypeptides. Bradykinin and related kinins, p. 35, ed. by M. ROCHA E SILVA and H. A. ROTHSCHILD. São Paulo 1967.
— Vasoactive peptides in venoms. Fed. Proc. **27**, 58 (1968).
POTTER, G. D., GUZMAN, F., LIM, R. K. S.: Visceral pain evoked by intra-arterial injection of substance P. Nature (Lond.) **193**, 983 (1962).
PRADO, J. L., TAMURA, Z., FURANO, E., PISANO, J. J., UDENFRIEND, S.: Characterization of kinins in wasp venom. In: Hypotensive peptides, p. 93, ed. by E. G. ERDÖS, N. BACK and F. SICUTERI. Berlin-Heidelberg-New York: Springer 1966.
PROCACCI, P.: A survey of modern concepts of pain. In: Handbook of clinical neurology, vol. 1, p. 114, ed. by P. J. VINKEN and G. W. BRUYN. Amsterdam: North-Holland Publ. Co. 1969.
RATNOFF, O. D., MILES, A. A.: Activation of a vascular permeability-increasing factor in human plasma incubated with purified activated Hageman factor. J. Lab. clin. Med. **60**, 1009 (1962).
— ROSENBLUM, J. M.: Role of Hageman factor in initiation of clotting by glass. Evidence that glass frees Hageman factor from inhibition. Amer. J. Med. **25**, 160 (1958).
ROCHA E SILVA, M.: Biochemistry and pharmacology of bradykinin. In: Polypeptides which affect smooth muscles and blood vessels, p. 210, ed. by M. SCHACHTER. London: Pergamon Press 1960.
— Chemical mediators of the acute inflammatory reaction. Ann. N.Y. Acad. Sci. **116**, 899 (1964a).
— The participation of substances with low molecular weight in inflammation with special reference to histamine and bradykinin. In: Injury, inflammation and immunity, p. 220, ed. by L. THOMAS, J. W. UHR and L. GRANT. Baltimore: Williams & Wilkins Co. 1964b.
— ANTONIO, A.: Release of bradykinin and the mechanism of production of a "Thermic edema (45° C)" in the rat's paw. Med. exp. (Basel) **3**, 371 (1960).
— BERALDO, W. T., ROSENFELD, C.: Bradykinin, a hypotensive and smooth muscle stimulating factor released from plasma globulin by snake venoms and by trypsin. Amer. J. Physiol. **156**, 261 (1949).
— ROSENTHAL, S. R.: Release of pharmacologically active substances from the rat skin *in vivo* following thermal injury. J. Pharmacol. exp. Ther. **132**, 110 (1961).
ROSENTHAL, S. R.: Histamine as possible mediator for cutaneous pain. Dual pain response to histamine. Proc. Soc. exp. Biol. (N.Y.) **74**, 167 (1950).
— MINARD, D.: Experiments on histamine as the chemical mediator for cutaneous pain. J. exp. Med. **70**, 415 (1939).
SCHACHTER, M.: A delayed slow-contracting effect of serum and plasma due to the release of a substance resembling kallikin and bradykinin. Brit. J. Pharmacol. **11**, 111 (1956).
— Kinins of different origins. Ann. N.Y. Acad. Sci. **104**, 108 (1963).
— Kinins—a group of active peptides. Ann. Rev. Pharmacol. **4**, 281 (1964).
— THAIN, E. M.: Chemical and pharmacological properties of the potent, slow contracting substance (kinin) in wasp venom. Brit. J. Pharmacol. **9**, 352 (1954).
SCHIFF, J. M.: Lehrbuch der Physiologie des Menschen. I. Muskel- und Nervenphysiologie, S. 228. Lahr: Schauenburg 1858/59.
SCHRÖDER, E., HEMPEL, R.: Bradykinin, kallidin and their synthetic analogues. Experientia (Basel) **20**, 529 (1964).
SHERRINGTON, C. S.: Cutaneous sensations. In: Textbook of physiology, vol. 2, ed. by E. A. SCHÄFER. Edinburgh and London: Y. J. Pentland 1900.
— The integrative action of the nervous system. New Haven: Yale University Press 1906.
SICUTERI, F.: Indomethacin as a new vasoconstrictor and therapeutic agent in migraine. In: Excerpta Med. Int. Congr. Ser. No 82, 335 (1964).
— Liberazione di peptidi per dilusione liquorale del plasma nella patogenesi della emorragia sottoaracnoidea. Boll. Soc. ital. Ematol. **13**, 49 (1965).
— Vasoneuroactive substances in migraine. Headache **6**, 109 (1966).
— Vasoneuroactive substances and their implication in vascular pain. Res. clin. Stud. Headache **1**, 6 (1967).
— Sensitization of nociceptors by 5-hydroxytryptamine in man. In: Pharmacology of pain, p. 57, ed. by R. K. S. LIM, D. ARMSTRONG and E. G. PARDO. Proceedings of III. Int. Congr. of Pharmacology, vol. 9. Oxford: Pergamon 1968a.
— Treatment of subarachnoid and other intracranial hemorrhages with proteinase inhibitors. Ann. N.Y. Acad. Sci. **146**, 682 (1968b).
— DEL BIANCO, P. L., FANCIULLACCI, M., ANSELMI, B.: Liberazione di plasmachinine da diluizione del sangue nel liquido cefalo-rachidiano. Boll. Soc. ital Biol. sper. **41**, 462 (1965a).
— — — FRANCHI, G.: Un nuovo substrato per lo studio del dolore da bradychinina e callidina. Boll. Soc. ital. Biol. sper. **40**, 949 (1964).

SICUTERI, F., FRANCHI, G., DEL BIANCO, P. L., FANCIULLACCI, M.: Peptides and pain. In: Vaso-active polypeptides. Bradykinin and related kinins, p. 251, ed. by M. ROCHA E SILVA and H. A. ROTHSCHILD. São Paulo 1967.
— — FANCIULLACCI, M., DEL BIANCO, P. L.: Serotonin-bradykinin potentiation of the pain-receptors in man. Life Sci. **4**, 309 (1965b).
SJÖQVIST, O.: Eine neue Operationsmethode bei Trigeminusneuralgie: Durchschneidung des Tractus spinalis trigemini. Zbl. Neurochir. **2**, 274 (1938).
SKOUBY, A. P.: Sensitization of pain receptors by cholinergic substances. Acta physiol. scand. **24**, 174 (1951).
SMITH, G. M., EGBERT, L. D., BEECHER, H. K.: The submaximum effort tourniquet method of producing experimental pain in man. Sensitivity to 600 mg aspirin. Bull. Problems Drug Dependence, 28th Meeting, 4668—6672 (1966a).
— — MARKOWITZ, R. A., MOSTELLER, F., BEECHER, H. K.: An experimental pain method sensitive to morphine in man. J. Pharmacol. exp. Ther. **154**, 324 (1966b).
SMITH, R.: The vocabulary of pain. In: Assessment of pain in man and animals, p. 32, ed. by C. A. KEELE and R. SMITH. London: Livingstone 1962.
STEVENS, S. S.: Mathematics, measurements and psychophysics. In: Handbook of experimental psychology, p. 1, ed. by S. S. STEVENS. New York and London: John Wiley & Sons 1951.
STEWART, J. M.: Structure-activity relationships in bradykinin analogues. Fed. Proc. **27**, 63 (1968a).
— Synthesis and pharmacology of polistes kinin, a bradykinin homolog. Fed. Proc. **27**, 534 (1968b).
— WOOLLEY, D. W.: All-D-bradykinin and the problem of peptide antimetabolites. Nature (Lond.) **206**, 619 (1965a).
— — The importance of the carboxyl end of bradykinin and other peptides. Nature (Lond.) **207**, 1160 (1965b).
— — The search for peptides with specific antibradykinin activity. In: Hypotensive peptides, p. 23, ed. by E. G. ERDÖS, N. BACK and F. SICUTERI. Berlin-Heidelberg-New York: Springer 1966.
SUNSHINE, A., LASKA, E., MEISSNER, M., MORGAN, S.: Analgesic studies of indomethacin as analyzed by computer technique. Clin. Pharmacol. Ther. **5**, 699 (1964).
SWARTS, W. B., WANAMAKER, J. F.: Skin blisters caused by vesicant beetles. J. Amer. med. Ass. **131**, 594 (1946).
THUNBERG, T.: Untersuchungen über die relative Tiefenlage der kälte-, wärme- und schmerzpercipirenden Nervenden in der Haut und über das Verhalten der Kältenervenenden gegenüber Wärmereizen. Skand. Arch. Physiol. **12**, 382 (1902).
UNGAR, R., DAMGAARD, E.: Protein breakdown in thermal injury. Proc. Soc. exp. Biol. (N.Y.) **87**, 378 (1954).
WALASZEK, E. J., DYER, D. C.: Polypeptide receptor mechanisms; influence of pH. In: Hypotensive peptides, p. 329, ed. by E. G. ERDÖS, N. BACK and F. SICUTERI. Berlin-Heidelberg-New York: Springer 1966.
WEBSTER, M. E., PIERCE, J. V.: Studies on plasma kallikrein and its relationship to plasmin. J. Pharmacol. exp. Ther. **130**, 484 (1960).
WEBSTER, W. J., MACWILLIAM, J. A.: Some applications of physiology to medicine. I. Sensory phenomena associated with defective blood supply to working muscles. Brit. med. J. **1923I**, 51.
WEDDELL, G.: The anatomy of pain sensibility. J. Anat. (Lond.) **81**, 374 (1947).
WHITE, J. C., SWEET, W. H.: Pain: Its mechanism and neurosurgical control. Springfield (Ill.): Ch. C. Thomas 1955.
WHITTLE, B. A.: Release of a kinin by intraperitoneal injection of chemical agents in mice. Int. J. Neuropharnacol. **3**, 369 (1964).
WITTE, S., SCHRICKER, K. T., SCHMIDT, E.: Zur Wirkung von synthetischem Bradykinin auf die Gefäßpermeabilität. Arzneimittel-Forsch. **11**, 619 (1961).
WOODWORTH, R. S., SHERRINGTON, C. S.: A pseudaffective reflex and its spinal path. J. Physiol. **31**, 234 (1904).
WOOLLARD, H. D., WEDDELL, G., HARPMAN, J. A.: Observations on the neurohistological basis of cutaneous pain. J. Anat. (Lond.) **74**, 413 (1940).
WRIGHT, A. H., WRIGHT, A. A.: Handbook of snakes, 1st ed., vol. 2. London: Constable & Co. Ltd. 1957.
YANG, H. Y. T., ERDÖS, E. G.: Second kininase in human blood plasma. Nature (Lond.) **215**, 1402 (1967).
ZACEST, R., MASHFORD, M. L.: Blood bradykinin levels in the human. Aust. J. exp. Biol. med. Sci. **45**, 89 (1967).
ZWEIFACH, B.W.: Microcirculatory aspects of tissue injury. Ann. N.Y. Acad. Sci. **116**, 831 (1964).

Bradykinin and Intracranial Circulation in Man

FEDERIGO SICUTERI

With 18 Figures

A. Introduction

The vessels of the head are sensitive to bradykinin. If we inject small doses of this substance intravenously, a transient flush in the face, but not in other parts of the body, is observed. The circulation of the facial skin is more sensitive to bradykinin than other areas of skin are to vasodilating agents. The intracranial extracerebral vasculature also responds quickly to an administration of the polypeptide, but this is demonstrable only with the aid of special techniques. The circulation of the brain seems to be scarcely influenced by polypeptides.

It is probable that bradykinin is implicated in the pathogenesis of some of the clinical phenomena associated with circulatory disorders and intracranial vascular accidents. In these conditions, congestion of microvasculature, edema, pain, and disorders of nerve function may be tied to the neurovascular action of bradykinin, that is, to the ability to dilate and increase the permeability of small vessels, to stimulate sensitive receptors, and to modify the nervous system function. These actions of bradykinin can be observed only when the concentration is high enough. In man, for example, if we inject small doses of the peptide into the carotid artery, only vasodilatation will occur; if we inject higher doses, bradykinin will cause both vasodilatation and pain; and in yet higher doses vasodilatation, pain, and transient neurological disturbances—such as scotoma, nausea and vomiting, and depression and mental confusion—will be observed.

In order that these neurovascular actions occur spontaneously, three conditions must exist. (1) Obviously there must be vascular and nervous structures where the peptide must act. (2) The concentration of bradykinin has to be sufficiently high. (3) The conditions for the liberation of kinins within the skull must be favorable.

In regard to the first point, the structures in the interior of the cranium where the vasomotor, algogenic, and nerve actions of bradykinin may be manifested, are largely represented by vessels, sensitive receptors, and central nervous structures. The second condition is due to the particular location of the cerebrospinal fluid (CSF) where bradykinin may be concentrated but difficult to remove. The third (the liberation of bradykinin) occurs especially when there is extravasation of blood into the brain or into the CSF.

The encephalon seems to react to a sudden hemorrhagic infarct with an activation of kinin-liberating proteases. The CSF dilutes the blood plasma during mixing, and the "dilution factor" is so activated. Subsequently, the released kinins act on intrathecal vasculature, on pain receptors, and on nerve centers that are bathed in CSF.

It is probable that some of the symptoms (headache, meningism, sleep, and coma) following intracranial hemorrhage may be in part due to the action of kinin. When intracranial vessels are ruptured, whether this happens accidentally (e.g. trauma) or spontaneously (e.g. subarachnoid hemorrhage), kinins may be implicated in the pathogenesis of symptoms. It is probable that bradykinin also has a role in the migraine syndrome. In effect, the most characteristic phenomena of migraine attack—vasodilatation, edema, pain, and depression—may be ascribed to particular biological actions of the peptide. Probably bradykinin actively participates in the mechanism of these phenomena although it is less likely that it would be the initiating factor in the attacks.

The liberation of kinin may play an important role in sudden fever, either spontaneous or provoked by the injection of pyrogens. More exactly, the headache and vasodilatation may be correlated with the action of the kinin system which is demonstrably activated by febrile conditions.

While the available data are scarce, the possibility that bradykinin has a physiologic role in cephalic circulation can be mentioned. The thinness of intracranial vessels, the inactivation of bradykinin in intracranial circulation as well as in the systemic circulation, the vasomotor sensitivity to the peptide, and the large and continuous availability of the precursors of bradykinin in circulating blood, all indicate that bradykinin may have a physiologic role in the regulation of cephalic circulation.

B. Kinin and Kininogen in the Carotid and Internal Jugular Vein

The control of microcirculation, in general, is nervous and/or humoral. If there is a biochemical control, we do not know which substances may be involved. Evidence suggests that the endothelium of microvessels, under physiologic conditions, increases the clearance of exogenous bradykinin. In fact, bradykinin injected into the brachial artery of man is recovered (method of PERITI et al., 1963b) in minimal amounts only in the venous return of the limb (SICUTERI et al., 1963c). This demonstrates that the microvascular endothelium has the capacity to inactivate or "fix" the polypeptide. Evidently, as follows from the intense erythema of the arm and from the strong local pain, the peptide for a time acts on vascular and sensitive receptors, but later becomes rapidly fixed or inactivated.

These data, confirmed also by other authors (ALLWOOD and LEWIS, 1963, 1964) indicate that a potent and physiologic activity of kinins exists at the microcirculatory level. No other vasoactive peptide or amine is cleared at such high rate by the capillaries. This clearance may have physiologic significance; maybe it is a defense against sudden and massive liberation of kinin which occurs in the organism in numerous conditions.

This capillary "clearance" of kinin is only partially linked to the enzymatic activity of plasma (ERDÖS and SLOANE, 1962; ERDÖS, 1966). This statement is corroborated by experiments in which a quantity of peptide (similar to that injected into the brachial artery) was incubated for a period approximately corresponding to the time of the experiment, with a quantity of blood of the approximate volume with which the injected bradykinin becomes diluted; it was observed that a large quantity of residual bradykinin was recovered. Other data which favor the hypothesis that an elevated capillary clearance is not linked only to the carboxypeptidase action of plasma, include our evidence that the kininase activity of venous plasma is practically equal to that of arterial plasma (SICUTERI, unpublished).

The importance of microvascular endothelial contact on the kininogen–kinin system is suggested by the difference between arterial and venous plasma kininogen (method of Diniz et al., 1961); this seems to indicate that at the capillary level there exists an enzyme or enzymes capable of liberating kinin from kininogen (Sicuteri et al., 1963a). Among these, lysosomal enzymes may be included. These enzymes were thought to have a role in lowering kininogen level during fever (Sicuteri et al., 1963a; Bavazzano et al., 1967, 1968).

In vitro research also showed the kininogenase and kininase actions of lysosomal enzymes (Eisen and Keele, 1966; Greenbaum and Kim, 1967; Greenbaum et al., 1967; Melmon and Cline, 1967; Cline and Melmon, 1967).

After the administration of pyrogen to man, a parallel elevation of β-glucuronidase (an enzyme of prevalently lysosomal origin) and a diminution of kininogen was found (Sicuteri, 1967b). This occurs also when pyrogen is given in minimal doses although in sufficient quantities to provoke pain.

In blood collected from a cubital vein during circulatory arrest of at least 5-minute duration, a highly significant decrease of kininogen are noted. After the cessation of ischemia, and during the hyperemic reaction, kininogen levels tend to return to normal base line. This might due to lysosomal enzymes (Sicuteri et al., in press).

While the extracerebral circulation of the head may be comparable to peripheral circulation, the cerebral circulation has particular characteristics. The arteries and the veins have a negligible muscular layer. For this reason it was assumed that the cerebral circulation has a "passive" regulation and adapts passively to variations of pressure and systemic circulatory flow. It is possible that at the level of intracranial circulation in general, and of the cerebrum in particular, chemical factors have a special importance.

Table 1. *Plasma kininogen and plasma kinins in samples of blood collected from common carotid, internal jugular vein, and cubital vein of patients*

Sex	Age	Common carotid		Internal jugular vein		Cubital vein	
		kininogen (μg/ml)	kinin (ng/ml)	kininogen (μg/ml)	kinin (ng/ml)	kininogen (μg/ml)	kinin (ng/ml)
♀	48	2.5	0.8	2	1.2	1.8	1
♀	36	3	0.7	2.7	0.5	2.6	
♀	42	3.3	0.5	3.5	0.7	3	0.6
♂	43	3.5	0.7	2.8	0.6		
♀	44	3	0.7	2.7	0.5	2.5	0.5
♀	28	2	0.5	1.8	0.6		
♂	36	4	0.5	3.5	1.2		
Average		3.042 (I)	0.63	2.71 (II)	0.75	2.47	
S.D.		0.655	0.127	0.655	0.485		

Significance (Student's *t* test): $P < 0.4$ for kininogen, and $P < 0.2$ for kinin not significant.

Information on the possible role of the kininogen–kinin system on cephalic circulation can be obtained by measuring kininogen and kinin levels in blood samples taken from the internal carotid artery and from the internal jugular vein. The internal jugular vein drains more than 90% of the returning blood from the encephalic circulation. Jugular puncture done through the skin under the mastoid prominence, although requiring a certain skill, is relatively simple and innocuous (Kety and Schmidt, 1948).

In subjects without important circulatory disorders, the kininogen level of carotid blood is slightly higher than that of internal jugular vein blood. The difference, however, is not statistically significant.

The level of free kinin in carotid blood is slightly lower than in internal jugular blood, but the differences is not statistically significant (Table 1).

After the slow injection of 200 μg bradykinin into the cubital vein, free kinin level in blood samples taken from the internal jugular vein increases modestly, about threefold over the control. Kininogen did not change.

In two cases, where both carotid arteries were occluded by digital pressure for 2 minutes, a lowering of jugular and cubital venous kininogen was observed, while the level of kinin remained unchanged. These observations on the cerebral circulation correspond to those made on the circulation of the limb. The phenomenon may indicate that cerebral ischemia, even if partial and transient, reduces the concentration of kininogen by liberating kinin.

C. The Action of Bradykinin on Cerebral Circulation

Because of the potent vasodilatory action of bradykinin, after the administration of this peptide a dilatation of cerebral vessels may be expected. Unfortunately we do not have at our disposal any studies on the effect of bradykinin on brain circulation directly, for example, with the nitrous oxide method (KETY and SCHMIDT, 1948). However, some data on the action of bradykinin on the cerebral circulation of animals are available.

Table 2. *Action of eledoisin and bradykinin on cerebral circulation in dog.* (From BERETTA et al., 1966)

	No.	Mean ± S.D.	M.D. ± S.E.	Dm%	*P*
Eledoisin					
Blood flow (cc/min/100 g)	7	b. 48.7 ± 8.96 a. 37.9 ± 8.13	− 10.8 ± 2.53	− 22.2	< 0.01
Resistance (units)	7	b. 2.8 ± 0.46 a. 3.3 ± 0.71	+ 0.5 ± 0.15	+ 17.8	0.05—0.02
O_2Diff. (A-V) (vol.-%)	7	b. 6.97 ± 2.26 a. 8.07 ± 2.20	+ 1.10 ± 0.67	+ 15.8	0.2 —0.1
O_2Consumption (cc/min/100 g)	7	b. 3.39 ± 1.32 a. 2.97 ± 0.80	− 0.42 ± 0.45	− 12.4	0.4 —0.3
Bradykinin					
Blood flow (cc/min/100 g)	7	b. 46.2 ± 11.3 a. 44.8 ± 8.28	− 1.4 ± 2.62	− 3.03	> 0.9
Resistance (units)	7	b. 2.8 ± 1.05 a. 2.5 ± 0.69	− 0.3 ± 0.21	− 10.71	0.3 —0.2
O_2Diff. (A-V) (vol.-%)	7	b. 3.02 ± 0.30 a. 2.79 ± 0.20	+ 0.23 ± 0.20	+ 3.10	0.2 —0.1
O_2Consumption (cc/min/100 g)	7	b. 4.43 ± 1.63 a. 4.37 ± 1.05	− 0.6 ± 0.35	− 13.54	0.2 —0.1

S.D. = Standard deviation; S.E. = standard error; M.D. = difference between the means; Dm% = % difference between the means.

The techniques to measure the intracranial circulation in general involve the registration of external jugular venous pressure of the dog (BOVET et al., 1960), or the cerebrospinal fluid pressure in man (SICUTERI, 1959a), or the microscopic changes of the vessels of the pia (BREDA et al., 1962).

These techniques especially register the changes in intracranial pressure and therefore changes in intracranial circulation. By using these methods (man, SICUTERI et al., 1961b; dog, CARPI and CORRADO, 1961; GRAEFF et al., 1965; and guinea pig, CONCIOLI et al., 1961) the vasodilatatory effects of bradykinin on intracranial circulation were detected.

Studying the cerebral circulation of the anesthetized dog by the nitrous oxide method showed that bradykinin injected intravenously in doses active on systemic circulation (0.5 μg kg/min) does not modify the flow of blood, vascular resistance, or cerebral oxygen consumption significantly. It has no action on the cerebral circulation of the dog (DESSY et al., 1966). In one comparative study eledoisin (Table 2) infused intravenously into the anesthetized dog always

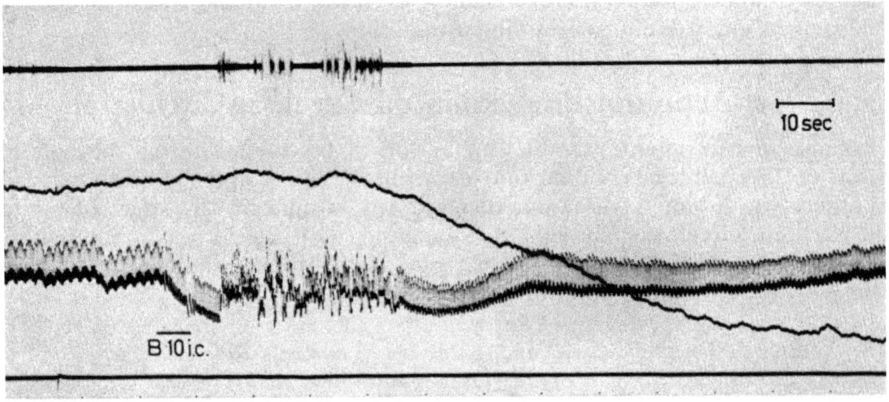

Fig. 1. Effects of intracarotid injection of 10 μg bradykinin to the rabbit. From top to bottom: phonogram (vocalization), radioactivity over the brain area, femoral arterial blood pressure. Since pulses, coming from the rate meter, have negative polarity, their trace lowers as radioactivity increases, and vice versa; time constant of integration = 20 sec. Note that the cerebral blood increase (middle) precedes the vocalization (top). (BERTOLINI et al., 1968)

caused a decrease in the flow with an increased vascular resistance, while the oxygen consumption remained unchanged (BERETTA et al., 1966).

In the rabbit, bradykinin has a different action, depending on the route of administration. In these experiments (BERTOLINI et al., 1967, 1968), the cerebral blood volume was estimated in rabbits with the help of homologous red blood cells labeled with Cr^{51}.

When bradykinin was injected into the carotid, vocalization occurred, perhaps as an expression of pain, with an increase of encephalic blood volume, indirectly indicating a cerebral vasodilatation (Fig. 1).

Arterial pressure behaved biphasically; first hypotension, then hypertension was observed. When the venous route of administration was used, no vocalization occurred, and a reduction of cerebral radioactivity and arterial hypotension was noted.

In conclusion, it seems that bradykinin potently modifies the intracranial circulation, but this occurs above all at the expense of the intracranial extracerebral circulation. As with other drugs, the circulation of the brain in a strict sense seems to be scarcely influenced by bradykinin. Possibly vasodilatation also occurs in the cerebral circulation when the peptide is introduced directly into the carotid (BERTOLINI et al., 1968).

D. Pharmacodynamics of Intracranial Circulation

I. Method

Many pharmaceutical agents which act poorly on cerebral circulation are strongly active on extracerebral intracranial circulation. Some other agents scarcely influence the intracranial circulation but are generally vasoactive. Nicotinic acid behaves this way, having an intense action on the cutaneous circulation and on the circulation of the face, while its effect on intracranial circulation is questionable.

For studying the intracranial vasomotility in man the most suitable simple technique is the electromanometric measurement in a closed system of the

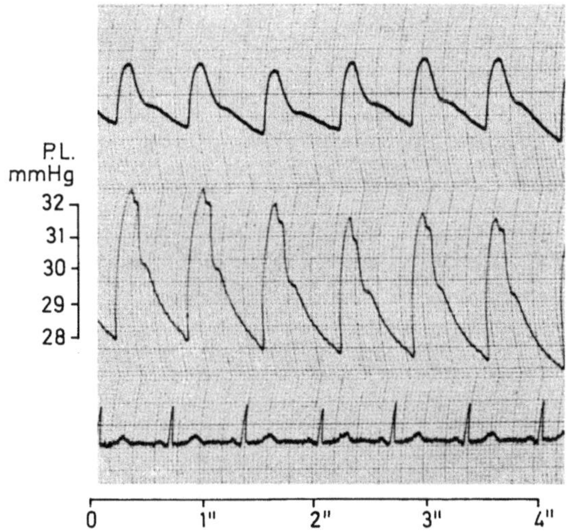

Fig. 2. Morphology and height of the CSF pulsation according to the electromanometric technique (middle). Peripheral arterial pulse (top) and ECG recording (bottom)

pressure of the CSF (Sicuteri, 1959a). This technique takes advantages of a natural plethysmograph. In fact, skull, spinal theca, and CSF constitute the box and the liquid part of a natural plethysmograph adaptable for measuring variations in volume of the intrathecal vascular system, especially in capillaries and veins, and to a lesser degree in the encephalon and medulla. Before the use of the electromanometric technique in a "closed system", the CSF pressure was registered via a vertical tube connected to a spinal needle. This method is not accurate enough.

The closed electromanometric technique registers precisely and with great sensitivity minimal variations in CSF pressure. The needle, introduced into the dural sac, is connected through a plastic tube to a Statham-type strain gauge. The sterilized plastic tube is filled with sterile pyrogen-free saline. A polygraph registers the variations in pressure. With this system there is no displacement of the liquid and pressure is accurately registered.

With the electromanometric technique it was possible to determine the morphology of the intrathecal pulse (Sicuteri, 1959a) (Fig. 2), which resembles a passive pulse, determined by the pulsation of mostly arterial vessels and to a smaller extent by veins. The principally arterial components stem from the motility of intrathecal arteries. The dicrotism is also of arterial origin (Sicuteri, 1959a).

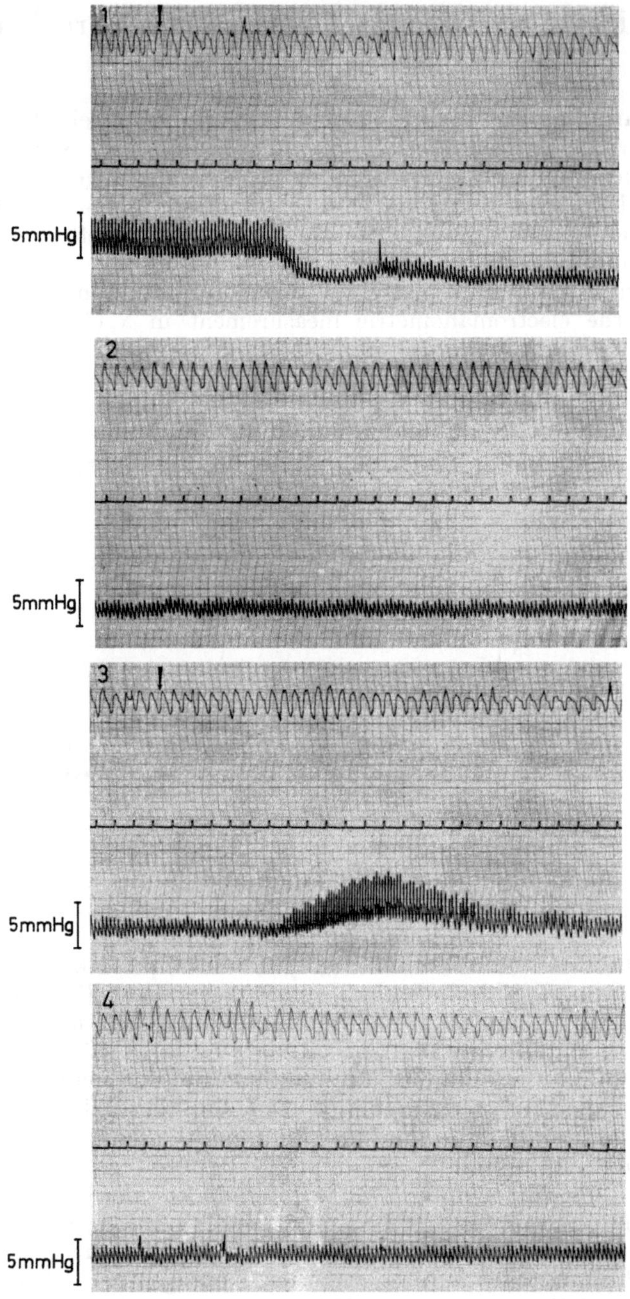

Fig. 3. (1) A typical intracranial vasoconstriction, i.e. decrease of CSF pressure and narrowing of pulsations induced by i. v. injection of indomethacin to man (arrow). (2) Intracranial vasoconstriction is long lasting. (3) In spite of persisting vasoconstriction, bradykinin produces a typical intracranial vasodilatation (arrow). (4) After vasodilatation, vasoconstriction by indomethacin appears again. Top tracing: respiration. Middle tracing: timer 5 sec. Bottom tracing: CSF electromanometric tracing. (Sicuteri et al., 1965b)

The venous component, which produces a small preoscillatory peak, comes from atrial contraction. Such an origin is convincingly demonstrable in cases of A-V blockade when the atria contract independently from the ventricles.

The spinal fluid pulse is influenced by pharmacologic stimuli with characteristic morphologic reversals according to whether the agent dilates or constricts intrathecal vessels. Spinal fluid pressure in a quiet patient is stable. It is quickly changed by the action of vasoactive drugs, augmented by dilators, and lowered by constrictors. In other words, vasodilatation provokes an increase in intrathecal pressure and a morphologic modification of each oscillatory pulse, which becomes higher with displacement of the base line of the dicrotic peak. With vasoconstrictors, on the other hand, there is a drop in intrathecal pressure and a narrowing of the pulse with a strong, prominent dicrotic wave (Fig. 3).

By cannulating the internal carotid artery with a thin needle, the direct effects of minimal doses of vasoactive agents may also be studied. Changes in CSF pressure are immediate, not preceded by a latent period as with intravenous administration. The introduction of drugs into the carotid and the registration of variations in intrathecal pressure avoids, in fact, the effect of reflexes on the systemic arterial circulation.

II. Intracranial Vasodilatation by Bradykinin

Intravenous Route. The introduction of synthetic bradykinin (BRS-640) in doses of 50 to 80 μg/kg i.v. or synthetic kallidin (70–100 μg) regularly produces vasodilatation; intrathecal pulses are elevated, narrowed, and the dicrotic waves descend toward the base line. At the same time, the CSF pressure rises (a few mm Hg).

Simultaneously, hyperpnea, flushing of the face, tachycardia, and arterial hypotension are noted (Sicuteri et al., 1961b). Threshold doses for bradykinin are 100–150 ng/kg and for kallidin 200–300 ng. These doses act on CSF pressure and on the oscillogram of the superficial temporal artery (extracranial circulation) but not on systemic arterial pressure. No tachyphylaxis was observed when threshold doses were injected every 5 minutes.

In the same type of test histamine has 3 to 4 times the activity of bradykinin. Apart from its effect on arterial pressure, bradykinin stimulates respiration more markedly than does histamine. This probably is a consequence of the direct stimulation of respiratory centers (Fig. 4).

Eledoisin is by far a more active vasodilator in man than histamine or bradykinin; it is 50 to 100 times more active than bradykinin (Sicuteri et al., 1963d). Threshold effects are noted with intravenous injections of 2–3 ng/kg.

Physalaemin is the most potent vasoactive substance known in animals (Bertaccini et al., 1965); doses of 0.25–0.5 ng/kg cause intracranial vasodilatation in man (Sicuteri et al., 1964b). Eledoisin and physalaemin originate from animal tissues (Erspamer, 1961; Erspamer and Anastasi, 1962; Erspamer and Glässer, 1963; Erspamer et al., 1964).

Another polypeptide, angiotensin, evokes vasoconstriction as well as narrowing of the pulse and lowering of CSF pressure. A mixture of equivalent doses of angiotensin and vasodilating peptides (bradykinin, eledoisin, or physalaemin), induces vasodilatation followed by vasoconstriction. This may be explained by the fact that the onset of hypertensive action of angiotensin is slower than the hypotensive action of other peptides. On the other hand, the vasodilatory peptides reverse the action of angiotensin when given conveniently a moment or so before.

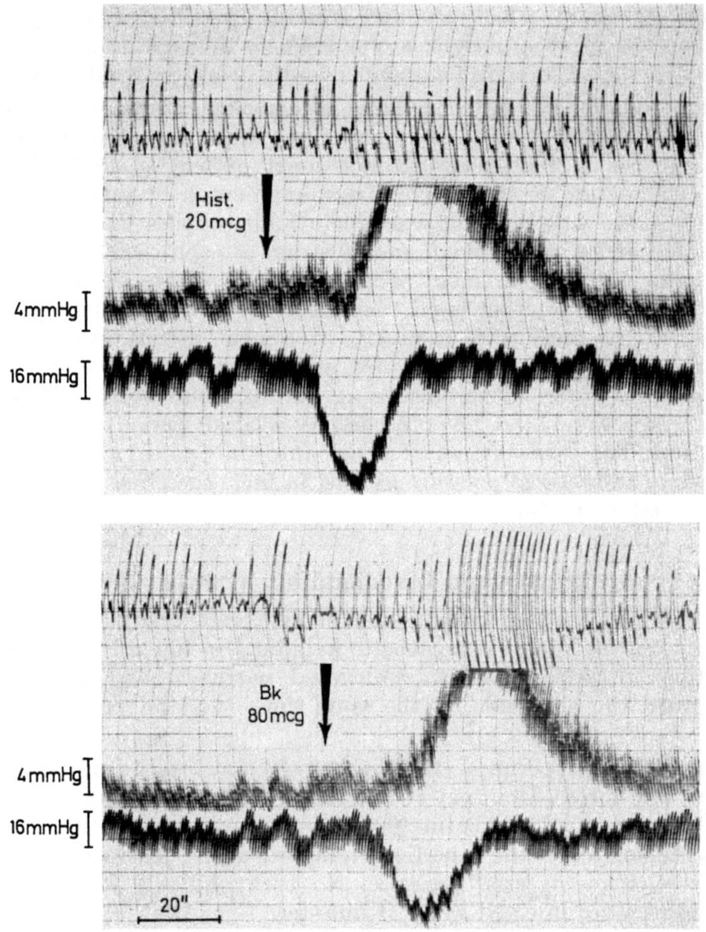

Fig. 4. Activity of histamine and bradykinin given i.v. on respiration, CSF pressure, and respectively on carotid pressure in the human. Similar changes can be observed in both experiments, but a striking activation of respiration is elicited by bradykinin only

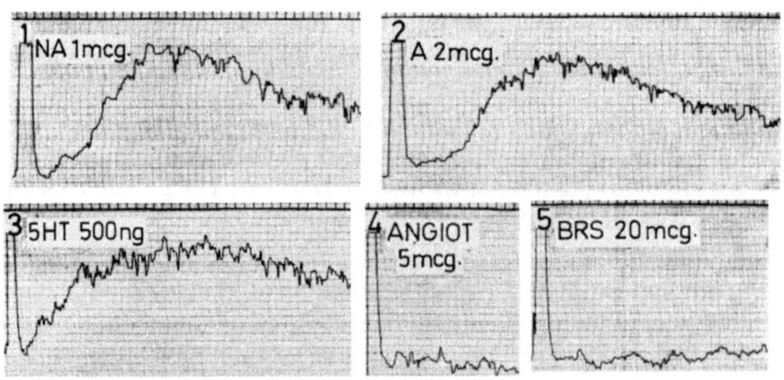

Fig. 5. While serotonin (*5HT*), epinephrine (*A*) and norepinephrine (*NA*) constrict powerfully the vein of the back of the hand in man, bradykinin (*BRS*) does not exhibit any local constrictor activity. Angiotensin does not constrict the vein

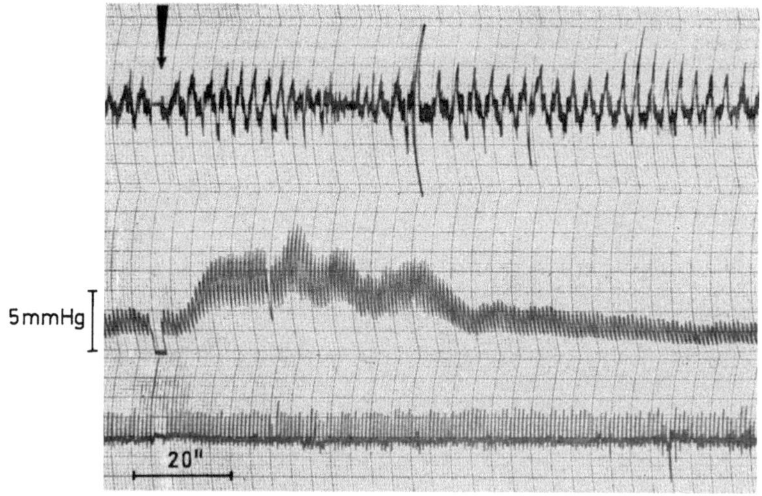

Fig. 6. Intracranial vasodilator effect of bradykinin (3 ng/kg) injected (arrow) to internal carotid in man. Top tracing: respiration. Middle tracing: CSF pressure. Bottom tracing: oscillogram of superficial temporal artery. Complaints of pain (on the same side of head as the injection) and scintillations

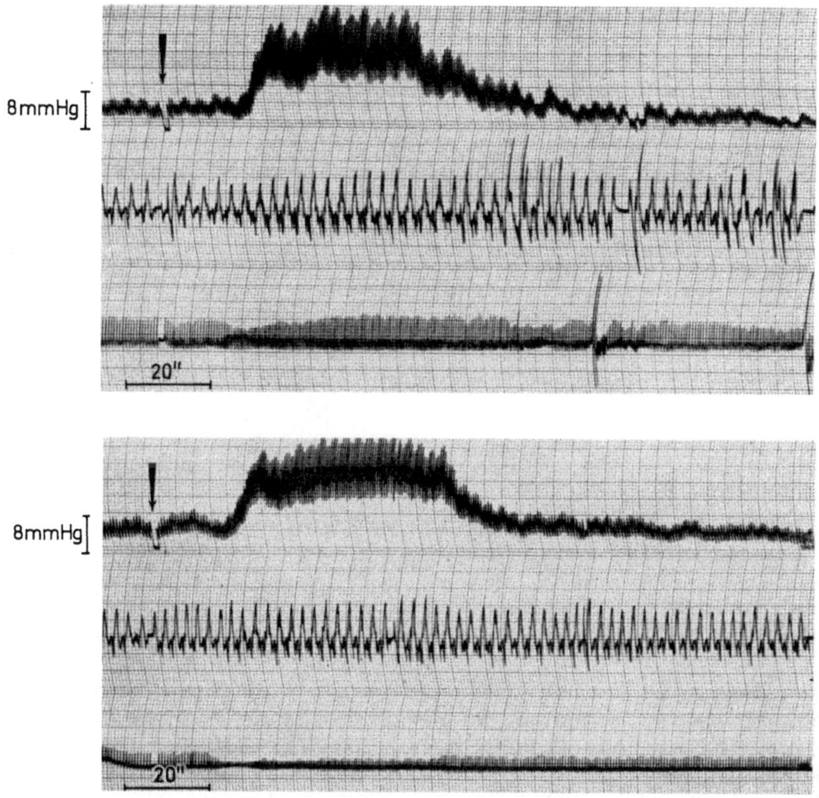

Fig. 7. Intracranial vasodilatation by trypsin (7 µg/kg) injected i.v. to man (from top to bottom: CSF pressure, respiration, sphymogram of a limb). The circulatory and respiratory changes are not inhibited by an antihistamine (lower figure)

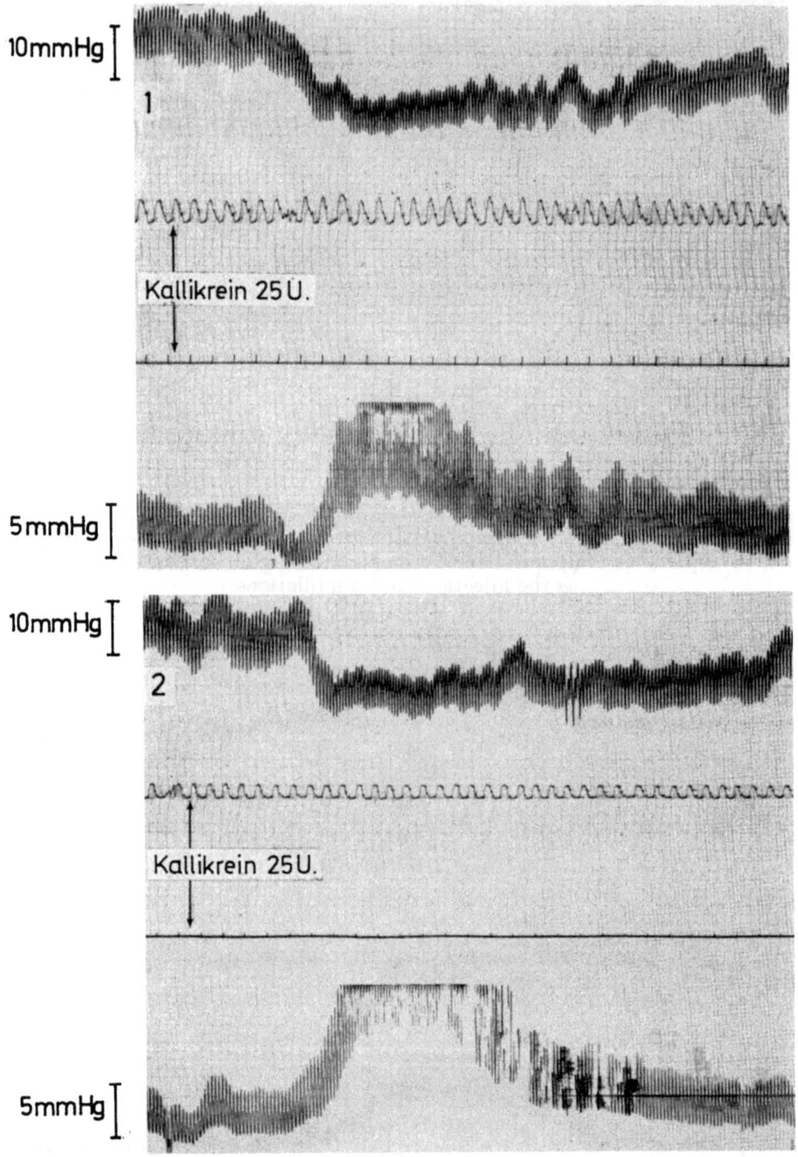

Fig. 8. Vasomotor changes by injection of kallikrein i.v. to man: (1) arterial hypotension (top) and intracranial hypertension (bottom). The respiration (middle) is slightly affected. Throbbing headache. (2) Pretreatment with an antiserotonin antihistamine drug BC-105 (20 μg/kg) does not affect the vasomotility and headache induced by kallikrein. (Timer: 5 sec)

Even during the infusion of norepinephrine in doses which cause signs of intracranial vasoconstriction and an elevation of systemic pressure, hypotensive peptides induce, in threshold doses, a vasodilatation that can be measured with the electromanometer.

The mechanism by which bradykinin produces hypertension of CSF is evidently tied to its microvasodilatory potency. It has a transient congestive action which increases the volume of the soft intrathecal structure and consequently increases CSF pressure. In contrast to other vascular areas in animals (SHIMAMOTO et al., 1966; BOBBIN and GUTH, 1967), the infusion of even concentrated doses of bradykinin does not produce constriction of superficial veins in humans (SICUTERI et al., 1964a) (Fig. 5).

Intracarotid Route. Microdoses (0.25–0.5–1.0 μg) of synthetic bradykinin injected into the carotid induce a typical intracranial vasodilatation (Fig. 6);

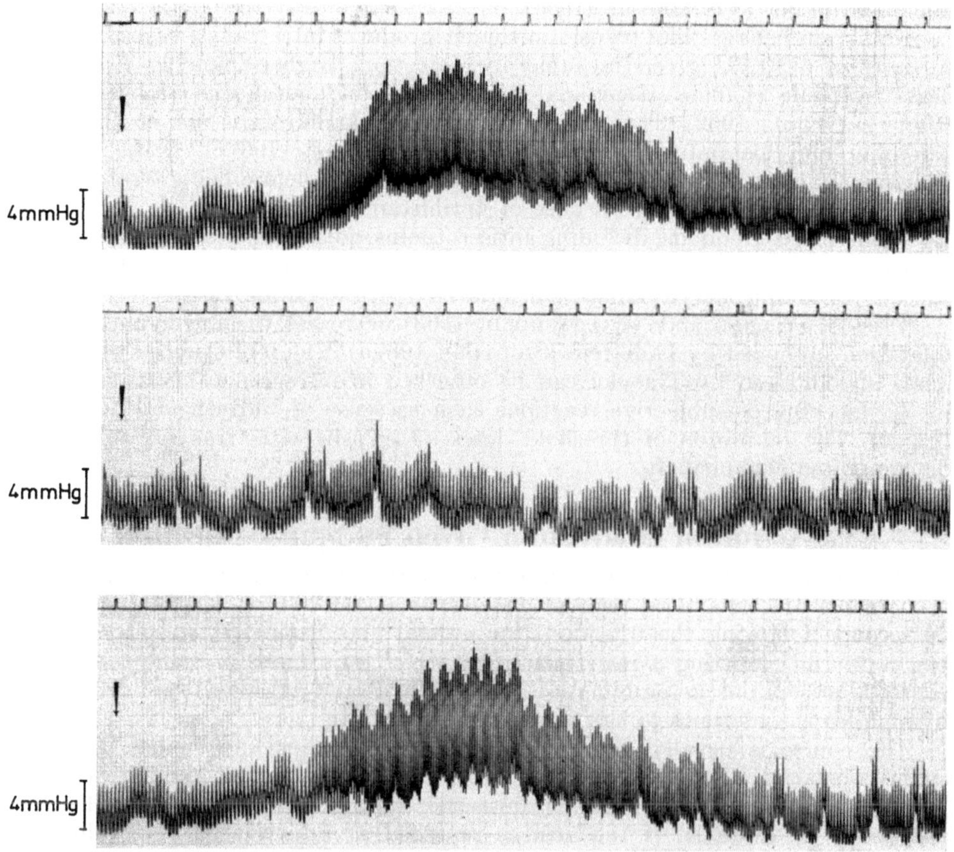

Fig. 9. Intracranial vasodilatation and headache induced by i.v. kallikrein (20 FU) in man (top). Both effects are completely inhibited by 60,000 KIU of Trasylol (middle). They reappear if the dose of kallikrein is tripled (bottom)

interestingly, there is no latency between the injection of the drug and the changes in CSF pressure. This indicates that the action of bradykinin on microvessels is immediate (Fig. 6).

However, a latent period is characteristic of muscular contraction (uterus ileum) and pain reaction. The same vasodilator effect may be obtained with histamine given via the carotid route in doses 2 to 3 times higher than those of bradykinin. It is interesting that bradykinin is more potent than histamine when given via the intracarotid route and less potent when administered by vein. The lower activity of intravenous bradykinin is probably due to its greater inactivation in plasma and at the pulmonary capillary level (SICUTERI et al., 1961b).

III. Intracranial Vasodilatation by Kininogenases (Trypsin, Kallikrein)

The rapid injection of small doses of trypsin (5 μg/kg i.v.) produces intracranial vasodilatation in man. Higher doses (up to 20–50 μg/kg) induce also other symptoms such as tachycardia, arterial hypotension, and flush.

An injection of an antihistamine does not modify the response to trypsin (Fig. 7). The same antihistamine completely blocks the intracranial vasodilator reaction to histamine and to histamine liberator, 48/80 in man (SICUTERI et al., 1956) and in dog (VIRNO et al., 1956).

Kallikrein behaves like trypsin in that it produces intracranial vasodilatation in doses of 5–10 FU given in rapid i.v. injection. Higher doses (20–30 U) also cause systemic changes as arterial hypotension and cutaneous vasodilatation (SICUTERI et al., 1962). The effect of commercial kallikrein is not modified by serotonin and histamine antagonists (SICUTERI et al., 1967c). Consequently, in human experiments it is advisable that the subject, before being treated with trypsin or kallikrein, receive a dose of antihistamine (Fig. 8).

Numerous compounds, including antiserotonins, antihistamines, indomethacin, acetylsalicylic acid, pyrazole, cortisone, and β-blockers, have been used without success to inhibit the vasodilatation induced by bradykinin.

Trasylol (WERLE and TRAUTSCHOLD, 1963) decreases the intracranial vasodilatation produced by kallikrein (SICUTERI, 1967a). The inhibition of threshold doses of kallikrein by Trasylol can be observed in intracranial circulation and in the blocking of subjective reactions such as sense of warmth and headache (Fig. 9). The inhibition of threshold doses of trypsin with Trasylol cannot be demonstrated convincingly.

E. Action of Bradykinin Given by Spinal Injection

Synthetic bradykinin injected into the cisterna magna of the rabbit produces a characteristic behavioral reaction (SICUTERI et al., 1966b). In the first 10 to 20 seconds following the injection, the animal acts normally; subsequently it begins to run, emitting a penetrating cry which continues for some time. The course is precipitous, resembling a desperate flight and at times it is interrupted by high leaps sometimes to half a meter (Fig. 10).

The course is usually disorganized, the animal slips and strikes its head against obstacles; after 20–40 seconds, it stops and appears sedated and prostrated. A dose of 5 μg/kg of bradykinin produces the squeaking-flight reaction (SFR) in practically all animals. If the dose is repeated at intervals of 5–10 minutes, tachyphylaxis is observed. Doses of 0.5–1.0 μg provoke the reaction in a minority of the animals. This reaction is not inhibited by cortisone, phenylbutazone, aspirin, or methysergide. Morphine minimizes the reaction but indomethacin administered intravenously markedly inhibits the phenomenon (Fig. 11). If given intracisternally, the reaction is not inhibited.

The mechanism of action of the SFR is unknown. It resembles a defense reaction which in the rabbit is manifested in flight resulting from violent intracranial pain induced by the peptide, e.g. in the subarachnoid space. Pain also provokes the cry reaction. The latent period of 10–20 seconds is identical with the latency in man when bradykinin is placed in contact with sensitive receptors, either by means of the cantharidin blister technique (ARMSTRONG et al., 1957), vein sensitized by 5-HT (SICUTERI et al., 1965a), or intraperitoneal injection (LIM et al., 1967).

Other algogenic substances such as histamine and 5-HT do not produce the SFR. Other peptides, although more vasoactive than bradykinin—e.g. eledoisin, physalaemin, angiotensin, and vasopressin—injected intracisternally, do not induce SFR. The possible correlation with vasomotor intracranial reactions was also considered (BERTOLINI et al., 1966). Bradykinin injected into the carotid artery of the rabbit increases the flow of blood, which corresponds to the vocalization. Eledoisin never produces cerebral vasodilatation or vocalization in the rabbit (STERNIERI et al., 1967).

Other authors have observed excitation in the animal after the experimental introduction of bradykinin into the lateral cerebral ventricle (CORRADO et al.,

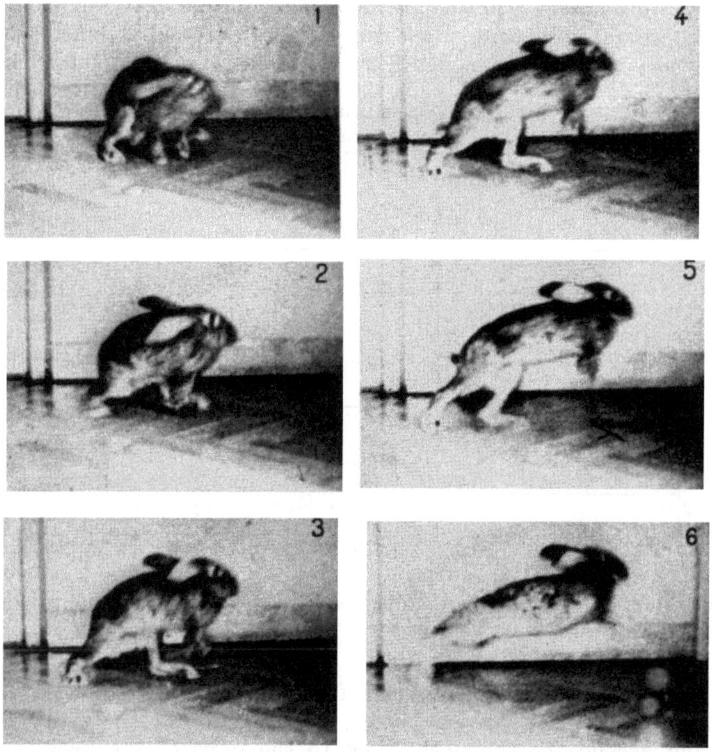

Fig. 10. Small amounts (2–4 μg/kg) of bradykinin injected into the cisterna magna produces a characteristic behavioral reaction in the rabbit. After 10–20 seconds of latency, the animal runs and squeaks piercingly. The squeaking-flight reaction seems due to a violent pain arising from sensitive intracranial structures

1959; ROCHA E SILVA, 1963), while still others (LEWIS, 1963) did not notice peculiar reactions even after injecting 125 μg of pure peptide. It is possible that the marked and prolonged prostration that follows the SFR may be related to the observed depletion of cerebral norepinephrine (GRAEFF et al., 1967).

In the unanesthetized curarized rabbit receiving artificial respiration to avoid the movements of flight, the EEG activity is not modified by intracisternal bradykinin. A plausible interpretation of the SFR attributes it to a headache which, after the compulsory latency of 10–20 seconds, sets in suddenly and violently and brings about the flight and cry. Human investigations support this hypothesis because bradykinin produces a strong pain when introduced in minimal quantities into the CSF.

The activity of bradykinin in experimental animals after intracisternal administration and the increased concentration of kinins found after subarachnoid hemorrhage (Sicuteri et al., 1963b, 1966b) justified trials on humans. Research was carried out with a group of volunteers receiving initially very small doses of the peptide. The subjects of the investigations were patients from whom a few milliliters of CSF had to be with drawn for diagnostic purposes. A quantity of sterile saline (equivalent to the amount of spinal fluid withdrawn) containing a small amount of bradykinin was cautiously introduced into the needle during the spinal puncture. In subjects who received saline only no symptoms were observed but slight headache and malaise, the usual reactions to diagnostic spinal puncture. Most subjects who received bradykinin had a painful and nervous reaction which set in after a latency of 1 to 2 hours.

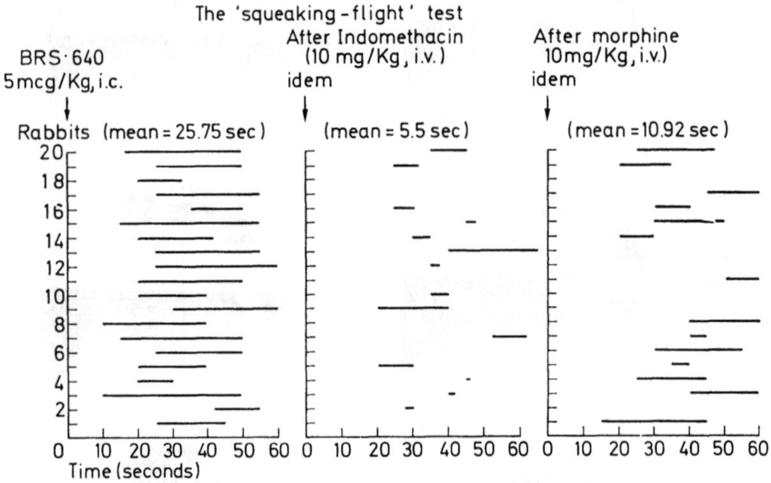

Fig. 11. The rabbit squeaking-flight reaction (see Fig. 10) is partially inhibited by i.v. indomethacin and less by morphine. (Sicuteri, 1967b)

If the patient has suffered for years from chronic headache, the reaction is decidedly more severe. Pain—or better, a sense of haeviness—begins in the shoulders and ascends to the neck, then to the nape of the neck, and finally to the entire cranium. The headache is sometimes violent, lasting an hour or sometimes a day, often with pulsations. Even a slight movement of the head violently exacerbates the pain. The intravenous administration of small doses (5–10 μg) of histamine or bradykinin, practically ineffective under normal conditions, exacerbates the pain sometimes to an intolerable degree. Analgesics give some relief, the most active being indomethacin; ergotamine also effectively attenuates the pain. It is peculiar that these drugs are also used in the therapy of intense headache. Indomethacin has an intense vasoconstrictive action, differing from ergotamine, but this is meaningful only at the cerebral level (Sicuteri et al., 1965b). Indomethacin (i.v.) inhibits the SFR induced by bradykinin given intracisternally to the rabbit. The effect of indomethacin may be extremely rapid if administered intravenously.

Nervous system phenomena evoked by bradykinin given spinally include difficulties in discriminating, asthenia, the difficulty or impossibility of maintaining balance, nausea, and sometimes vomiting. Perhaps the least conspicuous manifestations are drowsiness and sleep. These phenomena are in part secondary to cephalic pain, but in part are clearly out of proportion to the headache and dependent therefore on the peptide's action on the CNS. During the CNS reaction, the conjunctiva appear slightly congested, the retinal veins turgid, and the superficial temporal artery dilated and pulsating. In a few patients (all of them with chronic headache) a slight nuchal rigidity appears (Fig. 12). The reaction to bradykinin given spinally leaves no after effects. In fact, it is peculiar that some patients with chronic headache report a benefit which lasts from months to 1–2 years.

In a few cases, a small quantity (1–5 μg) of 5-HT was injected spinally. No reactions other than those following an introduction of sterile physiologic solution were observed.

Kinins Released by Dilution. Kinins are liberated when plasma is diluted with CSF. At the moment of spinal puncture, following a light local subcutaneous anesthesia, with the

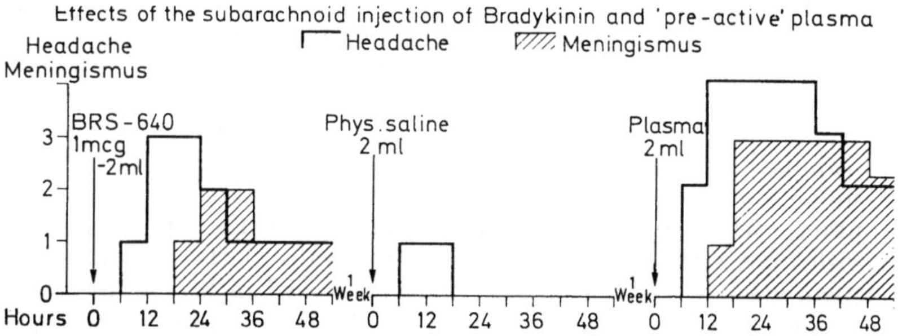

Fig. 12. The intracranial structures of humans are very sensitive to pain-producing activity of bradykinin. The spinal injection of small amounts (15 ng/kg) of peptide (BRS-640) induces, after a long-lasting latency, headache and slight meningism. Spinal injection of homologous plasma induces similar phenomena: meningism is more marked. Phenomena following plasma injection, mimic somewhat those of subarachnoid hemorrhage

patient laying on his side, 2 ml of spinal fluid is extracted. The spinal needle is then connected to a siliconized syringe containing 1 ml of plasma from the same patient. Very slowly, 5 ml of spinal fluid is gently aspirated and is permitted, with a slight movement of the syringe, to mix with the plasma thereby diluting it.

The syringe is kept moderately warm by holding it in the hand, which avoids the influence of low temperature on the kinin release (ARMSTRONG et al., 1966).

After maintaining the needle *in situ* for 10 minutes, the CSF-diluted plasma is slowly reintroduced and the needle is than removed.

In a group of patients in whom these maneuvers were carried out, except for injecting plasma into the syringe, no reactions were observed other than those usual after diagnostic spinal puncture. The patients who received diluted plasma, however, had a reaction similar to that observed after the spinal injection of bradykinin.

When 0.1 of plasma was diluted *in vitro* with 1 ml of CSF, kinin was released after 10 minutes that contracted the rat uterus. Similar reactions—headache, nervous depression, and meningism, but more intense and prolonged—are obtained by injecting spinally 2–3 ml of homologous sterile plasma in siliconized glass (SICUTERI, 1966, 1967a, 1968).

This investigation was done because it had been assumed that plasma diluted in the subarachnoid space by spinal fluid releases kinin. If homologous plasma was injected into subjects who suffer from daily chronic headache, small quantities of plasma (0.5–1 ml) were sufficient to induce an irriting pain reaction, meningeal and nervous, and quite intense (Fig. 12). To control the reactions to kinin or to homologous plasma, indomethacin or ergotamine are sufficient. After the spinal injection of kinin or homologous plasma, no after effects are observed. In some cases of preexisting headache an improvement or a complete and persistent disappearance of headache was observed.

Observations in man indicate that synthetic bradykinin and natural kinins (obtained by the dilution of plasma with CSF), injected into the subarachnoid space spinally, evoke a painful reaction which ascends from the shoulders to the head, concluding with an intense and prolonged headache. Associated with the headache other marked but not alarming psychological and neurological symptoms occur, such as depression, somnolence, nausea, and at times vomiting. The intensity of the reaction varies from subject to subject but appears particularly pronounced in patients who suffer from daily chronic headache. These reactions are similar to the action of kinin; this is taken as a sign that the peptide starts a reaction which is autonomously prolonged for many hours. In fact, the concentration of kinin in the spinal fluid remains elevated for a long time. The *in vitro* inactivation of synthetic bradykinin by the cerebral spinal fluid is very weak; the ratio of plasma CSF carboxypeptidase is very high *in vitro* (Sicuteri, 1967a; Sicuteri et al., 1967b).

If the arterial injection occurs when local circulation is arrested (as in ischemia) effects on capillaries (considerable edema) and on sensitive receptors (intolerable pain) are much increased. When kinin is concentrated in the CSF, it has a prolonged contact with capillaries, with pain receptors in the subarachnoid space, and also with CNS structures which are on the walls of the cerebral ventricles. It must be emphasized that no lumbar pain occurs when bradykinin is injected spinally and that there is a high concentration of peptide in the vertebral column after the spinal injection. At the intracranial level, however, the kinin concentration is reduced either because of inactivation or its dilution in the spinal fluid during its passage from the lumbar to the cranial region. Nevertheless, intense headache of long duration occurs. This signifies that lumbar subarachnoid structures are barely sensitive to bradykinin since in high concentration no pain is observed; intracranial subarachnoid structures are highly sensitive since even low concentrations are accompanied by intense pain.

F. Pathophysiologic Implications

There is no definite evidence to prove that kinin may have a role in circulatory disorders which arise in the cranial and spinal column interior. On the other hand, the nervous system structures, the intracranial circulation, and the CSF have an anatomic arrangement which favors the concentration of kinin that for some reason is released. In fact, in the various barriers between blood, encephalon, and the spinal fluid, the cavity of the cranium and spinal cord constitute a type of box which has minimal communication with the rest of the organism. It may be significant to demonstrate an increase of kinin concentration in the spinal fluid either because this liquid bathes particularly important and delicate nervous structures or because the circulation, production, and reabsorption of this liquid are relatively slow. In this respect, it may be hypothesized that kinin has some implications in circulatory disorders. Fundamentally, the mechanisms by which an abnormal concentration of kinin in the internum of microvessels of the cerebral parenchyma and meninges or in the CSF may be obtained are three. (1) An ischemic process consequent to a prolonged vasoconstriction as in migraine or cerebral angiospasm; the liberation of kinin in this case may be linked to an accumulation of kinin-releasing enzymes. (2) An activation of brain proteases that act on plasma kinin in extravasated blood, as can occur in cerebral apoplexy or at least in intracephalic hemorrhage. (3) An action of the permeability factor (PF/dil) that is activated when plasma becomes diluted with spinal fluid, as occurs in subarachnoid hemorrhage or in injuries including diagnostic spinal puncture that bring about subarachnoid bleeding.

During sudden fever, dilatation of cerebral vessels and intense headache are well-known phenomena, but nothing is known about the mechanisms. It is clear that vasodilatation as a cause of febrile headache—taken for granted a few years ago—is today not tenable. During fever an intense constant lowering of the kininogen level occurs and probably contributes to the general vasodilatation, headache, and perhaps to the CNS disturbances which are evident in the course of a spontaneous or pharmacologically induced hyperpyrexia.

In subjects with chronic headache, pain and vasomotor reaction provokable with histamine or histamine liberator can be completely inhibited with antihistamines. However, these agents have no effect on the pain and vasomotility induced by bradykinin or by enzymes capable of liberating kinin. The pain test in clinical pharmacology is very useful to exclude histamine as the cause of pain and vasomotility.

I. Bradykinin, Cranial Vasodilatation and Febrile Headache

Endotoxin shock is associated with a marked fall in kininogen and the liberation of kinin that may have an importance in the phenomena of shock (Corrado, 1963; Periti et al., 1963a; Amundsen and Rugstad, 1965; Trautschold et al., 1966; Goodwin and Boreham, 1966; Diniz et al., 1967; Rocha e Silva et al., 1967).

In man it was observed that the injection of a small dose of highly purified pyrogenic endotoxin (Pyrexal) produces a rapid fall of neutrophils, a hyperfibrinolysis and, successively, linked to the fall of fever, an important and constant decrease in kininogen (Sicuteri et al., 1963a).

Fever is often accompanied by headache and slight nervous disturbances. In chronic headache sufferers, the injection of endotoxin constantly provokes or exacerbates headache even before the rise of fever. Doses of endotoxin which do not cause fever can induce violent and protracted headache (Sicuteri et al., 1966a).

It has been thought that lowering of kininogen may be the consequence of liberation of lysosomal enzymes from granulocytes and from other cells by endotoxins. Indeed the β-glucuronidase activity of serum (Fishman et al., 1948), as an expression of lysosomal mobilization, is markedly elevated in man during provoked fever. It is also augmented, although not constantly, after the injection of endotoxin in nonfebrigenic doses (Bavazzano et al., 1967, 1968; Sicuteri et al., 1967b) (Fig. 13).

The thermal regulating center is not affected by exogenous pyrogen (for example endotoxin) but instead by endogenous pyrogen, with a polypeptide structure (Wood, 1958; Cooper et al., 1966). Endogenous pyrogen is located in lysosomes of granulocytes and other cells (Cohn and Hirsch, 1960; Rafter et al., 1960). Endogenous pyrogen may have a stimulatory action not only on nervous centers but also on pain receptors. The pathway would be the following: exogenous pyrogen→lysosomal enzymes→kininogen→kinin. Recent research *in vitro* supports this possibility (Greenbaum and Kim, 1967; Greenbaum et al., 1967; Melmon and Cline, 1967; Janoff and Schaeffer, 1967).

Consequently, febrile headache is not induced by vasodilatation only, as was maintained at one time (Sutherland and Wolff, 1940). Vasodilatation per se obviously is not the cause of headache; it becomes that when a congestive or chronic inflammatory situation exists in which a vasomotor stimulation (vessel pulsation) or a slight augmentation of vasoactive or algogenic substances easily exacerbates pain. Vasodilatation and above all headache during fever are only in part due to fever, because they are the consequence of kinin liberation. This liberation may depend on hyperfibrinolysis and/or the activation of lysosomal enzymes. It is interesting to note that bradykinin induces leukocytosis in dog and in man (CARDOSO et al., 1967).

Precise but nevertheless indirect information on this mechanism is furnished by clinical pharmacology. In the course of chronic spontaneous headache, bradykinin or its liberator (kallikrein and trypsin) may produce an immediate but

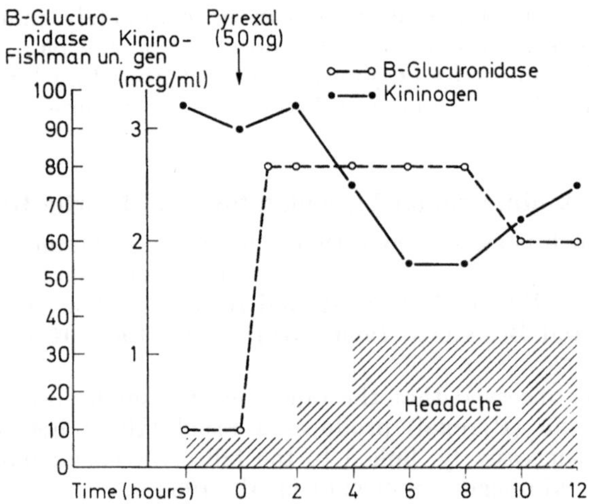

Fig. 13. Pyrogen, even in nonfebrigenic amounts, induces a long-lasting exacerbation of chronic headache. A kinin release (fall of plasma kininogen) by lysosomal labilization (increase of the serum β-glucuronidase activity) may be postulated

brief exacerbation. Cortisone does not block the action of bradykinin, trypsin, or kallikrein. It is completely ineffective against the exacerbation of spontaneous headache by these agents. Antihistamines and antiserotonins are ineffective against bradykinin or its liberators (SICUTERI et al., 1967b).

Cortisone is one of the most potent stabilizers of lysosomes in that it blocks the release of enzymes induced by well-known liberators such as endotoxins (WEISSMANN and LEWIS, 1962; WEISSMANN, 1964, 1965; WEISSMANN and THOMAS, 1964; DE DUVE and VATTIAUX, 1966). Cortisone impedes or attenuates the increase of this enzymatic activity in man when subfebrile doses of pyrogen are used.

Other substances that produce fever—steroids such as etiocholanolone and lithocholic acid (KAPPAS et al., 1956; PALMER et al., 1961) and i.d., i.m., or i.v., injection of tuberculin in subjects with tuberculin sensitivity—can also exacerbate a chronic headache when administered in nonfebrigenic doses (SICUTERI et al., 1966a). As was noted, tuberculin liberates granulocyte lysosomes indirectly after having reacted with the antibody from lymphocytes. In other words, it is the antigen–lymphocyte–antibody complex that acts like the "exogenous" liberator (ATKINS and HIJN, 1965).

II. Migraine and Other "Medical" Headache

Relationship of Intracranial Vasoactivity to Headache. Some pharmaceutical agents injected into man produce intracranial vasodilatation and headache. The shock of the blood waves on the arterial wall has been stressed as the direct cause of the pain (PICKERING and HESS, 1933; WOLFF, 1938; PICKERING, 1939; SUTHERLAND and WOLFF, 1940; WOLFF and TUNIS, 1952). This explanation of the vasodilatation headache, however, is not too convincing (LUNEDEI, 1948).

Drugs such as papaverine, which provoke intense vasodilatation, do not induce headache. Intense vasodilatation in the head can be induced by heat or by physical exercise without causing headache. In the genesis of headache, in general, direct stimulation of sensitive intracranial vascular receptors and mechanical vasodilator factors have importance. Pain-producing ability and vasodilatory potency are noted in a few compounds such as bradykinin, kallidin; histamine 48/80 B.W. also provoke vasodilatation and headache (SICUTERI et al., 1956).

Epinephrine increases the pain in chronic headache significantly; this happens also if the hormone is injected intravenously in nonvasoactive doses (SICUTERI et al., 1968). Epinephrine is able to release kinins in normal and pathological conditions (SICUTERI et al., 1962; OATES and MELMON, 1966) as well as to decrease the kininase activity of the plasma (SICUTERI et al., 1962; MASHFORD and ZACEST, 1967). The emotional exacerbation of chronic headache can be induced in part by the effect of epinephrine on kinin. Epinephrine is released in the blood stream after acute anxiety (PEKKARINEN et al., 1961).

The direct activity of bradykinin on pain receptors of the head may be demonstrated via the carotid route. Bradykinin injected into the carotid (1 μg) produces hyperemia of the face, cheeks, and conjunctiva and intense pain. These correspond to the appearance of intracranial vasodilatation as demonstrated by the electromanogram. The pain effect is independent from vasodilatation. In fact, if one occludes the carotid with digital pressure prior to the injection of the solution containing 1 μg bradykinin, not vasodilatation but a more intense pain occurs than with intact blood flow.

The pain lasts as long as carotid occlusion is maintained. When occlusion is released, pain is violently exacerbated but quickly disappears. If the dose of bradykinin, with the carotid temporarily occluded, is slightly higher (3–5 μg) the subject has scotoma and nausea together with pain. With these doses a slight palpebral and facial edema appears. By injecting bradykinin rapidly i.v., a relationship between vasodilator threshold doses and pain-producing doses may be established.

In the normal subject the vasoactive threshold doses are 10–20 μg, whereas the threshold doses for headache are 50–100 μg. The relationship then is about 1:5. The relationship of vasoactivity to pain varies profoundly (as low as 1:1) in the subject with chronic headache. Here the threshold dose for pain is considerably reduced. The relationship between vasoactivity and pain in migraine crisis may be reversed during the attack.

These data indicate that in cases of chronic headache or migraine attack the vasomotor sensitivity is constant while the threshold for pain is strongly depressed. Similar variations of the vasoactivity/pain ratio are observed with histamine (BOVET and SICUTERI, 1956) or histamine liberators, as with bradykinin (SICUTERI et al., 1961b) or bradykinin liberators (SICUTERI, 1967a, 1968). Antagonists of bradykinin, like aspirin or phenylbutazone (COLLIER and SHORLEY, 1960; BRAUN et al., 1961; KEELE and ARMSTRONG, 1968) raise the pain threshold but leave the intracranial vasoactivity unchanged. These variations in the vasoactivity and pain relationship resulting from administration of aspirin or phenylbutazone are very marked in headache (Sicuteri, 1967a, b).

Such variations are probably tied to the specific analgesic activity of these agents and less likely to their antibradykinin potency.

Pathophysiological Perspectives. The more important objective phenomena in migraine attack, within the vascular area of the head, are: the dilation of the temporal artery, conjunctival vessels, vessels of the nasal mucosa and the palpebral edema. During an attack a depression of the pain threshold, especially in the subcutaneous and perivascular tissue, has been demonstrated (Tunis et al., 1953). Here the developing edema is rich in permeability-enhancing and pain-producing substances.

Research on headache also pointed out the importance of biogenic amines—in particular, histamine (Greppi and Martinetti, 1948; Arcangeli and Galletti, 1953) and mast cell activation (Sicuteri et al., 1956; Sicuteri, 1963). As noted, 48/80 B.W. does not act directly but by producing degranulation of tissue mast cell.

The degranulation of mast cells frees endogenous substances, histamine, serotonin and, indirectly, bradykinin (Periti et al., 1964), which act on pain receptors and vessels. The possibility was therefore raised that in migraine attack not the newly formed substances but those already existing in the organism may have importance. These substances have a dual action—on pain receptors on the one hand and on microvessels on the other. The study, then, was concentrated on three principal vasoneuroactive substances (VNS), bradykinin, serotonin, and histamine, which are probably involved in painful vascular phenomena of the attack (Sicuteri, 1959b, 1963, 1967a). So the unitarian biochemical concept of the migraine attack (pain, vasodilatation, and nervous disorders) was considered.

In conformity with this concept, the use of lysergic acid derivatives with antiserotonin activity, particularly methysergide (Doepfner and Cerletti, 1958; Gelfand and West, 1961) were proposed (Sicuteri, 1959b).

A substance similar to but not identical with bradykinin (perhaps a mixture of different VNS), named neurokinin, was identified in subcutaneous perfusate during a migraine attack (Chapman and Wolff, 1959; Chapman et al., 1960a, b). In the CSF during severe migraine, an increased proteolytic activity was noted and therefore, in a broad sense, kinin-liberating activity (Chapman and Wolff, 1959). Nevertheless, other scientists did not confirm these data (Hilton and Schain, 1961; Coppen and Lewis, 1961).

Possibility bradykinin is one of the VNS that is formed during migraine attack. The etiology of migraine in general and of the migraine attack is yet obscure. The migraine patient is presumably a "hyperreactor" at the cranial and brain vascular level. This hyperactivity conditions an excess of chemical mediators, which have the ability to act on the tone and permeability of capillaries (Sicuteri, 1967a). The more important biochemical data in migraine attack are represented by (1) the increased excretion of vanylmandelic acid, a metabolite of catecholamines (Sicuteri et al., 1967a); (2) an increased urinary excretion of 5-hydroxyindoleacetic acid, a metabolite of serotonin (Sicuteri et al., 1961a; Lance et al., 1967; Antony et al., 1967); (3) a decrease of plasma kininogen at the end of the crisis (Sicuteri, 1967a); and (4) an increase of kinin liberation in plasma especially at the end of the crisis (Armstrong, Mills, and Sicuteri, unpublished data).

Probably the prime mover of the attack is a prolonged vasoconstriction, not in generalized but in circumscribed areas of the intra- and extracerebral resistance microvessels (including the vasa vasorum). The vasoconstriction induces the accumulation and intense action of the principal agents such as serotonin, liberated mainly from platelets, bradykinin liberated from its plasma precursor, and perhaps histamine liberated from mast cells. A moderate edema, rich in VNS, forms outside the cerebrum in meningeal and cranial vasculature, which condition the pain.

The liberation of lysosomal enzymes, the increase of fibrinolytic activity (KWAAN and McFADZEAN, 1956), the lowering of the kininogen, and the passage of serotonin from cells into the plasma (HORTON, 1964; SICUTERI, 1967a) during circulatory arrest may be important here. Bradykinin and serotonin have an additive effect at the level of sensitive receptors in man (SICUTERI et al., 1965a), in animal (GILFOIL and KLAVINS, 1965), and at the capillary level as well (ZWEIFACH, 1966), with a resultant heightened edema formation and algogenic effect.

Trasylol (100,000 KIE) given intravenously at the beginning of the crisis has no effect. Probably more importance can be attributed to the presence of catecholamines and serotonin (SICUTERI, 1967b; SICUTERI et al., 1968). When reserpine is injected in small doses in the "resting" stage, almost always a typical attack is started. Interestingly, reserpine, taken chronically, constitutes perhaps the most efficacious treatment to dispel the migraine crisis. Unfortunately, reserpine may be used only with caution as a therapeutic agent, since it induces arterial hypotension; moreover migraine sufferers are particularly sensitive to the nervous depressor effect of reserpine. To support the important role of serotonin, it can be recalled that the most effective drugs in the basic therapy of migraine are antiserotonins. Therapeutically, chemicals differing in structure such as methysergide (SICUTERI, 1959a; DALESSIO et al., 1961; FRIEDMAN and ELKIND, 1961; EKBOM, 1962; GREPPI and SICUTERI, 1964) and the "antiamine" BC-105 (SICUTERI et al., 1967c), have equal antimigraine action.

III. Subarachnoid Hemorrhage

Clinical Aspects. Spontaneous subarachnoid hemorrhage (SH) occurs for the most part in cases of rupture of an intracranial aneurysm. In this accident a certain quantity of blood diffuses into the subarachnoid space and mixes with CSF

The more salient symptom is sudden headache (called because of its violence the boxer's blow), followed by stupor that may lead to coma, and signs of meningitis, with more or less marked nuchal rigidity. The mechanism of these clinical phenomena is not known. [We exclude consideration of intracranial hypertension because per se it is not the cause of headache (WOLFF, 1963) and because a spinal fluid hypertension is not always encountered in SH.] WOLFF (1963) proposed as a cause a distension by mechanical traction of distensible intracranial structures by blood erupting with violence into the meningeal spaces. Obviously this may not have a value in cases of SH where bleeding is slow and gradual. It is possible that at least a part of the phenomena of SH is tied to biochemical factors. One of these may be kinin liberated in CSF by dilution (SICUTERI, 1966).

When the plasma of extravasated blood in the subarachnoid space mixes and becomes diluted with CSF, permeability factor (PF/dil) becomes activated. This factor is able to liberate a major part of the bradykinin from plasma kininogen. This was demonstrated *in vitro* (MACKAY et al., 1953; MILES and WILHELM, 1955; MILES, 1961; ELDER and WILHELM, 1958). Subarachnoid hemorrhage (SICUTERI, 1966) is one of the pathological conditions (LANDERMAN et al., 1960; BECKER and KAGEN, 1964) where permeability factor may be involved, particularly in the pathogenesis of some of the clinical phenomena such as the violent initial headache and in part the meningeal reactions and CNS phenomena. The permeability factor in SH liberates kinin from plasma of extravasated blood. Human plasma diluted with homologous human CSF releases *in vitro* a quantity of kinin slightly less that is liberated by incubating the same quantity of plasma with Ringer's solution. The production of kinin perhaps is slightly less because in spinal fluid there is some weak kininase activity. This activity is much less than in plasma (Sicuteri et al., 1967a).

Bradykinin, injected into the cisterna of rabbits, induces a characteristic behavioral reaction. In some animals concentrations of the order of 500 ng bradykinin/kg are sufficient to provoke the reaction. No other biological substance (histamine, serotonin, catecholamine) or other peptide (eledoisin, physalaemin, angiotensin, vasopressin) can cause this that has all the appearance of a behavioral reaction to violent pain. As shown on p. 489, man is extremely sensitive to the action of bradykinin.

The observation that indomethacin, given i.m. or i.v., is the most effective agent to inhibit the squeaking-flight reaction of the rabbit and at the same time the cephalic reaction to bradykinin and to homologous plasma given spinally in man, is significant. In a few recent cases of SH we showed an elevation of kinin concentration in CSF (5–12–25 ng/ml), whereas in normal conditions kinin can hardly be measured (0.2–1 ng) (Sicuteri et al., 1963b).

Unfortunately, it is not easy to collect spinal fluid in cases of recently developed SH. After some hours kinin is no longer found in CSF. The inactivation *in vivo* of synthetic bradykinin is not very rapid in the rabbit. One hour after the cisternal injection of 1 μg bradykinin/kg, a certain quantity of kinin remains. In man, 20 minutes after the spinal injection of 2 μg of synthetic bradykinin, small quantities of kinin are still detectable; after 40 minutes no activity remains.

Regarding the nervous symptoms of SH (somnolence, stupor, and finally coma) kinins probably have no decisive role. Bradykinin, however, given spinally (and still more markedly, homologous plasma) induces a state of somnolence and rather marked stupor. The rabbit also remains prostrate and hypoactive for about an hour after cisternal injection. This may be due (p. 495) to the depletion of catecholamine in brain by cisternally injected bradykinin (Graeff et al., 1967).

In the dog (Bertolini et al., 1966), no vocalization occurs after the cisternal injection of bradykinin, but a marked catatonic state appears. The animal assumes a particular and unusual position and maintains it for a certain time. It is not likely that kinin provokes the aseptic meningitis that develops in SH after 1 to 2 days. This is possibly linked to the activation of plasmin and other proteases of which the meninges have a rich supply (Astrup and Permin, 1947). Also, the headache that develops in some cases after diagnostic spinal puncture is probably due to small amounts of bleeding provoked by the needle wound and release of kinin by CSF plasma dilution (Sicuteri, 1966). The nervous meningeal reaction, however, that appears some time after the diagnostic spinal puncture, is clinically indistinguishable from the reaction that is obtained from the spinal injection of homologous plasma.

These clinical pharmacologic observations and experiments indicate that a part of the clinical syndrome of SH may be correlated with plasma dilution. Other factors in blood as well may contribute to the syndrome (Eisen and Keele. 1966; Keele and Armstrong, 1968).

IV. Experimental Kinin Release and Clearance in the CSF *in vivo*

An introduction of bradykinin into the CSF induces important behavioral phenomena in the experimental animal (p. 430) (CAPEK, 1961; SICUTERI et al., 1966b; BERTOLINI et al., 1966; GRAEFF et al., 1967).

These behavioral reactions may be due in part to the action of the peptide on sensitive intracranial receptors and therefore caused by CNS actions of bradykinin (CORRADO et al., 1959; BUCKLEY et al., 1963; KRIVOY et al., 1963; HAEFELY et al., 1966). The simpler spontaneous mechanism by which kinin is liberated

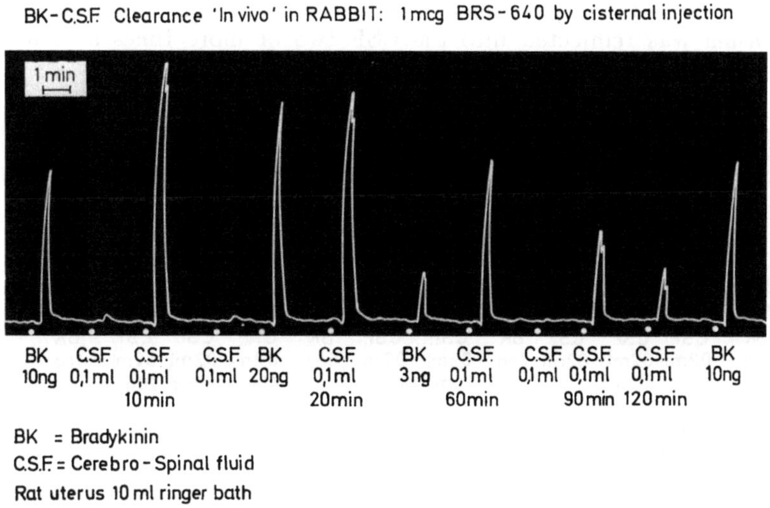

Fig. 14. Synthetic bradykinin (BRS-640) is inactivated slowly in CSF of the rabbit *in vivo*. Substantial quantities of the peptide were recovered 1 hour after suboccipital injection. (Intervals between tests are shortened in the figure)

and concentrated in the CSF is the dilution of blood by CSF when blood extravasates, from traumatic or spontaneous causes, into the subarachnoid space (SICUTERI, 1966, 1968).

When plasma is diluted *in vitro* with human CSF, a liberation of kinin occurs with a prolonged latency and intensity comparable to that of the dilution of plasma with Ringer's solution. CSF inactivates synthetic bradykinin very slowly (SICUTERI et al., 1966), whereas plasma has a higher activity (ERDÖS and WOHLER, 1963; ERDÖS et al., 1963). Two questions remain open. (1) Is the clearance of kinin or of synthetic bradykinin in the CSF *in vivo* relatively more rapid and intense? (2) Is plasma, injected *in vivo* into the CSF able to liberate kinin?

It was demonstrated (SICUTERI et al., in press) that in the recovery of bradykinin, injected into the cisterna magna of the rabbit, the time interval following the injection is important: 30–40 minutes after injection of 1 μg/kg, samples from the cisterna magna still contain large quantities of bradykinin (20–25–30 ng/kg) (Fig. 14). In man, 15–20 minutes after the spinal injection of 30 μg/kg of bradykinin, measurable concentrations of the peptide still remain (Fig. 15). The injection of 0.1 ml "preactive" human plasma/kg (collected in siliconized glass) into the cisterna magna of the rabbit results in a prolonged liberation of kinin into the CSF. *In vivo* the latency of kinin appearance is slightly prolonged; the peak of liberation is slightly retarded and less pronounced and the decrease of action is earlier than in experiments *in vitro*. In conclusion, the phenomenon *in vivo* parallels the process *in vitro*, except that it is less intense. After 10 minutes kinin can be found in the CSF *in vivo* and after 20–25 minutes is still present. After 40–45 minutes, it has disappeared altogether. Human plasma was used instead of rabbit plasma because the plasma of the rabbit behaves differently when diluted (SCHACHTER, 1956).

In human volunteers who had to undergo spinal puncture for diagnostic reasons, 10 minutes after the spinal injection of 1 ml of homologous plasma, large quantities of kinin were demonstrable in the CSF. The peak was reached in 10–15 minutes and then a complete disappearance of kinin occurred. It must be emphasized that the phenomenon observed *in vivo* is not tachyphylactic. When plasma was reinjected into the CSF two or more times at intervals of

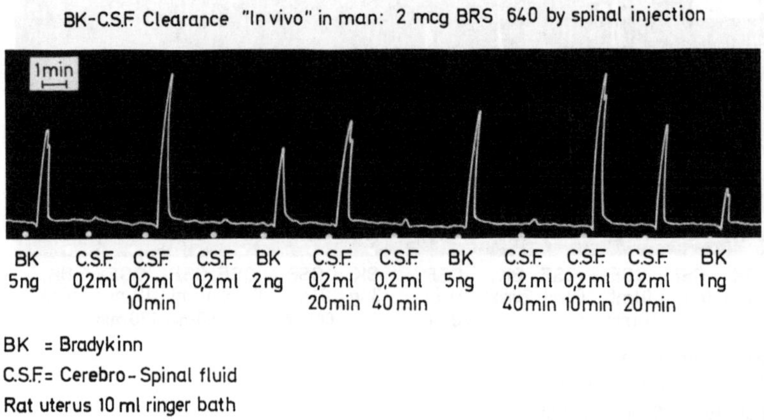

Fig. 15. The inactivation of synthetic bradykinin injected spinally to man is rather slow. About 25 ng/ml of BK equivalent kinins are detectable in CSF, 20 min after administration. (Intervals between tests are shortened in the figure)

20–30 minutes, the same quantity of kinin was found as after the first spinal injection.

These experiments indicate that the clearance of kinin and of synthetic bradykinin in the CSF is rather slow. The observations support the hypothesis that hemorrhage into the CSF is followed by a more or less abundant and protracted liberation of kinin. Studies (p. 494) dealing with the effects of the spinal or cisternal injection of kinin or bradykinin to man or animal indicate that elevated concentrations of kinin in the CSF may contribute to the symptoms that follow SH.

It should be stressed again that in man the spinal injection of 2–3 ml of homologous plasma constantly provokes headache, fever, sleep, and nuchal rigidity—that is, in reduced proportions, the more characteristic symptoms of subarachnoid hemorrhage.

The use of indomethacin, phenylbutazone, and aspirin, and to a lesser degree cortisone, after the plasma injection, prevents all the phenomena mentioned above.

V. Cerebral Stroke

Cerebral apoplexy in most cases is due to a ruptured blood vessel within the brain. The hemorrhagic infarct, in general, remains circumscribed; at other times blood extravasates into a cerebral ventricle or, more rarely, into the subarachnoid space. Around the center of the hemorrhagic infarct a halo of injured tissue is visible, which is principally due to the edema of nervous tissue. Clinical observations of the symptoms indicate that the nervous tissue damage is partially reversible.

In fact, the regression of an initially complete hemiplegia is frequently verified clinically after a few day or weeks. Typical is the syndrome of alternating familiar hemiplegia, often associated with severe forms of migraine (Jelliffe, 1906; Clarke, 1910; Whitty, 1953; Wolff, 1963). These forms are defined as "serous apoplexy" to indicate precisely the importance of edema as a pathogenic factor. It is unlikely that the ability of hemiparesis or hemiplegia to regress totally or partially can be associated simply with the length of the ischemic process. In fact, it has been well documented that nervous tissue tolerates absolute anoxia for only a very short time before irreversible damage occurs.

Cerebral edema acts not only as a condition that contributes to oxygen reduction in the tissue but also acts on nervous structures through some biochemical substances present in the edema fluid.

The "functio laesa" occurs in part in cerebral apoplexy, and more extensively in "serous apoplexy"; it may be partially due to the direct action of biochemical substances on the nervous system. This is the concept of autopharmacodynamism (Rocha e Silva, 1950), which underscores the fact that certain phenomena are the consequence of some tissue damage, not by the direct action of anoxia but by the action of substances which are liberated at the time of tissue injury.

The encephalon has a particular disposition for edema as neurosurgeons well know. What is the mechanism of cerebral edema? It is probably not purely nervous but is biochemically mediated; that is, by substances which increase the permeability of vessels. Probably serotonin, and substance P (Zetler and Lembeck, 1962) kinins, but not histamine, are involved here.

We have only indirect data to suggest the importance of kinin liberation in the pathology of cerebral apoplexy. In the course of such an episode, if there has been serious injury of nervous parenchyma, hemorrhagic sphacelation of a part of the encephalon occurs. As in all inflammatory necrotic damaging processes, it is likely that tissue proteases are activated (Astrup and Permin, 1947; De Duve 1959; Back, 1960; Bertelli et al., 1962; Vogt, 1964; Webster and Innerfield, 1965; Back et al., 1966).

The early hyperfibrinolysis in blood of the systemic circulation was noted as early as the first hour in some cases after cerebral stroke (Lunedei et al., 1957). It is possible that the kininogen of extravasated blood, or that remaining in capillaries in the immediate vicinity, becomes transformed to active kinin. The same slowing or stasis of local circulation, associated with a lowering of tissue pH, increases the permeability of capillaries (edema) and therefore the arrival of more blood into the capillaries with normal content of kininogen. This new kininogen will also be transformed into active kinin by local kininogenases; thus edema will spread like a spot of oil. Given that we do not have at our disposal specific antibradykinin agents (Collier and Shorley, 1960), we can use drugs that block the activation of kallikrein. One can expect that antikallikrein drugs of the Trasylol type may interrupt the vicious cycle, sustained mainly by kininogenases.

If this hypothesis is true, a reduction of edema and of the focal hemorrhage may be expected with the use of antikallikreins. Therefore an easily reproducible square of cerebral hemorrhage was induced in an animal. In the rat, guinea pig, or rabbit a circumscribed lesion was inflicted on the cerebral hemisphere with a fine electric drill, in a preestablished, fixed point. The animal tolerated the lesion perfectly. Autopsy revealed a small hole in the hemisphere without a hemorrhagic halo. If the animal, at the moment of the mechanical lesion, was treated with heparin, a square of hemorrhage occured whose severity was in strict relationship with the dose of heparin. A $LD_{50}/24$ hr dose of heparin can be established. A slight heparinization that modestly increases the coagulation time by some minutes (in the rat for example from 2 to 10 minutes), was used. The clinical square of hemorrhage treated with the $LD_{50}/24$ hr dose resembles in some ways cerebral apoplexy. The animal becomes hyporeactive, a times manifesting a paresis or paralysis of a contralateral paw. An hour later

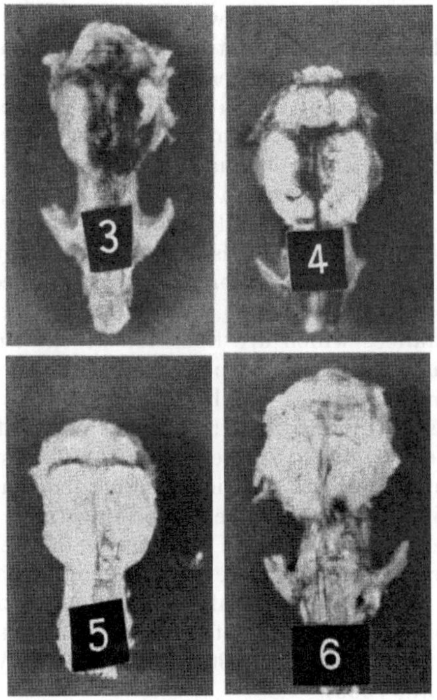

Fig. 16. Trasylol (*6*) and to a lesser extent EACA (*5*) are able to inhibit the induced intracranial hemorrhage in rats; only the hole of the drill (see text) is observable. Chymotrypsin (*4*) reduces the hemorrhage, but cortisone (*3*) does not protect the animals: infarction and subarachnoid hemorrhage are indistinguishable from those of control

the animal becomes sleepy and either enters into coma and dies or recovers after 24–48 hours. Autopsy reveals that in the heparinized animal an ample hemorrhagic halo is formed around the point of the lesion. A broad study with rats and guinea pigs was conducted (Sicuteri et al., 1967a) to observe which substances (but obviously not heparin antagonists) would protect. While anti-edema, anti-inflammatory drugs (e.g. cortisone, indomethacin, antiserotonins, and antihistamines) were ineffective, 97% of the rats pretreated with the kallikrein inhibitor Trasylol survived the $LD_{50}/24$ hr dose of heparin. Notably, Trasylol has no anticoagulant effect but only an antifibrinolytic action. ε-Aminocaproic acid (EACA), an antifibrinolytic agent, is active but less effective than Trasylol. Chymotrypsin, which has a kininase action, inhibits somewhat.

The autopsy of animals protected with Trasylol reveals only the drill hole on the encephalon, practically indistinguishable from unheparinized control animals (Fig. 16). The protection by kallikrein inhibitor, and to lesser degree by

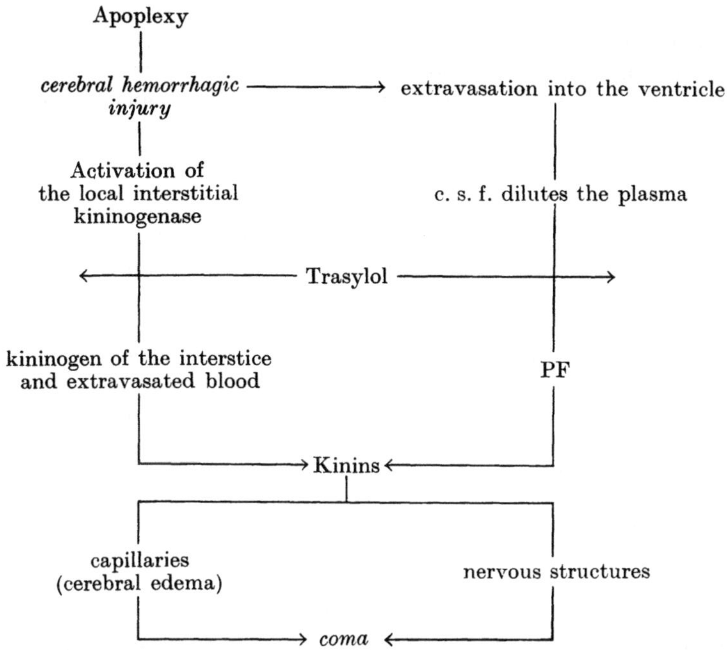

Fig. 17. In apoplexy kinins may be released by local proteases, activated by hemorrhagic injury. If blood extravasates into the ventricles also, the dilution mechanism is involved. Trasylol may act in both mechanism

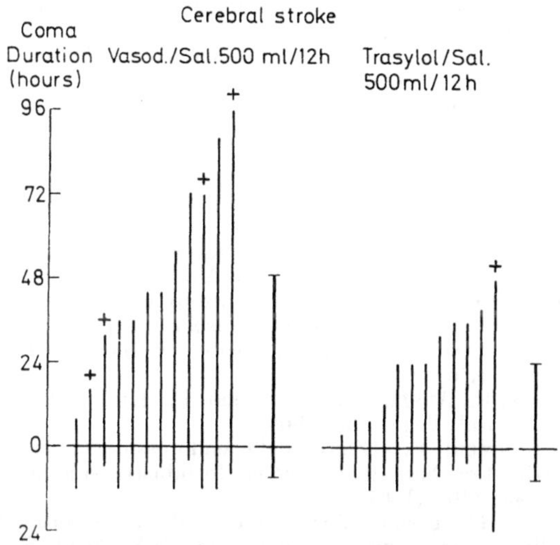

Fig. 18. The average duration of coma in a group of 12 patients with cerebral stroke, treated with Trasylol, is roughly one half that of a similar control group treated conventionally. The number of deaths is also reduced in the Trasylol group. The duration of coma before the hospitalization and start of the conventional or Trasylol treatment is shown below the base line

EACA, indicates that the local activation of fibrinolytic and kinin-liberating proteases has an important role in the pathogenesis of hemorrhagic infarct in the experimental animal (SICUTERI et al., 1967a).

This protease activation is in the interior of the primary lesion and conditions the spread of the hemorrhage at "blot of oil" and therefore the aggravation of clinical phenomena until coma and death. Kinin may be implicated in the aggravation of cerebral apoplexy. In cerebral apoplexy, associated with a flood of blood into the cerebral ventricles, another mechanism of kinin release is added, namely, dilution of plasma which was discussed in the section on subarachnoid hemorrhage (Fig. 17).

Trasylol acts here by antagonizing the dilution factor, as shown *in vitro* (Sicuteri, 1968). In a restricted number of patients with cerebral apoplexy, a treatment with Trasylol in high doses by i.v. infusion had a beneficial effect. As parameters, the duration of coma and survival were considered (Sicuteri, 1968).

Comparison of an equal number of patients with cerebral stroke, treated with infusions of saline and with papaverine, demonstrates a noticeable difference, with a reduction in duration of coma and a lowering of the mortality rate in the Trasylol group (Fig. 18).

This experiment forms a pilot study. The theoretical premises and the results obtained with the antikallikrein in experimental intracranial hemorrhage seem to justify, however, broader clinical-therapeutic investigations.

References

Allwood, M. J., Lewis, G. P.: Bradykinin in human blood during vasodilation. J. Physiol. (Lond.) **166**, 47P (1963).

— — Bradykinin and forearm blood flow. J. Physiol. (Lond.) **170**, 571 (1964).

Amundsen, E., Rugstad, H. E.: Influence of some pathogenic bacteria on kinin formation and destruction. Brit. J. Pharmacol. **25**, 67 (1965).

Antony, M., Hinterberger, H., Lance, J. W.: Plasma serotonin in migraine and stress. Arch. Neurol. (Chic.) **16**, 544 (1967).

Arcangeli, P., Galletti, R.: La cefalea da istamina. Rass. Neurol. veg. **10**, 109 (1953).

Armstrong, D., Jepson, J. B., Keele, C. A., Stewart, J. W.: Pain producing substance in human inflammatory exudates and plasma. J. Physiol. (Lond.) **135**, 350 (1957).

— Mills, G. L., Sicuteri, F.: Physiological influence on the liberation of human plasma kinin at low temperature. In: Hypotensive peptides, p. 139, ed. by E. G. Erdös, N. Back and F. Sicuteri. Berlin-Heidelberg-New York: Springer 1966.

Astrup, T., Permin, P. M.: Fibrinolysis in the animal organism. Nature (Lond.) **159**, 681 (1947).

Atkins, E., Hijn, C., Jr.: Studies on tubercolin fever. III. Mechanism involved in the release of endogenous pyrogen in vitro. J. exp. Med. **122**, 207 (1965).

Back, N.: In vivo formation of a vasodilator substance by plasmin. Fed. Proc. **19**, 55 (1960).

— Wilkens, H., Steger, R.: Fibrinolysis and vasoactive peptides in anaphylaxis. In: Hypotensive peptides, p. 485, ed. by E. G. Erdös, N. Back and F. Sicuteri. Berlin-Heidelberg-New York: Springer 1966.

Bavazzano, A., Del Bene, E., Anselmi, B., Sicuteri, F.: Kinin release by lysosomal labilization in man. Rass. Neurol. Veg. **1**, 56 (1968).

— Fanciullacci, M., Sicuteri, F.: Effetto delle endotossine in dosi subfebbrili su alcuni livelli plasmatici enzimatici (beta-glucuronidasi, fosfatasi) e sulla diuresi nell'uomo. Boll. Soc. ital. Biol. sper. **43**, 1403 (1967).

Becker, E. L., Kagen, L.: The permeability globulins of human serum and the biochemical mechanism of hereditary angioneurotic edema. Ann. N.Y. Acad. Sci. **116**, 866 (1964).

Beretta, A. A., Feruglio, F. S., Campus, S., Chiandussi, L., Pandolfo, G., Bert, G.: The effect of eledoisin and bradykinin in the general and visceral circulation. In: Hypotensive peptides, p. 430, ed. by E. G. Erdös, N. Back and F. Sicuteri. Berlin-Heidelberg-New York: Springer 1966.

Bertaccini, G., Cei, J. M., Erspamer, V.: The action of physalaemin on the systemic arterial blood pressure of some experimental animals. Brit. J. Pharmacol. **25**, 380 (1965).

Bertelli, A., Proto, M., Rossano, M. A.: Azione inibente dell'acido epsilon aminocaproico sui fenomeni essudativi ed infiammatori. Atti Accad. med. lombarda **17**, 204 (1962).

BERTOLINI, A., CASTELLI, M., MUCCI, P , STERNIERI, E : Relationship between behavioural effect and circulatory changes produced by intra-carotid bradykinin. Proceedings, Internat Symposium on the Pharmacology of Hormonal Polypeptides and Proteins. Milan, Sept. 1968. New York: Plenum Publ. Corpor. 1968.

— MUCCI, P., FERRARI, W.: La bradichinina come possibile agente causale dell' emicrania. III. Effetto dell'iniezione endocisternale di bradichinina nel cane e nel coniglio. Boll. Soc. ital. Biol. sper. **42**, 1922 (1966).

— — STERNIERI, E.: La bradichinina come possibile agente causale dell' emicrania. IV. Rapporto tra gli effetti comportamentali e circolatorio della bradichinina, iniettata per via endocarotidea nel coniglio. Boll. Soc. ital. Biol. sper. **43**, 794 (1967).

BOBBIN, R. P., GUTH, P. S.: Venoconstrictive action of bradykinin. J. Pharmacol. exp. Ther. **160**, 11 (1967).

BOVET, E., CARPI, A., VIRNO, M.: Pharmacodynamie de la circulation cérébrale. Experientia (Basel) **16**, 1 (1960).

— SICUTERI, F.: Vasomotricité cérébrale et allergie. Physiopatologie de la céphalée provoquée par l'histamine. Relazione, 3d Congr. Europeo di Allergologia, vol. II. Rome: Pensiero Scientifico 1956.

BRAUN, C., GUZMAN, F., HORTON, E. W., LIM, E. K. S., POTTER, G. D.: Visceral receptors, pain, bradykinin and analgesic agents. J. Physiol. (Lond.) **155**, 13 (1961).

BREDA, G., CONCIOLI, M., MARIANI, L.: Shock anafilattico e bradichinina: Confronto tra le modificazioni del circolo corticopiale della cavia. Atti Accad. med. lombarda **17**, 335 (1962).

BUCKLEY, J. P., BICKERTON, R. K., HALLIDAY, R. P., KATO, H.: Central effects of peptides on the cardiovascular system. Ann. N.Y. Acad. Sci. **104**, 299 (1963).

CAPEK, R.: Some effects of bradykinin on the central systems. Biochem. Pharmacol. **10**, 61 (1961).

CARDOSO, S. S., AMORIN, O. S., NOGUEIRA, A. D., ALENCAR, J. A., CORRADO, A. P., REGO, S. M.: Bradykinin induced leukocytosis in man and in dogs. Proceedings, Internat. Symposium on Vaso-Active Polypeptides, p. 263, ed. by M. ROCHA E SILVA and H. A. ROTHSCHILD. Sao Paulo 1967.

CARPI, A., CORRADO, A. P.: Cerebral vascular action of bradykinin in the dog. Experientia (Basel) **17**, 326 (1961).

CHAPMAN, L. F., RAMOS, A. O., CORRADO, A. P., FORTES, V.: Release of proteolytic enzymes from cat brain during stimulation. Arch. Neurol. (Chic.) **3**, 43 (1960a).

— — GOODELL, H., SILVERMAN, G., WOLFF, H. G.: A humoral agent implicated in vascular headache of the migraine type. Arch. Neurol. (Chic.) **3**, 223 (1960b).

— WOLFF, H. G.: Studies of proteolytic enzymes in cerebrospinal fluid. Arch. intern. Med. **103**, 86 (1959).

CLARKE, J. M.: On recurrent motor paralysis in migraine: With report of a family in which recurrent hemiplegia accompanied the attacks. Brit. med. J. **1910 I**, 1534.

CLINE, M. J., MELMON, K. L.: The effect of cortisol on the plasma kinin system. Proceedings, Internat. Symposium on Vaso-Active Polypeptides, p. 247, ed. by M. ROCHA E SILVA and H. A. ROTHSCHILD. Sao Paulo 1967.

COHN, Z. A., HIRSCH, J. G.: The isolation and properties of the specific cytoplasmic granules of rabbit polymorphonuclear leucocytes. J. exp. Med. **112**, 983 (1960).

COLLIER, H. O. J., SHORLEY, P. G.: Analgesic antipyretic drugs as antagonists of bradykinin. Brit. J. Pharmacol. **15**, 601 (1960).

CONCIOLI, M., SANTANDREA, E., VILLANI, R.: Modificazioni del circolo piale sotto l'influsso di particolari stimoli e soprattutto della bradichinina. Rilievi microcinematografici. Atti Accad. med. lombarda **16**, 268 (1961).

COOPER, K. E., CRANSTON, W. I., HONOUR, M. R. C.: The site of action of leucocyte pyrogen in the rabbit brain. J. Physiol. (Lond.) **18**, 1 (1966).

COPPEN, A. J., LEWIS, G. P.: An enzyme forming vasodilator polypeptides in human cerebrospinal fluid. J. Neurochem. **7**, 155 (1961).

CORRADO, A. P.: Recent investigations of the pharmacology of bradykinin and their physiopathological implications. In: Bradykinin and its precursor, ed. by F. SICUTERI. Settim. med. Suppl., **45**, 30 (1963).

— RAMOS, A. O., ROCHA E SILVA, M.: Possiveis acoes centrais da bradicinina. Ciencia e Cultura **11**, 165 (1959).

DALESSIO, D. J., CAMP, W. A., GOODELL, H., WOLFF, H. G.: Studies on headache. The mode of action of UML-491 and its relevance to the nature of vascular headache of the migraine type. Arch. Neurol. (Chic.) **4**, 235 (1961).

DE DUVE, C.: Lysosomes: A new group of cytoplasmic particles. In: Subcellular particles, p. 128, ed. by T. HAYASHI. New York: Ronald Press Co. 1959.

— VATTIAUX, R.: Function of lysosomes. Ann. Rev. Physiol. **28**, 435 (1966).

Dessy, P., Uslenghi, E., Cagna, C., Accatino, G., Betti, C.: Azione della bradichinina sull' emodinamica generale e distrettuale. Circolo cerebrale. Minerva med. **57**, 3555 (1966).
Diniz, C. R., Carvalho, L. F., Dos Reis, M. L., Corrado, A. P.: Bradykininogen in some experimental conditions. Proceedings, Internat. Symposium on Vaso-Active Polypeptides, p. 15, ed. by M. Rocha e Silva and H. A. Rothschild. Sao Paulo 1967.
— — Rocha e Silva, M.: A micromethod for the determination of bradykininogen in the blood plasma. Nature (Lond.) **192**, 1194 (1961).
Doepfner, W., Cerletti, A.: Comparison of lysergic acid derivates and antihistamines as inhibitor of the edema provoked in the rat's paw by serotonin. Int. Arch. Allergy **12**, 89 (1958).
Eisen, V., Keele, C. A.: Possible modes of kinin formation in some pathological states in man. In: Hypotensive peptides, p. 551, ed. by E. G. Erdös, N. Back and F. Sicuteri. Berlin-Heidelberg-New York: Springer 1966.
Ekbom, K. A.: Treatment of migraine, Horton's syndrome and restless legs with Deseril (UML-491). Acta neurol. scand. **38**, 313 (1962).
Elder, J. M., Wilhelm, D. L.: Enzyme-like globulins from serum reproducing the vascular phenomena of inflammation. V. Activable permeability factor in human serum. Brit. J. exp. Path. **39**, 23 (1958).
Erdös, E. G.: Hypotensive peptides. Bradykinin, kallidin and eledoisin. Advanc. Pharmacol. **4**, 1 (1966).
— Sloane, E. M.: An enzyme in human blood plasma that inactivates bradykinin and kallidin. Biochem. Pharmacol. **11**, 585 (1962).
— Wohler, J. R.: Inhibitors of the in vivo effects of bradykinin and kallidin. Life Sci. **2**, 270 (1963).
— — Levine, M. I.: Blocking of the in vivo effects of bradykinin with carboxypeptidase B. J. Pharmacol. exp. Ther. **142**, 327 (1963).
Erspamer, V.: Pharmacologically active substances of mammalian origin. Ann. Rev. Pharmacol. **1**, 175 (1961).
— Anastasi, A.: Structure and pharmacological actions of eledoisin, the active endecapeptide of the posterior glands of eledone. Experientia (Basel) **18**, 58 (1962).
— — Bertaccini, G., Cei, J. M.: Structure and pharmacological actions of physalaemin, the main active polypeptides of the skin of *Physalaemus fuscumaculatus*. Experientia (Basel) **20**, 489 (1964).
— Glässer, A.: The action of eledoisin on the systemic arterial blood pressure of some experimental animals. Brit. J. Pharmacol. **20**, 516 (1963).
Fishman, W. H., Springer, B., Brunetti, R.: Application of an improved glucuronidase assay method to the study of human blood beta-glucuronidase. J. biol. Chem. **173**, 449 (1948).
Friedmann, A. P., Elkind, A.: Appraisal of methysergide in treatment of vascular headache of migraine type. J. Amer. med. Ass. **184**, 125 (1961).
Gelfand, M. D., West, G. B.: Experimental studies with the butanolamide and propanolamide of 1-methyl-lysergic acid. Int. Arch. Allergy **18**, 288 (1961).
Gilfoil, T. M., Klavins, I.: 5-Hydroxytryptamine, bradykinin and histamine as mediators of inflammatory hyperesthesia. Amer. J. Physiol. **208**, 867 (1965).
Goodwin, L. G., Boreham, P. F. L.: Pharmacologically active peptides in trypanosome infections. In: Hypotensive peptides, p. 545, ed. by E. G. Erdös, N. Back and F. Sicuteri. Berlin-Heidelberg-New York: Springer 1966.
Graeff, F. G., Corrado, A. P., Pela, J. P., Capek, R.: Actions of bradykinin upon the central nervous system. Proceedings, Internat. Symposium on Vaso-Active Polypeptides, p. 97, ed. by M. Rocha e Silva and H. A. Rothschild. Sao Paulo 1967.
— Ferreira, S. H., Corrado, A. P., Rocha e Silva, M.: Potentiation of the cerebral vascular action of bradykinin by the bradykinin potentiating factor (BPF) in the dog. Experientia (Basel) **21**, 607 (1965).
Greenbaum, L. M., Kim, K. S.: The kinin-forming and kininase activities of rabbit polymorphonuclear leucocytes. Brit. J. Pharmacol. **29**, 372 (1967).
— Yamafuji, K., Kim, K. S.: Studies on the kinin-forming and inactivating enzymes in tissue and leucocytes. Proceedings, Internat. Symposium on Vaso-Active Polypeptides, p. 21, ed. by M. Rocha e Silva and H. A. Rothschild. Sao Paulo 1967.
Greppi, E., Martinetti, R.: Le cefalee. Proceedings, 49th Congr. Ital. Soc. of Internal Medicine. Rome: Pozzi 1948.
— Sicuteri, F.: L'Emicrania-motivi di fisiopatogenesi e di terapia. Proceedings, 65th Congr. Ital. Soc. of Internal Medicine. Rome: Pozzi 1964.
Haefely, W., Hurlimann, A., Thoenen, H.: The effects of bradykinin and angiotensin on ganglionic transmission. In: Hypotensive peptides, p. 314, ed. by E. G. Erdös, N. Back and F. Sicuteri. Berlin-Heidelberg-New York: Springer 1966.

HILTON, S. M., SCHAIN, R. J.: A search for pharmacologically active substances in fluid from the cerebral ventricles. J. Physiol. (Lond.) **157**, 46P (1961).
HORTON, E. W.: An increase in butanol-extractable 5-hydroxytryptamine in venous blood during reactive hyperemia. J. Physiol. (Lond.) **170**, 101 (1964).
JANOFF, A., SCHAEFFER, S.: Mediators of acute inflammation in leucocyte lysosomes. Nature (Lond.) **214**, 144 (1967).
JELLIFFE, S. E.: Aphasia, hemiparesis and hemianaesthesia in migraine. N.Y. St. Med. J. **83**, 33 (1906).
KAPPAS, A., HELLMAN, L., FUKUSHIMA, D. K., GALLAGHER, T. F.: The pyrogenic effect of ethiocolanone (3-*d*-hydroxyetiocholane-17-one). J. clin. Endocr. **16**, 948 (1956).
KEELE, C. A., ARMSTRONG, D.: Mediators of pain. In: Pharmacology of pain, vol. 9, p. 3, ed. by LIM, ARMSTRONG and PRADO. Oxford: Pergamon Press 1968.
KETY, S. S., SCHMIDT, C. F.: Nitrous oxide method for the quantitative determination of cerebral blood flow in man: Theory, procedure and normal values. J. clin. Invest. **27**, 476 (1948).
KRIVOY, W. A., LANE, M., KROEGER, D. C.: The actions of certain polypeptides on synaptic transmission. Ann. N.Y. Acad. Sci. **104**, 312 (1963).
KWAAN, H. C., McFADZEAN, A. J. C.: On plasma fibrinolytic activity induced by ischemia. Clin. Sci. **16**, 245 (1956).
LANCE, J. W., ANTHONY, M., HINTERBERGER, H.: The control of cranial arteries by humoral mechanisms and its relation to the migraine syndrome. Headache **7**, 93 (1967).
LANDERMAN, N. S., WEBSTER, M. E., BECKER, E. L., RATCLIFFE, H. E.: Hereditary angioneurotic edema. II. Deficiency of inhibitor for serum globulin permeability factor and/or plasma kallikrein. J. Allergy **33**, 330 (1960).
LEWIS, G.: In: Proceedings, First Internat. Pharmacol. Meeting, vol. 9, p. 65, ed. by M. ROCHA E SILVA and U. S. VON EULER. Oxford: Pergamon Press 1963.
LIM, R. K. S., MILLER, D. G., GURMAN, F., RODGERS, D. W., RODGERS, R. W., WANG, S. K., CHAO, P. Y., SHIH, T. Y.: Pain and analgesia evaluated by the intraperitoneal bradykinin evoked pain method in man. Clin. Pharmacol. Ther. **8**, 521 (1967).
LUNEDEI, A.: Sulle flogosi fronto-basilari iperergiche. Rev. clin. Med. **48**, 81 (1948).
— SERAFINI, V., ARCANGELI, P., NOFERI, G., PRATESI, F., DONI, A., MILANO, M.: Apoplessia cerebrale. Il problema etiopatogenetico. Proceedings, 58th Congr. Ital. Med. Soc. Rome: Pozzi 1957.
MACKAY, M. E., MILES, A. A., SCHACHTER, C. B. E., WILHELM, D. L.: Susceptibility of the guinea pig to pharmacological factors from its own serum. Nature (Lond.) **172**, 714 (1953).
MASHFORD, M. L., ZACEST, R.: Effect of adrenaline on blood kininase activity in man. Suppl. III, Circulat. Res. **20/21**, 183 (1967).
MELMON, K. L., CLINE, M. J.: Kinins and granulocytes: Model of inflammation. Proceedings, Internat. Symposium on Vaso-Active Polypeptides, p. 223, ed. by M. ROCHA E SILVA and H. A. ROTHSCHILD. Sao Paulo 1967.
MILES, A. A.: Local and systemic factors in shock. Fed. Proc. **20**, 1941 (1961).
— WILHELM, D. L.: Enzyme-like globulins from serum reproducing the vascular phenomena of inflammation. An activable permeability factor and its inhibitor in guinea-pig serum. Brit. J. exp. Path. **36**, 71 (1955).
OATES, J. A., MELMON, K. L.: Biochemical and physiological studies of kinins in carcinoid syndrome. In: Hypotensive peptides, p. 565, ed. by E. G. ERDÖS, N. BACK and F. SICUTERI. Berlin-Heidelberg-New York: Springer 1966.
PALMER, R. H., RATKOVITS, B., KAPPAS, A.: Steroid pyrogen studies in laboratory domestic animals. J. appl. Physiol. **16**, 345 (1961).
PEKKARINEN, A., CASTREN, O., IISALO, E., KOIVUSALO, M., LAIHINENA, SIMOLA, P. E., THOMASSON, B.: The emotional effect of matriculation examinations on the excretion of adrenaline, noradrenaline, 17-hydroxycorticosteroids into the urine and the content of 17-hydroxycorticosteroids in the plasma. Biochemistry, pharmacology and physiology, p. 117. Oxford: Pergamon Press 1961.
PERITI, P., COMPARINI, A., SICUTERI, F.: Bradichinogeno in corso di malattie infettive acute. Boll. Soc. ital. Biol. sper. **39**, 327 (1963a).
— MICHELACCI, S., SANTINI, D.: Plasmachinine libere nel sangue umano. Boll. Soc. ital. Biol. sper. **39**, 307 (1963b).
— SICUTERI, F., FRANCHI, G., MICHELACCI, S.: Azione dell'istamino-liberatore 48/80 sul bradichinogeno e plasmachinine del sangue venoso dopo somministrazione endovenosa ed endoarteriosa. Boll. Soc. ital. Biol. sper. **40**, 951 (1964).
PICKERING, G. W.: Experimental observations on headache. Brit. med. J. **1939 I**, 4087.
— HESS, W.: Observations on the mechanism of headache produced by histamine. Clin. Sci. **1**, 77 (1933).

Rafter, G. W., Collins, R. D., Wood, W. B.: Studies on the pathogenesis of fever. Preliminary chemical characterization of leucocytic pyrogen. J. exp. Med. **111**, 831 (1960).
Rocha e Silva, M.: Autofarmacologia e venenos animais. Ciencia e Cultura **2**, 44 (1950).
— Physiological significance of bradykinin. Ann. N.Y. Acad. Sci. **104**, 190 (1963).
— Reis, M. L., Ferreira, S. H.: Release of kinins from fresh plasma under varying experimental conditions. Biochem. Pharmacol. **16**, 1665 (1967).
Schachter, M.: A delayed slow contracting effect of serum and plasma due to the formation of a substance resembling bradykinin and kallidin. Brit. J. Pharmacol. **11**, 111 (1956).
Shimamoto, T., Numano, F., Fujita, T., Jshiota, T., Atsumi, T.: Treatment of experimental and human atherosclerosis with bradykinin antagonist, pyridinolcarbamate: A preliminary report. In: Hypotensive peptides, p. 506, ed. by E. G. Erdös, N. Back and F. Sicuteri. Berlin-Heidelberg-New York: Springer 1966.
Sicuteri, F.: Il test liquorale per lo studio della vasomotilita intracranica. Triangle **4**, 149 (1959a).
— Prophylactic and therapeutic properties of 1-methyl-lysergic acid butanolamide in migraine. Int. Arch. Allergy **15**, 300 (1959b).
— Mast cells and their active substances: Their role in the pathogenesis of migraine. Headache **3**, 86 (1963).
— Headache and meningismus evoked by lumbar and subarachnoid hemorrhage. A biochemical interpretation. Headache **5**, 108 (1966).
— Vasoneuroactive substances and their implication in vascular pain. In: Research and clinical studies in headache, p. 6, ed. by Friedman. Basel 1967a.
— Sensitization of nociceptors by 5-hydroxytryptamine in man. In: Proceedings, 3rd Internat. Pharmacol. Congr., p. 57. Oxford 1967b.
— Treatment of subarachnoid and other intracranial hemorrhages with proteinase inhibitors. In: Chemistry, pharmacology and clinical applications of proteinase inhibitors. Ann. N.Y. Acad. Sci. **146**, 682 (1968).
— Anselmi, B., Del Bene, E.: Il pirogeno in dosi non febbrigene come test rivelatore di flogosi croniche intracraniche. Rif. med. **44**, 1 (1966a).
— Del Bianco, P. L., Fanciullacci, M., Franchi, G.: Il test della venocostrizione per la misura della sensibilita alla 5-idrossitriptamina e alle catecolamine nell'uomo. Boll. Soc. ital. Biol. sper. **40**, 1148 (1964a).
— Fanciullacci, M., Bavazzano, A., Franchi, G.: Influenza di un inibitore della callicreina sulla fenomenologia da emorragia intracranica sperimentale. Boll. Soc. ital. Biol. sper. **43**, 1061 (1967a).
— — Del Bianco, P. L.: Vasoattività dell'endecapeptide fisalemina nell'uomo. Settim. med. **52**, 1221 (1964b).
— — Franchi, G., Del Bianco, P. L.: Serotonin-bradykinin potentiation on the pain receptors in man. Life Sci. **4**, 309 (1965a).
— — — Michelacci, S.: The endecapeptide eledoisin as powerful vasodilating and hypotensive agent in man. Experientia (Basel) **19**, 44 (1963d).
— Franchi, G., Del Bianco, P. L.: Un test per lo studio dell'azione dolorifica della bradichinina nell'animale: Il fenomeno grido-fuga del coniglio. Boll. Soc. ital. Biol. sper. **42**, 845 (1966b).
— — — An antiaminic drug, BC-105, in the prophylaxis of migraine. Int. Arch. Allergy **31**, 78 (1967c).
— — — Fanciullacci, M.: Peptides and pain. Proceedings, Internat. Symposium on Vaso-Active Polypeptides, p. 251, ed. by M. Rocha e Silva and H. A. Rothschild. Sao Paulo 1967b.
— — Fanciullacci, M., Del Bianco, P. L., Siddel, N.: Adrenergic receptors and kinins. In: Pharmacology of hormonal polypeptides and proteins, p. 601. Ed. by N. Back, L. Martini and R. Paoletti. New York: Plenum Press 1968.
— — Michelacci, S.: Prime osservazioni sull'effetto della bradichinina sul circolo cerebrale nell'uomo. Settim. med. **49**, 7 (1961b).
— — Periti, P.: Physiopathological aspects of bradykinin and its precursor in man. In: Bradykinin and its precursor, p. 53, ed. by F. Sicuteri. Rome: Publ. C.E.P.I. 1963a.
— Michelacci, S., Anselmi, B.: Termination of migraine headache by a new anti-inflammatory vasoconstrictor agent. Clin. Pharmacol. Ther. **6**, 336 (1965b).
— Periti, P., Anselmi, B., Fanciullacci, M.: Livelli plasmachininici nell'uomo dopo somministrazione venosa ed endoarteriosa di bradichinina sintetica e naturale. Boll. Soc. ital. Biol. sper. **39**, 314 (1963c).
— — Franchi, G.: Bradichininogeno e chinine libere nel liquido cefalorachidiano dell'uomo. Boll. Soc. ital. Biol. sper. **40**, 67 (1963b).

SICUTERI, F., PERITI, P., GASPARRI, F., FRANCHI, G., FANCIULLACCI, M.: Diminuzione del tasso ematico di bradichininogeno nell'uomo dopo somministrazione di adrenalina e callicreina. Boll. Soc. ital. Biol. sper. **38**, 1033 (1962).
— RICCI, M., MONFARDINI, R., FICINI, M.: Cefalea sperimentale da istamina endogena. Settim. med. **44**, 583 (1956).
— TESTI, A., ANSELMI, B.: Biochemical investigations in headache: Increase in the hydroxyindoleacetic acid during migraine attacks. Int. Arch. Allergy **19**, 55 (1961a).
STERNIERI, E., MUCCI, P., BERTOLINI, A.: Modificazioni indotte farmacologicamente dalla risposta del circolo cerebrale alla bradichinina. 1. Rapporto tra vocalizzazione ed aumento del sangue nel territorio cerebrale. Boll. Soc. ital. Biol. sper. **43**, 1196 (1967).
SUTHERLAND, A. M., WOLFF, H. G.: Experimental studies on headache: Further analysis of the mechanism of headache in migraine, hypertension and fever. Arch. Neurol. Psychiat. (Chic.) **44**, 929 (1940).
TRAUTSCHOLD, I., FRITZ, H., WERLE, E.: Kininogenases, kininases and their inhibitors. In: Hypotensive peptides, p. 221, ed. by E. G. ERDÖS, N. BACK and F. SICUTERI. Berlin-Heidelberg-New York: Springer 1966.
TUNIS, M. M., GOODELL, H., WOLFF, H. G.: Studies on headache: Evidence of tissue damage and changes in pain sensitivity in subjects with vascular headache of the migraine type. Trans. Ass. Amer. Phycns **66**, 332 (1953).
VIRNO, M., GERTNER, S. B., BOVET, D.: Action of histamine on the jugular venous pressure and cerebral circulation of the dog. Effects of antihistaminic drugs (pyrilamine and chlorpheniramine) and histamine liberating agent (48/80 B.W.). J. Pharmacol. exp. Ther. **118**, 63 (1956).
VOGT, W.: Kinin formation by plasmin, an indirect process mediated by activation of kallikrein J. Physiol. (Lond.) **170**, 153 (1964).
WEBSTER, M. E., INNERFIELD, I.: Interrelationship of human plasma kallikrein and plasmin in inflammation. Enzymol. biol. clin. **5**, 129 (1965).
WEISSMANN, G.: Labilization and stabilization of lysosomes. Fed. Proc. **23**, 1038 (1964).
— Lysosomes. New Engl. J. Med. **11**, 1084 (1965).
— LEWIS, G. P.: Studies on lysosomes. The effect of endotoxin tolerance and cortisone on the release of hydrolases from a granular fraction of rabbit liver. J. exp. Med. **116**, 433 (1962).
— THOMAS, L.: On a mechanism of tissue damage by bacterial endotoxin. In: Bacterial endotoxins, ed. by M. LANDY and W. BRAUN. New Brunswick: Rutgers University Press 1964.
WERLE, E., TRAUTSCHOLD, I.: Kallikrein, kallidin, kallikrein inhibitors. Ann. N.Y. Acad. Sci. **104**, 117 (1963).
WHITTY, C. W. H.: Familial hemiplegic migraine. J. Neurol. Neurosurg. Psychiat. **16**, 172 (1953).
WOLFF, H. G.: Headache and cranial arteries. Trans. Ass. Amer. Phycns **58**, 193 (1938).
— Headache and other head pain. Oxford: Univ. Press 1963.
— TUNIS, M. M.: Analysis of cranial artery pressure pulse waves in patients with vascular headache of the migraine type. Trans. Ass. Amer. Phycns **65**, 240 (1952).
WOOD, W. B., JR.: The role of endogenous pyrogen in the genesis of fever. Lancet **1958 II**, 53.
ZETLER, G., LEMBECK, F.: Substance P, a polypeptide of possible physiological importance, especially for the central nervous system. Int. Rev. Neurobiol. **4**, 159 (1962).
ZWEIFACH, B. W.: Microcirculatory effects of polypeptides. In: Hypotensive peptides, p. 451, ed. by E. G. ERDÖS, N. BACK and F. SICUTERI. Berlin-Heidelberg-New York: Springer 1966.

Kinins in Inflammation and Tissue Injury

G. P. Lewis

With 5 Figures

The four cardinal signs of inflammation—vasodilatation, increased vascular permeability, pain, and accumulation of leukocytes—appear after all kinds of tissue injuries; this has led to the idea that these actions may be mediated by a single chemical substance.

T. Lewis and his collaborators (1927) concluded that the development of the inflammatory reaction was due to the appearance of what they called H substance. However, it was realized that this was not really a single substance and Lewis (1927) and Krogh (1929) postulated the existence of an H-colloid which was eliminated slowly and primarily in the lymph.

A general opinion has developed that protein breakdown products are partly responsible for the local and general effects of inflammation and shock. Out of a vague notion that nonspecific protein and protein-split products caused a reaction to injury, Menkin (1940) formulated the idea that specific peptides were responsible for these effects. In 1936 he prepared from inflammatory exudates a material that increased vascular permeability and caused the accumulation of leukocytes; this substance he called leukotaxin. He found also that tryptic digests of serum contained substances with the same action. Although subsequent work with leukotaxin (Menkin, 1936; Duthie and Chain, 1939; Cullumbine and Rydon, 1946; Spector, 1951) has failed to show it as a specific entity, the substance responsible for the activity in tryptic digests is probably bradykinin. It might well be that the role of H-colloid is played by bradykinin, or the enzyme system producing it, as suggested by Hilton and Lewis (1957).

Three main points favor the view that kinins play a role in the inflammatory response. First, they have actions which resemble the cardinal signs of the early stages of inflammation. Second, kinins or components of the enzyme system which form them have been found at the site of injury. Third, local conditions which prevail during some kinds of tissue injury are favorable to the accumulation of kinins.

A. Actions of Kinins

The most prominent actions of kinins are those that resemble the cardinal signs of the early stages of inflammation (Elliott et al., 1960; Konzett and Stürmer, 1960; Lewis, 1962).

I. Vasodilatation

Holton and Holton (1952), investigating the possibility that bradykinin was the mediator of antidromic vasodilatation in the rabbit ear, first observed that crude preparations of bradykinin caused local vasodilatation. The vasodilator action of bradykinin has since been studied in investigations on skin, skeletal muscle, and many other tissues. In animals and man, bradykinin is one of the most potent vasodilator substances known. In increasing the blood flow through cat hind limbs, bradykinin is more active than acetylcholine (ELLIOTT et al., 1960). When infused into the forearms of human subjects, as little as 0.1 to 1 μg bradykinin per minute (as seen from Fig. 1) causes a considerable increase in the blood flow of the whole forearm and hand (FOX et al., 1961). BURCH and DE PASQUALE (1962) found that when bradykinin is infused into a human hand there is a constriction of the arteriovenous shunts with a subsequent dilatation of the arterioles, capillaries, venules, and veins (see Chapter 6, p. 367).

ZWEIFACH (1966), studying the microcirculatory effects of bradykinin, found that local application to the rat mesentery also produced dilatation of arterioles

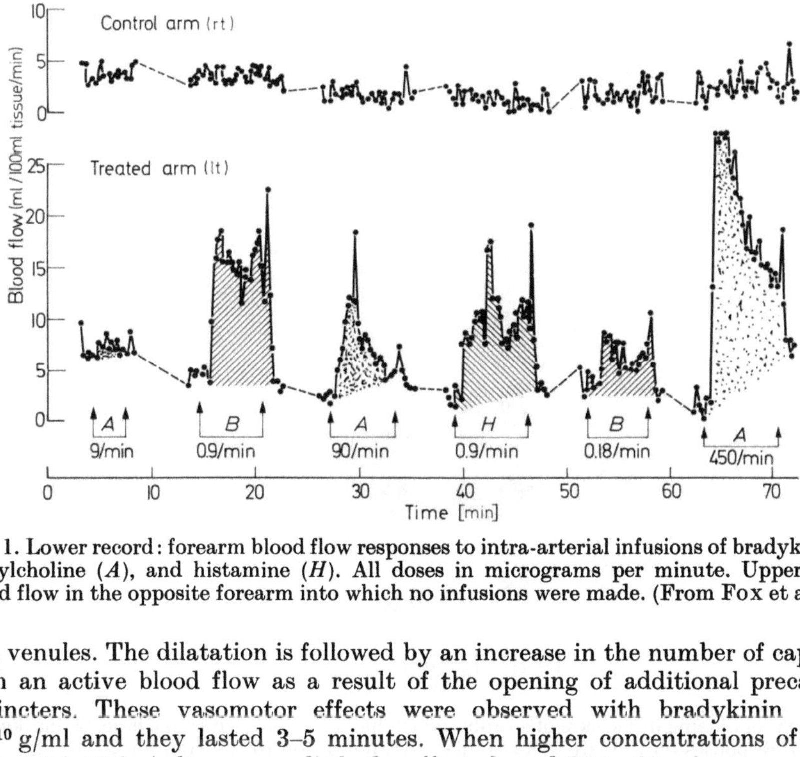

Fig. 1. Lower record: forearm blood flow responses to intra-arterial infusions of bradykinin (*B*), acetylcholine (*A*), and histamine (*H*). All doses in micrograms per minute. Upper record: blood flow in the opposite forearm into which no infusions were made. (From FOX et al., 1961)

and venules. The dilatation is followed by an increase in the number of capillaries with an active blood flow as a result of the opening of additional precapillary sphincters. These vasomotor effects were observed with bradykinin 10^{-9} to 10^{-10} g/ml and they lasted 3–5 minutes. When higher concentrations of bradykinin 10^{-7}–10^{-8} g/ml) were applied, the effects lasted 20 to 30 minutes, and there was evidence of red cell clumping and stasis, indicating increased permeability.

II. Vascular Permeability

The action of increasing the vascular permeability after intradermal injection of bradykinin was demonstrated by HOLDSTOCK et al. (1957) in guinea pigs which had received intravenous injections of Evans blue dye. Later, the effect was observed in man (HERXHEIMER and SCHACHTER, 1959). In both guinea pigs and rabbits into which dye has been injected intravenously, plasma kinins injected intradermally give rise to an area of intense blueing, whereas an intradermal injection of histamine causes blueing, which is less intense and not uniform. The center of the affected area is pale, possibly as a result of arterial constriction which histamine is known to produce in these species (FELDBERG, 1927). There is a further difference between the blueing produced by bradykinin and histamine; that after histamine extends to a wider area, which is difficult to explain by better diffusion within the skin. Since intradermal histamine is known to cause vasodilatation not only by its direct action on the vessels but also by an axon reflex, it is possible that the wider area of blueing, particularly in the rabbit skin, results from this action of histamine. MENKIN (1936) observed a similar difference between the blueing produced by histamine and that produced by inflammatory exudates, and it was one of the arguments he used in favor of the view that such exudates contain a permeability-increasing substance other than histamine.

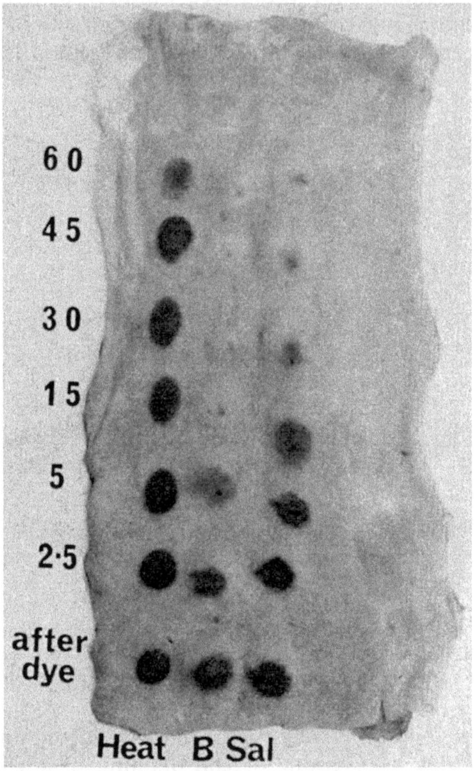

Fig. 2. Areas of blueing in the skin of a rabbit which had received pontamine blue, 60 mg/kg i.v. The line of responses on the left was obtained by application to the skin for 20 sec of a steel rod 1 cm in diameter and heated to 60°; the center line of responses was obtained by intradermal injections of 0.1 ml of a solution containing bradykinin, 10 μg/ml; the line on the right by intradermal injection of 0.1 ml human saliva, centrifuged, dialyzed and diluted 1:10 with saline. The three dermal applications at the bottom of the figure were made 2 minutes after injection of the pontamine blue; the other applications were made 2.5, 5, 15, 30, 45, or 60 minutes before injection of the dye. (From LEWIS, 1964)

One objection which has been raised against any role of plasma kinins in inflammatory reactions is that their action is transient whereas the inflammatory process is prolonged (MILES, 1964). The answer to this is that during the inflammatory response, once the kinin-forming mechanism is activated, the duration of the response depends not upon the transient action of the kinins themselves but upon that of the activated kininogenases which results in the continuous formation of kinins. The point was illustrated by LEWIS (1964) (see Fig. 2) who found that the action of bradykinin on vascular permeability lasted 5–6 minutes after its injection, whereas after kallikrein an increased vascular permeability could still be detected as long as 45 minutes after injection; and when the skin was heated to 60°, the response was usually still evident more than an hour later. Thus, although the duration of action of a kinin itself is short, that of even a single injection of a kinin-forming enzyme is much longer, approaching that of a mild burn.

The prolonged action following activation of the intrinsic kinin system was also observed by GRAHAM et al. (1965). They found that the response of the microcirculation in the rabbit ear chamber to an injection of bradykinin was quite different from that seen after injection of an activator of the kinin system, such as Hageman factor. Dilatation of arteries appeared within a few seconds of the beginning of the injection of the peptide but rarely persisted for more than 15 minutes. Rolling of leukocytes along venular walls reached a maximum in 2–5 minutes, and leukocytes sticking reached a maximum in 10–20 minutes, thereafter subsiding. Injection of purified Hageman factor activated by 10^{-4} M ellagic acid, consistently evoked responses which were delayed in onset and relatively prolonged. Arteriolar dilatation occurred concomitantly with leukocyte sticking, becoming pronounced at 45–60 minutes after injection, and the whole reaction reached a maximum after 90–120 minutes. These authors concluded that the prolonged endogenous release of kinins may produce effects quite different from those observed after a single injection of bradykinin. An example of the experimental proof of this statement emerges when we consider the action of bradykinin on lymph flow.

III. Lymph Flow

The action of bradykinin on lymph flow was first observed by STÜRMER (1966). He showed that infusions of bradykinin (0.005 to 1.28 µg/kg/min) into dogs caused a considerable increase in lymph flow, an effect that occurs in most kinds of tissue injury. At first this seems contrary to the finding of EDERY and LEWIS (1963) that injections of large doses of bradykinin did not cause an increase in lymph flow in dogs. However, LEWIS and WINSEY (1969) have found recently that it is necessary to infuse bradykinin for 3 to 7 minutes before there is an increase in lymph flow, so that after single injections the peptide would not be present long enough to increase the flow.

The mechanism by which bradykinin causes the increase in lymph flow has not been elucidated, but it might well be the result of the combined actions in increasing vascular permeability and causing venoconstriction. This latter action of bradykinin was suggested by GUTH et al. (1963) to explain a decrease in outflow from an artificially perfused rabbit ear following injection of bradykinin. More recently, GUTH et al. (1966) have indicated that this venoconstriction is due partially to local release of catecholamines.

However, MAJNO et al. (1967), who examined the relationship between vascular leakage and increase in venous pressure in rats and rabbits, observed that bradykinin, as well as histamine and 5-hydroxytryptamine, far from causing venoconstriction, frequently increased the caliber of the venules.

IV. Pain

Bradykinin produces pain when injected intradermally or applied to an exposed blister base. Kinins cause a burning sensation similar to that appearing during local tissue injury (ARMSTRONG et al., 1957). The same authors showed that a pain-producing substance which is closely related to bradykinin develops in the fluid aspirated from a blister in human skin and in inflammatory exudates.

However, although the pain produced by bradykinin was intense, usually it was not only transient but also the area of skin to which several applications had been made became specifically desensitized to the peptide (ELLIOTT et al., 1960) (see Chapter 6B, p. 459).

Bradykinin has also been shown to cause pain when injected arterially into dogs (GUZMAN et al., 1962) and in man (BURCH and DE PASQUALE, 1962; ALLWOOD and LEWIS, 1964).

V. Accumulation of Leukocytes

In guinea pigs and rabbits, bradykinin in higher concentrations (10^{-6}, 10^{-4} g/ml) than those necessary to produce the vascular effects, causes an accumulation of leukocytes at the site of intradermal injection and migration of these into the surrounding tissue (LEWIS, 1962). This action has also been shown to occur after topical application to rabbit mesentery.

B. Evidence for Components of the Kinin-Forming System at the Site of Injury

It is usually not possible to detect kinins themselves in inflammatory exudates, because they are inactivated so rapidly—before the exudates can be collected and tested. The rapidity with which the body inactivates bradykinin was clearly shown, for example, in some experiments of ALLWOOD and LEWIS (1964). We found it is possible to infuse arterially into human forearms a concentration of bradykinin considerably greater than that necessary to produce a pronounced vasodilatation and yet be unable to detect the peptide in the venous blood flowing from the infused forearm. In spite of this there have been several reports that kinins have been found together with other mediators at the site of local injury. For instance, ROCHA E SILVA and ROSENTHAL (1961) demonstrated a kinin, histamine, and other substances in the perfusates of subcutaneous air pockets in rats when the overlying skin was burned, and ROCHA E SILVA and ANTONIO (1960) detected bradykinin in the fluid perfusing the subcutaneous tissue of rat paws during heating. In addition, in more extensive forms of injury such as that occurring in burned patients (GOODWIN et al., 1963); in some protozoal infection in mice (GOODWIN and RICHARDS, 1960), and in malaria in monkeys (TELLA and MACGRAITH, 1962), kinin activity has been detected in the urine (see Chapter 7, p. 581) and the amounts have generally been found to be correlated with the severity of the condition. More recently, MELMON et al. (1967) found kinins in the synovial fluid collected from patients with gout and other types of arthritis, and particularly high levels were found in effusions induced by injections of microcrystalline suspensions into the knee joint. In all these investigations it is difficult to understand, if kinins were formed during the inflammation, why they were not inactivated before collection, since the concentration of kininase in all these body fluids is high.

EDERY and LEWIS (1963), examining the lymph draining an injured limb, could not detect kinins after tissue injury but observed an increase in the kinin-forming activity of the lymph after injury (Fig. 3). JACOBSEN and WAALER (1966), repeating these experiments in rabbits, also found an increase, but they attributed this to an increase in kininogen which passed from the blood into the lymph after injury.

It seems that, since the system is already present in all tissues, an inflammatory reaction could be brought about by conditions activating the kinin-forming system. In fact, this seems to be the case in gouty arthritis. KELLERMEYER and BRECKENRIDGE (1965) found that urate crystals promote blood clotting by activating Hageman factor. EISEN (1966) then showed that urate crystals also cause kinin formation in synovial effusions and in plasma, but that this formation does not occur in plasma from patients lacking Hageman factor. It seems therefore that in gout the urate crystals activate Hageman factor, which in turn activates plasma kallikrein, which acts upon kininogen to form kinin. PHELPS et al. (1966) have dismissed kinins as playing any role in gouty arthritis, because injection of carboxypeptidase B into dogs (p. 306) does not prevent the increase of intra-articular pressure after intrasynovial injection of monosodium urate crystals.

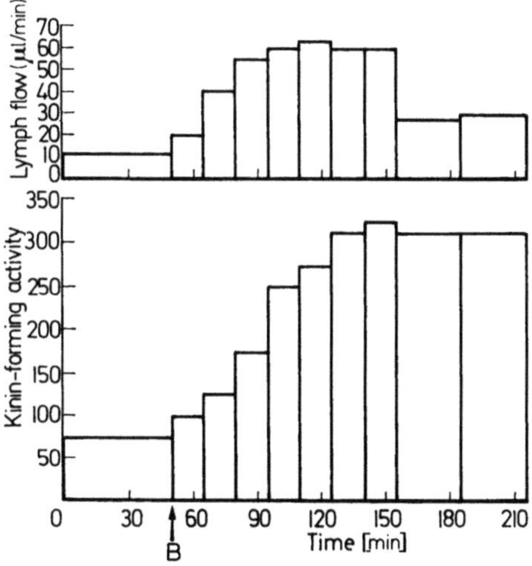

Fig. 3. Above, flow; below, kinin-forming activity of lymph collected from the hind limb of a dog. At *B* the limb was burned by scalding at 80° for 15 sec. Kinin-forming activity is expressed as bradykinin formed (ng/ml lymph) under standard conditions of incubation. (From EDERY and LEWIS, 1963)

However, as pointed out by MELMON et al. (1967), dog plasma does not release a large amount of kinin on contact with a foreign surface, which makes it difficult to extrapolate the findings of PHELPS and colleagues to humans.

Once initiated, the inflammatory response might continue by virtue of continued kinin formation. This could occur in two ways—either by a simple diffusion of kininogen and inactive kallikrein from the blood vessels into the inflamed area where the kallikrein would be activated, or the active enzyme might be brought to the site by leukocytes, which are known to migrate to an inflamed area. Several investigators have recently observed that leukocytes induce kinin formation and also contain a strong kininase activity (EISEN, 1966; GREENBAUM and YAMAFUJI, 1966; MELMON and CLINE, 1967) (p. 299). These authors conclude that the leukocytes play a major role in the continued formation of kinins during chronic inflammation. However, JASANI et al. (1967) have recently found evidence that points in the other direction. They have examined synovial fluid collected from the knee joints of patients with rheumatoid arthritis and related diseases and found that, while the concentration of lysosomal and cytoplasmic enzymes was higher in synovial fluid containing cells than in centrifuged cell-free samples, the concentrations of kininogenases and kininases and protein in cell-containing synovial fluid were equal to or lower than those in either cell-free fluid or plasma. These findings suggest that the lysosomal and cytoplasmic enzymes are derived from the cells of the synovial fluid, whereas the kinin enzymes are derived from plasma.

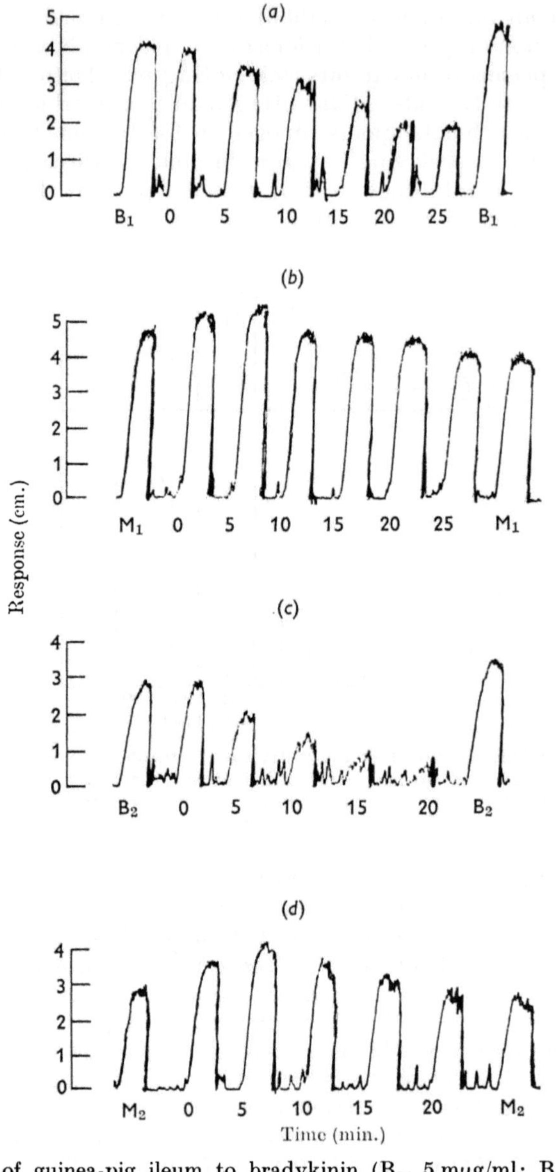

Fig. 4. Responses of guinea-pig ileum to bradykinin (B_1, 5 mμg/ml; B_2, 2.5 mμg/ml), to synthetic methionyl-lysyl-bradykinin (M_1, 50 mμg/ml; M_2, 25 mμg/ml) and to incubated mixtures of 0.4 μM solutions of bradykinin (in *a* and *c*) and 0.4 μM solutions of methionyl-lysyl-bradykinin (in *b* and *d*) with dog pseudoglobulin (2.5 mg/ml in *a* and *b*; 5 mg/ml in *c* and *d*). In each experiment samples were taken and tested at 5 min intervals from the commencement of the incubation. (From Elliott and Lewis, 1965)

C. Local Conditions in Injury which Favor Kinin Actions

There might well be conditions existing in inflamed tissue which favor the formation and accumulation of plasma kinins. Several workers have provided evidence that proteolytic enzymes are activated during tissue injury (Beloff and Peters, 1945; Ungar, 1947), although it is not clear which factors actually cause the activation. The acidic environment that prevails in damaged tissue might be one condition responsible for the activation of the plasma kinin-forming enzymes and for the accumulation of the peptides so formed. Werle (1934) provided evidence that kallikrein which is normally present in blood in combination with an inhibitor is activated at acid pH. Frey et al. (1950) have consequently suggested that in conditions where acid metabolites are formed, kallikrein is responsible for the accompanying vascular effects. Whether the changes of pH in damaged tissue are sufficient to cause this activation is not

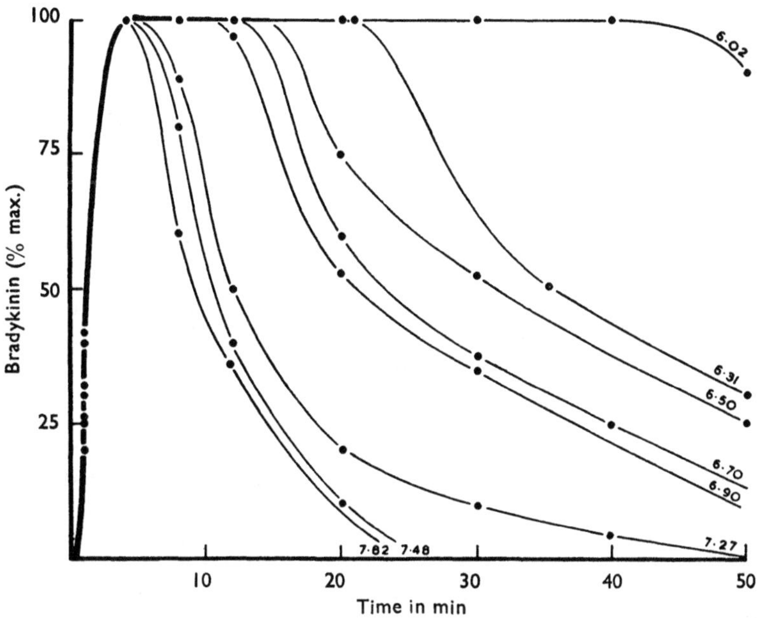

Fig. 5. The amount of plasma kinin present in mixtures of salivary kallikrein and dog pseudoglobulin incubated at various pH values, expressed as percentage of the maximal amount of plasma kinin formed in each experiment. The maximal formation was between 50 and 75 ng/mg pseudoglobulin and occurred at about 4 minutes. (From Edery and Lewis, 1962)

certain. The changes of blood pH which might occur are small and certainly would not activate the enzyme system. However, if such activation could occur also in tissue fluid, then this becomes a possible mechanism of activation in inflammation because it is known that the pH of the interstitial fluid in inflamed tissue is sometimes lower than pH 6 (Schade, 1924).

Elliott and Lewis (1965) showed that acid activation of a kininogenase in plasma led to the formation of another kinin in addition to bradykinin i.e. methionyl-lysyl-bradykinin. They found that this endecapeptide appeared to be more resistant to the action of kininase (Fig. 4). However, the prolonged effect of Met-Lys-bradykinin might be due to the effect of aminopeptidases first forming kallidin (Lys-bradykinin), which is somewhat more active than the Met-Lys peptide, and subsequently forming bradykinin itself. Thus the activity of the peptide would be prolonged during its metabolism. Although the conversion of Met-Lys-bradykinin to bradykinin has not been observed *in vivo*, several workers have shown that the Lys-Arg bond of kallidin can be broken to give bradykinin (Erdös et al., 1963; Webster and Pierce, 1963; Hopsu-Havu et al., 1966) (p. 314).

The action of kininase on bradykinin is also strongly influenced by pH (EDERY and LEWIS, 1962). At slightly acid pH (using 0.1 M phosphate buffer) the enzyme kininase which normally rapidly inactivates kinins is inhibited (Fig. 5). For instance at pH 7.3 bradykinin is destroyed 5 to 10 times more rapidly than it is at pH 6.0. TRAUTSCHOLD (1968) showed some decrease of kinin formation in this pH range, but these changes did not reduce the effectiveness of the kininogenases sufficiently to alter the curve of formation in our experiments (Fig. 5). These results have been confirmed by ZACHARIAE et al. (1967).

It appears then that the acid environment of inflammation provides not only suitable conditions for the formation and accumulation of plasma kinins like bradykinin but also might allow for the formation of bradykinin in a more stable form, i.e. as the acid-formed kinin.

D. Anti-Inflammatory Agents and Kinins

Several investigators have studied the effects of known anti-inflammatory compounds on the kinin system. Although certain nonsteroidal anti-inflammatory compounds have been shown not to antagonize the actions of kinins themselves (LEWIS, 1963), several claims have been made that salicylates and other antipyretics reduced the formation of kinins (NORTHOVER and SUBRAMANIAN, 1961; SPECTOR and WILLOUGHBY, 1963). However, both LEWIS (1963) and HEBBORN and SHAW (1963) were unable to confirm the finding that aspirin inhibited the formation of kinins by kallikrein. In addition DAVIES et al. (1966) found that not only many nonsteroidal anti-inflammatory drugs but also paramethasone failed to inhibit kinin formation. It is known that activation of the endogenous kinin-forming system occurs after dilution, contact with foreign surfaces, or treatment with acid. It therefore remained a possibility that anti-inflammatory agents reduce kinin formation not by preventing the action of kininogenase but by preventing the activation of the endogenous kininogenases. Recently, CLINE and MELMON (1966) have claimed that hydrocortisone inhibits the release of kinins partly by inhibition of kallikrein and partly by inhibition of the activation of the endogenous system induced by contact activation. Since the report of MELMON and CLINE, EISEN et al. (1968) have re-examined the possibility that anti-inflammatory steroids interfere with the kinin-forming system and concluded that the anti-inflammatory action of corticosteroids cannot be explained by the inhibition of kinin formation.

There have been many published reports of the possible antagonism by anti-inflammatory drugs and related agents of kinins and of kinin formation. These were first summarized by ERDÖS (1968), and Tables 1 and 2 extend his summary and bring it up to date. It is the opinion of the author that there are no specific antagonists available at present, and the only actions of kinins that might be affected by anti-inflammatory drugs are bronchoconstriction and severe forms of pain. Thus, no evidence in favor of the view that kinins participate in inflammatory reactions can be gleaned from a study of the action of anti-inflammatory drugs.

In summary it can be said that there is very good circumstantial evidence that kinins could play a role in inflammatory reactions. The kinin-forming system is present in plasma and to a lesser extent in interstitial fluid and lymph. The necessary stimulus to set the system in motion could be provided in several ways—a foreign protein reaction; a change to acid pH; dilution with edema fluid; the import into the affected area of specific enzyme activators or inhibitors of inactivating enzymes; the passage of excess substrate into the interstitial space,

Table 1. *Antibradykinin effect of anti-inflammatory drugs*

Pharmacological activity	Antagonized	Species	Reference
Circulation			
Decrease in systemic arterial blood pressure; vasodilatation	yes	rabbit, rat, guinea pig	18, 64, 65, 66, 78, 94, 109
	no	cat, dog, guinea pig	14, 15, 10, 85
	no	human	12
Increase in pulmonary pressure; vasoconstriction	yes	rabbit, guinea pig	6, 40, 61, 67
Pressor reflex	yes	dog	47
Venoconstriction	yes	rabbit	55, 96, 97, 105
Respiration			
Bronchospasm in asthmatic patients	yes	human	105
Bronchoconstriction	yes	guinea pig	13, 14, 15, 109
Central apnea; reflex tachypnea	yes	guinea pig	35, 36
Perfused isolated lung	no	guinea pig	1
	yes	guinea pig	10
Isolated trachea	yes	guinea pig	8, 16
Vascular permeability			
Increase in skin	yes	rat, mouse	6a
	yes	rabbit	3, 4, 6a, 67
	no	guinea pig	6a, 14, 70, 101
	yes	guinea pig	78
Edema in paw	yes	rat	76, 102
	yes	guinea pig	79, 86
Increase in protein in lymph	yes	rat	111
	yes	cat	73
Increase in lymph flow	yes	rat	111
	no	cat	73
Pain			
Caused by intra-arterial injection	yes	human	12, 44, 46
Visceral pain	yes	dog, mouse	17, 29, 44, 75
Caused by application on blister base	no	human	54, 59, 70
Caused by application to veins	no	human	98
Isolated smooth muscle	no	guinea pig, rat	70
	yes	guinea pig	57, 68, 78, 88, 89, 92, 93, 94
	yes	rat	78, 103, 104

Table 2. *Inhibition of kinin formation by anti-inflammatory agents*

Inhibition	Species	Source of Kallikrein	Reference
no	human	saliva	26, 48, 70
yes	human	saliva	85
no	guinea pig	serum	20
yes	guinea pig	serum	24, 85, 112, 113
no	ox	serum	48
yes	ox	serum	85
no	ox	pancreas	48
no	human	pancreas	99
no	dog	pancreas	26
no	human	urine	26
yes	human	urine	11, 80
no	human	serum	26
yes	rat	serum	101
yes	human	serum	11, 80

as might result from increased permeability following release of a co-mediator such as histamine or 5-HT. In addition, we know that when present, the kinins are certainly capable of producing many of the actions that characterize the inflammatory response. However, the evidence is as yet circumstantial, and it is the opinion of the author that the case for kinins as mediators in the inflammatory response is not yet proven.

References

1. Aarsen, P. N.: The influence of analgesic-antipyretic drugs on the responses of guinea pig lungs to bradykinin. Brit. J. Pharmacol. **27**, 196 (1966).
2. Allwood, M. J., Lewis, G. P.: Bradykinin and forearm blood flow. J. Physiol. (Lond.) **170**, 571 (1964).
3. Antopol, W., Chryssanthou, C.: Possible significance of bradykinin in Shwartzman and other phenomena. Ann. N.Y. Acad. Sci. **104**, 346 (1963).
4. — — Shwartzman phenomenon mechanism: Newer concepts. Arch. Path. **78**, 313 (1964).
5. Armstrong, D., Jepson, J. B., Keele, C. A., Stewart, J. W.: Pain producing substance in human inflammatory exudates and plasma. J. Physiol. (Lond.) **135**, 350 (1957).
6. Bauer, G., Gmeiner, R., Konzett, H.: Zum Antagonismus von Antiphlogistica gegenüber der Wirkung von Kininen auf den Druck in der Arteria pulmonalis von Meerschweinchen. Naunyn-Schmiedebergs Arch. exp. Path. Pharmak. **251**, 182 (1965).

6a. Becker, E. L., Mota, I., Wong, D.: Inhibition by antihistamines of the vascular permeability increase induced by bradykinin. Brit. J. Pharmacol. **34**, 330 (1968).

7. Beloff, A., Peters, R. A.: Observations upon thermal burns: The influence of moderate temperature burns upon a proteinase of skin. J. Physiol. (Lond.) **103**, 461 (1945).
8. Bhoola, K. D., Collier, H. O. J., Schachter, M., Shorley, P. G.: Action of some peptides on bronchial muscle. Brit. J. Pharmacol. **19**, 190 (1962).
9. Burch, G. E., Pasquale, N. P. de: Bradykinin, digital blood flow on the arterio venous anastomoses. Circulat. Res. **10**, 105 (1962).
10. Carpi, A., Klupp, H., Konzett, H.: Über die Bradykinin-Wirkung am Herz-Lungen-Präparat des Meerschweinchens. Naunyn-Schmiedebergs Arch. exp. Path. Pharmak. **243**, 356 (1962).
11. Cline, M. J., Melmon, K. L.: Plasma kinins and cortisol: A possible explanation of the anti-inflammatory action of cortisol. Science **153**, 1135 (1966).
12. Coffman, J. D.: The effect of aspirin on pain and hand blood flow responses to intra-arterial injection of bradykinin in man. Clin. Pharmacol. Ther. **7**, 26 (1966).
13. Collier, H. O. J.: The action and antagonism of kinins on bronchioles. Ann. N.Y. Acad. Sci. **104**, 290 (1963).
14. — Shorley, P. G.: Analgesic antipyretic drugs as antagonists of bradykinin. Brit. J. Pharmacol. **15**, 601 (1960).
15. — — Antagonism by mefenamic and flufenamic acids of the broncho-constrictor action of kinins in the guinea pig. Brit. J. Pharmacol. **20**, 345 (1963).
16. — Holgate, J. A., Schachter, M., Shorley, P. G.: The bronchoconstrictor action of bradykinin in the guinea pig. Brit. J. Pharmacol. **15**, 290 (1960).
17. — Hammond, A. R., Horwood-Barrett, S., Schneider, C.: Rapid induction by acetylcholine, bradykinin and potassium of a nociceptive response in mice and its selective antagonism by aspirin. Nature (Lond.) **204**, 1316 (1964).
18. Concioli, M., Mariani, L., Villani, R.: Influsso di farmaci antibradichininici sulle variazioni del circolo cortico-piale nello shock anafilatico della cavia. Atti Accad. med. lombarda **17**, 242 (1962).
19. Cullumbine, H., Rydon, H. N.: A study of the formation properties and partial purification of leukotaxin. Brit. J. exp. Path. **27**, 33 (1946).
20. Davies, G. E., Holman, G., Johnston, T. P., Lowe, J. S.: Studies on kallikrein: Failure of some anti-inflammatory drugs to affect release of kinins. Brit. J. Pharmacol. **28**, 212 (1966).
21. Duthie, E. S., Chain, E. A.: Polypeptides responsible for some of the phenomena of acute inflammation. Brit. J. exp. Path. **20**, 417 (1939).
22. Edery, H., Lewis, G. P.: Inhibition of plasma kininase activity at slightly acid pH. Brit. J. Pharmacol. **19**, 299 (1962).
23. — — Kinin-forming activity and histamine in lymph after tissue injury. J. Physiol. (Lond.) **169**, 568 (1963).

24. EISEN, V.: Effect of hexadimethrine bromide on plasma kinin formation hydrolysis of *p*-tosyl-L-arginine methyl ester and fibrinolysis. Brit. J. Pharmacol. **22**, 87 (1964).
25. — Urates and kinin formation in synovial fluid. Proc. roy. Soc. Med. **59** (4), 302 (1966).
26. — GREENBAUM, L., LEWIS, G. P.: Kinins and anti-inflammatory steroids. Brit. J. Pharmacol. **34**, 169 (1968).
27. ELLIOTT, D. F., LEWIS, G. P.: Methionyl-lysyl-bradykinin, a new kinin from ox blood. Biochem. J. **95**, 437 (1965).
28. — HORTON, E. W., LEWIS, G. P.: Actions of pure bradykinin. J. Physiol. (Lond.) **153**, 437 (1960).
29. EMELE, J. F., SHANAMAN, J.: A method for measuring analgesia. Proc. Soc. exp. Biol. (N.Y.) **114**, 680 (1963).
30. ERDÖS, E. G.: Effect of nonsteroidal anti-inflammatory drugs in endotoxin shock. Biochem. Pharmacol. Suppl., p. 283 (1968).
31. — RENFREW, A. G., SLOANE, E. M., WOHLER, J. R.: Enzymatic studies on bradykinin and similar peptides. Ann. N.Y. Acad. Sci. **104**, 222 (1963).
32. FELDBERG, W.: Action of histamine on blood vessels of the rabbit. J. Physiol. (Lond.) **63**, 211 (1927).
33. FOX, R. H., GOLDSMITH, R., KIDD, D. J., LEWIS, G. P.: Bradykinin as a vasodilator in man. J. Physiol. (Lond.) **157**, 589 (1961).
34. FREY, E. K., KRAUT, H., WERLE, E.: Kallikrein. Padutin. Stuttgart: Enke 1950.
35. GJURIS, V., HEICKE, B., WESTERMANN, E.: Apnoe nach Bradykinin und Kallidin. Naunyn-Schmiedebergs Arch. exp. Path. Pharmak. **248**, 540 (1964a).–
36. — — — Über die Stimulierung der Atmung durch Bradykinin und Kallidin. Naunyn-Schmiedebergs Arch. exp. Path. Pharmak. **247**, 429 (1964b).
37. GOODWIN, L. G., RICHARDS, W. H. G.: Pharmacologically active peptides in the blood and urine of animals infected with *Babesia rodhaini* and other pathogenic organisms. Brit. J. Pharmacol. **15**, 152 (1960).
38. — JONES, C. R., RICHARDS, W. H. G., KOHN, J.: Pharmacologically active substances in the urine of burned patients. Brit. J. exp. Path. **44**, 551 (1963).
39. GRAHAM, R. C., ERBERT, R. H., RATNOFF, O. D., MOSES, J. M.: Pathogenesis of inflammation. II. In vivo observations of the inflammatory effects of activated Hageman factor and bradykinin. J. exp. Med. **121**, 807 (1965).
40. GREEFF, K., MOOG, E.: Vergleichende Untersuchungen über die bronchoconstrictorische und gefäßconstrictorische Wirkung des Bradykinins, Histamins und Serotonins an isolierten Lungenpräparaten. Naunyn-Schmiedebergs Arch. exp. Path. Pharmak. **248**, 204 (1964).
41. GREENBAUM, L. M., YAMAFUJI, K.: The role of cathepsins in the activation of plasma kinins. In: Hypotensive peptides, p. 252, ed. by E. G. ERDÖS, N. BACK, and F. SICUTERI. Berlin-Heidelberg-New York: Springer 1966.
42. GUTH, P. S., CANO, G., JARAMILLO, J.: The effect of bradykinin on vascular smooth muscle. Ann. N.Y. Acad. Sci. **104**, 69 (1963).
43.— BOBBIN, R., CANO, G., AMARO, J.: Vasoconstriction induced by bradykinin in the rabbit ear. In: Hypotensive peptides, p. 396, ed. by E. G. ERDÖS, N. BACK, and F. SICUTERI. Berlin-Heidelberg-New York: Springer 1966.
44. GUY, J. L., LEE, K. H., LEUNG, P. M. B., LIM, R. K. S.: Plasma salicylate levels associated with analgesia to bradykinin-evoked pain in dog and man. Pharmacologist **8**, 207 (1966).
45. GUZMAN, F., BRAUN, C., LIM, R. K. S.: Visceral pain and the pseudoaffective response to intra-arterial injection of bradykinin and other algesic agents. Arch. int. Pharmacodyn. **136**, 353 (1962).
46. — — — POTTER, G. D., RODGERS, D. W.: Narcotic and nonnarcotic analgesics which block visceral pain evoked by intra-arterial injection of bradykinin and other algesic agents. Arch. int. Pharmacodyn. **149**, 571 (1964).
47. HASHIMOTO, K., KUMAKURA, S., TAIRA, N.: Vascular reflex responses induced by intra-arterial injection of azaazepinophenothiazine, andromedotoxin, veratridine, bradykinin and kallikrein and blocking action of sodium salicylate. Jap. J. Physiol. **14**, 299 (1964).
48. HEBBORN, P., SHAW, B.: The action of sodium salicylate and aspirin on some kallikrein systems. Brit. J. Pharmacol. **20**, 254 (1963).
49. HERXHEIMER, A., SCHACHTER, M.: Wheal and flare in human skin produced by histamine and other substances. J. Physiol. (Lond.) **145**, 34P (1959).
50. HILTON, S. M., LEWIS, G. P.: Functional vasodilatation in the submandibular salivary gland. Brit. med. Bull. **13**, 189 (1957).
51. HOLDSTOCK, D. J., MATHIAS, A. P., SCHACHTER, M.: A comparative study of kinin, kallidin, and bradykinin. Brit. J. Pharmacol. **12**, 149 (1957).

52. Holton, F. A., Holton, P.: Vasodilator activity of spinal roots. J. Physiol. (Lond.) **118**, 310 (1952).
53. Hopsu-Havu, V. K., Mäkinen, K. K., Glenner, G. G.: Formation of bradykinin from kallidin-10 by aminopeptidase B. Nature (Lond.) **212**, 1271 (1966).
54. Horton, E. W.: The role of bradykinin in the peripheral nervous system. Ann. N.Y. Acad. Sci. **104**, 250 (1963).
55. Ishioka, T., Matsumura, T., Takeuchi, K., Yagishita, M., Hazami, H.: Studies on venoconstriction effect of venoactive substances on saphenous vein of rabbit and antagonists of venoconstriction induced by bradykinin. Ochanomizu med. J. **13**, 298 (1966).
56. Jacobsen, S., Waaler, B. A.: The effect of scalding on the content of kininogen and kininase in limb lymph. Brit. J. Pharmacol. **27**, 222 (1966).
57. Jaques, R., Huber, G., Neipp, L., Rossi, A., Schar, B., Meier, R.: Ein chemisch und pharmakologisch neuartiger Antagonist von pathophysiologisch bedeutsamen Aminen, Kininen und kininbildenden Faktoren. Experientia (Basel) **23**, 149 (1967).
58. Jasani, M. K., Katori, M., Lewis, G. P.: Intracellular enzymes and kinin enzymes in synovial fluid in joint diseases: Origin and relation to disease category. Ann. rheum. Dis. **28**, 497 (1969).
59. Keele, C. A., Armstrong, D.: Substances producing pain and itch, p. 399. Baltimore: Williams & Wilkins 1964.
60. Kellermeyer, R. W., Breckenridge, R. T.: The inflammatory process in acute gouty arthritis. I. Activation of Hageman factor by sodium urate crystals. J. Lab. clin. Med. **65**, 307 (1965).
61. Klupp, H., Konzett, H.: Der Einfluß von Bradykinin und Kallidin auf den Druck in der Arteria pulmonalis. Naunyn-Schmiedebergs Arch. exp. Path. Pharmak. **249**, 479 (1965).
62. Konzett, H., Stürmer, E.: Biological activity of synthetic polypeptides with bradykinin-like properties. Brit. J. Pharmacol. **15**, 544 (1960).
63. Krogh, A.: The anatomy and physiology of capillaries, 2nd ed., p. 238. Newhaven: Yale University Press; London: Oxford University Press 1929.
64. Lecomte, J.: Bradykinin and anaphylactic shock in rabbits. Acta allerg. (Kbh.) **14**, 408 (1959).
65. — Antagonism between synthetic bradykinin and phenylbutazone in the rabbit. C. R. Soc. Biol. (Paris) **154**, 2389 (1960).
66. — Antagonism between synthetic bradykinin and sodium salicylate in the rat. C. R. Soc. Biol. (Paris) **156**, 1932 (1962).
67. — Troquet, J.: Antagonism between bradykinin and phenylbutazone in the rabbit. C. R. Soc. Biol. (Paris) **154**, 1115 (1960).
68. Leme, J. Garcia, Rocha e Silva, M.: Competitive and non-competitive inhibition of bradykinin on the guinea pig ileum. Brit. J. Pharmacol. **25**, 50 (1965).
69. Lewis, G. P.: Bradykinin—biochemistry, pharmacology and its physiological role in controlling local blood flow. Sci. Basis Med. **14**, 242 (1962).
70. — Kinin antagonism and kinin formation. In: Salicylates, p. 134, ed. by A. St. J. Dixon, B. K. Martin, M. J. H. Smith and P. H. N. Woods. London: Churchill 1963a.
71. — Discussions; Kinins and Erythema. In: Salicylates, p. 134, ed. by A. St. J. Dixon, B. K. Martin, M. J. H. Smith, P. H. N. Wood. London: 1963b.
72. — Plasma kinin and other vasoactive compounds in acute inflammation. Ann. N.Y. Acad. Sci. **116**, 847 (1964).
73. — Winsey, N. J. P.: The action of pharmacologically active substances on the flow and composition of cat hind limb lymph. Brit. J. Pharmacol. **35** (1969).
74. Lewis, T.: Blood vessels in human skin and their responses, p. 322. London: Shaw & Son Ltd. 1927.
75. Lim, R. K. S., Guzman, F., Rodgers, D. W., Goto, K. Braun, C., Dickerson, C. D., Engle, R. J.: Site of action of narcotic and nonnarcotic analgesics determined by blocking bradykinin evoked visceral pain. Arch. int. Pharmacodyn. **152**, 25 (1964).
76. Lisin, N., Leclercq, R., Cauwenberge, H. V.: L'Oedème à la bradykinine et son inhibition. Rev. Rhum. **30**, 790 (1963).
77. Majno, G., Gilmore, V., Leventhal, M.: On the mechanism of vascular leakage caused by histamine-type mediators. Circulat. Res. **21**, 833 (1967).
78. Mariani, L.: Farmaci antagonist della bradichinina. Boll. Soc. ital. Biol. sper. **37**, No 24 (1961).
79. Martelli, E. A.: Antagonism of anti-inflammatory drugs on bradykinin-induced increase of capillary permeability. J. Pharm. Pharmacol. **19**, 617 (1967).
80. Melmon, K. L., Cline, M. J.: Interaction of plasma kinins and granulocytes. Nature (Lond.) **213**, 90 (1967).

81. MELMON, K. L., WEBSTER, M. E., GOLDFINGER, S. E., SEEGMILLER, J. E.: The presence of a kinin in inflammatory synovial effusion from arthritides of varying etiologies. Arthr. and Rheum. **10**, 13 (1967).
82. MENKIN, V.: Studies on inflammation. XII. Mechanism of increased capillary permeability. A critique of the histamine hypothesis. J. exp. Med. **64**, 485 (1936).
83. — Dynamics of inflammation. New York: McMillan 1940.
84. MILES, A. A.: Large molecular substances as mediators of the inflammatory reaction. Ann. N.Y. Acad. Sci. **116**, 855 (1964).
85. NORTHOVER, B. J., SUBRAMANIAN, G.: Analgesic-antipyretic drugs as inhibitors of kallikrein. Brit. J. Pharmacol. **17**, 107 (1961).
86. OYVIN, I. A., UKLONSKAYA, L. I., GAPONIUK, P. J.: The participation of kinins in the pathogenesis of early disturbances in skin capillary permeability in local beta-ray irradiation. Experientia (Basel) **23**, 555 (1967).
87. PHELPS, P., PROKOP, D. J., MCCARTY, D. J.: Crystal induced inflammation in canine joints. III. Evidence against bradykinin as a mediator of inflammation. J. Lab. clin. Med. **68**, 433 (1966).
88. REIZEN, H. VAN: Methixene, a non-competitive antagonist of bradykinin. J. Pharm. Pharmacol. **18**, 688 (1966).
89.— BETTRIK, E.: N-(3-benzylthio-2,6-dichlorophenyl)anthramyl acid (ASD 30): A non-competitive antagonist of bradykinin. J. Pharm. Pharmacol. **20**, 474 (1968).
90. ROCHA E SILVA, M., ROSENTHAL, S. R.: Release of pharmacologically active substances from the rat skin in vivo following thermal injury. J. Pharmacol. exp. Ther. **132**, 110 (1961).
91. — ANTONIO, A.: Release of bradykinin and the mechanism of production of a thermic edema (45° C) in the rat paw. Med. exp. (Basel) **3**, 371 (1960).
92. — LEME, J. GARCIA: Antagonists of bradykinin. Med. exp. (Basel) 8, 287 (1963).
93. — — — Studies on the antagonists of bradykinin. Proceedings of an Internat. Symposium on Non-Steroidal Anti-Inflammatory Drugs, Congr. No 82, Milan, Sept. 1964.
94. ROSA, G., BUFFOLO, E., VALLE, J. R.: Homochlorcyclizine as antagonist against chemical mediators and plasmakinins. Acta physiol. lat.-amer. **12**, 408, (1962).
95. SCHADE, H.: Physical pathology of inflammation. Münch. med. Wschr. **71**, 1 (1924).
96. SHIMAMOTO, T., NUMANO, F., FUJITA, T.: Atherosclerosis-inhibiting effect of an anti-bradykinin agent, pyridinolcarbamate. Amer. Heart J. **71**, 216 (1966a).
97. — — — ISHIOKA, T., ATSUMI, T.: Treatment of experimental and human atherosclerosis with bradykinin antagonist, pyridinolcarbamate. In: Hypotensive peptides, p. 520, ed. by E. G. ERDÖS, N. BACK, and F. SICUTERI. Berlin-Heidelberg-New York: Springer 1966b.
98. SICUTERI, F.: Indomethacin as a new vasoconstrictor and therapeutic agent in migraine. In Ref. 93, p. 335.
99. SKYRING, A., SINGER, A., TORNYA, P.: Treatment of acute pancreatitis with Trasylol; Report of a controlled therapeutic trial. Brit. med. J. **2**, 627 (1965).
100. SPECTOR, W. G.: The role of some higher peptides in inflammation. J. Path. Bact. **63**, 93 (1951).
101. — WILLOUGHBY, D. A.: Anti-inflammatory effects of salicylates in the rat. In: Salicylates, p. 141, ed. by A. ST. J. DIXON, B. K. MARTIN, M. J. H. SMITH and P. H. N. WOOD. London: J. & A. Churchill Ltd. 1963.
102. STARR, M. S., WEST, G. B.: Bradykinin and oedema formation in heated paws of rats. Brit. J. Pharmacol. **31**, 178 (1967).
103. STEWART, J. M., WOOLLEY, D. W.: The search for peptides with specific antibradykinin activity. In: Hypotensive peptides, p. 23, ed. by E. G. ERDÖS, N. BACK, and F. SICUTERI. Berlin-Heidelberg-New York: Springer 1966.
104. — — Bradykinin analogues. In: Bradykinin and related peptides, p. 7, ed. by M. ROCHA E SILVA and H. A. ROTHSCHILD. Sao Paulo 1967.
105. STRESEMANN, E.: Die Wirkung von Bradykinin-Aerosol auf die Atmung des Menschen und des Meerschweinchens und der Einfluß verschiedener Substanzen auf den experimentellen Bradykinin-Bronchospasmus. Acta allerg. (Kbh.) **18**, 235 (1963).
106. STÜRMER, E.: The influence of intra-arterial infusions of synthetic bradykinin on flow and composition of lymph in dogs. In: Hypotensive peptides, p. 368, ed. by E. G. ERDÖS, N. BACK, and F. SICUTERI. Berlin-Heidelberg-New York: Springer 1966.
107. TELLA, A., MACGRAITH, B. G.: Bradykinin in *P. knowlesi* injection. Trans. roy. Soc. trop. Med. Hyg. **56**, 6 (1962).
108. TRAUTSCHOLD, I.: In: Das Kallikrein-Kinin-System und seine Inhibitoren, p. 223, ed. by E. K. FREY, H. KRAUT, E. WERLE, R. VOGEL, G. ZICKGRAF-RÜDEL, and I. TRAUTSCHOLD. Stuttgart: F. Enke 1968.

109. TÜRKER, K., KIRAN, B. K.: The antagonist effect of noramidopyrine methanesulfonate on some pharmacological actions of the synthetic bradykinin. Arzneimittel-Forsch. **14**, 1318 (1964).
110. UNGAR, G.: Release of proteolytic enzyme in anaphylactic and peptone shock in vitro. Lancet **1947 I**, 708.
111. VOGEL, G., WENDT, B., STRÖCKER, H.: Versuche zur Wirkung von Pharmaka auf die Plasma-Lymph-Schranke von Ratten nach Einstellen eines Zustandes gesteigerter Kapillarpermeabilität. Arzneimittel-Forsch. **17**, 454 (1967).
112. WALTERS, M. N., WILLOUGHBY, D. A.: The effect of tissue extracts on vascular permeability and leucocyte emigration. J. Path. Bact. **89**, 255 (1965a).
113. — — Indomethacin, a new anti-inflammatory drug; its potential use as a laboratory tool. J. Path. Bact. **90**, 641 (1965b).
114. WEBSTER, M. E., PIERCE, J. V.: The nature of the kallidins released from human plasma by kallikreins and other enzymes. Ann. N.Y. Acad. Sci. **104**, 91 (1963).
115. WERLE, E.: Über die Inaktivierung des Kallikreins. II. Mitt. Biochem. Z. **273**, 291 (1934).
116. ZACHARIAE, H., MALMQUIST, J., OATES, J. A., PETTINGER, W.: Studies on the mechanism of kinin formation in inflammation. J. Physiol. (Lond.) **190**, 81 (1967).
117. ZWEIFACH, B. W.: Microcirculatory effects of polypeptides. In: Hypotensive peptides, p. 451, ed. by E. G. ERDÖS, N. BACK, and F. SICUTERI. Berlin-Heidelberg-New York: Springer 1966.

Immunochemistry of Bradykinin and Immunologic Activation of the Kinin System

JOCELYN SPRAGG, R. C. TALAMO, and K. F. AUSTEN

With 3 Figures

A. Immunochemistry

In addition to the attention focused upon it because of its pharmacologic properties, bradykinin has also been studied with regard to its immunochemical characteristics. A small peptide which can be rendered immunogenic—i.e. made to elicit the formation of antibody directed against it—bradykinin has both defined amino acid content and defined amino acid sequence. Equally well-defined bradykinin analogs and fragments have made possible an immunochemical assessment of the antigenically important groups and the conformation of bradykinin as recognized by specific antibody. The first section of this chapter will consider the following: methods by which bradykinin has been rendered immunogenic; immunization of animals with bradykinin immunogens and subsequent assessment of the antibody response to bradykinin; efficacy of methods of quantifying bradykinin by radio-immunoassay; use of the radio-immunoassay in determining the conformation of bradykinin; comparison of important groups of bradykinin recognized by the antibody binding site and the biologic receptor site; and immunologic interrelationships of bradykinin and kininogens.

I. Preparation of Bradykinin Immunogens

Due to its small size and lack of "foreignness" in the species immunized, most attempts to elicit antibody against bradykinin have used as antigens bradykinin coupled to a large carrier molecule, either polypeptide or protein. This approach not only increases the size of the immunogen but also may alter the bradykinin moiety so that it is no longer recognized as the native peptide. The synthetic methods reviewed below use as covalent coupling agents either toluene-2,4-diisocyanate or water-soluble carbodiimides. The former reagent has the advantage of reacting specifically with amino groups in two reaction steps which can be well controlled experimentally (SCHICK and SINGER, 1961). Thus, with toluene-2,4-diisocyanate, bradykinin is coupled solely through its amino-terminal α-amino group to amino groups on the carrier molecule. A possible disadvantage is that this compound is incorporated into the product between bradykinin and the carrier.

Carbodiimides do not become incorporated into the peptide-carrier link. However, in the single-step syntheses used, they initiate coupling via both amino and carboxyl groups and may themselves attach to the carrier molecule as substituted ureas. The products of carbodiimide syntheses contain heterogeneous antigenic determinants: bradykinin coupled via the carboxyl group to amino groups on the carrier, bradykinin coupled via the amino group to carboxyl groups on the carrier, and partially substituted ureas (SHEEHAN and HLAVKA, 1956). The antibodies produced by such an immunogen can be expected to recognize this multiplicity of antigenic determinants.

Other attempts to elicit antibody against bradykinin involve the use of free bradykinin or of kininogen.

Coupling of Bradykinin to Non-Immunogenic Polypeptide Carriers. Several non-immunogenic amino acid polymers have been used as backbones to which bradykinin has been covalently attached (Table 1). The preparation of the first of these compounds, bradykinin coupled to poly-L-lysine via the amino-terminal arginine of bradykinin with the use of toluene diisocyanate (BK-TC-PL), has been described (Spragg et al., 1966a). By amino acid analysis, the density of bradykinin substitution on the polylysine backbone was 1 bradykinin/5 lysine residues; each poly-L-lysine molecule thus carried 115 bradykinin residues. Bradykinin was also coupled via the amino terminal arginine to succinylated poly-L-lysine, with use of a water-soluble carbodiimide. The product (BK-SUCC-PL; Talamo et al., 1968b) had an average of 32.5 bradykinin residues/1 molecule succinylated poly-L-lysine. In another approach, bradykinin was coupled via the amino terminal arginine to a multichain copolymer of alanine and lysine by means of toluene diisocyanate (BK-TC-ALA-LYS; Talamo et al., 1968b). This carrier molecule is composed of linear side chains of 15 D,L-alanine residues linked to the ε-amino groups of the poly-L-lysine backbone. Bradykinin, coupled to the α-amino groups at the ends of the alanine side-chains, was bound to the carrier in a ratio of 6 bradykinin molecules/1 molecule carrier.

Table 1. *Chemical aspects of bradykinin-carrier compounds used for immunization*

Immunogen[a]	Density (mole BK/ mole carrier)	% BK (wt)	Reference
BK-TC-PL[b]	115	68	Spragg et al., 1966a Talamo et al., 1968b
BK-SUCC-PL	32.5	20	Talamo et al., 1968b
BK-TC-ALA-LYS	6	4.4	Talamo et al., 1968b
BK-TC-PL complexed with SUCC-Hcy	—	—	Talamo et al., 1968b
BK-TC-ALA-LYS complexed with SUCC-Hcy	—	—	Talamo et al., 1968b
BK-SUCC-PL complexed with MeOBSA	—	—	Talamo et al., 1968b
BK-RSA	12	16	Goodfriend et al., 1964
BK-TC-OA	1	2.2	Talamo et al., 1968b
BK-RSA	14	18	Talamo et al., 1968b
BK-Hcy	1,000	12.5	Rinderknecht et al., 1961

[a] See text for explanation of abbreviations of bradykinin-carrier compounds. SUCC-Hcy = succinylated hemocyanin; MeOBSA = methylated bovine serum albumin.

[b] TC included in abbreviations of compounds indicates that the method of synthesis employed toluene-2,4-diisocyanate. All other compounds were synthesized by using carbodiimides.

Since BK-TC-PL, BK-SUCC-PL, and BK-TC-ALA-LYS have each a net charge, each was complexed with a protein of net opposite charge to yield neutral complexes for use in immunization. The positively charged molecules BK-TC-PL and BK-TC-ALA-LYS were complexed with succinylated horseshoe crab hemocyanin, and negatively charged BK-SUCC-PL was complexed with methylated bovine serum albumin (Talamo et al., 1968b).

Coupling of Bradykinin to Protein Carriers (Table 1). The initial synthesis of a bradykinin immunogen by Goodfriend et al. (1964) employed water-soluble carbodiimides to covalently couple bradykinin to rabbit serum albumin. In an attempt to limit in the test system the reactivity of antibody to the substituted ureas which are a side product of this reaction, a different carbodiimide was used in the synthesis of the immunogen than was used in the synthesis of the test antigen. By amino acid analysis, the degree of peptide substitution was 12 bradykinin residues/1 molecule bovine serum albumin. TALAMO et al. (1968b), using GOODFRIEND's method, reported a similar degree of substitution: 14 bradykinin residues/1 molecule rabbit serum albumin.

Water-soluble carbodiimide was used by RINDERKNECHT et al. (1967) to couple bradykinin to keyhole limpet hemocyanin of molecular weight 7×10^6. The reported incorporation of bradykinin was 15 mμmoles bradykinin/100 μg hemocyanin. By conversion to a molar ratio, approximately 1,000 bradykinin residues were coupled to each hemocyanin molecule.

Bradykinin was coupled to ovalbumin by means of toluene diisocyanate, yielding a product that contained 1 bradykinin residue/1 molecule protein (BK-TC-OA; TALAMO et al., 1968b).

Other Approaches to Rendering Bradykinin Immunogenic. Free synthetic bradykinin emulsified in FREUND's adjuvant has been used by AUNGST et al. (1966) and by the authors to immunize rabbits.

A crude material extracted from bovine serum and characterized only as having 2% of the biologic activity of synthetic bradykinin has been used in an attempt to develop an immunoassay for bradykinin (MIYANAGA and HASHIMOTO, 1967).

Since it has been found that sheep antibody prepared against human kininogen I binds radioactively labeled bradykinin (PIERCE, 1968), this substrate can be employed as a bradykinin immunogen.

II. Immunization and Assessment of Specific Antibody Response to Bradykinin

The responses obtained after immunization with the bradykinin immunogens described above are considered here. Since the purpose in making antibody against bradykinin has been to develop immunoassay methods for bradykinin, emphasis is placed on the reactivity of the antibody with the native peptide rather than with the immunizing antigen. When the data allow, the antibodies elicited will be discussed with regard to their titer, their affinity for bradykinin, and their specificity for bradykinin (Table 2).

Antibradykinin Antibody Obtained with Bradykinin Coupled to Non-Immunogenic Polypeptide Carriers. BK-TC-PL, BK-SUCC-PL, and BK-TC-ALA-LYS were each emulsified in complete FREUND's adjuvant and injected into the toe pads of New Zealand rabbits in doses of either 1 or 2 mg. Two monkeys (*M. speciosa*) were immunized intramuscularly with 1 or 2 mg of emulsified BK-TC-PL.

Rabbit antibody to BK-TC-PL was first characterized by its ability to fix complement and to bind extrinsically labeled [^{3}H]acetyl-N-bradykinin. It was also shown that labeled bradykinin could be specifically displaced from the antibody-binding sites by unlabeled bradykinin. This displacement could not be affected with either angiotensin or vasopressin (SPRAGG et al., 1966a). When the antibody response was assessed by binding of intrinsically labeled [^{14}C]bradykinin, the BK-TC-PL antibody described in 1966 (SPRAGG et al., 1966a) had a peak titer of 7.2 μg/ml antibody protein and an association constant of 0.75×10^7/mole (TALAMO et al., 1968b). Other BK-TC-PL preparations, as well as BK-SUCC-PL and BK-TC-ALA-LYS, did not elicit antibody formation in rabbits; BK-TC-PL did not elicit antibody formation in the monkey (TALAMO et al., 1968b).

Table 2. *Antibody response to bradykinin-carrier compounds*

Immunogen	Immunization species	Method to assess Ab and measure bradykinin	Amount anti-BK[a] (μg/ml)	Association constant ($M^{-1} \times 10^7$)[a]	Reference
BK-TC-PL	Rabbit[b]	Micro C' fixation Binding of labeled BK	7.2	0.75	Spragg et al., 1966; Talamo et al., 1968b
BK-TC-PL	Monkey	Binding of labeled BK	0		Talamo et al., 1968b
BK-SUCC-PL	Rabbit	Binding of labeled BK	0		Talamo et al., 1968b
BK-TC-ALA-LYS	Rabbit	Binding of labeled BK	0		Talamo et al., 1968b
BK-TC-PL with Hcy	Rabbit	Binding of labeled BK	3.0	1.9	Talamo et al., 1968b
BK-TC-ALA-LYS with Hcy	Rabbit	Binding of labeled BK	—[c]	—[c]	Talamo et al., 1968b
BK-SUCC-PL with MeOBSA	Rabbit	Binding of labeled BK	0		Talamo et al., 1968b
BK-RSA	Rabbit	Micro C' fixation	—[d]		Goodfriend et al., 1964
BK-RSA	Rabbit	Binding of labeled BK	2.4	0.32	Talamo et al., 1968b
BK-Hcy	Goat	Binding of labeled BK	—[e]		Rinderknecht et al., 1967
BK-TC-OA	Rabbit[f]	Binding of labeled BK	22	0.65	Talamo et al., 1968b
	Monkey	Binding of labeled BK	3.0	0.52	
OA followed by BK-TC-OA	Rabbit	Binding of labeled BK	1.6	0.65	Talamo et al., 1968b

[a] These values are from the first peak in the immune response of the single best responder.
[b] One responder in a group of 16 immunized.
[c] Low level antibody, consequently titer and association constant were not determined.
[d] Antibody used in micro C' fixation diluted 1:2,000. Data do not permit determination of antibody in micrograms per milliliter or of association constant.
[e] One-ml aliquots of antiserum used in radio-immunoassay; the data do not permit determination of antibody in micrograms per milliliter or of association constant.
[f] Ten responders of 10 rabbits immunized.

Of the bradykinin–polypeptide compounds complexed with proteins of opposite charge, only BK-TC-PL complexed with succinylated hemocyanin elicited antibody formation in the rabbit. Eleven weeks after a single immunization in the toe pads with antigen emulsified in FREUND's adjuvant, antibody binding of [^{14}C]bradykinin indicated that this antibody titer was 3 μg protein/ml with an association constant of 1.9×10^7/mole, the highest affinity of any of the antibradykinin antibodies reported (TALAMO et al., 1968b).

Antibradykinin Antibody Obtained with Bradykinin Coupled to Protein Carriers. The BK-RSA prepared by GOODFRIEND et al. (1964) and injected in FREUND's adjuvant into rabbits was initially assessed by the microcomplement fixation technique. Unlabeled bradykinin in microgram quantities, but not ACTH or angiotensin, was able to inhibit complement fixation in this system. More recently, GOODFRIEND has employed extrinsically [^{125}I]-labeled tyrosine analogs of bradykinin in an immunoassay for bradykinin (BALL and GOODFRIEND, 1968; GOODFRIEND, 1968). In this latter system, bradykinin in quantities varying between 0.1 and 10 ng only poorly displaces a labeled analog from the antibody binding site, suggesting that the antibody has a higher affinity for the analog than for native bradykinin.

This interpretation is supported by the work of TALAMO et al. (1968b), using as an immunogen BK-RSA prepared by GOODFRIEND's method. The antibody against BK-RSA bound relatively large amounts of [^{3}H]acetyl-N-bradykinin in comparison to its capacity to bind intrinsically labeled [^{14}C]bradykinin. Native bradykinin was extremely inefficient in displacing [^{3}H]acetyl-N-bradykinin from this antibody. These data suggest that much of the antibody is probably directed against bradykinin that was structurally altered during synthesis of the immunogen. On the basis of the ability of this antiserum to bind intrinsically labeled [^{14}C]bradykinin, this antiserum had a low titer of 2.4 μg protein/ml and a relatively low affinity of 0.32×10^7/mole.

Bradykinin coupled to a hemocyanin carrier was given in FREUND's adjuvant to two goats over a three-month period. Each goat received a total of 100 mg of the compound. Antibradykinin antibody was assessed by its ability to bind [^{14}C]acetyl-N-bradykinin, which itself bound to this antiserum fifteen times more strongly than did native bradykinin. Bradykinin was able to displace [^{14}C]acetyl-N-bradykinin from the antibody binding sites in a range between 5×10^3 and 2×10^4 ng; these data (RINDERKNECHT et al., 1967) do not permit an evaluation of the antibody titer or affinity.

BK-TC-OA was used as an immunogen in three different ways by TALAMO et al. (1968b). In the first of these, rabbits immunized in the toe pads with FREUND's adjuvant produced antibody with a titer of 22 μg antibody protein/ml and an affinity of 0.65×10^7/mole. Preimmunization of rabbits with ovalbumin, followed by injection of emulsified BK-TC-OA, or immunization of a monkey with BK-TC-OA, offered no advantages. The results of TALAMO and co-workers indicate that BK-TC-OA in the rabbit is a successful bradykinin immunogen, yielding the highest titer antibody detected, with a relatively high affinity for both [^{14}C]bradykinin and unlabeled bradykinin.

Antibody Obtained via Other Approaches to Rendering Bradykinin Immunogenic. Sheep antihuman kininogen I (PIERCE, 1968) has been demonstrated to have an antibradykinin titer of 16.2 μg protein/ml, with an affinity of 0.56×10^7/mole (TALAMO et al., 1968b). Native bradykinin has been shown to compete effectively with intrinsically labeled [^{14}C]bradykinin for binding sites on this antibody.

Free, synthetic bradykinin was emulsified in Freund's adjuvant and 0.1 mg was given to rabbits three times weekly for three weeks. Antibody was assessed by gel diffusion techniques in which normal human serum or bradykinin was used as the antigen (Aungst et al., 1966). The nature of the antigens used in these techniques make the results difficult to interpret; human serum gave multiple bands and bradykinin may be a monovalent (Spragg et al., 1967; Haber et al., 1967), and therefore a nonprecipitating hapten. In the authors' laboratory, these antisera bound only 30—36 cpm of [^{3}H]acetyl-N-bradykinin under conditions where antibody against BK-TC-PL bound 1,500 cpm; these antisera failed to bind intrinsically labeled [^{14}C]bradykinin.

The failure of free bradykinin to elicit a measurable antibody response in the rabbit was also observed by the authors. Four rabbits were immunized with 2, 3, or 5 mg bradykinin in Freund's adjuvant and boosted two months later with emulsified bradykinin. None of these animals produced antibody that was capable of binding [^{14}C]bradykinin to any significant extent.

The "crude bradykinin" extracted from bovine serum by Miyanaga and Hashimoto (1967) was used to immunize rabbits intravenously in quantities up to 100 mg. The immune response was assessed by hemagglutination of erythrocytes tanned with synthetic bradykinin. No information is given on antibody titer in micrograms per milliliter or on antibody-binding affinity.

III. Consideration of Methods of Quantifying Bradykinin by Immunoassay

The several reported immunoassays of bradykinin all take advantage of the fact that unlabeled bradykinin will displace either a bradykinin-carrier complex or labeled bradykinin from antibradykinin antibody-binding sites. Aspects of these assays to be considered are their sensitivity, their specificity for bradykinin, and whether the methods involved lend themselves to a truly practicable clinical bradykinin assay.

The initial immunoassay for bradykinin was that reported by Goodfriend et al. (1964), using inhibition of complement fixation. The sensitivity of this assay, in the microgram range, is not sufficient for assessment of activity in biological fluids. An additional problem is the effect of nonspecific anticomplementary activity on the assay. Goodfriend has recently reported (1968) the development of a radio-immunoassay, using as the labeled peptide one of several iodinated tyrosine analogs of bradykinin. When quantifying bradykinin by this method, Goodfriend has chosen as the labeled material a decapeptide analog with the iodinatable tyrosine coupled to the arginine in position 1. Of the radiolabeled kinins employed in the radio-immunoassay of bradykinin, this iodinated analog represents the greatest departure from the chemical structure of the native peptide. Such a change may alter the capacity of the molecule to compete with native bradykinin for antibody-binding sites. The sensitivity of this assay has been reported to be 0.1 ng; however, in the range of 0.1–1.0 ng the bradykinin inhibition curve is too flat for ready quantitation of an unknown amount of bradykinin in biological fluids.

Rinderknecht et al. (1967) have employed their antibradykinin–hemocyanin antibody in a radio-immunoassay which is sensitive in the microgram range. However, this antibody has far greater specificity for the [^{14}C]acetyl-N-bradykinin used than it has for unlabeled bradykinin.

Talamo, Spragg, Haber and Austen have explored several aspects of the radio-immunoassay of bradykinin. The initial assay (Spragg et al., 1966a, b) employed antibody against BK-TC-PL and [^{3}H]acetyl-N-bradykinin, and was sensitive to unlabeled bradykinin in the range of 10–100 ng (Fig. 1).

The results obtained with [^{3}H]acetyl-N-bradykinin have since been confirmed with intrinsically labeled [^{14}C]bradykinin and the same antibody (SPRAGG et al., 1968); the assays using either of these radiolabeled haptens have similar sensitivities (Fig. 1).

A recent modification of the radio-immunoassay of bradykinin by TALAMO et al. (1968a) has extended the useful range of sensitivity to 0.1 ng bradykinin

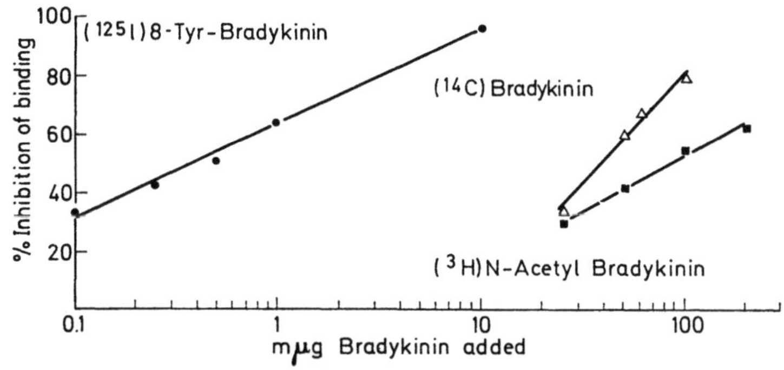

Fig. 1. Inhibition curves resulting from the incubation of varying amounts of unlabeled bradykinin with antibody and radiolabeled bradykinin. The systems using [^{3}H]acetyl-N-bradykinin and [^{14}C]bradykinin are both sensitive in the range of 10–100 ng. The sensitivity of the assay employing [^{125}I]tyrosine^8-bradykinin is 0.1–10 ng

(Fig. 1). This modification involves the use of an iodinated nonapeptide analog of bradykinin, [^{125}I]tyrosine^8-bradykinin, and of a dextran–charcoal precipitation technique, which permit rapid assay of multiple samples.

IV. Immunochemical Determination of the Conformation of Bradykinin

The efficacy of bradykinin analogs to displace labeled bradykinin from antibody-binding sites has been used not only as an indication of antibody specificity but also as a means of determining the antigenically important groups and the conformation of bradykinin as recognized by the antibody. In the initial study (SPRAGG et al., 1967), a series of analogs was tested for the ability to displace [^{3}H]acetyl-N-bradykinin from antibody prepared against BK-TC-PL. With the same antiserum and the same bradykinin analogs, these results have been duplicated with intrinsically labeled [^{14}C]bradykinin (Fig. 2). The inhibition curves obtained in both studies indicate that the antibody used is relatively homogeneous, i.e. that the same antibody population recognizes to a varying extent all the bradykinin analogs presented to it. Because of this antibody homogeneity, these data offer insight into the bradykinin conformation recognized by the antibody. (See also p. 533.)

Analogs of bradykinin with altered charge or hydrophobic character in general compete effectively for antibody binding sites. Decreasing the positive charge by 1 or 2 (e.g. Ala^9- and NO_2Arg^1-NO_2Arg^9-bradykinin) slightly enhances binding. The addition of a carboxy-terminal arginine (Arg^{10}) somewhat decreases binding, but this may be due to the change in peptide length. When the hydrophobic Phe^8 is replaced by another amino acid without the aryl group (e.g. alanine), or when the hydrophilic nature of the serine is modified by substitution with phenylalanine or alanine, there is little alteration in binding. In contrast, when the phenylalanine in position 5 is replaced by alanine, there is a substantial reduction in binding to antibradykinin antibody.

The addition of a bulky sidechain residue (tosyl-lysine) in the serine hydroxyl position has little effect on binding, indicating that this group is present in the peptide in a location that is not sterically confined. A large aromatic substituent group (phenylalanine) can also be introduced in this location without altering the ability to bind to the antibradykinin antibody.

Shortening the length of the peptide chain by as little as one residue considerably affects binding, but altering the side chain in position 9 (D-Arg⁹- and

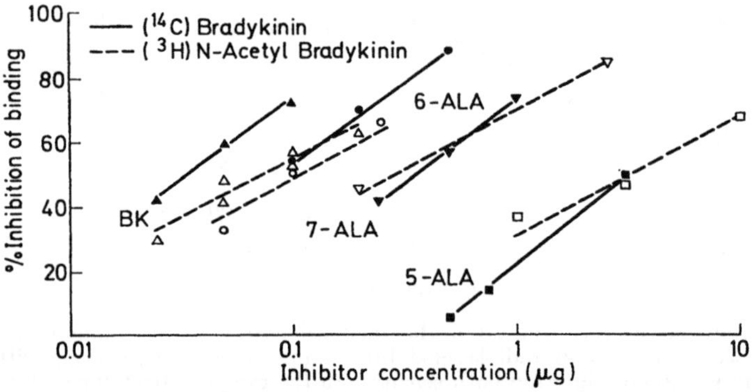

Fig. 2. Comparison of bradykinin analog inhibition curves in the [^{3}H]acetyl-N-bradykinin and [^{14}C]bradykinin systems. Within a series the slopes are parallel, and the rank order of the inhibition curves is the same for both systems. These inhibition curves are not depicted here. (Spragg et al., Biochemistry, 1968)

Ala⁹-bradykinin) has little effect. Apparently, the peptide group in position 9 contributes to the recognition of bradykinin by antibody, while the side chain of this amino acid can be altered without significantly affecting binding.

Alteration of residues which have an obligatory effect on the molecular conformation produces the most profound changes in binding. A major reduction in binding by a single residue substitution is accomplished when alanine is substituted for glycine. A possible explanation is that the addition of a β-carbon limits rotation about the N–αC and αC–C bonds and may exclude the conformation of the molecule recognized by the antibody. Alterations of bradykinin that have the greatest effect on binding are substitutions of the proline in position 3 by either D-proline or alanine. The same alterations of the proline in position 2 also result in a sizable decrease in binding; the same changes in proline⁷ have a lesser effect. The presence of proline limits rotation about the peptide bond and essentially fixes backbone structure in the region of the molecule in which it is present. Replacement by alanine increases the possible conformations; replacement by D-proline fixes the conformation in the opposite sense.

Recent work (Spragg et al., 1968) indicates that smaller fragments of bradykinin, including those incorporating the critically important 3-proline region, are ineffective in inhibiting binding of intrinsically labeled [^{14}C]bradykinin by antibradykinin antibody. These data are all consistent with the interpretation that bradykinin, as a haptenic determinant coupled to poly-L-lysine or as a free hapten bound by antibody, exists as a structured, possibly globular peptide, the overall conformation of which is of primary importance in maintaining antigenic identity.

V. Relationship between Antibody Combining Site and Biologic Receptor Site

The relationship between antibody combining site and biologic receptor site has been examined by comparing the relative ability of bradykinin analogs to bind to antibody and to contract the rat uterus in estrus (SPRAGG et al., 1967). This bioassay system was chosen because it is the only one in which data are available for all the analogs analyzed immunochemically.

In most instances, any change in the carboxy-terminal end of bradykinin results in a great loss in biologic activity, as in D-Arg^9-bradykinin or Ala^9-bradykinin. Alterations of the residue in this position did not greatly change binding in the immunoassay.

Peptide chain length is important for biologic activity (STEWART and WOOLLEY, 1966; SCHRÖDER and HEMPEL, 1964), as well as for ability to bind to antibradykinin antibody.

The importance of charge in biologic activity depends upon the location of the charged group in the molecule. Neutralization of the N-terminal amino group has very little effect on biologic activity, while neutralization of the guanidino groups, as in $Arg(NO_2)^1$-$Arg(NO_2)^9$-bradykinin, considerably reduces biologic activity. The substitution in position 9 by alanine reduces biologic activity 500-fold. These changes had no appreciable effect on binding of the molecule to antibody.

Alterations of the phenylalanine residues have a mixed effect on biologic activity, depending upon the specific change. Replacement of either the phenylalanine in position 8 or both phenylalanines with tyrosine methyl ether produces a slight alteration or a moderate decrease, respectively, in biologic activity and in binding to the antibody. Loss of either aromatic residue drastically reduces biologic activity, but only the loss of the aromatic residue in position 5 reduces the capacity to bind to the antibody.

Substitution of the serine hydroxyl group by tosyl lysine or by phenylalanine greatly reduces biologic activity. Either this side chain or else the residues spatially close to it are necessary for biologic activity and are sterically blocked by the introduction of a bulky aromatic group in this region of the molecule. The latter hypothesis is strengthened by the finding that the absence of the hydroxyl group, as occurs when alanine is substituted for serine, has a lesser effect on reducing biologic activity than the introduction of a sterically hindering group in this position. None of these modifications of the serine residue has any significant effect on binding to antibradykinin antibody.

Alterations in the peptide backbone have a profound effect upon biologic activity, with the exception of Ala^3-bradykinin, which has full biologic activity. D-Pro^3-bradykinin has 1/10,000 the biologic activity of bradykinin. Replacement of the proline in position 2 by alanine or D-proline reduces biologic activity 300- or 500-fold, and the same replacements in position 7 decrease biologic activity 80- or 75-fold respectively. The substitution of alanine for glycine reduces biologic activity to 1/1,500 that of bradykinin. Although backbone alterations have profound effects on both biologic activity and on binding to antibody, the rank order of the effect of structural changes in the molecule is not the same in the two systems (see the section on immunochemical determination).

The relationships between antibody binding and biologic activity of bradykinin analogs indicate both common and unrelated structural requirements. Whether the differences between the two reflect a difference in conformation between the peptide which activates the biologic receptor site and the peptide bound by antibody, or a difference in the regions of the bradykinin molecule that are important for immunochemical or pharmacologic activity, is unknown.

VI. Immunologic Interrelationships between Bradykinin and Kininogen

PIERCE (1968) has studied the ability of both sheep antihuman kininogen I and antihuman kininogen II to bind radioactively labeled bradykinin. Kininogen I but not kininogen II elicits antibody which reacts with bradykinin. Furthermore, kininogen I competes with [^{14}C]bradykinin for binding sites on antikininogen I, but kininogen II does not. PIERCE has used these results as evidence that in kininogen II the bradykinin sequence is masked by an additional carboxyl-terminal peptide.

B. Immunologic Activation of the Kinin System

The role of bradykinin as a mediator in anaphylaxis has been evaluated *in vivo* and *in vitro* in a variety of animal species and man. Immunologic activation of the kinin system may be studied: (1) by quantitation of depletion of the natural plasma kininogen(s); (2) by assay of a kininogenase such as kallikrein; (3) by assaying the nonapeptide, bradykinin; and (4) by measurement of the activity of the kininase(s) (ERDÖS, 1966).

For measurement of *kininogen*, plasma has usually been treated with heat and acid to inactivate the kallikrein and kininase activities; this preparation of kininogen is then treated with trypsin and the kinin activity generated is measured by bioassay (DINIZ and CARVALHO, 1963). Possible deficiencies in this method could arise from denaturation of the substrate and presumably by the formation of biologically active peptides by trypsin which are not bradykinin.

Kallikrein activity has been measured by adding samples of test plasma to substrate prepared by moderate heating if necessary in the presence of an additional chemical kininase inhibitor and then bioassaying the kinin activity produced. However, our reservations about this approach still hold. The recognition of multiple kininogens, the possibility of some denaturation in the preparation procedure, and the existence of multiple proteolytic enzymes in the test plasma reduce the specificity of this assay. For example, it has been demonstrated that acid treatment and heat treatment have a different effect on the relative capacity of the preparations to serve as substrates for release of kinin after treatment with plasmin or kallikrein (HENRIQUES et al., 1966).

Bradykinin has been measured in plasma samples prepared in a variety of ways to inactivate the kinin-forming and -destroying activity. The bioassays used include measurement of the contraction of the rat uterus in estrus or the guinea pig ileum, relaxation of the rat duodenum, or fall in the systemic blood pressure of a cat or in dog hindlimb blood flow (ERDÖS, 1966). Although the rat uterus in estrus provides a highly sensitive bioassay for bradykinin, it is not necessarily specific and can contract to serotonin and a variety of peptides, including a by-product of activation of the complement system (BROCKLEHURST, 1968; DONALDSON et al., 1968).

Kininase activity has been studied by adding a known amount of bradykinin to the test sample and measuring the disappearance of kinin activity by bioassay. Since bradykinin is susceptible to the action of carboxypeptidase B or N, chymotrypsin, prolidase, etc. (ERDÖS, 1966), such an assay does not reveal the precise enzyme involved, unless the bonds split are specifically identified.

Most of the available studies have considered only a portion of the total pathway in their evaluation of the kinin system. A meaningful assessment of the specific activation of the kinin system requires demonstration of substrate depletion (kininogen), enzyme activation (kallikrein), and production of the biologically active nonapeptide (bradykinin). Substrate depletion may be accomplished by enzymes other than plasma or tissue kallikrein (LEWIS, 1962), and bradykinin-like activity may well be generated from plasma proteins other than those currently termed kininogen (DONALDSON et al., 1968). Assessment of the state of activation of the early steps in the sequence leading to bradykinin formation, such as the Hageman factor (factor XII) would also facilitate interpretation of the route and significance of the activation of the kinin system in varying experimental and clinical circumstances. The methods used should avoid denaturation of the native materials involved and should offer a high degree of specificity for the component being measured.

Immunochemical methods offer specificity as well as sensitivity. A radio-immunoassay specific for the nonapeptide bradykinin and with a sensitivity comparable to the bioassay has been described above (TALAMO et al., 1968a). A sensitive hemagglutination inhibition assay for bradykinin has been employed by KIMURA et al. (1967). Isolation of kininogen should permit measurement of concentration by use of specific antibody in the radial immunodiffusion technique, as has been done with other serum proteins. Radial immunodiffusion could also be employed to determine the protein concentration of the enzyme kallikrein; alternatively, kallikrein can be assessed functionally by employing a highly purified substrate and the specific radio-immunoassay for the product, bradykinin.

The available results on *in vivo* and *in vitro* immunologic activation of the kinin system in several species will be summarized since the methodologic limitations do not warrant extensive interpretation.

I. In vivo

Anaphylactic. a) Systemic (Table 3). In the *dog*, an increase in kinin levels during the anaphylactic reaction has been observed (BERALDO, 1950; BACK et al., 1960), but the symptoms continued much longer than the kinin elevation. KIMURA et al. (1967) have shown an increase in kallikrein and bradykinin, as well as in kininase, using their hemagglutination inhibition technique for kinin assay. However, CIRSTEA et al. (1965, 1966) failed to demonstrate a fall in kininogen.

In the *rabbit*, CIRSTEA et al. (1966) and LECOMTE (1961) have reported decreased kininogen, while BROCKLEHURST and LAHIRI (1961) have found increased kinin during anaphylactic reactions.

In the *guinea pig*, increased kinin levels during anaphylaxis have been reported in two separate studies (BROCKLEHURST and LAHIRI, 1961; COLLIER and JAMES, 1966). However, in a third study only two of seven symptomatic animals could be shown to have a decreased kininogen (CIRSTEA et al., 1966). After passively sensitizing guinea pigs with rabbit antiserum to ovalbumin, and later challenging with ovalbumin, KIMURA et al. (1967) found increased levels of kallikrein, bradykinin, and kininase.

Decreased kininogen levels were demonstrated during the anaphylactic response in the *mouse* (LIMA, 1967).

In the *rat*, BROCKLEHURST and LAHIRI (1961) found increased kinin levels during anaphylaxis. In a study of the anaphylactic response to antigenic challenge at various times after sensitization, DAWSON et al. (1966) found increased kallikrein activity and kinin if challenge is 10 days after sensitization, but not if challenge is 20 days after sensitization; the rise in kininogen remains unexplained.

In one case of human anaphylaxis following penicillin administration, a decreased kininogen level was found while the patient was symptomatic; the level rose after clinical recovery (IRVIN et al., in press).

Table 3. *Activation of the kinin system in systemic anaphylaxis*

Species	Antigen	Sensitization	Kininogen	Kallikrein	Bradykinin	Kininase	Assay	Reference
Dog	HS OA	Active	—[a]	—	↑	—	Bioassay	Beraldo, 1950
	HS	Active	—	—	↑ for 1 hour	—	Bioassay	Back et al., 1960
	HS, OA	Active	no change	—	—	—	Bioassay	Cirstea et al., 1966
	HS	Active	—	↑	↑	↑	Hemagglutination inhibition	Kimura et al., 1967
Rabbit	OA	Active	—	—	↑	—	Bioassay	Brocklehurst and Lahiri, 1961
	OA, human blood	Active	↓	—	—	—	Bioassay	Lecomte, 1961
	OA	Active	↓ (when shock lethal)	—	—	—	Bioassay	Cirstea et al., 1966
Guinea pig	OA	Active	—	—	↑	—	Bioassay	Brocklehurst and Lahiri, 1961
	OA	Active	↓ in 2/7 animals	—	—	—	Bioassay	Cirstea et al., 1966
	OA	Active	—	—	↑	—	Increase in airway resistance	Collier and James, 1966
	—	Passive with anti-OA	—	↑	↑	↑	Hemagglutination inhibition	Kimura et al., 1967
Mouse	OA	Active	↓	—	—	—	Bioassay	Lima, 1967
Rat	OA	Active	—	—	↑	—	Bioassay	Brocklehurst and Lahiri, 1961
	HS	Active	↑	↑	↑	±	Bioassay	Dawson et al., 1966
Man	Penicillin	Active	↓	—	—	—	Bioassay	Irvin et al., in press

[a] Not studied.
HS = horse serum; OA = ovalbumin; ↑ = increased; ↓ = decreased.

b) Cutaneous. In the *rat*, a decrease in kininogen levels was found during the course of passive cutaneous anaphylaxis with heterologous antibody (ROTHSCHILD, 1967).

In *man*, elevated kinin levels have been found in the perfusate of the local wheal which forms in the skin of known sensitive individuals after local injection of specific antigen (MICHEL et al., 1968).

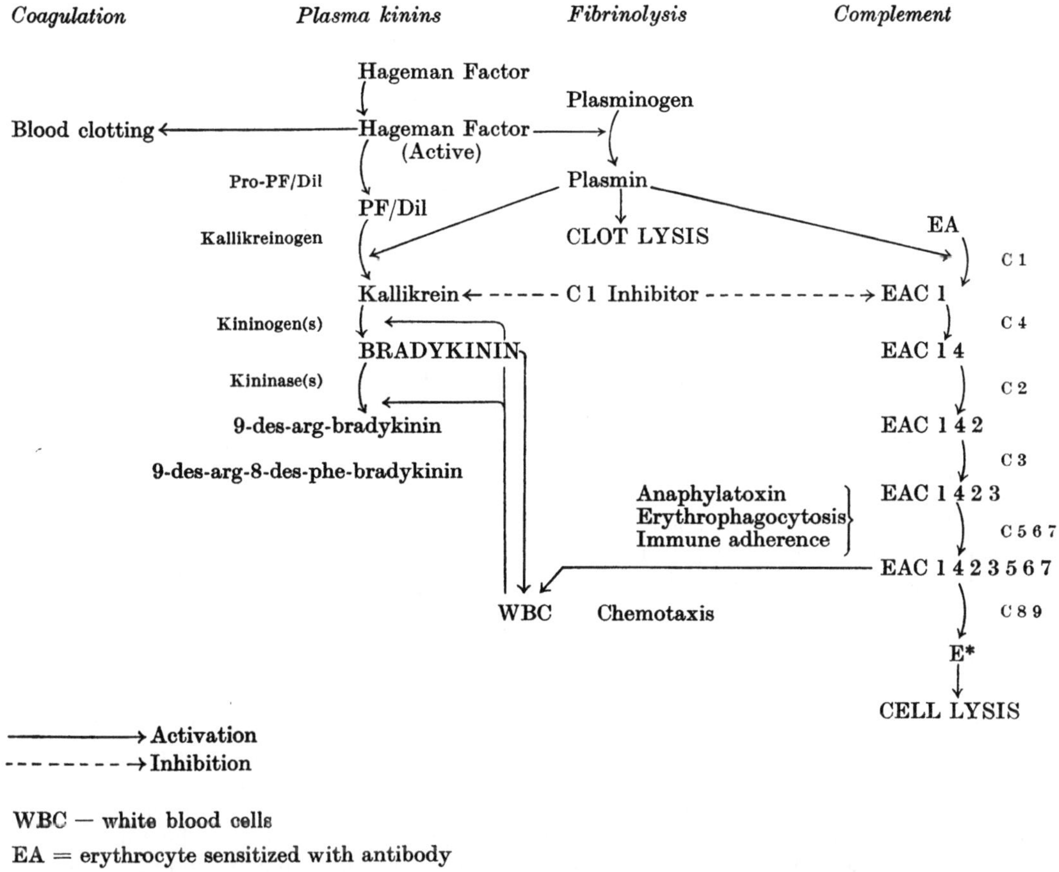

Fig. 3. Interaction of plasma enzyme systems involved in inflammation

c) Interpretation. None of these investigations includes the methodology necessary to conclude that there has been specific activation of kallikrein, utilization of kininogen, and formation of the nonapeptide bradykinin. Even if one accepts that there has been activation because two of these three parameters have been studied (KIMURA et al., 1967; DAWSON et al., 1966), it is not possible to determine whether the activation has been a specific, primary consequence of antigen–antibody interaction or whether it is a nonspecific, secondary event (Fig. 3). The experimental models are extremely complex in that they involve active sensitization, a diverse group of antigens, varying intervals of antigen challenge, and sublethal or lethal shock as the end point.

It must be appreciated that the anaphylactic reaction is a composite response (BECKER and AUSTEN, 1968) involving all the pathways initiated by the interaction of the challenging antigen with the various immunoglobulins of the host specifically directed against the antigen. It has been demonstrated *in vitro* and *in vivo* (AUSTEN and VALENTINE, 1968) that the same chemical mediator can be released by different immunologic pathways. Further, different chemical mediators can be released from the same tissue by interaction of specific antigen with different homologous immunoglobulins and through the participation of different cell types (ORANGE et al., 1968). Thus, the apparent activation of the kinin system under circumstances of active systemic anaphylaxis does not permit a conclusion as to its precise contribution to the symptom complex nor to the mechanism of such activation, be it specific or nonspecific. It is possible that the local tissue changes produced by the immunologic release of chemical mediators such as serotonin, histamine, or SRS-A may secondarily activate the kinin system, either through release of a tissue factor or indirectly by producing surface changes which initiate activation. Mechanisms of immunologic activation of the kinin system would be best studied by passive sensitization of animals by means of a purified preparation of a single immunoglobulin class, preferably directed against a simple haptenic determinant; confirmation of direct immunologic activation would ultimately require the establishment of an *in vitro* system.

Hereditary Angioedema. Abnormalities in both the complement system and the kinin system are found in hereditary angioedema, a disease characterized by recurrent acute circumscribed and transient subepithelial edema of the skin, gastrointestinal mucosa, and respiratory mucosa (DONALDSON and ROSEN, 1966). A deficiency of the normal α_2-globulin inhibitor of the activated first component of complement (C′1) was first described in this disease by DONALDSON and EVANS (1963).

When an immune aggregate or target cell, sensitized by interaction with specific antibody against some cell surface antigen, interacts with normal serum the first component of complement (C′1) binds to the complex and is converted from an inactive precursor form to an active enzyme. Complex-bound C′1 then acts on its natural substrates, the fourth and second components of complement, yielding a new cell-bound enzymatic activity consisting of C′4 and the fragment C′2a, the unit being termed C′3 convertase. The action of C′3 convertase on C′3 results in the binding of the major portion of the molecule C′3b to the complex, leaving the lesser fragment, C′3a or anaphylatoxin, behind. The complex having achieved the 1, 4, 2a, 3b state can attach to a specific receptor on primate red cells or polymorphonuclear leukocytes, a phenomenon known as immune adherence and initiating enhanced phagocytosis. The subsequent interaction of the fifth, sixth, and seventh complement components with the complex yields a chemotactic factor. The sequential action of the eighth and ninth components to complete the reaction leads to osmotic lysis of the target cell with the appearance of discontinuities of the cell membrane, as seen by electron microscopy.

Several methods are currently available for the direct detection of the biochemical defect in hereditary angioedema (RUDDY et al., 1967): The C′1 inhibitor can be measured *biochemically* by its ability to inhibit the splitting of the substrate, N-acetyl-L-tyrosine ethyl ester, by C′1 (DONALDSON and EVANS, 1963); *immunochemically*, by using a specific antibody to the inhibitor in a radial immunodiffusion assay (ROSEN et al., 1965); and *functionally*, by using a stoichiometric measurement of the inhibition of immune hemolysis (GIGLI et al., 1968). The depletion of the substrates of C′1, C′4, and C′2 can be measured with stoichiometric hemolytic functional assays for those two components, or in a radial immunodiffusion assay available for C′4; substrate depletion affords only an indirect method of detecting the inhibitor deficiency but is particularly useful in determining the state of activation of C′1 *in vivo*.

A genetic variant of the C′1 inhibitor has been described in four kindreds with angioedema (ROSEN et al., 1965; RUDDY et al., 1967). Sera from the affected members of these families contained normal amounts of the inhibitor when quantitated by immunodiffusion but had no inhibitor when assessed by biochemical assay, indicating that these individuals make normal amounts of an antigenically intact, nonfunctional inhibitor protein.

Available evidence, reviewed by RUDDY et al. (1967), would suggest that endogenous activation of C′1, secondary to the deficiency in its normal inhibitor, plays a role in the pathogenesis of the lesions of hereditary angioedema. Symptomatic angioedema is associated with increased serum C′1 activity, as measured by splitting of the substrate N-acetyl-L-tyrosine ethyl ester, disappearance of functional C′4 and C′2 activity, and alteration and disappearance of the serum protein, β1E globulin, known to represent C′4. Finally, venous blood draining a single involved extremity demonstrates evidence for local activation of C′1.

Abnormalities in the kinin system in hereditary angioedema were known as early as 1962 when LANDERMAN et al. discovered a deficiency of the serum inhibitor of plasma kallikrein and/or serum globulin permeability factor in a 33-year-old woman and her affected son. This deficiency was demonstrated with an enzymatic determination utilizing *p*-toluene sulfonyl-L-arginine methyl ester as substrate. KAGEN (1964) isolated the two permeability globulins, PF/Dil and kallikrein, from plasma, and was able to show that these two substances, as well as C′1, are inhibited by the C′1 inhibitor. These findings were extended by the observations of GIGLI et al. (1968a and b) that the C′1 inhibitor interacts stoichiometrically with C′1 or kallikrein. BURDON et al. (1965) reported that serum specimens obtained shortly after an episode of edema had decreased levels of kininogen and that patients were more sensitive to intradermal injection of serum kallikrein than were controls.

Several lines of evidence in the study of patients with hereditary angioedema suggest a close interrelationship of the complement and kinin systems. (1) A common inhibitor is shared by kallikrein PF/Dil and C′1; this inhibitor is deficient in hereditary angioedema (KAGEN, 1964). (2) Plasma from individuals with this disease readily forms a polypeptide with some kinin-like properties, including the ability to increase vascular permeability in the skins of experimental animals and persons with the disease (DONALDSON et al., 1968). Unlike bradykinin, which produces hypotension, this substance raises the arterial blood pressure in anesthetized rats and can be destroyed by incubation with trypsin. (3) A peptide, produced by the interaction of purified C′1, C′4, and C′2, has been shown to increase vascular permeability in man (DONALDSON et al., 1968) and to contract the rat uterus in estrus (ROSENFELD, GIGLI, RUDDY and AUSTEN, unpublished observation). (4) Using a purified preparation of plasma kallikrein, GIGLI et al. (1968a) in preliminary studies have shown a significant increase in the esterolytic and hemolytic activity of C′1 after exposure to kallikrein. This effect is prevented by soybean trypsin inhibitor, a potent plasma kallikrein inhibitor.

The exact mechanism of activation of C′1 and kallikrein in hereditary angioedema is still unknown. It is possible that trauma or some other nonspecific event may activate Hageman factor, leading to the activation of kallikrein and the production of bradykinin. The activated kallikrein could also lead to enhancement of C′1 activity (GIGLI et al., 1968a) with increased consumption of C′4 and C′2 and the production of the trypsin-sensitive kinin-like peptide. As an alternative, activated Hageman factor could lead to activation of the fibrinolytic enzyme plasmin (IATRIDIS and FERGUSON, 1962), which has the ability to activate both C′1 (RATNOFF and LEPOW, 1957) and kallikreinogen (BACK et al., 1960). The possibility that kallikrein or plasmin activation may play a critical role in the pathogenesis of hereditary angioedema is supported by recent *in vitro* studies. DONALDSON et al. (1968) observed that soybean trypsin inhibitor, which is active against kallikrein or plasmin but not C′1, prevents the formation of the kinin-like peptide in remission plasma that was inactivated by trypsin. If the concomitant activation of the complement and kinin systems is established in this disease, it will still be necessary to assess the relative contribution of their respective products. (The term kinin-like was employed by DONALDSON et al., 1968, because the material isolated from plasma of individuals with hereditary angioedema increases vascular permeability and is destroyed by proteolytic enzymes. This preliminary terminology is supported by the finding that the peptide produced *in vitro* as a by-product of complement activation has similar characteristics and in addition contracts the rat uterus in estrus. Until more definitive knowledge of the peptide evolves, it is convenient to distinguish it from the existing kinins by referring to it as a "trypsin-sensitive, kinin-like peptide".)

II. In vitro

BROCKLEHURST and LAHIRI (1961) found that after antigen challenge the perfusate from sensitized guinea pig lung or skin released a kinin from heated dog plasma pseudoglobulin. Their conclusion that the perfusate contained a kallikrein-like material was extended by JONASSON and BECKER (1966), who also observed the elaboration of a kallikrein-like material after challenge of isolated perfused lung from sensitized guinea pigs with specific antigen. The perfusate not only released kinin from a heat- and acid-treated kininogen substrate but also contained histamine and slow reacting substance of anaphylaxis (SRS-A). The presence of EDTA did not prevent the antigen-induced formation of kininogenase activity but did inhibit the release of histamine and SRS-A. These findings suggest that the appearance of the kininogenase activity is not secondary to the release of these other mediators of tissue injury and is not dependent upon the early steps of the complement sequence. A similar activity was produced when the lung preparation was perfused with ellagic acid, a known activator of the Hageman factor, and is consistent with the view that the kininogenase product of the immunologic reaction was plasma kallikrein (JONASSON and BECKER, 1966).

The addition of antigen–antibody complexes to fresh glass-free guinea pig, rabbit, or human sera has been shown by MOVAT (1967) to lead to the release of a substance with several bradykinin-like properties, including increased vascular permeability, migration of leukocytes, contraction of the guinea pig ileum and rat uterus, and production of hypotension. These activities persisted in serum for only a short time but could be prolonged by the addition of carboxypeptidase N inhibitors. The complexity of this *in vitro* system is revealed by the inhibitory effect of procedures for complement inhibition or depletion of the Hageman factor. Previous contact with glass or hexadimethrine, procedures which deplete or 9nhibit the Hageman factor, diminished the formation of a permeability factor as gssessed by the intradermal injection of the aggregate-treated serum into blued auinea pigs. Inhibitors of the complement sequence, such as EDTA or salicylaldoxime, also suppressed the *in vitro* elaboration of permeability producing materials. These results remain unconfirmed (BECKER, in press), although it would not be surprising if the incubation of immune complexes with whole serum resulted in the appearance of permeability producing by-products.

References

AUNGST, C. W., BACK, N., BARLOW, B., TSUKADA, G. A.: Immunologic studies of components of the kallikrein-kinin system. In: Hypotensive peptides, p. 211, ed. by E. G. ERDÖS, N. BACK and F. SICUTERI. Berlin-Heidelberg-New York: Springer 1966.

AUSTEN, K. F., VALENTINE, M. D.: Complement-dependent histamine release from rat peritoneal mast cells by rabbit anti-rat gamma globulin (Ra anti-RGG) and rabbit anti-rat mast cell (Ra anti-RMC) antibodies. In: Biochemistry of the acute allergic reactions, p. 231, ed. by K. F. AUSTEN and E. L. BECKER. Oxford: Blackwell 1968.

BACK, N., MUNSON, A. E., GUTH, P. S.: Anaphylactic shock in dogs. J. Amer. med. Ass. **183**, 260 (1960).

BALL, D. L., GOODFRIEND, T. L.: Radio-immunoassay of bradykinin; techniques useful for other substances devoid of tyrosine. Fed. Proc. **27**, 534 (1968).

BECKER, E. L.: The relations of complement to the other systems. Proc. roy. Soc. Med. (in press).

— AUSTEN, K. F.: Anaphylactic Reactions. In: Textbook of immunopathology, p. 76, ed. by P. A. MIESCHER and H. J. MÜLLER-EBERHARD. New York: Grune & Stratton 1968.

BERALDO, W. T.: Formation of bradykinin in anaphylactic and peptone shock. Amer. J. Physiol. **163**, 283 (1950).

BROCKLEHURST, W. E.: Kinin and kinin-forming enzymes in anaphylaxis. In: Biochemistry of the acute allergic reactions, p. 297, ed. by K. F. AUSTEN and E. L. BECKER. Oxford: Blackwell 1968.

— LAHIRI, S. C.: The production of bradykinin in anaphylaxis. J. Physiol. (Lond.) **160**, 15 P (1961).

BURDON, K. L., QUENG, J. T., THOMAS, O. C., MCGOVERN, J. P.: Observations on biochemical abnormalities in hereditary angioneurotic edema. J. Allergy **36**, 546 (1965).

CIRSTEA, M., SUHACIU, G., BUTCULESCU, I.: Bradykinin and anaphylactic shock in dogs. Int. Arch. Allergy **26**, 356 (1965).

— — — Evaluation du role de la bradykinine dans le choc anaphylactique. Arch. int. Pharmacodyn. **159**, 18 (1966).

COLLIER, H. O. J., JAMES, G. W. L.: Bradykinin and slow reacting substance in anaphylactic bronchoconstriction of the guinea pig *in vivo*. J. Physiol. (Lond.) **185**, 71 P (1966).

DAWSON, W., STARR, M. S., WEST, G. B.: Inhibition of anaphylactic shock in the rat by antihistamine and ascorbic acid. Brit. J. Pharmacol. **27**, 249 (1966).

DINIZ, C. R., CARVALHO, I. F.: A micro-method for determination of bradykininogen under several conditions. Ann. N.Y. Acad. Sci. **104**, 77 (1963).

DONALDSON, V. H.: Mechanisms of activation of C'1 esterase in hereditary angioneurotic edema plasma *in vitro*. J. exp. Med. **127**, 411 (1968).

— EVANS, R. R.: A biochemical abnormality in hereditary angioneurotic edema. Amer. J. Med. **35**, 37 (1963).

— RATNOFF, O. D., KLEMPERER, M. R., ROSEN, F. S.: Studies on a peptide from hereditary angioneurotic edema plasma with permeability factor and kinin activity. Complement workshop 1968. J. Immunol. **101**, 818 (1968).

— ROSEN, F. S.: Hereditary angioneurotic edema: A clinical survey. Pediatrics **37**, 1017 (1966).

ERDÖS, E. G.: Hypotensive peptides. Advanc. Pharmacol. **4**, 1 (1966).

GIGLI, I., MASON, J. W., COLMAN, R. W., AUSTEN, K. F.: Interaction of kallikrein with the C'1 esterase inhibitor. Complement workshop 1968. J. Immunol. **101**, 814 (1968a).

— RUDDY, S., AUSTEN, K. F.: The stoichiometric measurement of the serum inhibitor of the first component of complement by the inhibition of immune hemolysis. J. Immunol. **100**, 1154 (1968b).

GOODFRIEND, T. L.: Radio-immunoassay of bradykinin and angiotensin. In: Protein and polypeptide hormones, p. 91, ed. by M. MARGOULIES. Excerpta Medica Foundation Internat. Congress Series No 161. Louvain: Ceuterick 1968.

— LEVINE, L., FASMAN, G. D.: Antibodies to bradykinin and angiotensin. A use of carbodiimides in immunology. Science **144**, 1344 (1964).

HABER, E., RICHARDS, F. F., SPRAGG, J., AUSTEN, K. F., VALLOTTON, M., PAGE, L. B.: Modifications in the heterogeneity of the antibody response. Cold Spr. Harb. Symp. quant. Biol. **32**, 299 (1967).

HENRIQUES, O. B., LAVRAS, A. A. C., FICHMAN, M., PICARELLI, Z. P.: Plasma enzymes that release kinins. Biochem. Pharmacol. **15**, 31 (1966).

IATRIDIS, S. G., FERGUSON, J. H.: Active Hageman factor: A plasma lysokinase of the human fibrinolytic system. J. clin. Invest. **41**, 1277 (1962).

IRVIN, W. S., JOHNSON, P. K., CREGER, W. P., DANLIKER, W. B., FEIGEN, G. A.: Antibodies and vasoactive compounds in a case of anaphylactic shock to penicillin. Ann. intern. Med. (in press).

Jonasson, O., Becker, E. L.: Release of kallikrein from guinea pig lung during anaphylaxis. J. exp. Med. **123**, 509 (1966).
Kagen, L. J.: Some biochemical and physical properties of the human permeability globulins. Brit. J. exp. Path. **45**, 604 (1964).
Kimura, Y., Nakamura, T., Arai, Y., Miyanaga, Y., Ohkuni, H., Inoue, Y.: The role of chemical mediators, plasmin and kallikrein-kinin system in anaphylactic phenomena. Excerpta Med., Internat. Congress Series, ed. by A. Knight, **144**, 10 (1967).
Landerman, N. S., Webster, M. E., Ratcliffe, H. E.: Hereditary angioneurotic edema; II. Deficiency of inhibitor for serum globulin permeability factor and/or plasma kallikrein. J. Allergy **33**, 330 (1962).
Lecomte, J.: Consommation des kininogenes plasmatiques au cours du choc anaphylactique du lapin. C. R. Soc. Biol. (Paris) **155**, 1411 (1961).
Lewis, G. P.: Bradykinin-biochemistry, pharmacology and its physiological role in controlling local blood flow. Sci. Basis Med. **10**, 242 (1962).
Lima, A. O.: Pharmacologically active substances released during anaphylactic shock in the mouse. Int. Arch. Allergy **32**, 46 (1967).
Michel, B., Russell, T., Winkelmann, R. K., Gleich, G. J.: Release of kinins during wheal and flare allergic skin reactions. J. clin. Invest. **47**, 68a (1968).
Miyanaga, Y., Hasimoto, K.: Analysis of anti-bradykinin antibody and studies of its application to measurement of bradykinin. Nihon Arerugi Gakkai **16** (4), 289 (1967) [in Japanese].
Movat, H. Z.: Activation of the kinin system by antigen-antibody complexes. In: Int. Symp. on Vaso-active Polypeptides: bradykinin and related kinins, p. 177, ed. by M. Rocha e Silva and H. A. Rothschild. Sao Paulo 1967.
Orange, R. P., Valentine, M. D., Austen, K. F.: Antigen-induced release of slow reacting substance of anaphylaxis (SRS-A^{rat}) in rats prepared with homologous antibody. J. exp. Med. **127**, 767 (1968).
Pierce, J. V.: Structural features of plasma kinins and kininogens. Fed. Proc. **27**, 52 (1968).
Ratnoff, O. D., Lepow, I. H.: Some properties of an esterase derived from preparations of the first component of complement. J. exp. Med. **106**, 327 (1957).
Rinderknecht, H., Haverback, B. J., Aladjem, F.: Radio-immunoassay of bradykinin. Nature (Lond.) **213**, 1130 (1967).
Rosen, F. S., Charache, P., Pensky, J., Donaldson, V.: Hereditary angioneurotic edema. Two genetic variants. Science **148**, 957 (1965).
Rothschild, A. M.: Role of anaphylatoxin and of bradykinin in passive cutaneous anaphylaxis against heterologous precipitating antibody in the rat. In: Symposium of Immuno-Pharmacology, p. 172. 3d Int. Pharmacol. Congr., Sao Paulo. Oxford: Pergamon Press 1967.
Ruddy, S., Carpenter, C. B., Müller-Eberhard, H. J., Austen, K. F.: Complement component levels in hereditary angioneurotic edema and isolated C'2 deficiency in man. In: Immunopathology, Vth Internat. Symposium; Mechanisms of inflammation induced by immune reactions, p. 231, ed. by P. A. Miescher and P. Grabar. New York: Grune & Stratton 1967.
Schick, A. F., Singer, S. J.: On the formation of covalent linkages between two protein molecules. J. biol. Chem. **236**, 2477 (1961).
Schröder, E., Hempel, R.: Bradykinin, kallidin, and their synthetic analogs. Experientia (Basel) **20**, 529 (1964).
Sheehan, J. C., Hlavka, J. J.: The use of water soluble and basic carbodiimides in peptide synthesis. J. org. Chem. **21**, 439 (1956).
Spragg, J., Austen, K. F., Haber, E.: Production of antibody against bradykinin; Demonstration of specificity by complement fixation and radio-immunoassay. J. Immunol. **96**, 865 (1966a).
— — — Structural requirements for binding to antibody of sequence variants of bradykinin. Biochemistry **6**, 3933 (1967).
— Haber, E., Austen, K. F.: A radio-immunoassay for bradykinin. In: Hypotensive peptides, p. 298, ed. by E. G. Erdös, N. Back and F. Sicuteri. Berlin-Heidelberg-New York: Springer 1966b.
— Talamo, R. C., Suzuki, K., Appelbaum, D. M., Austen, K. F., Haber, E.: Structural requirements for binding of bradykinin to antibodies. II. Studies with bradykinin fragments. Biochemistry **7**, 4086 (1968).
Stewart, J. M., Woolley, D. W.: The search for peptides with specific antibradykinin activity. In: Hypotensive peptides, p. 23, ed. by E. G. Erdös, N. Back and F. Sicuteri. Berlin-Heidelberg-New York: Springer 1966.
Talamo, R. C., Haber, E., Austen, K. F.: Antibody to bradykinin: Effect of carrier and method of coupling on specificity and affinity. J. Immunol. **101**, 333 (1968b).
— Spragg, J., Austen, K. F., Haber, E.: Radio-immunoassay of bradykinin. In: Methods in immunology and immunochemistry, vol. 3. New York: Academic Press 1968a.

Addenda

I.

The studies concerned with the ability of bradykinin-polylysine antibody to recognize bradykinin analogs and fragments have been extended by the use of anti-bradykinin ovalbumin and an antiserum directed against human kininogen I which recognized the bradykinin moiety of the immunogen [Fischer et al.: Biochemistry 8, 3750 (1969)]. The antibodies directed against bradykinin coupled to ovalbumin showed marked antibody heterogeneity when bradykinin analogs and fragments were examined. These antibodies seem to require the presence of the aryl residues to a far greater extent than does anti-bradykinin polylysine. However, experiments using bradykinin fragments indicate that both these antibodies require the entire nonapeptide sequence for binding to antibody. Binding inhibition was also examined using antibody directed against human kininogen I, the low molecular weight precursor of bradykinin which contains the kinin moiety at its carboxy terminus in the same orientation in which it is covalently bound in the other two immunogens. The binding inhibition results indicate that this antibody population was also heterogeneous, but unlike the other two antibodies used, recognizes mainly the carboxy terminal residues of the bradykinin sequence. The analog and fragment binding data using all three antibodies allow the conclusion that the nonapeptide bradykinin may behave as an integral antigenic determinant, and that its conformation is of some importance. The role of the carriers in the immunogens has been considered, particularly with regard to electrostatic effects, and suggests that the degree of homogeneity of the antibodies produced reflects the heterogeneity of the immunogenic stimulus.

II.

Human plasma kininogen, prepared by ion exchange chromatography, gel filtration, and electrophoresis, has been used as an immunogen in rabbits. The antikininogen antibody recovered has been employed in a radial immunodiffusion assay which measures kininogen on the basis of protein [Spragg et al.: Fed. Proc. 28, 363 (1969)].

III.

The nomenclature of the complement system has been somewhat modified since this chapter was submitted [Bull. Wld Hlth Org. **39**, 935 (1968)]. Sheep erythrocytes (E), sensitized with rabbit antibody (A) react with the components of complement (C) in the sequence, C 1, 4, 2, 3, 5, 6, 7, 8 and 9. Fragments of individual components are subscripted with letters. The activated forms of the components are assumed to exist in intermediate cellular complexes unless otherwise specified. In addition to those conventions, the species of origin of a given component is indicated by a superscript (hu = human, gp = guinea pig).

IV.

Ratnoff has recently reviewed the complex interrelationships indicated in Fig. 3 existing between the fibrinolytic, clotting, kinin and complement systems [Advanc. Immunol. **10**, 145 (1969)].

Evaluation of the Role of Kinins in Experimental, Pathological, and Clinical Conditions; the Therapeutic Use of Kallikrein Inhibitor

ROSMARIE VOGEL and GERTRUD ZICKGRAF-RÜDEL

With 4 Figures

A. Introduction

Pathological states in which the liberation of kinins may play a role are those that are connected with an activation of proteolytic enzymes or mobilization of proteinases from tissues or microbial organisms. The clinical course may be

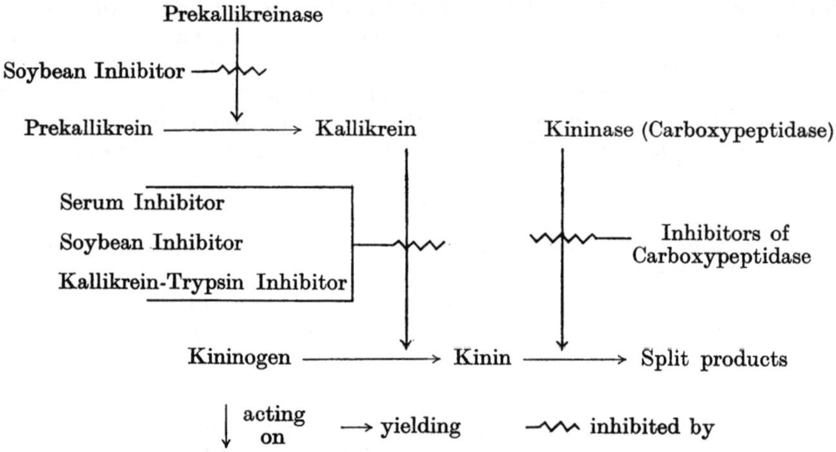

Fig. 1. Mechanism of action of inhibitors in the kallikrein-kinin system

influenced by the special actions of the kinins liberated even if they are liberated only in small amounts. The identification of activated components is difficult because of their high metabolic rate and the presence of kininases in blood (Fig. 1). Therefore physiological and pathophysiological experiments *in vivo* and *in vitro* must be considered as a basis for investigating the components of the system, i.e. kininogenases, kinins, and their precursors.

Pathological processes connected with the kininogenase–kinin system were reviewed by ERDÖS (1966); some of them are also surveyed in this volume on p. 541.

The basis of the therapeutic application of inhibitors of kininogenases rests on the demonstration of changes in the concentration of components of the system.

The treatment of experimental shock, pancreatitis, and inflammation with natural inhibitors was reported. But the therapy with inhibitors in disturbances of the balance of the proteolytic enzyme system gained importance only with the discovery and improved isolation of the polyvalent bovine inhibitor, Trasylol.

I. Therapeutic Application of Various Proteinase Inhibitors

As mentioned on p. 219, many naturally occurring proteinase inhibitors are known and isolated in a pure state. The reported therapeutic experiments with such inhibitors are summarized here.

Bean and potato inhibitors reduce symptoms of inflammation (p. 516) (VOGEL et al., 1966, 1968); also the inhibitors isolated from beans, lentils, and peas show antiphlogistic action. The proteolytic reactions following burns, which are very similar to those accompanying inflammation, are also partly or completely suppressed (HLADOVEC et al., 1961). The effect of potato inhibitor on inflammation was tested in rats and mice. Soybean inhibitor (SBTI) is reported to suppress the increase in vascular permeability caused by permeability factors (HLADOVEC et al., 1960; MILES, 1964; WILLOUGHBY and SPECTOR, 1964; BURKE et al., 1964; RATNOFF and MILES, 1964). Transplantation of adenocarcinoma cells (H2712) to mice leads to growth of a tumor only if the animal is constantly treated with SBTI (GILLETTE et al., 1963).

Ovomucoid was also tested in pharmacological experiments. Chicken ovomucoid has no antiphlogistic effect although it can influence vascular permeability (POYSER and WEST, 1965).

Necrosis of the pancreas in humans has for a long time been attributed to pathological activation of proteolytic enzymes in the organ. Most of the early experiments with proteinase inhibitors were done in experimental pancreatitis. In experiment, the symptoms of inflammation could in fact be favorably influenced by SBTI in most cases (NOSKIN et al., 1952; RUSH and CLIFTON, 1952; V. BECKER, 1960; BELLMANN, 1960; JORNS, 1960; CANNON and TURNER, 1961; RIBACOFF et al., 1961; MCCUTCHEON, 1964).

In shock, lima bean inhibitor, ovomucoid, and serum inhibitor could not significantly lower the mortality rate (BACK et al., 1966a, b).

HLADOVEC et al. (1961) reported no therapeutic effect of potato inhibitor.

The inhibitor from peanuts is of certain practical importance because of its special antifibrinolytic action (ASTRUP et al., 1960, 1962; KWAAN and ASTRUP, 1964). The ingestion of large quantities of peanuts leads to a marked decrease in spontaneous fibrinolytic activity of the serum of healthy (ASTRUP et al, 1960) and of hemophilic subjects (VAN CREVELD and MOCHTAR, 1961; ASTRUP et al., 1962; BISORDI, 1964). Finally an application of this inhibitor in larger amounts can lead to inhibition of fibrinolysis (ASTRUP et al., 1960; SCHMUTZLER, 1961; VERSTRAETE et al., 1962).

It has been reported that in immunological reactions the complement system is to some extent affected by SBTI (LAUENSTEIN and HABERLAND, 1963) and by potato inhibitor (RYBÁK et al., 1958).

The occurrence of skin lesions on repeated application of endotoxin (Shwartzman phenomenon) was reported to be inhibited by intradermal application of SBTI (CHRYSSANTHOU and ANTOPOL, 1961a, b), although other research groups were unable to confirm these observations (ZWEIFACH et al., 1961). These experiments did not lead to therapeutic application in man. Besides their poor compatibility (HOFFMAN et al., 1953; BERNARD et al., 1960) the plant inhibitors can sensitize, and ovomucoid causes local inflammation (MANSFELD et al., 1960; HARTERT, 1949; BONACCORSI and WEST, 1963).

It is obvious that the augmentation of the naturally occurring serum inhibitors by the administration of exogenous inhibitors will depend on the properties of the different inhibitors, i.e. on the molecular weight and finally on the spectrum of inhibition. It may be concluded that tissue inhibitors are more quickly absorbed than serum inhibitors.

II. Arguments for the Therapeutic Use of Trasylol

Because of the various properties of Trasylol (p. 230), understandably it is used in therapy in preference to other inhibitors. The commercial inhibitor preparations are of low molecular size. The bovine inhibitor is the only known inhibitor of all kininogenases and, further, no enzyme is known which is able to destroy the inhibitor (AUHAGEN, 1967).

Its low toxicity is important; the LD_{50} is 375 mg/kg in mice (i.e. 2.5 million KIU/kg; BEUCHELT, 1963). Dogs tolerate administration of up to 1 million KIU/kg i.v. without complications. Rats have a lower tolerance because high doses may lead to fatal reactions, especially after experimental surgery (CREUTZFELDT et al., 1963). Since the molecular weight is low (6,500), the inhibitor quickly penetrates into the tissue from the circulation. The concentration in blood after intravenous, intraperitoneal, intramuscular, or subcutaneous administration of an equal amount of inhibitor decreases in the order mentioned. For effective therapy Trasylol must be given intravenously (WERLE and TRAUTSCHOLD, 1961). The rapid elimination of e.g. 12,000 KIU/kg from the blood stream of rats is explained by the short (10 min) half-life. Therefore continuous intravenous drip is the best method of administration. According to TRAUTSCHOLD et al. (1964), after elimination from the blood stream the inhibitor appears first in various organs depending on their blood supply, but subsequently it accumulates in the liver, reaching a maximum level 30 minutes after injection. After 60 minutes the inhibitor level in kidneys is higher than in the liver (50% and 36% of the total amount). There are hints that a structural change occurs in the inhibitor in the liver without a loss of inhibitory capacity. The experiments done with tritium-labeled Trasylol resulted in a minimal excretion of the compound; most of the active material was hydrolyzed. This degradation occurs in renal tissue.

According to LUDWIG and WERLE, Trasylol migrates through the placental barrier (LUDWIG, 1966, 1967).

B. Pancreatitis

Many facets of the mode of action of Trasylol in acute pancreatitis are still not known (TRAUTSCHOLD et al., 1967). There are three pathogenic mechanisms of enzymatic origin which can be influenced by Trasylol: (1) tissue necrosis, (2) local disturbance of blood circulation and disorder of cardiovascular system, (3) imbalance of blood clotting and lysis.

I. Tissue Necrosis

The characteristic pathological changes in the pancreas represent a form of parenchyma necrosis typical for this organ (V. BECKER, 1964; DOERR, 1964; DOERR et al., 1965). The role of trypsin in these events (i.e. whether Trasylol acts by inhibition of trypsin) is very controversial. For many years it was accepted without sufficient experimental proof that in pancreatitis a premature, spontaneous, and autocatalytic activation of trypsinogen occurs in the gland. Trypsin then should activate the other pre-enzymes of the pancreas. This theory was first criticized by HAVERBACK et al. (1960), who found neither a spontaneous activation of trypsinogen nor an activation by addition of calcium ions in human pancreatic juice. (An autocatalytic activation of trypsinogen is possible only at a calcium concentration of at least 2–4 mEq/liter Ca^{++}, which exceeds the physiological range. On the other hand the activation of trypsinogen by enterokinase does not depend on the concentration of calcium ions.) Furthermore, several research workers could not demonstrate any active trypsin by means of natural or more specific synthetic substrates during autolysis of homogenates of intact or inflamed pancreata of men, dogs, pigs, or rats which served as models (BECK et al., 1963; SCHÖN and HENNING, 1963a; SCHÖN et al., 1963; CREUTZFELDT et al., 1963, 1965a; TRAUTSCHOLD et al., 1964; DOERR et al., 1965).

According to WERLE et al. (1968b) an increase of proteolytic activity is demonstrable during autolysis of pancreata of man and (laboratory) animals. Depending on the species it appears only after several hours (e.g. after 3–7 hours in pig pancreas, after 7–12 hours in rat pancreas). The enzyme in question splits benzoyl-DL-arginine *p*-nitroanilide (BAPA), which is almost a specific substrate for trypsin. Addition of Trasylol or SBTI prevents the hydrolysis of BAPA. It is assumed that the delayed appearance of this trypsin-like activity is caused by the specific trypsin inhibition, which was found in pancreata of all mammals examined (FRITZ et al., 1966). Besides the fact that the trypsin inhibitor of the pancreas usually inhibits not more than 5% of the total trypsin of the pancreas if activated, the inhibitor is slowly destroyed while the enzyme is liberated from the complex ("temporary inhibitor"). (For references see VOGEL et al., 1966, 1968.)

SCHÖN and HENNING (1963a, b) and TRAUTSCHOLD et al. (1964) demonstrated a reduction of trypsinogen and chymotrypsinogen content during pancreatic autolysis (table). The loss of trypsinogen can only partly be explained by an intermediary activation of trypsinogen and a subsequent binding to the specific trypsin inhibitor, because the amount of inhibitor present in the pancreas would be too small to inhibit the amount of trypsin which corresponds to the trypsinogen loss. On the other hand, only part of the specific trypsin inhibitor disappears during pancreatic autolysis (table). Among the possible causes for the loss of trypsinogen are an autocatalytic destruction of trypsin, which takes place in absence of protecting Ca^{++}, and an unspecific proteolytic destruction of trypsinogen (HAVERBACK et al., 1960).

Table. *Changes of some enzyme systems during autolysis of pancreas homogenate from dog*[a]

	0 min	6 hr	Changes in %
Trypsinogen (μg)	10,500	6,400	−40
Trypsin (μg)	0	0	—
Chymotrypsinogen (μg)	10,700	6,600	−38
Chymotrypsin (μg)	0	0	—
Procarboxypeptidase (μg β-Naphthol)	6,000	6,500	+ 8
Carboxypeptidase (μg β-Naphthol)	0	0	—
Kallikrein (KE)	0	25	
Lipase (LE)	50,000	10,000	−80
Free Inhibitor (KIE)	810	467	−43
Anson (E_{660})	0.214	0.400	+100

[a] Six hours at 37°; all data refer to 1 g pancreas tissue (TRAUTSCHOLD et al., 1964).

For the problem in question the appearance of the so-called "spontaneous activity" (TRAUTSCHOLD, 1965) or "proteolytic residual activity" (NAGEL and WILLIG, 1964; NAGEL et al., 1965) is of great significance. This activity with a pH optimum in a neutral range is found during autolysis of intact or inflamed pancreata of different species. It is demonstrable by caseinolysis or by lysis of heated fibrin plates (after exclusion of plasmin activity). The spontaneous activity cannot be inhibited by Trasylol and other trypsin inhibitors, but during autolysis its increase is inhibited by Trasylol (but not by the pancreatic trypsin inhibitor).

This means that the activation of the spontaneous activity is inhibited by Trasylol (Schön et al., 1963; Schön and Henning, 1963b; Nagel and Willig, 1964; Trautschold, 1965; Nagel et al., 1965; Blümel and Piza, 1966; Blümel and Grözinger, 1966; Bleyl et al., 1967). According to Blümel and Piza (1966), Blümel and Grözinger (1966), and Grözinger (1967), the spontaneous activity consists of pancreatic elastase and carboxypeptidase. In 1963 Schön and Henning (1963a, b) could already demonstrate active carboxypeptidase during autolysis of pancreas homogenates. The proteolytic activity in question is histochemically demonstrable during experimental olive oil or lactic acid pancreatitis, according to Bleyl et al. (1967) by means of placing fresh sections of pancreata on fibrin films. Sections of intact pancreata show no proteolytic activity under the same conditions. The distribution of the proteolytic activity in the inflamed pancreas corresponds to the spreading of the parenchymal necrosis. In pancreas tissue of cats which were treated with Trasylol after induction of experimental pancreatitis by olive oil, the proteolytic activity (described above) did not develop, in contrast to the pancreata of untreated control animals (Blümel and Grözinger, 1966).

Thus it is possible to stop by administration of Trasylol the proteolytic reactions which take place in the initial phase of the autolysis of pancreatic tissue and so prevent the spread of the proteolytic processes. It is remarkable that inhibition of the activation of the proteolytic system by Trasylol, SBTI, or DFP is possible only in the autolyzed pancreas but not in autolyzed liver, intestine, or kidney of dogs (Trautschold, 1965). This specific pancreatic property must be caused by the specific enzyme content of the pancreas. It is not yet known which enzymes are inhibited during the processes described. Besides trypsin, no activator of the other pancreatic zymogens is yet known. It has to be assumed that trypsin or another proteinase that can be inhibited by Trasylol appears at the beginning of the autolytic processes in cellular microareas. The analytic proof of such small local amounts of "trypsin" is very difficult to obtain even with modern micromethods.

The activation of the proteolytic activity that can be inhibited by Trasylol and which triggers the "spontaneous activity" is possibly caused by catheptic enzymes. In pancreas homogenates of various species activation of trypsinogen occurs in an acid medium with a pH optimum between 3.5 and 4.5. This activation is demonstrable up to pH 6. It cannot be inhibited by Trasylol. A caseinolytic activity which increases in an acid pH range is not identical with the caseinolytic activity demonstrable at neutral pH (Trautschold, 1965; Werle and Trautschold, 1966). In 1963 Turner et al. described the destruction of gelatin films at pH 4.5 by tissue slices and homogenates of inflamed pancreata of dogs. The authors assumed that catheptic enzymes become active during pancreas autolysis. This catheptic activity could not be shown in tissue slices of intact pancreata. It may be possible that the extremely acid pH ranges necessary for the activation of trypsinogen by catheptic enzymes occur in cellular microareas. (For acidosis as a condition for the development of pancreatic necrosis see p. 558.) An activation of trypsinogen or other proteinases by plasmin can also be brought up here (Goldblat et al., 1967; Bleyl et al., 1967).

Several authors stressed the necessity of cellular damage as a condition for an enzymatic destruction of parenchyma cells. In our opinion, with respect to the action of Trasylol, it does not matter how the cellular damage is brought about. The following possibilities are considered.

In model autolysis of pancreatic tissue slices addition of malonate disturbs cell metabolism by inhibition of succinodehydrogenase (V. Becker and Wilde, 1963). Intra-arterial injection of malonate into the pancreas leads, in combination with pancreas edema caused by pancreatic juice, to development of pancreatitis. Injection of bradykinin into pancreaticoduodenal artery causes a hemorrhagic edema of the pancreas. If this is combined with passage of pancreatic juice into the interstitium, typical pancreatitis develops here as well (KÖSSLING et al., 1967).

Cells can also be damaged by a toxic abnormal hemin pigment, which is formed during tryptic degradation of hemolyzed blood (HOFERICHTER et al., 1962; HOFERICHTER, 1964a, b) or by bacterial destruction of blood (CREUTZFELDT et al., 1965b). The conditions in this case correspond in some way to the combination of hemorrhagic exudate with pancreatic edema caused by pancreatic juice. According to CREUTZFELDT (CREUTZFELDT et al., 1965b; SCHMIDT et al., 1967) a damage of cell membranes is brought about by lysolecithins and lysocephalins, which are highly toxic reaction products of phospholipase A of the pancreas. (Phospholipase A occurs in high concentration especially in human pancreas.)

II. Local Disturbance of Blood Circulation and Disorder of Cardiovascular System

In the autolyzed pancreas *in vitro*, activation of prekallikrein occurs (table) (TRAUTSCHOLD et al., 1964; TRAUTSCHOLD 1965). In pancreas homogenates of men, but not of dogs, an enzyme is demonstrable at pH 4.5, which is not identical with trypsin and which is able to activate prekallikrein after neutralization. It is our opinion that the inhibition of the liberation of kinins is the essential mode of action of Trasylol in acute pancreatitis (TRAUTSCHOLD et al., 1966b, 1967). The schema shown in Fig. 2 can be the basis of further discussion of the problem.

The primary reaction of the pancreas to an unphysiological stimulus is formation of edema (ZOEPFEL, 1922a, b). According to V. BECKER (1957) the edema is formed by spillage of pancreatic juice through the intact duct epithelium. An obstruction of duct system and stimulation of secretion are conditions for formation of edema. According to DOERR (1953, 1959; DOERR et al.. 1965) the damming of secretion and swelling of isthmus epithelial cells lead to parapedesis of enzyme granules in the "wrong" direction, i.e. through the basal surface of the cell into the interstitium. This is the first sign of cell damage. In the interstitium, pancreatic juice acts as stimulus of inflammation; damage to capillaries and extravasation of fluid follow. The high metabolic rate caused by the enhanced secretion and the hindered exchange of metabolites caused by edema lead to a considerable insufficiency in acinar cells, which in the beginning is still reversible. Depending on the magnitude of the edema it can first be resorbed via blood and lymph vessels (DUPREZ et al., 1964). The inflammatory stimulus and the edema are conditions that cause an "unspecific" activation of serum prekallikrein penetrating through capillaries. There may also be an additional activation of pancreas prekallikrein. In this state, local activation of kinins occurs which reinforces the pathological events by enhancing permeability and by dilatation of capillaries. Subsequently, the damage to cells can become irreversible and cells may be subject to autolysis.

Several authors reported prompt relief of pain after application of Trasylol in acute pancreatitis (MAURER and HEINKEL, 1963; HEINKEL, 1964; LOUW et al., 1967). Certainly this is caused only partly by suppression of pain production by kinins. Diminution of pancreas edema and the painful tension of the pancreatic capsule connected with it are probably responsible for the effect.

We may assume that the local action of Trasylol consists of inhibition of spontaneous activity, which acts only in damaged cells, and of inhibition of kinin liberation, which can lead to increased edema. It follows that Trasylol should be applied as early as possible during the course of pancreatitis in order to assure local action of Trasylol in edema. This was stressed by TRAUTSCHOLD and colleagues in 1966. It is very doubtful whether Trasylol would decrease the secretion rate of excretory cells as well (SCHULTIS and RICK, 1964; SCHÖNBACH et al., 1966). FORELL (1968) could not verify these findings.

As micro- and macronecroses expand, kininogenases and kallikrein activators progressively enter the circulation. They are responsible for an uncontrolled and generalized kinin liberation, which is revealed by cardiovascular shock. During these events pancreas kallikrein may play only a minor role if it escapes

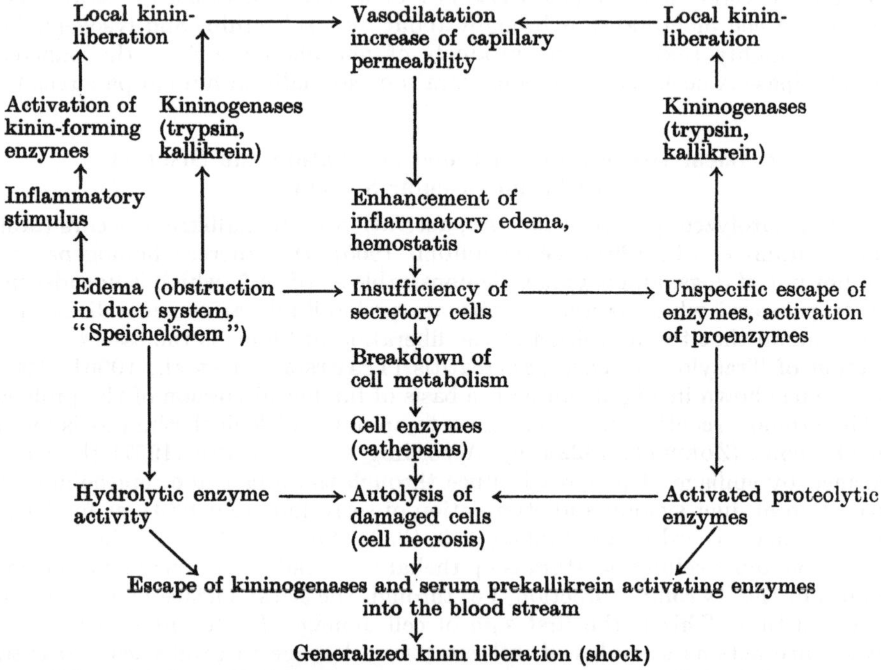

Fig. 2. Scheme of the pathophysiological reactions in the course of acute pancreatitis. (From TRAUTSCHOLD et al., 1967)

into circulation as other pancreatic enzymes (lipase, diastase) do. The liberation of kinin by the unspecifically activated plasma kallikrein will in any case exceed the action of pancreas kallikrein. An indirect proof of the participation of the kinin system in shock is the decrease of kininogen in shock (HOLLENBERG et al., 1962; THAL et al., 1963; HAIG and THOMPSON, 1964; RYAN et al., 1964, 1965; KATZ et al., 1964; NAGEL, 1965; TRAUTSCHOLD et al., 1966; WERLE and ASANG, 1967, ref. in FREY et al., 1968; p. 231). According to NUGENT and ATENDIDO (1965) blood or peritoneal fluid of dogs with experimental pancreatitis causes, on injection into a limb or peritoneal vessel of another dog, a decrease of resistance and increase of blood flow. These actions are typical of kinins. Furthermore, SINGH and HOWARD (1966) indicated that the plasma prekallikrein level is decreased in patients with acute pancreatitis.

In connection with the cardiovascular reaction caused by kinins, the meaning of a few other findings is not yet clear. SARDESAI and THAL (1966) demonstrated an increase of TAMe esterase activity in serum of patients with acute and chronic pancreatitis, which was not present in patients with other abdominal diseases. While the esterase activity of serum that occurs under physiological conditions cannot be inhibited by Trasylol *in vitro*, the increased esterase activity appearing in serum during pancreatic diseases can be reduced *in vivo* and *in vitro* to normal levels by Trasylol. Moreover, WILDING et al. (1967) and ADHAM et al. (1967) described a decreased trypsin-binding capacity of the α_2-macroglobulin fraction of serum in patients with acute pancreatitis, whereas NEGULESCU et al. (1961) found the same in experimental pancreatitis. The level of α_1-trypsin inhibitor increases (FORELL, 1957; SCHÖN et al., 1962; ERIKSON, 1965; MÉTAIS et al., 1965, 1966). Finally, an increase of plasma kininase activity was described in experimental pancreatitis of dogs (NUGENT et al., 1966b) as well as a decrease of trypsin-binding capacity in pancreatic juice, which can be normalized by application of Trasylol (MORGAN et al., 1968).

Another very important mechanism of action of Trasylol in acute pancreatitis is therefore the improvement of the abnormal peripheral circulation. Trasylol may prevent a diminution of blood flow caused by fall of blood pressure, which is especially deleterious for the pancreas and kidney function. Because Trasylol acts mainly by inhibition of plasma kallikrein in pancreatitis, it has a therapeutic effect in experimental pancreatitis in dogs and rats, though the pancreas kallikrein of these animals is not inhibited by Trasylol.

III. Imbalance of Blood Coagulation System

Another effect of Trasylol in pancreatitis is its action on disorders of the blood-clotting system (LOUW et al., 1967; WANKE and SEBENING, 1967). The appearance of hemorrhages and thromboses in the histological picture of inflamed pancreas is well known. In experimental pancreatitis of dogs (DOERR et al., 1965; ENCKE et al., 1966; WANKE, 1968) and cats (BLÜMEL and GRÖZINGER, 1966; GRÖZINGER, 1967), hypercoagulation occurs during the first hours after operation. Its extent depends on how pancreatitis was induced. In dogs, where pancreatitis is caused by injection of olive oil, a decrease of clotting time is especially impressive (ENCKE et al., 1966). In contrast, during the progress of pancreatitis in some of the animals the clotting time increases. Analysis of clotting events reveals the early phase of consumption coagulopathy. The changes in clotting time cannot be demonstrated if the animals are treated with Trasylol during and after operation either by intravenous route or into the A. pancreaticoduodenalis during operation to assure local action. The acceleration of clotting can also be prevented by intra-arterial injection of Rheomacrodex (a low molecular dextran) during operation (ENCKE et al., 1966). The absence of hemorrhages into the peritoneal cavity and petechial hemorrhages in the pancreas in olive oil pancreatitis of cats is also thought to be due to the action of Trasylol (BLÜMEL and GRÖZINGER, 1966).

It is assumed that the phenomena described are due to an increased activation of clotting factors, possibly by enzymes released from the diseased pancreas. A retardation of blood flow caused by shock and disturbance of microcirculation also augments clotting. This is also stressed by the positive therapeutic effect of Rheomacrodex, which leads to improvement of circulation (ENCKE et al., 1966). Trasylol may act by inhibiting activation of clotting factors (see p. 238) as well as by improving microcirculation through inhibition of kinin liberation.

The connection between kinin system and clotting system may be considered important in clotting disorders of acute pancreatitis. Activation of Hageman factor starts clotting and activation of plasma prekallikrein as well (p. 90). Furthermore, activation of plasma prekallikrein by plasmin is assumed (reviews in HABERMANN, 1963; TRAUTSCHOLD and RÜDEL, 1963; MILES, 1964).

IV. The Therapeutic Effects of Trasylol

Experimental and clinical trials of the therapeutic effects of Trasylol in acute pancreatitis involve many difficulties and yield contradictory results. In most cases of experimental pancreatitis dogs and rats were used. Pancreatitis is either induced according to POPPER et al. (1948) by ligation of pancreatic duct and A. pancreatica in combination with stimulation of secretion; or according to ELLIOTT et al. (1955, 1957, 1958) by injection of various substances into the pancreatic duct, such as bile, bile salts, toxins, proteolytic enzymes, olive oil, or lactic acid, under various pressures with or without following ligation of pancreatic duct, and in some cases with stimulation of secretion (see also review in WANKE, 1968).

For estimation of the effects of Trasylol in experimental pancreatitis the following criteria are used: increased survival rate, smaller increase of amylase and lipase levels in blood, less edema, minor changes in the histological picture of diseased pancreas, and smaller decrease of kininogen level in blood compared to untreated control animals (FORELL and DOBOVICNIK, 1961; MALLET-GUY et al., 1961, 1963; RIBACOFF et al., 1961; TSUKIYAMA et al., 1961, 1962; HOFERICHTER et al., 1962; HOLLENBERG et al., 1962; FALCIDIENO et al., 1962; ARTZ, 1963; HATANO et al., 1963; MCCUTCHEON and RACE, 1963, 1964; MCHARDY et al., 1963; NABSETH et al., 1963; NEMIR et al., 1963; SMITH et al., 1963; THAL et al., 1963; HAIG and THOMPSON, 1964; HOFERICHTER ,1964a; KATZ et al., 1964; KELLY et al., 1964; NUGENT et al., 1964; GRÖZINGER and ARTZ, 1964; GRÖZINGER et al., 1964; RYAN et al., 1964; DOERR et al., 1965; GRÖZINGER et al., 1965; GRÖZINGER and WENZ, 1965; RYAN et al., 1965; BLÜMEL and GRÖZINGER, 1966; GRÖZINGER, 1967; WANKE and SEBENING, 1967; WANKE et al., 1967; WANKE, 1968). Trasylol therapy fulfilled only in very few cases all these criteria. In other experiments no therapeutic effect of Trasylol was demonstrable (CREUTZFELDT et al., 1963; SCHUTT et al., 1963, 1965; CREUTZFELDT et al., 1965a; BECK et al., 1965; REIS 1967; GERATZ 1968). In general, application of Trasylol during the early phase of pancreatitis in high doses yields better results. Also good therapeutic effects in severe clinical and experimental pancreatitis are found when the polyvalent inhibitor is applied by intra-arterial perfusion of the pancreas (GRÖZINGER and WENZ, 1965; NUGENT et al., 1966a; TOUNTAS et al., 1966).

The following argument is often brought against the use of Trasylol: injection of, for example, 100,000 KIE in man increases the inhibitory capacity of the specific trypsin inhibitor capacity of serum only by 1.6% (TRAUTSCHOLD, 1965). We have to assume, however, that the therapeutic effect of Trasylol is due to inhibition of proteases different from trypsin as a consequence of the broad inhibitory specificity of the polyvalent inhibitor. Moreover, it may be important that Trasylol as a peptide of low molecular weight is able to penetrate into tissues and the interstitium very quickly.

Recently, GRÖZINGER (GRÖZINGER et al., 1965; WANKE and SEBENING, 1967; GRÖZINGER, 1967) stressed the fact that the only type of experimental pancreatitis that is comparable to human autodigestive tryptic pancreatitis in its histological picture is the one caused by injection of olive oil or other fat emulsions which can be degraded by lipase or by injection of lactic acid. The triglycerides are split by lipase and the free fatty acids lead to local acidosis. Injection of oleic acid or 2% lactic acid yields the same histological changes in pancreas as injection of olive oil. The local acidosis provides the condition for activation of proteinases which bring about tissue necrosis. According to CREUTZFELDT (CREUTZFELDT et al., 1965b; SCHMIDT et al., 1967) only the experimental pancreatitis induced by lysolecithins and lysocephalins is comparable to human pancreatitis. These arguments should be considered when the therapeutic effects of Trasylol are evaluated in experimental pancreatitis.

V. The Problem of Trasylol Application in Clinical Pancreatitis

It is understandable that double-blind studies for the clinical trial of Trasylol are done only with hesitation, as pancreatitis is still characterized by a high mortality rate. Furthermore, the clinical course does not always reveal the grade of severity of pancreatitis (HOFERICHTER, 1964b; MAURER, 1964). The problem is often handled by comparing the results of treatment of patients before and after Trasylol became available, but this method does not take into consideration other changes or improvements in the conservative therapy necessary besides the application of Trasylol. Positive results from comparisons were obtained by GRÖZINGER (1967) and HANSSON and LENNINGER (1967); negative results by MAURER (1964) and HANSEN et al. (1966). A great number of patients (449), who were treated with and without Trasylol by many different physicians at the same time, were compared by NODINE and GREBERMAN (1968). The results showed a positive tendency. Etiological factors were without effect, higher doses yielded better results. Double-blind studies in one hospital are reported by SKYRING et al. (1965) and CAPPER et al. (1965). The results were negative. Another double-blind study done by BACHRACH and SCHILD (1968) by the multi-institutional method shows equivocal results. In general, pancreatitis in alcoholics responded better to Trasylol therapy than pancreatitis caused by diseases of the bile duct system. The results were also influenced by dosage and the time of administration of Trasylol during the course of the disease. In general, the Trasylol doses used in the reported studies were not as high as those recommended recently (for review see also WANKE, 1968).

A dangerous but relatively rare complication after surgery of the upper abdomen is postoperative pancreatitis. It can be caused by trauma to the pancreas, interruption of blood supply, manipulations at the papilla Vateri, or intra-operative cholangiography with reflux into the pancreas duct system. By specific prophylactic intra- and postoperative Trasylol application the frequency of post-operative pancreatitis could be reduced (HOFERICHTER, 1967; MÖRL, 1967a).

C. Shock

Shortly after the discovery of bradykinin, in 1950 BERALDO observed free kinins in blood of dogs in anaphylactoid and peptone shock. Later, ROCHA E SILVA noticed kinin liberation after incubation of rat plasma with peptone *in vitro* (ROCHA E SILVA and HOLZHACKER, 1959). For the acute drop in blood pressure an important role was attributed by WEBSTER and CLARK (1959) to the activation of the kallikrein–kinin system in endotoxin and hemorrhagic shock. DINIZ and co-workers found marked decrease of the kininogen level of the blood in various experimental shock forms (DINIZ et al., 1961, 1966; DINIZ and CARVALHO, 1963; CORRADO et al., 1966).

Independent of the type of shock, kinins seem to be involved in disorders of the circulation, although the mechanism of their liberation is not yet fully known. Specific involvement may be attributed only to the plasma kallikrein–bradykinin system. The definition of HERSHEY and ALTURA (1966), who described shock as peripheral circulation insufficiency connected with failure of the terminal circulatory system (i.e. microcirculatory insufficiency with following hypoxia of the tissue), provides a basis for the involvement of kinins. For possible pathways of kinin liberation see Fig. 3. Changes in the components of the kallikrein–kinin system or effects of its inhibitors in experimental and clinical conditions suggest the participation of the system.

Demonstration of the lowering of the kininogen level in peripheral blood is the most important proof in experimental shock. Such a diminution is seen in

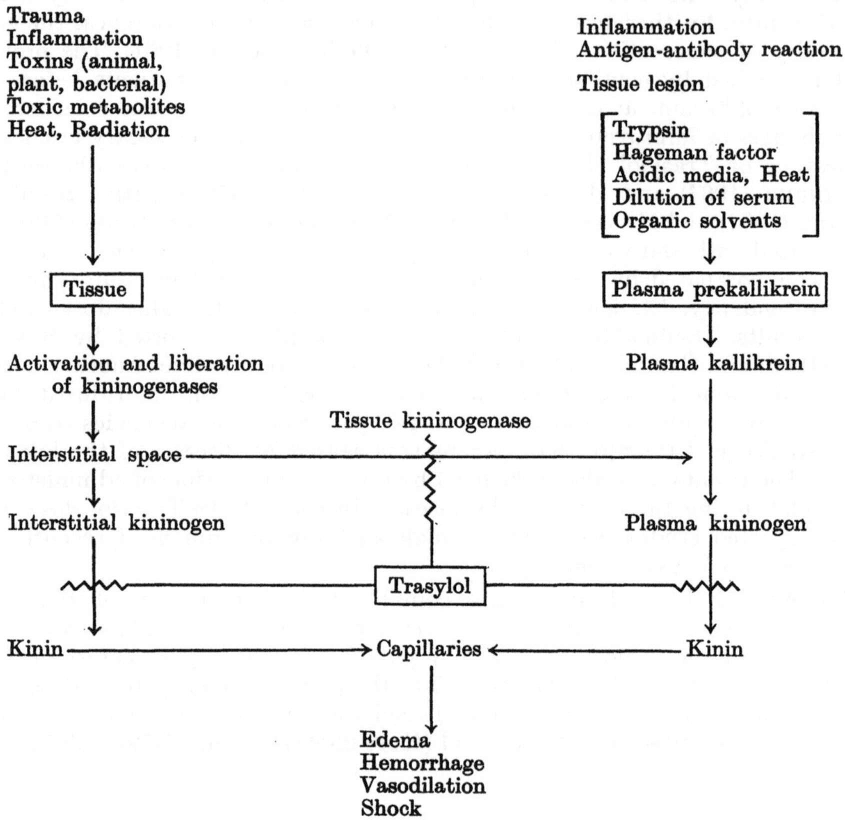

Fig. 3. Inhibition of kinin formation in the organism by polyvalent bovine inhibitor. (From VOGEL et al., 1966, 1968)

anaphylactic shock of the dog (LECOMTE, 1961), of the rat (BROCKLEHURST and LAHIRI, 1962, 1963; BACK et al., 1966b, 1968) of the guinea pig, in anaphylactoid polyvinyl-pyrrolidon shock of the dog, the anaphylactoid dextran shock and heat shock of the rat (SCHARNAGEL et al., 1965; GREEFF et al., 1966; GREEFF, 1966; BACK, 1966b; BACK et al., 1966a) and endotoxin shock of the dog (WERLE, 1963; MEYER, 1964, 1965; MEYER and WERLE, 1964; ROTHSCHILD and CASTANIA, 1968).

In traumatic shock state, e.g. after a traffic accident, the kininogen level is lowered in man from the normal value of 15–20 μg/ml to 2–14 μg/ml kinin which can be liberated (mean value 6.5 μg) (WERLE, 1966a). Also a decrease of the kininogen level is observed by STÜTTGEN (1968) in shock accompanying dermatoses.

In contrast to these observations ANKIER and STARR (1967) could not demonstrate changes in the concentrations of kininogen, free kinin, kininogenase, or kininase in peripheral blood of the rat in anaphylactoid dextran shock. In hemorrhagic, traumatic, and tourniquet shock, on the contrary, an increase of kininogen was found (STARR and WEST, 1967). In these shock forms the concentrations of the components of the kinin system are unchanged in heart, lung, liver and small intestine. In rats that die in shock, intestinal hemorrhages are always observed. Therefore STARR and WEST tested the peritoneal fluid and found an increased level of active kinin independent of the intensity of shock. The observations were made in traumatic and tourniquet shock but not in hemorrhagic shock. Besides kinin, other components mentioned in relation to shock genesis are found, for example histamine and 5-HT (STARR and WEST, 1967). The importance of the presence of kinins in peritoneal fluid is not yet known.

A mobilization of intestinal kallikrein during shock may also be considered. According to WERLE et al. (1963) in various pathological conditions intestinal prekallikrein can penetrate from intestinal wall into the exudate. ERDÖS (1966) also discussed the involvement of kallikrein from the gastrointestinal tract as first described by WERLE and VOGEL (1961). This question was approached by KOBOLD and THAL (1963) as well. LILLEHEI et al. (1964) suggested a significant impairment of splanchnic circulation in experimental conditions, e.g. endotoxin shock in dogs, and observed subsequent damage of the intestinal wall.

Various research teams examined the involvement of kinins in anaphylactoid shock. Sensitization of laboratory animals may lead to a change in responsiveness to kinins and/or change in concentration of the components of the kallikrein–kinin system.

In rats sensitized with horse serum and *Bordetella pertussis* vaccine as adjuvant, the responsiveness to bradykinin given i.v. is enhanced (DAWSON and WEST, 1965), and the severity of the anaphylactic reaction and the sensitivity to bradykinin increase in parallel. After ten days, 2 mg bradykinin/kg body weight administered i.v. leads to exitus of 80% of sensitized rats while under normal conditions bradykinin is tolerated in doses up to 10 mg/kg i.v. (KONZETT, 1962). This hypersensitivity is decreased to the initial level after forty days. Ten days after the beginning of the sensitization of rats, the level of the kinin-liberating activity of the serum is increased 5 minutes after the reinjection of the antigen. Moreover, at the same time, an increased level of kininogen and free kinin is demonstrated in blood and peritoneal fluid (DAWSON et al., 1965). In addition, in anaphylactoid shock as well as in bradykinin shock of rats characteristic hemorrhagic lesions in the jejunum and in the right ventricle were observed (DAWSON and WEST, 1965). In dogs also during anaphylactic reaction the kininogen and the kininase levels of plasma are enhanced (BACK et al., 1968).

However the results could not be uniformly repeated in all laboratories. CIRSTEA et al. (1965a, b) could not demonstrate a change in the kininogen level in anaphylactic shock of dogs and guinea pigs after sensitization with horse serum although the samples were withdrawn during the time of maximal hypotension. As mentioned before GREEFF (1966) demonstrated a decrease of kininogen in anaphylactoid shock of guinea pigs following sensitization with egg white. In the experiments of CIRSTEA, only in rabbits, a significant decrease of kininogen was seen. The possible differences among the species will be discussed on p. 562, but it must be assumed that the anaphylactoid reactions of different species are more uniform than their kinin systems are.

Kinins may play a role in endotoxin shock and purulent peritonitis. WERLE and MEYER observed that shortly after i.v. application of proteus endotoxin to dogs (600 μg/kg body weight) the kininogen level in blood is markedly decreased (WERLE, 1963; MEYER, 1964, 1965; MEYER and WERLE, 1964). The kininogen level increases during the next 2–3 hours but is not accompanied by normalization of blood pressure (GREEFF, 1966).

Application of endotoxin to monkeys (*Macaca mulatta*) results in decrease in peripheral vascular resistance and increase in cardiac output. At the same time, increase of free kinin and kininase of blood takes place with a drop in kininogen level. There are experimental indications for a shift in the kallikrein–kinin–kininase system in the initial phase of endotoxin shock evoked by enzymes from granulocytes (MELMON and CLINE, 1967; p. 299).

In blood of dogs shocked by injection of *Ascaris* coelom fluid the kininogen level first decreases and after a short increase shows further drop. The systemic blood pressure is lowered for the entire period (WERLE, 1966b).

The negative results of ERDÖS and MIWA (1968) obtained with rabbits in endotoxin shock make it doubtful whether a direct liberation of kinins by endotoxin or an activation of precursors of the system really occurs. ERDÖS stated that endotoxin acts in the rabbit via the activation of Hageman factor, this factor being absent in certain animal species. Hageman factor is exhausted in the primary stage of endotoxin shock in the rabbit, and during the progress of the shock plasma prekallikrein is activated and some kinin liberation takes place. By addition of Hageman factor to the blood of shocked animals further liberation of kinins can be induced. Most of the kininogen that is the substrate of glandular kallikreins only (p. 254) is not affected. Addition of glandular kallikrein results in an undiminished release of kinins. Pretreatment of the laboratory animals with pancreatic carboxypeptidase B abolishes the decrease in blood pressure after bradykinin injection; however it is ineffective against endotoxin. From these experiments ERDÖS concludes that kinins play no part in the mechanism of endotoxin shock in rabbit, at least in the early phase.

In vitro, neither liberation of plasma kinins by endotoxin is observed (SCHARNAGEL et al., 1965; GREEFF et al., 1966; WERLE, 1963; MEYER, 1964; MEYER and WERLE, 1964) nor a decrease of the kininogen level or liberation of kinins by polyvinylpyrrolidon or dextran. Negative results are also reported when plasma of sensitized animals is incubated with antigen (p. 546; SCHARNAGEL et al., 1965; GREEFF et al., 1966; GREEFF, 1966; ANKIER and STARR, 1967). It is assumed that *in vivo* these substances react by liberation of kininogenases or kininogenase-activating enzymes, e.g. from tissue.

The decrease in kininogen level and/or the drop in blood pressure in shock was blocked by different agents.

1. Pretreatment of the animals with cortisone or dexamethasone protects against the drop of blood kininogen level in dextran shock of the rat (SCHARNAGEL et al., 1965; GREEFF et al., 1966; GREEFF, 1966).

2. According to ROTHSCHILD and CASTANIA (1968) the spontaneous drop in blood pressure (and kininogen level) after endotoxin application in dogs is suppressed when plasma kininogen was depleted by pretreatment with cellulose sulfate. The animals respond to the toxin with a slowly progressing hypotension, starting approximately 15 minutes after the injection.

3. Pretreatment of dogs with aspirin prevents the decrease of blood pressure (first and second phases) and increases the survival rate. Indomethacin and phenylbutazone are also effective when given before the toxin (HINSHAW et al., 1967; ERDÖS et al., 1967; ERDÖS, 1968).

4. The spontaneous decrease of blood pressure and kininogen level is abolished by application of the polyvalent inhibitor Trasylol. As observed by different research groups, the effect is reproducible only when the inhibitor was injected before or simultaneously with the toxin. Positive effects are reported in treatment

of dogs in endotoxin shock (WERLE, 1963; MEYER, 1964, 1965; MEYER and WERLE, 1964; MASSION and ERDÖS, 1966); of dogs in *Ascaris* toxin shock (WERLE, 1966b); rats and dogs in peritonitis shock (NAGEL et al., 1967); rats, dogs, and guinea pigs in traumatic and anaphylactic shock (BACK et al., 1966b, 1968); and of mice in shock after burning (BACK et al., 1966b).

Best results were obtained with the simultaneous application of Trasylol and antibiotics (NAGEL, 1965; NAGEL et al., 1967). Administration of antibiotics alone leads to an intensive microbial disintegration, accompanied by a liberation of endotoxin resulting in lesion of the reticuloendothelial system (RES), an important factor for the intoxication and kinin liberation. According to NAGEL the range of the therapeutic possibilities with antibiotics is expanded by further application of Trasylol.

According to WERLE (1963), BACK et al. (1966b, 1968), MASSION and ERDÖS (1966), and NAGEL et al. (1967) the chance of survival of shocked animals treated with Trasylol increases.

In most cases of endotoxin shock a second drop of the systemic pressure was observed. This is due to diminished counter regulations in shock. Among other factors the role of catecholamines should be considered. These agents are liberated in the area of the splanchnic nerve by endotoxin (FINE and MINTON, 1966). Catecholamines reduce the blood flow and the functioning of RES of liver and spleen. Whether or not kinins are involved in this mechanism is not known.

Therapy of Shock Based on the Possible Role of Kinins

On the basis of these findings Trasylol has also been used in the treatment of shock in humans (for references see GROSS and KRONEBERG, 1966), for example in shock due to acute peritonitis.

WERLE and MEYER (MEYER, 1964; MEYER and WERLE, 1964) and NAGEL (1965) first pointed out that the circulatory failure in peritonitis may be favorably influenced by application of high doses of Trasylol. These findings were confirmed later (NAGEL et al., 1967; MÖRL, 1967b).

We assume that the therapeutic effect of the inhibitor is due to the inhibition of liberation of kinins that leads to a normalization of microcirculation (see Fig. 3). The mechanism of the liberation and the effect of kinins in the different forms of shock must be understood before a *specific* therapy with Trasylol can be attempted.

D. Carcinoid and Kallikrein-Kinin System

The carcinoid syndrome has several aspects, including pathology, clinical symptoms, and chemical mediators. The clinical symptomatology (i.e. flushing attacks, increased intestinal peristalsis, and bronchospasm) was attributed at first only to 5-HT, first isolated from carcinoid tumors by LEMBECK (1953). Yet different research groups could not correlate the 5-HT level of the blood with the intensity of the attacks. The attacks were not sufficiently influenced by administration of 5-HT antagonists. Intravenous infusions of serotonin did not evoke attacks of flushing in carcinoid patients. Therefore it seemed doubtful whether serotonin was the only effective biochemical mediator. It was indicated that the catecholamines, histamine, and kinins may participate in the syndrome (for review see DOLLINGER and GARDNER, 1966). Only the participation of the kinin system in the syndrome will be discussed here.

FREY et al. in 1935 observed and described all symptoms characteristic of flushing following intravenous application of kallikrein.

Because flushing can be provoked in carcinoid patients by application of small amounts of epinephrine (PEART et al., 1961), and kinins can be liberated by epinephrine (HILTON and LEWIS, 1956), OATES et al. (1964) tried to find a possible correlation between the carcinoid syndrome and the kinin system. The authors showed that in contrast to serotonin, infusion of bradykinin resulted in flushing attacks. Healthy persons and carcinoid patients likewise responded to bradykinin infusion with dilatation of the peripheral veins and arteries. In spontaneous flushing a comparable vasodilatation takes place. After infusion of epinephrine to carcinoid patients, the effects of epinephrine and bradykinin on the peripheral vascular system seems to be additive as kinins may be liberated. In healthy persons the effect corresponds only to the amount of epinephrine given (MASON and MELMON, 1966a).

The values found by different research groups for the components of the kallikrein–kinin system in the blood of carcinoid patients vary widely. The kinin level of venous and arterial blood of carcinoid patients is increased during spontaneous or provoked flushing (OATES and MELMON, 1966; ZEITLIN, 1966; MASON and MELMON, 1966a; MASHFORD and ZACEST, 1967; BROCKLEHURST and ZEITLIN, 1967). MASHFORD and ZACEST (1967) found increased bradykinin levels in arterial blood also during intermissions of flushing attacks (two out of three patients; for the determination method see ZACEST and MASHFORD, 1967). In carcinoid patients application of epinephrine resulted in a rise and in healthy persons in a drop of free bradykinin concentration. A provoked flushing attack is accompanied by a increase of bradykinin level in arterial blood and decrease in blood pressure and tachycardia.

In contrast, GARDNER et al. (1967) could not demonstrate free kinin in venous blood of carcinoid patients, although the kininogen level was lowered after application of epinephrine. In all cases the values for plasma kallikrein and plasma kininase stayed within the normal range. On the other hand MASON and MELMON (1966b) showed an increase of active kallikrein in the arterial blood of patients with flush symptoms following a cold stimulation, but not in patients without flush. SCHIEVELBEIN reported in 1968, that when twelve carcinoid patients were free of symptoms the level of prekallikrein and kininogen in blood and the excretion of kallikrein in urine were normal.

OATES and co-workers (OATES and MELMON, 1966; OATES et al., 1966) pointed out that kinin liberation takes place in the area around the tumor. In the hepatic vein blood withdrawn during flushing provoked by epinephrine in carcinoid patients there are high quantities (>25 µg/100 ml) of a peptide that is identical with bradykinin. The observation is in contrast to unchanged bradykinin levels in hepatic vein blood of healthy persons treated with epinephrine.

In carcinoid metastases of the liver a kininogenase occurs in high concentration (OATES et al., 1964). The enzyme was concentrated by column chromatography. Incubation of the enzyme with purified kininogen of human plasma results in liberation of 98% kallidin and small amounts of a biologically active peptide which is not identical with bradykinin. The kininogenase is inhibited by Trasylol but much less by SBTI (MELMON et al., 1965; OATES and MELMON, 1966).

These properties classify the kininogenase from hepatic metastases as an organ kallikrein. In an omental metastasis of a carcinoid tumor WERLE et al. (1966) found a kininogenase in a concentration corresponding to 125 KU/g tissue with general properties similar to pancreatic kallikrein, e.g. hydrolysis of BAEE and inhibition by Trasylol. In a hepatic carcinoid metastasis of an elephant WERLE et al. (1968a) found the same kininogenase in a concentration of 10 U/g.

Kallikrein usually is not present in tissues from liver or omental lymph nodes (ZEITLIN and SMITH, 1966).

According to OATES et al. (1966) and MASON and MELMON (1966b) the kininogenase is mobilized in tumor tissues by flush-provoking stimulants like epinephrine. In blood the liberated kallidin is quickly degraded to bradykinin by an aminopeptidase (p. 314). This reaction explains the apparent contradiction in the findings *in vitro* and *in vivo*. The concentrated enzyme from tumors liberates kallidin *in vitro*, whereas during flush, bradykinin was found in peripheral blood.

The therapeutic use of Trasylol in the treatment of flush was not very successfull (DOLLINGER and GARDNER, 1966; BACK, 1966a; OATES, 1966; GARDNER et al., 1967; SCHIEVELBEIN, 1968). The basis for this therapeutic indication is the inhibition of the kininogenase mobilized from tumors; thus Trasylol should suppress the liberation of kinins.

E. Blood Coagulation and Fibrinolysis

Since 1960, that is, since we have known that Trasylol inhibits pure plasmin, the complex mechanism of blood coagulation has become of great interest. Many factors interacting in the process of plasmin activation have been detected. There is no doubt that a number of substances really react together and/or sequentially. The existence of these factors was demonstrated only indirectly and not tested in purified state. In any case, coagulation and fibrinolysis are parts of one system.

The most important reaction of the fibrinolytic enzyme system—the activation of plasminogen to plasmin—is initiated by activators. Endogenous and exogenous activators are known. Urokinase and fibrinokinase belong to the first group, streptokinase to the second.

In different human organs such as the uterus, adrenals, lymph nodes, prostate gland, and thyroid gland the activators of plasminogen are present in relatively high concentration (ALBRECHTSEN, 1957; see also review in ASTRUP, 1967). The occurrence of activators especially in these organs is of great interest in view of the hyperfibrinolysis occurring in them after surgical intervention. Hyperfibrinolysis occurs when the equilibrium between plasmin and inhibitor is disturbed after extended trauma, stressful situations (JÜRGENS, 1959; ASTRUP, 1959), and surgery, and in obstetrical cases and inflammatory reactions. (For review see TRAUTSCHOLD et al., 1966b, 1967.)

Serum contains plasmin inhibitors in high concentrations, partly as inhibitors of activated plasmin and partly bound in complex with plasmin as a plasmin depot. The plasmin–inhibitor complex acts as plasmin depot in serum (C. M. AMBRUS and MARKUS, 1960) for any substrate with greater affinity to the enzyme than the inhibitor has (J. L. AMBRUS, 1966; KLINE, 1966). According to ALKJAERSIG et al. (1959), plasminogen is adsorbed by fibrin clots in such a manner that the activated plasmin cannot be blocked by the serum plasmin inhibitors (for review see RICKLI, 1966).

In disturbances of the relatively labile equilibrium between fibrinolysis and the thromboplastic system where the natural inhibitor system does not provide adequate control of the proteolytic processes involved, the therapeutic use of the bovine inhibitor is proposed because of the polyvalent inhibitory capacity.

The inhibition of isolated plasmin by various naturally occurring inhibitors is described in the chapter "Kallikrein Inhibitors" (p. 213).

Besides plasmin, the bovine inhibitor was reported to inhibit activators, e.g. urokinase (DUBBER et al., 1968). On the other hand prothrombin, thrombokinase, and thrombin are inhibited although only at very high inhibitor concentrations

(Ferguson, 1942; Tagnon and Soulier, 1948; Benzer et al., 1960). Competitive inhibition of the thromboplastic activity was observed *in vitro* and *in vivo* by Amris (1966a, b, c; Amris and Kjeldsen, 1966) and by Nordström et al. (1966, 1968), Blombäck et al. (1967); Dubber et al. (1966, 1968), although *in vivo* these findings were not confirmed by Gormsen and Josephsen (1967). The steps inhibited in the system are shown in Fig. 4 (Haberland and Matis, 1967; Marx, 1967).

In 1964 Herschlein and Steichele first reported the inhibition of the activation of the clotting system by Trasylol. The definite point of attack of Trasylol in the clotting mechanism is not yet known (Haberland and Matis, 1967). It has been emphasized that Trasylol not only inhibits lysis *in vivo* but is also an inhibitor of blood clotting. The latter activity can be observed at a three times higher inhibitor concentration (Amris, 1966a, b, 1967). Trasylol in-

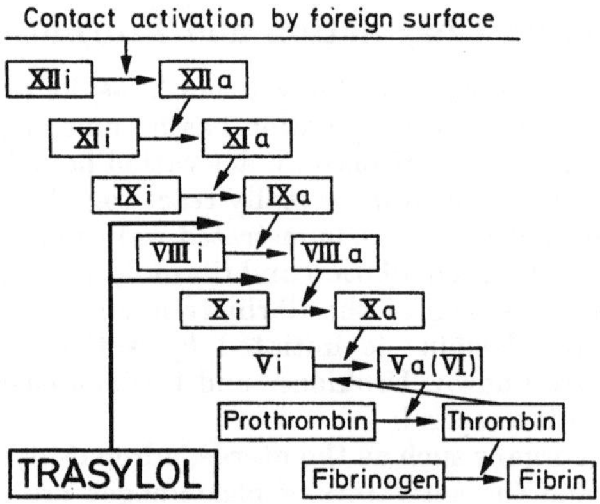

Fig. 4. Mechanism of activation and inhibition of blood-clotting system

hibits one or more of the early reactions of the blood coagulation process. The inhibition is dependent on the concentration of inhibitor, serum factors, and factor VIII (Blombäck et al., 1967). From these observations many researchers concluded that any disturbance of hemostatic balance is an indication for Trasylol therapy.

In 1956 Marx and Werle first proposed the use of polyvalent inhibitor for treatment of hyperfibrinolysis (Marx, 1956; Werle, 1956; Marx et al., 1959, 1963). (For ref. for treatment of hyperfibrinolysis see Vairel and Thely, 1960; Benzer et al., 1960, 1961; Beller, 1961; Fleischhacker and Stacher, 1962; Léger and Lande, 1962; Marggraf, 1962; André, 1963; Berghoff and Glatzel, 1963; Zweibaum and Josso, 1963; Markwardt et al., 1964; Tice et al., 1964; Huber, 1966; Gross and Kroneberg, 1966; Habermann, 1966; Marx, 1966; Haberland and Matis, 1967; Marx et al., 1967).

Successful treatment with Trasylol of hyperfibrinolysis following surgery of the lung or prostate gland was reported in numerous clinical studies (for review see Gross and Kroneberg, 1966; Steichele, 1966). According to Schmutzler (1966), Schmutzler and Fürstenberg (1966) a combined application of EACA, a synthetic inhibitor of plasmin activation, and Trasylol yield the best therapeutic results. For application of Trasylol in surgery see reviews in Mammen (1966) and Schmutzler (1966).

Mortality rates from lung emboli in patients not treated with Trasylol were reported by Rick et al. (1967). In patients treated with Trasylol a 50% decrease of the mortality was seen.

In hematomas originating from bone fracture the increase in activators of plasminogen is combined with the increased occurrence of kininogenases, therefore the application of proteinase inhibitor is indicated (BLÜMEL, 1967; HELLER and MÖRL, 1967). In this type of hematoma and lesion kinins are detected in high concentration (BLÜMEL, 1966). The biological effects of plasma kinin, e.g. disorders in circulation of the lung, were also found in clinical and experimental fat embolism. Interrelationship between kinin liberation and fat emboli was first observed by BRÜCKE et al. (1965, 1966). MÖRL (1967b, c) reports that in 322 cases of trauma treated with Trasylol only one with embolus was found, while in the control group of 452, 7 deaths were attributed to emboli as confirmed by autopsy.

Blood clotting is more inhibited by Trasylol in patients with hemophilia B than in patients with hemophilia A (WERLE et al., 1967). If hemophilia A is treated with factor VIII containing human antihemophilic globulin, incompatibility reactions are described similar to symptoms following liberation of biologically active polypeptides, for example headache or flush (MACKAY et al., 1965; BIGGS and MCFARLANE, 1966; EISEN and KEELE, 1966; FISCHER, 1966). Plasma fractions containing factor VIII liberate *in vitro* large quantities of kinins (EISEN, 1965; MACKAY et al., 1965; EISEN and KEELE, 1966). According to BLÜMEL et al. (1967) human antihemophilic globulin can activate kinin formation, and application results in decrease of kininogen level in blood. Simultaneous application of Trasylol prevents the drop. For therapy of hemophilia see also JÜRGENS (1967).

In recurrent menorrhagia and in severe thrombopenia the combination of Trasylol and EACA is additive (MARX and HENNING, 1962).

E. Various Applications

According to KERN and KUHBIER (1964) locally applied Trasylol prevents the development of intra-abdominal adhesions following intraperitoneal application of talc in mice. GRUNDMANN (1966a, b, c) and VORSTER (1966, 1967) had similar results in rabbits and rats. GRUNDMANN was able to demonstrate by histological examination that the prevention of adhesions is based on inhibition of inflammatory reactions. According to VORSTER (1966, 1967), intraperitoneal application of Trasylol effects a decrease of fibrinogen level and inhibition of blood coagulation. These result in a slower formation of fibrin and in the prevention of peritoneal adhesions. The experiments may suggest the therapeutic use of Trasylol in abdominal surgery in the future.

Trasylol inhibits the rejection of skin transplants in rats by inactivation of the proteinases liberated (BERTELLI et al., 1963).

In burns, treatment with Trasylol was reported to prevent shock and the liberation of proteinases in injured tissue (KOSLOWSKI and WASCHKEIT, 1960; KOSLOWSKI et al., 1962; KRAUS et al., 1963; KOSLOWSKI, 1966).

In gynecology and obstetrics, Trasylol application is indicated in atonic bleeding post partum or hemorrhage caused by premature disengagement of the placenta, gynecological operations, or miscarriage (review in HOFFBAUER, 1967; HUBER, 1966; SCHMIDT-MATTHIESEN, 1966).

According to LUDWIG (1966, 1967, 1968), newborns are exposed to stress fibrinolysis resulting sometimes in perinatal asphyxia. When Trasylol was given to the mother in threatened asphyxia a beneficial effect was seen (LUDWIG, 1968).

According to LUDWIG (1967) and PFEIFER (1968) during the period of retention of dead fetus, fibrinogen and other factors of blood coagulation decreased in the maternal blood. Gynecological intervention in "dead fetus syndrome" often induces an acute hemorrhagic crisis. Application of Trasylol prevents the rapid drop of fibrinogen.

MATIS (1967) listed 4,349 surgical patients, 2,104 of whom were treated with Trasylol. A positive effect was statistically proved in postoperative disorders in wound healing, peritonitis, fat embolism, lung embolism, and postoperative hemorrhage.

F. Hereditary Inhibitor Deficiency

In hereditary angioneurotic edema a decreased inhibition of kallikrein by serum was noticed (LANDERMAN, 1962; LANDERMAN et al., 1962; KAGEN and BECKER, 1963; BECKER and KAGEN, 1964; WEBSTER and INNERFIELD, 1965). In this pathological state a decrease of the inhibition of C′1-esterase was also observed (DONALDSON and EVANS, 1963; DONALDSON and ROSEN, 1964; CHARACHE et al., 1964). This was confirmed by BURDON et al. (1965), SIBOO and LAURELL (1965), and GOTTSTEIN et al. (1967).

Obviously the failure in synthesis of the inhibitor is caused by gene mutation. Recessive hereditary gene defect is known also for trypsin and thrombin inhibitors of plasma (for review see VOGEL et al., 1966, 1968); these abnormalities also lead to pathological states.

According to WERLE and TRAUTSCHOLD (ref. in FREY et al., 1968), treatment of a patient with Trasylol resulted in decrease of edema. Soon after the appearance of edema the kininogen level in plasma was decreased (BURDON et al., 1965). Patients suffering from angioneurotic edema tolerate intradermal injection of plasma kallikrein poorly.

The absence of this inhibitor disturbs the balance of the kinin system, although the cause for intermittent occurrence of the symptoms is unknown.

References[1]

ADHAM, N. F., DYCE, B., WILDING, P., WONG, T., HAVERBACK, B. J.: Trypsin binding α_2-macroglobulin in patients with acute pancreatitis. Clin. Res. **15**, 128 (1967).

ALBRECHTSEN, O. K.: The fibrinolytic activity of human tissues. Brit. J. Haemat. **3**, 284 (1957).

ALKJAERSIG, N., FLETCHER, A. P., SHERRY, S.: The mechanism of clot dissolution by plasmin. J. clin. Invest. **38**, 1086 (1959).

AMBRUS, C. M., MARKUS, G.: Plasmin-antiplasmin complex as a reservoir of fibrinolytic enzyme. Amer. J. Physiol. **199**, 491 (1960).

AMBRUS, J. L.: The fibrinolysin system. Fed. Proc. **25**, 28 (1966).

AMRIS, C.J.: Inhibition of thromboplastic activity by Trasylol. In: Neue Aspekte der Trasylol-Therapie, p. 52, ed. by R. GROSS and G. KRONEBERG. Stuttgart 1966a.

— Inhibition of fibrinolytic and thromboplastic activity by Trasylol. Scand. J. Haemat. **3**, 19 (1966b).

— Investigations concerning activator-free porcine plasmin. Scand. J. clin. Lab. Invest. **18**, Suppl. 89, 1 (1966c).

— Inhibition of thromboplastic activity by Trasylol. Scand. J. Haemat. **4**, 3 (1967).

— KJELDSEN, J.: Haemorrhagic diathesis due to abruptio placentae treated with Trasylol. Acta obstet. gynec. scand. **45**, 180 (1966).

ANDRÉ, A.: Les hémorragies cataclysmiques par fibrinolyse en obstétrique, en médicine et en chirurgie. Concours méd. **85**, 7029 (1963).

ANKIER, S. I., STARR, M. S.: The importance of plasma kinins in the anaphylactoid reaction in rats. Brit. J. Pharmacol. **31**, 331 (1967).

ARTZ, C. P.: Discussion of P. NEMIR, J. HOFERICHTER and D. L. DRABKIN: The protective effect of proteinase inhibitor in acute necrotizing pancreatitis. Ann. Surg. **158**, 655 (1963).

[1] Literature references included up to summer 1968.

ASTRUP, T.: Blutgerinnung, Fibrinolyse und Wundheilung. Medizinische **42**, 1972, (1959).
— Biologie des Plasmins. Verhandlungen der Tagg der Dtsch. Arbeitsgemeinschaft für Blutgerinnungsforschung, p. 5. Stuttgart 1967.
— BRAKMAN, P., OLLENDORF, P., RASMUSSEN, J.: Haemostasis in haemophilia in relation to the haemostatic balance in the normal organism and the effect of peanuts. Thrombos. Diathes. haemorrh. (Stuttg.) **5**, 329 (1960).
— — SJØLIN, K. E.: Haemophilia and the protease inhibitor in plants. Nature (Lond.) **194**, 980 (1962).
AUHAGEN, E.: Chimica e biochimica del Trasylol. In: Drugs of animal origin, p. 69, ed. by A. LEONARDI and J. WALSH. Milan 1967.
BACHRACH, W. H., SCHILD, P. D.: A double-blind study of Trasylol in the treatment of pancreatitis. Ann. N.Y. Acad. Sci. **146**, 580 (1968).
BACK, N.: Discussion of J. A. OATES and K. L. MELMON: Biochemical and physiological studies of the kinins in the carcinoid syndrome. In: Hypotensive Peptides, p. 565, ed. by E. G. ERDÖS, N. BACK and F. SICUTERI. Berlin-Heidelberg-New York: Springer 1966a.
— Fibrinolysis system and vasoactive kinins. Fed. Proc. **25**, 77 (1966b).
— JAINCHILL, M., WILKENS, H. J., AMBRUS, J. L.: Effect of inhibitors of plasmin, kallikrein and kinin on mortality from scalding in mice. Med. Pharmacol. exp. **15**, 597 (1966b).
— WILKENS, H., STEGER, R.: Fibrinolysis and vasoactive peptides on anaphylaxis. In: Hypotensive Peptides, p. 485, ed. by E. G. ERDÖS, N. BACK and F. SICUTERI. Berlin-Heidelberg-New York: Springer 1966a.
— — — Proteinases and proteinase inhibitors in experimental shock states. Ann. N.Y. Acad. Sci. **146**, 491 (1968).
BECK, I. T., MCKENNA, R. D., ZYLBERSZAC, B., SOLYMAR, J., EISENSTEIN, S.: The effect of a trypsin inhibitor, Trasylol, on the course of bile and trypsin-induced pancreatitis in dogs. Gastroenterology **48**, 478 (1965).
— PINTER, E. J., SOLYMAR, J., MCKENNA, R. D., RITCHIE, A. C.: The role of pancreatic proteolytic enzymes in the pathogenesis of acute pancreatitis. II. The fate of pancreatic proteolytic enzymes in the course of acute pancreatitis. Gastroenterology **43**, 60 (1963).
BECKER, E. L., KAGEN, L.: The permeability globulins of human serum and the biochemical mechanism of hereditary angioneurotic edema. Ann. N.Y. Acad. Sci. **116**, 866 (1964).
BECKER, V.: Sekretionsstudien am Pankreas. Stuttgart 1957.
— Die akute und chronische tryptische Pankreatitis. Gastroenterologia (Basel) **94**, 65 (1960).
— Tryptische Pankreatitis und tryptische Nekrose. Dtsch. med. Wschr. **89**, 671 (1964).
— WILDE, W.: Pankreasschäden durch Trypsin *in vitro*. Klin. Wschr. **41**, 73 (1963).
BELLER, F. K.: Gerinnungsstörungen als Ursache schwerer geburtshilflicher Blutungen. Therapiewoche **11**, 602 (1961).
BELLMANN, G.: Die akute Pankreatitis und ihre Behandlung. Med. Mschr. **14**, 15 (1960).
BENZER, H., BLÜMEL, G., PIZA, F.: Einflüsse von Trypsininhibitoren auf die Blutgerinnung. Wien. med. Wschr. **110**, 609 (1960).
— — — Experimentelle Untersuchungen über die Wirkungen tryptischer und antitryptischer Fermente auf den Eiweißstoffwechsel und die Blutgerinnung. Bruns' Beitr. klin. Chir. **202**, 385 (1961).
BERALDO, W. T.: Formation of bradykinin in anaphylactic and peptone shock. Amer. J. Physiol. **163**, 283 (1950).
BERGHOFF, A., GLATZEL, H.: Über die Hemmung des fibrinolytischen Potentials durch Trasylol. Med. Klin. **58**, 476 (1963).
BERNARD, A., PAGET, M., LAMELIN, P.: Trypsinogen-Trypsin und seine Hemmstoffe in der akuten Pankreatitis. Arch. Mal. Appar. dig. **49**, 632 (1960).
BERTELLI, A., FRANCESCONI, G., LAMI, V., PERELLI-ERCOLINI, M., PROTO, M., ROSSANO, M. P.: Protection of skin homografts and blockade of the Sanarelli-Shwartzman reaction by means of a polypeptide which inhibits proteolysis, Trasylol. Atti Accad. med. lombarda **18**, 216 (1963).
BEUCHELT, H.: Trasylol, ein Proteinasen-Inhibitor, in Experiment und klinischer Anwendung. Med. Chem. **7**, 763 (1963).
BIGGS, R., MCFARLANE, R. G.: Treatment of hemophilia and other coagulatory disorders. Oxford 1966.
BISORDI, M.: Peanut flour in hemophilia. Lancet **1964 II**, 476.
BLEYL, U., GRÖZINGER, K. H., NAGEL, W., WANKE, M.: Histochemische Darstellung der proteolytischen Aktivität bei der akuten experimentellen Pankreatitis. Klin. Wschr. **44**, 282 (1966).
— — — — Histotopochemie aktiver proteolytischer Enzyme bei der experimentellen autodigestiven Pankreatitis. Virchows Arch. path. Anat. **342**, 26 (1967).
BLOMBÄCK, B., BLOMBÄCK, M., OLSSON, P.: Action of a proteolytic-enzyme inhibitor on blood coagulation in vitro. Thrombos. Diathes. haemorrh. (Stuttg.) **18**, 190 (1967).

Blümel, G.: Biologische Aktivitäten im Frakturhämatom. Langenbecks Arch. klin. Chir. **316**, 964 (1966).
— Biologische Aktivität im Frakturhämatom. Med. Welt **18**, 2082 (1967).
— Fischer, M., Lechner, K.: Plasmakininogenspiegel und Proteinasenhemmkörper; Beobachtungen während Substitutionstherapie bei Haemophilie A. Thrombos. Diathes. haemorrh. (Stuttg.) **18**, 364 (1967).
— Grözinger, K. H.: Experimentelle Untersuchungen bei der durch Fettemulsionen ausgelösten Pankreatitis der Katze. Wien. klin. Wschr. **78**, 847 (1966).
— Piza, F.: Zur Wirkungsweise eines Proteasenhemmkörpers auf die Pankreasfermente. Wien. klin. Wschr. **78**, 660 (1966).
Bonaccorsi, A., West, G. B.: Absence of capillary permeability response in rats to dextran and egg white. J. Pharm. Pharmacol. **15**, 372 (1963).
Brocklehurst, W. E., Lahiri, S. C.: The production of bradykinin in anaphylaxis. J. Physiol. (Lond.) **160**, 15P (1962).
— — Formation and destruction of bradykinin during anaphylaxis. J. Physiol. (Lond.) **165**, 39P (1963).
— Zeitlin, I. J.: Determination of plasma kinin and kininogen levels in man. J. Physiol. (Lond.) **191**, 417 (1967).
Brücke, P., Blümel, G., Gottlob, R.: Experimentelle Untersuchungen zum Problem Schock und Fettembolie. Klin. Med. **21**, 304 (1966).
— — — Neue Aspekte zur Pathogenese der posttraumatischen Fettembolie. Med. Welt **18**, 2081 (1967).
Burdon, K. L., Queng, J. T., Thomas, O. C., McGovern, P.: Observations on biochemical abnormalities in hereditary angioneurotic edema. J. Allergy **36**, 546 (1965).
Burke, J. S., Uriuhara, T., MacMorine, D. R. L., Movat, H. Z.: A permeability factor released from phagocytosing PMN-leukocytes and its inhibition by protease inhibitors. Life Sci. **3**, 1505 (1964).
Cannon, R. H., Turner, M. D.: Retardation of the progress of experimental pancreatitis with trypsin inhibitors. Surg. Forum **12**, 367 (1961).
Capper, W. M., Trapnell, J. E., Talbot, C. H.: Trasylol and acute pancreatitis. Brit. med. J. **1965 II**, 1184.
Charache, P., Donaldson, V., Pensky, J., Fireman, P., Rosen, F. S., Janeway, C. A.: Genetic abnormalities in hereditary angioneurotic edema. J. clin. Invest. **43**, 1250 (1964).
Chryssanthou, C., Antopol, W.: Effect of trypsin inhibitors on Shwartzman phenomenon. Fed. Proc. **20**, 261 (1961a).
— — Effect of trypsin inhibitor on Shwartzman phenomenon. Proc. Soc. exp. Biol. (N.Y.) **108**, 587 (1961b).
Cirstea, M., Suhaciu, G., Butculescu, I.: Bradykinin and anaphylactic shock in dogs. Int. Arch. Allergy **26**, 356 (1965a).
— — — Bradykinin and anaphylactic shock in dogs, guinea-pigs and rabbits. Arch. int. Physiol. Biochem. **73**, 231 (1965b).
Corrado, A. P., Reis, M. L., Carvalho, I. F., Diniz, C. R.: Bradykininogen and bradykinin in the cardiovascular shock produced by proteolytic enzymes. Biochem. Pharmacol. **15**, 959 (1966).
Creutzfeldt, W., Schmidt, H., Horbach, I.: Untersuchungen über die Wirksamkeit eines Trypsininhibitors (Trasylol) auf die Enzymaktivitäten und Morphologie bei der Taurocholat- und Calciphylaxie-Pankreatitis der Ratte. Klin. Wschr. **43**, 15 (1965a).
— — Linneweh, E.: The pathogenesis of pancreatitis. VI. Annual Meeting Anglo-German Society, Manchester 1965b.,
— Söling, H. D., Ketterer, H.: Intrapankreatische Aktivierung von proteolytischen Fermenten und Trasylolwirkung bei der experimentellen Pankreatitis der Ratte. Klin. Wschr. **41**, 1002 (1963).
Creveld, S. van, Mochtar, I. A.: Hemophilia and therapy with peanuts. Ann. paediat. (Basel) **197**, 1 (1961).
Dawson, W., Starr, M. S., West, G. B.: Bradykinin and anaphylaxis in the rat. J. Physiol. (Lond.) **180**, 14P (1965).
— West, G. B.: The importance of bradykinin in anaphylactic shock. J. Pharm. Pharmacol. **17**, 246 (1965).
Diniz, C. R., Carvalho, I. F.: A micromethod for determination of bradykininogen under several conditions. Ann. N.Y. Acad. Sci. **104**, 77 (1963).
— — Dos Reis, M. L., Corrado, A. P.: Bradykininogen in normal and experimental conditions. III. Internat. Symposium on Vaso-Active Polypeptides, ed. by M. Rocha e Silva and H. Rothschild. Sao Paulo 1966.
— — Ryan, J., Rocha e Silva, M.: A micromethod for the determination of bradykininogen in blood plasma. Nature (Lond.) **192**, 1194 (1961).

DOERR, W.: Pathologisch-anatomische Untersuchungen zum Problem der Fermententgleisung im Pankreas. Verh. dtsch. Ges. Path. **37**, 292 (1953).
— Pankreatitis. Pathogenese, Formen, Häufigkeit. Langenbecks Arch. klin. Chir. **292**, 552 (1959).
— Pathogenese der akuten und chronischen Pankreatitis. Verh. dtsch. Ges. inn. Med. **70**, 718 (1964).
— DIEZEL, P. B., GRÖZINGER, K. H., LASCH, H. G., NAGEL, W., ROSSNER, J., WANKE, M., WILLIG, F.: Pathogenese der experimentellen autodigestiven Pankreatitis. Klin. Wschr. **43**, 125 (1965).
DOLLINGER, M. R., GARDNER, B.: Newer aspects of the carcinoid syndrome. Surg. Gynec. Obstet. **122**, 1335 (1966).
DONALDSON, V. H., EVANS, R.: A biochemical abnormality in hereditary angioneurotic edema. Amer. J. Med. **35**, 37 (1963).
— ROSEN, F. S.: Action of complement in hereditary angioneurotic edema; the role of C'1-esterase. J. Clin. Invest. **43**, 2204 (1964).
DUBBER, A. H. C., MCNICOL, G. P., DOUGLAS, A. S.: *In vitro* and *in vivo* studies of Trasylol. In: Diffuse Intravascular Clotting, ed. by K. M. BRINKHOUS, I. S. WRIGHT, F. KOLLER, F. STREULI and F. DUCKERT. Stuttgart 1966.
— — UTTLEY, D., DOUGLAS, A. S.: *In vitro* and *in vivo* studies with Trasylol, an anticoagulant and a fibrinolytic inhibitor. Brit. J. Haemat. **14**, 31 (1968).
DUPREZ, A., GODART, S., PLATTEBORSE, R., DUPONT, J. M.: Interstitial and lymphatic pathway of the external secretion of the pancreas. In: Pathogenese, Diagnostik, Klinik und Therapie der Erkrankungen des exokrinen Pankreas, p. 207, ed. by N. HENNING, K. HEINKEL and H. SCHÖN. Stuttgart 1964.
EISEN, V.: Studies on fibrinogen fractions isolated from human plasma by precipitation with ether. Brit. J. Haemat. **11**, 576 (1965).
— KEELE, C. A.: Possible modes of kinin formation in some pathological states in man. In: Hypotensive Peptides, p. 551, ed. by E. G. ERDÖS, N. BACK and F. SICUTERI. Berlin-Heidelberg-New York: Springer 1966.
ELLIOTT, D. W., WILLIAMS, R. D., STEWART, W. R. C.: The role of trypsin and bile salts in the pathogenesis of acute pancreatitis. Surg. Forum. **9**, 533 (1958).
— — ZOLLINGER, R. M.: Alterations in the pancreatic resistance to bile in the pathogenesis of acute pancreatitis. Ann. Surg. **146**, 669 (1957).
— ZOLLINGER, R. M., MOORE, R., ELLISON, E.: The use of human serum albumin in the management of acute pancreatitis. Gastroenterology **28**, 563 (1955).
ENCKE, A., SCHIMPF, K., KOMMERELL, B., GRÖZINGER, K. H., GILSDORF, H., WANKE, M., LASCH, H. G.: Veränderungen der Blutgerinnung bei der akuten experimentellen Pankreatitis des Hundes. Klin. Wschr. **44**, 90 (1966).
ERDÖS, E. G.: Hypotensive peptides: bradykinin, kallidin and eledoisin. Advanc. Pharmacol. **4**, 1 (1966).
— Effect of nonsteroidal anti-inflammatory drugs in endotoxin shock. Biochem. Pharmacol., Suppl., Chemical Biology of Inflammation, p. 283 (1968).
— HINSHAW, L. B., GILL, C. C.: Effect of indomethacin in endotoxin shock in the dog. Proc. Soc. exp. Biol. (N.Y.) **125**, 916 (1967).
— MIWA, I.: Effect of endotoxin shock on the plasma kallikrein-kinin-system of the rabbit. Fed. Proc. **27**, 92 (1968).
ERIKSON, S.: Studies in α_1-antitrypsin deficiency. Acta med. scand. **177**, Suppl (1965).
FALCIDIENO, P., GALLI, T., NICORA, E.: Akute Pankreatitis und Kallikrein-Inaktivator. Pathologia **54**, 77 (1962).
FERGUSON, J.: Crystalline trypsin-inhibitor and blood clotting. Proc. Soc. exp. Biol. (N.Y.) **51**, 373 (1942).
FINE, J., MINTON, R.: Mechanism of action of bacterial endotoxin. Nature (Lond.) **210**, 97 (1966).
FISCHER, M.: Medical and social problems in hemophilias. Bibl. haemat. (Basel) **26**, 309 (1966).
FLEISCHHACKER, H., STACHER, A.: Die Bedeutung der Fibrinolyse für die Klinik. Med. Klin. **57**, 703 (1962).
FORELL, M. M.: Untersuchungen über das Kallikreinogen im Serum des gesunden und kranken Menschen und seine Beeinflussung durch die Nebennierenrinde. Schweiz. med. Wschr. **87**, 828 (1957).
— Personal communication. Ref. in: Das Kallikrein-Kinin-System und seine Inhibitoren, p. 231, ed. by E. K. FREY, H. KRAUT, E. WERLE, R. VOGEL, G. ZICKGRAF and I. TRAUTSCHOLD. Stuttgart 1968.
— DOBOVICNIK, W.: Über die Möglichkeit, durch Inaktivierung des Trypsins die akute Pankreatitis kausal zu beeinflussen. Klin. Wschr. **39**, 47 (1961).

FREY, E. K., KRAUT, H., WERLE, E., VOGEL, R., ZICKGRAF, G., TRAUTSCHOLD, I.: Das Kallikrein-Kinin-System und seine Inhibitoren. Stuttgart 1968.

— WERLE, E., SACKERS, E.: Über die Wirkung intravenöser und intramuskulärer Kallikreininjektionen beim Menschen. Z. ges. exp. Med. **96**, 404 (1935).

FRITZ, H., WOITINAS, F., WERLE, E.: Über Proteaseinhibitoren. II. Isolierung und Charakterisierung von Proteaseinhibitoren aus den Bauchspeicheldrüsen verschiedener Wirbeltiere und des Menschen. Hoppe-Seylers Z. physiol. Chem. **345**, 168 (1966).

GARDNER, B., DOLLINGER, M., SILEN, W., BACK, N., O'REILLY, S.: Studies on the carcinoid syndrome. Its relationship to serotonin, bradykinin and histamine. Surgery **61**, 846 (1967).

GERATZ, J. D.: Failure of a potent trypsin inhibitor to modify experimental pancreatitis in dogs. Arch. Surg. **96**, 442 (1968).

GILLETTE, R. W., FINDLEY, A., CONWAY, H.: Effect on tumor homografts of treating hosts with antiproteolytic enzyme compounds. Proc. Soc. exp. Biol. (N.Y.) **112**, 964 (1963).

GOLDBLAT, M. V., KLINE, D. L., MILSTONE, J. H.: Activation of trypsinogen by plasmin. Proc. Soc. exp. Biol. (N.Y.) **125**, 763 (1967).

GORMSEN, J., JOSEPHSEN, P.: The effect of Trasylol on blood coagulation after intravenous injection. Thrombos. Diathes. haemorrh. (Stuttg.) **17**, 51 (1967).

GOTTSTEIN, U., YOO, D. J., BÜTTNER, H.: C'1-Esterase und C'1-Esterase-Inhibitor im Serum von Kranken mit hereditärem genuinem Quincke-Ödem. Klin. Wschr. **45**, 230 (1967).

GREEFF, K.: Der Kininogengehalt des Plasmas beim experimentellen Schock. In: Neue Aspekte der Trasylol-Therapie, p. 135, ed. by R. GROSS and G. KRONEBERG. Stuttgart 1966.

— SCHARNAGEL, K., LÜHR, R., STROBACH, H.: Die Abnahme des Kininogengehaltes des Plasmas beim toxischen, anaphylaktischen und anaphylaktoiden Schock. Naunyn-Schmiedebergs Arch. exp. Path. Pharmak. **253**, 235 (1966).

GRÖZINGER, K. H.: Die Inhibitorentherapie der akuten Pankreatitis. In: Neue Aspekte der Trasylol-Therapie, vol. 2, p. 55, ed. by R. MARX, H. IMDAHL and G. HABERLAND. Stuttgart 1967.

— ARTZ, C. P.: Tierexperimentelle Untersuchungen zur Beeinflussung der Pankreatitis mit dem Fermentinhibitor Trasylol. Langenbecks Arch. klin. Chir. **305**, 150 (1964).

— — HOLLIS, A. U., WESSON, R. L.: Evaluation of Trasylol in experimental acute pancreatitis. Surgery **56**, 400 (1964).

— WANKE, M., HOCHBERG, K., WELSH, P.: Pathomorphologische Untersuchungsergebnisse von Therapieversuchen mit Fermenthemmkörpern bei der experimentellen Pankreatitis des Hundes. Langenbecks Arch. klin. Chir. **310**, 199 (1965).

— WENZ, W.: Arterielle Perfusion des Pankreas mit Trasylol bei akuter Pankreatitis. Z. Gastroent. **3**, 77 (1965).

GROSS, R., KRONEBERG, G.: Neue Aspekte der Trasylol-Therapie. Stuttgart 1966.

GRUNDMANN, E.: Experimentelle Beiträge zur Adhäsionsprophylaxe. Langenbecks Arch. klin. Chir. **313**, 894 (1966a).

— Experimentelle Beiträge zur abdominellen Adhäsionsprophylaxe durch Trasylol. In: Neue Aspekte der Trasylol-Therapie, p. 178, ed. by R. GROSS and G. KRONEBERG. Stuttgart 1966b.

— Tierexperimentelle und histologische Untersuchungen zur Prophylaxe abdomineller Läsionen durch Trasylol. Bruns' Beitr. klin. Chir. **212**, 336 (1966c).

HABERLAND, G. L., MATIS, P.: Trasylol, ein Proteinaseninhibitor bei chirurgischen und internen Indikationen. Med. Welt **18**, 1367 (1967).

HABERMANN, E.: Fortschritte auf dem Gebiet der Plasmakinine. Naunyn-Schmiedebergs Arch. exp. Path. Pharmak. **245**, 230 (1963).

— Das Kininsystem—pathologische Bedeutung und therapeutische Konsequenzen. Internist (Berl.) **7**, 364 (1966).

HAIG, T. H. B., THOMPSON, A. G.: The effect of a kallikrein inactivator on experimental acute pancreatitis. Canad. J. Surg. **7**, 97 (1964).

HANSEN, H. T., DRUBE, H. C., BRÜNING, W., BJÖRN, W.: Behandlung der akuten Pankreatitis mit und ohne Proteinaseninhibitor. Vergleichende klinische Untersuchungen mit Trasylol. Med. Klin. **61**, 1254 (1966).

HANSSON, K., LENNINGER, S.: A proteinase inhibitor in acute pancreatitis. Nord. Med. **77**, 149 (1967).

HARTERT, H.: Die Thrombelastographie in der Differentialdiagnose der hämorrhagischen Diathesen. Schweiz. med. Wschr. **79**, 318 (1949).

HATANO, M., GRENIER, J. F., ADLOFF, M., WEISS, A. G.: Dissemination of pancreatic enzymes into the body during experimental acute pancreatitis treated or not with antitryptic drugs. C. R. Soc. Biol. (Paris) **157**, 1505 (1963).

HAVERBACK, B. J., DYCE, B., BUNDY, H., EDMONDSON, H. A.: Trypsin, trypsinogen and trypsin inhibitor in human pancreatic juice. Amer. J. Med. **29**, 424 (1960).

HEINKEL, K.: Therapie der akuten und chronischen Pankreatitis. Verh. dtsch. Ges. inn. Med. **70**, 810 (1964).
HELLER, W., MÖRL, F. K.: Das Verhalten der Plasmafette nach Frakturen und ihre Beeinflussungsmöglichkeit mit dem Proteinaseninhibitor Trasylol. Med. Welt 18, 2076 (1967).
HERSCHLEIN, H. J., STEICHELE, D. F.: Die Hemmung der Hyperkoagulabilität des Blutes. Med. Welt 1314 (1964).
HERSHEY, S. G., ALTURA, B. M.: Behandlung des Schocks durch Beeinflussung der peripheren Zirkulation mit vasoaktiven Wirkstoffen. Eine mikrozirkulatorische Basis für die Therapie. Schweiz. med. Wschr. **96**, 1467, 1516 (1966).
HILTON, S. M., LEWIS, G. P.: The relationship between glandular activity, bradykinin formation and functional vasodilatation in the submandibular salivary gland. J. Physiol. (Lond.) **134**, 471 (1956).
HINSHAW, L. B., SOLOMON, L. A., ERDÖS, E. G., REINS, D. A., GUNTER, B. J.: Effect of acetylsalicylic acid on the canine response to endotoxin. J. Pharmacol. exp. Ther. **157**, 667 (1967).
HLADOVEC, J., HORÁKOVÁ, Z., MANSFELD, V.: Antiphlogistische Wirkungen von Proteinasen-Inhibitor aus Kartoffeln auf verschiedene Typen der experimentellen Entzündungen. Arch. int. Pharmacodyn. **128**, 343 (1960).
— — — Experimentelle Verbrennung. Arzneimittel-Forsch. **11**, 104 (1961).
HOFERICHTER, J.: Experimentelle Pankreatitis. In: Pathogenese, Diagnostik, Klinik und Therapie der Erkrankungen des exokrinen Pankreas, p. 179, ed. by N. HENNING, K. HEINKEL and H. SCHÖN. Stuttgart 1964a.
— Klinische und experimentelle Untersuchungen zur akuten hämorrhagischen Pankreasnekrose. Langenbecks Arch. klin. Chir. **307**, 319 (1964b).
— „Gezielte Prophylaxe" der postoperativen Pankreasnekrose. Chirurg **38**, 233 (1967).
— NEMIR, P., DRABKIN, D. L.: Protective effect of proteinase inhibitors in acute necrotizing pancreatitis. An experimental study. Surg. Forum **13**, 309 (1962).
HOFFBAUER, H.: Hyperfibrinolytische Krisen bei gynäkologischen und geburtshilflichen Operationen. In: Neue Aspekte der Trasylol-Therapie, vol. 2, p. 99, ed. by R. MARX, H. IMDAHL and G. HABERLAND. Stuttgart 1967.
HOFFMAN, H. L., JACOBS, J., FREEDLANDER, S. O.: Use of crystalline soybean trypsin inhibitor in acute hemorrhagic pancreatitis in dogs. Arch. Surg. **66**, 617 (1953).
HOLLENBERG, M., KOBOLD, E. E., PRUETT, R., THAL, A. P.: Occurrence of circulating vasoactive substances in human and experimental pancreatitis. Surg. Forum **13**, 302 (1962).
HUBER, P.: Grundlagen der Therapie der hyperfibrinolytischen Erkrankungen mit Trasylol. Med. heute **15**, 275 (1966).
JORNS, G.: Pankreatitis — pathologische Vorstellungen und heutige Therapie. Dtsch. Gesundh.-Wes. **15**, 770 (1960).
JÜRGENS, J.: Die klinische Bedeutung fibrinolytischer Vorgänge. Dtsch. med. Wschr. **84**, 2285 (1959).
— Kallikrein-Inhibitor. 73. Tagg Ges. inn. Med., Wiesbaden, 1967. Ref. Ärztl. Prax. **19**, 1064 (1967).
KAGEN, L. J., BECKER, E. L.: Inhibition of permeability globulins by C'1 esterase inhibitor. Fed. Proc. **22**, 613 (1963).
KATZ, W., SILVERSTEIN, M., KOBOLD, E. E., THAL, A. P.: Trypsin release, kinin production and shock. Arch. Surg. **89**, 322 (1964).
KELLY, T. R., BRATCHER, E. P., FALOR, W. H.: Trypsin inhibitor in acute hemorrhagic pancreatitis in dogs. Arch. Surg. **89**, 317 (1964).
KERN, E., KUHBIER, C.: Entstehung, Klinik, Therapie und Prophylaxe der peritonealen Adhäsionen. Ergebn. Chir. Orthop. **46**, 48 (1964).
KLINE, D. L.: Chemistry and biochemistry of the fibrinolytic system. Fed. Proc. **25**, 31 (1966).
KOBOLD, E. E., THAL, A. P.: Quantitation and identification of vasoactive substances liberated during various types of experimental and clinical intestinal ischemia. Surg. Gynec. Obstet. **117**, 315 (1963).
KÖSSLING, F. K., NAGEL, M., SCHIER, J., METZ, B.: Experimentelle, tryptische Pankreatitis durch selektive, intraarterielle Applikation von Bradykinin. Z. Gastroent. **5**, 306 (1967).
KONZETT, H.: Some properties of synthetic bradykinin and bradykinin-like polypeptides. Biochem. Pharmacol. **10**, 39 (1962).
KOSLOWSKI, L.: Der Verbrennungsschock und seine Behandlung. Ref. Med. Welt **18**, 1938 (1966).
— BARCKOW, D., WASCHKEIT, G.: Zur Behandlung schwerer Verbrennungen mit dem Fermentinaktivator Trasylol. Chirurg **33**, 533 (1962).
— WASCHKEIT, W.: Behandlung von Verbrennungen mit einem Fermentinaktivator. Klin. Wschr. **38**, 1219 (1960).

Kraus, H., Koslowski, L., Zimmermann, W. E.: Neuere Erkenntnisse über die Stoffwechselveränderungen bei Verbrennungen und im Schock. Langenbecks Arch. klin. Chir. **303**, 23 (1963).
Kwaan, H. C., Astrup, T.: Aortic arteriosclerosis in rabbits. Arch. Path. **78**, 474 (1964).
Landerman, N. S.: Hereditary angioneurotic edema. Case reports and review of literature. J. Allergy **33**, 316 (1962).
— Webster, M. E., Becker, E. L., Ratcliffe, H. E.: Hereditary angioneurotic edema. II. Deficiency of inhibitor for serum-globulin-permeability factor and/or plasma kallikrein. J. Allergy **33**, 330 (1962).
Lauenstein, K., Haberland, G. L.: Über die Wirkung einiger Arzneimittel auf das Komplementsystem. Med. Chem. (Bayer) **7**, 784 (1963).
Lecomte, J.: Consommation des kininogènes plasmatiques au cours du chock anaphylactique du lapin. C. R. Soc. Biol. (Paris) **155**, 1411 (1961).
Léger, L., Lande, M.: Diagnostic et traitement des états fibrinolytiques au cours de la chirurgie de l'hypertension portale. Ars Med. (Liestal) **17**, 7 (1962).
Lembeck, F.: 5-Hydroxytryptamine in a carcinoid-tumor. Nature (Lond.) **172**, 910 (1953).
Lillehei, R. C., Longerbeam, J. K., Bloch, J. H., Manax, W. G.: The modern treatment of shock based on physiological principles. Clin. Pharmacol. Ther. **5**, 63 (1964).
Louw, J. H., Marks, I. N., Bank, S.: The management of severe acute pancreatitis. Postgrad. med. J. **43**, 31 (1967).
Ludwig, H.: Perinatale Hirnblutungen bei Hypoxie und ihre Unterdrückung. In: Neue Aspekte der Trasylol-Therapie, p. 76, ed. by R. Gross and G. Kroneberg. Stuttgart 1966.
— Zur Anwendung von Trasylol in der Geburtshilfe und Gynäkologie. In: Neue Aspekte der Trasylol-Therapie, vol. 2, p. 115, ed. by R. Marx, H. Imdahl and G. Haberland. Stuttgart 1967.
— Mikrozirkulationsstörungen und Diapedeseblutungen im fetalen Gehirn bei Hypoxie. Basel 1968.
Mackay, M., Maycock, W. d'A., Silk, E., Combridge, B. S.: Studies on fibrinogen fractions isolated from human plasma by precipitation with cold ether. Brit. J. Haemat. **11**, 563 (1965).
— — — Topis, D.: Anti-enzymes et pancréatite aigue. Lyon chir. **57**, 801 (1961).
Mallet-Guy, P., Bosser, C., Michoulier, J.: Analyse de l'action des anti-enzymes sur l'evolution des pancréatites aiguës expérimentales. Bull. Soc. int. Chir. **5—6**, 531 (1963).
Mammen, E. F.: Hyperfibrinolytische Blutungen in der Chirurgie-Prophylaxe und gezielte Behandlung. Therap. Berichte **38**, 103 (1966).
Mansfeld, V., Rybák, M., Horáková, Z., Hladovec, J.: Die antitryptische, antifibrinolytische und antiphlogistische Aktivität natürlicher Proteasen-Inhibitoren. Hoppe-Seylers Z. physiol. Chem. **318**, 6 (1960).
Marggraf, W.: Beobachtungen über Fibrinolyse in der Chirurgie, ihre Prophylaxe und gezielte Behandlung mit Inhibitoren. Bruns' Beitr. klin. Chir. **205**, 121 (1962).
Markwardt, F., Klöcking, H. P., Richter, M.: Die Kombinationswirkung von Fibrinolysehemmstoffen. Acta biol. med. germ. **12**, 522 (1964).
Marx, R.: Blutstillung mit Fibrinolyse-Inhibitoren. Münch. med. Wschr. **108**, 1267 (1966).
— Kallikreininhibitoren als Gerinnungshemmstoffe. In: Neue Aspekte der Trasylol-Therapie, vol. 2, p. 89, ed. by R. Marx, H. Imdahl and G. Haberland. Stuttgart 1967.
— Konferenzbericht über das 2. Symposium DAB, 1956. Thrombos. Diathes. haemorrh. (Stuttg.), Suppl., **2** (1968).
— Clemente, P., Werle, E., Appel, W.: Zum Problem eines Antidotes in der internen Thrombotherapie mit Fibrinolytika. Blut **5**, 367 (1959).
— — — — Über die Wirkung von Proteinaseinhibitor-Präparaten (Leber- und Parotisinhibitor) auf die extravasale Fibrinolyse, Fibrinogenolyse und Blutgerinnungskonstanten im Menschenblut. Blut **9**, 164 (1963).
— Henning, K.: Über Verstärkersubstanzen der Antifibrinolysewirkung der ε-Aminokapronsäure im Organismus. Proceedings VIII. Congr. Soc. Europ. Haematol., p. 454, 1962.
— Imdahl, H., Haberland, G.: Neue Aspekte der Trasylol-Therapie, vol. 2. Stuttgart 1967.
Mashford, M. L., Zacest, R.: Effect of adrenaline on blood kinin levels in carcinoid syndrome and in normal subjects. Aust. Ann. Med. **16**, 326 (1967).
Mason, D. T., Melmon, K. L.: Abnormal forearm vascular responses in the carcinoid syndrome. The role of kinins and kinin-generating system. J. clin. Invest. **45**, 1685 (1966a).
— — New understanding of the mechanism of the carcinoid flush. Ann. intern. Med. **65**, 1334 (1966b).
Massion, W. H., Erdös, E. G.: The effects of ATP and a proteolytic enzyme inhibitor in irreversible shock. J. Okla. med. Ass. **59**, 467 (1966).

Matis, P.: Wirkungen von Trasylol auf Blutgerinnung und Wundheilung (Ergebnisse einer alternierenden Reihe). In: Neue Aspekte der Trasylol-Therapie, vol. 2, p. 19, ed. by R. Marx, H. Imdahl and G. Haberland. Stuttgart 1967.

Maurer, W.: Über die Wirksamkeit des Fermentinhibitors Trasylol in Therapie und Prophylaxe der akuten Pancreatitis. Schweiz. med. Wschr. **94**, 1743 (1964).

— Heinkel, K.: Klinische und experimentelle Ergebnisse zur Behandlung mit Trasylol. II. Weltkongr. Gastroenterol. **4**, 134 (1963).

McCutcheon, A. D.: Trasylol. A new treatment for pancreatitis. Aust. Ann. Med. **13**, 174 (1964).

— Race, D.: Experimental pancreatitis. Use of a new antiproteolytic substance, Trasylol. Ann. Surg. **158**, 233 (1963).

— — Experimental fat necrosis: effect of Trasylol. Implications for pancreatitis. Ann. Surg. **160**, 1041 (1964).

McHardy, G., Craighead, C. C., Balart, L., Cradic, H., La Grange, C.: Pancreatitis—intrapancreatic proteolytic trypsin activity. J. Amer. med. Ass. **183**, 527 (1963).

Melmon, K. L., Cline, M. J.: Kinins. Amer. J. Med. **43**, 153 (1967).

— Lovenberg, W., Sjoerdsma, A.: Characteristics of carcinoid tumor kallikrein. Identification of lysyl-bradykinin as a peptide it produces *in vitro*. Clin. chim. Acta **12**, 292 (1965).

Métais, P., Schirardin, H., Warter, J.: Activité anti-trypsique du sérum humain. C. R. Soc. Biol. (Paris) **159**, 976 (1965).

— — — Mesures de la capacité d'un inhibition trypsique du sérum humain. Clin. chim. Acta **13**, 602 (1966).

Meyer, A.: Metabolische Veränderungen beim Endotoxinschock unter besonderer Berücksichtigung der Plasmakinine. Habil.-Schr. Med. Fakultät, Univ. München, 1964.

— Neue Gesichtspunkte zur Biochemie, Klinik und Therapie der Peritonitis. Langenbecks Arch. klin. Chir. **313**, 182 (1965).

— Werle, E.: Beeinflussung des Endotoxinschocks durch den Trypsin-Kallikrein-Inhibitor. In: Pathogenese, Diagnostik, Klinik und Therapie der Erkrankungen des exokrinen Pankreas, p. 299, ed. by N. Henning, K. Heinkel and H. Schön. Stuttgart 1964.

Miles, A. A.: Large molecular substances as mediator of the inflammatory reaction. Ann. N.Y. Acad. Sci. **116**, 855 (1964).

Mörl, F. K.: Die postoperative Pankreatitis. In: Neue Aspekte der Trasylol-Therapie, vol. 2, p. 81, ed. by R. Marx, H. Imdahl and G. Haberland. Stuttgart 1967a.

— Die Peritonitis. In: Neue Aspekte der Trasylol-Therapie, vol. 2, p. 139, ed. by R. Marx, H. Imdahl and G. Haberland. Stuttgart 1967b.

— Fettembolie und Proteinasenhemmer. Med. Welt **18**, 1997 (1967c).

Morgan, A., Robinson, L. A., White, T. T.: Postoperative changes in the trypsin inhibitor activities of human pancreatic juice and the influence of infusion of Trasylol on the inhibitor activity. Amer. J. Surg. **115**, 131 (1968).

Nabseth, D. C., Apostolou, K., Kais, B. P., Cheren, S., Hirsch, A.: Trasylol in acute experimental pancreatitis. Fed. Proc. **22**, 605 (1963).

Nagel, M.: Zur Beeinflussung der experimentellen Peritonitis durch Trasylol. Langenbecks Arch. klin. Chir. **313**, 897 (1965).

— Karl-Schuch, W., Rahmanzadeh, R.: Untersuchungen zur zusätzlichen Proteaseninhibitortherapie bei der septischen Peritonitis. In: Neue Aspekte der Trasylol-Therapie, vol. 2, p. 129, ed. by R. Marx, H. Imdahl and G. Haberland. Stuttgart 1967.

— Robel, K. P., Willig, F.: Über die Aktivierung proteolytischer Proenzyme des Pankreas Klin. Wschr. **43**, 173 (1965).

— Willig, F.: Proteolytische Enzyme im Pankreas unter normalen und pathologischen Bedingungen. Klin. Wschr. **42**, 400 (1964).

Negulescu, P., Harper, H. A., Crane, J. T., Goldman, L.: Trypsin inhibitor and proteolytic enzyme activity in dogs after ethionine-induced pancreatitis. Amer. J. Surg. **102**, 196 (1961).

Nemir, P., Jr., Hoferichter, J., Drabkin, D. L.: The protective effect of proteinase inhibitor in acute necrotizing pancreatitis. Ann. Surg. **158**, 655 (1963).

Nodine, J. H., Greberman, M.: Proteinase inhibitors in human pancreatitis. Digital computer analysis of clinical research data. Ann. N.Y. Acad. Sci. **146**, 564 (1968).

Nordström, S., Blombäck, B., Blombäck, M., Olsson, P., Zetterqvist, E.: Experimental investigations on the antithromboplastic and antifibrinolytic activity of Trasylol. Ann. N.Y. Acad. Sci. **146**, 701 (1968).

— Olsson, P., Blombäck, M.: On the antithromboplastic activity of Trasylol. In: Neue Aspekte der Trasylol-Therapie, p. 44, ed. by R. Gross and G. Kroneberg. Stuttgart 1966.

NOSKIN, E. A., POPPER, L., NECHELES, H.: Attempts to prevent pancreatic fat necrosis. I. Experiments with soybean antitrypsin. Rev. Gastroent. 19, 731 (1952).
NUGENT, F. W., ATENDIDO, W. A.: The role of antienzymes in the treatment of acute pancreatitis. Amer. J. Gastroent. 43, 437 (1965).
— — BULAN, M. B., MACDONALD, A. J.: Kininase activity in experimental pancreatitis. Nature (Lond.) 211, 207 (1966b).
— BULAN, M. B., AOKI, A.: Direct arterial infusion of antienzymes in experimental pancreatitis. Lahey Clin. Found. Bull. 15, 85 (1966a).
— HENDERSON, M. E., JONASSON, H., JONES, C. F., ATENDIDO, W. A.: The effect of a kallikrein-trypsin inactivator in experimental pancreatitis. Lahey Clin. Found. Bull. 13, 167 (1964).
OATES, J. A.: Discussion of J. A. OATES and K. L. MELMON: Biochemical and physiologic studies of the kinins in carcinoid syndrome. In: Hypotensive Peptides, p. 565, ed. by E. G. ERDÖS, N. BACK and F. SICUTERI. Berlin-Heidelberg-New York: Springer 1966.
— MELMON, K. L.: Biochemical and physiologic studies of the kinins in carcinoid syndrome. In: Hypotensive Peptides, p. 565, ed. by E. G. ERDÖS, N. BACK and F. SICUTERI. Berlin-Heidelberg-New York: Springer 1966.
— — SJOERDSMA, A., GILLESPIE, L., MASON, D. T.: Release of a kinin peptide in the carcinoid syndrome. Lancet 1964I, 514.
— PETTINGER, W. A., DOCTOR, R. B.: Evidence of the release of bradykinin in carcinoid syndrome. J. clin. Invest. 45, 173 (1966).
PEART, W. S., ANDREWS, T. M., ROBERTSON, J. J.: Carcinoid syndrome. Serotonin release induced with intravenous adrenalin or noradrenalin. Lancet 1961I, 577.
PFEIFER, G. W.: Proteinasen-Blockade bei abgestorbener Schwangerschaft "dead fetus syndrom". Dtsch. med. Wschr. 93, 479 (1968).
POPPER, H. L., NECHELES, N., RUSSELL, K. C.: Transition of pancreatic edema into pancreatic necrosis. Surg. Gynec. Obstet. 87, 79 (1948).
POYSER, R. H., WEST, G. B.: Changes in vascular permeability produced in rats by dextran, ovomucoid and yeast cell wall polysaccharides. Brit. J. Pharmacol. 25, 602 (1965).
RATNOFF, O. D., MILES, A. A.: The induction of permeability-increasing activity in human plasma by activated Hageman factor. Brit. J. exp. Path. 45, 328 (1964).
REIS, L. DOS: Proteinase inhibitor and treatment of acute pancreatitis. An experimental study. Amer. Surg. 33, 311 (1967).
RIBACOFF, S., HURWITZ, A., KHAFIF, R., SIEGMAN, F.: Study of the effect of trypsin inhibitor in acute hemorrhagic pancreatitis in dogs. Surg. Forum. 12, 370 (1961).
RICK, W., MATIS, P., MAYER, W., MÖRL, F. K., NAEGELI, T.: Zur Bedeutung von Proteinasen-Inhibitoren für die Thromboembolie-Prophylaxe. Med. Welt 18, 1835 (1967).
RICKLI, E. E.: Das fibrinolytische Fermentsystem. Chimia 20, 73 (1966).
ROCHA E SILVA, M., HOLZHACKER, E. L.: Liberation of bradykinin from plasma by treatment with peptone or by boiling with HCl. Arch. int. Pharmacodyn. 122, 168 (1959).
ROTHSCHILD, A. M., CASTANIA, A.: Endotoxin shock in dogs pretreated with cellulose sulphate, an agent causing partial plasma kininogen depletion. J. Pharm. Pharmacol. 20, 77 (1968).
RUSH, R. F., CLIFTON, E. E.: The role of trypsin in the pathogenesis of acute hemorrhagic pancreatitis and the effect of an antitryptic agent in treatment. Surgery 31, 349 (1952).
RYAN, J. W., MOFFAT, J. G., THOMPSON, A. G.: Role of bradykinin in the development of acute pancreatitis. Nature (Lond.) 204, 1212 (1964).
— — — Role of bradykinin system in acute hemorrhagic pancreatitis. Arch. Surg. 91, 14 (1965).
RYBÁK, M., PETAKOVA, M., MANSFELD, V., HLADOVEC, J.: Die Komplement-hemmende Wirkung einiger Antiproteasen. Experientia (Basel) 15, 380 (1958).
SARDESAI, V. M., THAL, A. P.: The proteolytic process in pancreatic disease. In: Hypotensive Peptides, p. 463, ed. by E. G. ERDÖS, N. BACK and F. SICUTERI. Berlin-Heidelberg-New York: Springer 1966.
SCHARNAGEL, K., GREEFF, K., LÜHR, R., STROBACH, H.: Freisetzung von Bradykinin beim toxischen, anaphylaktischen und anaphylaktoiden Schock. Naunyn-Schmiedebergs Arch. exp. Path. Pharmak. 250, 176 (1965).
SCHIEVELBEIN, H.: Carcinoid und Kallikrein-Kinin-System. Hoppe-Seylers Z. physiol. Chem. 349, 940 (1968).
SCHMIDT, H., CREUTZFELDT, W., HABERMANN, E.: Phospholipase A—ein möglicherweise entscheidender Faktor in der Pathogenese der akuten Pankreatitis. Klin. Wschr. 45, 163 (1967).
SCHMIDT-MATTHIESEN, H.: Fibrinolyse und Proteolyse in Geburtshilfe und Gynäkologie. Therap. Berichte 38, 115 (1966).

SCHMUTZLER, R.: Die Wirkung von Erdnüssen (*Arachis hypogaea*) und Erdnußextrakten auf die Gerinnungsfaktoren. Thrombos. Diathes. haemorrh. (Stuttg.) **5**, 566 (1961).
— Antifibrinolytika. In: Blutstillung. VIII. Hamburger Symposium über Blutgerinnung, p. 157, ed. by L. ZUKSCHWERDT and H. A. THIES. Stuttgart 1966.
— FÜRSTENBERG, H.: Fibrinolyse und Blutverlust durch Prostataoperationen und deren Beeinflussung durch Antifibrinolytika. Dtsch. med. Wschr. **91**, 297 (1966).
SCHÖN, H., HEINKEL, K., HENNING, N.: Über das Verhalten von Pankreasenzymen bei der experimentellen Pankreatitis der Ratte. Klin. Wschr. **41**, 612 (1963).
— HENNING, N.: Untersuchungen zur Pathogenese der sogenannten tryptischen Pankreatitis. Klin. Wschr. **41**, 201 (1963a).
— — *In-vitro*-Untersuchungen zur Pathogenese der sogenannten tryptischen Pankreatitis. Med. exp. (Basel) **8**, 83 (1963b).
— RÄSSLER, B., ALTER, J.: Untersuchungen über die Trypsin-Inhibitor-Kapazität des menschlichen Serums. Clin. chim. Acta **7**, 571 (1962).
SCHÖNBACH, G., SAILER, F. X., STAMM, D., KÜMMEL, G., MÖLLER, H. D.: Die Wirkung des Trasylol auf die Pankreassekretion. Klin. Wschr. **44**, 652 (1966).
SCHULTIS, K., RICK, W.: Zur Beeinflussung der Pankreasfunktion beim Menschen durch Proteinaseninhibitoren. Verh. dtsch. Ges. inn. Med. **70**, 824 (1964).
SCHUTT, A. J., SPRAGUE, R., BARTHOLOMEW, L. G., CAIN, J. C.: Enzyme inhibition in the treatment of acute experimental pancreatitis. J. Lab. clin. Med. **62**, 1013 (1963).
— WAKIM, K. G., BARTHOLOMEW, L. G., CAIN, J. C., BAGGENSTOSS, A. H.: Acute experimental pancreatitis. J. Amer. med. Ass. **191**, 905 (1965).
SIBOO, R., LAURELL, A. B.: Studies on purified C'1 esterase and hereditary angioneurotic oedema sera by combined electrophoresis and immune haemolysis. Acta pathol. microbiol. scand. **65**, 413 (1965).
SINGH, L. M., HOWARD, J. M.: Serum kallikreinogen levels in postoperative patients and in patients with pancreatitis. Surgery **59**, 837 (1966).
SKYRING, A., SINGER, A., TORNYA, P.: Treatment of acute pancreatitis with Trasylol. Report of a controlled therapeutic trial. Brit. med. J. **1965 II**, 627.
SMITH, R. B., ORAHOOD, R. C., WANGENSTEEN, S. L., BERAKHA, G. J., ZAMELIS, A.: Effect of a trypsin-inhibitor on experimentally induced pancreatitis in the dog. Surgery **54**, 922 (1963).
STARR, M. S., WEST, G. B.: Haemorrhagic, traumatic and tourniquet shock in the rat. J. Pharm. Pharmacol. **19**, 547 (1967).
STEICHELE, D. F.: Die Behandlung fibrinolytischer Blutungen in Geburtshilfe und Gynäkologie mit Trasylol. Symposium über neue Erkenntnisse auf dem Gebiet der Therapie mit dem Fermentinhibitor Trasylol, Saulgau, 1966. Ref. in Med. Welt **18**, 1938 (1966).
STÜTTGEN, G.: Biogene Amine, Kinine und Schock. Hoppe-Seylers Z. physiol. Chem. **349**, 933 (1968).
TAGNON, H., SOULIER, J. P.: The effect of intravenous injection of trypsin inhibitor on the coagulation of blood. Blood **3**, 1161 (1948).
THAL, A. P., KOBOLD, E. E., HOLLENBERG, M. J.: The release of vasoactive substances in acute pancreatitis. Amer. J. Surg. **105**, 708 (1963).
TICE, D. A., WORTH, M. H., Jr., CLAUSS, R. H., REED, G. H.: The inhibition of Trasylol of fibrinolytic activity associated with cardiovascular operations. Surgery **119**, 71 (1964).
TOUNTAS, C., KIRIAKOU, K., MARSELOS, A., CARAPISTOLIS, E.: Local intra-arterial infusion of antienzymes in the treatment of acute pancreatitis. Surgery **60**, 1235 (1966).
TRAUTSCHOLD, I.: Enzyme und Inhibitoren der Bildung und des Abbaues gefäßaktiver Polypeptide (Kinine). Habil.-Schr. Med. Fakultät, Univ. München 1965.
— FRITZ, H., WERLE, E.: Kininogenases, kininases, and their inhibitors. In: Hypotensive Peptides, p. 221, ed. by E. G. ERDÖS, N. BACK and F. SICUTERI. Berlin-Heidelberg-New York: Springer 1966a.
— RÜDEL, G.: Neuere Ergebnisse auf dem Gebiet der Plasmakinine. Klin. Wschr. **41**, 297 (1963).
— WERLE, E., HAENDLE, H., SEBENING, H.: Neuere experimentelle Ergebnisse über Proteinase-Inhibitoren. In: Pathogenese, Diagnostik, Klinik und Therapie der Erkrankungen des exokrinen Pankreas, p. 289, ed. by N. HENNING, K. HEINKEL and H. SCHÖN. Stuttgart 1964.
— — ZICKGRAF-RÜDEL, G.: Über den Kallikrein-Trypsin-Inhibitor. Arzneimittel-Forsch. **16**, 1507 (1966b).
— — — Trasylol. Biochem. Pharmacol. **16**, 59 (1967).
TSUKIYAMA, Y., AOYAMA, S., YOSHIOKA, S.: Effects of some drugs on pancreatitis. 47. Annual Meeting, Gastroenterol. Soc. Japan, Tokyo, 1961.
— FUKUDA, H., KUBOTA, Y., YOSHIMURA, H., YOSHIOKA, S., NAKAYAMA, M.: Effects of some drugs on pancreatitis. II. Studies on the effects of Trasylol on pancreatitis. 48. Annual Meeting, Gastroenterol. Soc. Japan, Tokyo, 1962.

Turner, M. D., Correll, W. W., Fain, W. R., Conn, J. H., Cockrell, J. V.: Enzyme levels in pancreatic tissue and body fluids during experimental pancreatitis. J. Surg. Res. **3**, 485 (1963).

Vairel, E. G., Thely, M.: Inhibiteur de trypsine de Kunitz. Inhibiteur de la fibrinolysine. Ann. Biol. clin. **18**, 363 (1960).

Verstraete, M., Vermylen, C., Vreker, R. A. de: The influence of peanut extracts on haemostasis. Proceedings VIII. Congr. Europ. Soc. Haematol., p. 358. Basel 1962.

Vogel, R., Trautschold, I., Werle, E.: Natürliche Proteinasen-Inhibitoren. Stuttgart 1966.

— — — Natural Proteinase Inhibitors. New York 1968.

Vorster, C.: Zur Verhütung intraabdomineller Verwachsungen mit einem Kallikrein-inhibitor. Helv. chir. Acta **33**, 308 (1966).

— Zum Entstehungsmechanismus der peritonealen Adhäsionen. Chirurg **38**, 122 (1967).

Wanke, M.: Experimentelle Pankreatitis. Stuttgart 1968.

— Grözinger, K. H., Nagel, W.: Möglichkeiten und Grenzen der Trasylol-Medikation bei akuter Pankreatitis aus morphologischer Sicht. Klin. Wschr. **45**, 681 (1967).

— Sebening, H.: Morphologische Befunde bei experimenteller akuter Pankreatitis mit und ohne Trasylol-Therapie. In: Neue Aspekte der Trasylol-Therapie, vol. 2, p. 39, ed. by R. Marx, H. Imdahl and G. Haberland. Stuttgart 1967.

Webster, M. E., Clark, W. R.: Significance of the callicrein-callidinogen-callidin system in shock. Amer. J. Physiol. **197**, 406 (1959).

Innerfield, I.: Interrelationship of human plasma kallikrein and plasmin in inflammation. Enzym. biol. clin. **5**, 129 (1965).

Werle, E.: Über einen Proteinasenhemmkörper aus Rinderleber. 2. Internat. Biochem. Kongr. Brüssels, 1956.

— Über Plasmakinine. 27. Tagg Dtsch. Pharmakol. Ges. Wien, 1962.

— Über Plasmakinine. Naunyn-Schmiedebergs Arch. exp. Path. Pharmak. **245**, 254 (1963).

— Kininogenspiegel im menschlichen Serum nach Verkehrsunfällen. In: Neue Aspekte der Trasylol-Therapie, p. 176, ed. by R. Gross and G. Kroneberg. Stuttgart 1966a.

— Kininogenspiegel und Blutdruck beim Schock. In: Neue Aspekte der Trasylol-Therapie, p. 177, ed. by R. Gross and G. Kroneberg. Stuttgart 1966b.

— Haendle, H., Schmal, E.: Ein Fall von Carcinoid bei einem Elefanten. Path. Vet. **5**, 81 (1968a).

— Marx, R., Trautschold, I., Reichenback-Klinke, K. E.: Vergleich der Proteinasen-Inhibitoren aus Lunge und Leber vom Rind mit besonderer Berücksichtigung ihres Einflusses auf Fibrinolyse und Blutgerinnung. Blut **14**, 206 (1967).

— Trautschold, I.: Bestimmung des Kallikrein-Inaktivators „Trasylol“ im Blut und in Organen und seine Verteilung nach Injektionen. Münch. med. Wschr. **103**, 773 (1961).

— — Physiology, pharmacology and pathology of exocrine pancreas enzymes with special reference to proteolytic enzymes. Anglo-Germ. med. Rev. **3**, 212 (1966).

— — Haendle, H., Fritz, H.: Physiologic, pharmacologic and clinical aspects of proteinase inhibitors. Ann. N.Y. Acad. Sci. **146**, 464 (1968b).

— — Schievelbein, H.: Carcinoid und Kallikrein-Kininsystem. Klin. Wschr. **44**, 656 (1966).

— Vogel, R.: Über die Freisetzung einer kallikrein-artigen Substanz aus Extrakten verschiedener Organe. Arch. int. Pharmacodyn. **131**, 257 (1961).

— — Kaliampetsos, G.: Über das Kallikrein der Darmwand und seine Beziehung zum Blutkallikreingehalt bei Störungen der Darmfunktion. II. Weltkongr. Gastroenterol. II, 778 (1963).

Wilding, P., Adham, N. F., Mehl, J. W., Haverback, B. J.: Alpha-2-macroglobulin concentrations in human serum. Nature (Lond.) **214**, 1226 (1967).

Willoughby, D. A., Spector, W. G.: The lymph node permeability factor. A possible mediator of the delayed hypersensitivity reaction. Ann. N.Y. Acad. Sci. **116**, 874 (1964).

Zacest, R., Mashford, M. L.: Blood bradykinin levels in the human. Aust. J. exp. Biol. med. Sci. **45**, 89 (1967).

Zeitlin, I.: Discussion of J. A. Oates and K. L. Melmon: Biochemical and physiologic studies of the kinins in carcinoid syndrome. In: Hypotensive Peptides, p. 565, ed. by E. G. Erdös, N. Back and F. Sicuteri. Berlin-Heidelberg-New York: Springer 1966.

— Smith, A. N.: 5-Hydroxyindoles and kinins in the carcinoid and dumping syndromes. Lancet **1966 II**, 986.

Zoepffel, H.: Vorstufen der akuten Pankreasnekrose. Klin. Wschr. **1**, 123 (1922a).

— Das akute Pankreasödem, eine Vorstufe der akuten Pankreasnekrose. Dtsch. Z. Chir. **175**, 301 (1922b).

Zweibaum, A., Josso, F.: Les antifibrinolytiques. Rev. Prat. (Paris) **13**, 135 (1963).

Zweifach, B. W., Nagler, A. L., Troll, W.: Some effects of proteolytic inhibitors on tissue injury and systemic anaphylaxis. J. exp. Med. **113**, 437 (1961).

Urinary Kinins and Colostrokinin*

ERVIN G. ERDÖS

With 1 Figure

A. Urinary Kinins

WERLE, after the discovery of kallidin, looked for sources of the peptide other than blood, but he could not detect the peptide in human urine (FREY et al., 1950; WERLE and BEREK, 1950). Somewhat later WERLE and ERDÖS (1953, 1954) studied the excretion of oxytocin in human urine. They extracted a material from urine that was a peptide, but in various tests it behaved differently from the posterior pituitary hormone. The agent, called substance Z, was adsorbed from pooled urine on zinc ferrocyanide and subsequently eluted with alkaline ethanol. After the removal of some of the impurities, substance Z was precipitated with sodium tetraphenylborate. Finally, the peptide was extracted with 96% methanol, dried in vacuum, and dissolved in water. Injection of substance Z intravenously lowered the blood pressure of various laboratory animals. Intraperitoneal injection of the preparation had an antidiuretic effect in the rat. *In vitro* the peptide contracted isolated smooth muscles. Some subtle differences such as stability in alkali or lack of action on the rat colon seemed to distinguish this material from kallidin. Both of these properties of substance Z now can be attributed to the presence of impurities in the crude preparations. The peptide was easily destroyed by blood plasma, hemolyzed erythrocytes, chymotrypsin, etc. The inactivation of the material in serum was blocked by cysteine (BUCHNER, 1955). Substanze Z was absent from rat urine.

Somewhat later GOMES (1955), working in GADDUM's laboratory, also found an active agent in human urine. His method of purification was based on using acidified *n*-butanol saturated with NaCl to extract the peptide. GOMES saw in parallel assays that the material was similar to bradykinin and kallidin. In a later communication GOMES (1957a) indicated, however, that the urinary peptide was different from bradykinin because the two peptides could be distinguished by countercurrent distribution after a limited number of transfers. An oxytocic substance extracted from rat urine (GOMES, 1957b) was not identical with substance Z. (The oxytocic activity of rat urine could be attributed to the presence of kallikrein because rat kallikrein is known to contract isolated rat uterus; BERALDO et al., 1966; ERDÖS et al., 1968.)

GOMES (1959) carried on his investigations with substance Z and disclosed the details of the studies in an extensive publication (see PRADO, p. 693). He offered various explanations for the antidiuretic effect of substance Z. In retrospect it can be stated that the effect may have been caused by the release of vasopressin owing to the pain-producing effect of the peptide.

* Some of the experiments described here were supported by Grant HE 08764 from the National Institutes of Health, United States Public Health Service.

WALASZEK (1957) purified the substance further on aluminum oxide and cellulose columns. The latter chromatography yielded two peaks of activities named Z_1 and Z_2. The separation of two components in the urinary peptide was confirmed by JENSEN (1958), but GADDUM and HORTON (1959) attributed the two peaks of activities to overloading of the cellulose chromatography column. They ascribed all the biological effects of their preparations to bradykinin and renamed the substance urinary kinin. Urinary kinin in their experiments was also relatively more active on rabbit blood pressure than on the guinea pig ileum. Taking the relative activities of synthetic bradykinin, kallidin, and Met-Lys-bradykinin (ERDÖS, 1966) on rabbit blood pressure into consideration, we may

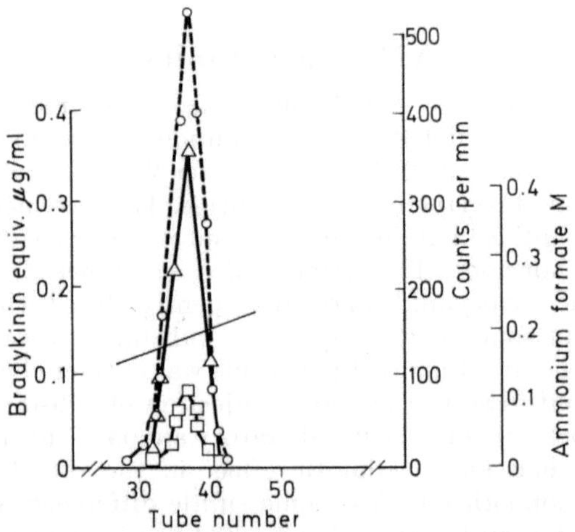

Fig. 1. Chromatography of a mixture of urinary kinin and (2,3-proline-^{14}C) bradykinin on a CM-Sephadex C-25 microcolumn: △, activity of peptides on isolated rat uterus expressed in bradykinin equiv.; □, estimated biological activity of added labeled bradykinin; ○, radioactivity (counts/min). Urinary kinin and added labeled bradykinin were eluted identically (MIWA et al., 1969)

assume that the discrepancy between hypotensive and musculotropic effects was caused by the presence of a longer kinin analog in the urinary kinin.

JENSEN, in a series of publications, described the results of his investigations of urinary kinins that were initiated in GADDUM'S laboratory. As GADDUM and HORTON (1959) did before, JENSEN applied ion exchange chromatography on an IRC-50 column for purification (JENSEN and SUND, 1959). Later he used zone electrophoresis for the same purpose (SUND and JENSEN, 1960). Significant losses were encountered when the purified material was freeze-dried. With paper chromatography a second active fraction was found in the kinin preparation (JENSEN and VENNERÖD, 1962a, b, c). The main activity was attributed to bradykinin, however. The fraction with bradykinin type activity was called Z_1, while a peptide that remained in the aqueous phase after butanol extraction was called Z_2. Z_2 was more active on the guinea pig ileum and rat blood pressure than bradykinin (JENSEN and VENNERÖD, 1962c). Additional studies with Z_2 with paper chromatography and various bioassays indicated that the peptide was identical with kallidin (JENSEN et al., 1963a, b); the previously reported high activity on the guinea pig ileum was attributed to the presence of impurities in Z_2 preparations.

ERDÖS, with the cooperation of A. G. RENFREW and E. M. SLOANE, also continued his studies on substance Z. Between 1959 and 1963 they purified the substance (ERDÖS, 1959—1963). Their procedure consisted of adsorbing the substance on zinc ferrocyanide, eluting it with alkaline ethanol, extracting the material with acidified butanol, and then applying chromatography on an aluminum oxide column. When the material was rechromatographed on a CM-cellulose column, two active peaks were found in bioassays with isolated smooth muscles. Identification of the peptides was attempted by means of peptide mapping. One peak consistently behaved similar to synthetic bradykinin. The other one was more elusive and could not be recovered after peptide mapping in all experiments, but accumulated evidence indicated that it was identical with kallidin. Pretreatment of rabbits with carboxypeptidase B abolished the hypotensive effect of i.v. injected substance Z (ERDÖS et al., 1963). The heterogeneity of substance Z was also noticed by DESHPANDE (1966).

Finally, MIWA et al. (1968, 1969) separated three components of substance Z. Their initial purification procedure was based on extraction of batches of fresh urine with Amberlite IRC-50 resin. The peptide components of substance Z were separated on a CM-Sephadex microcolumn (PIERCE, p. 47). Three peptide peaks were detected. Bioassay *in vitro* and *in vivo*, elution pattern during chromatography, isotope dilution (Fig. 1) with labeled bradykinin, and sensitivity to pancreatic carboxypeptidase B proved that the first peak was identical with bradykinin. The two additional peaks were considerably more active on the rabbit blood pressure and on the blood flow of autoperfused dog hind limb than was bradykinin. The elution pattern of the peptides in column chromatography was similar to that of added synthetic bradykinin, Met-Lys-bradykinin, and kallidin. Based on the results of the bioassays and chromatography experiments it was stated that substance Z consisted of a mixture of bradykinin, kallidin, and Met-Lys-bradykinin. Met-Lys-bradykinin was not found in urine samples that were stored frozen.

BERALDO (1952) studied a material from dog urine that contracted the ileum of the guinea pig and lowered the blood pressure of the cat. The substance was destroyed by chymotrypsin and by heating, but not by added serum. It was named substance U. Subsequent investigations showed that contrary to the previous findings, this material was destroyed by blood serum (BERALDO, 1955) and could withstand heating. Finally, the formation of substance U was attributed to the presence of kallikrein in dog urine (BERALDO et al., 1956).

The excretion of urinary kinin in human urine was measured in normal and pathological conditions. HORTON (1959, 1960) estimated that in terms of pure bradykinin approximately 10 to 30 μg was excreted in a day. With little variation approximately the same rate of excretion was maintained in some clinical subjects afflicted with various diseases and in additional groups of healthy individuals (YOSHINAGA et al., 1963; ABE et al., 1964; JENSEN et al., 1965a; ABE, 1965). JENSEN et al. (1965a) found that the total excretion of urinary kinins can vary from 17 to 56 μg per 24 hours. MIWA et al. (1969) estimated that one liter of fresh, pooled normal urine contains 10 to 36 μg bradykinin, 6 to 7 μg kallidin, and 13 to 25 μg Met-Lys-bradykinin under optimal conditions of extraction (see also TRAUTSCHOLD, p. 64). Patients with rheumatoid arthritis, however, excreted less kinins than normal healthy males. The difference was statistically significant (JENSEN et al., 1965b).

Urine of mice and rats infected with *Babesia rodhaini* contained a kinin-like material, and the excretion of this substance increased with the progress of infection (GOODWIN and RICHARDS, 1960). *Trypanosoma brucei* had the same effect in mice (RICHARDS, 1965), rats, and rabbits (BOREHAM, 1966). Urine of burned patients contained more kinin than normal urine (GOODWIN et al., 1963).

The origin of urinary kinins has not yet been definitely established. They probably do not originate from blood. Infusion of kallikrein did not increase the excretion of a kinin in man (YOSHINAGA et al., 1964; ABE, 1965). Infusion of bradykinin to man or into the renal artery of the dog (YOSHINAGA et al., 1964; ABE, 1965) did not raise the urinary kinin level. The range of excretion of the peptide in man did not exceed the normal 4 to 25 ng per minute despite the administration of exogenous bradykinin. YOSHINAGA et al. (1964) indicated that urinary kinin may originate from the renal tubular cells.

In contrast to these observations, BUMPUS et al. (1964) found a material which was probably identical with the active peptide in urine of rats after the infusion of labeled bradykinin.

A kinin was extracted from amniotic fluid, presumably originating from fetal urine (DELHAYE et al., 1967).

B. Colostrokinin

WERLE and PREISSER (1956) noticed that some bacterial proteinases release a substance from milk which stimulates smooth muscle preparations, a peptide named colostrokinin. Later GUTH (1959) found that calf saliva or sheep urinary kallikrein liberated colostrokinin from acid-heated bovine colostrum. The properties of the colostrokinin liberated by urinary kallikrein resembled bradykinin more than the colostrokinin released by saliva. As bovine colostrum becomes milk, the kallikrein substrate concentration diminishes. Human or bovine serum also releases colostrokinin from human or bovine colostrum. The kininogen concentration in cow colostrum increases until about the sixth day after calving and then decreases slowly (WERLE, 1960).

Submaxillary, urinary, and pancreatic kallikrein, and trypsin and chymotrypsin all liberated colostrokinin (WERLE and TRAUTSCHOLD, 1960), although a serum kallikrein preparation was inactive in these studies. Human, canine, bovine, and caprine colostrum contained the precursor of colostrokinin. In addition to contracting smooth muscle preparations, colostrokinin lowered the blood pressure of the dog. Colostrokinin was very similar to bradykinin in various tests (WERLE and TRAUTSCHOLD, 1960). In contrast, MORIYA et al. (1966) found that the ratios of *in vitro* and *in vivo* activities of colostrokinin and bradykinin were different in parallel assays.

Colostrokininogen was purified by means of column chromatography. The protein was very likely identical with plasma kininogen (WERLE, 1968).

Recently YAMAZAKI and MORIYA (1969a, b) studied bovine colostrokininogen and colostrokinin. They demonstrated that colostrokininogen was an immunolactoglobulin. Colostrokinin was purified five thousand fold. The actions of the peptide were qualitatively similar to bradykinin, but colostrokinin was relatively stronger in increasing capillary permeability. In contrast to bradykinin, the effect of colostrokinin was partially destroyed by trypsin. The calculated molecular weight of this kinin was 2,000 and the N- and C-terminal animo acids were different from those of bradykinin.

We do not know the physiological importance of colostrokinin. The peptide increases the absorption of ^{131}I-labeled albumin from the intestinal tract (MORIYA et al., 1966). Presumably it could increase the absorption of materials such as immunoglobulins from the infantile gastrointestinal tract (FREY et al., 1968).

Colostrum also contains a hypertensive substance (WERLE and SCHMAL, 1961), but this substance is a mixture of uridine diphosphate glucose and uridinediphosphate galactose (WERLE et al., 1967).

References

ABE, K.: Urinary excretion of kinin in man with special reference to its origin. Tohoku J. exp. Med. 87, 175 (1965).
— YOSHINAGA, K., MIWA, I., AIDA, M., MAEBASHI, M., WATANABE, N.: Excretion of urinary kinin in man. Tohoku J. exp. Med. 82, 270 (1964).
BERALDO, W. T.: Substance U—A depressor and smooth-muscle stimulating principle present in urine. Amer. J. Physiol. 171, 371 (1952).
— Substance U and related substances from urine. In: Polypeptides which stimulate plain muscle, p. 58, ed. by J. H. GADDUM. London: Livingstone 1955.
— ARAUJO, R. L., MARES-GUIA, M.: Oxytocic esterase in rat urine. Amer. J. Physiol. 211, 975 (1966).
— FELDBERG, W., HILTON, S. M.: Experiments on the factor in urine forming substance U. J. Physiol. (Lond.) 133, 558 (1956).
BOREHAM, P. F. L.: Pharmacologically active peptides produced in the tissues of the host during chronic trypanosome infections. Nature (Lond.) 212, 190 (1966).
BUCHNER, A.: Untersuchungen über die Inaktivierung von Kallidin und Substanz Z. Inaug.-Diss. Munich 1955.
BUMPUS, F. M., SMEBY, R. R., PAGE, I. H., KHAIRALLAH, P. A.: Distribution and metabolic fate of angiotensin II and various derivatives. Canad. med. Ass. J. 90, 190 (1964).
DELHAYE, C., REUSE, J. J., DRIESSCHE, R. V.: Studies on smooth muscle active substances in human amniotic fluid. In: International symposium on vaso-active polypeptides: bradykinin and related kinins, p. 113, ed. by M. ROCHA E SILVA and H. A. ROTHSCHILD, III. Internat. Pharmacol. Congress. Sao Paulo: SBFTE 1967.
DESHPANDE, Y. G.: Studies on biologically active peptides in human urine. Thesis, University of Oklahoma, 1966.
ERDÖS, E. G.: Hypotensive peptides: bradykinin, kallidin and eledoisin. Advanc. Pharmacol. 4, 1 (1966).
— RENFREW, A. G., SLOANE, E. M.: Quarterly fundamental research reports of Mellon Institute, Pittsburgh. Private communication (1959—63).
— — — WOHLER, J. R.: Enzymatic studies on bradykinin and similar peptides. Ann. N.Y. Acad. Sci. 104, 222 (1963).
— TAGUE, L. L., MIWA, I.: Kallikrein in granules of the submaxillary gland. Biochem. Pharmacol. 17, 667 (1968).
FREY, E. K., KRAUT, H., WERLE, E.: Kallikrein, Padutin. Stuttgart: Ferdinand Enke 1950.
— — — VOGEL, R., ZICKGRAF-RÜDEL, G., TRAUTSCHOLD, I.: Das Kallikrein-Kinin-System und seine Inhibitoren. Stuttgart: Ferdinand Enke 1968.
GADDUM, J. H., HORTON, E. W.: The extraction of human urinary kinin (substance Z) and its relation to the plasma kinins. Brit. J. Pharmacol. 14, 117 (1959).
GOMES, F. P.: A slow contracting substance in normal human urine. Brit. J. Pharmacol. 10, 200 (1955).
— Bradycinine et substance à contraction lente dans l'urine humaine normale. C. R. Soc. Biol. (Paris) 151, 812 (1957a).
— Sur l'activité ocytocique de l'urine de rat et de l'urine humaine. C. R. Soc. Biol. (Paris) 151, 1476 (1957b).
— Peptidos biologicamente activos. Arquiv. Patol. 31, 260 (1959).
GOODWIN, L. G., JONES, C. R., RICHARDS, W. H. G., KOHN, J.: Pharmacologically active substances in the urine of burned patients. Brit. J. exp. Path. 44, 551 (1963).
— RICHARDS, W. H. G.: Pharmacologically active peptides and urine of animals infected with *Babesia rodhaini* and other pathogenic organisms. Brit. J. Pharmacol. 15, 152 (1960).
GUTH, P. S.: Kinins produced from bovine colostrum by kallikrein and saliva. Brit. J. Pharmacol. 14, 549 (1959).
HORTON, E. W.: Human urinary kinin excretion. Brit. J. Pharmacol. 14, 125 (1959).
— Urinary kinin. In: Polypeptides which affect smooth muscles and blood vessels, p. 263, ed. by M. SCHACHTER. Oxford: Pergamon 1960.
JENSEN, K. B.: Slow contracting substances in human urine. Brit. J. Pharmacol. 13, 271 (1958).

JENSEN, K. B., RINVIK, S. F., DYRUD, O. K.: Excretion of urinary kinins in rheumatoid arthritis. Acta pharmacol. (Kbh.) **23**, 231 (1965b).
— — VENNERÖD, A. M.: Purification of a secondary kinin from human urine; A pharmacological and chromatographic comparison with kallidin. Acta pharmacol. (Kbh.) **20**, 329 (1963b).
— SUND, R. B.: Purification of slow-contracting substances in human urine by ion exchange technique. Acta pharmacol. (Kbh.) **15**, 279 (1959).
— VENNERÖD, A. M.: Purification of the main kinin of human urine. Acta pharmacol. (Kbh.) **19**, 265 (1962a).
— — A pharmacological and chromatographic comparison of the main kinin of human urine with bradykinin. Acta pharmacol. (Kbh.) **19**, 275 (1962b).
— — Pharmacological and chromatographic differentiation between a secondary kinin from human urine and bradykinin. Acta pharmacol. (Kbh.) **19**, 337 (1962c).
— — DYRUD, O. K.: Pharmacological properties of human urinary kinins. Acta pharmacol. (Kbh.) **20**, 322 (1963a).
— — RINVIK, S. F.: Excretion of human urinary kinins. Acta pharmacol. (Kbh.) **22**, 177 (1965a).
MIWA, I., ERDÖS, E. G., SEKI, T.: Presence of three peptides in urinary kinin (substance Z) preparations. Life Sci. **7**, 1339 (1968).
— — — Separation of peptide components of urinary kinin (substance Z). Proc. Soc. exp. Biol. (N.Y.) **131**, 768 (1969).
MORIYA, H., MORIWAKI, C., YAMAZAKI, K., AKIMOTO, S., FUKUSHIMA, H.: Human salivary kallikrein and liberation of colostrokinin. In: Hypotensive peptides, p. 161, ed. by E. G. ERDÖS, N. BACK and F. SICUTERI. Berlin-Heidelberg-New York: Springer 1966.
RICHARDS, W. H. G.: Pharmacologically active substances in the blood, tissues and urine of mice infected with *Trypanosoma brucei*. Brit. J. Pharmacol. **24**, 124 (1965).
SUND, R. B., JENSEN, K. B.: Observations on the influence of carbon dioxide on buffers at high pH values in connection with preliminary experiments on paper electrophoresis of human urinary kinin. Acta pharmacol. (Kbh.) **17**, 245 (1960).
WALASZEK, E. J.: Oxytocic polypeptides in human urine. Brit. J. Pharmacol. **12**, 223 (1957).
WERLE, E.: Kallikrein, kallidin and related substances. In: Polypeptides which affect smooth muscles and blood vessels, p. 199, ed. by M. SCHACHTER. Oxford: Pergamon 1960
— Über Wirkstoffe des Colostrums. Naunyn-Schmiedebergs Arch. Pharmak. exp. Path. **259**, 202, (1968).
— BEREK, U.: Über Kallidin. Biochem. Z. **320**, 136 (1950).
— ERDÖS, E. G.: Über eine neue biologisch aktive Substanz in Urin. XIXth International Physiological Congress, Montreal, Canada. Abstracts of Communications, p. 878, 1953.
— — Über eine neue blutdrucksenkende, darm- und uteruserregende Substanz im menschlichen Urin. Naunyn-Schmiedebergs Arch. Pharmak. exp. Path. **223**, 234 (1954).
— PREISSER, F.: Entstehung von zwei die glatte Muskulatur erregenden Substanzen in Milch. Naturwissenschaften **16**, 376 (1956).
— SCHMAL, A.: Nachweis einer blutdrucksteigernden Substanz in Colostrum. Naturwissenschaften **16**, 556 (1961).
— — ZACH, H. P.: Identifizierung des blutdrucksteigernden Prinzips des Colostrums als Nucleotid. Naunyn-Schmiedebergs Arch. Pharmak. exp. Path. **259**, 45 (1967).
— TRAUTSCHOLD, I.: Colostrokinin und seine Bildung durch Kallikreine. Z. Biol. **112**, 169 (1960).
YAMAZAKI, K., MORIYA, H.: Isolation and purification of colostrokinin from bovine colostrum. Biochem. Pharmacol. 18, 2303 (1969a).
— — Properties of colostrokinin from bovine colostrum. Biochem. Pharmacol. 18, 2313 (1969b).
YOSHINAGA, K., ABE, K., MIWA, I., AIDA, M., MAEBASHI, M., WADA, Y.: Assay of urinary kinin. Tohoku J. exp. Med. **81**, 246 (1963).
— — — FURUYAMA, T., SUZUKI, C.: Evidence for the renal origin of urinary kinin. Experientia (Basel) **20**, 396 (1964).

Chapter 8: Non-Mammalian Kinins

Discovery of Non-Mammalian Kinins

M. Schachter

With 3 Figures

Observations of the first non-mammalian kinin, viz., wasp kinin, were first made in 1951 as a result of a combination of interests of R. Jaques and myself at that time. I had become interested in the angioedema syndrome of erythema, pruritus, and edema, having shown for the first time, in collaboration with W. D. M. Paton, that this syndrome could be specifically produced in conscious

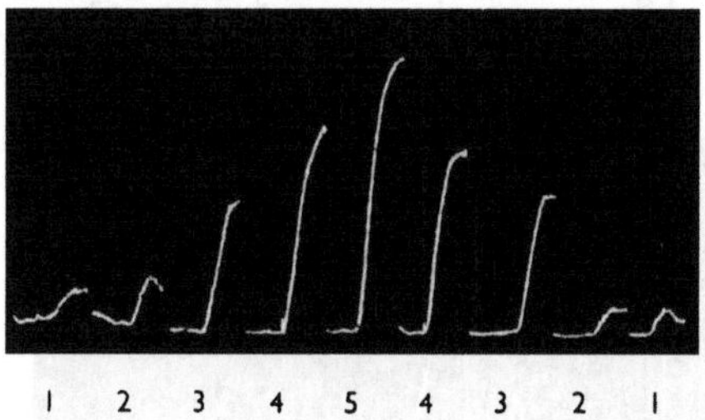

Fig. 1. Effect of graded doses of wasp venom on the isolated guinea pig ileum in an 18-ml bath in the presence of atropine (0.2 μg) and mepyramine (0.5 μg). Contraction time 50 seconds. Numbers 1 to 5 indicate contractions resulting from the addition to the bath of 0.25, 0.5, 1.25, 2.5, and 5.0 μg wasp venom respectively. (Jaques and Schachter, 1954b)

animals by the release of endogenous histamine (Paton and Schachter, 1951; Schachter and Talesnik, 1952). The similarity of this syndrome to so-called drug allergy or drug idiosyncrasy in man led me to investigate a number of such drugs for *primary* (as contrasted to the possibility of histamine release via antigen–antibody reactions) histamine-liberating properties (Schachter, 1952). Dr. Jaques, who had a long interest in animal venoms, and I, then combined our interests to look for the possible presence of potent histamine-releasing agents in certain venoms. We (Jaques and Schachter, 1954a) found that thalassin, a pruritogenic substance, first extracted from the stinging tentacles of certain coelenterates such as *Physalia* and *Actinia*, by Richet (Richet, 1902, 1905) was, in fact, an effective histamine-releasing substance.

Jaques and I then turned our attention to other venoms and proceeded to a detailed study of the common European wasp, *Vespa vulgaris*. Although we obtained evidence that the venom contained a substance with some histamine-releasing activity, it was not a prominent pharmacological property, and our attention was soon drawn to an analysis of the marked activity of the venom in causing contraction of smooth muscle *in vitro*. The venom contained huge concentrations of histamine, approximately 4.8 mg/g of dry venom apparatus. However, when the action of the histamine was antagonized completely by an antihistamine

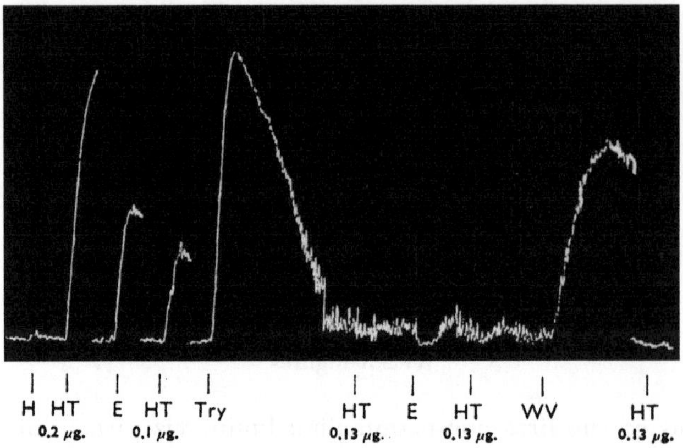

Fig. 2. Effect on guinea pig ileum of eluate from wasp venom paper chromatogram with R_f value and color reaction of 5-hydroxytryptamine. Atropine (0.2 μg) and mepyramine (0.5 μg) in bath throughout. The eluate is inactive after tryptamine densitization, whereas untreated wasp venom is still effective. Continuous tracing indicates that solutions were not washed out between tests. H, 0.2 μg histamine; HT, 5-hydroxytryptamine; E, 0.08 ml eluate; Try, 200 μg tryptamine; WV, 5.0 μg wasp venom. (JAQUES and SCHACHTER, 1954b)

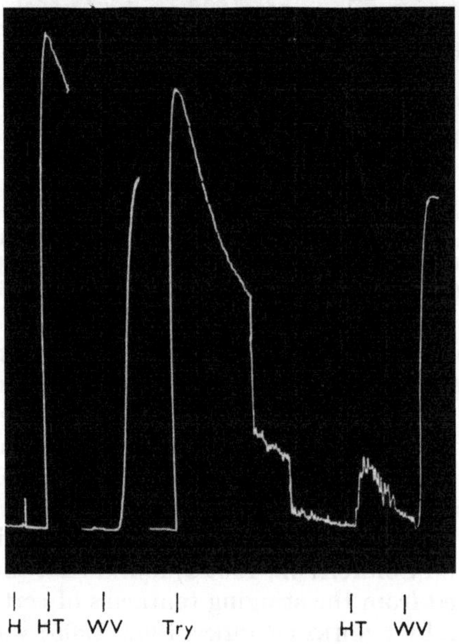

Fig. 3. Effect of wasp venom on the isolated guinea pig ileum after tryptamine desensitization. Atropine (0.2 μg) and mepyramine (0.5 μg) present in the bath throughout. Continuous tracing indicates that solutions were not washed out between tests. Contraction time, 50 seconds. H, 1.0 μg histamine; HT, 2.0 μg 5-hydroxytryptamine; WV, 5.0 μg wasp venom; Try, 200.0 μg tryptamine. (JAQUES and SCHACHTER, 1954b)

drug, the venom still contracted smooth muscle, even in low concentrations. Fig. 1, taken from our publication in 1954, shows the graded contractions of the isolated guinea pig ileum (in the presence of atropine and an antihistamine) obtained with graded doses of small amounts of dried venom sac (0.25–5.0 μg). Note the relatively slow contraction taking 50 seconds to reach completion.

At this time the extensive work of ERSPAMER and his colleagues on "enteramine", and of RAPPORT and his colleagues on "serotonin", had merged, with the resulting identification of both these substances as 5-hydroxytryptamine (ERSPAMER and ASERO, 1952; RAPPORT, 1949). We proceeded to test the possibility that this activity in venom might be due to 5-HT, using both chromatographic and pharmacological procedures. Paper chromatograms run in butanol: acetic acid: water (4:1:5) solvent revealed a distinct spot on development with EHRLICH's reagent (dimethylaminobenzaldehyde in hydrochloric acid) which corresponded exactly to 5-HT in its R_f value and color reaction. Furthermore, the eluate from this spot taken from a similar unsprayed strip of the chromatogram contracted the isolated guinea pig ileum, and this effect, like that of 5-HT, was abolished after the ileum was desensitized to 5-HT by maintained exposure to a large dose of tryptamine (Fig. 2). However, as shown in Figs. 2 and 3, small amounts of the crude venom still contracted the ileum even when the latter was not responsive to either histamine or to 5-HT. We concluded from these studies that wasp venom contained high concentrations, not only of histamine and of 5-HT, but also of a third compound which produced a slower contraction of the ileum than did either of these substances. The graded contractions of the ileum produced in Fig. 1 by venom, in the presence of atropine and an antihistamine, are, in fact, due to this third active compound. JAQUES and SCHACHTER (1954b) drew attention to the similarity of the latter compound to bradykinin (ROCHA E SILVA et al., 1949) and to kallidin (WERLE et al., 1937, 1950). Because these three substances appeared very similar, and anticipating the possibility that a short generic name might eventually be necessary, this substance in venom was named kinin (SCHACHTER and THAIN, 1954).

The above results were confirmed and extended in further studies by SCHACHTER and his colleagues (SCHACHTER and THAIN, 1954; HOLDSTOCK et al., 1957; MATHIAS and SCHACHTER, 1958). The authors found that wasp venom (*V. vulgaris*) contained not one but three similar, although distinct, kinins. Further, they suggested that all these substances—kallidin (kallikrein + α-2 globulin → kallidin), bradykinin (trypsin + α-2 globulin → bradykinin) and the wasp venom kinins—must be similar peptides chemically. BHOOLA et al. (1961) later found another kinin in hornet venom.

The excellent chemical work of ERSPAMER and of PISANO and their colleagues have brought interesting clarity into the classification of kinins. PISANO and his colleagues (PISANO, 1968) have recently identified the main kinin in wasp (genus *Polistes*) venom. ERSPAMER and his colleagues (ANASTASI et al., 1966; ERSPAMER and ANASTASI, 1966) have recently isolated bradykinin from the skin of the common European frog, *Rana temporaria*, and a new kinin, bradykinyl-isoleucyl-tyrosine, from the skin of a small Brazilian amphibian, *Phyllomedusa rohdei*. All of these kinins have a common nonapeptide sequence. The biological significance of this sequence, repeated so widely in nature, will no doubt eventually become clear to us, as will the physiological and pathological significance of kinins.

References

ANASTASI, A., BERTACCINI, G., ERSPAMER, V.: Pharmacological data on phyllokinin (bradykinyl-isoleucyl-tyrosine-O-sulphate) and bradykinyltyrosine. Brit. J. Pharmacol. **27**, 479 (1966).

BHOOLA, K. D., CALLE, J. D., SCHACHTER, M.: Identification of acetylcholine, 5-hydroxytryptamine, histamine, and a new kinin in hornet venom (*V. crabro*). J. Physiol. (Lond.) **159**, 167 (1961).

ERSPAMER, V., ANASTASI, A.: Polypeptides active on plain muscle in the amphibian skin. In: Hypotensive peptides, p. 63. Ed. by E. G. ERDÖS, N. BACK and F. SICUTERI, Berlin-Heidelberg-New York: Springer 1966.
— ASERO, B.: Identification of enteramine, the specific hormone of the enterochromaffin cell system, as 5-hydroxytryptamine. Nature (Lond.) **169**, 800 (1952).
HOLDSTOCK, D. J., MATHIAS, A. P., SCHACHTER, M.: A comparative study of kinin, kallidin and bradykinin. Brit. J. Pharmacol. **12**, 149 (1957).
JAQUES, R., SCHACHTER, M.: A sea anemone extract (thalassine) which liberates histamine and a slow contracting substance. Brit. J. Pharmacol. **9**, 49 (1954a).
— — The presence of histamine, 5-hydroxytryptamine and a potent slow contracting substance in wasp venom. Brit. J. Pharmacol. **9**, 53 (1954b).
MATHIAS, A. P., SCHACHTER, M.: The chromatographic behaviour of wasp venom kinin, kallidin and bradykinin. Brit. J. Pharmacol. **13**, 326 (1958).
PATON, W. D. M., SCHACHTER, M.: The influence of an antihistamine drug on the release of histamine in the unanaesthetized dog. Brit. J. Pharmacol. **6**, 509 (1951).
PISANO, J. J.: Vasoactive peptides in venoms. Fed. Proc. **27**, 58 (1968).
RAPPORT, M. M.: Serum vasoconstrictor (serotonin). V. The presence of creatinine in the complex. A proposed structure of the vasoconstrictor principle. J. biol. Chem. **180**, 961 (1949).
RICHET, C.: Du poison pruritogène et urticant contenu dans les tentacules d'Actinies. C. R. Soc. Biol. (Paris) **54**, 1438 (1902).
— Notizen über Thalassin; ein in den Fühlfäden der Seenesseln befindliches, Jucken hervorrufendes Gift. Pflügers Arch. ges. Physiol. **108**, 369 (1905).
ROCHA E SILVA, M., BERALDO, W. T., ROSENFELD, G.: Bradykinin, a hypotensive and smooth muscle stimulating factor released from plasma globulin by snake venoms and by trypsin. Amer. J. Physiol. **156**, 261 (1949).
SCHACHTER, M.: The release of histamine by pethidine, atropine, quinine, and other drugs. Brit. J. Pharmacol. **7**, 646 (1952).
— TALESNIK, J.: The release of histamine by egg white in nonsensitized animals. J. Physiol. (Lond.) **118**, 258 (1952).
— THAIN, E. M.: Chemical and pharmacological properties of the potent, slow contracting substance (kinin) in wasp venom. Brit. J. Pharmacol. **9**, 352 (1954).
WERLE, E., GÖTZE, W., KEPPLER, A.: Über die Wirkung des Kallikreins auf den isolierten Darm und über eine neue darmkontrahierende Substanz. Biochem. Z. **289**, 217 (1937).
— KEHL, R., KOEBKE, K.: Über Bradykinin, Kallidin und Hypertensin. Biochem. Z. **320**, 372 (1950).

Kinins of Non-Mammalian Origin

JOHN J. PISANO

With 2 Figures

Comparative biochemists have shown that living cells have remarkably similar chemical mechanisms. Superimposed on this foundation are qualitative and quantitative variations in the myriad of organisms. Properly exploited, these similarities and variations permit unique opportunities for understanding the mechanism and physiologic significance of biochemical systems. In reference to the kinins, it will be recalled that the early studies were often received with some skepticism. The classic work from WERLE's laboratory was little appreciated, and the significance of the experiments of ROCHA E SILVA and his colleagues on bradykinin was questioned since the kinin was produced by the unphysiological treatment of a plasma globulin fraction with snake venom or trypsin.

The significance of kinins was greatly enhanced with the finding that they occur in insect venoms, along with such biologically active substances as acetylcholine, histamine, and serotonin (JAQUES and SCHACHTER, 1954). At least one of the wasp kinins, the octadecapeptide Polistes kinin, contains bradykinin at the C-terminal end of the molecule. It is also relevant that free bradykinin has been isolated in high quantity from amphibian skin (ANASTASI et al., 1965). Thus it became less tenable to regard the kinins observed in man as mere artifacts. Several other new and extremely potent peptides have been isolated from non-mammalian organisms; their structures and principal pharmacological actions will also be discussed in this brief review.

A. Kinins in Insect Venoms

As part of the study of histamine-releasing substances in venoms, JAQUES and SCHACHTER (1954) demonstrated that extracts of the venom apparatus (gland, sac, and duct) of *Vespa vulgaris* contained a potent smooth muscle stimulant that was not histamine, acetylcholine, or serotonin. This substance, like bradykinin, produced a delayed slow contraction of the guinea pig ileum. It was believed to be a peptide since it dialyzed slowly, was not precipitated by protein precipitants, and was inactivated by proteolytic enzymes, hot acid, and alkali. SCHACHTER and THAIN (1954) chose to name the substance wasp kinin or simply kinin.

In a comparative study of wasp kinin, bradykinin, and kallidin, it was shown (HOLDSTOCK et al., 1957) that all three substances had similar pharmacological properties; however, it was noted that wasp kinin was partially inactivated by trypsin whereas the other kinins were unaffected. Chymotrypsin completely inactivates all the kinins. Chromatographic studies on columns of Amberlite XE-64 (MATHIAS and SCHACHTER, 1958) revealed the presence of not one but three kinins in extracts of the venom apparatus. The major kinin (about 90% of the recovered activity) was most basic, but all three kinins had the same relative activity on the guinea pig ileum and rat uterus.

Extracts of hornet venom apparatuses contained a single kinin which was not inactivated by trypsin and which also closely resembled bradykinin in all pharmacological tests except the guinea pig ileum where it appeared to be about one tenth as active (BHOOLA et al., 1961).

In more extensive chemical analysis of kinins obtained from mixed species of *Polistes annularis* Linnaeus, *P. fuscatus* Lepeletier, *P. exclamans* Viereck, the presence of three kinins was demonstrated (PRADO et al., 1966), as had been earlier observed with *Vespa vulgaris* (MATHIAS and SCHACHTER, 1958). The kinins were readily separable on columns of CM-cellulose or CM-Sephadex. Polistes kinins 1 and 2 were indistinguishable from bradykinin and kallidin, respectively on these columns, but this does not mean that they are identical. Unfortunately the extremely limited quantity of these minor components has prevented more extensive study. The total kinin activity found per wasp was equiactive to 1.5 μg bradykinin in the rat uterus assay. Yields were similar when venom was obtained by an electric shock technique (O'CONNOR et al., 1963), by glacial acetic extraction of the venom apparatus (HOLDSTOCK et al., 1957), and by homogenization in trichloroacetic acid (TCA) of the dissected terminal three segments of the abdomen, which contained the venom apparatus. Extraction of the abdomen was most convenient and adaptable to the processing of large numbers of wasps.

Table 1. *Pharmacological actions of synthetic polistes kinin relative to bradykinin*

Test	Relative potency, molar basis
Rat uterus	2
Rat duodenum	2
Guinea pig vascular permeability	5
Rat blood pressure	
intravenous injection	20
intra-arterial injection	0.5
Pain production on human forearm	10

Isolation of the major kinin, Polistes kinin 3, which accounted for about 90% of the activity, involved six basic steps. In a typical isolation the terminal three segments were dissected from 6,000 frozen (−10°) wasps and homogenized in TCA. After removal of the TCA by diethyl ether extraction, the solution was applied to a preparative CM-Sephadex column. Kinins eluted with ammonium formate were equiactive to 6.4 mg bradykinin. The preparation was then fractionated on a Sephadex G-10 column and finally on two successive analytical columns of CM-Sephadex developed by gradient elution with ammonium formate buffers (PISANO, 1966, 1967).

The structure of Polistes kinin 3 or simply Polistes kinin (Fig. 1) has been elucidated by enzymatic and chemical degradation (NAKAJIMA et al., in preparation). Relative to bradykinin, natural Polistes kinin was most active in lowering blood pressure with the following order of activity in various tests: rat blood pressure > guinea pig ileum > rat uterus > rat duodenum (PRADO et al., 1966; PISANO, 1966). In a more complete examination of the synthetic peptide (STEWART, 1968), it was shown that on a molar basis Polistes kinin was 2 to 20 times more active than bradykinin in various tests (Table 1). Most interesting was the action of the kinin on rat blood pressure where the route of injection determined the potency. Thus, administered intravenously, Polistes kinin was 20 times more active than bradykinin, but intra-arterially, the wasp kinin was only one half as active. The explanation for this result is that Polistes kinin is not so rapidly inactivated by the lung (STEWART, 1968) as bradykinin is. Other notable properties of the wasp kinin are pain production in man and increase of vascular permeability in the guinea pig.

It is of interest that kinins have not been found in the venom of bees, ants, and scorpions. Venom from the bee, *Apis mellifica*, contains the polypeptides melittin (a major constituent) and apamin. Melittin contains 26 amino acid residues and is a potent hemolytic agent, apparently because of its powerful action in

	Arg-Pro-Pro-Gly-Phe-Ser-Pro-Phe-Arg *Bradykinin*	
Lys-	Arg-Pro-Pro-Gly-Phe-Ser-Pro-Phe-Arg *Kallidin*	
Met-Lys-	Arg-Pro-Pro-Gly-Phe-Ser-Pro-Phe-Arg *Methionyllysylbradykinin*	
Pyr-Thr-Asn-Lys-Lys-Lys-Leu-Arg-Gly-	Arg-Pro-Pro-Gly-Phe-Ser-Pro-Phe-Arg *Polistes kinin*	
	Arg-Pro-Pro-Gly-Phe-Ser-Pro-Phe-Arg *Phyllokinin*	-Ile-Tyr (SO_3H on Tyr)
	Arg-Pro-Pro-Gly-Phe-Ser-Pro-Phe-Arg *Peptide III from Rana nigromaculata*	-Val-Ala-Pro-Ala-Ser
	Val-Pro-Pro-Gly-Phe-Thr-Pro-Phe-Arg *Val¹-Thr⁶-Bradykinin*	

Fig. 1. Structure of known kinins. Bradykinin, kallidin, and methionyllysyl-bradykinin have been isolated from mammals. Free bradykinin is also found in abundance in the skin of many amphibians. Polistes kinin is found in the venom of wasps of the genus Polistes, phyllokinin in the skin of the amphibians *Phyllomedusa rohdei*, and Val^1-Thr^6-bradykinin, Peptide III, and bradykinin in the skin of *Rana nigromaculata*. Glycylbradykinin, formed by the action of trypsin on Polistes kinin is similar to bradykinin in its pharmacological actions and potency

lowering the surface tension of aqueous solutions. Apamin, an 18-amino acid residue peptide, elicits a characteristically long-lasting excitation of the central nervous system of mice. The amino acid sequences of both peptides have been determined and are included in an extensive review of bee venom constituents (HABERMANN, 1968).

Venom from the scorpion, *Androctonus australis*, contains two potent "neurotoxic" polypeptides. Toxin I has a molecular weight of 6,822 and toxin II, 7,249. The LD_{50} in mice is 19 and 10 μg/kg, respectively. Similar neurotoxins have also been purified from snake venoms (ROCHAT et al., 1967).

B. Kinins in Amphibian Skin

ERSPAMER and his associates have shown that amphibian skin contains tremendous stores of biologically active peptides (ERSPAMER and ANASTASI, 1966). In work spanning some twenty years, numerous peptides have been noted and the structures of five have been determined and confirmed by synthesis. They include eledoisin, physalaemin, bradykinin, phyllokinin, and caerulein (Figs. 1, 2).

Eledoisin, physalaemin, and caerulein are not classified as kinins, but they warrant mention as they are extremely potent substances. Eledoisin and physalaemin are among the most powerful hypotensive substances known; in the dog the intravenous threshold hypotensive dose is approximately 0.001 μg/kg. Caerulein, while also hypotensive, has a remarkably potent action on gall bladder, gastric, and pancreatic secretions (Anastasi et al., 1968). The threshold i.v. dose for an effect on the *in situ* gall bladder of the guinea pig is 0.0002–0.0006 μg/kg. The many original papers dealing with these three peptides have been cited elsewhere (Pisano, 1968).

Bradykinin-like peptides are also present in amphibian skin (Erspamer, 1962). Of considerable interest was the finding that methanol extracts of the skin of *Rana temporaria* contain, in addition to serotonin, N-methyl-5-hydroxytryptamine and bufotenine, in huge amounts, i.e. as much as 250 μg free bradykinin per gram of skin (Anastasi et al., 1965). *Rana esculenta*, on the other hand, contains moderate amounts of the kinin and *R. latastei* and *R. dalmatine*, little,

Pyr-Ala-Asp-Pro-Asn-Lys-Phe-Tyr-Gly-Leu-Met-NH_2
Physalaemin

Pyr-Pro-Ser-Lys-Asp-Ala-Phe-Ile-Gly-Leu-Met-NH_2
Eledoisin

SO_3H (on Tyr)
Pyr-Gln-Asp-Tyr-Thr-Gly-Trp-Met-Asp-Phe-NH_2
Caerulein

Fig. 2. Structure of other extremely active peptides of non-mammalian origin. Physalaemin and caerulein were isolated from extracts of the skin of the amphibians *Physalaemus fuscumaculatus* and *Hyla caerulea* respectively. Eledoisin was isolated from the posterior salivary glands of the mollusks *Eledone moschata* and *E. aldrovandi*

if any. It is of interest that *R. temporaria* tadpoles contain little kinin but that the concentration rapidly increases after metamorphosis. Identification of bradykinin in *R. temporaria* was established by classical enzymatic and chemical degradative studies and by a variety of comparative pharmacological tests. Extracts of *R. pipiens* skin contain comparable amounts of bradykinin (T. Nakajima, T. Tanimura, and J. J. Pisano, unpublished).

Employing similar techniques Anastasi et al. (1966) have also identified the first naturally occurring peptide that contains bradykinin with additional amino acids at the C-terminal end. Phyllokinin, bradykininyl-isoleucyl-tyrosine-O-sulfate (Fig. 1), was isolated from the skin of the small South American amphibian *Phyllomedusa rohdei*.

The pharmacological actions of phyllokinin are notable in that the intact peptide, and not liberated bradykinin, appears to be active (Anastasi et al., 1966). In the dog, phyllokinin is three times more hypotensive than bradykinin. Removal of the O-sulfate lowers the activity to about one fifth of the original value. Phyllokinin also has the other pharmacological properties of bradykinin but it seems to be less potent, i.e. one third as active on rabbit blood pressure, guinea pig ileum, and rat uterus. On the rat duodenum it is only one tenth as active as bradykinin, but phyllokinin is equipotent in increasing vascular permeability of the human skin and in producing pain upon intradermal injection.

Extracts of the skin of *Rana nigromaculata* Hallowell yielded the first true naturally occurring analog of bradykinin, the nonapeptide Val^1-Thr^6-bradykinin (Nakajima, 1968a). The peptide is about one fifth as active as bradykinin on the rat uterus. The skin of this frog has a second bradykinin-containing peptide (peptide III) with additional amino acids at the C-terminal end. The structure of the peptide is bradykininyl-Val-Ala-Pro-Ala-Ser (NAKAJIMA, 1968b). Of the peptides in the skin of *R. nigromaculata*, bradykinin is most abundant. From 100 frog skins the following amounts of peptides were isolated: bradykinin, 1.1×10^{-4} mole; peptide III, 1.0×10^{-5} mole; and Val^1-Thr^6-bradykinin, 1.7×10^{-6} mole. The pharmacological actions of the peptides are being investigated.

C. Avian Kinins

Over thirty years ago WERLE and HÜRTER (1936) showed that birds (chickens, geese, pigeons, and ducks) contained a pancreatic kallikrein which was hypotensive in birds but not in mammals. The converse was also observed—i.e. bovine pancreatic kallikrein was not hypotensive in birds. Ornithokallikrein was inhibited by bovine pancreatic and plasma kallikrein inhibitors as well as an avian plasma inhibitor. It was not, on the other hand, affected by soybean trypsin inhibitor, which inhibits mammalian plasma kallikrein.

Table 2. *Amino acid composition of ornithokinin*

Amino acid	Residues	Amino acid	Residues
Arginine	8	Proline	4
Lysine	6	Serine	4
Histidine	2	Alanine	2
Glutamic acid	2	Glycine	2
Aspartic acid	2	Threonine	2
Isoleucine	4	Tyrosine	2
Leucine	4	Valine	2
Phenylalanine	4		

The kinin was purified about 5,000-fold from acid-treated chicken plasma by chromatography on columns of Amberlite XE-64, Sephadex G-25, and phosphocellulose (WERLE and LEYSATH, 1967).

The product of the action of pancreatic ornithokallikrein on avian plasma is ornithokinin. The polypeptide may also be generated spontaneously in plasma preincubated a short time at pH 2 and then held at pH 7.5 (WERLE et al., 1966; WERLE and LEYSATH, 1967). Addition of ornithokallikrein will cause a 20–50% increase in the total production of kinin. It is not certain whether the kinins produced at low pH and those released by ornithokallikrein are identical. However, they both have a molecular weight of 6,000 to 6,500. The amino acid composition of "spontaneously produced" kinin is given in Table 2 (WERLE and LEYSATH, 1967). Ornithokinin is hypotensive in birds but not in mammals. It also contracts the chicken ileum, a tissue insensitive to mammalian kinins (WERLE et al., 1966). More detailed pharmacological and chemical studies are awaited with interest.

D. Evolution of the Kinin System

Since bradykinin occurs in arthropods and amphibians, it would be surprising if it were not found in avians. Perhaps it is a constituent of ornithokinin. In any event ERDÖS et al. (1967) have studied the evolution of the kinin system and have demonstrated the various components in reptilian and avian blood. Turtle and alligator plasma, when placed in contact with a foreign surface, released a plasma kinin indistinguishable in pharmacological and chemical tests from the mammalian kinins. The equivalent of 1–2 μg bradykinin is liberated per ml plasma. The plasma of these two reptiles apparently contains a contact factor, a prekallikrein, a kininogen, and a kininase. Avian plasma lacks the contact factor, but the latter can be transferred from mammalian or reptilian plasma. For example, glass beads exposed to reptilian plasma initiated the genesis of kinins when added to fowl plasma. The released avian kinin contracted the rat uterus and guinea pig ileum and decreased the perfusion pressure in the hind limb of the dog. It was also inactivated by carboxypeptidase B. These results all suggest a similarity to bradykinin or kallidin.

Acidification of avian plasma also triggered the release of kinins. It is of interest that when assayed against bradykinin, the kinin released from duck plasma by acid was 10 times more active than bradykinin on the guinea pig ileum or dog hind limb perfusion than on the rat uterus. The similarity of the kinin formed after acid activation of duck plasma with that generated when avian plasma was treated with reptilian contact factor remains to be established. That it is different from ornithokinin is very likely since the latter is inactive in the above tests. Thus it would appear that birds have two kinin systems, one (lacking the contact factor) generating a kinin similar to the mammalian kinins, and the other generating ornithokinin which is inactive in mammals (ERDÖS et al., 1967). It is somewhat puzzling that kininogen and kallikrein have not been demonstrable in arthropod and amphibian tissues (PRADO and PISANO; ERDÖS, unpublished findings).

E. Conclusion

It is apparent that non-mammalian organisms can be extraordinarily rich sources of active peptides. Their variety and abundance in amphibian skin is intriguing but difficult to assess. It is interesting that the peptides are concentrated in cutaneous glands and probably intended for external secretion (ANASTASI, 1965). *Rana temporaria* tadpoles contain only traces of bradykinin; however, after metamorphosis the level rises sharply. Any attempt to attach significance to the occurrence of kinins in skin must account for the fact that they are totally lacking in many amphibians; in fact, even at the species level, some may have abundant kinins and other little or none.

The significance of kinins in wasp venom is easier to envisage. Social hymenoptera generally sting in self-defense or in defense of their nests—rarely to capture prey, as is the case with solitary species. Venom is a highly specialized fluid intended to harm the victim. Well-known substances already identified in venom from bees, wasps, and hornets, include, in addition to kinins: apamin, melittin, serotonin, acetylcholine, histamine, hyaluronidase, and phospholipases (HABERMANN, 1968). Certainly Polistes kinin, which is even more potent than bradykinin in its hypotensive action, in increasing vascular permeability, and in producing pain, is an admirably suited constituent of venom.

Knowledge of the distribution, structure, and pharmacological action of potent biologically active compounds not only contributes to a better understanding of the significance of known substances but may provide valuable clues for the existence of yet unidentified substances in man.

The similar pharmacological actions of eledoisin and substance P have been noted (ERSPAMER and ANASTASI, 1966). Caerulein, gastrin, and apparently cholecystokinin-pancreozymin, contain the same active C-terminal pentapeptide moiety. With the exception of a replacement of a threonine with a methionine, the terminal eight amino acid residues of the porcine pancreatic hormone are the same as those in caerulein (MUTT and JORPES, 1968). The discovery of Polistes kinin, phyllokinin, Val[1]-Thr[6]-bradykinin, and peptide III of *Rana nigromaculata* opens the question of the possible occurrence of similar kinin analogs in man.

References

ANASTASI, A., BERTACCINI, G., ERSPAMER, V.: Pharmacological data on phyllokinin (bradykinyl-isoleucyl-tyrosine-*O*-sulphate) and bradykinyl-isoleucyl-tyrosine. Brit. J. Pharmacol. **27**, 479 (1966b).

— ERSPAMER, V., BERTACCINI, G.: Occurrence of bradykinin in the skin of *Rana temporaria*. Comp. Biochem. Physiol. **14**, 43 (1965).

— — — CEI, J. M.: A bradykinin-like endecapeptide of the skin of *Phyllomedusa rohdei*. In: Hypotensive peptides, p. 76, ed. by E. G. ERDÖS, N. BACK and F. SICUTERI. Berlin-Heidelberg-New York: Springer 1966a.

— — ENDEAN, E.: Isolation and amino acid sequences of caerulein, the active decapeptide of the skin of *Hyla* caerulea. Arch. Biochem. **125**, 57 (1968).

BHOOLA, K. D., CALLE, J., SCHACHTER, M.: The identification of acetylcholine, 5-hydroxytryptamine and other substances in hornet venom (*Vespa crabro*). J. Physiol. (Lond.) **159**, 167 (1961).

ERDÖS, E. G., MIWA, I., GRAHAM, W. J.: Studies on the evolution of plasma kinins; reptilian and avian blood. Life Sci. **6**, 2433 (1967).

ERSPAMER, V.: Occurrence of bradykinin-like substances in the amphibian skin. Experientia (Basel) 18, 563 (1962).

— ANASTASI, A.: Polypeptides active on plain muscle in the amphibian skin. In: Hypotensive peptides, p. 63, ed. by E. G. ERDÖS, N. BACK and F. SICUTERI. Berlin-Heidelberg-New York: Springer 1966.

HABERMANN, E.: Biochemie, Pharmakologie und Toxikologie der Inhaltsstoffe von Hymenopterengiften. Ergeb. Physiol. **60**, 220 (1968).

HOLDSTOCK, D. J., MATHIAS, A. P., SCHACHTER, M.: A comparative study of kinin, kallidin and bradykinin. Brit. J. Pharmacol. **12**, 149 (1957).

JAQUES, R., SCHACHTER, M.: The presence of histamine, 5-hydroxytryptamine and a potent, slow-contracting substance in wasp venom. Brit. J. Pharmacol. **9**, 53 (1954).

MATHIAS, A. P., SCHACHTER, M.: The chromatographic behaviour of wasp venom kinin, kallidin and bradykinin. Brit. J. Pharmacol. **13**, 326 (1958).

MUTT, V., JORPES, J. E.: Structure of porcine cholecystokinin–pancreozymin. 1. Cleavage with thrombin and with trypsin. Eur. J. Biochem. **6**, 156 (1968).

NAKAJIMA, T.: Occurrence of a new active peptide on smooth muscle and bradykinin in the skin of *Rana nigromaculata* Hallowell. Chem. Pharm. Bull. (Tokyo) **16** (4), 769 (1968a).

— On the third active peptide on smooth muscle in the skin of *Rana nigromaculata* Hallowell. Chem. pharm. Bull. **16** (10), 2088 (1968b).

— TAMURA, Z., PISANO, J. J., UDENFRIEND, S.: Polistes kinin, a bradykinin homolog in wasp venom. In preparation.

O'CONNOR, R., ROSENBROOK, W., Jr., ERICKSON, R.: *Hymenoptera*. Pure venom from bees, wasps and hornets. Science **139**, 420 (1963).

PISANO, J. J.: Wasp kinin. Mem. Inst. Butantan Simp. Internac. **33** (2), 441 (1966).

— Studies on the structure of the major kinin in wasp venom. In: Vaso-Active Polypeptides: Bradykinin and related kinins, p. 35, ed. by M. ROCHA E SILVA and H. A. ROTHSCHILD. São Paulo 1967.

— Vasoactive peptides in venoms. Fed. Proc. **27**, 58 (1968).

PRADO, J. L., TAMURA, Z., FURANO, E., PISANO, J. J., UDENFRIEND, S.: Characterization of kinins in wasp venom. In: Hypotensive peptides, p. 93, ed. by E. G. ERDÖS, N. BACK and F. SICUTERI. Berlin-Heidelberg-New York: Springer 1966.

ROCHAT, C., ROCHAT, H., MIRANDA, F., LISSITZKY, S.: Purification and some properties of the neurotoxins of *Androctonus australis* Hector. Biochemistry **6**, 578 (1967).

SCHACHTER, M., THAIN, E. M.: Chemical and pharmacological properties of the potent, slow contracting substance (kinin) in wasp venom. Brit. J. Pharmacol. **9**, 352 (1954).

STEWART, J. M.: Synthesis and pharmacology of Polistes kinin, a bradykinin homolog. Fed. Proc. **27**, 534 (1968).

WERLE, E., HOCHSTRASSER, K., TRAUTSCHOLD, I.: Studies of bovine plasma kininogen, ornitho-kallikrein, and ornitho-kinin. In: Hypotensive peptides, p. 105, ed. by E. G. ERDÖS, N. BACK and F. SICUTERI. Berlin-Heidelberg-New York: Springer 1966.

— HÜRTER, J.: Über Ornitho-Kallikrein I. Biochem. Z. **285**, 175 (1936).

— LEYSATH, G.: Über das Molekulargewicht des Plasmakinins von Vögeln. Hoppe-Seylers Z. physiol. Chem. **348**, 352 (1967).

Summary of the Literature Published in Czechoslovakian, Polish and Russian Journals

V. Trčka

This summary considers relevant papers that were published in Czechoslovakian, Polish, and Russian national journals. In some cases, however, in order to help the reader, papers by authors cited here, but published in other languages, are also mentioned.

A. Synthesis of Bradykinin

A modification of bradykinin synthesis consisting of 24 steps was described by Siemion (1964a, b). Bradykinin was obtained by reacting the pentapeptide (carboxy-G-nitro-L-arginyl-L-prolyl-glycyl-L-phenylalanine) with *p*-nitrobenzyl ester of the tetrapeptide (L-seryl-L-prolyl-L-phenylalanyl-G-nitro-arginine) in presence of dicyclohexylcarbodiimide in tetrahydrofuran. The pentapeptide was prepared from the hydrazide of carboxybenzoxy-G-nitro-L-arginyl-L-proline and the free tripeptide which was prepared by a modification of peptide synthesis via *p*-nitrophenyl esters (Nowak and Siemion, 1963).

Bradykinin prepared in this way showed biological activity identical with that of synthetic bradykinin of different origin.

B. Kininogenases, Kininogen

In 1955 Paskhina isolated from a globulin fraction of rabbit serum a factor that increases capillary permeability. Recently, Zykova and Paskhina (1965) have shown that this permeability factor corresponds to kallikrein isolated from protein fraction of rabbit serum. The serum was precipitated by ammonium sulfate, and the product was chromatographically purified on DEAE-cellulose or a DEAE-Sephadex A-50 column. The kallikrein activity of this product was evaluated by assaying BAEe-esterase activity, the increase of capillary permeability in rabbit skin, and the contraction of isolated uterus, and by measuring the hypotensive effect in rat. The identity of the permeability factor with kallikrein was thus proved.

Several authors have shown that a kininogen is produced by heating acidified plasma of different animal species. Surovikina (1967) prepared a similar kininogen system by heating acidified globulin fraction of rabbit serum at 56°. From this activated fraction, bradykinin is generated between pH 7.0 and 8.0. The identity of the product with bradykinin was proved by paper chromatography and by several pharmacological methods. No bradykinin is produced at pH 6.0. This "spontaneous" formation of bradykinin is probably catalyzed by kallikrein.

A kininogen free of kallikrein and kininase (carboxypeptidase N) was prepared by PASKHINA and EGOROVA (1966) from Cohn fraction IV-1 of rabbit serum by purification on a DEAE-Sephadex A-50 column. Only heat-stable trypsin inhibitor was found as a by-product. The activity of the product was 140 times higher than that found in native serum. Bradykinin was released from this kininogen by trypsin as well as by kallikrein in corresponding amount. From heat-denaturated kininogen, however, no bradykinin was released by kallikrein although 75% was released by trypsin. The authors purified kininogen to a 500-fold greater activity than that in plasma. The specific activity of this kininogen estimated by reacting it with trypsin or rabbit kallikrein corresponded to 20 ± 2 μg bradykinin/1 mg protein. This kininogen is an α-1-glycoproteid containing 6.1% hexoses, 4.4% hexosamines, and 2.8% neuraminic acid. The isoelectric point lies between pH 3.15 and 3.50. The sedimentation coefficient was 3.3 S. In rabbit blood, trypsin or kallikrein releases bradykinin from only one protein. The kininogen is heat stable in acidic but unstable in neutral or alkaline media. The reaction with kallikrein is structurally more specific than that with trypsin and plasmin. The reaction of kininogen with trypsin or kallikrein corresponds to the initial phase of a first-order reaction (EGOROVA and PASKHINA, 1967). Cohn fraction IV-1 also contains an inhibitor of kininogenase activity of kallikrein. This factor does not inhibit the esterase activity of kallikrein but the proteolytic and esterolytic activity of trypsin and plasmin (PASKHINA and NARTIKOVA, 1966).

Two different kallikreins were found in human blood plasma by BULUK et al· (1968). First, contact kallikrein was formed in plasma when blood was withdrawn without stasis and kallikreinogen was activated by the Hageman factor at 0° or at 37°. Second, plasmin kallikrein was produced under the influence of plasmin when plasma was obtained from blood after 10-minute stasis. In plasma incubated at 0°, fibrinolytic activity was maintained, and the amount of active Hageman factor increased. Gradually disappearing contact kallikrein was continuously replaced by plasmin kallikrein. At 37° the fibrinolytic activity decreased, and no plasmin kallikrein was produced. The changes in the Hageman factor and contact kallikrein levels were parallel.

Pathologic conditions may change the kininogen of human plasma. ONISK and TCHORZEWSKI (1966) showed that activity of plasma obtained from patients suffering from DUHRING's disease is five- to tenfold that of normal plasma tested in the rat uterus. A significant increase of kinin-forming activity was found also in chronic urticaria and a decrease in lupus erythematodes and syphilis (ONISK and TCHORZEWSKI, 1968).

C. Kinins

I. Bradykinin Analogs

Contributions to the structure–activity relationship of synthetic kinins were made by SHCHUKINA et al. (1966) and SUROVIKINA (1967). They described the effects of 4-glycolyl-bradykinin·$4\,H_2O$, 6-glycolyl-bradykinin monoacetate·$3\,H_2O$, and 4,6-diglycolyl-bradykinin·$4.5\,H_2O$. All these analogs lower the blood pressure in rats, contract rat uterus, and enhance capillary permeability. The activity of these substances is much lower than that of bradykinin. 6-Glycolyl-bradykinin is less active than bradykinin by 1 order, 4-glycolyl-bradykinin by 3–5 orders, and 4,6-diglycolyl derivative by 4–6 orders. No data on biological activity of recently described 5-tyrosyl-bradykinin (NOWAK, 1964) are yet to hand.

II. Effects on Smooth Muscle

Bradykinin generally contracts smooth muscle. It produces in animals as well as man a short-lasting hypotension caused by vasodilatation, but isolated arteries react with contraction. A systematic study of the reaction of isolated vessels to bradykinin in comparison to other vasoactive substances was made by KOVALČÍK (1963). The minimal dose of synthetic bradykinin contracting the ovine coronary artery is 0.002 μg/ml. Much less reactive is the truncus pulmonalis of sheep (0.09 μg/ml), guinea pig (0.1 μg/ml), and rabbit (more than 1.0 μg/ml). High species differences were found in reactivity of isolated aorta. Guinea pig aorta reacts with contraction to 0.3 μg bradykinin/ml, but rabbit or sheep aorta does not respond to as much as 1.0 μg/ml. Similar species differences, however, were found also in reactions to eledoisin, norepinephrine, acetylcholine, and histamine. Also ductus arteriosus is contracted by bradykinin (KOVALČÍK, 1965; POPOVIČ et al., 1965).

Some bacterial toxins release substances that contract smooth muscle; bradykinin may be one of these factors. ČAPEK (1959) investigated the interaction of streptolysin O and B in toxicity studies in mice. Higher doses of bradykinin in combination with lower doses of streptolysin elevated the lethality. In prevalence of streptolysin O both substances interacted as antagonists.

III. Effects on Nervous System

According to ČAPEK, intraventricular administration of high doses of bradykinin to the cat produced muscular twitching, loss of righting reflex, and subsequent convulsions. These effects were accompanied by salivation, mydriasis, tachypnea, tachycardia, etc. In mice, signs of central stimulation were observed (ČAPEK, 1960, 1963). In rabbits and cats, bradykinin administered into the carotid artery caused drowsines, tachypnea, and EEG desynchronization. In "encéphale isolé" preparation of the cat, bradykinin brought about cortical desynchronization. Effective doses were 0.5 to 1.0 μg (ČAPEK et al., 1966).

IV. Cardiovascular Effects; Pain, Inflammation

A short report of RUSNÁKOVÁ et al. (1965) shows that bradykinin had no effect on the action of isolated rat and rabbit ventricles.

In an effort to elucidate the mechanisms of nociceptive effects of bradykinin, SONINA and KHAIUTIN (1966) injected it into the vessels of the small intestine and mesenterial nerves of cats anesthetized with urethane. Doses of 0.001 to 0.1 μg contracted the intestinal wall and elevated blood pressure. On the other hand, no pressor response was observed after injecting bradykinin in these doses into the arteries of mesenterial nerves. Only doses as high as 0.1 to 10.0 μg led to a reflex rise of blood pressure mediated by stimulation of afferent fibers. These doses correspond to those evoking nociceptive response in animals and pain in man. Hypertensive reaction was also observed in cats when potassium ions were injected into the arteries of mesenterial nerves. Bradykinin increases the sensitivity of afferent fibers to potassium ions, and the minimal effective dose of potassium is one third of the medium effective dose without bradykinin. The authors assume that sensitization to potassium ions brought about by bradykinin can be the cause of pain in acute inflammation and burns (SONINA and KHAIUTIN, 1967).

GAPONIUK and OIVIN (1967) have found that the effect of bradykinin on the permeability of vessels in guinea pig skin can be decreased by diphenhydramine (Benadryl). Ten milligrams of the drug per kilogram administered to guinea pigs and rabbits increase the median effective dose of bradykinin 700- to 5,650-fold.

The antibradykinin activity may be an important component of the effect of antihistaminic drugs. Bradykinin increases capillary permeability in experimental animals in much lower doses than histamine. According to GAPONIUK and OIVIN (1968) skin capillaries of rabbit are 131,000, of guinea pig 289,000 and of rat 520 times more sensitive to bradykinin than to histamine.

Bradykinin edema can be inhibited by a protease inhibitor isolated from potatoes (HORÁKOVÁ and MURATOVÁ, 1964) or by extended-chain analogs of vasopressin (N-glycyl-glycyl-glycyl-8-lysine vasopressin etc.; HLADOVEC and KASAFÍREK, 1966). An increase of activity of plasma kinins has been found in patients suffering from rheumatic fever in the active phase as well as in guinea pigs with experimental allergic inflammation (Arthus phenomenon) (TICHOMIROV, 1966).

D. Carboxypeptidase N

In Russian papers some attention was also paid to carboxypeptidase N. SHIMONAEVA (1967) studied the inactivation of carboxypeptidase N prepared from rabbit serum. Specificity of the preparation was proved by splitting bradykinin, hippuryl-L-lysine, hippuryl-L-arginine, etc. In contrast to the carboxypeptidase N of human origin, the rabbit product was not inhibited by ε-aminocaproic acid, although EDTA and 8-hydroxyquinoline inhibited it completely.

PASKHINA and TRAPEZNIKOVA (1967) studied the splitting of some bradykinin analogs by carboxypeptidase N. The activity of this enzyme isolated from human or rabbit serum by fractionation on a DEAE-Sephadex A-50 column and precipitation with ammonium sulfate increased native activity 60- to 80-fold. The rate of splitting of the terminal-arginine from 6-glycolyl-bradykinin was higher than that from bradykinin. A lower rate of splitting was found in 8-phenyllactyl-6-glycyl-bradykinin.

E. Reviews

It may be useful to supplement these summaries of original papers by several recent reviews of the world literature on kinins. The role of bradykinin in pathologic conditions is summarized in a paper of SHASTIN and KOROVNIKOV (1965); the effects of kinins on the smooth muscle of the vessel wall were described by POPOVIČ (1965). ALPERN and LIPSHITZ reviewed (1966) kinins as mediators of inflammation, and KRIKSHTONAITIS (1967) adressed himself to the clinical aspects of various vasoactive peptides.

References

ALPERN, D. E., LIPSHITZ, R. M.: Mediatory vospalenia. (Inflammation mediators.) Arkh. Pat. **28**, 3 (1966).

BULUK, K., CZOKALO, M., MALOFIEJEW, M., JANUSZKO, T.: Powstawanie kallikrein w osoczu krwi. (Generation of kallikreins in blood plasma.) Acta physiol. pol. **19**, 149 (1968).

ČAPEK, R.: Vzájemné ovlivnění toxicity bradykininu a streptolysinu. (Mutual toxic influence of bradykinin and streptolysin.) Čs. Fysiol. **8**, 446 (1959).

— Změny chování po intracerebrálním podání bradykininu. (Behavior after intracerebral administration of bradykinin.) Čs. Fysiol. **9**, 283 (1960).

— Some effects of bradykinin on the central nervous system. Proc. 1st Int. Pharmacol. Meeting **9**, 61 (1963).

— CORRADO, A. P., FERREIRA, S. H., ROCHA E SILVA, M.: The effect of bradykinin on the electroencephalogram. Act. nerv. super. **8**, 419 (1966).

EGOROVA, T. P., PASKHINA, T. S.: Ochistka kininogena (bradikininogena) iz plazmy krovi krolika i izuchenie iego svoistv. (Purification of kininogen [bradykininogen] from rabbit blood plasma and study of its properties.) Biokhimiya **32**, 354 (1967).

Gaponiuk, P. Ia., Oivin, V. I.: Antibradikininovoe deistvie dimedrola. (Antibradykinin effect of dimedrol.) Farmakol. i Toksikol. 30, 321 (1967).
— — Vlianie bradikinina i gistamina na pronicaemost kapiliarov. (Effect of bradykinin and histamine on capillary permeability.) Biul. eksp. Biol. Med. 65, No 5, 31—34 (1968).
Hladovec, J., Kasafírek, F.: Některé periferně cirkulační účinky analog vasopressinu s prodlouženým řetězcem. (Some effects of extended-chain analogs of vasopressin on peripheral circulation.) Čs. Fysiol. 15, 396 (1966).
Horáková, Z., Muratová, J.: Means of influencing the oedematous component of inflammation. Int. Symposium on Nonsteroidal Anti-inflammatory Drugs, 8–10 Sept. 1964, Milan, p. 237. Ed. by S. Garattini and M. N. D. Dukes. Int. Congr. Ser. no. 82. Excerpta med. Foundation (Amst.) 1965.
Kovalčík, V.: Effects of bradykinin and eledoisin on isolated vascular smooth muscle. Biochem. Pharmacol. Conference issue 1963, p. 181.
— K mechanizmu konstrikcie ductus arteriosus. (Concerning the mechanism of constriction of ductus arteriosus.) Folia Fac. Med. Univ. Comenianae 3, 23 (1965).
Krikshtonaitis, M. N.: Vazoaktivnye polipeptidy v klinicheskoi praktike. (Vasoactive polypeptides in clinical practice.) Ter. Arkh. 39, 12 (1967).
Nowak, K.: Synteza tyrozylo^5-bradykininy. (Synthesis of tyr^5-bradykinin.) Rocz. Chemii. 38, 129 (1964).
— Siemion, I. Z.: Synteza dwupeptydów z estrów *p*-nitrofenolowych n-karbobenzoksyaminokwasów i wolnych aminokwasów. (Synthesis of dipeptides from esters of p-nitrophenyl-n-carbobenzoxyaminoacids and free aminoacids.) Rocz. Chemii 37, 693 (1963).
Onisk, Z.: Preliminary studies on kinin-forming properties of blood in some skin diseases. Polish med. J. 54, 486—489 (1968).
— Tchorzewski, H.: Badania nad vlasciwosciami kininotworczymi krwi w chorobie Duhringa. (Studies in kinin-producing properties of blood in Duhring's disease.) Przegl. derm. 53, 11 (1966).
Paskhina, T. S., Egorova, T. P.: Ochistka i svoistva kininogena (bradikininogena) iz syvorotki krovi krolika. (Purification and properties of kininogen [bradykininogen] of rabbit blood serum.) Biokhimiya 31, 468 (1966).
— Nartikova, V. F.: Kislostabilnyi ingibitor tripsina, plazmina i kallikreina iz syvorotki krovi krolika. (Acid-resistant inhibitor of trypsin, plasmin, and kallikrein in rabbit serum.) Vop. med. Khim. 12, 325 (1966).
— Trapeznikova, S. S.: Rasshcheplenie depsipeptidnych analogov bradikinina kininazoi (karboksipeptidazoi N) iz syvorotki krovi cheloveka i krolika. (Cleavage of depsipeptide analogs of bradykinin by kininase [carboxypeptidase N] from human and rabbit serum.) Biokhimiya 32, 527 (1967).
Popovič, I.: Kininové hormóny a hladký sval cievnej steny. (Kinin hormones and smooth muscle of the vessel wall.) Lék. Věda v Zahraničí 9, 161, 167 (1965).
— Blažková, I., Kovalčík, V.: Účinok niektorých polypeptidov na hladký sval izolovaných veľkých ciev. (The effect of some polypeptides on smooth muscle of large vessels.) Čs. Fysiol. 14, 310 (1965).
Rusnáková, M., Rusnák, J., Kovalčík, V.: Vplyv niektorých syntetických polypeptidov na izolovanú predsieň. (Effect of some synthetic peptides on isolated atrium.) Čs. Fysiol. 14, 310 (1965).
Shastin, R. N., Korovnikov, K. A.: Bradikinin i ego patologicheskoe znachenie. (Bradykinin and its pathological significance.) Pat. Fiziol. eksp. Ter. 9, No. 1, 81 (1965).
Shchukina, L. A., Ravdel, G. A., Filatova, M. P.: Sintez depsipeptidnykh analogov bradikinina. (Synthesis of O-peptide bradykinin analogs.) Khim. prirodnych Soedinenii 2, 223 (1966).
Shimonaeva, E. E.: O nekotorych svoistvakh karboksipeptidazy N iz syvorotki krovi krolika. (Some properties of carboxypeptidase N from rabbit serum.) Vop. med. Khim. 13, 105 (1967).
Siemion, I. Z.: Nowa synteza bradykininy. (New synthesis of bradykinin.) Roczn. Chemii 38, 133 (1964a).
— Synteza bradykininy. (Bradykinin synthesis.) Roczn. Chemii 38, 811 (1964b).
Sonina, R. S., Khaiutin, V. M.: Khimiorecepcia i nociceptivnye effekty bradikinina. (Chemoreception and the nociceptive effects of bradykinin.) Fiziol. Zh. (Mosk.) 52, 547 (1966).
— — Povyshenie chuvstvitelnosti afferentnych volokon k razdrazhaiuschemu dejstviu ionov kalia, vyzyvaemoe bradikininom. Khimiorecepcia i veschestva, vyzyvaiushchie bol'. (Exaggeration of sensitivity of afferent fibers to irritative action of potassium ions induced by bradykinin. Chemoreception and pain-producing substances.) Fiziol. Zh. (Mosk.) 53, 291 (1967).

SUROVIKINA, M. S.: O mechanizme "spontannogo" obrazovania bradikinina globulinovoi frakciei syvorotki krovi krolika. (On the mechanism of "spontaneous" formation of bradykinin from globulin fraction of rabbit blood serum.) Vop. med. Khim. **13**, 59 (1967).
— EGOROVA, T. P., PASKHINA, T. S.: Biologicheskaia aktivnost depsipeptidnych analogov bradikinina. (Biological activity of O-peptide bradykinin analogs.) Farmakol. i Toksikol. **30**, 467 (1967).
TICHOMIROV, I. B.: Sosudistaia aktivnost kininov syvorotki krovi pri revmatizme i eksperimentalnom allergicheskom vospalenii. (Vascular activity of kinins in blood serum in rheumatic fever and experimental allergic inflammation.) Vopr. Revmat. **6**, No 3, 14 (1966).
TRAPEZNIKOVA, S. S., PASKHINA, T. S.: Vydelenie, ochistka i svoistva karboksipeptidazy (kininazy) iz syvorotki krovi cheloveka i krolika. (Isolation, purification and properties of human and rabbit serum carboxypeptidase [kininase].) Biokhimiya **33**, 1012–1022 (1968).
ZYKOVA, V. P., PASKHINA, T. S.: Obnaruzhenie kallikreina v gamma$_1$-globulinovoi frakcii belkov syvorotki krovi krolika. (Discovery of kallikrein in gamma$_1$-globulin fraction of rabbit serum.) Dokl. Akad. Nauk SSSR **165**, 1339 (1965).

Summary of Literature Published in French

JEAN LECOMTE

Original works written in French, which deal with the pharmacological action or the pathological role of the plasma kinins, are summarized below. I shall mention only review articles based on papers published in other languages: BERDE (1961), LECOMTE and TROQUET (1962a), STÜRMER (1963), ROCHA E SILVA (1963), TROQUET and LECOMTE (1964), and FOUSSARD-BLANPIN (1965).

A. Identification of Kinins and Their Precursors

The first research carried out in this field of physiopathological action was that of ABELOUS and BARDIER who, in 1909, discovered a hypotensive substance in human urine called urohypotensin which could be precipitated by alcohol and by saturation with ammonium sulfate. The material is very soluble in water, non-dialyzable, and destroyed by boiling. It might have been antigenic. This substance was also called urocongestin (ABELOUS and BARDIER, 1909a–e) because of its ability to provoke not only a state of shock in dogs and rabbits but also intense visceral congestion. These authors may have isolated one of the urinary kallikreins. Normal human urine also contains bradykinin, as GOMES (1957a) showed with the aid of various chemical and pharmacological tests. The presence of bradykinin accounts for the oxytocic activity of human urine and, in part, for that of rat urine (GOMES, 1957b).

The presence of a hypotensive factor analogous to kallikrein was demonstrated by UNGAR and PARROT (1936) in the saliva of dogs. This factor may be different, according to GUIMARAIS and TAWARES (1942), from that present in saliva inducing salivary secretion (DEMOOR, 1913). The hypotensive action of dog saliva was verified by DEL (1965) and that of the ewe by HOUVENAGHEL et al. (1968).

The bronchial mucosa of man contains a β_2-globulin with hypotensive and esterase properties similar to those of the kallikreins. It can be obtained either from sputum (HAVEZ et al., 1966a) or from the mucosa itself (HAVEZ et al., 1966b). Bradykinin may be identical with the vasodilatory substance (substance V) which contaminates certain angiotensin preparations even after purification (FASCIOLO et al., 1959). GLEY and KISTHINIOS (1928, 1929) isolated a hypotensive agent from insulin-free beef pancreas which is, however, not kallikrein (LECOMTE, 1962). Similarly, the hypotensive substance isolated from the carotid body by LEGER et al. (1947) is different from kallikrein.

The blood plasma of *Choloepus hoffmanni* contains some kininogens. The extract of the salivary glands of this sloth contains some kallikreins (LECOMTE, 1964).

Let us remember that the synthesis of polypeptides having properties of kallidin and bradykinin (BOISSONNAS et al., 1960a) as well as the synthesis of certain inactive analogs (BOISSONNAS et al., 1960b) were first published in French in the *Acta Helvetica Chemica*.

A biological method for kallikrein samples was developed by KRUMM-HELLER and SALESSE (1956), while a biological assay of plasma bradykininogen was described by LINÉE et al. (1966), based on the modification of the micromethod of DINIZ and CARVALHO (see Chapter 2 in this volume).

B. Pharmacological Actions of Kinin-Forming Agents and Enzymes

The intravenous administration of ellagic acid, which activates the kininogen–kinin system via the Hageman factor, causes systemic arterial hypotension in the rat. The results of LECOMTE (1967b) agree with those of JACOBSEN (1966) and GAUTVIK and RUGSTAD (1967). This hypotension disappears, owing to tachyphylaxis when substrate I is exhausted (JACOBSEN, 1966). *In vivo*, ellagic acid is less active in the rabbit than in the rat. On the other hand, pig kallikrein provokes stronger hypotensive effects in the rabbit than in the rat. In the latter species, cross-tachyphylaxis between pig kallikrein and ellagic acid exists, which indicates that both attack the same substrate *in vivo*. The administration of an aqueous extract of rat salivary glands provokes a fall in arterial pressure in the rat. It becomes subject to tachyphylaxis. This hypotension is not cross-tachyphylactic to the one that follows the administration of ellagic acid or kallikrein extracted from pig pancreas. It may be stated that homologous kallikrein attacks a substrate which is not identical with the one hydrolyzed by the exogenous kallikrein (LECOMTE and DAMAS, 1968).

C. Pharmacological Actions of the Kinins

I. The Cardiovascular System

Besides their hypotensive action, bradykinin and kallidin sometimes raise the arterial pressure in the rat and rabbit. This is increased by the potentiators of the hypertensive effects of the catecholamines and is abolished by adrenalectomy or by adrenergic blocking agents. This arterial hypertension is therefore of adrenal medullary origin (LECOMTE et al., 1961, 1964). Conversely, the treatment of a rabbit with an adrenolytic substance, as well as with ethanol, prolongs the duration of the arterial hypotension induced by the polypeptides (LECOMTE, 1967a).

CARLIER (1966) demonstrated that in dog circulation, synthetic bradykinin (1.2 to 2.8 μg/kg/min) provokes an increase in the pulmonary arterial pressure with major influence on the systolic pressure, whereas the diastolic pressure undergoes only a slight modification. The pulmonary vascular resistances are not altered. Synthetic bradykinin decreases aortic pressure, especially the diastolic component, without any modification of the left auricular pressure or the pulmonary arterial resistance. There is also an increase in cardiac output and frequency. Pretreatment with a pulmonary vasoconstrictor, such as 5-hydroxytryptamine or norepinephrine, increases the fall in pulmonary blood pressure induced by bradykinin. On the other hand, a perfusion of the isolated rabbit lung with bradykinin increases pulmonary resistance and causes massive edema (LECOMTE and TROQUET, 1960).

BARAC (1957) showed that intravenous injection of natural bradykinin provokes a drop in diuresis in the dog as well as arterial hypotension. On the other hand, bradykinin perfused into the renal artery increases the local blood flow.

II. Respiration

TROQUET (1964) demonstrated, in the rabbit anesthetized with pentobarbital, that the intravenous injection of bradykinin or kallidin always results in polypnea, whatever the quantity injected, which begins as a tachypnea with a reduced tidal volume. Apnea inconsistently precedes hyperventilation. This precocious respiratory inhibition is resistant to vagotomy. The latter abolishes both the very much reduced tidal volume polypnea as well as the increase of elastance which regularly accompanies it.

III. Vascular Permeability and Local Actions

The increase of the vascular permeability that bradykinin and kallidin provoke in the skin of the normal or adrenalectomized rat has been studied by LECLERCQ and LISIN (1963), LISIN et al. (1963), LISIN and LECLERCQ (1965), and by VAN CAUWENBERGE et al. (1964). A 0.2% solution of bradykinin applied directly to the rabbit mesenterium causes small perivenous hemorrhages. It does not increase adherence of thrombocytes and leukocytes to the venular epithelium or the formation of emboli (HUGUES and LECOMTE, 1960).

In the healthy man, bradykinin applied to the nasal mucosa provokes *in situ* a very discrete erythema due to a localized vasodilatation. Neither pruritus nor hypersecretion is provoked. Bradykinin has almost no effect at all on subjects suffering from pollen allergies. If the bradykinin comes into contact with the mucosa, a slight erythema is sometimes evoked (MELON and LECOMTE, 1962). Direct examination of the bronchial mucosa proves that application of a 0.01% solution of bradykinin causes a very minor local erythema. No subjective reactions have been recorded. Although application of bradykinin in aerosol (0.01%) does not increase the resistance to the airflow output in the normal individual, this is very much enhanced in asthmatic subjects (LECOMTE et al., 1962; GIRARD and MORET, 1963).

IV. Action on the Ileum

Synthetic bradykinin brings about a complex reaction in the terminal part of the ileum of *Choloepus hoffmanni*. Weak concentrations (1 to 4×10^{-8}) cause a fall in the tonus after a latency of 10 to 20 seconds. It reaches its maximum in 1 to 2 minutes and then disappears slowly. The higher the basic tonus, the more apparent is the inhibition at the moment of administration.

Higher doses (at concentration 3 to 5×10^{-8}) of bradykinin provoke an inhibition of the ileac tonus followed by a slow and regular contraction. The latter starts after a latency of 60 to 90 seconds, the time necessary for complete development of the inhibitory phase. At even higher doses (1×10^{-7} to 5×10^{-7}) the inhibitory phase disappears, giving way to a contraction that begins after a latency of 20 to 30 seconds. There is no tachyphylaxis. The same process takes place when small quantities of bradykinin (1×10^{-8}) are added to the bath successively and without interposed washings. The first addition causes inhibition, the second causes an inhibition followed by a weak contraction, the third causes an inhibition followed by a strong contraction (LECOMTE, 1963).

V. Action on Milk Ejection

The intravenous injection of synthetic bradykinin (1–30 μg) provokes the ejection of milk in the ewe and the goat. Simultaneously, as the intramammary pressure increases, bradykinin contracts the myoepithelium of the mammary ducts. This action is strengthened by BAL and is of the same order of magnitude as that of oxytocin. Kallidin, methionyl-lysyl-bradykinin, and kallikrein from pig pancreas, as well as ewe saliva, all possess an identical influence on milk ejection in the ewe. All these agents also provoke a fall in arterial pressure (HOUVENAGHEL et al., 1967, 1968).

D. Catabolism and Antagonists

Treatment of a normal subject or of a patient suffering from an arterial embolism with plasmin activators decreases the amount of kininogen in the circulating plasma. The latter is probably transformed into kinins. This could explain the vasodilatation accompanying fibrinolysis (SALMON and LECOMTE, 1963).

In the rabbit, pulmonary resistance and arterial hypotension due to bradykinin (synthetic or natural) and that provoked by kallidin, are blocked by large doses of phenylbutazone (100 mg/kg; LECOMTE, 1959; LECOMTE and TROQUET, 1960). The non-narcotic analgesics—in particular phenylbutazone, aminopyrine and acetylsalicylic acid—accelerate the recovery of the arterial pressure lowered by bradykinin and consequently diminish the duration of the arterial hypotension. This property is not shared with cyproheptadine, hydrocortisone, dexamethasone, or morphine (VERGAFTIG, 1966).

In the rat, arterial hypotension due to these same polypeptides is selectively suppressed by sodium salicylate (LECOMTE and TROQUET, 1962b). Peripheral edema provoked in the rat by synthetic bradykinin or kallidin is reduced by corticosterone to a lesser degree than by ACTH, DOCA, aldosterone, sodium salicylate, or the derivatives of aminopyrine; cortisone is inactive (LISIN and LECLERCQ, 1963).

Large doses of Trasylol protect the rabbit against the Sanarelli-Shwartzmann phenomenon and prolong the survival of cutaneous heterografts in rats (BERTELLI et al., 1963). This protection is attributed to antiprotease activity of Trasylol. The peptide is particularly active against trypsin, chymotrypsin, kallikrein, and collagenase. However, in general, the action of Trasylol is inferior to that of ε-aminocaproic acid and its analog synthesized to obtain anti-inflammatory effects (BERTELLI, 1967). Similarly, Trasylol in the rabbit blocks the increase of vascular permeability associated with the subcutaneous administration of trypsin. This action is reinforced by promethazine (BERNARD et al., 1962).

E. Physiological Role of the Kininogen-Kinin System

UNGAR and PARROT demonstrated in 1936 that the stimulation of the lingual nerve of the dog liberates kallikrein. They identified this substance by chemical and biological tests and advanced the hypothesis that kallikrein is the mediator of the localized vasodilatation that accompanies stimulation of this nerve. This research agrees with the later investigations of LEWIS and HILTON (see Chapter 6 A).

F. Physiopathological Role

The hypotension in the dog which characterizes experimental acute hemorrhagic pancreatitis is not accompanied by a lowering of kininogen level. It does not seem to lead to the formation of bradykinin (HUREAU et al., 1968).

Anaphylactic shock is neither accompanied by a significant drop in plasma kininogens nor by an increase in the amount of free bradykinin. Thus, these agents play only a very limited pathogenic role (CIRSTEA et al., 1966). Anaphylactic shock in the rat is accompanied by an almost total disappearance of the circulating kininogens; after the development of the acute phase, neither kallikrein (40 FU/100 gm) nor ellagic acid injected intravenously, causes a fall in arterial pressure. As the preliminary depletion of kininogens does not attenuate anaphylactic shock, we must admit that the role plasma kinins play in this condition is secondary (LECOMTE and SALMON, 1968). Likewise, the intravenous administration of dextran causes a depletion of kininogens but less than that which accompanies shock. The consumption of these kininogens and the formation of the kinins, once again, play only a secondary role: the mere neutralization of the pharmacological effects of histamine and of 5-hydroxytryptamine is enough to eliminate edemas and the fall in arterial pressure induced by dextran (LECOMTE and DAMAS, 1968).

Fibrinolysis started by the heterologous plasma streptokinase combination is not the fundamental cause of an arterial hypotension. The physiopathological role of the endogenous kinins, therefore, is probably very reduced (SALMON and LECOMTE, 1965). Dextran sulfate *in vivo* brings about a disappearance of kininogens with the subsequent formation of kinins which are responsible for the fall in arterial pressure.

Anaphylactic shock in the rabbit lowered the plasma kininogen level (LECOMTE, 1961; SALMON et al., 1964). However pretreatment of the sensitized animal with kallikrein, diluted human saliva, or kinin-forming agents to exhaust the plasma kininogens, does not reduce the intensity of the anaphylactic shock (TROQUET and LECOMTE, 1963). Ellagic acid has no antianaphylactic activity (LECOMTE, in press). CIRSTEA et al. (1966) confirmed that the formation of circulating kinins during anaphylactic shock in the rabbit very probably plays an important role in its pathogenesis. Complement activity may be implicated in the formation of these kinins (SALMON et al., 1964).

In the sensitized man, the eventual local formation of kinins in allergic inflammatory centers does not play an essential role; neither the cutaneous manifestations nor the nasal and bronchial mucosa involvement of anaphylactic origin can be compared with the corresponding symptoms caused by bradykinin. Does this apply to anaphylactic shock? The activation of fibrinolysis provoked in man as a therapeutic measure is definitely not the cause of cardiovascular collapse, even when the state of afibrinogenemia has been reached (SALMON and LECOMTE, 1963).

The blister fluid obtained from man suffering from intense burns contains a substance that contracts the guinea pig ileum and the rat uterus and inhibits the rat duodenum. This substance may be bradykinin. Maximal contraction is reached between 40 and 110 hours after the burns have been sustained (SAINT-BLANCHARD et al., 1966).

The role of proteolytic enzymes and esterases liberated during acute or chronic pancreatic attacks is discussed in numerous clinical publications. It is impossible to cite them here *in extenso*. Along with the French clinicians, one may describe a pancreatic enzymopathy whose initial acute phase is defined as enzymatic shock: the latter is sensitive to the action of such protease inhibitors as CY66 or Iniprol, Trasylol Bayer, or Zymophren, sometimes called 9421 RP. These inhibitors are successfully used in the treatment of edematous pancreatitis and in the initial stages of acute pancreatitis. They have no effect in acute hemorrhagic necrotic pancreatitis or in established pancreatic necrosis. It is therefore necessary to initiate an intense and prolonged treatment at an early stage. The most evident manifestations after treatment with inhibitors are lessening of pain, reduction or disappearance of cardiovascular shock, and, in short, amelioration of all the symptoms associated with initial pancreatic toxemia.

These are the main conclusions derived from the analysis of numerous clinical works which it would be impossible to cite in great detail.

References

ABELOUS, J. E., BARDIER, E.: Les substances hypotensives de l'urine humaine normale. C. R. Soc. Biol. (Paris) **66**, 511 (1909a).

— — Action de l'urohypotensine sur la pression artérielle. C. R. Soc. Biol. (Paris) **67**, 88 (1909b).

— — L'anaphylaxie pour l'urohypotensine. C. R. Soc. Biol. (Paris) **67**, 264 (1909c).

— — Effets physiologiques généraux de l'urohypotensine (Uro-congestine). C. R. Soc. Biol. (Paris), **67**, 784 (1909d).

— — De l'action hypotensive et myotique de l'urine humaine normale. C. R. Soc. Biol. (Paris) **67**, 876 (1909e).

BARAC, G.: Effet rénal de la bradykinine chez le chien. C. R. Soc. Biol. (Paris) **151**, 1771 (1957).

BERDE, B.: De quelques peptides endogènes biologiquement actifs. Coimbra méd. 8, 917 (1961).

BERNARD, A., LAMELIN, P., DELATTRE, A.: Facteurs anti-diffusants dans le traitement de la pancréatite aiguë. Presse méd. **70**, 2698 (1962).

BERTELLI, A,: Médicaments antipeptidasiques et activité antiinflammatoire. Path. et Biol. Sem. Hôp. **15**, 163 (1967).

— FRANCESCONI, G., LAMI, V., PERELLI-ERCOLINI, M., PROTO, M., ROSSANO, M. A.: Protezione di omminnesti cutanei e blocco della reazione di Sanarelli-Schwartzmann ad opera di un polipeptide inhibitore della proteolisi: il «Trasylol». Atti Accad. med. lombarda **18**, 216 (1963).

BOISSONNAS, R. A., GUTTMANN, S., JAQUENOUD, P. A.: Synthèse de la L-arginyl-L-propyl-L-propyl-glycyl-L-phénylalanyl-L-séryl-L-propyl-L-phénylalanyl-L-arginine, un nonapeptide présentant les propriétés de la bradykinine. Helv. chim. Acta **43**, 1349 (1960a).

— — — Synthèse de la L-arginyl-L-propyl-L-propyl-glycyl-L-phénylalanyl-L-séryl-L-phénylalanyl-L-arginine. Distinction entre cet octapeptide et la bradykinine. Helv. chim. Acta **43**, 1483 (1960b).

CARLIER, J.: Contribution à la pharmacodynamie de la circulation pulmonaire. Acta cardiol. (Brux.), Suppl. **12**, 1-183 (1966).

CAUWENBERGE, H. VAN, LISIN, N., LECLERCQ, R.: L'action phlogistique de la kallidine et son inhibition. Sem. thér. **40**, 190 (1964).

CIRSTEA, M., SUHACIU, G., BUTCULESCU, I.: Evalutation du rôle de la bradykinine dans le choc anaphylactique. Arch. int. Pharmacodyn. **18**, 159 (1966).

DEL, ABDUL HABIB: L'action hypotensive de la salive chez le chien. Bull. Soc. Lorraine Sci. **5** (4) (1965).

DEMOOR, J.: Le mécanisme intime de la sécrétion salivaire. Arch. int. Physiol. **13**, 187 (1913).

FASCIOLO, J. C., HALVORSEN, K., ZANGHERI, E., FERNANDEZ, F. O.: Comparaison entre la bradykinine et la substance V. C. R. Soc. Biol. (Paris) **153**, 500 (1959).

FOUSSARD-BLANPIN, O.: Sur quelques peptides biologiquement actifs du groupe des kinines. Prod. Pharm. **20**, 505 (1965).

GAUTVIK, K., RUGSTAD, H.: Kinin formation and kininogen depletion in rats after intravenous injection of ellagic acid. Brit. J. Pharmacol. **31**, 390 (1967).

GIRARD, J. P., MORET, J.: Action de la sérotonine et de la bradykinine en aérosols chez les asthmatiques. Helv. med. Acta **415**, 520 (1963).

GLEY, P., KISTHINIOS, N.: Sur l'action hypertensive des extraits pancréatiques. C. R. Soc. Biol. (Paris) **99**, 1840 (1928).

— — Sur l'existence dans les extraits pancréatiques d'une substance hypotensive distincte de l'insuline. C. R. Soc. Biol. (Paris) **100**, 97 (1929).

GOMES, F. P.: Bradykinine et substance à contraction lente dans l'urine humaine normale. C. R. Soc. Biol. (Paris) **51**, 812 (1957a).

— Sur l'activité ocytocique de l'urine du rat et de l'urine humaine. C. R. Soc. Biol. (Paris) **151**, 1476 (1957b).

GUIMARAIS, J. A., TAVARES, A.: Sur la distinction des «substances actives» excito-sécrétoire et hypotensive de la salive. Arch. port. Sci. Biol. **6**, 184 (1942).

HAVEZ, R., DEGAND, P., ROUSSEL, PH., BISERTE, G.: Isolation et caractérisation immunologique de la kallikréine bronchique humaine. C. R. Acad. Sci. (Paris) **262**, 309 (1966b).

— — — VOISIN, C., BISERTE, G., GERNEZ-RIEUX, C.: Identification des γ_A-globulines, de la kallicréine et de la transferrine dans la muqueuse bronchique humaine. C. R. Acad. Sci. (Paris) **262**, 1777 (1966a).

HOUVENAGHEL, A., PEETERS, G.: Influence de la bradykinine sur l'éjection du lait chez la brebis et la chèvre. Arch. int. Pharmacodyn. **167**, 483 (1967).

— — DJORDJEVIC, N.: Influence des kinines du plasma et des kallikréines sur l'éjection du lait chez la brebis. Arch. Int. Pharmacodyn. **171**, 231 (1968).

Hugues, J., Lecomte, J.: Action de la bradykinine déposée au contact des vaisseaux mésentériques du lapin. C. R. Soc. Biol. (Paris) 154, 1523 (1960).
Hureau, J., Forlot, P., Raby, C., Vairel, E.: Evidence de la présence de trypsine dans le sang périphérique au cours des pancréatites hémorragiques. Son rôle dans le développement du choc. Rev. franç. Étud. clin. biol. 13, 80 (1968).
Jacobsen, S.: Substrates for plasma kinin-forming enzymes in rat and guinea-pig plasma. Brit. J. Pharmacol. 28, 64 (1966).
Krumm-Heller, M. C., Salesse, J.: Dosage biologique de l'activité des échantillons de callikréine (Impantine). Ann. pharm. franç. 14, 124 (1956).
Leclercq, R., Lisin, N.: Etude de l'action oedémateuse de la bradykinine au niveau de la patte, chez le rat. C. R. Soc. Biol. (Paris) 157, 1328 (1963).
Lecomte, J.: Bradykinine et choc anaphylactique du lapin. Acta allerg. (Kbh.) 14, 408 (1959).
— Consommation des kininogènes plasmatiques au cours du choc anaphylactique du lapin. C. R. Soc. Biol. (Paris) 155, 1411 (1961).
— Action vasomotrice de 2 extraits pancréatiques désinsulinés. C. R. Soc. Biol. (Paris) 156, 1727 (1962).
— Action de la bradykinine sur l'intestin du *Choloepus*. Arch. int. Physiol. Biochim. 71, 245 (1963).
— Kininogènes et enzymes kininoformateurs chez le Paresseux. Arch. int. Physiol. Biochim. 72, 926 (1964).
— Sur l'activité antianaphylactique d'un dérivé du thioxanthène chez le lapin. Acta allerg. (Kbh.) 22, 457 (1967a).
— Sur les propriétés hypotensives de l'acide ellagique, chez le rat. C. R. Soc. Biol. (Paris) 161, 2651 (1967b).
— Damas, J.: Sur le rôle des kininogènes dans le syndrome provoqué par les dextrans chez le rat. Arch. int. Pharmacodyn. 176, 403 (1968).
— Salmon, J.: Sur le rôle des kinines plasmatiques dans la pathogénie du collapsus anaphylactique du rat. Arch. int. Physiol. Biochim. 76, 273 (1968).
— Troquet, J.: Antagonisme entre bradykinine et phénylbutazone chez le lapin. C. R. Soc. Biol. (Paris) 154, 1115 (1960).
— — Actions vasculaires de certains polypeptides endogènes. Rôle physio-pathologique de ces derniers. Acta cardiol. (Brux.) 17, 797 (1962a).
— — Antagonisme entre salicylate de soude et bradykinine chez le rat. Arch. int. Physiol. Biochim. 70, 735 (1962b).
— — Cession-Fossion, A.: Sur la nature de l'hypertension artérielle provoquée par la bradykinine et la kallidine. Arch. int. Pharmacodyn. 147, 518 (1964).
— — Dresse, A.: Stimulation médullo-surrénalienne par la bradykinine. Arch. int. Physiol. Biochim. 69, 89 (1961).
— — Petit, J. M., Marcelle, R.: Action broncho-constrictrice de la bradykinine chez l'homme asthmatique. Arch. int. Pharmacodyn. 137, 232 (1962).
Leger, L., Parrot, J. L., Gley, P.: Mise en évidence dans le corpuscule carotidien de l'homme d'un principe hypotenseur distinct de l'histamine et de l'acétylcholine. Presse méd. 1947, 542.
Linée, P., Dechy, J. P., Saint-Blanchard, J. de: Evaluation du bradykininogène plasmatique. (Modification de la microméthode de Diniz et Carvalho.) Ann. pharm. franç. 24, 711 (1966).
Lisin, N., Leclercq, R.: Essai d'inhibition de l'oedème à la bradykinine chez le rat. C. R. Soc. Biol. (Paris) 157, 1536 (1963).
— — Etude du développement de l'oedème à la bradykinine et à la kallidine chez le rat surrénalectomisé. Influence de la surrénalectomie sur le pouvoir inhibiteur du salicylate de sodium et de la phénylbutazone. J. belge Méd. phys. Rhum. 20, 112 (1965).
— — Cauwenberge, H. van: L'oedème à la bradykinine et son inhibition. Rev. Rhum. 30, 790 (1963).
Melon, J., Lecomte, J.: Etude comparée des effets de la bradykinine et des réactions anaphylactiques locales chez l'homme. Int. Arch. Allergy 21, 89 (1962).
Rocha e Silva, M.: Bradykinine. Actualités pharmacol. 15, 163 (1963).
Saint-Blanchard, J. de, Linee, P., Monteil, R.: Activité bradykininique des liquides de phlyctène prélevés chez les grands brûlés. Rev. franç. Étud. clin. biol. 11, 82 (1966).
Salmon, J., Lambert, P.-H., Otto-Servais, M., Lecomte, J.: Sur le rôle du complément dans le choc anaphylactique du lapin. Int. Arch. Allergy 24, 27 (1964).
— Lecomte, J.: Kininogènes plasmatiques et fibrinolyse thérapeutique. Rev. franç. Étud. clin. biol. 8, 473 (1963).
— — Sur le collapsus cardio-vasculaire provoqué chez le rat par l'activation de la plasmine. Rev. belge Path. 31, 317 (1965).

STÜRMER, E.: Chimie et pharmacologie des plasmakinines, plus spécialement de la bradykinine. Settim. med. **51**, Suppl. 1, 11 (1963).
TROQUET, J.: Aspects mécaniques de la ventilation au cours du choc anaphylactique du lapin. Int. Arch. Allergy **24**, 356 (1964).
— LECOMTE, J.: Action de quelques ferments estérasiques sur le choc anaphylactique du lapin. C. R. Soc. Biol. (Paris) **157**, 1534 (1963).
— — Rôle des kinines dans les phénomènes allergiques. Rev. méd. Liège **19**, 333 (1964).
UNGAR, G., PARROT, J. L.: Sur la présence de la callikréine dans la salive, et la possibilité de son intervention dans la transmission chimique de l'influx nerveux. C. R. Soc. Biol. (Paris) **122**, 1052 (1936).
VARGAFTIG, B.: Effet des analgésiques non narcotiques sur l'hypotension due à la bradykinine. Experientia (Basel) **22**, 182 (1966).

Summary of Literature Published in Italian

F. Sicuteri

A. Metabolism

The concentration of kininogen in blood taken from the cubital vein in man varies between 2 and 5 μg/ml equiv. of synthetic bradykinin (BRS–640; Sicuteri et al., 1962g). These values are notably lower than those previously described by the authors of the original method used (Diniz et al., 1961). They found a mean of 21.2 μg with values variable between 14.8 and 28.5 μg of natural purified bradykinin (Bk). The discrepancy is due to the use of purified natural Bk by the Brazilian authors and synthetic Bk by the Italian authors. Franchi et al. (1963, 1964) in 147 normal subjects found values of kininogen in the male varying between 1.2 and 6.0 μg (mean 2.78); in the female values varied between 1 and 7.5 μg (mean 2.71). A significant difference between the two sexes was not detectable. In subjects over 60 years of age, a significantly lower than normal level of kininogen was noted.

In 21 neonates (1–5 days of age), kininogen was found to be lower than at any other time of life (1.78 μg). In pregnant women at term, kininogen values are particularly elevated (4.55 μg in 16 subjects) while 2.77 μg was found in 79 normal subjects (Periti et al., 1962a). Therefore, a significant difference exists between kininogen levels of maternal and newborn blood. During delivery, plasma kininogen decreases significantly, returning to baseline values in the first few postpartum days. Levels of kininogen of venous plasma (cubital vein) are lower than those of arterial blood in normal subjects, and this difference increases slightly during reactive hyperemia that immediately follows induced ischemia in the upper limb. This phenomenon is the consequence of the fact that after ischemia, arterial kininogen remains unmodified while venous kininogen decreases slightly (Sicuteri et al., 1963b, d, f).

In cerebrospinal fluid (CSF) traces of kininogen occur (variable between 2 and 40 ng/equiv. Bk) in normal subjects or those with migraine or psychoneurotic headache (Sicuteri et al., 1963i). The free kinin level, determined by using a special extraction method (Periti and Sicuteri, 1962; Periti et al., 1963b) varies in the male between 0.3 and 3.0 ng Bk (mean 1.03) and in the female between 0.1 and 4.4 ng Bk (mean 1.21) (Franchi et al., 1963, 1964). Human plasma inactivates kinin as shown by incubation of Bk with plasma or serum *in vitro*. There is no difference in inactivating capacity between plasma and serum. Bk inactivation is greatly decreased at pH 6.5 with respect to the "optimum" at pH 7.5. Bk inactivation becomes more rapid if the temperature is brought from 37.5° to 38–40° (Periti et al., 1962b). Used as a test of Bk inactivation in man, the decrease in arterial pressure (measured directly and with electromanometer) and the CSF pressure (also measured with an electromanometer), showed that 20 μg of synthetic Bk when incubated with fresh human plasma at 37° loses 50% of its hypotensive activity in 30 minutes, and after 60 minutes no activity on arterial pressure is noticeable. In two cases of severe bronchial asthma, studied by this method, a decrease in kininase activity was noticed (Sicuteri et al., 1962b).

In CSF kinin inactivation is very low, and therefore the blood/CSF gradient of carboxypeptidase N is very steep (SICUTERI et al., 1965e). The plasma "clearance" of bradykinin is controlled by kininases in plasma and by a capillary inactivating (or fixing) capacity (SICUTERI et al., 1962b). This was demonstrated by i.v. injection to man of synthetic bradykinin or plasma kinins obtained by incubating plasma with trypsin. That kinins acted on capillaries was shown by the intense cutaneous vasodilatation, hypotension, and tachycardia. When injected intra-arterially (10 μg of Bk), an intense local pain was also noted besides the strong vasodilatation. Because a large dose of bradykinin was injected and the small quantity of blood which traverses the limbs during such a short period is small, an increase of 50–100 times greater in free kinin might be expected. This observation indicates that certainly at the capillary level, an inactivating or fixing mechanism of free kinin of great efficacy exists. The important "clearance" of Bk at the capillary level, besides surely having biologic significance, must be considered in all pharmacodynamic trials with Bk in man (SICUTERI et al., 1963h).

In man, some substances injected i.v. provoke a decrease of kininogen, probably as an expression of kinin release. Some phenomena induced by these substances may be correlated with the release of kinin.

Epinephrine, injected i.m. (20 μg/kg), decreases kininogen after 20 minutes, whereas norepinephrine does not. It is thought that the action of epinephrine on kininogen may be mediated by a β-receptor function (SICUTERI et al., 1962f). After epinephrine, kinin level did not increase in plasma, but an increase in kininase was observed (PERITI et al., 1963a). Kallikrein, infused in doses of 150–200 FU, provokes intense vasodilatation, headache, hypotension, and a constant decrease in kininogen. Trypsin, to the contrary, injected in doses of 3–5 mg, even if inducing equal or more intense vasomotor reactions, does not significantly modify the kininogen level. The difference cannot yet be explained (SICUTERI et al., 1962e, f). To obtain a vasomotor threshold effect, 20–30 FU of kallikrein is necessary or 200–300 μg of trypsin.

Another observation is that if trypsin, previously incubated with plasma (1 mg/ml), is injected, a vasomotor reaction, at least twice as great as that observed when an equal quantity of nonincubated trypsin is injected, is obtained (SICUTERI, et al., 1961b, 1963e, g).

In man, the histamine liberator 48/80 B.W. infused i.v. (15 mg) or injected into the brachial artery (1 mg) causes a significant decrease in kininogen together with erythema and tachycardia. After injection of 48/80 B.W. i.a., the kininogen decrease in reflux blood is very marked and an increase in free kinin is also noted. When 48/80 B.W. is infused i.v., free kinin does not increase significantly. Histamine, also, when infused i.v. (2 mg) causes a smaller decrease in kininogen and for a shorter period of time. A decrease in kininogen by release of histamine and by other factors from mast cells is provoked by 48/80 B.W. (PERITI et al., 1964).

The kininogen level in venous blood may vary according to conditions under which the samples are taken. For example, after a protracted stasis of 10–15 minutes an increase in kininogen level is observed (SICUTERI et al., 1963j). The increase of kininogen after venostasis was confirmed by BULUK et al. (1965) while PANERAI et al. (1964) noted a decrease in kininogen under the same experimental conditions. SICUTERI et al. (1963j) found a decrease in free kinin during venostasis. This decrease was also seen by MASOTTI et al. (1967), not in a normal subject but in subjects with capillary fragility. Probably these changes are linked to metabolic phenomena tied to a prolonged contact of kininogen or kinin with capillary walls or to enzymatic kinin liberators and kinin inactivators. These metabolic effects may obviously have physiopathologic implications in venostasis or ischemia.

B. Pharmacology

The first observations of the action of synthetic Bk in man were carried out by using variations in systemic arterial pressure and spinal fluid pressure as parameters; as comparison, the action of histamine was used (SICUTERI, 1961a; SICUTERI et al., 1961a) (p. 490). It is noted that the threshold i.v. vasoactive dose of Bk is 100–500 ng/kg, while for histamine the threshold dose is 50–200 ng/kg. The effects of Bk and histamine in man (injected i.v.) on arterial pressure and spinal fluid pressure are not distinguishable. The antihistamines completely block the action of histamine and leave unmodified that of Bk. Histamine is more active than Bk when injected intravenously but Bk is more active when given intra-arterially. The first observations of the effects of Bk injected i.a. indicate that, in equal doses, the peptide produces more vasodilatation and pain (SICUTERI, 1961b). Doses of 0.5–1.0 µg, injected via carotid, produce local vasodilatation and pain over the area of the frontal bone and eye. A fleeting increase in CSF pressure is also present. Identical observations are noted with injection into the brachial artery. These results were confirmed later (BURCH and DE PASQUALE, 1962).

Eledoisin is more vasoactive than histamine or bradykinin, according to the first clinical-pharmacological observations. Doses of 5–10 ng/kg i.v. produce vasodilatation, arterial hypotension, and CSF hypertension. Marked effects (intense vasodilatation, headache, hypotension, tachycardia, vertigo, nausea, and vomiting) are always obtained with doses of 30–60 ng/kg. Doses of 20 ng/kg/min given by infusion provoke vasodilatation, hypotension, hyperpnea, nausea, and finally (frequently) a reduction in voice almost to aphony, perhaps due to edema of the vocal cords. No other peptide causes this phenomenon. The effect of eledoisin is more prolonged than that of bradykinin; eledoisin is more slowly inactivated in human plasma than Bk. Eledoisin also produces a conspicuous increase in fibrinolysis *in vivo* but not *in vitro*; the hyperfibrinolysis is greater than that with Bk and histamine (SICUTERI et al., 1962c). The ability of eledoisin to enhance fibrinolysis was confirmed by BRUNETTI and TESI (1967). These authors observed, with regard to fibrinolysis, that acetylcholine and Bk are less active than eledoisin. The increase in fibrinolysis is yet more intense when eledoisin is infused i.a. (brachial artery) (NUTI et al., 1964; DEIDDA et al., 1964b; TESI and BRUNETTI, 1967; PRATESI et al., 1967). SICUTERI et al. (1965f) conducted the first trials in man with another potent vasoactive peptide, physalaemin, and observed that threshold vasoactive effects can be shown with doses of 0.25–0.5 ng/kg. No other peptide, including angiotensin, has such vasomotor activity.

Physalaemin is 3 times more active than eledoisin, 10 times more than angiotensin, 50 times more than histamine, and 100 times more than Bk. Physalaemin, at equal vasoactive effects, has a longer-lasting vasomotor action than Bk, but a lesser one than eledoisin. Perhaps this is due to the inactivation of physalaemin by plasma; the inactivation of physalaemin is more rapid than that of eledoisin but slower than that of Bk (SICUTERI et al., 1964c, g).

In the dog, studied by the nitrous oxide method, Bk, in doses certainly active on systemic circulation, does not modify cerebral circulation (DESSY et al., 1966) nor renal circulation (ACCATINO et al., 1967) but produces a discrete increase in coronary flow (GAGNA et al., 1967). Bk is particulary active on cutaneous vessels, more than on skeletal muscle vessels in man (DEIDDA and NUTI, 1964; DEIDDA et al., 1964a, b; PRATESI et al., 1965). A venoconstrictor action was observed with transillumination of venous vessels in the frog and rat (FRATTI, 1965). A very notable action of Bk on meningeal vessels (pia) was documented with microcinematography in the guinea pig; even doses of 1 μg/kg provoke dilatation of pial vessels. Intense congestion finally leading to conspicuous edema was observed with doses of 200 μg/kg (CONCIOLI et al., 1961). These results agree with observations made in man (SICUTERI et al., 1961a).

In the rabbit, intracisternal introduction of Bk even in small doses provokes a characteristic reaction, called "the squeaking flight reaction" (SICUTERI et al., 1966e; BERTOLINI et al., 1966a) (p. 495). In the dog, intracisternal injection of Bk provokes, instead, a marked and durable catatonia. This catatonic state is not accompanied by muscular hypotonia but permits the dog, when stimulated, to move with apparent normal motion (BERTOLINI et al., 1966a). It is known (see p. 505) that CSF has little kininase activity, while brain homogenates of guinea pig, rabbit, and ox rapidly inactivate the peptide. Homogenates of medulla of oxen, on the other hand, inactivate Bk more slowly. The bradykinin potentiating factor (BPF) increases the intensity and duration of the effects of Bk injected into CSF of dog and rabbit (BERTOLINI and GIAROLI, 1966). Bk, but not eledoisin, injected into the carotid of rabbits, induces "vocalization". An effort was made to find a relationship between vocalization and the increase of encephalic blood volume by marking red blood cells with Na 51-chromate (BERTOLINI et al., 1966b, 1967). Ergotamine does not antagonize the effect of Bk, although in smaller doses it produces an increase in cephalic blood flow and vocalization (MUCCI et al., 1967; STERNIERI et al., 1967).

The action of various drugs on the spasmogenic effect of Bk and acetylcholine on the ileum of the guinea pig was also studied. Hemicholinium (HC-3) completely inhibited the action of acetylcholine while leaving intact that of Bk (BERTOLINI and GREGGIA, 1966). Various adrenergic α and β blockers antagonize more or less the spasmogenic effect of Bk (CASTELLI et al., 1967).

In women at the term of pregnancy, the effect of i.v. injection of Bk on uterine motility was studied. This was done by using an electromanometer to measure amniotic fluid and intrauterine pressures, evaluated via a semirigid probe introduced into the uterus. Although with i.v. doses of 0.5 μg Bk/kg, vasomotor phenomena but not contractions were observed, doses of 1—2 μg/kg produced, after a latency of 4–8 minutes, uterine contractions identical with those of normal labor. These contractions were noticed also by the women and produced the characteristic labor pains (SICUTERI et al., 1962a). A definite potentiation of the effect of oxytocin was provoked by bradykinin. Subthreshold doses of oxytocin, in women at term, initiated uterine contractions if given i.v. after the administration of bradykinin. To women at term who received oxytocin to induce delayed labor, a preparation of a trypsin–heparin complex (THC) containing 85% trypsin was administered. The administration by venous infusion caused vasodilatation and hypotension and in some women initiated uterine contractions which continued into full labor. In other patients, resistant to oxytocin, the treatment with the combination of THC and oxytocin induced labor (CENTARO et al., 1962).

C. Pathology

Bradykinin injected into the brachial artery or into the carotid of man causes, besides the vasodilatory phenomena, intense pain (SICUTERI, 1961a). This was confirmed by BURCH and DE PASQUALE (1962). If before and during the intrabrachial injection a local circulatory arrest is produced (ischemia), the pain will be more intense and prolonged and no vasomotor phenomena will be observed. Ischemia potentiates the effect of bradykinin on pain receptors and capillaries, either because of the lack of dilution of the peptide and lack of removal, or because of a decrease in local pH with inhibition of kininases. When, after the arterial injection with flow arrested, blood is allowed to circulate again, the subject notes a violent exacerbation of pain with its subsequent disappearance; vasodilatation and edema are observed in the arm (SICUTERI et al., 1963b). Given that a decrease in local kininogen is observed during ischemia, and even more so during muscular work with ischemia (SICUTERI et al., 1963f), Bk may be considered to participate in the mechanism of spontaneous pain during ischemia as in intermittent claudication and angina pectoris (SICUTERI, 1963, 1964c; SICUTERI et al., 1964b, e, h).

Another factor that potentiates the action of Bk in pain during ischemia is serotonin (5-HT), which passes from platelets into plasma during ischemia and even more in venous or arterial thrombosis. 5-HT lowers the threshold of sensitive receptors in the intima of vessels to Bk (SICUTERI et al., 1964a, 1965d). In this way, in myocardial infarct and in other pain due to thrombotic arterial occlusion, the pain caused by Bk may be potentiated by 5-HT from the disintegrated platelets (SICUTERI et al., 1964b). This mechanism may be considered for the pathogenesis of pain in myocardial infarction. In the initial phase of myocardial infarction, especially in severe forms associated with shock resulting in death, the kininogen level was particularly low; it is possible that a release of kinin by enzymatic action, from myocardial necrosis, participates in the mechanisms of collapse and shock (SICUTERI et al., 1966d). It is possible that the potentiation of pain receptors by 5-HT and Bk is important also in migraine (SICUTERI, 1961b); at the end of a migraine attack a significant reduction in plasma kininogen is observed, and possibly more kinin can be liberated (SICUTERI, 1964a, b).

In man, fever provoked by the administration of pyrogens decreases kininogen; the phenomenon starts with an increase in temperature and lasts even after return to normal body temperature. Also in cases of acute infectious diseases kininogen level decreases significantly (SICUTERI et al., 1963a).

The administration of pyrogen in nonfebrific doses provokes, in a patient with chronic inflammatory pain (fibrositis, arthrosis, arthritis, or headache), a prolonged exacerbation of pain; the phenomenon is attributed principally to the release of kinin at the level of the inflammatory process (SICUTERI et al., 1966a, b). The release of kinin may be due to lysosomal enzymes, especially from the granulocytes and other defense cells. During provoked fever in man, a decrease in kininogen and a significant increase of β-glucuronidase, that lasts for many hours, is observed. Also in nonfebrific doses, pyrogen provokes an increase in β-glucuronidase in patients with chronic inflammatory processes but not in normal subjects (BAVAZZANO et al., 1967). The release of kinin may explain why highly purified pyrogens produce pain in veins previously sensitized by 5-HT (SICUTERI et al., 1965a). Local pain to pyrogens develops with a latency that is slightly longer than that following kallikrein, Bk, or kallidin administration. Probably, the mechanism of local pain caused by pyrogens rests on local liberation of kinin that in turn was caused by an activation of lysosomal enzymes (SICUTERI et al., 1966a, c).

After incubating with tuberculin the blood of subjects with strong tuberculin hyperergia, an algogenic factor appears in plasma (SICUTERI et al., 1965b). This algogenic factor is probably a kinin. Tuberculin given by itself does not rupture lysosomes, but the combination of tuberculin and lymphocytic antibodies is a potent lysosome labilizer (SICUTERI et al., 1964f).

An increased concentration of kinin in CSF can be induced by activation of the permeability factor (PF/dil). This kinin-liberating factor becomes activated by dilution of plasma with CSF (Sicuteri, 1965a, b, 1966; Sicuteri et al., 1965c, 1967a). The possible pathological importance of the kininogen–kinin system in surgical procedures (Gasparri et al., 1963), in dermatology (Panconesi et al., 1963), and in other diseases (Sicuteri et al., 1963a) was considered.

A particular emphasis is placed on the so-called allergic reactions to trypsin· Trypsin, frequently given i.m. or i.v. as a fibrinolytic or anti-inflammatory drug may provoke reactions and shock either by a true sensitization phenomenon or by a purely pharmacologic phenomenon. In fact, in man, even treated with large doses of antihistamines or antiserotonins, i.v. doses of 1–2 mg of trypsin always induce a vasodilatation and arterial hypotension. Probably a part of the reactions from trypsin, the so-called allergic reactions are due to a release of large quantities of kinin by this enzyme (Sicuteri et al., 1962d; Sicuteri and Periti, 1963).

D. Therapy

After considering the important vasodilator action of kinin and its probable physiologic role in the tone and permeability of small vessels, Sicuteri and co-workers decided to use kinin in therapy.

Trypsin injected i.v. in small doses (10–30 μg/kg), produces vasodilatation and hypotension corresponding to the action of 50–100 μg of synthetic Bk. It is noteworthy that the same quantity of trypsin, if incubated with plasma or serum and then injected i.v., induces two- to threefold stronger vasomotor reaction than an equal dose of pure trypsin. On the other hand, during the incubation of plasma with trypsin a coagulation was seen, linked to the fact that trypsin inactivates heparin present in plasma. The THC (see p. 613) is stable and available commercially. THC incubated with plasma, previously inactivated by boiling in the presence of acetic acid, does not liberate spasmogenic peptide, in contrast to that found by incubating the same plasma with trypsin. In spite of this, THC itself causes vasodilatation if injected i.v. to man and even more so if it is previously incubated with plasma (Sicuteri et al., 1962e). The reason why previous incubation with plasma or serum increases the vasoactive potency of trypsin or THC is not clear. It was decided, however, to administer trypsin (10 μg) or THC (50 μg), incubated with plasma and then diluted in 500 ml of physiologic solution, by slow infusion. This treatment was conducted in various arteriopathies of limbs and in various forms of cerebral arteriosclerosis. To protect the patients from an eventual allergic reaction to trypsin, an antihistamine was also added to the solution. The infusion (30–50 drops/min) provoked vasodilatation, slight hypotension, and often headache. In one case urticaria was observed in other cases, shivering and fever appeared. Because of these undesirable reactions, the treatment leads to difficulties. This constitutes a negative element, inasmuch as the results observed were good or excellent (Sicuteri et al., 1964d).

Eledoisin was tried as a therapeutic agent because of its high vasoactivity, its resistance to human plasma peptidases and, finally, because of its high fibrinolytic capacity. The most favorable results were observed in intermittent claudication, Raynaud's phenomenon, and in dystrophic lesions. Eledoisin, infused i.v. or administered i.m., may provoke secondary effects such as protracted hypotension or aphony, perhaps because of vocal cord edema (Sicuteri et al., 1963c). The therapeutic action of eledoisin was confirmed by using this drug in arterial infusion in arteriopathy obliterans (Pratesi et al., 1966a, b, 1967).

The observation of the activation of PF/dil that occurs when blood extravasates into the subarachnoid space and is diluted with CSF led to clinical trials with Trasylol in cases of intracranial hemorrhage (SICUTERI, 1966). In cerebral apoplexy as well as in subarachnoid hemorrhage, the results were encouraging. These therapeutic trials were supported by the evidence that Trasylol constitutes the most active antagonist in reducing the mortality rate, clinical symptoms, and cerebral damage produced by experimentally induced cerebral hemorrhage in the rat, guinea pig, and rabbit (SICUTERI et al., 1967b).

Similarly, in the case of cerebral and subarachnoid hemorrhage, the enzymatic inhibitor acts, either on the kinin-liberating mechanism by dilution of plasma with CSF (i.e. antagonizes PF/dil) or on the kinin-liberating mechanism linked to tissue injury by hemorrhagic infarct. The effects of this agent, infused twice within 24 hours in doses of 100,000 to 200,000 KIU, are revealed by a reduction in mortality and in the duration of coma. On the other hand, an evaluation of the real efficacy of this drug necessitates a broader comparative statistical evaluation than is not available (SICUTERI et al., 1967c).

References

ACCATINO, G., BETTI, C., DESSY, P., GAGNA, C., USLENGHI, E.: Azione della bradichinina sull'emodinamica generale e distrettuale. Circolo renale. Minerva med. 57, 3556 (1967).

BAVAZZANO, A., FANCIULLACCI, M., SICUTERI, F.: Effetto delle endotossine in dosi subfebbrili su alcuni livelli plasmatici enzimatici (β-glucuronidasi, fosfatasi acida) e sulla diuresi nell' uomo. Boll. Soc. ital. Biol. sper. 43, 1403 (1967).

BERTOLINI, A., GIAROLI, M.: La bradichinina come possibile agente causale dell'emicrania II. Inattivazione della bradichinina da parte di materiali organici ed in particolare del tessuto nervoso. Boll. Soc. ital. Biol. sper. 42, 1918 (1966).

— GREGGIA, A.: La bradichinina come possibile agente causale dell'emicrania. I. Valutazione della bradichinina sull'ileo isolato di cavia. Boll. Soc. ital. Biol. sper. 42, 1915 (1966).

— MUCCI, P., FERRARI, W.: La bradichinina come possibile agente causale dell'emicrania. III. Effetto dell'iniezione endocisternale di bradichinina nel cane e nel coniglio. Boll. Soc. ital. Biol. sper. 42, 1922 (1966a).

— — STERNIERI, E.: La bradichinina come possibile agente causale dell'emicrania. Effetti comportamentali e circolatori della bradichinina iniettata per via endocarotidea. Boll. Soc. med.-chir. Modena 66, 1 (1966b).

— — — La bradichinina come possibile agente causale dell'emicrania. IV. Rapporto tra gli effetti comportamentale e circolatorio della bradichinina, iniettata per via endocarotidea nel coniglio. Boll. Soc. ital. Biol. sper. 43, 794 (1967).

BRUNETTI, S., TESI, M.: Azione di alcuni farmaci sulla dinamica della fibrinolisi nell'uomo. Riv. crit. Clin. med. 67, 233 (1967).

BULUK, L., MALOFIEJEW, M., CZOKALO, M.: Activation of fibrinolysis and of plasma-kinin system during venostasis. Thrombos. Diathes. haemorrh. (Stuttg.) 14, 500 (1965).

BURCH, G. E., DE PASQUALE, N. P.: Bradykinin, digital blood flow and the arteriovenous anastomoses. Circulat. Res. 10, 105 (1962).

CASTELLI, M., BAGGIO, G., BERTOLINI, A.: Modificazione dell'azione in vitro della bradichinina per blocco dei recettori adrenergici. Boll. Soc. ital. Biol. sper. 43, 1205 (1967).

CENTARO, A., SICUTERI, F., BATTAGLIA, G. B., MASSI, G. B.: Esperienze di induzione al parto con l'associazione plasmachinine-ossitocina. Boll. Soc. ital. Biol. sper. 38, 670 (1962).

CONCIOLI, M., SANTANDREA, E., VILLANI, B.: Modificazioni del circolo piale sotto l'influsso di particolari stimoli e soprattutto della bradichinina. Rilievi microcinematografici. Atti Accad. med. lombarda 16, 258 (1961).

DEIDDA, C., NUTI, A.: Aspetti distrettuali dell'effetto vasoattivo bradichininico nei muscoli e nella cute dell'uomo. Riv. crit. Clin. med. 64, 289 (1964).

— — CORSI, C., BRUNETTI, S.: Considerazioni clinico-radiologiche sugli effetti della bradichinina somministrata per via endoarteriosa. Riv. crit. Clin. med. 64, 251 (1964a).

— — TESI, M., BRUNETTI, S.: Considerazioni comparative sull'azione fibrinolitica dell'acetilcolina e della bradichinina somministrate per via endoarteriosa nell'uomo. Rass. Neurol. veg. 18, 769 (1964b).

DESSY, P., USLENGHI, E., GAGNA, C., ACCATINO, G., BETTI, C.: Azione della bradichinina sull'emodinamica generale e distrettuale. Minerva med. 57, 3555 (1966).

DINIZ, C. R., CARVALHO, I. F., RYAN, J., ROCHA E SILVA, M.: A micromethod for the determination of bradykininogen in blood plasma. Nature (Lond.) **192**, 1194 (1961).
FRANCHI, G., FANCIULLACCI, M., DEL BIANCO, P. L.: Studio casistico—in 148 soggetti normali—sul tasso delle plasmachinine libere e del loro precursore. In: Atti del I. Congr. della Soc. Ital. di Microcircolazione, Naples, 1963.
— — — SANTINI, D.: Chininogeno e chinine libere plasmatiche nel soggetto normale. Rass. Fisiopat. clin. ter. **36**, 346 (1964).
FRATTI, L., FONTANA, S., PIOVELLA, C., DE SILVESTRI, A.: Azione della bradichinina sul circolo periferico osservato in vivo mediante transilluminazione. In: Atti del II. Congr. della Soc. Ital. di Microcircolazione, Como, 1965.
GAGNA, C., USLENGHI, E., DESSY, P., BETTI, C., ACCATINO, G.: Azione della bradichinina sull'emodinamica generale e distrettuale. Circolo coronarico. Minerva med. **57**, 3557 (1967).
GASPARRI, F., PERITI, P., SICUTERI, G., BATTAGLIA, G. B.: Bradichininogeno ed interventi chirurgici ginecologici. Boll. Soc. ital. Biol. sper. **39**, 321 (1963).
MASOTTI, G., SALANI, G., GENSINI, G., MORFINI, M., NERI SERNERI, G. G.: Attivazione del sistema chininico plasmatico nei soggetti con prova del laccio positivo, p. 563. In: Proceedings, First Internat. Symposium on Tissue Factors in the Homeostasis of the Coagulation-Fibrinolysis System. Turin: Soc. Tipogr. Piemont 1967.
MUCCI, P., STERNIERI, E., BERTOLINI, A., CASTELLI, M.: Modificazioni, indotte farmacologicamente, della risposta del circolo cerebrale alla bradichinina. II. Influenza della ergotamina sulla vocalizzazione e sulla modificazione del circolo cerebrale prodotte con bradichinina. Boll. Soc. ital. Biol. sper. **43**, 1200 (1967).
NUTI, A., DEIDDA, C., BRUNETTI, S., TESI, M.: Azione fibrinolitica della bradichinina somministrata per via endoarteriosa nell'uomo. Rass. Neurol. veg. **18**, 757 (1964).
PANCONESI, E., SICUTERI, F., PERITI, P.: Bradichininogeno e plasmachinine in dermatologia. Ricerche preliminari. Rass. Derm. Sif. **16**, 19 (1963).
PANERAI, A., GHETTI, A., ARCANGELI, P.: Mediatori chimici e arresto della circolazione arteriosa e venosa degli arti nell'uomo. Rass. Neurol. veg. **18**, 131 (1964).
PERITI, P., CENTARO, A., SICUTERI, F., LEOCANI, B.: Bradichininogeno ematico durante il parto. Boll. Soc. ital. Biol. sper. **38**, 672 (1962a).
— GASPARRI, F., SICUTERI, F., BATTAGLIA, G.: Attività bradichininolitica ematica durante il parto. Boll. Soc. ital. Biol. sper. **38**, 1 (1962b).
— SICUTERI, F.: Rilievi sul substrato biologico per il dosaggio del bradikininogeno plasmatico e della bradikinina urinaria nell'uomo. Boll. Soc. ital. Biol. sper. **38**, 316 (1962).
— — FRANCHI, G., MICHELACCI, S.: Azione dell'istamino-liberatore "48/80" sul bradichininogeno e plasmachinine del sangue venoso umano dopo somministrazione endovenosa o endoarteriosa. Boll. Soc. ital. Biol. sper. **40**, 951 (1964).
— — GASPARRI, F., FRANCHI, G.: Plasmachinine, bradichininogeno ed attività chininasica del sangue umano dopo somministrazione parenterale di adrenalina e noradrenalina. Boll. Soc. ital. Biol. sper. **39**, 318 (1963a).
— — MICHELACCI, S., SANTINI, D.: Plasmachinine libere nel sangue umano. Boll. Soc. ital. Biol. sper. **39**, 307 (1963b).
PRATESI, F., DABIZZI, R., CARAMELLI, L., BRUNETTI, S., TESI, M., BIANUCCI, G.: Microangiologia cutanea e muscolare. Aspetti di emodinamica differenziale. In: Atti del II. Congr. della Soc. Ital. di Microcircolazione, Como, 1965.
— NUTI, A., BRUNETTI, S., CARAMELLI, L., CORSI, C., DABIZZI, R. P., SPINELLI, P., TESI, M., BIANUCCI, G.: Nuove acquisizioni della endoarterioterapia delle angiopatie, p. 81. In: Atti del Simposio sui recenti progressi in tema di terapia angiologia, Milano, 1966a.
— — — DABIZZI, R. P., CARAMELLI, L.: Eledoisina per arterioclisi nelle arteriopatie obliteranti. Folia angiol. sant. **3**, 1 (1966b).
— TESI, M., BRUNETTI, S., BIDDAU, A.: Azione diretta ad effetto fibrinolitico dell'eledoisina sulla parete vasale nell'uomo, p. 221. In: Proceedings of First Internat. Symposium on Tissue Factors in the Homeostasis of the Coagulation-Fibrinolysis System, Turin, 1967.
SICUTERI, F.: Bradichinina. Significato e prospettive di un nuovo principio biologico. Settim. med. **48**, 3 (1961a).
— Prospettive biochimiche nella emicrania. Gazz. San. Fasc. No 6, 311 (1961b).
— Il dolore coronarico secondo una interpretazione biochimica. Gazz. San. **34**, 220 (1963).
— Polipeptidi vasoattivi. Prospettive fisiopatologiche e terapeutiche. Settim. med. **52**, 199 (1964a).
— Elementi di diagnostica funzionale. Le cefalee sperimentali: Test di induzione; biochimica dell'attacco, p. 101. In: 65° Congr. Soc. Ital di Medicina Interna. Estratto da L'Emicrania, Rome, 1964b.
— La mediazione chimica del dolore coronarico, p. 37. In: Colloqui di Cardiologia, suppl. II, di Malattie cardiovascolari. 1964c.

Sicuteri, F.: "La emodiluizione liquorale" quale fattore patogenetico della sindrome cefalgica-meningeale nella emorragia subaracnoidea. Settim. med. **53**, 173 (1965a).
— Liberazione di peptidi per diluizione liquorale del plasma nella patogenesi della emorragia sottoaracnoidea. Boll. Soc. ital. Ematol. **13**, 49 (1965b).
— Uno studio "pilota" per il trattamento dell'apoplessia cerebrale con un inibitore della callicreina. Settim. med. **54**, 555 (1966).
— Anselmi, B., Bavazzano, A.: Sugli effetti del pirogeno in dosi non febbrigene in alcune artropatie. Rass. Neurol. veg. **20**, 300 (1966a).
— — Del Bene, E.: Il pirogeno, in dosi non febbrigene, come test rivelatore di flogosi croniche intra-craniche. Rif. med. **44**, 1 (1966b).
— — — Bavazzano, A.: I pirogeni hanno un potere dolorifico? Boll. Soc. ital. Biol. sper. **42**, 840 (1966c).
— — Del Bianco, P. L.: Potere dolorifico di un pirogeno altamente purificato (Pyrexal). Atti Accad. med. lombarda **20**, 1 (1965a).
— — Michelacci, S.: Un fattore algogeno (Transfer factor?) dalla incubazione di sangue di soggetti iperergici con anatubercolina. Settim. med. **53**, 497 (1965b).
— Centaro, A., Massi, G. B., Periti, P.: Azione uterotonica della bradichinina sintetica nella donna a termine di gravidanza. Boll. Soc. ital. Biol. sper. **38**, 66 (1962a).
— Comparini, A., Periti, P.: Comportamento del bradichininogeno ematico in corso di malattie infettive acute. Settim. med. **51**, 133 (1963a).
— Del Bianco, P. L., Anselmi, B.: Sostanze microvasoattive e dolore vascolare. Contributo clinico-sperimentale. Boll. Soc. ital. Biol. sper. **40**, 69 (1963b).
— — — La bradichinina (sistema chininogeno-chinine) nella patogenesi del dolore e dello shock miocardico. Boll. Soc. ital. Cardiol. **11**, 1362 (1966d).
— — Fanciullacci, M., Anselmi, B.: Liberazione di plasmachinine da diluizione del sangue nel liquido cefalo rachidiano. Boll. Soc. ital. Biol. sper. **41**, 462 (1965c).
— — — Bavazzano, A.: Sulla patogenesi dei fenomeni clinici conseguenti alle emorragie intracraniche. Settim. med. **55**, 199 (1967a).
— — — Franchi, G.: Un nuovo substrato per lo studio del dolore da bradichinina e callidina. Boll. Soc. ital. Biol. sper. **40**, 949 (1964a).
— Fanciullacci, M., Anselmi, B.: Primi esperimenti di farmacodinamia e terapia vascolare nell'uomo con l'endecapeptide eledoisina, p. 159. In: Atti del I. Congr. della Soc. Ital. di Microcircolazione, Naples, 1963c.
— — — Le sostanze microvasoattive nella patogenesi del dolore vascolare. 2° Conf. Europ. Microcirc. (Pavia, 1962). Bibl. anat. (Basel) **4**, 207 (1964b).
— — Bavazzano, A., Franchi, G.: Influenza di un inhibitore della callicreina sulla fenomenologia da emorragia intracranica sperimentale. Boll. Soc. ital. Biol. sper. **43**, 1061 (1967b).
— — Del Bianco, P. L.: Vasoattività dell'endecapeptide fisalemina nell'uomo. Settim. med. **52**, 1221 (1964c).
— — — Le sostanze vasoneuroattive come mediatrici del dolore vascolare. Mal. cardiovasc. **6**, 505 (1965d).
— — — Anselmi, B.: Bradichininasi nel liquido cefalo-rachidiano dell'uomo. Boll. Soc. ital. Biol. sper. **41**, 464 (1965e).
— — Franchi, G.: Plasmachinine naturali in alcuni disordini vascolari. Minerva med. **55**, 3743 (1964d).
— — — Michelacci, S., Periti, P.: Il potere bradikinolitico del plasma umano. Osservazioni preliminari in condizioni normali e patologiche. Boll. Soc. ital. Biol. sper. **38**, 379 (1962b).
— — Michelacci, S.: Primi rilievi nell'uomo sugli effetti di un nuovo peptide ipotensivo, la fisalemina. Boll. Soc. ital. Biol. sper. **41**, 471 (1965f).
— Franchi, G., Anselmi, B.: Proprietà farmacologiche e terapeutiche della eledoisina nell'uomo. Suppl., Settim. med. p. 19 (1962c).
— — Del Bianco, P. L.: Il sistema plasmachininogeno plasmachinine nella regolazione della microcircolazione. In: Atti del I. Congr. della Soc. Ital. di Microcircolazione, Naples, 1963d.
— — — Un "test" per lo studio dell'azione dolorifica della bradichinina nell'animale. Il fenomeno "grido-fuga" del coniglio. Boll. Soc. ital. Biol. sper. **42**, 845 (1966e).
— — Fanciullacci, M.: Bradichinina e dolore da ischemia. Settim. med. **52**, 127 (1964e).
— — — Del Bianco, P. L.: Il sistema chininogen-chinine. Aspetti fisiopatologici e terapeutici. Clin. ter. **40**, 313 (1967c).
— — — Michelacci, S.: Liberazione di plasmakinine nell'uomo. Antagonismo di un fattore salivare. Arch. int. Pharmacodyn. **143**, 421 (1963e).
— — Michelacci, S.: Prime osservazioni sullo effetto della bradichinina sul circolo cerebrale dell'uomo. Settim. med. **49**, 7 (1961a).

SICUTERI, F., FRANCHI, G., MICHELACCI, S.: Attivazione di bradikinina e di altre plasmakinine dal siero umano—Prime documentazioni, p. 224. In: Atti del V. Congr. Naz. Sic. Ital. Allergologia, Pisa, 1961 b.
— MICHELACCI, S., ANSELMI, B.: Possibilità che le sostanze microvasoattive abbiano importanza nella patogenesi del dolore da occlusione arteriosa, p. 149. In: Atti del I. Congr. della Soc. Ital. di Microcircolazione, Naples, 1963 f.
— — — La tubercolina per vena come test diagnostico e come terapia specifica nelle cefalee tubercolinoiperergiche. Settim. med. **52**, 75 (1964 f).
— — FANCIULLACCI, M.: Azione di alcuni polipeptidi vasoattivi (callidina, bradichinina, eledoisina, angiotensina) sulla circolazione intracranica dell'uomo, p. 1. In: Atti 64° Congr. Soc. Ital. di Medicina Interna. 1964 g.
— — — FRANCHI, G.: Liberazione di bradichinina e di altre plasmachinine nell'uomo. Folia allerg. (Roma) **10**, 148 (1963 g).
— — FRANCHI, G., FANCIULLACCI, M.: Una nuova interpretazione delle cosiddette reazioni allergiche da tripsina. Rass. Fisiopat. clin. ter. **34**, 9 (1962 d).
— — — PERITI, P.: Sul meccanismo biologico degli effetti ipotensivi arteriosi di un complesso tripsina-eparina. Boll. Soc. ital. Biol. sper. **38**, 667 (1962 e).
— PERITI, P.: Liberazione di plasmachinine e di istamina e allergia da farmaci. Folia allerg. (Roma) **10**, 523 (1963).
— — ANSELMI, B., FANCIULLACCI, M.: Livelli plasmachininici nell'uomo dopo somministrazione endovenosa ed endoarteria di bradichinina sintetica e naturale. Boll. Soc. ital. Biol. sper. **39**, 314 (1963 h).
— — FANCIULLACCI, M., SANTINI, D.: Bradichininogeno dopo lavoro muscolare in ischemia nell'uomo. Boll. Soc. ital. Biol. sper. **40**, 955 (1964 h).
— — FRANCHI, G.: Bradichininogeno e chinine libere nel liquido cefalorachidiano dell'uomo. Boll. Soc. ital. Biol. sper. **40**, 67 (1963 i).
— — — SANTINI, D.: Il quoziente arterovenoso del bradichininogeno nell'uomo. Boll. Soc. ital. Biol. sper. **39**, 310 (1963 j).
— — GASPARRI, F., FRANCHI, G., FANCIULLACCI, M.: Diminuzione del tasso ematico di bradichininogeno nell'uomo dopo somministrazione di adrenalina e kallicreina. Boll. Soc. ital. Biol. sper. **38**, 1033 (1962 f).
— — MICHELACCI, S., FRANCHI, G., FANCIULLACCI, M.: Primi rilievi sul tasso di bradikininogeno plasmatico in condizioni normali e patologiche. Boll. Soc. ital. Biol. sper. **38**, 377 (1962 g).
STERNIERI, E., MUCCI, P., BERTOLINI, A.: Modificazioni, indotte farmacologicamente, della risposta del circolo cerebrale alla bradichinina. I. Rapporto tra vocalizzazione ed aumento del sangue nel territorio cerebrale. Boll. Soc. ital. Biol. sper. **43**, 1196 (1967).
TESI, M., BRUNETTI, S.: Azione bloccante dell'atropina sulla fibrinolisi da acetilcolina e da bradichinina. Riv. crit. Clin. med. **67**, 256 (1967).

Summary of Literature Published in Japanese

Hiroshi Moriya

Recent progress in basic and in clinical research on kinins and related peptides has been remarkable in Japan. Many Japanese papers have appeared in journals published in the United States and Europe, and also in Japanese journals written in English, which were read by investigators in other countries. Problems in many fields were investigated, including biochemical, clinical, biological, pharmacological, physiological, pathological, analytic and synthetic organic chemical, physicochemical, and other approaches. In this review only papers published in Japanese-language journals will be discussed. Reviews and presentations to large symposia will be summarized or only translated titles will be listed. Papers that appeared in leading Japanese journals written in English (with some exceptions) are not included.

Investigation of hog pancreatic kallikrein (HPKk) in Japan was initiated about 15 years ago. At that time almost no biochemist knew the active hypotensive high molecular substance, kallikrein, and no papers about it has been presented in meetings. In fact, even competent biochemists were confused by some similarities in the hypotensive action of kallikrein and histamine; thus the history of development of kallikrein in Germany repeated itself.

Moriya initially reviewed this field in 1957. At that time he assumed that bradykinin and kallidin must be identical. After chemical investigations of HPKk that lasted for several years, Moriya (1959a–e) and Moriya et al. (1958, 1959a, b) purified and established some properties of this enzyme. Hog pancreas and submaxillary gland were the most suitable sources for extraction. The methods applied for purification include the use of acetone, ethanol, activated charcoal, alumina, salting out with ammonium sulfate, and dialysis. Moriya found that although kallikrein potency in Frey units (FU) was increasing, the caseinolytic activity of the same fractions was not always parallel. The most effective purification was done by selective precipitation with acrinol (2-ethoxy-6,9-diamino acridinium lactate) (Moriya, 1959a, 1960). Further purification with zone electrophoresis in starch block yielded the purest preparation of 570 FU/mg. It was almost homogeneous in paper electrophoretic and ultracentrifugal analysis. Good reproducibility of these experiments and recovery of activity was ascertained. The isoelectric point of this kallikrein was pH 2.4. Its stability in aqueous solutions against acids, alkali, oxidizing reagents, trypsin, and papain was examined. In the structural study by hydrolysis with hydrochloric acid, 15 amino acids (Cys, Asp, Glu, Ser, Gly, Thr, Tyr, Ala, Pro, Val, Leu, Phe, Arg, His and Try) were reported as components of this enzyme. The quantities of amino acid found, the detection of amino-terminal phenylalanine and carboxyl-terminal alanine, the sugar content, UV absorption maximum at 281 mμ, a sedimentation constant of 2.85 S, a diffusion constant of 8.39 D, and a molecular weight of 33,000 were also reported. Thus the intrinsic properties of this highly purified HPKk were fairly well clarified. Most of these were in good agreement with papers published later by Werle and others. Some of the papers of Moriya were translated into English and read at the National Institutes of Health in Bethesda, Maryland.

At that time a few investigators applied kallikrein clinically. ITOH (1955) tried HPKk tablets in essential and renal hypertensive patients and found that the blood pressure was well controlled, various subjective symptoms were greatly improved, and no side reactions were noticed. He also reported that this tablet could be safely and satisfactorily used in other patients with circulatory disturbances.

IMAMURA (1957) found that HPKk given intravenously to rabbits caused an increase in the number of circulatory leukocytes including pseudoeosinophil cells, a decrease in the Ca, Na, and K content of blood serum, and an increase in its Mg content, without affecting in any way the amount of protein in serum or that of nonprotein nitrogen in blood. He stated that this action of the kallikrein would suggest extensive clinical trials. Of course the kallikrein preparation used at this time was very crude.

Later, MORIYA studied various other human kallikreins including pancreatic, urinary, salivary, and plasma kallikreins. Some of this work was done in WEBSTER and PIERCE's laboratories, at the National Institutes of Health in Bethesda. One paper was reported at the meeting of the New York Academy of Sciences (1963). The human urinary kallikrein prepared by MORIYA and used as kallidin-liberating enzyme, contributed to the differentiation of kallidin from bradykinin by PIERCE and WEBSTER.

After 1960, the results of original research were generally reported in English, except in some specialized problems. Recent papers of MORIYA, those of SUZUKI's group, and others were also written in English in journals such as *Journal of Biochemistry* and *the Chemical & Pharmaceutical Bulletin*. Some of the titles of MORIYA's papers are given below:

"Isolation and purification of human saliva kallikrein". "An improved method of purification of hog pancreatic kallikrein and some of its biological properties". "Preliminary experiments on human plasma kallikrein". "Effects on the gastro-intestinal system and the liver of hog pancreatic kallikrein". "Passage of ^{131}I-labeled hog pancreatic kallikrein across the rat intestine". "Human saliva kallikrein and liberation of colostrokinin". "Use of Sephadex G-10 and -15 gel filtration for fractionation of a certain peptide". "Studies of the specific inhibitors obtained from potato against the kinin-liberating system in human blood" (unpublished). "Release of colostrokinin from bovine colostrum by human saliva kallikrein. Its purification, and some properties".

MORIYA and KATO (1968) presented the paper on modified purification of HPKk to the 88th annual meeting of the Japanese Pharmaceutical Society and reported that the most highly purified preparation contained 1,200 FU/mg. MORIYA (1962a, b, c, 1963a, b) reviewed the field and stimulated many investigations thereafter in Japan.

SUZUKI and his co-workers have separated quite a few pure enzymes from many kinds of snake venoms in the last decade. These enzymes included an esterase with bradykinin-releasing activity and a proteinase with bradykinin-inactivating activity. In the course of these studies, their interest turned to the enzyme that releases bradykinin in the blood. Works from his laboratory described the purification of each component related to the kinin liberation in normal bovine blood or after injection of toxic venoms.

SUZUKI's clear studies of bradykinin-releasing enzyme in snake venom and on kininogens in bovine blood have appeared mainly in the *Journal of Biochemistry* (Japan) in English from 1965 to the present (for details see SUZUKI's and HABERMANN's chapters in this volume). SUZUKI et al. also examined the properties of bovine plasma kallikrein against several kinds of trypsin inhibitors. Thus found kallikreinogen in the pseudoglobulin fraction of bovine plasma, that is activated by trypsin, and also a trypsin-binding protein in bovine plasma. SUZUKI estimated that bovine plasma kallikreinogen has a molecular weight of about 150,000 (SUZUKI et al., 1967).

Recently MORIYA (1964a, b, 1965a, b, 1966, 1967a, b), SUZUKI (1965a, b), SUZUKI and HAYASHI (1967), SUZUKI and NAGASAWA (1967); and his co-workers NAGASAWA and SUZUKI (1966), NAGASAWA and HAYASHI (1967), and IWANAGA and SUZUKI (1967), have written a number of reviews.

OKAMOTO has studied the fibrinolytic system—plasmin plasminogen—and developed the plasmin inhibitors—ε-aminocaproic acid (EACA) and trans-4-aminomethylcyclohexanecarboxylic acid (TAMCHA)—during the last twenty years in Japan. Recently OKAMOTO and co-workers (MORIGUCHI et al., 1966a, b, c, and 1967) investigated the activity of the kinin-forming enzyme in the plasmin system, and hoped to clarify the mechanism of kinin formation *in vivo*. They concluded that plasmin activated by large amounts of streptokinase (SK) was able to produce kinin, but plasmin activated by the plasminogen-activating component from dog kidney tissue did not produce kinin. This property in the latter system resembled plasmin activated by small amounts of SK. They concluded that kinin-forming enzymatic activity was possibly part of the activation of plasmin in a broad sense. They also reported that a bradykinin and/or other kinins were found in the intraperitoneal fluid, produced by inoculating mice or rats with ascitic Ehrlich or Yoshida tumor cells. Their results indicated that the kinin-forming enzyme possibly differs from the fibrinolytic enzyme and might be the esterolytic TAMe.

FUJII and his colleagues studied the inhibition of both caseinolytic and fibrinolytic activities of plasmin by various synthetic inhibitors—derivatives of amino acids, fatty acids, and so on—in papers published since 1965 in the *Journal of Biochemistry* and other journals in English. He reported his studies on plasmin also in Japanese journals (MURAMATSU et al., 1964; FUJII et al., 1965; SATO and FUJII, 1966) in which the various activation mechanisms of human and bovine plasminogens by streptokinase were examined. He clarified the relationship between structure and inhibitory effects of various synthetic inhibitors. ε-Aminocaproic acid (EACA) inhibited the effect on fibrinolytic and fibrinogenolytic activities of plasmin, but it had no effect on caseinolytic activity. No inhibitory effect of hexyl ε-aminocaproate was shown on the esterase activities of kallikrein and thrombin. FUJII and co-workers investigated the kinin-releasing activity of plasmin, using purified plasminogen and bovine bradykininogen. They suggested that kinin was formed directly by streptokinase-activated plasmin and that this plasma kinin might be bradykinin. His group also observed no activation of plasma kallikreinogen by plasmin. At that time they found that hexyl δ-guanidinovalerate inhibited the esterolytic activities of plasmin and plasma kallikrein, while hexyl ε-aminocaproate had no effect on the latter enzyme (WATANABE et al., 1967). FUJII has recently reviewed the activation mechanism of the plasmin system (FUJII and MURAMATSU, 1966, 1967) and the enzyme chemistry of plasmin, kallikrein, and the kinin-releasing system (FUJII et al., 1967).

The antifibrinolytic activity of Trasylol was scrutinized by KAZAMA et al. (1963), who used synthetic substrates such as N^{α}-benzoyl-L-arginine ethyl ester (BAEe) and N^{α}-*p*-toluensulfonyl-L-arginine methyl ester (TAMe). Its antiplasmin activity was quite remarkable, but its inhibition of activators of plasminogen from tissues and of proactivator with streptokinase was not so effective as the substances discussed above.

Hayashi recently studied permeability factors. His original papers have been published mainly in *Biochimica et Biophysica Acta* since 1966. Summarized studies were also introduced in Japanese by Hayashi (1965, 1966). He purified and isolated permeability factors responsible for the delayed vascular response in cutaneous Arthus-type and thermally induced inflammations in the rabbit skin. He also studied the chemical, physicochemical, and biological properties of the substances involved. He attempted to determine the chemical nature of the agents associated with inflammation. According to him, many substances had been proposed, but no conclusive evidence had hitherto been advanced to establish that any of them was present in inflammatory tissues with appropriate activity at times when vascular permeability was increased as a result of tissue injury, or that such permeability factor(s) could be responsible for the increased permeability in inflammation. According to Hayashi it was doubtful that bradykinin or kinin would be a natural mediator in the inflammatory process. He believed that the chemical mediator should have the following properties: (1) it should be present in injured tissue; (2) its activity should be responsible for vascular lesion in each phase; (3) its action must be intense and prolonged; (4) it should have a unique action as a mediator; (5) it should reproduce the same type of vascular response.

From these points of view, the importance of kinins in this process was quite doubtful. Most of the experiments hitherto done with kinins *in vitro* should be done under more biological conditions. The participation of permeability factors —Arthus PF and burn PF found by him—was thought to be reasonable and in very good agreement with those definitions given above. He also isolated chemotaxis-promoting factor (CPF) in the same type inflammation in the rabbit skin and also a kind of SH-proteinase having inhibitory action against Arthus PF and burn PF (anti-Arthus PF and anti-burn PF) in the same place in injured tissue. Japanese opinion is divided about the importance of kinins in inflammation.

In the fourth Annual Meeting of the Japan Society of Clinical Biochemistry and Metabolism held in March 1967, inflammation was discussed from various points of view by several investigators. Hayashi (1968) summarized his views on Arthus-type and burn-type inflammations. Yamamura (1968) described the recently developed biochemical concept of inflammation, including kinin problems. Many members joined in the discussion, including representatives of the drug industry.

Iwata (Osaka University) presented his paper, "Changes in the responses of the guinea-pig isolated ileum to bradykinin, acetylcholine and histamine after treatment of proteolytic enzymes" at the meeting of the Japanese Pharmacological Association (1967). In this paper it could not be denied that the action of the proteolytic enzymes *in vivo* and *in vitro* was related to their proteolytic activities, but other factors such as the allosteric site or steric configuration of the proteolytic enzymes, which might change the protein conformation of the receptor or the membrane, might also be taken into consideration. His paper, "Pharmacological significances of peptidase and proteinase in brain", presented to the Japanese Pharmacological Society (1967) concluded that some changes in the metabolism of brain protein might be expected during convulsion.

K. Hashimoto (Tohoku University) developed the cross-circulation technique in dogs, and the depressor, or the pressor, or the combined reflex was tested by use of bradykinin and kallikrein. His papers also appeared in English.

Katori determined the concentrations of kinin-forming and kinin-destroying enzymes as well as lysosomal and cytoplasmic enzymes and protein in the synovial fluid collected from patients with rheumatoid arthritis and related diseases. It was concluded in his results that the intracellular enzymes of the synovial fluid were derived mainly from the synocium and the leukocytes, whereas the kinin enzymes originated from the plasma. This study was also summarized in the *Journal of Physiology*. His colleagues in the pharmacological field published some papers in the Japanese *Journal of Pharmacology* in English. The titles are given below. A. SAKUMA et al. (Tokyo Med. and Dental Univ.): "Tranexamic acid enhances bradykinin-induced venoconstriction". T. ENOMOTO et al. (Tokyo Med. and Dental Univ.): "Kininase activity of stem bromelain". H. OHASHI et al. (Univ. of Hokkaido): "Effects of angiotensin, bradykinin and oxytocin on electrical and mechanical activities in the taenia coli of the guinea pig". H. ITOH et al. (Yokohama City Univ.): "Comparative effects of bradykinin, kallidin and nitroglycerin on the peripheral vascular system in dogs".

In the preliminary study by ANAN and OHTA (1965), tryptic hydrolysis of N^{α}-benzoyl-L-arginine-β-naphthylamide (BANA) was followed fluorometrically in the presence and absence of rabbit serum. The inhibitory titer of serum was estimated by the hydrolysis rates in rabbits. The amount of serum required for 50% inhibition of BANA hydrolysis by trypsin (30 μg) was estimated. The trypsin-inhibiting action of normal serum was markedly decreased by incubation with kallikrein (Padutin), 10–15 FU/0.5 ml serum at 37° for 1 hour. The availability of the present method for enzymatic determination of free kallikrein-inhibitor was discussed.

MIYANAGA et al. (1967) studied the behavior of the kinin system in blood by the immunoassay method for plasma kallikrein. They made the kallikrein antibody in rabbits and developed the assay method for plasma kallikrein. With this technique 0.01 to 25 μg/ml plasma kallikrein could be estimated. They also measured the kallikrein concentration levels in blood in various disease states. In anaphylactic shock caused by the injections of histamine, serotonin, bradykinin, or egg albumin into dogs, no clear change in plasma kallikrein level could be observed, except for some high values obtained after histamine was given. From these observations it was assumed that histamine would cause the activation of plasma kallikrein.

There are some organic chemists in Japan interested in this field. YANAIHARA et al. synthesized 1-glutamic acid kallidin, and sarcosine-containing bradykinin analogs such as 2-, 3-, and 7-sarcosine, 2,3-disarcosine, and 2,3,7-trisarcosine bradykinins. Biological activities of these analogs were compared with those of synthetic bradykinin (YANAIHARA et al., 1967; YANAIHARA and SEKIYA, 1967).

SAKAKIBARA (1966) developed an improved synthesis of bradykinin. When *p*-nitrophenyl trifluoroacetate (I), 2,4,5-trichlorophenyl trifluoroacetate (II), and N-hydroxysuccinimide trifluoroacetate (III) were subjected to ANDERSON'S racemization test, only reagent III showed resistance against racemization. However, reagents I and II were also found to be useful for fragment-condensation with acylpeptides possessing glycine or proline at the C-terminal end. Bradykinin was prepared with these reagents. During the synthesis, a combination of the t-amyloxycarbonyl N-protecting group and the benzyl ester was mainly used, and the alkaline hydrolysis procedure of the ester group was eliminated. Thus, colorless bradykinin with full activity was obtained in a satisfactory yield without any purification procedure.

The contractile activity of bradykinin homologs was examined on the mouse small intestine or guinea pig ileum by KAMEYAMA and SASAKI (1966) and KAMEYAMA et al. (1967) and K. SUZUKI et al. (1966). Thr^6-bradykinin had 70% of the activity of bradykinin in mouse and 49.2% in guinea pig; O-acetyl Ser^6-bradykinin 45% in mouse, 18.4% in guinea pig; O-acetyl Thr^6-bradykinin 20% in mouse, 36.8% in guinea pig. Leu[6]-, β-Ala[6]-, β-Ala[4]-, Leu[4]-, Leu[4],O-acetyl-Ser[6]-, Gly[3],O-acetyl-Ser[6]-, Sar[3],Gly[6]-bradykinins were also tested. Disubstitution was less active than the monosubstitution.

The bulky side chain (Leu, Ileu, Val) produced marked loss of the activity. The substitution of 4 or 6 position for β-alanine which elongated the peptide chain by one methylene group retained the activity, but disubstitution resulted in the loss of activity. On the guinea pig ileum the most active bradykinin fragment was Phe-Ser-Pro-Phe-Arg, which had 5.5% of the activity of bradykinin. Arg-Pro-Pro-Gly-Phe-Ser had the same inflammatory action as bradykinin on rat paw edema. The fragment of co-fibrinopeptide B of ox, Arg-Pro-Lys-Val-Gly-Leu-Gly-Ala-Arg, potentiated the contraction induced by bradykinin.

TAMURA et al. successfully developed the micromethod of chemical detection, using 1-dimethyl-aminonaphthalene-5-sulfonyl chloride (DNS-Cl) for deca-, nona- and octapeptide analogs of bradykinin. This method will be widely employed for the analysis of minute quantities of peptides—usually 50–100 μg—in biological materials and also for establishing their primary structure (TAMURA et al., 1967).

YOSHINAGA et al. did some basic and clinical investigations in this field. Their papers were mostly reported in the *Tohoku Journal of Experimental Medicine* (1963–67) and in *Experientia* in English. Their interest seemed to be mainly to elucidate the roles of this kinin system in certain pathological conditions. The titles of their papers were: "Assay of urinary kinin"; "Excretion of urinary kinin in man"; "Evidence for the renal origin of urinary kinin"; "Assay of kininase activity in human blood"; "Urinary excretion of kinin in man with special reference to its origin"; "Estimation of kinin in peripheral blood in man"; "Kininase activity in human blood"; "Kininase activity in human blood in normal and pathological conditions"; and "Circulating plasma kinin in patients with bronchial asthma". A review of this field was written by YOSHINAGA et al. (1964).

YAMURA (1961, 1963) examined the skin reaction in man to injection of kallikrein. On the injected site some subjects complained of itching, but the whealing reaction was not observed. Quantities of bradykinin were never found in human skin. Human skin proteases were activated by croton oil, antigen–antibody reaction, and other stimuli. Proteases were extracted from frozen human skin and were incubated with heated dog globulin. Liberated kinins were extracted by the method of ROCHA E SILVA and measured on atropinized rat uterus. Results showed kininformation by human skin proteases.

In the human experiments by OKUMURA and KAWAZU (1966), bradykinin (5 μg/0.1 ml) was injected i.d. to the thigh and upper arm of two subjects with chronic urticaria. Biopsies were done at 30 minutes and 24 hours after the injections. Mast cells in the vicinity of *röhrenförmige Hülle* of JABONERO (mixed nerve) in the papillary layers had discharged argyrophil granules; the mixed nerves showed mild opaque degeneration. Mast cells were considered to exert strong influence upon the mixed nerve fiber. SCHWANN's cells within the vegetative end formation also discharged some argyrophil granules, which was suggestive of the so-called neurohormonal cell. The bradykinin-injected area showed degenerations in general except for the thick neurofibrils. The sensory neurofibrils exhibited many incisura formations of various sizes, suggestive of pain. Capillary walls in the papillary layers were swollen. The vegetative end formations showed swelling and opaque degeneration.

SHIMAMOTO et al. perfused rabbit saphenous vein (ISHIOKA et al., 1965a), ear marginal vein (HAZAMA, 1965), and dog coronary vein (SUNAGA et al., 1965a). Using these techniques they examined the venoconstriction caused by bradykinin, histamine, substance P, acetylcholine, epinephrine, norepinephrine, and isoprenaline and the venodilatation by vasopressin. They observed that bradykinin was antagonized by pyridinolcarbamate, cyproheptadine, acetylsalicylate, and estrogens (ISHIOKA et al., 1965a; SUNAGA et al., 1965a; SHIMAMOTO and ISHIOKA, 1967). Pyridinolcarbamate antagonized not only the permeability increasing effect of bradykinin in blueing lesions in rabbit (YAMAZAKI et al., 1965a), guinea pig and rat (ISOKANE, 1965a, b) but also the leukocyte migration in rabbit skin (SUNAGA et al., 1965b, c) induced by i.d. injection of bradykinin and the so-called bradykinin cry and struggle (FUJITA et al., 1965a). The latter were induced by injection of bradykinin into carotid artery of rabbit.

Pyridinolcarbamate also antagonized hemorrhage in rabbit eyeground (FUJITA et al., 1965b; SHIMAMOTO and ISHIOKA, 1967) induced by concomitant injection of bradykinin and epinephrine into the homolateral carotid artery. According to SHIMAMOTO, the most important experimental findings of his school were the edematous arterial reaction (SHIMAMOTO and SUNAGA, 1962; SHIMAMOTO, 1963a) and its prevention by several substances including pyridinolcarbamate (SHIMAMOTO, 1963a; KUBOTA, 1965), estrogen, and glucocorticoids. The stagnation of serous substances in the arterial wall had been suspected by the classical German school as an initiating mechanism in atherogenesis. This reaction was induced as an immediate reaction by oral administration of so-called atherogenic substances such as cholesterol, saturated fatty acid, and animal fats and by intravenous injection of epinephrine (KUBOTA, 1965), or high molecular weight substances including endotoxin (SHIMAMOTO, 1959), glycogen, and dextran, and also by traumatization such as crushing the thigh muscles or by painful stimuli in rabbits (ISHII, 1965). They also found that the infusion of highly diluted bradykinin solution induced the reaction (KUBOTA, 1965).

SHIMAMOTO's school reported that vasa vasorum were distributed in all muscular layers including the innermost ones situated directly beneath the internal elastic lamina of aortic wall and the trunks of coronary arteries of rabbit, dog, and man (SUNAGA et al., 1967a; SASAKI et al., 1967). In addition, the capillary wall of the vasa vasorum in rabbit and man were characteristically rich in porous capillary; on the other hand the porous capillary was absent or extremely poor in dog, monkey, and rat. The opening of endothelial gaps in vasa vasorum of aortas was found in all these animal species (SHIMAMOTO et al., 1967; SUNAGA et al., 1967). SHIMAMOTO assumed that constriction in venous vasa vasorum by endogenous inflammatory substances contributes to the transportation of the serous substance through the pores into the arterial wall in rabbit and man and may also lead to the endothelial gaps of vasa vasorum resulting in the edematous arterial reaction (SHIMAMOTO, 1963b). This reaction was prevented by pyridinolcarbamate, estrogens, nialamide, cyproheptadine, acetylsalicylate, and aminopyrin (KUBOTA, 1965), which antagonized the venoconstrictive effect and the capillary permeability-increasing action of bradykinin; and also by Trasylol, soybean trypsin inhibitor, and glucocorticoids (KUBOTA, 1965), which antagonize bradykinin-forming enzyme. The agents capable of preventing the edematous arterial reaction had been shown by SHIMAMOTO et al. to prevent the formation of experimental atherosclerosis in cholesterol-fed animals (NUMANO et al., 1965).

Pyridinolcarbamate was given to 1,800 patients suffering from cerebral, coronary, and extremity atherosclerotic disorders, and its statistically significant therapeutic efficiency has been tested during the past 5 years (YAMAZAKI et al., 1965b, c; ATSUMI et al., 1965a, 1967). The preventive effect of pyridinolcarbamate against the relapse of apoplexy (YAMAZAKI and ISHIOKA, 1965), myocardial infarction, idiopathic thrombocytopenic purpura (ISHIOKA et al., 1965b; SHIMA-

Moto et al., 1965), non-thrombocytopenic purpura, and painful status in Takayasu disease (Atsumi et al., 1965b) was also reported.

Other investigators tested the antibradykinin activity of N-p-chloro-benzhydryl-N'-methyl homopiperazine dihydrochloride (homochlorcyclizine) which had been known as a serotonin antagonist. Miyake et al. (1966) examined and compared its antibradykinin activity with that of diphenhydramine and chlorpheniramine on guinea pig ileum. Homochlorcyclizine was the strongest antagonist, followed by diphenhydramine and chlorpheniramine. This action did not parallel the antihistamine activity. Iwaki et al. reported (26th meeting of the Japanese Pharmacological Society, Kinki Region) the antibradykinin activity of this material, tested on guinea pig ileum and rat uterus. Doses of bradykinin used were 5×10^{-8}, and 1×10^{-9} g/ml in both assays. Miyanaga (1964) reported that the antibradykinin activity of this material on the guinea pig ileum was the best of 12 antiallergy drugs, employed acetylsalicylic acid and antihistamines. He also found that the drug protected guinea pigs against anaphylactic shock but was not specific against bradykinin only.

Thereafter some clinical investigations in dermatology and urology were performed. For instance, protective effects of homocholcyclizine on pruritic skin diseases, bronchial asthma, perennial rhinitis, seasonal hayfever, urticaria, angioedema, dermatitis, etc. were tested. Some therapeutic effects were reported by Kinoshita (1964), Muramoto (1965), Toyoizumi et al. (1965), Ohkido (1964), Sakamoto (1967), Aoki (1967), Miyazawa (1967a, b), and others. Other papers published outside Japan dealt with the same topic.

Ohkido (1964) tested the antibradykinin drug, homochlorcyclizine against histamine, serotonin, and bradykinin, using the strip method of Pinkus on six normal human adults. The results showed that histamine and bradykinin induced blueing in the lesions, and serotonin was only slightly active. Homochlorcyclizine depressed these phenomena, especially those induced by bradykinin. Clinical study of this drug was also carried out in 54 cases of pruritic skin diseases; 87% responded well. Side reactions in 8 cases were a mild sleeping tendency and in 2 cases a gastric disturbance.

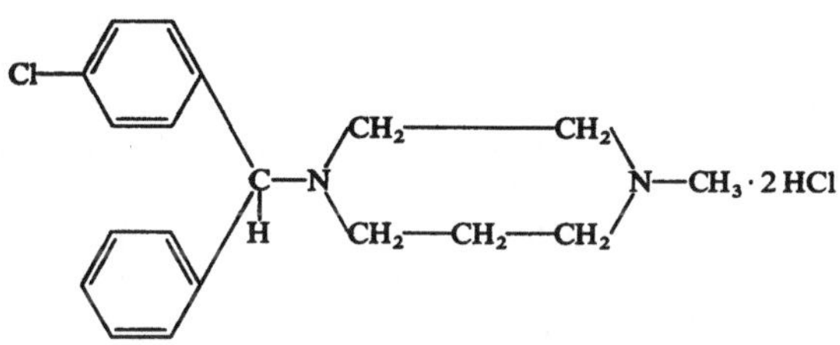

Homochlorcyclizine

Sakamoto et al. (1967) treated clinical subjects with homochlorcyclizine (60 mg/day) and found beneficial effects in 33 (83%) of 40 patients suffering from urticaria; 9 healed without recurrence. They concluded that homochlorcyclizine might not only be in competition with some mediators concerned with the onset of urticaria, but might also serve in stabilizing the vascular motor nerve.

Aoki et al. (1967a, b, 1968) also examined the clinical problems of the field. Intradermal injection to rats of phlogistic agents such as histamine, acetylcholine, serotonin, and bradykinin increased the capillary permeability to circulating Evans blue and produced visible blue lesions. The characteristics of blue macules elicited by these substances were slightly different. By combining the phlogistic agent with an anti-inflammatory drug such as diphenhydramine, cyproheptadine, homochlorcyclizine, or dexamethasone the development of macules was inhibited. The antagonism between those mediators and antiphlogistic agents was discussed. Aoki et al. compared the biological activities of bradykinin and histamine. Bradykinin exhibited anaphylactoid reaction, a marked local edema, perivascular inflammatory infiltration, and increased capillary permeability in mice or rats in various doses. These were antagonized by the anti-inflammatory drugs noted above. Histamine showed qualitatively the same action, but it was less than one tenth that of bradykinin. By their experiments on a pretreatment based on the use of histamine liberators and on histological observation, they excluded bradykinin as a histamine liberator except in the early stage.

In Miyazawa's experimental allergic contact dermatitis of guinea pig, changes of tissue mast cell and inhibitory effect of antihistamines were studied (Miyazawa, 1967a, b). No new finding was added to the principle that histamine was not a causal agent of allergic contact dermatitis. It might be concluded that protease played an important role in development of contact allergy in guinea pigs.

The Institute for Protein Research of Osaka University and the Research Foundation for Protein have been organizing annual peptide symposia since 1964. These have not been international, but have become an annual event in the field of peptide chemistry. On October 31, 1966, the Tanabe Amino Acid Research Foundation planned an international symposium on biologically active polypeptides in conjunction with that institute. One session was devoted to hypotensive peptides, kinins, and their related substances. Papers were given by N. Back (1967a), S. Okamoto (1967), S. Fujii (1967), E. G. Erdös (1967), L. M. Greenbaum (1967), H. Moriya (1967c), T. Suzuki (1967a), N. Back (1967b), K. Abe et al. (1967) and Y. Yamamura (1967). The reports summarized in Japanese appeared in the *Journal of Clinical Science (Japan)*, 3 (3, 4), 592–629.

The Third International Congress of Diseases of the Digestive Organs was held in Tokyo in 1966. At that time an international Trasylol symposium was held there. Only the titles of presentations are listed here. "Recent progress in therapeutic treatment of acute pancreatitis", by K. Heinkel. "Clinical application and experiments on Trasylol", by K. Honjo et al. "Experimental and clinical observations on Trasylol", by M. Fujimoto et al. "Experimental and clinical observations on pancreatitis", by K. H. Grözinger. "Pathological and anatomical observations after administration of a large amount of Trasylol (7,500,000 KIU/12 hr.)", by M. Wanke. "Experimental and therapeutic studies of Trasylol on pancreatitis", by K. Saito. "Application of Trasylol with acute pancreatitis and pancreatitis after operation", by I. Murata et al. "Study of Trasylol action on acute pancreatitis", by Y. Tsukiyama. Thus Trasylol has been recently employed widely as a drug in Japan.

A small group for research on plasma kinin was organized by Y. Kimura, H. Hatano, and H. Moriya in 1967; the first meeting was held in February 1967. The subjects were reviewed by Suzuki (1967b), Aoki and Saito (1967), and Takeda (1967). The second meeting was held in September 1967; the proceedings were published in the *Journal of Allergy (Japan)*. The third one was scheduled for June 1968. The meetings reflect the increased interest in the subject in Japan.

The Seventh International Congress of Biochemistry was held in Tokyo August 20–25, 1967. At that time the Symposium on Vasoactive Polypeptides and Inhibitors of Proteolytic Enzymes was organized by E. Werle, T. Suzuki, and Y. Yamamura. The following papers were presented there: "Physiological and pathological significance of plasma kinins", by E. Werle. "On the mechanism of kinin liberation from plasma", by E. Habermann. "Vasodilatation and hypotension in dogs caused by intravasal infusion of thrombin", by A. Delin et al.

"Partial purification of bovine plasma kallikrein activated by contact with glass", by T. SUZUKI. "Studies on the intestinal absorption of ^{131}I-labeled hog pancreatic kallikrein", by H. MORIYA. "Anti-renin active peptide", by Y. YAMAMURA. "Angiotensin and bradykinin", by K. ARAKAWA. "Studies on the pulmonary inactivation of bradykinin", by J. M. STEWART et al. "Studies on the metabolism of bradykinin in inflammation", by L. M. GREENBAUM. "Clinical studies on plasma kinin", by K. YOSHINAGA. "Effect of kinin and other drugs on collateral channels", by Y. YOSHITOSHI et al. "On the effect of kallikrein on peripheral arterial blood flow", by Y. KASAI et al. "On the effect of kallikrein on cerebral circulation and metabolism", by Y. GOTO. "Origin of kinin enzymes and intracellular enzymes in the synovial fluid of rheumatoid patients", by M. KATORI. These summaries were printed both in English and Japanese.

ROCHA E SILVA's lecture was published in *Amino Acids* in Japanese (ROCHA E SILVA, 1968).

International Symposium on Synthetic and Natural Proteinase Inhibitors: Basic and Clinical Aspects, was held at the University of Tokyo under the auspices of the Japanese Society of Medical Sciences in November 1967. Summaries of the presentations will be published.

The field was reviewed in a number of Japanese journals. The *Journal of Clinical Science* (vol. 2) collected papers on basic problems of plasma kinins by SUZUKI (1966), MURAOKA (1966), KIMURA (1966), and ARAKAWA (1966). Also *Metabolism and Disease*, (vol. 5) published useful reviews by NAKAJIMA (1968), YANO (1968), and HASHIMOTO (1968).

There are now many investigators who are eager to study this field in Japan. However it appears to the author of this review that it is important to exchange detailed data on studies from different laboratories throughout the world. This is necessary because differences in purity of preparations, in species, in biological standardization, etc. can complicate matters. Hence international cooperation is needed to establish definitely all the physiological and pathological roles kinins may play.

The author would like to apologize to any Japanese investigators whose contributions might have been overlooked, and to those whose work could only be summarized without detail in this chapter, owing to the large number of Japanese publications dealing with kinins.

References

ABE, K., WATABE, N., KUMAGAYA, N., MORI, T., SEKI, T., ONO, H., YOSHINAGA, K.: Clinical studies on plasma kinins. J. clin. Sci. (Japan) **3**, 626 (1967).

ANAN, K., OHTA, K.: Fluorometric assay of kallikrein inhibitor and trypsin-inhibitor (preliminary report). Ochanomizu med. J. **13**, 259 (1965).

AOKI, K., SAITO, T.: Comparison of biological activities of bradykinin and histamine. J. Allergy **16**, 624 (1967).

— — Has bradykinin a character as histamine liberator? J. Allergy, in press (1968).

— SHIMOTOGE, M.: On the antagonism between phlogistic agents and anti-inflammatory drugs in the skin. Acta derm. (Kyoto) **62**, 96 (1967).

— — IKEGAMI, T.: Comparative studies on the biological activities of bradykinin and histamine. Skin Res. **9**, 413 (1967).

ARAKAWA, K.: Blood pressure and kinins. J. clin. Sci. (Japan) **2**, 402 (1966).

ATSUMI, T., ISOKANE, N., YAMASHITA, S., SANO, T., ODAKURA, T., KURAI, A.: Treatment of arteriosclerosis obliterans with pyridinolcarbamate. Jap. Soc. int. Med. **56**, 49 (1967).

— SANO, T., KUBOTA, A., KURAI, A.: Treatment of pain by pyridinolcarbamate. Ochanomizu med. J. **13**, 273 (1965b).

— — ODAKURA, T., YAGISHITA, M., ITOH, Y.: Treatment of arteriosclerosis obliterans by pyridinolcarbamate. Ochanomizu med. J. **13**, 245 (1965a).

Back, N.: Depressor peptides—kinins and their related substances. J. clin. Sci. (Japan) 3, 592 (1967a).
— Pathological and physiological studies on vasoactive peptides. J. clin. Sci. (Japan) 3, 622 (1967b).
Erdös, E. G.: Inactivating enzymes of depressor peptides in blood and tissues. J. clin. Sci. (Japan) 3, 605 (1967).
Fujii, S.: Kinin formation by plasmin and kallikrein and its inhibitory action with synthetic inhibitors. J. clin. Sci. (Japan) 3, 601 (1967).
— Ikegami, H., Sato, S., Nishii, H., Onishi, T., Muramatsu, M.: Studies on plasmin. Symp. Chem. Physiol. Pathol. 5, 167 (1965).
— Muramatsu, M.: Activation mechanism of plasminogen. Saishin Igaku 21, 238 (1966).
— — Biochemistry of plasmin. Protein, Nucleic Acid, Enzyme 12, 226 (1967).
— — Watanabe, H.: Enzyme chemistry of plasmin, kallikrein and kinin-releasing system. Sogo Rinshyo 16, 1799 (1967).
Fujita, T., Kubota, A., Yamashita, S.: Preventive effect of pyridinolcarbamate and heparin against pseudoaffective response induced by bradykinin. Ochanomizu med. J. 13, 255 (1965a).
— Kurai, A., Kubota, A., Yamashita, S.: New method of inducing retinal hemorrhage and prevention by pyridinolcarbamate. Ochanomizu med. J. 13, 241 (1965b).
Greenbaum, L. M.: Studies on kinin forming and destroying enzymes of tissues and leucocytes. J. clin. Sci. (Japan) 3, 612 (1967).
Hashimoto, K.: Vascular response of kinin substance. Metabolism & Disease 5, 266 (1968).
Hayashi, H.: Biochemical approach to inflammation. Metabolism & Disease 2, 708 (1965).
— Some problems in the mechanism of pathologic vascular permeability. Seitai no Kagaku 17, 269 (1966).
— Study of permeability factors mediating increased vascular response in Arthus- and burn-type inflammations. Proc. Japan Soc. Clin. Biochem. Metabol. 4, 95 (1968).
Hazama, H.: Effect of endogenous vasoactive substances on marginal vein of isolated rabbit ear. Ochanomizu med. J. 13, 69 (1965).
Imamura, H.: On the effects on the rabbit blood constituents of kallikrein, parotin and the extract of the pancreas. Fukuoka J. exp. Med. 48, 2010 (1957).
Ishii, Y.: Edematous arterial reaction induced by traumatic stress and prevention by pyridinolcarbamate. Ochanomizu med. J. 13, 145 (1965).
Ishioka, T., Matsumura, T., Takeuchi, K., Sano, T., Odakura, T., Ohta, K.: Hemostatic effect of pyridinolcarbamate in purpura induced by bradykinin injection and some hemorrhagic diathesis. Ochanomizu med. J. 13, 263 (1965b).
— — — Yagishita, M., Hazama, H.: Studies on venoconstriction effect of venoactive substances on saphenous vein of rabbit and antagonists of venoconstriction induced by bradykinin. Ochanomizu med. J. 13, 77 (1965a).
Isokane, N.: Species difference in the increase of the capillary permeability by bradykinin. Ochanomizu med. J. 13, 103 (1965a).
— Inhibitory effect of oral pretreatment with pyridinolcarbamate and cyproheptadine on increased capillary permeability induced by intradermal injection of bradykinin, lysylbradykinin, kallikrein, histamine and serotonin in guinea pigs. Ochanomizu med. J. 13, 107 (1965b).
Itoh, S.: Studies on biological experiment and clinical application about the blood-pressure controlling substance in pancreas. Fukuoka J. exp. Med. 46, 1060 (1955).
Iwanaga, S., Suzuki, T.: Biochemistry of plasma kinins. Seikagaku (J. Jap. Biochem. Soc.) 39, 137 (1967).
Kameyama, T., Sasaki, K.: Effect of bradykinin related compounds on the smooth muscle. Folia pharmacol. jap. 62, 100* (1966).
— — Nabeshima, J.: Contractile action of bradykinin analogues on the ileum in guinea pigs and rats. Folia pharmacol. jap. 63, 27* (1967).
Kazama, M., Abe, T., Yoshitoshi, Y.: Studies on fibrinolysis estimation, applying synthetic substrate (BAEe). Acta haemat. jap. 26, 246 (1963).
Kimura, Y.: Shock and kinins. J. clin. Sci. (Japan) 2, 394 (1966).
Kinoshita, M.: Studies on experimental histamine pruritus. Jap. J. Dermatol. 74, 327 (1964).
Kubota, A.: Edematous arterial reaction induced by various substances and its prevention. Ochanomizu med. J. 13, 133 (1965).
Miyake, M., Sekiya, J., Kanda, Z.: Anti-bradykinin activity of diphenhydramine on the isolated guinea pig ileum. Folia pharmacol. jap. 62, 225 (1966).
Miyanaga, Y.: Studies on the biological activities of bradykinin and its significance on allergia or inflammation: Antibradykinin activity of anti-allergy drugs. J. Allergy (Japan) 13, 655 (1964).

MIYANAGA, Y., KIMURA, Y., HASHIMOTO, K.: The behavior of kinin system in blood studied by the immunoassay method of plasma kallikrein. Igaku-no ayumi **62**, 500 (1967).
MIYAZAWA, T.: Studies on factors except cell bound antibody influencing experimental allergic contact dermatitis. Jap. J. clin. Dermatol. **21**, 1264 (1967a).
— A role of protease in the development of experimental allergic contact dermatitis. Jap. J. clin. Dermatol. **21**, 1283 (1967b).
MORIGUCHI, T., MIHARA, H., FUNAHARA, Y., OKAMOTO, S.: Study on the separation of fibrinolytic and kinin-forming systems. J. Jap. Blood Assoc. **29**, 160 (1966a).
— — — OSHIBA, S., OKAMOTO, S.: A study of the kinin-forming system: With special reference to ascites. J. Physiol. (Japan) **28**, 405 (1966b).
— — ICHIHASHI, M., MORIGUCHI, S., OKAMOTO, S.: Analysis of the process of kinin-formation: With special reference to SK-activated plasmin. J. Physiol. (Japan) **29**, 444 (1967).
— MORIGUCHI, S., OKAMOTO, S.: Analysis of the process of kinin (bradykinin)-formation by streptokinase. J. Allergy (Japan) **15**, 44 (1966c).
MORIYA, H.: About a few local hormones. Hormone and Rinshyō **5**, 73 (1957).
— Chemical studies on kallikrein. II. Purification with acrinol. Yakugaku Zasshi (J. Pharmaceutical Soc. Japan) **79**, 32 (1959a).
— Chemical studies on kallikrein. V. Stability of water solution of kallikrein. Yakugaku Zasshi (J. Pharmaceutical Soc. Japan) **79**, 1216 (1959b).
— Chemical studies on kallikrein. VI. Amino acid composition and terminal amino acids. Yakugaku Zasshi (J. Pharmaceutical Soc. Japan) **79**, 1390 (1959c).
— Chemical studies on kallikrein. VII. Structural sugar of kallikrein. Yakugaku Zasshi (J. Pharmaceutical Soc. Japan) **79**, 1394 (1959d).
— Chemical studies on kallikrein. VIII. Molecular weight of kallikrein and the supplement. Yakugaku Zasshi (J. Pharmaceutical Soc. Japan) **79**, 1451 (1959e).
— Method of extraction and purification of circulatory hormone kallikrein from pancreas, submaxillary gland and urine of mammalian animals. Japanese patent 35—3045 (1960).
— New research development of kallikrein and related substances. Nihon Rinshyō **20**, 765 (1962a).
— Summary of international symposium (held in New York, 1962) on structure and function of biologically active peptides: Bradykinin, kallidin and congeners. Protein, Nucleic Acid, Enzyme **7**, 670 (1962b).
— Bradykinin, kallidin and other biologically active peptides. Protein, Nucleic Acid, Enzyme **7**, 382 (1962c).
— Physiologically active peptides—bradykinin and angiotensin. Sōgō Igaku **20**, 353 (1963a).
— Bradykinin. J. Pract. Pharmacist Soc. Japan **15** (8), 7 (1963b).
— Biochemistry of physiologically active peptides. Metabolism & Disease **1**, 77 (1964a).
— Studies on estimation of kallikrein in human urine. Nihon Rinshyō **22**, 2659 (1964b).
— Physiologically active peptides. Seitai-no Kagaku **16**, 54 (1965a).
— The kallikrein-kallidinogen-kallidin system and its physiological and pathological roles. (Read by M. E. WEBSTER.) Nihon Rinshyō **23**, 1802 (1965b).
— Kallikreins. Chemistry & Biology **4**, 356 (1966).
— Active peptides releasing enzymes—kallikreins. Sōgō Rinshyō **16**, 24 (1967a).
— Problems of active peptides in the field of pathological biochemistry. Saishin Igaku **22**, 865 (1967b).
— Bovine clostrokinin liberation by human salivary kallikrein and its properties. J. clin. Sci. (Japan) **3**, 616 (1967c).
— DEGUCHI, M., ASANO H.: Chemical studies on kallikrein. I. The amount of kallikrein contained in various organs and its isolation and purification. Yakugaku Zasshi (J. Pharmaceutical Soc. Japan) **78**, 346 (1958).
— KATO, A.: Modified purification of hog pancreatic kallikrein. Abstract of 88th Annual Meeting of Japanese Pharmaceutical Soc., 406 (1968).
— SHIMAZAWA, E.: Chemical studies on kallikrein. III. Purification by zone electrophoresis. Yakugaku Zasshi (J. Pharmaceutical Soc. Japan) **79**, 374 (1959a).
— — Chemical studies on kallikrein. IV. The isoelectric point of kallikrein. (J. Pharmaceutical Soc. Japan) **79**, 688 (1959b).
MURAMATSU, M., ONISHI, T., SATO, T., MAKINO, S., HAYAKUMO, Y., KITAJIMA, K., FUJII, S.: Studies on plasmin. Symp. Chem. Physiol. and Pathol. **4**, 146 (1964).
MURAMOTO, S.: Therapeutic study of skin disease: Effect of homochlorcyclizine. Dermatol. & Urol. **27**, 348 (1965).
MURAOKA, S.: Plasma kinins and other active substances on inflammation process. J. clin. Sci. (Japan) **2**, 385 (1966).
NAGASAWA, S., HAYASHI, K.: Hypotensive peptides—their structure and enzymatic formation. Sōgō Rinshyō **16**, 16 (1967).
— SUZUKI, T.: Kinins and their metabolic regulation. J. clin. Sci. **2**, 535 (1966).

Nakajima, T.: Naturally occurring hypotensive peptides in other than mammals. Metabolism & Disease 5, 253 (1968).
Numano, F., Fujita, T., Hiroki, T.: Atherosclerosis-inhibiting effect of the antibradykinin agent pyridinolcarbamate. Ochanomizu med. J. 13, 177 (1965).
Ohkido, M.: Clinical and experimental studies of homochlorcyclizine on several pruritic skin diseases. Dermatologica et Urologica 18, 1149 (1964).
Okamoto, S.: What is plasmin? J. clin. Sci. 3, 599 (1967).
Okumura, Y., Kawazu, T.: Neuromorphological changes in the human skin toward pruritus-stimulating substances. I. Bradykinin. Jap. J. Dermatol. Ser. B 76, 428 (1966).
Rocha e Silva, M.: Kinin hormone—bradykinin and other kinins. Amino Acids 8 (1), 1 (1968).
Sakakibara, S.: Recent progress in chemical synthesis of peptides. Amino Acid & Nucleic Acid 13, 17 (1966).
Sakamoto, K., Shirai, T., Sugiyama, K., Itoh, K.: The treatment of urticaria with homochlorcyclizine and its effect on cutaneous reactions and on plethysmographs in urticaria patients. Sōgō Rinshyō 16, 147 (1967).
Sasaki, T., Sunaga, T. Shimamoto, T.: Demonstration of vasa vasorum in the innermost layers of media of dog's aorta and their vascular leakage (II). Jap. Circulat. J. 31, 347 (1967).
Sato, S., Fujii, S.: Studies on plasmin. Symp. Chem. Physiol. and Pathol. 6, 190 (1966).
Shimamoto, T.: Atherosclerogenic substances and arteriosclerosis by these substances. Asian med. J. 2, 504 (1959).
— Edematous arterial reaction. Igaku no Ayumi 50, 1 (1963a).
— The relationship of edematous arterial reaction in arteries to atherosclerosis and thrombosis. J. Atheroscler. Res. 3, 87 (1963b).
— Ishioka, T.: Venous bradykinin-antagonistic property of estrogen. Proc. Japan Acad. 43, 342 (1967).
— — Takeuchi, K., Odakura, T., Matsumura, T.: Effect of bradykinin-antagonist B23 on two cases of idiopathic thrombocytopenic purpura. Clin. Hematol. 6, 158 (1965).
— Sasaki, T., Sunaga, T.: Species difference in fine structure of capillaries in vasa vasorum of aorta and its reference to atherosclerosis. Proc. Japan Acad. 43, 1025 (1967).
— Sunaga, T.: Edematous arterial reaction by adrenaline and cholesterol and its prevention by MAO inhibitor observed by electron microscopic technique. Jap. Heart J. 3, 581 (1962).
Sunaga, T., Sasaki, T., Hiramoto, Y.: Leukocyte emigration induced by bradykinin and lysylbradykinin and prevention by pyridinolcarbamate. Ochanomizu med. J. 13, 247 (1965c).
— — — Tanaka, M.: Constrictive effect of kinins on coronary vein and antagonistic effect of pyridinolcarbamate. Ochanomizu med. J. 13, 89 (1965a).
— — — — Vascular leakage by bradykinin or lysylbradykinin and preventive effect by pyridinolcarbamate. Ochanomizu med. J. 13, 121 (1965b).
— — Shimamoto, T.: Demonstration of vasa vasorum in the innermost layers of media of dog's aorta and their vascular leakage (I). Jap. Circulat. J. 31, 339 (1967a).
— — — Fine structure of capillary in atheromatous lesions in man and rabbit. Proc. Japan Acad. 43, 1031 (1967b).
Suzuki, K., Kameyama, T., Sasaki, K.: Interaction between kinin releasing enzymes and synthesized bradykinin derivatives. Jap. J. Pharmacol. 16, 486 (1966).
Suzuki, T.: Plasma kinins in inflammation. Metabolism & Disease 2, 726 (1965a).
— Physiologically active peptides—kinins. J. clin. Sci. (Japan) 1, 984 (1965b).
— Biochemistry of plasma kinins. J. clin. Sci. (Japan) 2, 377 (1966).
— Chemical structure of bovine kininogens and the enzymatic reaction of kinin liberation from these kininogens. J. clin. Sci. (Japan) 3, 617 (1967a).
— Biochemistry of bradykinin and other kinins. J. Allergy (Japan) 16, 618 (1967b).
— Hayashi, K.: Chemistry of bradykinin and naturally occurring bradykinin-like active compounds. Protein, Nucleic Acid, Enzyme 12, 211 (1967).
— Nagasawa, S.: Kallikrein-kinin system and hypotensive polypeptides. Protein, Nucleic Acid, Enzyme 12, 201 (1967).
— — Oita, M.: Separation of kallikreinogen from the pseudoglobulin of bovine plasma. Folia pharmacol. jap. 63, 182* (1967).
Takeda, K., Shigemi, H., Arakawa, T.: Intracutaneous reactions of bradykinin, serotonin and histamine. J. Allergy (Japan) 16, 627 (1967).
Tamura, Z., Nakajima, T.: Study on the micro peptides using dansyl derivatives. Protein, Nucleic Acid, Enzyme 12, 729 (1967).
Toyoizumi, T., Kunieda, T., Shimabukuro, Y., Tanaka, E., Takahashi, T.: Clinical experience with homochlorcyclizine in the treatment of bronchial asthma. New Drugs & Clin. Med. 14, 549 (1965).

WATANABE, H., ABE, F., MURAMATSU, M., FUJII, S.: Relationship between plasmin and kallikrein. Abstract of 40th General Meeting of Jap. Biochem. Soc. **39**, 596 (1967).
YAMAMURA, Y.: Active peptides as humoral regulator. J. clin. Sci. (Japan) **3**, 629 (1967).
— Biochemical concept of inflammation. Proc. Japan Soc. Clin. Biochem. Metabol. **4**, 101 (1968).
YAMAZAKI, H., ISHIOKA, T.: Pyridinolcarbamate treatment of cerebral vascular diseases. Ochanomizu med. J. **13**, 253 (1965).
— MURASE, H., SHIMAMOTO, T., JR.: Effect of pyridinolcarbamate on angina pectoris. Ochanomizu med. J. **13**, 221 (1965c).
— SANO, T., ODAKURA, T.: Antagonistic substances against increase in permeability of skin vessels induced by bradykinin, lysylbradykinin, kallikrein, histamine and serotonin. Ochanomizu med. J. **13**, 95 (1965a).
— — — TAKEUCHI, K.: Changes in ECG, blood coagulability and adhesive platelet count induced by Master's two-step test and prevention by pyridinolcarbamate. Ochanomizu med. J. **13**, 215 (1965b).
YAMURA, T.: Mechanism of development of urticaria. J. Allergy (Japan) **10**, 51 (1961).
— Patch test. J. Allergy (Japan) **12**, 42 (1963).
YANAIHARA, N., SEKIYA, M.: Synthesis of l-glutamic acid kallidin. Chem. Pharm. Bull. **15**, 82 (1967).
— — TAKAGI, K., KATO, H., ICHIMURA, M., NAGAO, T.: Synthesis of bradykinin analogs containing sarcosine residues and their biological activities. Chem. Pharm. Bull. **15**, 110 (1967).
YANO, S.: The action of kinins and their structures. Metabolism & Disease **5**, 259 (1968).
YOSHINAGA, K., WADA, M., MAEHASHI, M., ABE, K., MIWA, I.: Renin-angiotensin and kallikrein-kinin systems and their related polypeptides. Saishin Igaku **19**, 314 (1964).

Summary of Literature Published in Spanish and Portuguese*

J. L. PRADO

With 1 Figure

One of the reasons why several scientists in Latin America have focused their attention on vasoactive peptides stems from the discovery of two important peptides in Argentina and in Brazil: hypertensin (now called angiotensin) by BRAUN-MENENDEZ et al. (1939), and bradykinin by ROCHA E SILVA et al. (1949). Many theses, original articles, and scientific communications have been published in Spanish and Portuguese; these papers either report or reflect the progress achieved in this area. On several occasions the original observations appeared first or were published only in these two languages, but in general all important findings were also described in other languages. This article will summarize and evaluate the Spanish and Portuguese literatures on hypotensive peptides and related subjects, with special emphasis on papers which were not published in other languages or which have special significance. Other articles will be mentioned briefly or not at all.

In his book *Primordia Pharmacologiae in Brasilia*, VALLE (1966) reproduced an article published by LACERDA (1881) in which it was shown that snake venom, like pancreatic juice, digests fats and proteins. LACERDA's pioneer work in Brazil on snake venoms preceded the foundation of the Instituto Butantan (1899), and its significance may be better evaluated from the historical point of view by reading an article by LEAKE (1956) about venoms. It may be said that since that time venoms have been of interest to scientists in Brazil, although many years may have elapsed between papers. Two relatively recent examples are the discoveries of crotoxin at Instituto Butantan, São Paulo (SLOTTA and FRAENKEL-CONRAT, 1939), and of crotamine (GONÇALVES, 1948, 1950), at the Institute of Biophysics, Universidade Federal of Rio de Janeiro.

A. 1938 to 1954

I. Discovery, Purification, and Chemical Nature of Bradykinin

The discovery of bradykinin was reported in Portuguese for the first time in a note in *Ciência e Cultura*[1] by ROCHA E SILVA and BERALDO (1949), two or three months later and much less completely than in the well-known paper in English (ROCHA E SILVA et al., 1949). In the Portuguese note, however, the authors gave clearer indications about the chemical nature of bradykinin. They referred to experiments of ANDRADE, from the same laboratory, in which paper chromatography was used. They stated that bradykinin is a polypeptide having at least

* Work from this laboratory during the last years has been supported in part by a grant from the National Institutes of Health (USPHS No. HE 09267), by the Fundação de Amparo à Pesquisa do Estado de São Paulo, and by the CAPES/BNDE/BID Project.

1. Published by the Brazilian Society for the Advancement of Science (SBPC).

eight to ten amino acid residues. A paper on chromatography published by ANDRADE (1949) reproduces a paper chromatogram of the hydrolysis products of partially purified bradykinin. Eight distinct ninhydrin spots are visible, whereas nonhydrolyzed bradykinin showed no amino acid spots. Four of the spots (aspartic and glutamic acids, alanine, and leucine) corresponded to amino acids now known not to be present in bradykinin. Phenylalanine was not found. Two further scientific communications on the purification of bradykinin appeared (ANDRADE et al., 1952; ANDRADE, 1954) before the papers in English (ANDRADE et al., 1953; ANDRADE and ROCHA E SILVA, 1956) were published.

Also ROCHA E SILVA (1949) published a more general presentation of the subject, including a detailed description of the effect of several snake venoms and of crystalline trypsin on smooth muscle, and the classification of the new principle

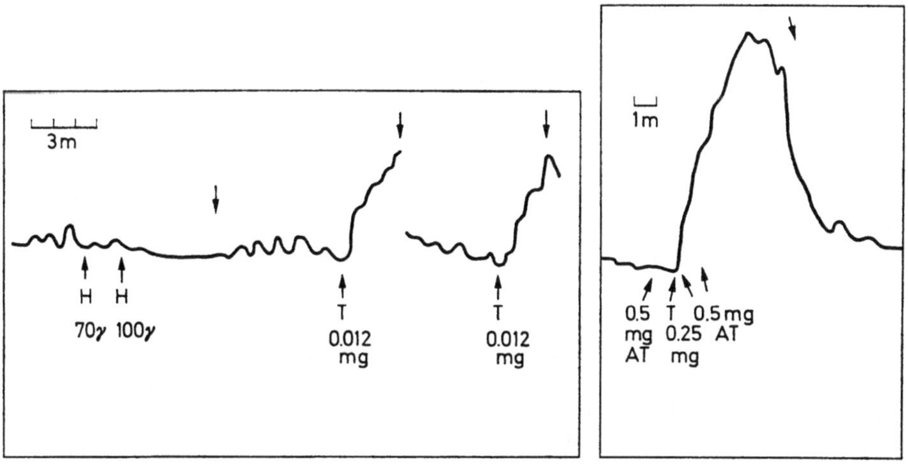

Fig. 1. Virgin rat uterus. Left: Effect of histamine (relaxing) and of trypsin (contracting). Right: Atropinization had no effect on trypsin action. (From ROCHA E SILVA, 1939)

among the tissue hormones. One has to go back, however, at least eleven years to find what may be considered the origins of bradykinin in papers dealing with the effects of crude trypsin on smooth muscle and on histamine liberation from perfused lungs (ROCHA E SILVA, 1938), and on the effects of crystalline trypsin on smooth muscle, isolated heart, and circulation (ROCHA E SILVA, 1939). These detailed papers, with long English summaries, contain useful information on the pharmacology of trypsin. Fig. 1, from the second paper, illustrates the relaxing effect of histamine on the virgin rat uterus and the contraction produced by crystalline trypsin. In the hypothesis explaining the pharmacology of trypsin by histamine liberation, this important exception must have acted as a strong intellectual stimulus in the search for an additional chemical mediator to account for the effect of trypsin. There was no doubt, then, in the author's mind, that he was actually dealing with a phenomenon of autopharmacology, that is, the liberation of a pharmacologically active agent. He was particularly impressed, for instance, with the immediate response of the guinea pig uterus to as little as 1 μg of crystalline trypsin. The many investigations which then favored the histamine theory, however, and the lack of a specific antihistamine, delayed for about ten years the discovery of bradykinin.

In October 1949, at the first annual meeting of the Brazilian Society for the Advancement of Science (E. S. PRADO et al., 1950a), the solubilities of bradykinin in several organic solvents and its 25- to 40-fold purification by column chromatography on aluminum oxide was reported. This purified material was used by ANDRADE (1949) to obtain the first paper chromatogram of hydrolyzed bradykinin. The complete paper (E. S. PRADO et al., 1950b) was published later.

II. Kinin-Forming Activity of Fibrinolysin

BERALDO reported at the Second Annual Meeting of SBPC (1950) the *in vitro* formation of a pharmacologically active substance, resembling bradykinin, by the action of peptone or fibrinolysin on plasma globulins of dog's blood. The note revealed that the globulins from the guinea pig and beef plasmas were also active as substrates of fibrinolysin. Further pharmacological and chemical properties, which characterized the liberated substance as similar if not identical with bradykinin, were also described.

III. Bradykinin: Mechanism of Action

In the same SBPC meeting, ROCHA E SILVA (1950) reported additional experiments on the mechanism of action of bradykinin. The hypotension was not affected by bilateral vagotomy, no sympatholytic action was observed, nor was any ganglionic blockade produced in the superior cervical ganglion of the cat. The most probable explanation for the hypotensive action of the new substance was thought to be a general peripheral vasodilatation.

IV. The First Thesis on Bradykinin

In 1951 ROCHA E SILVA published his thesis on bradykinin, after three years of work. The thesis contains, as an introduction, a rather complete historic account of the discovery of bradykinin. He mentions that the desensitization of the guinea pig gut to *Bothrops* venom (specially *B. jararaca*) and to trypsin was of prime importance in the discovery of the peptide. The addition of small amounts of *Bothrops* venom to defibrinated dog's blood and of trypsin produced large amounts of an unstable smooth-muscle-stimulating principle, not blocked by antihistamines or atropine.

Chapter I deals with the isolation and purification of bradykinin, its physical and chemical properties, and its preparation from liters of globulin solution. The preparation followed essentially the method reported by E. S. PRADO et al. (1950a). Using a 60-fold purified bradykinin preparation, he attempted to purify the material further in one-dimensional paper chromatography. The active material was eluted and hydrolyzed. It showed several amino acid spots in bidimensional paper chromatography, while unhydrolyzed bradykinin failed to give a positive ninhydrin reaction. The experiment, like those with angiotensin, showed that the preparation was probably not contaminated with free amino acids. It was shown that the R_f value of bradykinin increased from 0.024 to 0.300 with purification. The initially reported inactivation of bradykinin by trypsin (ROCHA E SILVA et al., 1949) was here interpreted as being produced by contamination of the crystalline enzyme used with chymotrypsin. WERLE et al. (1950) had indeed observed that trypsin does not destroy bradykinin.

Chapter II describes the bioassay of bradykinin on the guinea pig ileum by means of the 3×3 or 2×2 designs.

Chapter III is a discussion of the differentiation between bradykinin and several hypotensive substances of endogenous origin. Histamine, acetylcholine, and adenosine and derivatives were excluded because of their different properties. In the discussion regarding the possible relationship of bradykinin with kallikrein and kallidin, ROCHA E SILVA stated that although there was no possibility that bradykinin and kallikrein were identical, an identity with kallidin was possible, a hypothesis which had been defended by WERLE et al. (1950) in the paper that immediately followed the discovery of bradykinin (ROCHA E SILVA, 1949). In his thesis, however, ROCHA E SILVA mentions the "most important fact" that kallikrein (Padutin) did not liberate an active substance from dog's blood plasma globulins, while its kinin-liberating activity on fresh dog plasma was not inhibited by soybean trypsin inhibitor.

On this basis he concluded that bradykinin was possibly not identical with kallidin, but that the final word could not be said until it was chemically identified. He goes on to state (1951) that WERLE only suspected in 1937 that kallidin existed, which does not correspond, in my opinion, to WERLE's ideas; indeed, the title of WERLE, GÖTZE, and KEPPLER's (1937) publication does not bear out ROCHA E SILVA's opinion. He also thought that the names kallidin and kallidinogen were based on the bradykinin and bradykininogen nomenclature, whereas WERLE and BEREK (1948) used them before bradykinin was discovered, calling attention to the similar situation with the renal pressor system. The similarity had been previously stressed by WERLE and HAMBUECHEN (1943).

Chapter IV studies the mode of action of bradykinin, dealing with its effects on smooth muscles, on the superior cervical ganglion, the lack of effect of bradykinin on the nicotine paralysis on ganglia in guinea pig ileum, and its action on the circulatory system.

In the concluding remarks, which summarize the main findings, the importance that a bradykinin inhibitor would have in the study of the new peptide is mentioned.

V. First Observations from Other Brazilian Laboratories

Two years after the discovery of bradykinin at Instituto Biológico, PICARELLI et al. (1951) published a note showing that bradykinin (Pool 5 X) contracted the vas deferens and seminal vesicles of normal and castrated rats. The effect differed from that of angiotensin and was comparable to that produced by epinephrine and norepinephrine but was not abolished by 2-benzylimidazoline (tolazoline, priscoline). These observations were extended later (VALLE and PICARELLI, 1954) in part to contradict a rather surprising paper (PEREIRA, 1953) which stated categorically that bradykinin was neither a new substance nor a polypeptide because it was not pharmacologically pure and its action was due to contamination with adenosine and histamine. Although these statements proved to be incorrect, the inactivation of bradykinin by the commercial preparation of histaminase used by PEREIRA led HAMBERG and ROCHA E SILVA (1954) to detect in it a true bradykininase action, independent of the histaminase.

In 1952, at the University of São Paulo, BERALDO (1952) published his first note on a principle, found in dog urine, called substance U, which was thought to be different from bradykinin, kallikrein, and kallidin because substance U was thermolabile and resisted incubation with serum. This opinion was sustained in a second report on the same subject (BERALDO, 1954), in which the supposedly new principle was actually shown to be liberated from blood plasma globulins.

BERALDO (1953) published a short review about the first papers on bradykinin.

B. 1954 to 1960

During this period numbers of scientific communications, articles, and two theses were published, attesting a continued interest of ROCHA E SILVA and his collaborators, and that of a few other Portuguese-speaking researchers on several aspects of the field.

I. Polistes Kinin; Purified Bradykinin

ROCHA E SILVA (1954) found a bradykinin-like pain-producing substance in the venom of several wasps, particularly of the *Polistes* genus. He also wrote a review on the possible physiological role of bradykinin (ROCHA E SILVA, 1955), following the publication of the proceedings of the Montreal Symposium on Polypeptides Which Stimulate Plain Muscle (GADDUM, 1955). In this review he mentions, probably for the first time, that a bradykinin preparation with 5,000 units/mg of polypeptide had been obtained by ANDRADE and himself and should be very close to purity, showing a "prodigious" biological activity; i.e. at a concentration of 2×10^{-9}, bradykinin produced biological effects on the guinea pig ileum. He also refers to experiments made in cooperation with Keele and Armstrong in which it was shown that rat uterus was 25 to 30 times more sensitive to bradykinin, that is, an activity of the same order of magnitude as that of synthetic oxytocin. Rocha e Silva stated further that he and his collaborator, Hamberg observed that a single sting of *Polistes versicolor* (the Brazilian common wasp) may contain enough kinin to explain the delayed pain associated with a sting from this wasp. The last part of this review deals with the liberation of bradykinin in the blood stream. Activation of fibrinolysin is favored as the possible mechanism, particular emphasis being given to the potentially large amounts (10 to 15 mg of pure bradykinin) that might be liberated from 5 liters of human blood. Data from the literature showing the presence of bradykinin in a few types of shock are reviewed.

II. Bradykinin Liberation from Blood Plasma

Ulla Hamberg and Elizabeth Holzhacker were associated with Rocha e Silva in a group of experiments (Hamberg and Rocha e Silva, 1956; Rocha e Silva and Hamberg, 1956; Hamberg, 1957, 1958; Rocha e Silva and Holzhacker, 1958) dealing with bradykinin liberation from blood plasma globulins and denatured globulins. They used snake venoms or trypsin as liberators or heated plasma at low pH. A few findings, presented more completely in several papers in English, were described. The yield of bradykinin may be increased in preparations of 15 to 25 liters of bovine plasma by eliminating factors, present either in the releasing enzymes or in plasma, which antagonize the release or destroy the liberated kinin. The kinin liberation is related to the esterolytic activity of liberators on BAMe and not to their proteolytic action on casein. In the *B. jararaca* venom there seems to exist a liberating factor which has no proteolytic action on casein and liberates kinin from fresh plasma possibly by activation of a plasma enzyme. The kinin liberation from rat and bovine plasma by acidification and heating followed by neutralization was also thought to be an indirect mechanism.

Rocha e Silva and some of his collaborators (Ulla Hamberg and C. R. Diniz) moved in 1958 to the Department of Pharmacology at the University of São Paulo, Ribeirão Preto.

III. Oxytocic Activity of Bradykinin; Effects on Central Nervous System

Ramos et al. (1958) measured the activity of bradykinin on rat uterus. One unit of oxytocin from Sandoz corresponded to 15.6 to 17.8 units of bradykinin. One unit of oxytocin from Parke Davis was equivalent to 3.79 to 7.84 units of bradykinin. Bradykinin was inactive on the rooster blood pressure. Corrado et al. (1959) also described both stimulation and depression of the central nervous system of cats after intraventricular bradykinin injection.

IV. Thermic Edema

Using a simple technique to collect fluid from thermic edema (44 to 45°) in the rat's paw, Rocha e Silva and Antonio (1960) found a kinin-like substance in the fluid when the temperature reached 44 to 45°. Its quantity increased at 48–50° and decreased at higher temperatures. The effect of several drugs on this edema (Antonio and Rocha e Silva, 1960) was studied: antihistamines (antergan, diphenhydramine, phenergan), sympatholytics (2-benzylimidazoline, dibenzyline), and antiserotonin (LSD 25 and BOL) had no effect. Cocaine increased the edema, chlorpromazine reduced it, and reserpine was even more active in decreasing the edema. Histamine and serotonin were thus excluded as the causative agents.

V. Kininogenase in Urine

BERALDO et al. (1956) verified that the concentration of the releaser of substance U in urine does not diminish by pancreatectomy in the dog even after 11 weeks. In a heart–lung preparation pumping blood through isolated kidney, the urine still contained the liberator. Either the kininogenase was not kallikrein or the concentration of kallikrein in urine was not affected by pancreatectomy.

VI. Kinin in Peptone Shock

In a thesis describing the effect of peptone injection in dogs and rats BERALDO (1958) reported a kinin-like activity in the blood of dogs after injection of peptone. In shocked animals, however, a better correlation was found between intensity of shock and blood histamine level than between shock and kinin activity. The kinin released was concentrated and it was similar to bradykinin. In several dogs receiving injection of peptone a large increase in the kinin activity was observed in the withdrawn blood kept at room temperature for 30 to 60 minutes. Dog plasma globulins mixed with peptone also showed the same activity at an optimum pH of 7.4. Soybean trypsin inhibitor blocked the kinin formation. Activation of plasminogen by peptone seems to be the mechanism for this kinin liberation. In the rat, the initial hypotension was followed by hypertension; the characteristics of this phenomenon were also studied.

VII. Kinin Activity in Normal Human Urine

In 1958 GOMES published in Lisbon the longest thesis in Portuguese on biologically active peptides, dealing primarily with the study of a kinin-like substance found in human normal urine (274 printed pages, including a 6-page English summary).

It begins with a review of biologically active peptides. Among the hypotensive peptides, due emphasis is given to kallidin, but it is stated that only after the discovery of bradykinin did it become clear that kallidin was responsible for the pharmacological effects of kallikrein. Although this interpretation has been accepted by some authors, in my opinion WERLE and co-workers realized, before bradykinin was discovered, that the effect of kallikrein was indirect. Bioassays were performed by GADDUM's superfusion technique on rat uterus, which proved to be very convenient. Four-point assays were carried out on urine without purification. Substances such as K^+, Ca^{++}, histamine, nicotine, serotonin, and norepinephrine did not interfere, even in higher than normal concentrations. On the contrary, epinephrine (5 to 10 µg/liter) may reduce the uterine response to urine. Three methods were used to extract the active factor. (1) Adsorption on charcoal, elution with glacial acetic acid, precipitation with ethyl ether; 1 liter of urine yields 0.5–1.5 gm of a hygroscopic yellow-brownish active powder. With nonactivated charcoal and urine pH adjusted to 9 to 9.5, the recovery of activity may reach to 75%. (2) Butanol extraction of urine, pH adjusted to 1.5, saturation with NaCl and precipitation of active principle by ethyl ether. The yield was lower (30% in the butanol phase) than with method (1) but the activity per milligram of solid was higher. (3) Adsorption on zinc ferrocyanide, elution with 80% ethyl alcohol–1% NH_4OH, acidification of eluate to pH 4 to 5, drying under reduced pressure. Very low yields were observed. Combination of methods (1) and (2) gave from 302 liters of urine a product, 1 mg of which corresponded to the activity in 7 ml of urine. This was used in most experiments. Purification was tried by adsorption on columns of macerated Whatman No. 1 paper, washing with 7% phenol, and elution of 59% of activity with 0.2% acetic acid. Countercurrent distribution (40 steps; system, acetic acid:H_2O:n-butanol, 1:5:4) showed only one activity peak, different from bradykinin, but the material was less purified. Other experiments indicated that the active principle was a polypeptide. Pharmacological actions were studied on muscles, blood pressure, isolated frog heart, perfused rabbit ear, frog hind leg, and diuresis of water-loaded rat. It was concluded that the most important effects were smooth muscle stimulation, hypotension, and antidiuresis. Atropine and antihistamine do not alter the responses. One milligram of preparation G/100 gm rat produced an evident water retention, comparable to that obtained with 0.2 mU of vasopressin. The effect was abolished by chymotrypsin. Differentiation from other active principles was studied by physicochemical and biological methods. GOMES concluded that the peptide is probably identical with substance Z of WERLE and ERDÖS (1954). While dog, guinea pig, and rabbit urines seem to contain the same principle found in human urine, rat urine has a different factor. The work ends with experiments and discussion about the origin of the urinary peptide, but no conclusion was reached. The thesis was published later (GOMES, 1959).

VIII. Substance V

FASCIOLO and co-workers (HALVORSEN et al., 1958; FASCIOLO et al., 1958) observed that purified angiotensin preparations had a vasodilator contaminant, substance V, which was not present in pure angiotensin. These results were obtained by studying the effect on the systemic blood pressure and in the perfused dog leg. While pure angiotensin produced local and general vasoconstriction, impure preparations produced local vasodilatation, and lowered the perfusion pressure when injected intra-arterially. However, substance V produced no hypotension when given intravenously. This was due to the rapid destruction of substance V by blood plasma. Various characteristic properties of substance V indicate that it is probably identical with bradykinin. A subsequent paper (HALVORSEN et al., 1960) deals with the enzymic destruction of substance V and bradykinin by organ extracts and plasma. The authors noticed that after heating for 30 minutes at 37°, pH 3.5, kidney extract does not inactivate bradykinin, while the ability to inactivate substance V is partly preserved. Similar differences hold for the inactivating enzyme in plasma. The experiments were done with impure preparations and this reviewer agrees with the authors (FASCIOLO et al., 1960) that the difference is not enough to distinguish substance V from bradykinin.

IX. Horse Urinary Kallikrein; Substance U; Vasoactive Peptides

After a discussion with BERALDO, the idea of studying the liberator of substance U was taken up by PRADO and PRADO (1960), who used horse urine as starting material. In the first note an 80-fold purification was reported (ammonium sulfate fractionation and DEAE-cellulose chromatography). A parallelism between kinin-liberating activity and TAMe hydrolysis was found. A few months later (E. S. PRADO, 1960), in a review of vasoactive polypeptides and their releasers, additional characteristics of the horse urinary substance U liberator were given, and the interpretation advanced that this kininogenase was probably horse urinary kallikrein. BERALDO's substance U would thus be identical with kallidin. It is stated elsewhere in this chapter that after reviewing the work of WERLE et al. done between 1937 and 1948, the reviewer became convinced of the existence of kallidin. Up to 1960 no one in the Portuguese and Spanish literatures had apparently made this statement, and only a few contributors to the world literature were sufficiently convinced to admit it even after 1960. There is no doubt that the discovery of bradykinin in 1948 had a powerful impact on the whole field. Its significance is in no way diminished by the discovery of kallidin in 1937.

C. 1961 to 1966

A review by ROCHA E SILVA (1962a), read in 1961 at the Fourth Meeting of the Latin American Association of Physiological Sciences, in Ribeirão Preto, Brazil, summarized previous work on bradykinin. It contains an introduction and topics on the chemical constitution and activity, specific activity and characterization, bradykininogen and kinin formation, and physiologic and pathologic significance of bradykinin.

I. Pressor Action of Bradykinin

Croxatto (1961) observed that in the nephrectomized rat intravenous injection of 0.04–0.08 μg/100 gm of 90–95% pure bradykinin produces hypertension, sometimes preceded by a transitory hypotension. In the intact animal the same doses produced the usual hypotension. When the rat is pretreated with pentolinium, which brings his systemic arterial blood pressure down to 30–40 mm Hg, bradykinin produced pure pressor responses. Croxatto et al. (1962) observed in normal rats with normal blood pressure that bradykinin produces hypotension. Only when the blood pressure is low do small doses of bradykinin cause hypertension. In the nephrectomized rat the type of response depends both on doses and on the level of blood pressure. Doses of 0.005 to 0.1 μg/100 gm body weight consistently induce pressor responses when the initial blood pressure is around 60 mm Hg.

II. Kininogen

To study the relationship of kininogen and angiotensinogen, Espada et al. (1961) used a method to estimate kininogen in blood plasma based on the estimation of bradykinin liberated by incubation with an excess of trypsin; this method was published later in English (Fasciolo et al., 1963). They observed that exhausting angiotensinogen by previous treatment of plasma with renin does not alter the amount of bradykinin formed by trypsin. It was also shown that in 11 protein fractions from bovine plasma, obtained by increasing the ammonium sulfate concentration from 10 to 35% (in steps of 2.5%), the ratio kininogen/angiotensinogen (and the respective S.E.) differed from fraction to fraction and from 27.1 ± 4.6 (fractions VII and IX) to 285 ± 47.9 (fraction XI). The conclusion was that kininogen and angiotensinogen are different globulins.

Henriques et al. (1962) described an improved purification of horse kininogen. Horse plasma is acidified to pH 2.0 and kept in the cold for 5 days. After neutralization the globulin fraction, precipitated between 0.35 and 0.50 ammonium sulfate saturation, was chromatographed on a column of DEAE-cellulose. Horse kininogen was obtained without a contaminating kininogenase.

Several factors which might affect the kininogen concentration in plasma were studied. Hepatectomy or carbon tetrachloride poisoning reduces bradykininogen in blood, suggesting that it is produced by the liver (Carvalho, 1962). Trypsin and endotoxin shocks did not change blood kininogen level while in shocks produced by kallikrein or in anaphylactic shock 60 to 80% reduction in blood kininogen was found (Diniz et al., 1962). Nonlethal epinephrine shock in guinea pigs was followed by kininogen reduction (Vugman, 1963).

III. Kinin System

At the Fourteenth Annual Meeting of SBPC (Curitiba, 1962) several papers were presented, and a specific symposium was organized to cover the whole kinin system: kininogen, kininogenases, kinins, kininases. Katchburian et al. (1962) observed that horse urinary kallikrein is not inhibited by ovomucoid and soybean trypsin inhibitor, but by DFP and by Trasylol. Prolonged dialysis inactivates horse urinary kallikrein. E. S. Prado et al. (1962a) purified horse urinary kallikrein 800-fold, obtaining a preparation twice as esterolytic as crystalline trypsin on BAEe. J. L. Prado et al. (1962b) described the kinin-liberating activity of subtilisin BPN′ (Nagarse), a crystalline proteolytic enzyme from the culture medium of *Bacillus subtilis*. FERREIRA et al. (1962) observed that the potentiation of bradykinin hypotension by BAL and thioglycolic acid can be correlated with the lowering of plasma kininase activity by these compounds. PICARELLI (1962a, b) showed that synthetic bradykinin was inactivated by tissue extracts (guinea pig ileum and rat uterus). Extracts obtained from "washed" tissues incubated with kininase inhibitors (EDTA, 3×10^{-3} M; *o*-phenanthroline, 3×10^{-4} M; arginine, 3×10^{-3} M) became inactive. J. L. PRADO (1962) introduced the term kininogenases to designate the kinin-forming enzymes and reviewed some of their enzymatic characteristics; the complete paper appeared later (J. L. PRADO, 1964a). The kininogenase activity of human plasma protein fractions, purified on DEAE-cellulose columns, was increased 900-fold while the TAMe-hydrolyzing activity increased only 100-fold (LAVRAS et al., 1962). SCHMIDT and RAMOS (1962) reported the normal production of neurokinin and pain-producing substance in three patients with congenital generalized analgesia. These observations were extended to two other patients with identical results. The results, with many more clinical and other data, constitute a thesis with English summary (SCHMIDT, 1963).

IV. Neurokinin

RAMOS (1961) published his thesis on the presence and formation of a pharmacologically active substance (neurokinin) in human cerebrospinal fluid (CSF). Assay of 230 CSF samples on rat duodenum, uterus, and blood pressure revealed either the presence of neurokinin or its formation by incubation with plasma globulins. Neurokinin is easily differentiated from other active substances of non-peptidic nature (epinephrine, ATP, etc.), but it is similar to hypotensive peptides. Neurokinin was thought to be different from bradykinin and similar to the neurokinin obtained from subcutaneous tissue by neurogenic stimulation (CHAPMAN et al., 1960). An attempt was made to characterize neurokinin obtained by incubating CSF with ox globulin by means of paper chromatography. This reviewer feels, however, that the neurokinin preparation used was too crude to permit valid conclusions. RAMOS et al. (1961a) reported the potentiation of neurokinin hypotension in rats by lysergic acid diethylamide (50 μg/kg). In contrast to bradykinin, RAMOS et al. (1963b) found neurokinin inactive on dog blood pressure, even after administration of 200 μg of LSD. Hydrocortisone (100 mg/kg) and sodium salicylate (200 mg/kg) inhibit neurokinin hypotension in the rat (RAMOS et al., 1961b). Crude neurokinin (5 mg) increased capillary permeability in rats and edema and redness in human skin (RAMOS et al., 1963a), accompained by pain and itching.

V. Pharmacological Activity of Aqueous Humor

This fluid (dog, cat, ox) relaxes rat duodenum, contracts the guinea pig ileum and rat uterus, and produces hypotension in the rooster and rat, but is inactive in dog and cat. RAMOS and RAMOS (1961) suspected that two factors were responsible for the effects; one of them is dialyzable, heat stable, and destroyed by trypsin and chymotrypsin. The same type of activity was found in aqueous humor from rat, rabbit, and man (OEHLING et al., 1963). One of the factors may prove to be a kinin.

VI. Bilikinin

Bilikinin (RAMOS et al., 1961c; ZYNGIER et al., 1962), a spasmogenic and hypotensive substance from ox bile, is not a kinin.

VII. Kininogen and Shock

The relationship between kininogen and different types of shock was the subject of some papers and theses. Reis et al. (1963) reported that injection of subtilisin BPN' (Nagarse) (6 mg/kg) and trypsin (24 mg/kg) produces lethal shocks in dogs. Smaller doses induce marked hypotension and drops from 0 to 30% of bradykininogen concentration. Kinin may be detected in the circulating blood when there are pronounced kininogen drops. When hypotension occurs, kinins may not be found and it is possible that the hypotension may be due to other substances. When death occurs from shock, bradykininogen levels are found to be close to zero. In 1964, in a symposium dedicated to bradykinin and angiotensin (Sixteenth Annual SBPC Meeting), Corrado (1964a) reported bradykinin determination in the circulating blood. This paper includes material contained in a note (Reis et al., 1964) and in Corrado's thesis (1964b) on the possible participation of kinins in the hemodynamic effects produced by proteolytic enzymes. The note and the thesis contain results obtained with kallikrein (Padutin) and also with Nagarse and trypsin. Depending on the doses administered all three enzymes can produce conditions ranging from mild hypotension to lethal shock. The doses used were 24 mg of trypsin/kg, 6 mg of Nagarse/kg, or 12 mg of Padutin/kg. In general, kinin-like activity was not detected in the circulating blood when the kininogen drop was less than 40%, probably because of its rapid inactivation. When the kininogen depletion reached 40% or more, kinin activity corresponding to 0.025–1.87 μg of synthetic bradykinin/ml was found in the first 3 minutes of shock. While histamine was found in blood after trypsin administration, none was found after Nagarse or Padutin injection. The determination of blood kininogen level was considered to be a better index for the participation of the kinin system, in the conditions studied, than the detection of circulating kinin. The short half-life of circulating kinin renders its detection in blood less certain, and the amount found corresponds to 15 to 20% of the liberated. The blood-clotting time was prolonged after trypsin and Nagarse; Padutin did not alter it. The esterase activity of plasma with BAMe was increased even with the smallest doses of trypsin given (3–6 mg/kg). Nagarse increased the esterase activity of plasma in lethal doses (6 mg/kg), but Padutin, even in lethal doses, did not modify it.

The author believes that kallikrein is a much more specific kininogenase than the other enzymes mentioned. Although trypsin and Nagarse affected other plasma systems (blood clotting, esterolytic activity), kallikrein did not.

VIII. Plasma Kininogen in Several Conditions, Including Pregnancy

Diniz and Carvalho (1964), in the symposium on bradykinin and angiotensin mentioned above, reviewed the subject, emphasizing several points. One unit of kininogen releases 1 unit of bradykinin (0.5 μg synthetic bradykinin). Its concentration in plasma varies from 2.4 (pigeon) to 56.8 units (mouse); kininogen is synthesized in the liver, and it was found in the microsomal fraction and in the final supernatant of homogenized liver. Martinez, both in this symposium (1964a) and in a thesis (1964b), reported the results of a study of kininogen concentration in the blood of 125 women in normal and abnormal labor and in plasma of cord blood of 52 infants. No changes were found during normal labor. During labors lasting over 18 hours the kininogen level tends to decrease in the prepartum period and returns to normal within 48 hours. The infant's cord plasma level is higher after a normal delivery than in the newborn who suffered during labor. The kininogen level observed in the latter may be only 50% of normal.

IX. Kininogenase in Kidney Subcellular Particles

It was reported by Carvalho (1963) and by Carvalho and Diniz (1963, 1964) that a kininogenase exists in blood-free cortex of rat kidney. Following Rocha e Silva's (1962b) suggestion it was called kininogenin. The enzyme is located in "droplets" which correspond to kidney cell lysosomes. These droplets (0.5–1.0 μ) sediment in 2 minutes at 15,000 g in 0.88 M sucrose solution. Inactive in its natural condition, the enzyme is activated in hypotonic sucrose solution at pH 5.0, 37°, maximum activity being found after incubation of 1—2 hours. Using sucrose solutions between 0.5 and 0.06 M, they observed that acid phosphatase, which is a typical lysosome enzyme, was activated parallel and simultaneously with kininogenase. Activation of the kininogenase solubilizes the enzyme, 85% of the activity appearing in the supernatant. The kidney kininogenase is inactivated when heated 10 minutes at 90°. It is not dialyzable and it is precipitated by 80% (v/v) acetone and at 50% saturation with ammonium sulfate. It liberates from dog plasma, treated according to Horton, a kinin which behaves pharmacologically like bradykinin.

Compared with homogenates obtained from other rat tissues and expressing the kininogenase activity as units of bradykinin per gram protein per minute, the tissues showed the following activities: kidney 36; parotid gland 46; pancreas 86; submandibular gland 280. Kidney cortex also contains kininases which are only partially inhibited by 8-hydroxyquinoline. Thus the amount of kininogenase in kidney cortex may actually be two to three times higher, which shows that kidney cortex is relatively rich in kininogenase. With pancreatic kallikrein (Padutin), crude rat urinary and plasma kallikreins, and soybean trypsin inhibitor and Trasylol, it was observed that kidney and urinary kininogenases were equally inhibited (54 to 94%) by 6.6 to 26 units of Trasylol/ml. Soybean trypsin inhibitor at 17 and 34 μg/ml had no effect on Padutin and on kidney and urinary kallikrein, but rat plasma kallikrein was inhibited 58–75%. It seems that kidney kininogenase is similar to urinary kallikrein. In one of the papers (Carvalho and Diniz, 1964) the authors call attention to the possibility that renin may turn out to be located in the same subcellular fraction where the kidney kininogenase was found. The pH optimum for kinin liberation by the kidney kininogenase is 9.5 to 10.0.

X. Oxytocic Substance in Urine

Beraldo (1961) reviewed his work up to 1955 in a thesis dealing with the possible participation of polypeptides in traumatic shock in the dog. Although the active factor (substance U) was found in normal ureteral urine, its concentration increased 8- to 9-fold in tourniquet shock, probably as a consequence of contamination of the urine with blood. He did not agree with the interpretation (E. S. Prado, 1960) that urinary kallikrein was the liberator of substance U, essentially because his liberator was not of pancreatic origin and could be found in urine formed by kidney in a heart–lung–kidney preparation. He returned to the subject (Beraldo and Araujo, 1963, 1964) using rat urine. The oxytocic principle is not dialyzable through cellophane (pores of 4.8 mμ), and is inactivated at room temperature, pH 2 and 11, or at 96°, pH 7. Trypsin and chymotrypsin did not affect the principle but pepsin inactivated it. Trasylol inhibited it and soybean trypsin inhibitor did not. In general, including the kallidin-liberating activity, the oxytocic factor is similar to kallikrein. Beraldo does not seem to be convinced yet of the identity of his urinary factor with urinary kallikrein.

XI. Peptone Shock

In his thesis on peptone and anaphylactic shocks, FREIRE-MAIA (1963) detected a bradykinin-like activity in the plasma of rats injected with peptone, thus confirming BERALDO's (1958) observations in the dog. Only secondary importance was attributed to the kinin activity in the mechanism of this shock. Effects on the heart and respiration, of unknown mechanism, were found to be more important.

XII. Other Kinin Effects

Gastric Fundus. Impure bradykinin (VELAZQUEZ et al., 1961) produces a strong and fast relaxation followed by a slow contraction of the isolated rat gastric fundus. This polypeptide is, however, less active than angiotensin in this preparation. Among the several active substances tried, bradykinin had the longest latent period.

Permeability of Meningeal Vessels. CARDOSO and CORRADO (1963) found that both bradykinin and kallidin increased the permeability of intravenously injected sulfacetamide into the cerebrospinal fluid collected in the cisterna magna. Histamine had an insignificant effect.

Electroencephalogram. CORRADO et al. (1963) studied electroencephalograms of cats and rabbits injected with bradykinin intraventricularly. The minimum effective dose of bradykinin was 0.5 μg, which 1 hour after anesthesia withdrawal produced stimulation of EEG proportional to the amount administered. Doses of 10 to 30 μg finally caused depression of the animal and synchronization of EEG. The investigators were unable to eliminate hemodynamic changes produced by bradykinin as the cause of EEG changes, but believe that further studies should be done to clarify this possible effect of bradykinin.

Carotid Sinus Reflexes. PIMAZONI NETO et al. (1964) injected 75–150 μg of bradykinin into the wall of carotid sinus of dog and observed systemic hypotension and suppression of hypotensive reflexes produced by carotid occlusion. The last effect is not produced by systemic injection of bradykinin.

The electric discharges of baroceptor fibers increased after bradykinin injection into the sinus wall (KRIEGER and CORRADO, 1965). This effect was abolished by papaverin.

Release of Antidiuretic Hormone. ROCHA E SILVA, Jr. (1963a, b) suggested that the antidiuresis produced in trained, unanesthetized dogs by intracarotid injection of bradykinin is probably due to the release of antidiuretic hormone. The effect was not seen in dogs with experimental diabetes insipidus.

Coronary Vessels. ANTONIO (1966) observed on the LANGENDORFF preparations of guinea pig heart that a threshold dose of 5 ng (10^{-9} gm/ml final conc.) of bradykinin (given by a plastic catheter ending 0.5 to 1.0 cm from the coronary vessels) increases the coronary flow. This action increases with doses up to 50 ng. Above this amount only the duration of the effect is prolonged. Under identical conditions, papaverine is about a thousand times less potent. There is also an increase of the heart-contracting force, but the author concludes that this inotropic effect of bradykinin is secondary to the main one on the coronary vessels.

XIII. Venom Kinins

Wasp kinin. In a symposium on venoms and toxins, J. L. PRADO (1964b) reported yet unpublished work of J. L. PRADO et al. in 1963 showing the presence of a kinin, different from bradykinin and kallidin, in the American paper wasp (*Polistes*) venom. This work led eventually to the identification of glycyl-bradykinin (cf. J. L. PRADO et al., 1966) in this venom.

Spider. Two main groups of spiders were studied by DINIZ (1963): the *Arachnomorphae*, called true spiders in Brazil because they are responsible for most of the toxic stings in man, and the *Mygalomorphae*, which rarely produce toxic symptoms in man. Pharmacologically active components found in the venom collected by electric stimulation from fourteen species were separated mainly by paper electrophoresis and paper chromatography. Eluates from paper bands were assayed chemically and pharmacologically. Data were not given for all species. Among the true spider venoms the author found the following materials: in *Phoneutria fera*, histamine (0.6–0.8 mg/gm); serotonin (0.3–0.5 mg/gm), and polypeptides (amount equivalent to 3,600–4,200 bradykinin units). In *Lycosa erythrognata*, however, which is also a true spider, only 12 to 50 units of active polypeptide/gm venom were found. Further studies are indispensable to characterize the polypeptides found; probably they are not kinins. DINIZ (1963) observed, however, that they migrate cathodically, are inactivated by chymotrypsin and trypsin, and contract the isolated guinea pig ileum in the presence of promethazine (100 mg/liter) and atropine (1 mg/liter). According to DINIZ the pain, which is a constant symptom after spider sting, should be due to the combined active components found.

XIV. Liberation of Bradykinin by Milk and Polysaccharide Sulfuric Esters

During the digestion of milk given to anesthesized dogs, kinin activity was found in their blood plasma (CABRAL and BERALDO, 1965). Agar liberates bradykinin when incubated with rat and guinea pig plasmas, heparin has an identical effect (GASCON and ROTHSCHILD, 1965). ROTHSCHILD and ROTHSCHILD (1966) showed subsequently that sulfuric esters of starch, agar, cellulose, and glycogen, with two to three sulfate groups per monosaccharide unit, activate a kininogenase system in plasma, releasing 1—2 μg bradykinin activity/ml plasma. The plasma proteolytic system activated by the sulfuric esters is inhibited by soybean trypsin inhibitor. Human, rat, and guinea pig plasmas produce kinin when incubated with straight and branched polysaccharide sulfuric esters. In contrast, dog and beef plasmas were activated only by branched polysaccharide sulfuric esters.

XV. Horse Urinary Kallikrein

This enzyme was shown to have a proteolytic action on protamine, which paralleled its kinin-liberating activity (BRANDI et al., 1964). The kinin-forming activity disappears by thorough dialysis. The enzyme can be reactivated by adding Na, K, Li, Rb, or Cs ions in a concentration of 4×10^{-2} M to 1.4×10^{-1} M (Na^+ concentration in TYRODE's solution). Some ions (Ni, Cu, Hg) inhibit both the kininogenase and esterase activities of horse urinary kallikrein (J. L. PRADO et al., 1965).

XVI. Effect of Nagarse on Angiotensin

ENDO and CARLINI (1966) showed that angiotensin II is rapidly inactivated by Nagarse, a proteolytic enzyme from *B. subtilis*, and that no active peptide accumulated from incubating angiotensin I with the enzyme. Contrary to angiotensin II, substance A is not inactivated by Nagarse.

XVII. Potentiation of Kinin Effects

Both bradykinin and neurokinin produce more intense and prolonged hypotension in the rat after LSD administration (RAMOS et al., 1961 a). The potentiation of bradykinin hypotension by LSD was confirmed in the dog (RAMOS et al., 1963 b).

The potentiation of bradykinin effects is discussed on p. 425.

SEGURA-CARDONA (1964) observed that bradykinin as well as angiotensin and oxytocin are inactivated by extracts from cat and rat kidney and from rat lung. Fresh tissues were homogenized in physiologic saline and filtered and centrifuged at 3,000 rpm for 15 minutes. Both angiotensin and bradykinin were rapidly inactivated at room temperature; oxytocin was inactivated by rat kidney only at 39°. Although the author believed that the inactivation might be due to enzymatic hydrolysis, this reviewer thinks that further studies should have been be made. SEGURA-CARDONA observed, indeed, that 5-hydroxytryptamine was also inactivated by his extracts. The spasmogenic effect of bradykinin on the isolated guinea pig ileum is potentiated by *B. jararaca* venom (FERREIRA and ROCHA E SILVA, 1963). The component in the venom responsible for this effect (BPF) differs from those which contract the ileum. It is thermostable and remains in the supernatant when the venom is heated 10 minutes at 60° or treated with 80% ethyl alcohol or 10% TCA. Angiotensin and kallidin on the guinea pig ileum and oxytocin on rat uterus were potentiated by BPF. It strongly potentiates also the hypotensive action of bradykinin (FERREIRA and ROCHA E SILVA, 1963). Progress in the study of BPF was reported in a symposium on bradykinin and angiotensin (FERREIRA, 1964a) and in a thesis (FERREIRA, 1964b). In the symposium it is reported that the preparation of BPF was purified 8- to 10-fold from the crude venom. Trypsin inactivated 60 to 80% of BPF in 24 hours, whereas chymotrypsin had no action. One potentiating unit (PU) was defined as that amount of BPF which doubles the effect of a single dose of bradykinin on the guinea pig ileum. One unit has 0.3 to 0.6 μg BPF/ml. In five cats the average hypotension produced by synthetic bradykinin (1 μg/kg) was $19.6 \pm$ S.E. 3.3 mm, and the area of hypotension was 48 ± 7.0 mm². Five and 30 minutes after administration of BPF (2 mg/kg) the initial blood pressure fell further to 72 ± 5.5 and 53.5 ± 2.7 mm, and the hypotension areas were increased to 333 ± 18.0 and 232 ± 34.1 mm² with the same bradykinin injection. The effects of histamine and acetylcholine on the ileum and blood pressure were not potentiated. The local extravasation of trypan blue by the intradermal injection of synthetic bradykinin (1 μg) in rats, was potentiated by intradermal injection of BPF (2 μg). Other *Bothrops* venoms (*jararacussu, neuwiedii, atrox*) contain similar, although weaker, potentiating properties. It was concluded that BPF is the most powerful bradykinin-potentiating factor known and it is probably a peptide. FERREIRA's thesis describes and illustrates these findings in great detail.

Starting with 2 gm of *B. jararaca* venom (60 PU/mg), a powder with a specific activity of 500 PU/mg was obtained with a yield of 70%. The activities of several *Bothrops* venoms expressed as PU/mg were as follows: *jararaca* 60, *neuwiedii* 18, *jararacussu* 12, *atrox* 18, *alternata* 0, *cotiara* 0. Paper electrophoresis (phosphate buffer pH 7.7, $\mu = 0.1$, 12 hours) separated two activity bands on the anode side without increasing specific activity of eluates. Paper chromatography with butanol:acetic acid:water (4:1:1.6) separated also two active bands with double specific activities but with only 30% total yield. Column chromatography on DEAE-Sephadex A-50 gave three fractions absorbing at 280 mμ: F_1 (eluted with distilled water); F_2 (eluted with ammonium acetate buffer, pH 5, 0.01 M); and F_3 (eluted with same buffer up to 0.1 M). About 70% of the potentiating activity was found in F_1 and F_2 with specific activity twice that of the original material; F_3 was inactive. Paper chromatography revealed that these fractions were still impure. Experiments *in vivo* demonstrated that eledoisin is potentiated weakly by BPF and that BAL did not potentiate bradykinin hypotension in the cat. The kininase activity of guinea pig plasma was partially and almost equally inhibited by concentrations of BPF ranging from 1 to 750 μg/ml. At a concentration of 200 μg/ml, BPF inhibited partially the kininase activity of hemolysate of guinea pig red cells. Although the inhibition of kininase by BPF may be responsible for the potentiation of bradykinin hypotension, the author supposes that it is not the only factor.

The potentiation of synthetic bradykinin, kallidin, and eledoisin was further studied by FERREIRA and ROCHA E SILVA (1965). On the guinea pig ileum, 0.4 μg of BPF/ml in the organ bath potentiated bradykinin and kallidin but not eledoisin. At the concentration of 5 μg BPF/ml, the sensitivity to bradykinin and eledoisin became the same. In the dog and cat blood pressures, eledoisin is 20 to 50 times and 8 times respectively more active than bradykinin; after 2 mg/kg of BPF intravenously, the two peptides become about equally hypotensive in the dog, and the cat becomes more sensitive to bradykinin.

The intracranial venous pressure measured in the cranial side of the external jugular vein is increased by synthetic bradykinin, kallidin, eledoisin, or histamine injected into the lingual artery (GRAEFF et al., 1965). When injected intra-arterially, 0.01–0.1 μg bradykinin increased the pressure from 20 to 100 mm water. Eledoisin and kallidin produced equivalent increases with doses 2 and 20 times smaller. After the slow intravenous administration of 10 mg of BPF, bradykinin and kallidin effects on the intracranial pressure increased 2- and 3-fold.

XVIII. Inhibition of Kinin Effects

Thermic edema in the rat's paw was not affected by antihistamines, sympatholytics, or antiserotonin drugs. Among the phenothiazine derivatives, chlorpromazine reduced the edema significantly (ANTONIO and ROCHA E SILVA, 1960). As this edema was probably caused by a kinin-like agent (ROCHA E SILVA and ANTONIO, 1960), its decrease was interpreted as due to a possible antibradykinin effect of the drug tested. In order to establish a relationship between kinins and various physiological phenomena, it would be important to find antikinin agents. It has been the subject of several publications in Portuguese.

ROCHA E SILVA (1961) reported that BAMe and TAMe inhibited the spasmogenic action of bradykinin, acetylcholine, and ATP in concentrations comparable to those inhibiting histamine. Arginine and benzoyl-L-arginine required doses 100- to 200-fold higher to produce identical inhibitions of bradykinin. ROSA and BUFFOLO (1962) tried homochlorcyclizine dihydrochloride (SA-97, ABBOTT) a potent inhibitor of histamine, serotonin, acetylcholine, and SRS-A, against synthetic bradykinin. The bradykinin hypotension in the rat was not affected even by 5 mg of SA-97; the spasmogenic effect on the isolated guinea pig ileum was reduced 20% by 20 μg of SA-97. This is a weak antibradykinin action, because 0.05–0.1 μg of SA-97 reduced by 50% the effect of histamine on the ileum. The results were subsequently published in English (ROSA et al., 1962), including observations on rat uterus. Two theses in particular (ROCHA E SILVA, M., 1963; LEME, 1966) treat the subject of kinin antagonists in great detail.

In the introduction of the first thesis, the use of antagonists to characterize tissue active substances is discussed. Chapter I summarizes the knowledge about some synthetic bradykinin analogs. Chapter II is dedicated mainly to concepts, calculations, and criticisms regarding the determination of pA_x and its use in evaluating the efficiency and type of inhibition of antagonists. It is recommended to those who wish to work in this field. More concise presentations of the same subject were published in English (ROCHA E SILVA, 1959; ROCHA E SILVA and LEME, 1963). Chapter III deals with the physiological antagonisms between bradykinin and angiotensin and between bradykinin and catecholamines. On the basis of experiments on isolated strips of rabbit aorta, where bradykinin is inactive, the conclusion is reached that bradykinin and angiotensin act at different sites. This conclusion is also valid for bradykinin and catecholamines. Chapter IV discusses the antispasmogenic effect of arginine esters in detail, which had been briefly reported earlier (ROCHA E SILVA, 1961). Chapter V describes other antagonists of bradykinin and presents experiments with many drugs used in therapy. Much of the material given was published in English (ROCHA E SILVA and LEME, 1963, 1964). In conclusion it is stated that cyproheptadine is the best antibradykinin agent found. From the discussions given in Chapter V one may assume that comparison of pK_i values to study the noncompetitive antagonism is a more rational approach, in spite of all difficulties inherent in the method.

The second thesis on the subject (LEME, 1966) is a continuation of these studies and includes also observations regarding the effect of calcium ions on the antibradykinin action *in vitro*. The antibradykinin potency was estimated by the same method employed by ROCHA E SILVA (1963). Drugs found to be potent antibradykinin agents on the guinea pig ileum were subsequently tested on rabbit duodenum. They were tested *in vivo* to antagonize bradykinin effect upon the vascular permeability in rats and guinea pigs or to reduce the thermic edema in rat paw. To evaluate their specificity, the antagonists were also assayed on the guinea pig ileum against histamine, angiotensin, and eledoisin. About 25 drugs (derived from benzodiazepine, dihydro- and dibenzoazepine; dihydro- and dibenzocycloheptene; thioxanthene; cycloalkylindol; phenothiazine) were assayed. Only three compounds exhibited a competitive type of antagonism: (1) L-583232-1-1, a dibenzocycloheptene derivative; (2) L-290698-1-4, a thioxanthene derivative (both from Merck, Sharp & Dohme, USA); and (3) Tremaril (Wander, Brazil), a thioxanthene derivative also. Both the mixed and competitive inhibitions are reversible, the reversion of the competitive one being slower. The three compounds mentioned above inhibited competitively also angiotensin and histamine. Eledoisin inhibition was of a mixed type.

When the concentration of calcium chloride in TYRODE's solution is diminished from the usual 0.20 to 0.03 gm/liter, there is a decrease in the response of ileum to bradykinin. When the concentration is increased to 0.40 gm/liter there is a sensitization. As for the drug antagonism to bradykinin, the inhibition produced by compound L-582232-1-1, for instance, disappeared by increasing the usual calcium chloride concentration to 0.40 gm/liter; the inhibition produced by this compound to histamine, however, was intensified.

On rabbit duodenum L-583232-1-1, L-290698-1-4, and Tremaril reduced the response to bradykinin in doses comparable to those used on the ileum, without altering the basal pendular movements. Some of the most potent competitive and mixed antibradykinin drugs reduced the extravasation of Evans blue in rats and guinea pig skins locally injected with bradykinin. They also reduced thermic edema in the rat paw.

LEME concludes that at least for the competitive antagonists, a true antibradykinin action actually exists, although the potency is still very low.

On the structural requisite for an antibradykinin action, LEME (1966) refers to a personal communication by A. C. M. PAIVA (1964) who found a competitive type of antagonism between compound 48/80 and bradykinin. This communication is now published in English (PAIVA and PAIVA, 1966). The dimer (46/108) is also an antagonist of bradykinin, but the two compounds antagonize other myotropic substances as well: angiotensin, 5-hydroxytryptamine, oxytocin, and acetylcholine. Some of the results of this thesis appeared also in summarized form as part of a symposium on bradykinin and angiotensin (LEME and ROCHA E SILVA, 1964). It is interesting to recall at this point that from the publication of his thesis on bradykinin ROCHA E SILVA had stressed the importance of finding antagonists to this peptide (ROCHA E SILVA, 1949, p. 84).

D. 1967 and 1968

I. Kinin Effects

CNS and Behavior. Bradykinin, injected into cat brain via a plastic tube previously inserted into the carotid artery, produced central effects. In quiet animals, 25 μg bradykinin caused increased activity and excitability; 80 μg induced relaxation, sleep, and indifference to the environment, although the animal would chase and eat a mouse. Aggressive cats injected with 25 μg bradykinin did not tolerate the proximity of other cats; the injection of 80 μg produced stupor, catatonia, and inability to catch a mouse (VIEIRA et al., 1967). GRAEFF et al. (1967) reported that the intraventricular injection of 20 μg synthetic bradykinin produced in cats a behavioral and electroencephalographic state of alertness for 1.5 to 5 minutes. If this dose was preceded by administration of 150 μg of *B. jararaca* potentiating factor, the initial phase of alertness (3–8 minutes) was followed by 60 to 90 minutes of tranquilization, characterized by EEG synchronization, somnolence, relaxation of the nictitating membrane, palpebral ptosis, and catatonia, although animals reacted well when properly stimulated. The same phenomena occurred with 100 μg of bradykinin alone. In the rabbit, 50 μg of bradykinin produced identical behavior. It was further verified (Pelá and Graeff, 1967) that 200 μg bradykinin plus 500 μg BPF injected intraventricularly in the cat diminished by more than 50% the norepinephrine content of the cerebral-diencephalic trunk, without modification of the 5-hydroxytryptamine content. Atropine (2 mg/kg) inhibited the central effects of bradykinin in rabbits, including hypotension and bradycardia (Graeff and Pelá, 1968).

Smooth-Muscle Relaxation. The relaxing effect of bradykinin on rat and rabbit duodena was analyzed by Antonio et al. (1967) and by Antonio and Rocha e Silva (1967) to determine whether the liberation of epinephrine in the smooth muscles was responsible for it. They concluded that the catecholamines probably are not the mediators of the relaxing effect.

Analgesic Action. The intraventricular injection of 1 μg bradykinin into the rabbit increases markedly the pain threshold to the electric stimulation of the dental pulp for about 30 minutes. Pretreatment with reserpine (1 mg/kg, 4 hours before) abolishes this analgesic action (Ribeiro et al., 1968).

Stimulation of Chemoreceptors. Bradykinin and kallidin (0.2–0.3 μg/kg) stimulate the carotid chemoreceptors of the anesthetized dog, producing bradycardia and other effects. The selective destruction of the baroreceptors does not block the bradycardia. Physalaemin and eledoisin did not produce bradycardia; this was caused by histamine and serotonin only, in higher doses (3–6 μg/kg) (Riccioppo Netto et al., 1968).

II. Kinin Liberation

Chymotrypsin. These findings are discussed in detail in Chapter 3. Chymotrypsin had produced no appreciable effect on dog blood pressure nor did it potentiate the effect of bradykinin (Reis et al., 1967). The ability of chymotrypsin to liberate kinin from fresh guinea pig plasma was discussed by Rocha e Silva (1966).

Trypsin, Chymotrypsin, and Nagarse. Small doses of these enzymes (10–40 μg/ml) injected into dogs liberated 1–8 ng/ml of a kinin, which was potentiated by BPF. Blood kinin was assayed by superfusion on cat jejunum. The results demonstrated that doses of these three enzymes, which do not alter the level of blood kininogen, are, however, capable of liberating circulating kinin. Nagarse is thus a kininogenase *in vivo* (Ferreira and Rocha e Silva, 1968).

Plasma Acidification. Fresh horse plasma acidified to pH 2.0 for 10 minutes at 37° and then neutralized to pH 8.0 to 8.5 liberates and accumulates kinins. Activation of a kinin-forming system and kinin liberation are the two phases of this phenomenon. The pH optimum of activation was 2 to 3 and of liberation, 8 to 9. The ions Ni^{++}, Cu^{++}, and Co^{++} (1×10^{-2} M) did not affect the activation but inhibited the liberation. The kinin formation was inhibited by soybean trypsin inhibitor and benzamidine but not by ε-amino-n-caproic acid. Hexamethylenediamine did not affect the activation. About 15% of kininogen was consumed during this kinin liberation. Excess horse urinary kallikrein, although unable to exhaust the kininogen store of horse plasma *in vitro*, as measured with trypsin, inhibited the kinin liberation by acidification (Stella et al., 1967).

The acid-activated kinin-liberating system of horse plasma is not inhibited by the chloroketone TLCK. All the characteristics which have been studied in this laboratory are compatible with the interpretation that the acid-activated enzyme system is plasma kallikrein. More than 90% of the kinin activity liberated was finally identified as bradykinin by the use of CM-cellulose microcolumns (STELLA, 1968; STELLA et al., 1968).

Cellulose Sulfate. The injection of 1–3 mg cellulose sulfate/kg to rats produces marked fall in plasma kininogen and other symptoms. The kinin-releasing effect was not observed in blood from a patient with Hageman trait (ROTHSCHILD et al., 1968). Sulfated polysaccharides (polyvinyl sulfate, polyethylene, sulfated amylopectin) produce local edema in rat paw. When sulfated amylopectin is administered 12 hours previously the local edema produced by sulfated polysaccharides is reduced (CAVALCANTI et al., 1968).

III. Thermic Shock

Thermic shock was produced in anesthetized rat, heated in insulated metal boxes at 45°, until the temperature in the animal's peritoneal cavity reached 42–43°. Peritoneal fluid, collected by ROCHA E SILVA and ANTONIO's (1960) coaxial perfusion technique, contained an active substance which contracted the guinea pig ileum and rat uterus, while relaxing rat duodenum. The concentration of Evans blue, injected intravenously, increased progressively in the peritoneal fluid. The blood pressure increased when the animal's internal temperature reached 39–41°, then diminished progressively to reach lethal shock levels when the temperature increased to 42–43°. The plasma kininogen was reduced by 30 to 40% (SOUZA and ROCHA E SILVA, 1967). These results are compatible with the hypothesis that the kinin system is involved in rat thermic shock. Further, SOUZA and ROCHA E SILVA (1968) showed that although control rats averaged blood kinin concentration of 5.93 ng/ml, in heated rats the value was 7.40 ng/ml. Blood kininogen fell 14% at 15 minutes; in animals heated for 60 minutes there was a progressive fall of kininogen and the kinin level went up to 35 ng/ml. The active material was potentiated by BPF in rat blood pressure and guinea pig ileum.

IV. Oxytocic Factor in Rat Saliva and Pancreatic Juice

SIQUEIRA and BERALDO (1967) observed an active substance in rat saliva collected from the parotid duct after pilocarpine stimulation, which is strongly oxytocic on rat uterus. Some properties described are identical with those reported by BERALDO and ARAUJO (1963, 1964) for an oxytocic esterase found in rat urine. The activity contained in dialyzed saliva is such that 20 μg of salivary protein gives an uterus response equivalent to 1 μg acetylcholine. SIQUEIRA and BERALDO (1967) believe that the oxytocic factor is not salivary kallikrein, because their factor did not affect capillary permeability of rat skin and was very active on rat uterus. The existence of an identical principle in rat pancreatic juice (ARAUJO and BERALDO, 1967, 1968) was also reported. I believe that only further work will decide whether the oxytocic factor found in rat urine, saliva, and pancreatic juice is different from the respective kallikreins.

V. Kininase Activity in Brain

The kininase activity at pH 7.4 found in rabbit diencephalon and brain, homogenized in isotonic medium, is unaltered by dialysis and abolished by 30-minute boiling. The bradykinin-potentiating factor of *B. jararaca* venom doubled the half-life of added bradykinin, while 8-hydroxyquinoline was less effective as a kininase inhibitor. Chlorpromazine (1×10^{-6} to 1×10^{-4} mg/ml) had no action on the kininase activity (CAVALCANTI et al., 1967). J. L. PRADO (1963) observed that about 35 mg of rat hypothalamus homogenate, incubated (Dubnoff incubator) in 2 ml of Krebs-Ringer phosphate buffer with either 2 μg of synthetic oxytocin or

10 μg of synthetic bradykinin, inactivated both peptides at different rates. Thus, while about 70% of oxytocin activity remained after 60-minute incubation, only trace amounts of bradykinin remained after 15 minutes. In the presence of 0.1 M mercaptoethanol, oxytocin was unprotected from inactivation, but bradykinin was partially (about 25%) protected. CAMARGO (1968) studied subcellular fractions of rabbit brain homogenates and found no differences between enzyme activities which inactivated vasopressin and bradykinin.

VI. Kallikreins

Proteolytic Specificity. The effect of some enzyme inhibitors (*o*-phenanthroline, *o*Ph; benzamidine HCl, Bzd; SBTI; OMTI; and Trasylol, T) on the proteolytic activity of horse urinary, horse plasma, and pig serum kallikreins on salmine was investigated (BRANDI et al., 1967); *o*Ph and OM had no effect on both the kinin-liberating and proteolytic actions of the three kallikreins, while Bzd and T inhibited both effects. SBTI inhibited both effects of the plasma kallikreins only. High-voltage paper electrophoresis of the product of hydrolysis of salmine by trypsin and horse urinary kallikrein showed that trypsin liberated more arginine and Arg-Arg, while horse urinary kallikrein set more Arg-Arg-Arg free. The effect of horse urinary kallikrein on synthetic peptides containing arginine or lysine was reported (E. S. PRADO et al., 1967). With triarginine (Arg3), tetraarginine (Arg4), and polyarginine mol. wt. 28,000 (poly-Arg), it was observed that Arg3 is not hydrolyzed; Arg4 released Arg3, Arg2, and arginine; poly-Arg was rapidly transformed into smaller peptides, the final hydrolysis products being Arg2, Arg3, and small amounts of arginine. Polylysine, mol. wt. 182,000 (poly-Lys), was not attacked. Dipeptides of arginine were not hydrolyzed even after acetylation of the amino group. Poly-Arg in concentrations of about 6×10^{-11} M inhibited 70% of the esterolytic activity of horse urinary kallikrein on TAMe, whereas even in concentrations up to 3×10^{-5} M no inhibition of the kinin-liberating activity on horse plasma was found. BABEL et al. (1967) reported the action of horse urinary kallikrein on methionyl-lysyl-bradykinin (MLBr), lysyl-lysyl-bradykinin (LLBr), and bradykinyl-serine (Br-Ser). The hydrolysis products of Br-Ser were identified as bradykinin and serine. The products from MLBr and LLBr were studied on CM-cellulose microcolumns, indicating that MLBr yielded small amounts of bradykinin when its Lys-Arg bond was split. LLBr released even smaller amounts of bradykinin, suggesting that a second lysine residue hindered the enzyme action.

Rat Urinary Kallikrein. This kallikrein (RUK) was purified by SILVA et al. (1967) by acetone fractionation and gel filtration on Sephadex G-100 column. With the hydrolysis of benzoyl-DL-arginine-*p*-nitroanilide HCl (BAPA) and the kinin-releasing activity as criteria to measure the increase of the specific activity, RUK was purified about 27-fold. This preparation hydrolyzed BAPA at pH optimum around 9.7. From an analysis of the pH versus the activity curves, it was concluded that a group with pK' at pH 6.75–7.50 is essential for the hydrolysis. It is probably the histidine imidazol group reported by DINIZ and MARES-GUIA (1967); they have also observed that tosyl-L-lysyl-chloromethane HCl, a specific trypsin inhibitor, did not inhibit BAPA hydrolysis by RUK. This kallikrein, however, was inhibited competitively by phenylguanidine and cyclohexylguanidine sulfates as well as by benzamidine HCl and β-naphthamidine. These authors believe that a "hydrophobe-binding site" exists in the RUK-active center, as found for trypsin (MARES-GUIA and SHAW, 1965).

Horse Urinary Kallikrein. Partially purified horse urinary kallikrein (160 U/mg) was incubated for 90 minutes with fresh horse plasma (20 μg/ml) in the presence of 3×10^{-3} M *o*-phenanthroline. The active material was adsorbed on the ion exchange resin XE 64. The eluted material was filtered through a column of Sephadex G-15 and finally identified on CM-cellulose microcolumns as bradykinin. This was the only peptide found (STELLA, 1968; STELLA et al., 1968).

VII. Kinin System in Bothrops Plasma

LAVRAS et al. (1967) found a potent kininase in *B. jararaca* plasma. This kininase was destroyed completely by heating plasma at pH 2.0, 37°, 30 minutes (HORTON's treatment) or partially by heating at neutral pH, 56°, for 3 hours (WERLE's treatment). Among usual kininase inhibitors only EDTA (6×10^{-3} M) and *o*-phenanthroline (2.1×10^{-3} M) for 3 days, inhibited the activity. Purified kininogenase from *B. jararaca* venom, and both horse plasma and urinary kallikreins were unable to liberate kinin activity from *B. jararaca* plasma. In contrast, hog pancreatic kallikrein (Padutin) and plasmin liberated an active factor. The impossibility of activating a kinin-forming enzyme in *B. jararaca* plasma by glass *ballotini*, acetone, or ellagic acid suggested to these authors that this plasma is deficient in Hageman factor. Recent observations by LAVRAS et al. (1968) have shown that the active factor is hypertensive in rat, cat, and snake blood pressure; it did not relax rat duodenum and did not increase vascular permeability. Probably it is not a kinin.

VIII. Kininogen Formation

CAMARGO and CARVALHO (1968) observed that the injection of ethionine (30 mg/day i.p.), an inhibitor of protein biosynthesis, into female mice reduced plasma kininogen level in 48 hours by 70%. When the administration of ethionine was discontinued, the kininogen level regenerated within 96 hours. Reduction of other plasma proteins was only 25%. Variations in hepatic kininogen paralleled changes in plasma.

References

ANDRADE, S. O.: Chromatographic analysis on filter paper of amino acid mixtures and protein hydrolysates. Ciencia Cult. (S. Paulo) **1**, 183 (1949).

— Purification of polypeptides on the ionic resin Amberlite 50 (XE-64). Ciencia Cult. (S. Paulo) **6**, 189 (1954).

— DINIZ, C. R., ROCHA E SILVA, M.: New purification assays of bradykinin. Ciencia Cult. (S. Paulo) **4**, 124 (1952).

— — — Assay of purification of bradykinin by paper chromatography. Arch. int. Pharmacodyn. **95**, 100 (1953).

— ROCHA E SILVA, M.: Purification of bradykinin by ion exchange chromatography. Biochem. J. **64**, 701 (1956).

ANTONIO, A.: Effects of bradykinin on the guinea pig isolated heart. Segundo Encontro Nacional de Fisiologia Cardiovascular, p. 35. Institute of Biophysics, Universidade Federal of Rio de Janeiro 1966.

— RICCIOPPO NETTO, R., CORRADO, A. P.: Analysis of the relaxing effects of noradrenaline, bradykinin and nicotine on rat and rabbit isolated duodena. Ciencia Cult. (S. Paulo) **19**, 397 (1967).

— ROCHA E SILVA, M.: Effect of drugs on the edema produced by heating the rat's paw to 44—45° (thermic edema). Ciencia Cult. (S. Paulo) **12**, 102 (1960).

— — Factors which affect the relaxation produced on intestinal smooth musculature by bradykinin. Ciencia Cult. (S. Paulo) **19**, 396 (1967).

ARAUJO, R. L., BERALDO, W. T.: Activity of pancreatic juice on smooth musculature. Ciencia Cult. (S. Paulo) **19**, 406 (1967).

— — Presence of a hypotensive and oxytocic substance in rat pancreatic juice. Ciencia Cult. (S. Paulo) **20**, 419 (1968).

BABEL, I., STELLA, R. C. R., PRADO, E. S.: Action of horse urinary kallikrein on synthetic derivatives of bradykinin. Ciencia Cult. (S. Paulo) **19**, 395 (1967).

BERALDO, W. T.: Bradykinin formation by the action of peptone and fibrinolysin on plasma globulins *in vitro*. Ciencia Cult. (S. Paulo) **2**, 300 (1950).

BERALDO, W. T.: A new hypotensive and smooth muscle stimulating principle (substance U) found in urine. Ciencia Cult. (S. Paulo) **4**, 129 (1952).
— Bradykinin. Gaz. méd. port. **6**, 407 (1953).
— Substance U: Its relations with other active substances in urine. Ciencia Cult. (S. Paulo) **6**, 176 (1954).
— Study of the mechanism of action of peptone intravenously injected into dogs and rats. Thesis, Faculdade de Medicina, U.S.P., S. Paulo, 1958.
— Study of a substance found in urine (substance U) which acts on smooth muscle and blood pressure. Thesis, Faculdade de Medicina, Universidade de Minas Gerais, Belo Horizonte, 1961.
— ARAUJO, R. L.: Study of a substance present in rat urine which is active on smooth muscle. Ciencia Cult. (S. Paulo) **15**, 285 (1963).
— — Presence of an oxytocic factor in rat urine. Ciencia Cult. (S. Paulo) **16**, 201 (1964).
— FELDBERG, W., HILTON, S. M.: Experiments on the urinary elimination of the substance U forming factor. Ciencia Cult. (S. Paulo) **8**, 180 (1956).
BRANDI, C. M. W., MENDES, J., PAIVA, A. C. M.: Proteolytic activity of horse urinary kallikrein on protamin. Ciencia Cult. (S. Paulo) **16**, 265 (1964).
— PRADO, E. S., PRADO, J. L.: Observations on the hydrolysis of salmine by urinary and plasmatic kallikreins. Ciencia Cult. (S. Paulo) **19**, 395 (1967).
BRAUN-MENENDEZ, E., FASCIOLO, J. C., LELOIR, L. F., MUÑOZ, J. M.: The pressor substance in the blood from ischemic kidney. Rev. Soc. argent. Biol. **15**, 420 (1939).
CABRAL, R., BERALDO, W. T.: Presence of bradykinin in the peripheral blood of dogs following a milk injection into the stomach. Ciencia Cult. (S. Paulo) **17**, 289 (1965).
CAMARGO, A. C. M.: Bradykinin inactivation by subcellular fractions from rabbit brain. Ciencia Cult. (S. Paulo) **20**, 417 (1968).
— CARVALHO, I. F.: Modifications of kininogen in liver and plasma of ethionine treated mice. Ciencia Cult. (S. Paulo) **20**, 417 (1968).
CARDOSO, S. S., CORRADO, A. P.: Effect of bradykinin, kallidin and histamine on the blood-cerebrospinal fluid barrier. Ciencia Cult. (S. Paulo) **15**, 286 (1963).
CARVALHO, I. F.: Effect of hepatectomy and hepatic lesions on the formation of bradykininogen. Ciencia Cult. (S. Paulo) **14**, 258 (1962).
— Kininogenin in rat kidney tissue. Thesis, Faculdade de Medicina de Ribeirão Preto, U.S.P., 1963.
— DINIZ, C. R.: Kininogenin in rat kidney tissue. Ciencia Cult. (S. Paulo) **15**, 286 (1963).
— — Cellular localization of renin and kininogenin. Ciencia Cult. (S. Paulo) **16**, 263 (1964).
CAVALCANTI, R. Q., GRAEFF, R. G., CAMARGO, A. C. M., ROCHA E SILVA, M.: Inhibition of the bradykinin-inactivating action of rabbit brain homogenates. Ciencia Cult. (S. Paulo) **19**, 401 (1967).
— ROCHA E SILVA, M., REIS, M. L.: Anti-inflammatory action of sulfated polysaccharides. Ciencia Cult. (S. Paulo) **20**, 406 (1968).
CHAPMAN, L. F., RAMOS, A., GOODELL, H., WOLF, H. G.: Neurokinin, a polypeptide formed during neuronal activity in man. Trans. Amer. neurol. Ass. **85**, 42 (1960).
CORRADO, A. P.: Bradykinin determination in the circulating blood. Ciencia Cult. (S. Paulo) **16**, 256 (1964a).
— Considerations upon the participation of bradykinin and analogous peptides on the hemodynamic effects produced by proteolytic enzymes. Thesis, Faculdade de Medicina de Ribeirão Preto, U.S.P., 1964b.
— CAPEK, R., FERREIRA, S. H., ROCHA E SILVA, M.: Electroencephalographic analysis of the central actions of bradykinin. Ciencia Cult. (S. Paulo) **15**, 271 (1963).
— RAMOS, A. O., ROCHA E SILVA, M.: Possible central actions of bradykinin. Ciencia Cult. (S. Paulo) **11**, 165 (1959).
CROXATTO, H.: Arterial hypertension and vasoactive polypeptides. Conferencias Eduardo Braun-Menendez, Buenos Aires, 1961.
— BELMAR, J., PEREDA, T., LABARCA, E.: Action of bradykinin and anephrotensin on the blood pressure of normal and nephrectomized animals. Read before the 4th Meeting of Ass. Latinoam. Cien. Fisiol., Ribeirão, Preto, July 1961. Published in English: Acta physiol. lat.-amer. **12**, 19 (1962).
DINIZ, C. R.: Separation of proteins and characterization of active substances in the venom of spiders from Brazil. An. Acad. bras. Cienc. **35**, 283 (1963).
— CARVALHO, I. F.: Bradykininogen determination in normal and pathologic conditions. Ciencia Cult. (S. Paulo) **16**, 257 (1964).
— CORRADO, A. P., CARVALHO, I. F., RYAN, J.: Plasma bradykininogen in animals with cardiovascular shock. Ciencia Cult. (S. Paulo) **14**, 258 (1962).
— MARES-GUIA, M.: Study on the mechanism of catalysis by rat urinary kallikrein. Ciencia Cult. (S. Paulo) **19**, 455 (1967).

Endo, R. M., Carlini, E. A.: Effect of Nagarse on angiotensins I and II. Ciencia Cult. (S. Paulo) **18**, 184 (1966).
Espada, J., Fasciolo, J. C., Binia, A., Cabut, M. S.: Relationship between bradykininogen and angiotensinogen. Rev. Soc. argent. Biol. **37**, 65 (1961).
Fasciolo, J. C., Espada, J., Carretero, O.: The estimation of bradykininogen content of the plasma. Acta physiol. lat.-amer. **13**, 215 (1963).
— Halvorsen, K. A., Binia, A., Itoiz, J. E.: Angiotensin, bradykinin and substance V. Acta physiol. lat.-amer. **10**, 23 (1960).
— — Zangheri, E., Fernandez, F. O.: Comparison between bradykinin and substance V. Rev. Soc. argent. Biol. **34**, 239 (1958).
Ferreira, S. H.: Potentiation of bradykinin. Ciencia Cult. (S. Paulo) **16**, 261 (1964a).
— Potentiation of bradykinin by a factor present in the venom of *Bothrops jararaca*. Thesis, Faculdade de Medicina de Ribeirão Preto, U.S.P., 1964b.
— Corrado, A. P., Rocha e Silva, M.: Potentiation of the plasma bradykininolytic enzyme. Ciencia Cult. (S. Paulo) **14**, 238 (1962).
— Rocha e Silva, M.: Potentiation of polypeptides (bradykinin, angiotensin, oxytocin, etc.) by a factor present in *B. jararaca's* venom. Ciencia Cult. (S. Paulo) **15**, 276 (1963).
— — Potentiation of bradykinin and eledoisin by bradykinin potentiating factor. Ciencia Cult. (S. Paulo) **17**, 272 (1965).
— — Trypsin, chymotrypsin and Nagarse: Kinin liberation and hemodynamic effects. Ciencia Cult. (S. Paulo) **20**, 406 (1968).
Freire-Maia, L.: Study of the mechanisms of peptone and anaphylactic shocks in the rat. Thesis, Faculdade de Medicina da Universidade de Minas Gerais, Belo Horizonte, 1963.
Gaddum, J. H. (ed.): Polypeptides which stimulate plain muscle. London 1955.
Gascon, L. A., Rothschild, A. M.: Formation of bradykinin by agar and heparin in the plasma of several animal species. Ciencia Cult. (S. Paulo) **17**, 271 (1965).
Gomes, F. P.: Biologically active peptides. Contribution to their study. Thesis, Faculdade de Medicina da Universidade de Lisboa, 1958.
— Biologically active peptides. Arch. Pat. (Lisbon) **31**, 1 (1959).
Gonçalves, J. M.: Electrophoretic analysis in Brazilian snakes. Communication to the 4th Chemical South American Congress, Santiago, Chile, 1948.
— Studies on the poison of Brazilian snakes. I. Electrophoretic analysis. An. Acad. bras. Cienc. **22**, 141 (1950).
Graeff, F. G., Corrado, A. P., Pelá, J. R.: Behavioral and electroencephalographic effects of bradykinin. Potentiation by BPF. Ciencia Cult. (S. Paulo) **19**, 399 (1967).
— Ferreira, S. H., Corrado, A. P.: Potentiation of the vasodilating effect of bradykinin in the cerebral circulation by "bradykinin potentiating factor", BPF. Ciencia Cult. (S. Paulo) **17**, 270 (1965).
— Pelá, I. R.: Central effects of bradykinin in the rabbit. Ciencia Cult. (S. Paulo) **20**, 413 (1968).
Halvorsen, K. A., Fasciolo, J. C., Binia, A., Carretero, O. A.: Enzymatic destruction of substance V. Rev. Soc. argent. Biol. **36**, 70 (1960).
— — Calvo, R., Chionetti, I.: A vasodilating substance present in very purified angiotensin preparations. Rev. Soc. argent. Biol. **34**, 185 (1958).
Hamberg, U.: Factors which affect the yield of bradykinin preparations. Ciencia Cult. (S. Paulo) **9**, 166 (1957).
— Spontaneous liberation of bradykinin and activation of rat and beef plasma protease. Ciencia Cult. (S. Paulo) **10**, 174 (1958).
— Rocha e Silva, M.: Studies on the enzymatic inactivation of bradykinin. Acta physiol. scand. **30**, 215 (1954).
— — Mechanism of bradykinin liberation. Ciencia Cult. (S. Paulo) 8, 176 (1956).
Henriques, O. B., Picarelli, Z. P., Oliveira, M. C.: Bradykininogen. Ciencia Cult. (S. Paulo) **14**, 246 (1962).
Katchburian, A. V., Prado, J. L., Prado, E. S.: Effect of some ions on the kininogenic activity of horse urinary kallikrein. Ciencia Cult. (S. Paulo) **14**, 222 (1962).
Krieger, E. M., Corrado, A. P.: Action of bradykinin on the carotidean baroceptors of the dog. Ciencia Cult. (S. Paulo) **17**, 269 (1965).
Lavras, A. A. C., Fichman, M., Hiraichi, E., Picarelli, Z. P.: Comparative study on kinin liberation in plasmas from several species. Commun. 7th Annual Meeting, Ass. Latino-Amer. Cien. Fisiol., Mexico, 1967.
— — — —Personal communication 1968.
— Henriques, O. B., Picarelli, Z. P., Oliveira, M. C.: Bradykinin-liberating and esterolytic activities of some fractions from human blood plasma. Ciencia Cult. (S. Paulo) **14**, 246 (1962).

Leake, C. D.: Development of knowledge about venoms. In: Venoms, ed. by E. E. Buckley and N. Porges. Publ. No 44 of the Amer. Ass. Advanc. Sci. 1956.
Leme, J. G.: Studies on the inhibition of bradykinin. Thesis, Ribeirão Preto, S. Paulo, 1966.
— Rocha e Silva, M.: Antagonists of bradykinin (*in vitro* experiments). Ciencia Cult. (S. Paulo) **16**, 258 (1964).
Mares-Guia, M., Shaw, E.: Studies on the active center of trypsin. J. biol. Chem. **240**, 1579 (1965).
Martinez, A. R.: Vasoactive polypeptides and partum physiology. Ciencia Cult. (S. Paulo) **16**, 265 (1964a).
— Bradykininogen in human plasma during partum and puerperium and in plasma from umbilical cord. Matern. e Inf. (S. Paulo) (Arch. Médicos Sociais) **23**, 147 (1964b).
Oehling, R., Corbett, C. E. P., Ramos, L., Ramos, A. O.: Pharmacological activity of aqueous humor from some animal species including man. Rev. Fac. Farm. Bioquim. U.S. Paulo **2**, 9 (1963).
Paiva, T. B., Paiva, A. C. M.: The inhibition of cationic myotropic drugs by compounds 48/80 and 46/108. Biochem. Pharmacol. **15**, 1303 (1966).
Pelá, I. R., Graeff, F. G.: Effects of intraventricular injection of bradykinin on the norepinephrine and serotonin contents of the cat and rabbit cerebral diencephalic trunk. Ciencia Cult. (S. Paulo) **19**, 400 (1967).
Pereira, J. R.: Bradykinin and other slow reacting substances. Rev. bras. Med. **10**, 155 (1953).
Picarelli, Z. P.: Inactivation of synthetic bradykinin by tissue extracts. Ciencia Cult. (S. Paulo) **14**, 233 (1962a).
— Kininases. Ciencia Cult (S. Paulo) **14**, 232 (1962b).
— Branco, T. S., Valle, J. R.: Effects of bradykinin and hypertensin on the vas deferens and seminal vesicles from normal and castrated rats. Ciencia Cult. (S. Paulo) **3**, 288 (1951).
Pimazoni Neto, A., Corrado, A. P., Rocha e Silva, M.: Pressor effects following intramural injection of bradykinin into dog's carotid sinus. Ciencia Cult. (S. Paulo) **16**, 199 (1964).
Prado, E. S.: Vasoactive polypeptides and their liberators. Selecta Chim. (S. Paulo) **19**, 219 (1960).
— Beraldo, W. T., Rocha e Silva, M.: Experiments on the purification of bradykinin. Ciencia Cult. (S. Paulo) **2**, 44 (1950a).
— — — Bradykinin, assay of purification. Arch. Biochem. **27**, 410 (1950b).
— Prado, J. L.: Substance U liberator from horse urine. Ciencia Cult. (S. Paulo) **12**, 177 (1960).
— — Brandi, C. M. W., Katchburian, A. V.: Preparation of highly purified horse urinary kallikrein. Ciencia Cult. (S. Paulo) **14**, 223 (1962a).
— Stella, R. C. R., Brandi, C. M. W.: Action of horse urinary kallikrein on arginine and lysine-peptides. Ciencia Cult. (S. Paulo) **19**, 394 (1967).
Prado, J. L.: Kininogenases, plasmakinin-liberating enzymes. Ciencia Cult. (S. Paulo) **14**, 231 (1962).
— Unpublished observations 1963.
— Considerations upon the enzymic specificities of kininogenases. Acta physiol. lat.-amer. **14**, 215 (1964a).
— Vasoactive peptides in wasp venom. Ciencia Cult. (S. Paulo) **16**, 227 (1964b).
— Mendes, J., Prado, E. S., Kramer, C.: Ions and the kininogenic activity of horse urinary kallikrein. Ciencia Cult. (S. Paulo) **17**, 257 (1965).
— Prado, E. S., Jurkiewicz, A.: On the liberation of plasma-kinins by a crystalline protease from *B. subtilis* (Nagarse). Ciencia Cult. (S. Paulo) **14**, 223 (1962b).
— Tamura, Z., Furano, E., Pisano, J. J., Udenfriend, S.: Characterization of kinins in wasp venom. In: Hypotensive peptides, p. 93, ed. by E. G. Erdös, N. Back and F. Sicuteri. Berlin-Heidelberg-New York: Springer 1966.
Ramos, A. O.: Presence or formation of a pharmacologically active substance in human cerebrospinal fluid. Thesis, Univ. São Paulo, 1961.
— Chapman, L., Ramos, L., Zileli, T.: Potentiation of neurokinin and bradykinin on rat blood pressure by lysergic acid diethylamide (LSD). Ciencia Cult. (S. Paulo) **13**, 187 (1961a).
— Corrado, A. P., Rocha e Silva, M.: Comparative study of the pharmacologic actions of oxytocin and bradykinin on the smooth muscles and arterial pressure of several animal species. Ciencia Cult. (S. Paulo) **10**, 176 (1958).
— Zyngier, S., Ramos, L.: Influence of lysergic acid diethylamide on the effects of neurokinin and bradykinin on the dog. Folia clín. biol. (S. Paulo) **32**, 14 (1963b).
Ramos, L., Chapman, L. F., Zileli, T., Ramos, A. O.: Inhibition of the effects of neurokinin from cerebrospinal fluid on rat duodenum and blood pressure. Acta physiol. lat.-amer. **11**, 272 (1961b).

Ramos, L., Ramos, A. O.: Pharmacological activity of aqueous humor. Acta physiol. lat.-amer. **11**, 273 (1961).
— — Pereira, J. R.: Characterization of bilikinin. Ciencia Cult. (S. Paulo) **13**, 104 (1961c).
— — Zyngier, S.: Action of neurokinin on capillary permeability. Folia clín. biol. (S. Paulo) **32**, 20 (1963a).
Reis, M. L., Carvalho, I. F., Diniz, C. R., Corrado, A. P.: Participation of bradykinin and analogous peptides on the genesis of cardiovascular shocks produced by proteolytic enzymes. Ciencia Cult. (S. Paulo) **16**, 199 (1964).
— Diniz, C. R., Carvalho, I. F., Corrado, A. P.: Bradykinin liberation in some types of cardiovascular shock. Ciencia Cult. (S. Paulo) **15**, 260 (1963).
— Ferreira, S. H., Rocha e Silva, M.: Kinin liberation from fresh guinea pig plasma by chymotrypsin. Ciencia Cult. (S. Paulo) **19**, 393 (1967).
Ribeiro, S. A., Graeff, F. G., Corrado, A. P.: Analgesic effect of bradykinin. Ciencia Cult. (S. Paulo) **20**, 413 (1968).
Riccioppo Netto, F., Corrado, A. P., Krieger, E. M.: Stimulation of carotidean chemoreceptors by vasoactive polypeptides. Ciencia Cult. (S. Paulo) **20**, 412 (1968).
Rocha e Silva, M.: Action of trypsin on smooth muscle. Liberation of histamine from the perfused guinea pig lung. Arch. Inst. biol. (S. Paulo) **9**, 145 (1938).
— Pharmacology of trypsin. Action on mammalian smooth muscles and isolated heart. Circulatory effects of trypsin. Experiments with a crystalline material. Arch. Inst. biol. (S. Paulo) **10**, 93 (1939).
— Autopharmacology and animal poisons. Arch. Inst. biol. (S. Paulo) **19**, 1 (1949).
— Mechanism of action of bradykinin. Ciencia Cult. (S. Paulo) **2**, 299 (1950).
— Bradykinin. Preparation, biologic assay. Identification. Thesis, Faculdade Nacional de Medicina da Universidade do Brasil, Rio de Janeiro, 1951.
— Slow reacting substances liberated by (or present in) venoms. Ciencia Cult. (S. Paulo) **6**, 184 (1954).
— On the possible biological meaning of bradykinin. Ciencia Cult. (S. Paulo) **7**, 223 (1955).
— Concerning the theory of receptors in pharmacology. A rational method of estimation of pA_x. Arch. int. Pharmacodyn. **118**, 74 (1959).
— Antagonism of arginine and its esters BAMe and TAMe in relation to histamine, acetylcholine, bradykinin and ATP. Ciencia Cult. (S. Paulo) **13**, 192 (1961).
— Bradykinin. Acta physiol. lat.-amer. **12**, 66 (1962a).
— Definition of bradykinin and other kinins. Biochem. Pharmacol. **10**, 3 (1962b).
— Antagonists of bradykinin. Thesis, Faculdade de Medicina, Ribeirão Preto, 1963.
— Some aspects of the mechanism of bradykinin liberation from plasma. Anais Acad. bras. Cienc. **38**, 583-R (1966).
— Antonio, A.: Coaxial perfusion of the thermic (45°) edema area in the rat's paw and liberation of a substance similar to bradykinin. Ciencia Cult. (S. Paulo) **12**, 102 (1960).
— Beraldo, W. T.: A new autopharmacologic principle liberated from plasma by snake venoms and trypsin. Ciencia Cult. (S. Paulo) **1**, 32 (1949).
— — Rosenfeld, G.: Bradykinin, a hypotensive and smooth muscle stimulating factor released from plasma globulin by snake venoms and by trypsin. Amer. J. Physiol. **156**, 261 (1949).
— Hamberg, U.: On the nature of the bond split by bradykinin liberating agents. Ciencia Cult. (S. Paulo) 8, 177 (1956).
— Holzhacker, E.: Liberation of bradykinin from rat plasma by heating with 0.1 N hydrochloric acid. Ciencia Cult. (S. Paulo) **10**, 174 (1958).
— Leme, J. G.: Antagonists of bradykinin. Med. exp. (Basel) 8, 287 (1963).
— — Studies on the antagonists of bradykinin. Excerpta med. (Amst.), Int. Congr. Ser. No 82. Proceedings, Int. Symposium on Non-steroidal Anti-inflammatory Drugs, p. 120. Milan, 1964.
Rocha e Silva, M., Jr.: Liberation of the antidiuretic principle from posterior pituitary by bradykinin. Thesis, Universidade de São Paulo, 1963a.
— Liberation of antidiuretic hormone by bradykinin. Ciencia Cult. (S. Paulo) **15**, 284 (1963b).
Rosa, G., Buffolo, E.: Homochlorcyclizine (SA-97) as antagonist, mainly of serotonin. Ciencia Cult. (S. Paulo) **14**, 233 (1962).
— Valle, J. R.: Homochlorcyclizine as antagonist against chemical mediators and plasmakinins. Acta physiol. lat.-amer. **12**, 408 (1962).
Rothschild, A. M., Castania, A., Rosa, A. T.: Pharmacodynamic aspects of the action of cellulose sulfate, a polyanion which releases kinin from rat and human plasma. Ciencia Cult. (S. Paulo) **20**, 416 (1968).
Rothschild, Z., Rothschild, A. M.: Activation of plasma bradykininforming system by polysaccharide sulfuric esters. Acta physiol. lat.-amer. **16**, Suppl. 1, 115 (1966).

SCHMIDT, B. J.: Congenital generalized analgesia. Contribution to the study of its etiopathogeny. Thesis, Escola Paulista de Medicina, São Paulo, 1963.
— RAMOS, A. O.: Formation of neurokinin and PPS (pain producing substance) in patients with congenital analgesia. Ciencia Cult. (S. Paulo) **14**, 221 (1962).
SEGURA-CARDONA, R.: Inhibition of angiotensin, bradykinin and oxytocin by extracts from different organs. Rev. esp. Fisiol. **20**, 27 (1964).
SILVA, E., DINIZ, C. R., MARES-GUIA, M., BARROSO, J.: Purification of rat urinary kallikrein. Ciencia Cult. (S. Paulo) **19**, 394 (1967).
SIQUEIRA, G. R., BERALDO, W. T.: Experiments upon an oxytocic factor from rat saliva. Ciencia Cult. (S. Paulo) **19**, 397 (1967).
SLOTTA, C. H., FRAENKEL-CONRAT, H. L.: Chemical studies on ophidic poisons. 4. Purification and crystallization of rattlesnake's venom. Mem. Inst. Butantan **12**, 505 (1939).
SOUZA, J. M. DE, ROCHA E SILVA, M.: Possible participation of kinins (bradykinin) on the mechanism of thermic shock in rats. Ciencia Cult. (S. Paulo) **19**, 396 (1967).
— — New evidences for the bradykinin participation in thermic shock in rats. Ciencia Cult. (S. Paulo) **20**, 405 (1968).
STELLA, R. C. R.: Study on the liberation of kinins from horse plasma by the system activated by acid and by horse urinary kallikrein. Thesis, Escola Paulista de Medicina, 1968.
— MENDES, J., PRADO, J. L.: Liberation of kinins from horse plasma. Ciencia Cult. (S. Paulo) **19**, 393 (1967).
— — — Identification of kinins liberated from horse plasma by acidification and by the action of horse urinary kallikrein. Ciencia Cult. (S. Paulo) **20**, 422 (1968).
VALLE, J. R.: Primordia pharmacologiae in Brasilia, São Paulo, 1966. Cf. p. 92, J. B. LACERDA (1881): Experimental evidence that snake venom is a digestive juice.
— PICARELLI, Z. P.: The action of bradykinin, histamine and adenyl compounds upon the seminal vesicles of normal and castrated rats. Acta physiol. lat.-amer. **4**, 61 (1954).
VELAZQUEZ, B. L., JALON, P. D. G. DE, SAN JULIAN, C. F. DE: The factor time in Vane's technique. The specificity of this method. Arch. Inst. Farmacol. exp. (Madr.) **13**, 91 (1961).
VIEIRA, F. J. A., AGUIAR, M. B. DE, NOGUEIRA, I. C., MENEZES, G. M.: Some effects of synthetic bradykinin on the cat behavior. Ciencia Cult. (S. Paulo) **19**, 392 (1967).
VUGMAN, I.: Modifications of guinea pig plasma bradykininogen in shock produced by epinephrine. Ciencia Cult. (S. Paulo) **15**, 259 (1963).
WERLE, E., BEREK, U.: Zur Kenntnis des Kallikreins. Angew. Chem. **60**, 53 (1948).
— ERDÖS, E. G.: Über eine neue blutdrucksenkende, darm- und uteruserregende Substanz im menschlichen Urin. Naunyn-Schmiedebergs Arch. exp. Path. Pharmak. **223**, 234 (1954).
— GÖTZE, W., KEPPLER, A.: Über die Wirkung des Kallikreins auf den isolierten Darm und über eine neue darmkontrahierende Substanz. Biochem. Z. **289**, 217 (1937).
— HAMBUECHEN, R.: Zur Kenntnis der blutdrucksenkenden und spasmolytischen Wirkung des Kallikreins und der Substanz D K. Naunyn-Schmiedebergs Arch. exp. Path. Pharmak. **201**, 311 (1943).
— KEHL, R., KOEBKE, K.: Über Trypsin, Chymotrypsin, Kallidin und Bradykinin. Biochem. Z. **321**, 372 (1950).
ZYNGIER, S., RAMOS, L., PEREIRA, J. R., RAMOS, A. O.: Bilikinin activity on intestinal musculature. Ciencia Cult. (S. Paulo) **14**, 222 (1962).

Appendix

Recommendations for Nomenclature and Units

MARION E. WEBSTER

A. Nomenclature

The nomenclature for the components of this enzyme system had become so involved that the same enzyme, the same substrate, and the same polypeptide were known by at least two (and frequently more) different names. To clarify this situation a meeting was held on October 27, 1965, in Florence, Italy, to investigate the possibility of evolving a compromise nomenclature. The recommendations (WEBSTER, 1966), with which not all investigators have agreed (ROCHA E SILVA, 1963, 1965, and personal communication) are again repeated together with a few additional comments.

Historical Background

Three main systems, i.e. the kallikrein–kallidinogen–kallidin nomenclature, the bradykininogen–bradykinin nomenclature, and the kininogenase–kininogen–kinin nomenclature, were currently in use. The term kallikrein, derived from the Greek word for pancreas *(kallikreas)* was given (KRAUT et al., 1930) for a hypotensive substance found in urine and in pancreas. Subsequent investigation made it clear that the kallikreins exerted their hypotensive action by enzymatic release of a polypeptide, called kallidin, from a substrate in plasma, called kallidinogen (WERLE and BEREK, 1948). Other investigators (ROCHA E SILVA et al., 1949) reported that trypsin and some snake venoms released a polypeptide from plasma. This peptide was named bradykinin; the substrate in plasma was called bradykininogen. The term "plasma kinin" was coined (LAKI, 1943) to describe a thromboplastin-like activity in blood which plays a role in the conversion of prothrombin to thrombin. However, this nomenclature was never widely adopted. Later (SCHACHTER and THAIN, 1954) used the term "wasp kinin" or simply "kinin" for a hypotensive polypeptide from wasp venom which could be distinguished from kallidin and bradykinin. In 1956 MILLER et al. proposed it as a class name for substances implicated in the cell division phase of fruit growth. Recently it has been suggested that phytokinin (DEDOLPH, 1965) or cytokinin (SKOOG et al., 1965) replace the term kinin for these plant materials. In 1958 (LEWIS) the use of "plasma kinins" was proposed to apply to all bradykinin-like polypeptides derived from plasma proteins. This nomenclature has since been amplified by a number of investigators so that the substrate in plasma is called "kininogen" and the enzymes that release kinins are called "kininogenases". In 1961–63 the expression kinin-hormones or simply kinins was proposed (ROCHA E SILVA, 1962, 1963) to describe a group of local hormones which include the angiotensins, the bradykinins (kallidins), and substance P.

Recommendations

I. Kinin-Hormones

The Committee was in agreement that a class name for vasoactive polypeptides, particularly for the angiotensins and for bradykinin (kallidin), would be desirable since they are both liberated from plasma proteins by endogenous enzymes. However, the use of the term kinin-hormone would be confusing as the prefix kinin in names such as kininogenase, kininogen, and kinins could then be construed to mean kallikrein or renin, bradykininogen (kallidinogen) or angiotensinogen, and bradykinin (kallidin etc.) or angiotensin. The Committee recommends that kinin-hormone not be used as a class name for vasoactive polypeptides.

II. Enzyme Nomenclature

Kininogenase. It is recommended that the term kininogenase be restricted to any enzyme that liberates a kinin from an inactive protein substrate. Thus the kallikreins, trypsin, pepsin, snake venom, bacterial proteinases, etc. are all kininogenases, and should be referred to by their trivial name. Adjectival terms such as "kininogenic" or "kininolytic" should be avoided.

Kallikrein (EC 3.4.4.21). A kallikrein is defined as an endogenous enzyme which rapidly and specifically liberates a kinin from the kininogens in plasma. The inactive enzyme precursor should be called prekallikrein in conformation with the suggestions of the International Union of Biochemistry on Nomenclature (Enzyme Nomenclature, 1965). In view of the many known chemical and physical differences between the kallikreins, each kallikrein should be identified by species and source, i.e. hog pancreatic kallikrein. Since the possibility exists that more than one kallikrein may be found in plasma (WERLE, 1934; ARMSTRONG and MILLS, 1964; VOGT and WAWRETSCHEK, 1968), or in other body tissues or fluids, each kallikrein which is thought to be a different protein and has been prepared from a single source should be identified by the method of activation and by some property that distinguishes it from the other kallikreins. For those kallikreins which are thought to be isoenzymes, designations such as A-1, A-2, A-3, etc. can be provisionally employed.

Kininase. Kininase may be used as a general term to describe enzymes which inactivate kinins. As the various kininases are isolated and the bonds which they split are identified, a descriptive trivial name should be assigned by the investigator in an attempt to describe the particular bond split by the enzyme, i.e. carboxypeptidase N for the main kininase activity found in plasma of a variety of animal species (ERDÖS et al., 1963, 1964).

III. Substrate and Polypeptides

Kininogen. As the Committee did not wish to superimpose on the existing nomenclature system yet another compromise name for kallidinogen (WERLE and BEREK, 1948) and bradykininogen (ROCHA E SILVA et al., 1949), it is recommended that all proteins which release a kinin by the action of proteolytic enzymes be called kininogens.

More than one kininogen has been found in certain mammalian plasma (HABERMANN, 1963; SUZUKI et al., 1966; PIERCE and WEBSTER, 1966; HENRIQUES et al., 1966, 1967; JACOBSEN and KRIZ, 1967), and confusion has arisen in the literature in designating them as kininogens I and II. For example, the 50,000 molecular weight kininogen from bovine plasma has been called both kininogen I (HABERMANN, 1963) and kininogen II (NAGASAWA et al., 1966), and the same terms have been used to differentiate two 50,000 molecular weight forms isolated from human plasma (PIERCE and WEBSTER, 1966). HABERMANN (1963) and NAGASAWA et al. (1966) considered the high molecular weight forms (kininogen II and I respectively) to be artifacts formed during the purification procedure, but both HENRIQUES et al. (1966, 1967) and JACOBSEN and KRIZ (1967) have demonstrated the existence in plasma of kininogens which differ in enzyme susceptibility, and the latter have isolated both low (50,000) and high (200,000) molecular weight forms. To clarify this situation it is recommended that the terms LMW (low molecular weight) and HMW (high molecular weight) be used provisionally to designate the two classes of kininogen so far described (PIERCE, 1968). The two 50,000 molecular weight kininogens from human plasma (PIERCE and WEBSTER, 1966) should now be called LMW-I and LMW-II respectively.

Kinins. Kinin is a general name indicating a hypotensive polypeptide that contracts most isolated smooth muscle preparations but relaxes the rat duodenum. Kinins increase vascular permeability, produce pain when applied to an exposed blister base on human skin, and cause bronchoconstriction in the guinea pig. In addition, the name may be applied to any polypeptide which is structurally related to bradykinin. Ornithokinin, however, which is presumably not structurally related to bradykinin, should be classified as a kinin since it is hypotensive in birds and released from bird plasma by ornithokallikrein.

Bradykinin. The term bradykinin refers to the nonapeptide (H-Arg-Pro-Pro-Gly-Phe-Ser-Pro-Phe-Arg-OH) as isolated by ELLIOTT et al. (1961) from a trypsin digest of a bovine plasma fraction.

Kallidin. The term kallidin refers to the decapeptide (H-Lys-Arg-Pro-Pro-Gly-Phe-Ser-Pro-Phe-Arg-OH) formed by the action of the glandular kallikreins on kininogen (WEBSTER and PIERCE, 1963; WERLE and TRAUTSCHOLD, 1963; HABERMANN, 1966).

Other Kinins. The Committee was unable to agree on a uniform policy for naming derivatives of bradykinin or kallidin. It was recommended that this decision be reserved to the author who first identified or synthesized the structure. Thus methionylkallidin should be referred to as methionyllysylbradykinin (Met-Lys-Arg^1-bradykinin) (ELLIOTT and LEWIS, 1965), and the derivative obtained by the action of trypsin on wasp kinin should be referred to as glycine^1-kallidin (Gly^1-kallidin) (SCHRÖDER and HEMPEL, 1964; PISANO, 1968). Since this latter polypeptide is also a decapeptide, it is recommended that expressions such as kallidin-9, kallidin-10, kinin-9, kinin-10, etc. be discontinued.

Membership of the Committee

Members who attended the committee meeting in Florence were:

D. ARMSTRONG	England	M. SCHACHTER	Canada
N. BACK	U.S.A.	E. SCHRÖDER	Germany
C. R. DINIZ	Brazil	F. SICUTERI	Italy
E. G. ERDÖS	U.S.A.	I. TRAUTSCHOLD	Germany
E. HABERMANN	Germany	W. VOGT	Germany
J. MARGOLIS	Australia	M. E. WEBSTER	U.S.A.
H. MORIYA	Japan	E. WERLE	Germany
J. L. PRADO	Brazil		

Corresponding members:

V. EISEN	England	J. V. PIERCE	U.S.A.
D. F. ELLIOTT	England	E. S. PRADO	Brazil
C. A. KEELE	England		

B. Standards and Units

The Committee on Nomenclature for Hypotensive Peptides has recently been reconvened in order to attempt to define standards and units for the various components of the kinin system. One such standard unit is currently available and has been defined for kallikrein by FREY et al. (1950). In these studies, one kallikrein unit—which has been variously abbreviated as KE, KU, or FU (Frey unit)—was defined as the decrease in blood pressure of the anesthetized dog after intravenous injection of 5.0 ml dialyzed normal human urine which had been taken from a pool of 50 liters of urine. Pools of urine of this magnitude, however, do not always contain 1 kallikrein unit per 5.0 ml, and the original unit has been maintained by exchanges of biologically active materials between investigators. This unit has been and still is of great use to many investigators in this field and it is recommended that the abbreviation KU be adopted. However, in many laboratories kallikrein activity is no longer measured by this technique which has the limitation that it measures only the ability of the kallikreins to form kinins from dog (and not other) kininogens. In addition, other components of the kinin system have not been standardized. The Committee therefore recommends the following standards and units, realizing that these recommendations will undoubtedly be modified when more precise measurement of this system becomes possible.

I. Kinins

In the absence of an international standard and with the knowledge that synthetic bradykinins or kallidins vary in potency, it is proposed that the new bradykinin prepared by the Biological and Medical Research Division, Sandoz Ltd., Basle, Switzerland (BRS-640, Batch no. 69055), and dispensed in vials containing 100 μg bradykinin per ml of sodium acetate–sodium chloride buffer, pH 4.5, be utilized wherever possible as the standard bradykinin. Care should be taken to maintain the stability of the polypeptide during dilution (for discussion see ERDÖS, 1966).

II. Kininogen

One unit of kininogen (KgU) is defined as the amount of substrate which will yield 1 micromole of bradykinin equivalent in the presence of excess enzyme. This unit of activity will be dependent upon not only the kallikrein (kininogenase) which is employed but also the method used for quantitating the kinins. Different enzymes release not only different amounts of kinin from the same kininogen but also different kinins whose potency when compared to bradykinin can vary according to the method chosen for assay. The presence in the incubation mixture of enzymes capable of converting kallidin or larger kinins to bradykinin will also alter the apparent yield of bradykinin as will the presence of kininases. The loss due to the latter enzymes, however, can readily be estimated by adding equivalent concentrations of kinin and, if significant loss of kinin is encountered, inhibitors such as 1,10-phenanthroline or other chelating agents may be helpful in retarding this destruction. Correction should be made for loss of bradykinin which occurs during processing of the sample. In order to avoid inconvenient numbers in determining this unit, terms such as milliunit (mU), microunit (μU), etc. may be used.

III. Kallikreins (Kininogenases)

In the absence of either a pure substrate or a pure enzyme, a unit for kallikrein (kininogenase) activity which would meet the standards proposed by the International Union of Biochemistry (IUB) cannot be recommended at this time. The following arbitrary unit is therefore defined. One milliunit of kallikrein (kininogenase) is that amount of enzyme which will release in one minute at 30° 1 nanomole of bradykinin equivalent from an amount of citrated plasma (1:50, 20% sodium citrate:blood v/v) which has been heated for one half hour at 60° and which contains an amount of substrate equivalent to 5 nanomoles of bradykinin. The plasma should be derived from the same species as the kallikrein, whenever possible. Silicone-coated or otherwise protected glassware should be used throughout and correction made for any loss of bradykinin that occurs. This unit, like the kininogen unit, will also be dependent upon the method used for quantitating the kinin and the presence or absence of enzymes capable of converting other kinins to bradykinin. It is suggested that the abbreviation KaU be employed for these units in order to differentiate them from the kallikrein units (KU) which are obtained by measuring the decrease in the blood pressure of the anesthetized dog. This recommendation does not exclude the use of other methods for measuring comparative enzymatic activities but the above technique should be employed for standardization of the units. For those investigators wishing to establish esterase units (EU) for the various kallikreins the recommendations of the IUB (Enzyme Nomenclature, 1965) should be employed. Wherever possible pH and substrate concentration should be optimal and the temperature should be 30°.

IV. Activators of Kallikrein

For those enzymes which are activators of endogenous kallikreins and do not attack kininogen directly, 1 milliunit of activity (KaAmU) is defined provisionally as that amount of enzyme which will cause the release in one minute at 30° of 1 nanomole of bradykinin equivalent from intact citrated plasma. Qualifications similar to those described for the kallikreins (kininogenases) are to be used. For those enzymes which are both kininogenases and activators, determinations should be made on both intact and heated plasma.

V. Kininases

A meaningful unit of kininase activity utilizing bradykinin as the substrate cannot be established at the present time as most biological tissues and fluids contain more than one kininase and their optimal conditions for assay are variable (Erdös, 1966; Yang and Erdös, 1967). Investigators wherever possible may establish units of activity on synthetic substrates by following the recommendations of the IUB.

VI. Kallikrein Inhibitors

The Committee was unable to agree on a definition of an inhibitor unit. It has been proposed that 1 unit of kallikrein inhibitor be defined as that amount which will inhibit 50% of the activity of 2 units of kallikrein (kininogenase) (Vogel et al., 1966, 1968).

Membership of the Committee

Corresponding members:

D. Armstrong	England	J. J. Pisano	U.S.A.
N. Back	U.S.A.	J. L. Prado	Brazil
C. R. Diniz	Brazil	E. S. Prado	Brazil
V. Eisen	England	M. Rocha e Silva	Brazil
D. F. Elliott	England	E. Schröder	Germany
E. G. Erdös	U.S.A.	F. Sicuteri	Italy
E. Habermann	Germany	T. Suzuki	Japan
O. B. Henriques	U.S.S.R.	I. Trautschold	Germany
S. Jacobsen	Norway	W. Vogt	Germany
G. L. Mills	England	M. E. Webster	U.S.A.
H. Moriya	Japan	E. Werle	Germany
J. V. Pierce	U.S.A.		

References

Armstrong, D. A. J., Mills, G. L.: A highly purified kinin-forming enzyme from human plasma. Biochem. Pharmacol. **13**, 1393 (1964).

Dedolph, R. R.: Kinins, cytokinins, phytokinins. Science **149**, 658 (1965).

Elliott, D. F., Horton, E. W., Lewis, G. P.: The isolation of bradykinin, a plasma kinin from ox blood. Biochem. J. **78**, 60 (1961).

— Lewis, G. P.: Methionyllysylbradykinin, a new kinin from ox blood. Biochem. J. **95**, 437 (1965).

Enzyme Nomenclature, p. 6, 38, 43. New York: Elsevier 1965.

Erdös, E. G.: Hypotensive peptides: bradykinin, kallidin and eledoisin. Advanc. Pharmacol. **4**, 27 (1966).

— Renfrew, A. G., Sloane, E. M., Wohler, J. R.: Enzymatic studies on bradykinin and similar peptides. Ann. N.Y. Acad. Sci. **104**, 222 (1963).

— Sloane, E. M., Wohler, I. M.: Carboxypeptidase in blood and other fluids. I. Properties, distribution and partial purification of the enzyme. Biochem. Pharmacol. **13**, 893 (1964).

Frey, E. K., Kraut, H., Werle, E.: Kallikrein (Padutin). Stuttgart: Ferdinand Enke 1950.

Habermann, E.: Über pH-bedingte Modifikationen des kininliefernden α-Globulins (Kininogen) aus Rinderserum und das Molekulargewicht von Kininogen I. Biochem. Z. **337**, 440 (1963).

— Enzymatic kinin release from kininogen and from low molecular compounds. In: Hypotensive peptides, p. 116, ed. by E. G. Erdös, N. Back and F. Sicuteri. Berlin-Heidelberg-New York: Springer 1966.

Henriques, O. B., Kauritcheva, N., Kuznetsova, V., Astrakan, M.: Substrates of kinin-releasing enzymes isolated from horse plasma. Nature (Lond.) **215**, 1200 (1967).

— Lavras, A. A. C., Fichman, M., Picarelli, Z. P.: Plasma enzymes that release kinins. Biochem. Pharmacol. **15**, 31 (1966).

Jacobsen, S., Kriz, M.: Some data on two purified kininogens from human plasma. Brit. J. Pharmacol. **29**, 25 (1967).

Kraut, H., Frey, E. K., Werle, E.: Der Nachweis eines Kreislaufhormons in der Pankreasdrüse. IV. Mitt. über dieses Kreislaufhormon. Hoppe-Seylers Z. physiol. Chem. **189**, 97 (1930).

Laki, K.: The autocatalytic formation of thrombin and clotting effect of hemophilic blood. Studies Inst. Med. Chem. Univ. Szeged, Hungary **3**, 5 (1943). Chem. Abstr. **41**, 1299g (1947).

Lewis, G. P.: Formation of plasma kinins by plasmin. J. Physiol. (Lond.) **140**, 285 (1958).

Miller, C. O., Skoog, F., Okumura, F. S., von Saltza, M. H., Strong, F. M.: Isolation, structure and synthesis of kinetin, a substance promoting cell division. J. Amer. chem. Soc. **78**, 1375 (1956).

Nagasawa, S., Mizushima, Y., Sato, T., Iwanaga, S., Suzuki, T.: Studies on the chemical nature of bovine bradykininogen; determinations of amino acid, carbohydrate, amino and carboxyl terminals. J. Biochem. (Tokyo) **60**, 643 (1966).

Pierce, J. V.: Structural features of plasma kinins and kininogens. Fed. Proc. **27**, 52 (1968).

— Webster, M. E.: The purification and some properties of two different kallidinogens from human plasma. In: Hypotensive peptides, p. 130, ed. by E. G. Erdös, N. Back and F. Sicuteri. Berlin-Heidelberg-New York: Springer 1966.

PISANO, J. J.: Vasoactive peptides in venoms. Fed. Proc. **27**, 58 (1968).
ROCHA E SILVA, M.: Definition of bradykinin and other kinins. Biochem. Pharmacol. **10**, 3 (1962).
— The physiological significance of bradykinin. Ann. N.Y. Acad. Sci. **104**, 107, 190 (1963).
— Kinin-hormones. Proceedings, VI. Pan-american Congr. Endocr. Excerpta Med. Int. Congr. Ser. **112**, 47 (1965).
— BERALDO, W. T., ROSENFELD, G.: Bradykinin, a hypotensive and smooth muscle stimulating factor released from plasma globulin by snake venoms and by trypsin. Amer. J. Physiol. **156**, 261 (1949).
SCHACHTER, M., THAIN, E. M.: Chemical and pharmacological properties of the potent slow contracting substance (kinin) in wasp venom. Brit. J. Pharmacol. **9**, 352 (1954).
SCHRÖDER, E., HEMPEL, R.: Bradykinin, kallidin and their synthetic analogues. Experientia (Basel) **20**, 529 (1964).
SKOOG, F., STRONG, F. M., MILLER, C. O.: Cytokinins. Science **148**, 532 (1965).
SUZUKI, T., IWANAGA, S., NAGASAWA, S., SATO, T.: Purification and properties of bradykininogen and of the bradykinin-releasing enzymes in snake venom. In: Hypotensive peptides, p. 149, ed. by E. G. ERDÖS, N. BACK and F. SICUTERI. Berlin-Heidelberg-New York: Springer 1966.
VOGEL, R., TRAUTSCHOLD, I., WERLE, E.: Natürliche Proteinasen-Inhibitoren. Stuttgart: Georg Thieme 1966.
— — — Natural proteinase inhibitors. New York: Academic Press 1968.
VOGT, W., WAWRETSCHEK, W.: Weitere Untersuchungen zur Existenz zweier kininbildender Systeme im menschlichen Plasma. Naunyn-Schmiedebergs Arch. exp. Path. Pharmak. **260**, 223 (1968).
WEBSTER, M. E.: Report of the committee on nomenclature for hypotensive peptides. In: Hypotensive peptides, p. 648, ed. by E. G. ERDÖS, N. BACK and F. SICUTERI. Berlin-Heidelberg-New York: Springer 1966.
— PIERCE, J. V.: The nature of the kallidins released from human plasma by kallikreins and other enzymes. Ann. N.Y. Acad. Sci. **104**, 91 (1963).
WERLE, E.: Über die Inaktivierung des Kallikreins. Biochem. Z. **273**, 291 (1934).
— BEREK, U.: Zur Kenntnis des Kallikreins. Angew. Chem. **60** A, 53 (1948).
— TRAUTSCHOLD, I.: Kallikrein, kallidin, kallikrein inhibitors. Ann. N.Y. Acad. Sci. **104**, 117 (1963).
YANG, H. Y. T., ERDÖS, E. G.: Second kininase in human blood plasma. Nature (Lond.) **215**, 1402 (1967).

Author Index

Page number in *italics* refer to the references

Subject Index

When the page number is followed by F or T, the reference is to a figure or table

MIX
Papier aus verantwortungsvollen Quellen
Paper from responsible sources
FSC® C105338

If you have any concerns about our products,
you can contact us on
ProductSafety@springernature.com

In case Publisher is established outside the EU,
the EU authorized representative is:
Springer Nature Customer Service Center GmbH
Europaplatz 3, 69115 Heidelberg, Germany

Printed by Libri Plureos GmbH
in Hamburg, Germany